Sure Success
COMED-K

Sure Success COMED-K

(Solved Papers from 2015 to 2004 with Explanations and References from Latest Editions of Various Textbooks)

Sixth Edition

B Ramgopal MBBS MS Ophth
Consultant Ophthalmologist
Bengaluru, Karnataka
India

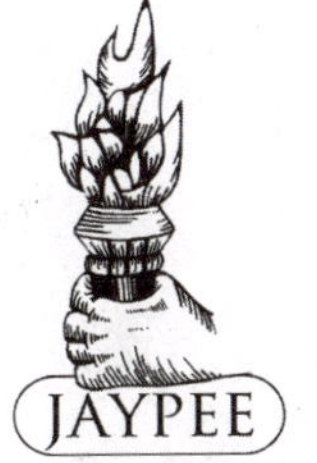

JAYPEE The Health Sciences Publisher

New Delhi | London | Philadelphia | Panama

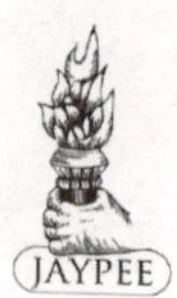

Jaypee Brothers Medical Publishers (P) Ltd

Headquarters

Jaypee Brothers Medical Publishers (P) Ltd
4838/24, Ansari Road, Daryaganj
New Delhi 110 002, India
Phone: +91-11-43574357
Fax: +91-11-43574314
Email: jaypee@jaypeebrothers.com

Overseas Offices

J.P. Medical Ltd
83 Victoria Street, London
SW1H 0HW (UK)
Phone: +44 20 3170 8910
Fax: +44 (0)20 3008 6180
Email: info@jpmedpub.com

Jaypee-Highlights Medical Publishers Inc
City of Knowledge, Bld. 237, Clayton
Panama City, Panama
Phone: +1 507-301-0496
Fax: +1 507-301-0499
Email: cservice@jphmedical.com

Jaypee Medical Inc
325 Chestnut Street
Suite 412, Philadelphia, PA 19106, USA
Phone: +1 267-519-9789
Email: jpmed.us@gmail.com

Jaypee Brothers Medical Publishers (P) Ltd
17/1-B Babar Road, Block-B, Shaymali
Mohammadpur, Dhaka-1207
Bangladesh
Phone: +08801912003485
Email: jaypeedhaka@gmail.com

Jaypee Brothers Medical Publishers (P) Ltd
Bhotahity, Kathmandu, Nepal
Phone: +977-9741283608
Email: kathmandu@jaypeebrothers.com

Website: www.jaypeebrothers.com
Website: www.jaypeedigital.com

Inquiries for bulk sales may be solicited at: jaypee@jaypeebrothers.com

Sure Success – COMED-K

First Edition: 2010
Second Edition: 2012
Third Edition: 2012
Fourth Edition: 2014
Fifth Edition: 2015
Sixth Edition: **2016**

ISBN 978-93-5250-135-9

Printed at Sanat Printers

Dedicated to

My Father
Late Sri KL Balu
and
All my Facebook and PG aspirant friends

PREFACE

A message for the PG aspirants

The COMED-K PG Entrance Examination, similar to the Karnataka PGET, is one of the most transparent entrance examinations in the country with the question paper being given out at the end of the examination and the answer key appearing soon on the website. This examination is held usually around February 1st week (for actual dates visit www.comedk.org the official website of the COMED-K).

Sure Success – COMED-K contains the solved question papers from the year 2015 to 2004 of COMED-K PG Entrance Examination with references and detailed explanations from the latest editions of standard textbooks. This book fulfills the need for an exclusive and high quality solved paper books for the COMED-K PG entrance aspirants.

Along with each answer, the related and relevant high yield information from each topic is given, so that any similar MCQ can be easily answered. The repeated questions and topics have been highlighted so that these can be given the due importance. Numerous flowcharts, tables and information boxes make this book more reader friendly.

As you know, Karnataka is one of the states with a large number of medical colleges. Many of these colleges are renowned teaching institutions with state-of-the-art facilities to learn and good patient load, so that, at the end of your PG course you are fully qualified and confident to practice. Hence, start preparing for the COMED-K PG Entrance Examination simultaneously with any other All India or State Level examinations you may be preparing for. By doing this, you will be automatically fully prepared by the time of COMED-K Examination.

Gear up and aim high for COMED-K PG Entrance, so that you come out in flying colors and grab the PG seat of your choice. This book is being released well in time for the 2016 COMED-K PG Entrance Examination to enable you to achieve this.

Wishing you the very best of luck and may God bless you!

B Ramgopal
Bengaluru
www.facebook.com/suresuccessramgopal
www.suresuccessramgopal.com
suresuccessinpg@gmail.com

ACKNOWLEDGMENTS

This book has been possible for so many years due to the best wishes of a lot of people, a few of whom I have mentioned below:

- My wife Dr BK Suma and daughter Ms Shriya Gopal, for their encouragement, patience and understanding.
- My mother Smt HR Padmini, for her persuasion and encouragement.
- My brother Mr Murli Balu, for always urging me to think BIG.
- All PG aspirants who keep encouraging me to continue my writing work and for their feedback.
- Shri Jitendar P Vij (Group Chairman), Mr Ankit Vij (Group President) and Mr Tarun Duneja (Director-Publishing) of M/s Jaypee Brothers Medical Publishers (P) Ltd, New Delhi, India, who always produce wonderful books.
- Mr Venugopal Vishnumurthy [Associate Director-South (Sales & Marketing)] of M/s Jaypee Brothers Medical Publishers (P) Ltd, Bengaluru, Karnataka, India, for his promptness, speed, inspiration and encouragement.
- All my friends and well-wishers.

CONTENTS

COMED-K 2015

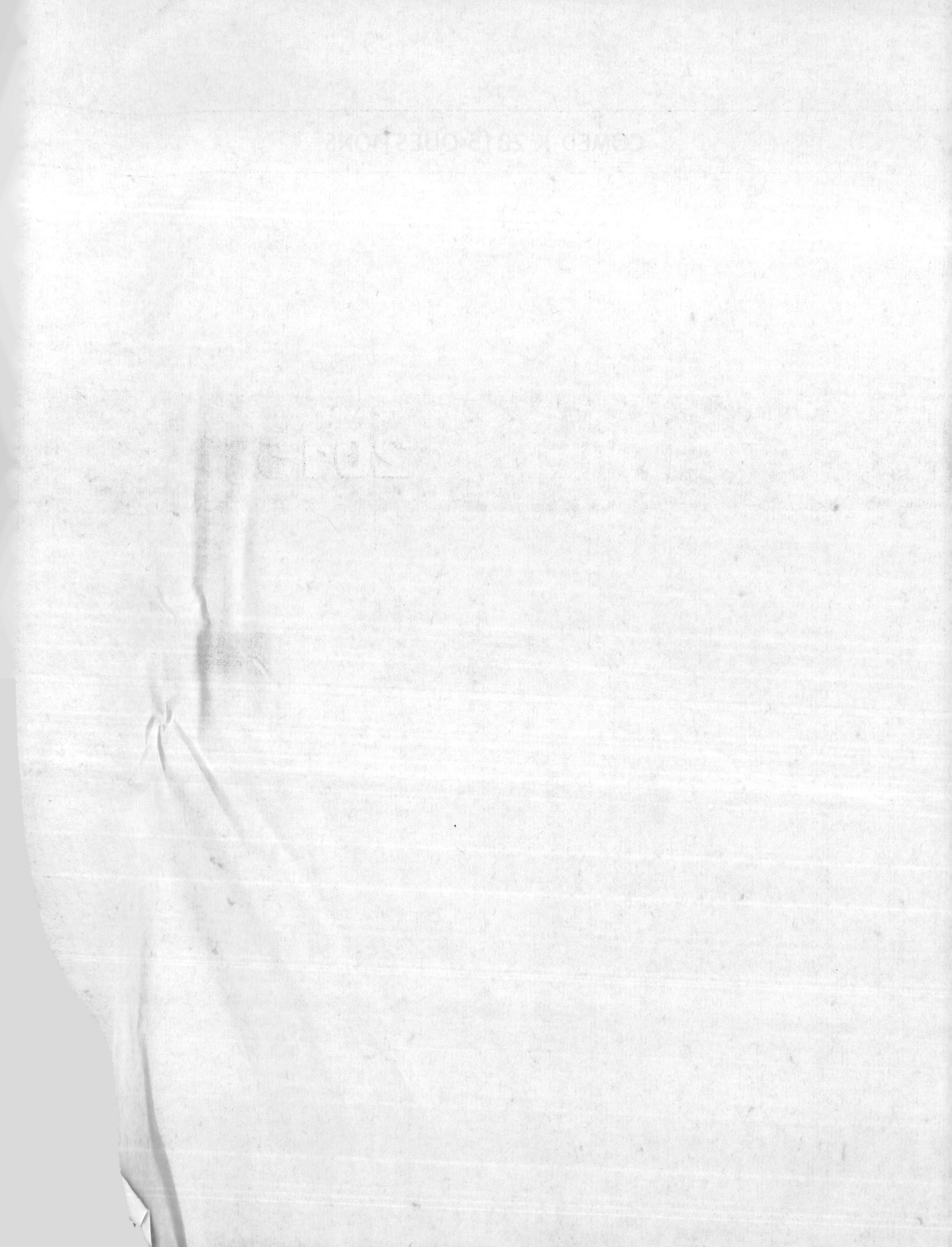

29. The etiology of primary lymphoedema includes all *EXCEPT*
(a) Lymphoedema tarda
(b) Nonne-Milroy disease
(c) Lymphoedema precox
(d) Primary lymphatic malignancy

30. The shelf life of stored whole blood is approximately
(a) 3 weeks
(b) 6 weeks
(c) 9 weeks
(d) 12 weeks

31. Toll-like receptors form a part of
(a) Innate immunity
(b) Active immunity
(c) Adoptive immunity
(d) Passive immunity

32. Chromoblastomycosis is caused by
(a) *Cryptococcus neoformans*
(b) *Cladosporium carrionii*
(c) *Claviceps purpurea*
(d) *Coccidioides immitis*

33. Which among these blocks vitamin B_{12} absorption?
(a) *Giardia lamblia*
(b) *Diphyllobothrium latum*
(c) *Hymenolepis nana*
(d) *Spirometra*

34. The specialized type of microscope, which enable quantitative measurements of the chemical constituents of cells is
(a) Optical microscope
(b) Interference microscope
(c) Phase contrast microscope
(d) Polarization microscope

35. Preformed toxin is seen in
(a) *Staphylococcus aureus*
(b) *Clostridium perfringens*
(c) *Escherichia coli*
(d) *Yersinia enterocolitica*

36. Clinically gender is NOT apparent until …… weeks of embryonic life
(a) 6
(b) 8
(c) 10
(d) 12

37. A woman's risk at birth of having ovarian cancer at some point in her lifetime is …………%
(a) 1–1.5
(b) 1.5–2
(c) 2–2.5
(d) 2.5–3

38. Endometrial cancer is responsible for ……..% of postmenopausal bleeding
(a) 15
(b) 30
(c) 45
(d) 60

39. The clinical finding that suggests insulin resistance
(a) Body mass index – 20
(b) Waist to hip ratio – 0.70
(c) Waist circumference – 65 cm
(d) Numerous acrochordons

40. The incorrect statement among the following regarding congenital bilateral absence of vas deferens (CBAVD)
(a) Transrectal ultrasound is not generally needed for CBAVD
(b) Renal imaging is not necessary in CBAVD
(c) Most men with CBAVD will have seminal vesicle agenesis
(d) At least two third of men with CBAVD have mutations of the cystic fibrosis transmembrane conductance regulator gene (CFTR)

41. Treatment for cerebral metastasis in gestational trophoblastic neoplasia
(a) Excision of the metastatic lesion
(b) Whole brain irradiation
(c) Intrathecal methotrexate
(d) Concurrent use of combination of chemotherapy and brain irradiation

42. The most common ovarian tumor of first decade of life
(a) Germ cell tumor
(b) Epithelial cell tumor
(c) Sex cord stromal tumor
(d) Krukenburg's tumor

43. The following gram positive bacteria account for the most of the organisms isolated from bacterial corneal ulcers *EXCEPT*

(a) Coagulase negative *Staphylococcus*
(b) *Staphylococcus aureus*
(c) *Corynebacterium*
(d) *Streptococcus*

44. A disease characterized by chronic bilateral inflammation of the conjunctiva that generally affects children and young adults, who have an atopic personal or family history and live in warm climates
(a) Atopic conjunctivitis
(b) Vernal keratoconjunctivitis
(c) Conjunctivochalasis
(d) Allergic conjunctivitis

45. A retinal disease is characterized by the features of progressive rod-cone dystrophy, retinal vessel attenuation and a pale optic disk. What is the fourth characteristic feature?
(a) Macular degeneration
(b) Bone spicule pigmentary change
(c) Preretinal hemorrhages
(d) Cotton-wool spots

46. The essential optic nerve head changes in glaucoma that need to be assessed are
i. Cup-to-disk ratio
ii. Neuroretinal rim area
iii. Retinal nerve fiber layer
iv. Optic disk size
(a) i and ii
(b) ii and iii
(c) i and iv
(d) i, ii and iii

47. In older children, which type of refractive error is most frequent?
(a) Myopia
(b) Hyperopia
(c) Astigmatism
(d) Presbyopia

48. The frequent cause of isolated III, IV and VI cranial nerve palsies in adults is
(a) Microvascular ischemia
(b) Oligodendroglioma
(c) Posterior intercerebellar artery aneurysm
(d) Brain stem infarction

49. Which of the following is FALSE regarding stress fractures?
(a) Commonly seen in military trainees
(b) Second metatarsal is one of the common site
(c) Fracture involves an abnormal bone
(d) Surgery is not usually required

50. In the cases of lumbar spondylolisthesis, which of the following is TRUE?
(a) Isthmic listhesis is not the commonest type
(b) Degenerative listhesis is usually high grades slip
(c) Beheaded scotty dog appearance indicates paralysis
(d) There is a defect in the spinous processes

51. Blount's disease involves
(a) Capital femoral epiphysis
(b) Medial tibial epiphysis
(c) Lateral tibial epiphysis
(d) Both distal femoral and proximal tibial epiphysis

52. The most effective treatment for hepatitis C is
(a) Interferon
(b) Deflazacort
(c) Acyclovir
(d) Peginterferon with ribavarin

53. The commonest location of a small foreign body in the lung in children is
(a) Left main bronchus
(b) Left lower lobe
(c) Right main bronchus
(d) Left middle lobe

54. A 1-year-old boy was admitted in pediatric ICU with history of fever for 2 days, altered sensorium and one episode of convulsion. He had no neck stiffness. CT brain revealed hemorrhage in temporal lobe and lumbar puncture revealed 25 lymphocytes with red blood cells. What is your diagnosis?
(a) Pyogenic meningitis
(b) Herpes simplex encephalitis
(c) Subarachnoid hemorrhage
(d) Cerebral abscess

55. In a child with simple febrile seizures
(a) Antiepileptic therapy, continuous or intermittent is generally not recommended
(b) Antipyretics are useful in preventing recurrence
(c) Non-benzodiazepine antiepileptics are effective
(d) EEG should be done with the first episode itself

56. If a patient with celiac disease develops an obstructive lesion in the small intestine, what is the most likely diagnosis?

(a) Crohn's disease
(b) T-cell lymphoma
(c) MALT lymphoma
(d) Tubulovillous adenoma

57. What is the name given to persistent vitelline duct remnant?

(a) Omphalocele
(b) Heister's diverticulum
(c) Rokitansky's diverticulum
(d) Meckel's diverticulum

58. Breast disorder which is most likely to occur during lactation and breastfeeding is

(a) Acute mastitis
(b) Chronic mastitis
(c) Fat necrosis
(d) Intraductal carcinoma

59. Hypopituitarism is NOT produced by

(a) Pituitary irradiation
(b) Chromophobe adenoma
(c) Sheehan's syndrome
(d) Basophil adenoma

60. von Recklinghausen disease of bone is characterized by

(a) Reduced bone resorption and diffuse skeletal sclerosis
(b) Multiple neural tumors in the bones
(c) Increased bone resorption, fibrosis and cystic brown tumors
(d) Defect in matrix mineralization, oseteopenia and susceptibility to fractures

61. *Plasmodium vivax* uses the following as receptors to penetrate red blood cells

(a) Rh antigens
(b) Lewis antigens
(c) Lutheran glycoproteins
(d) Duffy glycoproteins

62. All the following have a role in the pathogenesis of type 1 diabetes mellitus *EXCEPT*

(a) Presence of susceptibility HLA locus
(b) Autoimmunity mediated cell destruction
(c) Immune destruction of cells following viral infections
(d) Insulin resistance in peripheral tissue

63. A 20-year-old female came to the medical OPD with severe pain and redness over the dorsum of the foot. There was a past history of severe abdominal pain episodes. Peripheral smear showed anemia with the presence of poikilocytes. The likely diagnosis is

(a) Hemoglobin C disease
(b) Thalassemia minor
(c) Sickle cell disease
(d) G6PD deficiency

64. Which of the following is INCORRECT about Phenytoin?

(a) Dose-related ataxia
(b) Highly protein bound
(c) Dose-dependent elimination
(d) Intramascular (IM) injection preferred

65. A 55-year-old male presented with low mood, ideas of hopelessness, crying spells and death wishes. He also reported decrease sleep and appetite. He was been prescribed tablet Imipramine 150 mg/day by a general practitioner 2 weeks back. He presented with urinary retention, dizziness and dry mouth. Which of the following is correct statement?

(a) Continue imipramine at 150 mg/day
(b) Change to escitalopram 10 mg/day
(c) Addition of haloperidol 10 mg/day with the current medication
(d) Change to sodium valproate 500 mg/day

66. A 54-year-old obese patient with type 2 diabetes and a history of alcoholism probable should not receive metformin because it can increase his/her risk of

(a) Disulfiram-like reaction
(b) Excessive weight gain
(c) Hypoglycemia
(d) Lactic acidosis

67. Which of the following drugs has activity against many strains of *P. aeruginosa*, however, when use alone resistance emerges during the treatment. It cannot be used in patients who are allergic to penicillin and its activity is increased when combined with tazobactam?

(a) Amoxicillin
(b) Aztreonam
(c) Imipenam
(d) Piperacillin

68. Which antitumor monoclonal antibody is NOT indicated as a drug of choice in slowing the progression of neovascular macular degeneration?

(a) Alemtuzumab
(b) Bevacizumab
(c) Ranibizumab
(d) Pegaptanib

69. Mirtazepine is NOT a substrate for which CYP450 enzyme?

(a) CYP2D6
(b) CYP3A4
(c) CYP1A2
(d) CYP2C9

70. Skeletal muscle was stimulated with increasing frequency of stimulus. The force of contraction increase progressively and reached a plateau. The most likely mechanism responsible for this effect is

(a) Reduced sensitivity of troponin to calcium ions
(b) Reduced time for calcium reuptake into sarcoplasmic reticulum
(c) Increased calcium entry from interstitial fluid
(d) Phosphorylation of myosin light chain kinase

71. The following statements are true for apoptosis *EXCEPT*

(a) Gets rid of inappropriate clones of immunocytes
(b) Facilities removal of web between fingers
(c) Helps in regression of duct system in the course of sexual development
(d) Leads to neurodegenerative diseases and cancer

72. The mechanism of action of nitric oxide synthase during erection is

(a) Increase in the level of cAMP causing relaxation of smooth muscle enhancing blood flow
(b) Blocking phosphodiesterase to increase cGMP causing relation of smooth muscle enhancing blood flow
(c) Activating soluble guanylate cyclases to increase cGMP causing relaxation of smooth muscle enhancing blood
(d) Promoting formation of greater number of calcium-calmodulin complex

73. The only neurons in retina showing action potentials are

(a) Rods and cones
(b) Bipolar cells
(c) Amacrine cells
(d) Ganglion cells

74. The need for vitamin B_{12} and folic acid in the formation of red blood cells is related primarily to their effects on

(a) Synthesis and release of erythropoietin from the kidney
(b) Absorption of iron from the gut
(c) DNA synthesis in the bone marrow
(d) Hemoglobin formation in the red blood cell

75. Rapid eye movement sleep is also called paradoxical sleep because

(a) EEG shows low-voltage, high frequency waves
(b) Eye is moving rapidly
(c) There is dreaming during this state
(d) Muscle tone is grossly depressed

76. Syndrome characterized by an elaborate delusion that patient is passionately loved by another person is also known as

(a) Ekbom's syndrome
(b) De Clerambault's syndrome
(c) Querulous paranoia
(d) Othello syndrome

77. Which is TRUE of bipolar disorder?

(a) Genetic predisposition is significant
(b) Its onset is usually in the fifth decade of life
(c) Manic episodes occur twice as frequently as depressive episodes
(d) Mixed episodes are rare

78. Rapid eye movement sleep is characterized by all of the following features *EXCEPT*

(a) Presence of dreams
(b) Low amplitude mixed frequency EEG
(c) Absent of EMG activity
(d) Absence of activity on electro-oculogram

79. X-rays behave like

(a) Sound waves
(b) Particles only
(c) Electromagnetic waves and particles
(d) Electromagnetic waves only

80. Bronchiectasis is currently best diagnosed by

(a) Plain radiography
(b) Bronchography

(c) Bronchial angiography
(d) Computed tomography

81. Chest radiographs of children with foreign body aspiration
(a) Are always abnormal
(b) May show overinflation of the involved lung
(c) Always show the foreign body
(d) Commonly show pneumothorax

82. Interpret the following ABG – pH: 7.00; PaO_2: 60 mm Hg; $PaCO_2$: 80 mm Hg; HCO_3: 28
(a) Respiratory acidosis with normoxemia
(b) Metabolic acidosis with normoxemia
(c) Metabolic acidosis with hypoxemia
(d) Respiratory acidosis with hypoxemia

83. Which of the following antiretroviral agent interacts with rifampicin?
(a) Nevirapine
(b) Azidothymidine
(c) Ritonavir
(d) Efavirenz

84. An indication for ultrasonography of the thorax is
(a) Lobar pneumonia
(b) Pulmonary thromboembolism
(c) Pleural effusion
(d) Pulmonary TB

85. Following are true in choanal atresia *EXCEPT*
(a) Bilateral choanal atresia endangers newborn life
(b) Membranous atresia is common than bony atresia
(c) Presents with unilateral mucoid nasal discharge without air bubbles
(d) By persistence of primitive bucconasal membrane

86. Following are the features of laryngomalacia *EXCEPT*
(a) Collapse of supraglottic structures on inspiration
(b) Omega-shaped epiglottis
(c) Narrow interarytenoid cleft
(d) Aryepiglottic mucosal fold prolapsed into airway

87. Which is TRUE in fibrous dysplasia?
(a) Benign hamartomatous neoplasm of nasofacial region
(b) Presents in the first or second decade of life
(c) Classical X-ray finding of ground glass appearance
(d) Mandible is commonly affected

88. 'Rat-hole' appearance of entry wound of firearm is seen in
(a) Close range of rifles
(b) Contact range of shotguns
(c) Near range of rifles
(d) Near range of shotguns

89. Strychnine acts by inhibiting
(a) GABA
(b) Glycine
(c) Acetylcholine
(d) Dopamine

90. 'Declaration of Tokyo' deals with
(a) Abortion
(b) Torture
(c) Human experimentation
(d) Consumerism

91. Choking is seen in
(a) Revolver
(b) Pistol
(c) Shotgun
(d) Rifle

92. A young girl presents with arthralgias, hypertension and discrepancies in blood pressure of both upper limbs. Which of the following is the most likely diagnosis?
(a) Giant cell arthritis
(b) Takayasu's arteritis
(c) Polyarteritis nodosa
(d) Henoch-Schonlein purpura

93. A 50-year-old male who had fever since 5 days developed hypotension and desaturation. He was put on ventilator. Chest X-ray showed bilateral diffuse alveolar and interstitial opacities. Which of the following is the most probable diagnosis?
(a) Acute pulmonary edema
(b) Acute respiratory distress syndrome
(c) Lobar pneumonia
(d) Interstitial lung disease

94. 'Broadbent's sign' is seen in
(a) Constrictive pericarditis
(b) Restrictive cardiomyopathy
(c) Cardiac tamponade
(d) Right ventricular myocardial infarction

95. Tei index or 'TAPSE' is used in
(a) Cor pulmonale
(b) Left heart failure
(c) Myocardial infarction
(d) Angina pectoris

96. In Doppler echocardiography 'green' color superimposed indicates
(a) Blood flow towards transducer
(b) Blood flow away from transducer
(c) Turbulent blood flow
(d) None of the above

97. In nephronophthisis all are seen *EXCEPT*
(a) Retinitis pigmentosa
(b) Cerebellar ataxia
(c) Atrial septal defect
(d) Situs inversus

98. Which of the following is TRUE statement regarding silent thyroiditis?
(a) This condition is exclusively seen in pregnancy
(b) Glucocorticoids are the treatment of choice
(c) It is characterized by brief period of thyrotoxicosis
(d) ESR levels are high

99. Which of the following is NOT indicated in treatment of takotsubo cardiomyopathy?
(a) Nitrates
(b) Combined alpha and beta blocker
(c) Magnesium
(d) Anticoagulation

100. Kernohan-Woltman sign is seen in
(a) Uncal herniation
(b) Cental herniation
(c) Transfalcine herniation
(d) Foraminal herniation

101. All are true of Dent's diseases *EXCEPT*
(a) It is x-linked recessive nephrolithiasis
(b) Unusual form of Fanconi syndrome
(c) High-molecular-weight proteinuria
(d) Nephrolithiasis

102. Bone manifestation of secondary hyperparathyroidism in chronic kidney disease starts to occur at GFR level below
(a) 40 mL/min
(b) 60 mL/min
(c) 30 mL/min
(d) 15 mL/min

103. Fibrinolysis in pulmonary embolism can be done up to
(a) 6 hours
(b) 2 days
(c) 7 days
(d) 14 days

104. All of the following drugs are used in the treatment of acute myocardial infarction *EXCEPT*
(a) Streptokinase
(b) Aspirin
(c) Amlodipine
(d) Atorvastatin

105. Which of the following organisms are known to cause invasive diarrhea?
(a) *Vibrio cholerae*
(b) Enterotoxigenic *Escherichia coli*
(c) *Campylobacter jejuni*
(d) *Bacillus cereus*

106. Which of the following statements regarding adult polycystic kidney disease is TRUE?
(a) Inherited as an autosomal recessive trait
(b) Rarely causes end-stage renal failure
(c) Often fatal in early middle age
(d) Triad of loin pain, mass and attacks of renal colic

107. Parkland formula is useful in resuscitating burns patients. It is a
(a) Isotonic formula
(b) Hypertonic formula
(c) Colloid formula
(d) None of the above

108. Dieulafoy's disease is a
(a) Colonic arterial venous malformation
(b) Gastric arterial venous malformation
(c) Biliary arterial venous malformation
(d) Pancreatic arterial venous malformation

109. Which of the following DOES NOT form a boundary of the Calot's triangle?
(a) Cystic artery
(b) Cystic duct
(c) Inferior surface of the liver
(d) Common hepatic artery

110. The following statement is NOT true regarding congenital diaphragmatic hernia

(a) Hernias through the foramen of Morgagni are common at any age
(b) Hernias through the foramen of Morgagni are common on the right side
(c) About 80% of the hernias through the foramen of Bochdalek is on the left side.
(d) Newborns with congenital diaphragmatic hernia can have hypoplasia of both lungs.

111. Human genome project was completed in the year
(a) 1997
(b) 2001
(c) 2003
(d) 2005

112. Below mentioned is the etiology of dynamic intestinal obstruction and their relative frequencies. Choose the correct answer.
(a) Adhesions (40%), Obstructed hernia (12%), Inflammatory (15%), Fecal impaction (8%)
(b) Adhesions (40%), Obstructed hernia (15%), Inflammatory (8%), Fecal impaction (12%)
(c) Adhesions (40%), Obstructed hernia (8%), Inflammatory (12%, Fecal impaction (15%)
(d) Adhesions (40%), Obstructed hernia (12%), Inflammatory (8%), Fecal impaction (15%)

113. A patient comes to the casualty with complaints of pain due to wound in the leg. The intern gets ready to give intramuscular injection to the gluteal region. The injection should be ideally given in the
(a) Upper lateral quadrant
(b) Upper medial quadrant
(c) Lower lateral quadrant
(d) Lower medial quadrant

114. Net protein utilization (NPU) is
(a) Energy from protein/N_2 retained by body
(b) N_2 intake × 100/N_2 retained by body
(c) Product of digestibility coefficient and biological value divided by 100
(d) Measures of concentration of each amino acid in protein

115. Which of the following is FALSE regarding the immature skeleton?
(a) They are more malleable
(b) Periosteum is much thinner
(c) Fractures occurring close to the joint and in the plane of motion usually remodel well
(d) Nonunion of the fractures are less common compared to the mature skeleton

116. The commonest infective agent responsible for catheter related infection in children undergoing total parenteral nutrition is
(a) *Escherichia coli*
(b) *Pseudomonas aeruginosa*
(c) Coagulase negative *Staphylococcus*
(d) *Pneumocystis carinii*

117. The following is an example of a depot preparation of a long acting antipsychotic
(a) Olanzapine
(b) Thioridazine
(c) Ziprasidone
(d) Haloperidol

118. Salivary calculi are most commonly seen in the ducts of the
(a) Parotid gland
(b) Submandibular gland
(c) Sublingual gland
(d) Minor salivary gland

119. Cardiac resynchronization therapy (CRT) is indicated in heart failure patients with
(a) Patient's in sinus rhythm with an EF < 35% and a QRS < 120 ms
(b) Patient's in sinus rhythm with an EF < 35% and a QRS > 120 ms
(c) Patient's in sinus rhythm with an EF < 40% and a QRS < 120 ms
(d) Patient's in sinus rhythm with an EF < 45% and a QRS > 120 ms

120. Zollinger-Ellison syndrome is caused by a tumor located in
(a) Tail of pancreas
(b) Pyloric antrum
(c) Greater omentum
(d) Gastrinoma triangle

REGARDING RADIOGRAPHIC CONTRAST MEDIA

121. Which of the following elements is contained in a safe intravascular radiographic contrast medium
(a) Iodine
(b) Barium
(c) Bromine
(d) Fluorine

122. In water soluble radiological contrast, the iodine particle ratio is highest in
(a) Ionic monomers
(b) Non-ionic monomers
(c) Ionic dimmers
(d) Non-ionic dimers

123. Hypersomolar reactions due to intravenous iodinated contrast media are all *EXCEPT*
(a) Erythrocyte damage
(b) Endothelial damage
(c) Hypervolemia
(d) Hypovolemia

124. Which of the following groups of contrast agents may be safely injected intrathecally?
(a) Water soluble ionic monomers
(b) Water soluble non-ionic monomers
(c) Water soluble ionic dimmers
(d) Oil based iodinated contrasts

IN A RADIOLOGY DEPARTMENT THAT USES CONVENTIONAL FILM AND DARK ROOM TECHNIQUES

125. The dark areas in a conventional radiographic film are due to particulate deposits of which of the following?
(a) Carbon
(b) Iron
(c) Silver
(d) Copper

126. Safe lights in a radiographic darkroom are ideally light of which color?
(a) Red
(b) Blue
(c) White
(d) Yellow

127. In radiography regarding scattered radiation, which of the statements are TRUE?
(a) Improves image contrast
(b) Improves image resolution
(c) Reduces image contrast
(d) Reduces patient's radiation dose

128. X-rays behave like
(a) Sound waves
(b) Particles only
(c) Electromagnetic waves and particles
(d) Electromagnetic waves only

WITH REGARD TO MAGNETIC RESONANCE IMAGING

129. Images are based on the distribution on which of the following nulei in water and lipids?
(a) Carbon
(b) Calcium
(c) Phosphorous
(d) Hydrogen

130. Increased water content in a tissue results in
(a) High signal intensity on T1-weighted images
(b) High signal intensity on T2-weighted images
(c) Intermediate signal intensity on T1-weighted images
(d) Low signal intensity on T2-weighted images

131. Paramagnetic substances cause a
(a) Shortening of both T1 and T2 relaxation times
(b) Shortening of both T2 relaxation time only
(c) Shortening of T1 relaxation time only
(d) No effect on T1 or T2 relaxation times

132. One of the following elements is used as an intravenous contrast agent
(a) Lanthanum
(b) Gadolinium
(c) Terbium
(d) Strontium

Q. A 55-year-old male came for a routine medical health check up and his chest radiograph demonstrated a solitary calcific focus in the left upper lobe.

133. The following differential diagnosis can be included *EXCEPT*
(a) Tuberculosis
(b) Pulmonary hamartoma
(c) Varicella pneumonia
(d) Metastasis

134. Calcific pulmonary metastases may be seen in
(a) Osteogenic sarcoma and Ewing's sarcoma
(b) Ewing's sarcoma and chondrosarcoma
(c) Chondrosarcoma and osteogenic sarcoma
(d) Osteogenic sarcoma and mucinous ovarian carcinomas

135. Pulmonary harmatomas have
(a) Popcorn calcification and do not undergo malignant transformation
(b) Popcorn calcification and commonly undergo malignant transformation
(c) Lamellar calcification and commonly undergo malignant transformation
(d) Lamellar calcification and do not undergo malignant transformation

136. Eggshell calcification is seen in both
(a) Silicosis and asbestosis
(b) Tuberculosis and silicosis
(c) Sarcoidosis and blastomycosis
(d) Amyloidosis and asbestosis

Q. A child aged 3 years is brought to the pediatrician with a history of cough for 3 weeks treated at a local clinic conservatively. Serial radiographs of the chest reveal a large persistent right lower zone opacity with crowding of the ribs and a slight shift of the mediastinum to the same side.

137. Which of the possibilities is most likely?
(a) Collapse of the right lower lobe
(b) Consolidation of the right lower lobe
(c) Pleural effusion
(d) Sequestration

138. Chest radiographs of children with foreign body aspiration
(a) Are always abnormal
(b) May show overinflation of the involved lung
(c) Always show the foreign body
(d) Commonly show pneumothorax

139. Most common long-term sequel of an impacted bronchial foreign body include
(a) Emphysematous bulla
(b) Bronchiectasis
(c) Empyema
(d) Pneumothorax

140. Air trapping can be diagnosed by
(a) Inspiratory and expiratory radiographs
(b) Deep inspiratory radiography only
(c) Deep expiratory radiography only
(d) Lateral decubitus radiography

Q. A 58-year-old male visited a dermatologist with complaints of multiple eruptions on the skin all over the body. On examination, round to oval vesicles and bullae were seen on the scalp, face, chest, axilla and groin. Some of the vesicles had ruptured leaving erosions. A biopsy was performed and direct immunofluorescence showed fishnet-like pattern of IgG deposition in the squamous intercellular spaces in the lower epidermis.

141. What is your diagnosis?
(a) Bullous pemphigoid
(b) Epidermolysis bullosa
(c) Pemphigus vulgaris
(d) Dermatitis herpetiformis

142. The characteristic microscopic feature of bullous pemphigoid is
(a) Subepidermal non-acantholytic blister
(b) Subcorneal non-acantholytic blister
(c) Suprabasal acantholytic blister
(d) Subepidermal acantholytic blister

143. Intestinal celiac disease is associated with
(a) Bullous pemphigoid
(b) Epidermolysis bullosa
(c) Pemphigus vulgaris
(d) Dermatitis herpetiformis

144. Autoantibodies against desmoglenis 1 and 3 are seen in
(a) Bullous pemphigoid
(b) Bullous systemic lupus erythematosus
(c) Pemphigus vulgaris
(d) Pemphigus foliaceus

Q. A 5-year-old girl presents with recurrent itchy lesions on her face and limbs since the age of 6 months. The itching is worse in winter and there is a history of occasional oozing. It is temporarily relieved with topical steroids and emollient application. On examination, flexural areas are found to have lichenified skin and there is erythema and scaling in the face.

145. Lichenified skin has the following features *EXCEPT*
(a) Thickening
(b) Accentuation of normal skin markings
(c) Hyperpigmentation
(d) Wheal formation on stroking

146. An essential feature for diagnosis of atopic dermatitis is

(a) Pruritus
(b) Tendency towards cutaneous infections
(c) Xerosis
(d) Lichenification

147. Factors which have been implicated in the aggravation of atopic dermatitis include

(a) Sunlight
(b) Soya milk
(c) House dust
(d) Moisturizers

148. Treatment of atopic dermatitis includes any of the following *EXCEPT*

(a) Calcineurin inhibitors
(b) Phototherapy
(c) Cyclosporine
(d) Isotretinoin

Q. A 40-year-old well-nourished female working as a top level executive at a law firm presented to the surgical clinic with complaints of well-localized midepigastric abdominal pain. The pain was usually tolerable and frequently relieved by food. The pain was episodic, seasonal in the spring and fall, and relapsed during periods of emotional stress. Upon further enquiry she revealed that she had noticed that her stools were black tarry and foul smelling. She had undergone an upper GI endoscopy for the above complaints and was given medical management, which did provide her only symptomatic relief.

149. What is the most probable diagnosis in the above condition?

(a) Gastric ulcer
(b) Duodenal ulcer
(c) Cholelithiais
(d) Carcinoma stomach

150. This microorganism is known to cause 90% of the above condition. Which of the following is an invasive method for confirming the offending organism?

(a) ELIZA method
(b) Urea breath test
(c) Radioimmune assay
(d) Rapid urease assay

151. Physiological gastric acid secretion is stimulated by all of the below local stimuli *EXCEPT*

(a) Acetylcholine
(b) Gastrin
(c) Somatostatin
(d) Histamine

152. Which of the antisecretory drugs used to the treat the above condition is structurally related to heparin ………… does not have any anticoagulant effects?

(a) Cimetidine
(b) Pantoprazole
(c) Ranitidine
(d) Sucralfate

Q. A 60-year-old male, presented to the surgical clinic with complaints of passing blood in stool for about 2 months. He had not sought medical intervention as the symptoms did not alarm him. He jokingly mentioned that he consumes red meat regularly. He said he was often fatigued but could carry on his normal chores. He however, did not complain of abdominal pain. He mentioned that his trousers were loose and needed to wear a tight belt. He had undergone colonoscopy as advised by his physician and it revealed grade 1 hemorrhoids and an ulcer in the ascending colon. A diagnosis of colonic cancer was written on the pathology report.

153. What is the most likely pathological type of malignancy in this patient?

(a) Acinar cell carcinoma
(b) Adenocarcinoma
(c) Adenosquamous carcinoma
(d) Squamous cell carcinoma

154. The arc of Riolan is a collateral artery first described by Jean Riolan (1580–1657) that directly connects which two vessels?

(a) Proximal SMA with distal IMA
(b) Distal SMA with distal IMA
(c) Proximal SMA with proximal IMA
(d) Distal SMA with proximal IMA

155. What is the imaging modality of choice to assess the T stage of the above malignancy?

(a) Virtual colonoscopy
(b) Contrast enhanced CT
(c) Double contrast barium enema
(d) Colonoscopic ultrasound

156. Based on the clinical details available and assuming that there is no contraindication to resectional surgery, what is the most appropriate surgery for this patient?

(a) Left hemicolectomy
(b) Extended left hemicolectomy
(c) Extended right hemicolectomy
(d) Right hemicolectomy

IN A PATIENT WITH GOUT

157. Radiological changes are first seen
(a) 5–10 years before clinical symptoms
(b) At the onset of clinical symptoms
(c) 5–10 years after the onset of clinical symptoms
(d) 1–2 years after the onset of clinical symptoms

158. Typical site of involvement is the
(a) 1st MCP joint
(b) 1st MTP joint
(c) Sternoclavicular joint
(d) Knee joint

159. Can be secondary to
(a) Lymphoma
(b) Leukemia
(c) Myeloma
(d) All of the above

160. Typical radiographic findings include
(a) Joint space loss with periarticular osteopenia
(b) Diffuse sclerosis with joint debris
(c) Punched out periarticular erosion
(d) Radio-opaque periarticular tophi

Q. An adolescent male presents with hypertension, hyperkalemia and metabolic acidosis with normal renal function.

161. Diagnosis is
(a) Liddle's syndrome
(b) Gordon's syndrome
(c) Barter's syndrome
(d) Familial hypomagnesemia with hypercalciuria and nephrocalcinosis

162. Pathogenesis is located at
(a) DCT
(b) Cortical collecting duct
(c) Henle's loop
(d) PCT

163. Treatment for this is
(a) NSAID's Mg+2 repletion
(b) Amiloride
(c) Thiazide diuretic
(d) Loop diuretic

164. Mutation responsible for this condition is
(a) Claudin 16
(b) TRPM6
(c) WNK kinase 1 and 4
(d) NBC-1

Q. A child present with low molecular proteinuria, hypercalciuria, nephrocalcinosis and nephrolithiasis. Later he progresses to renal failure from interstitial fibrosis, tubular atrophy and glomerulosclerosis.

165. Diagnosis is
(a) Cystinuria
(b) Hartnup's disease
(c) Cystinosis
(d) Dent's disease

166. Pattern of inheritance of this disease is
(a) Autosomal dominant
(b) Autosomal recessive
(c) X-linked recessive
(d) Mitochondrial inheritance

167. Defective gene responsible is
(a) SLC 3AI and SLC 7AQ
(b) SLC 6AI9
(c) Cystnosin, a hydrogen ion driven transporter
(d) CLC-5

168. The site of lesion in this condition in kidney is
(a) PCT
(b) DCT
(c) Loop of Henle
(d) Collecting duct

Q. A 50-year-old lady presented with chronic sinusitis. She was also having cough with hemoptysis. Her chest X-ray shows multiple cavities involving lower lobes. Her urine examination shows numerous RCB and proteinuria.

169. What is the probable diagnosis?
(a) Microscopic polyangitis
(b) Granulomatosis with polyangitis (Wegner's)
(c) Churg Strauss syndrome
(d) Polyarteritis nodosa

170. Which of the following serological test helps an diagnosis?
(a) p-ANCA
(b) c-ANCA
(c) Anti-mitochondrial antibody
(d) Anti-centromere antibody

171. The histopathological features of the lung lesions will show all *EXCEPT*
(a) Granulomas
(b) Geographic patterns of central necrosis
(c) Leucocyte infiltrates and Giant cells
(d) Large vessel vasculitis

172. Which of the following is NOT used in the treatment of this condition?
(a) Cyclophosphamide
(b) Methotrexate
(c) Rituximab
(d) Plasmapheresis

Q. A 50-year-old lady, who was suffering from hypertension presented with sudden onset of severe headache and projectile vomiting. On examination she was drowsy with Glasgow coma scale of 7/14. Neck stiffness was present. There was no fever. Her CSF examination shows presence of xanthochromia.

173. Which is the probable diagnosis?
(a) Meningitis
(b) Subarchnoid hemorrhage
(c) Migraine
(d) Space-occupying lesion in brain

174. Which of the following grading scale is used to assess the severity?
(a) Hunt and Hess scale
(b) SOFA score
(c) PIRO score
(d) Mini-mental state examination score

175. Which of the following is useful in treatment?
(a) Amlodipine
(b) Nicardipine
(c) Nimodipine
(d) Nifedipine

176. Which of the following metabolic abnormality can be a delayed complication?
(a) Hypercalcemia
(b) Hypokalemia
(c) Hyponatremia
(d) Hypernatremia

Q. A 15-year-old boy presented with a history of jaundice and pain in the knee joints after an episode of fever in the winter. On examination, no hepatosplenomegaly was seen. His hemoglobin was 8 g/dL and the anemia was normocytic and normochromic. His father too was anemic.

177. What is the probable diagnosis?
(a) Thalassemia
(b) Hereditary spherocytosis
(c) Sickle cell anemia
(d) Cold autoimmune hemolytic anemia

178. The peripheral smear in this patient will show all the following *EXCEPT*
(a) Anisopoikilocytosis with target cells
(b) Oval cells with Howell-Jolly bodies
(c) Nucleated red blood cells
(d) Rouleaux formation

179. Which is the most common causative organism for osteomyelitis in such a patient?
(a) *Staphylococcus*
(b) *Salmonella*
(c) *Pseudomonas*
(d) *Klebsiella*

180. Aplastic anemia can develop in this patient due to
(a) Myelodysplasia
(b) Marrow fibrosis
(c) Autoantibodies
(d) Parvovirus B19 infection

COMED-K 2015

ANSWERS AND EXPLANATIONS

AUTHOR'S COMMENTS: The answers for this paper have been verified from the revised final answer key from the Comedk website (last accessed on 1st June 2015).

1. **Answer is c (End tidal CO_2).**
Ref: Anesthesiology Keywords Review, edited by Raj K Modak, Pg 605.

- Venous air embolism is the entrapment of air into the pulmonary circulation. It occurs in two settings:
  - When there is ***subatmospheric pressure with an open vein***
  - More risk when the ***wound is above the level of the heart.***
- *MC* in ***sitting craniotomies***.
- **Diagnosis** of air embolism:
  - Sudden ***decrease*** in ***$ETCO_2$***
  - Sudden ***increase*** in ***ETN_2*** (End tidal nitrogen)
  - Sudden ***attempts to self ventilate*** by patients, who are being mehcanically ventilated.
- Later signs of venous air embolism includes: Cardiac arrhythmias, hypotension, tachycardia, a 'mill wheel' murmur and cyanosis.
- ***Best method*** to ***confirm diagnosis*** is transesophageal echocardiography (*TEE*); next best method is *precordial Doppler U/S*.
- ***Treatment***: Flood surgical field with saline; deliver 100% oxygen; aspirate central venous catheter; give volume to increase CVP; treat hemodynamic changes appropriately.

2. **Answer is c (Circumoral numbness).**
Ref: Pocket Anesthesia, By Richard D Urman, Pg 2D-26.

- Toxicity of local anesthetics mainly affects the *CNS and CVS*.
- Progressive signs of ***local anesthetic toxicity*** are light headedness > ***circumoral numbness*** > facial tingling > tinnitues > slurred speech > seizures > unconsciousness > respiratory arrest > CVS depression > circulatory arrest.

3. **Answer is a [Biphasic, truncated, exponential (BTE)].**
Ref: Resuscitation: Translational Research, Clinical Evidence, Education, Guidelines, By Antonino Gullo, Giuseppe Ristagn, Pg 69.

- Earlier ***AEDs*** (Automated electric defibrillators) used monophasic waveforms, which deliver current to the patients in a single direction (unidirectional—from one electrode to another).
- Unlike monophasic waveforms, the biphasic waveforms are more effective due to a lesser tendency to reinitiate ventricular fibrillation (VF) in areas of residual charge left on the myocardium.
- The second phase of the biphasic shock is believed to neutralize virtual electrodes and tissue polarization residual from the first phase.
- The ***most widely used*** in the AED's now is the ***biphasic truncated exponential*** (BTE) waveform.
- The advanatage is that it has lower defirbillation threshold compared to monophasic defibrillation and could therefore allow the design of devices that are substantially smaller and lighter than the monophasic waveform.

4. **Answer is a (50:50).**
Ref: Oxford Handbook of Emergency Medicine, 4th edition Pg 278.

- A mix of ***nitrous oxide 50%*** and ***oxygen 50%*** is a medical analgesic gas, commonly known as ***Entonox*** (a registered trademark of BOC) or ***Nitronox***, or colloquially as 'gas and air'
- The ***Poynting effect*** involves the dissolution of gaseous O_2 when bubbled through liquid N_2O, with vaporization of the liquid to form a gaseous O_2/N_2O mixture

5. Answer is d (Tail).
Ref: Human Anatomy, Anand Mahindra Kumar, Pg 176.

- ***Tail of pancreas***: This is the ***narrow left end*** of pancreas.
- It ***lies in the lienorenal ligament*** together with ***splenic artery***.
- It is the ***most mobile part of pancreas***.

6. Answer is d (Neural crest).
Ref: Textbook of Clinical Embryology, By Vishram Singh, Pg 277.

Neural Crest Derivatives

Trunk neural crest cells	Cranial neural crest cells
– MelaNoCytes[Q],	– Pia and arachnoid mater
– SchwanN Cells	– Bones of cranium
– ***Adrenal medulla***[Q] (including chromaffiN Cells)	– Pharyngeal arch cartilage
– Dorsal root ganglia,	– ***Odontoblasts***[Q] (***dentin of teeth***[Q])
– Sympathetic chain ganglia; prevertebral sympathetic ganglia	– ***Parafollicular C cells***[Q] of thyroid
	– Aorticopulmonary septum and endocardial cushions
– ***Parasympathetic ganglia of the gut***[Q] (Meissner's and Auerbach's plexus, CN X)	– Sensory ganglia of CN V, CN VII, CN IX and CN X Ciliary (CN III), Pterygopalatine (CN VII), submandibular (CN VII) and Otic (CN IX) parasympathetic ganglia.
– Abdominal/Pelvic cavity parasympathetic ganglia	

7. Answer is b (Seventh).
Ref: Clinical Anatomy, Neeta Kulkarni, Pg 319.

- The ***stellate ganglion (or cervicothoracic*** ganglion) is a sympathetic ganglion formed by the fusion of the *inferior cervical ganglion and the first thoracic ganglion*, which exists in 80% of cases.
- Stellate ganglion is located at the level of ***C7 (7th cervical vertebrae)***, anterior to the transverse process of C7, superior to the neck of the first rib and just below the subclavian artery.

8. Answer is b (Flexor tendon of the digits).
Ref: Problem Solving in Musculoskeletal Imaging, By William B Morrison, Timothy G Sanders, Pg 482.

- The ***tendons of the flexor digitorum superficialis*** muscle have a ***split (Camper's Chiasm; chiasma tendineum)*** at the end of them through which the tendons of flexor digitorum profundus pass.

9. Answer is d (Ophthalmic veins).
Ref: Clinical Anatomy (A Problem-Solving Approach), 2nd Edition, By Neeta V Kulkarn, Pg 329.

- The ***dangerous area of the face*** is drained by the ***facial vein***.
- The facial vein communicates with the cavernous sinus through
  - ***Superior ophthalmic*** veins
  - ***Pterygoid venous plexus***.

- Infective thrombi from a boil on the dangerous area of the face spreads to the cavernous sinus causing cavernous sinus thrombosis.

10. Answer is b (Monoacylglycerol).
Ref: Textbook of Biochemistry, Vasudevan, 7th edition Pg 149.

- In order for the ***triglyceride to be absorbed***, two processes must occur:
  - Large aggregates of dietary triglyceride, which are virtually insoluble in an aqueous environment, must be broken down physically and held in suspension— a process called ***emulsification***.
  - Triglyceride molecules must be enzymatically digested to ***yield monoglyceride and fatty acids***, both of which can ***efficiently diffuse or be transported into the enterocyte.***

11. Answer is b (α-2 globulin).
Ref: Textbook of Biochemistry, Vasudevan, 7th edition Pg 384.

- ***Ceruloplasmin (Cp)*** is an **α-2 *globulin***.
- It is ***blue in color*** with a molecular weight of 16,000 Daltons.
- It contains 6–8 copper atoms per molecule.
- It is also called ***ferroxidase***, an enzyme, which helps in incorporation of iron into transferrin. It is an important ***anti-oxidant*** in plasma.
- ***Increased plasma Cp levels*** are seen in active hepatitis, biliary cirrhosis, hemochromatosis, obstructive biliary disease, pregnancy, estrogen therapy, collagen disorders and malignancies. Drugs increasing Cp levels are estrogen and contraceptives.
- In ***Wilson's disease, AR*** condition, ***reduced Cp*** levels are seen.

12. Answer is c (Acute intermittent porphyria).
Ref: Textbook of Biochemistry, Vasudevan, 7th edition Pg 274.

PORPHYRIAS

❖ ***Porphyrias*** are a group of inherited or acquired disorders of certain enzymes in the heme biosynthetic pathway (also called porphyrin pathway). Based on the site of the overproduction and accumulation of the porphyrins (or their chemical precursors), porphyrias are broadly classified as:
  - ***Acute***Q (***hepatic***) porphyrias: characterized by *acute* ***neurological attacks***Q (seizures, psychosis, extreme back and abdominal pain and an acute polyneuropathy).
  - ***Cutaneous***Q (***erythropoietic***Q) porphyrias: Present with ***skin problems***, usually a light-sensitive blistering rash and increased hair growth.
  - ***Variegate*** porphyria (***mixed*** porphyria) has both *neurological and skin features*.

❖ *Porphyrias* = Disease of 5PsQ = Pain abdomen, Psychological disturbances, Polyneuropathy, Purple urine, Precipitated by Pills.

Classification of human porphyrias

Condition	Enzyme defect
Hepatic porphyrias	
Acute intermittent porphyria (AD)	Porphobilinogen deaminase Q (uroporphyrinogen 1 synthaseQ)
Porphyria cutanea tarda (AD), MC	UroporphyrinogenQ decarboxylase
Hereditary coproporphyria (AD)	Coproporphyrinogen oxidaseQ
Erythropoietic porphyrias	
Congenital erythropoietic porphyria (Gunther's disease) (AR)	Uroporphyrinogen cosynthaseQ
Erythropoietic protoporphyria (AD)	FerrocheletaseQ (Heme synthase)
Mixed	
Vareigate porphyria (AD)	Protoporphyrinogen oxidaseQ

COMED-K 2015 ANSWERS

13. Answer is c (Glycine).
Ref: CMDT 2013, Pg 1429.

- ***Strychnine*** is a ***high-affinity competitive antagonist*** at the ***glycine receptor***.
- Strychnine *prevents the inhibitory effects of glycine* on the postsynaptic neuron. Therefore, action potentials are triggered with lower levels of excitatory neurotransmitters.
- When the inhibitory signals are prevented, the motor neurons are more easily activated and the victim will have spastic muscle contractions resulting in death by asphyxiation.

14. Answer is b (Lysosomes).
Ref: Cellular Organelles and the Extracellular Matrix, edited by Edward Bittar, Pg 15.

- Two different mechanisms exist for targeting of ***proteins to lysosomes***:
- The first is ***Mannose-6-phosphate*** dependent and ***targets the newly synthesized lysosomal hydrolases to the lumen of the lysosome***.
- The second mechanism is dependent on sequence features of the cytoplasmic domain, the cytoplasmic tail of newly synthesized lysosomal proteins.

15. Answer is a (Phospholipase A2).
Ref: Textbook of Biochemistry, Vasudevan, 7th edition Pg 90.

- ***Phospholipases*** are enzymes that hydrolyse phospholipids.
- The extracellular forms of ***phospholipases A2*** have been isolated from different ***venoms (snake, bee and wasp)***.

16. Answer is c (Midyear population).
Ref: Park, 23rd edition Pg 57.

- When analysis is planned to throw light on etiology, it is essential to use specific death rates.
- The ***denominator for all specific death rates*** is the ***mid-year population*** and the ***multiplier is 1,000***.
- Thus, ***specific death rate due to TB*** = Number of deaths from TB during a calendar year/midyear population × 1,000.

17. Answer is d [Tolerable upper intake level (UL)].
Ref: Park, 23rd edition Pg 632.

- ***Tolerable upper intake level (UL)***: The highest average daily nutrient intake level that is likely to pose no adverse health effects for almost all individuals in the general population.
- ***Recommended dietary allowance (RDA)***: The average daily dietary nutrient intake level sufficient to meet the nutrient requirement of nearly all (97–98%) healthy individuals in a particular life stage and gender group.
- ***Adequate intake***: A recommended average daily intake level based on observed or experimentally determined approximation or estimates of nutrient intake by a group (or groups) of apparently healthy people—used when RDA cannot be determined; in the Indian context, this is the 'acceptable intake'.
- ***Estimated average requirement (EAR)***: The average daily nutrient intake level estimated to meet the requirement of half of the healthy individuals in a particular life stage and gender group.

18. Answer is b (138).
Ref: http://www.nhp.gov.in/sites/default/files/anm_guidelines.pdf

- Birth rate = ***25/1,000*** population
- Population under the ***SubCenter = 5,000***
- Therefore, expected number of live births = (25 × 5,000)/1,000 = 125 births
- Correction factor (pregnancy wastage) = 10% of 125 (i.e. [10/100] × 125) = 13

Therefore, ***total no. of expected pregnancies*** in a year = ***125 + 13 = 138***

any month, the ANM should have about 69 pregnancies registered with her.

19. Answer is b (Specific).
Ref: Park, 23rd edition Pg 24.

- ***Health indicators***: Indicators are required to assess the health of a community and also to compare the health status of one community with the other. Also they are required to monitor and evaluate the success of health services and health programs.
- ***Characteristics of*** an ***ideal health indicator*** should be as below:
  - ***Valid***: It must measure what it is supposed to measure.
  - ***Reliable***: The answer should be the same if measured by different people in similar circumstances.
  - ***Sensitive***: They should be sensitive to changes in the situation concerned.
  - ***Specific***: They should reflect changes only in the situation concerned.
  - ***Feasible***: They should have the ability to obtain data needed
  - ***Relevant***: They should contribute to the understanding of the phenomenon of interest.

20. Answer is b [2(HRZE)3, 4(HR)3].
Ref: Park, 23rd edition Pg 188.

- There are three categories of treatment regimens for patients suffering from tuberculosis (pulmonary or extra-pulmonary). Each patient has a ***Patient Wise Box*** issued on his name with program registration number once(s) he starts treatment under DOTS at a DOT center. All the diagnosis and treatment with DOTS is done FREE of COST to all its patients through all *Diagnostic and treatment (DOT)* centers.

Category	Color of label on box
Category 1	Red
Category 2	Blue
Category 3	Green

Category of Treatment	Type of Patient	Regimen*
Category I	New sputum smear—positive New sputum smear—negative New extrapulmonary New others	2H3R3Z3E3+ 4H3R3
Category II	Sputum smear—positive relapse Sputum smear—positive failure Sputum smear—positive treatment after default, others	2H3R3Z3E3S3 + 1H3R3Z3E3 + 5H3R3E3
Category III	New sputum smear—negative, not seriously ill New extrapulmonary, not seriously ill	2H3R3Z3 + 4H3R3

- * - Number before the letters refers to the number of months of treatment. The subscript after the letters refers to the number of doses per week. H (Isoniazid) 600 mg; R (Rifampicin) 400 mg; Z (pyrazinamide) 1,500 mg; E (Ethambutol) 1,200 mg; S (streptomycin) 750 mg. Patients, who weigh more than 60 kg recieve additoinal rifampicin 150 mg. Patients more than 50 years recieve streptomycin 500 mg.
- Examples of ***seriously ill extrapulmonary TB = TB spine***, TB meningitis; TB peritonitis; TB pericarditis; Intestinal TB; genitourinary TB; TB pleurisy.

21. Answer is a (Work sampling).
Ref: Park, 23rd edition Pg 872.

- ***Work sampling*** is a systematic observation and recording of activities of one or more individuals carried out at predetermined or random intervals. It provides quantitative measurements of the various activities.

22. Answer is b (Coronary heart disease).
Ref: Park, 23rd edition Pg 80, 371.

- The ***Framingham study*** has played a major role in establishing the nature and relative importance of risk factors for coronary heart disease.
- The ***Framingham Heart Study*** is a long term, ongoing ***cardiovascular study*** on residents of the town of ***Framingham, Massachusetts***. The study ***began in 1948*** with 5,209 adult subjects from Framingham and is now on its third generation of participants.

23. Answer is b (Spectrum of health).
Ref: Park, 23rd edition Pg 18, 39.

- ***Spectrum of health***: Health and disease lie along a continuum and there is no single cut off point. The lowest point on the health disease spectrum is death and the highest point corresponds to the WHO definition of positive health.
- ***Spectrum of disease***: Is a graphic representation of the various manifestations of a disease—similar to the spectrum of light where the colors vary from one end to the other, but difficult to determine where one color ends and the other color begins.

24. Answer is b (Eligible couple).
Ref: Park, 23rd edition Pg 492.

- An ***'eligible couple'*** refers to a currently married couple wherein the wife is in the reproductive age (15–45 years). There will be at least 150–180 such couples for 1000 population in India.
- ***'Target couple'***: Include families with one child and even newly married couples with a view to develop the acceptance of family planning from the earliest stage.

25. Answer is c (Pterygium unguis).
Ref: CMDT 2013. Pg 144.

Nail changes in Lichen Planus
• Nail plate thinning causing ***longitudinal grooving and ridging;*** • ***Hyperpigmentation,*** • ***Subungual hyperkeratosis,*** • ***Onycholysis,*** • ***20-nail dystrophy***[Q] • ***Longitudinal melanonychia***[Q]. • Rarely, the matrix can be permanently destroyed with prominent ***pterygium***[Q] formation.

All about Lichen Planus (LP)

- **'5Ps'** = lesions are **Pruritic** (itchy), **Plain** (flat) topped, **Polygonal**, **Purple** (violaceous), **Papules**.
- Cell-mediated immune response of unknown origin.

Associations

- A/w ***Hepatitis C***[Q] infection; LP-like lesions have been seen after usage of ***drugs such as*** gold, antimalarials, diuretics, penicillamine, phenothiazines; allergy to mercury and in patients with skin lesions of *chronic graft versus host disease*

Clinically

- ***Common sites***[Q]: Inner aspects of ***wrists and ankles, flexor aspect of forearms, shins***, lower back (*lumbar region*), *genitalia* (as annular white lesion), ***oral mucosa*** (as white netlike/lacelike eruption).
- ***Wickham's striae***[Q]: Fine network of gray/white lines on the lesions.
- ***Koebner's phenomenon***[Q]: New lesions may appear at the site of trauma.
- ***Lichen planopilaris***[Q] ***(follicular LP)***: LP affecting hairy areas such as the scalp; MC in women; *scarring alopecia* may result
- ...*nant* transformation (squamous cell Ca)—in oral, genital and esophageal LP.

- *Vulvar* lesions can be *pruritic* and *painful.*
- ***Residual hyperpigmentation***Q and ***scarring***Q can occur.

Histology of LP
– Confirmation of diagnosis is by ***skin biopsy.***
– *Basal cell degeneration*Q (forming ***'colloid***Q', ***'Civatte*** **bodies**Q', ***'hyaline or cytoid***Q' in the epidermis),
– ***Heavy T-lymphocyte infiltration in the upper dermis*** (***'sawtooth***Q' ***rete ridges***);
– ***'Interface dermatitis***Q'
– ***Acanthosis***Q; ***hyperkeratosis***Q; ***orthokeratosis***Q (*i.e., hyperkeratosis without parakeratosis*) and a prominent granular layer (***wedge-shaped hypergranulosis***Q),
– ***'Liquefactive degeneration***Q' of the basal layer
– ***Pigment incontinence***Q *(responsible for postinflammatory hyperpigmentation)*
– ***IgM*** on the colloid body surface gives ***'bunch of grapes'*** immunofluorescent pattern;
– ***Max Joseph space***Q: Subepidermal clefts formed by acantholysis or hydropic degeneration of basal cells.

Treatment

- ***Spontaneous resolution***Q occurs in 6 months to 2 years; *topical* ***glucocorticoids***Q are the mainstay of therapy, antihistamines are used for pruritus; phototherapy (PUVA) maybe used; *Oral LP* is *more difficult to treat*Q and typically *lasts longer than skin lichen planus*; hydroxychloroquine for oral LP.

26. Answer is d (Lupus vulgaris).

Ref: Dermatology, By Otto Braun-Falco, Pg 136.

Lupus vulgaris

- ***MC form of skin TB***Q; seen in *previously infected/ sensitized persons;* ***MC*** **in *females***Q; often a/w *underlying active TB* in the lung or lymph nodes.
- *MC* in ***head and neck***Q and are red-brown plaques; ***'apple-jelly nodules***Q' on diascopyQ; ***scarring and SCC***Q can develop within the plaques.
- Cartilage (nose, ears) within the affected area is progressively destroyed (***lupus vorax***Q); *bone usually is spared.*

OTHER TUBERCULAR INFECTIONS OF SKIN

Scrofuloderma
– Skin TB that results from ***direct extension from underlying tuberculous focus***Q, i.e. infected lymph nodes, muscles or bones.
Tuberculous chancre
– Skin TB occurring in persons with ***NO previous infection and immunity***Q; infection ***follows an injury,*** usually in children.
– *Firm, NON-healing,* shallow, *NON-tender,* ***undermined***Q *ulcer* with a granulomatous base a/w *painless* ***regional lymphadenopathy***Q.
Tuberculosis verrucosa cutis (TVC)
– TVC occurs in ***previously infected individuals*** with a *high degree of immunity* and may be from *infected sputum* or due to *handling infected material.*
– MC seen on ***hands and legs***Q; warty papule often mistaken for verruca vulgaris (***Anatomist's / postmort-*** ***prosector's wart***Q); NO regional lymphadenopathy

Tuberculids
– Tuberculids are ***symmetric generalized exanthems***Q in the skin of tuberculous patients, possibly resulting from ***hypersensitivity***Q reactions to tubercle bacillus. Typically, patients with tuberculids are in relatively good healthQ and show (1) ***Strongly positive Mantoux test***Q (2) Tuberculous ***involvement***Q (usually inactive) of viscera or lymph nodes, (3) ***Absence of M. tuberculosis bacilli***Q in tissue by smear/culture and (4) ***Satisfactory therapeutic response*** of skin lesions to antitubercular treatment – *Currently only three entities are accepted as tuberculids* – ***Papulonecrotic tuberculid***Q, ***Lichen scrofulosorum***Q, ***Erythema induratum***Q ***(Bazin's disease***Q***)***
Swimming pool or fish-tank granuloma
– Caused by ***M. marinum***Q; after contact with contaminated ***tropical fish tanks***Q, ***swimming pools***Q ***or salt-water fish;*** a small *violet nodule* or pustule may appear at a site of *minor trauma;* ***lymphangitic spread*** with several nodules up the extremity in a *sporotrichoid fashion* may occur; lesions often *heal spontaneously* (Marine = water).
Buruli ulcer
– *Caused by* ***Mycobacterium ulcerans***Q; chronic, necrotizing ulcer, painless and occurs ***after penetrating skin trauma; spontaneously heal,*** but frequently result in chronic *lymphedema* and *disfiguring scarring;* Treat with *Excision* (Bur**ULi Ulcer** = M. **ULcer**ans).

27. Answer is c (*Corynebacterium tenuis*).
Ref: Dermatology, By Otto Braun-Falco, Pg 182.

- Trichomycosis axillaris is dense colonization of the axillary hair by *Corynebacterium tenuis,* which do not normally cause disease.
- Occurs in the presence of poor hygeine and hyperhidrosis.
- It is a misnomer (NOT a 'mycosis', but was thought to be a fungal infection).

28. Answer is b (Sebaceous glands).
Ref: Harrison's, 19th edition Pg 127, 240.

- ***Fordyce spots***Q: **Ectopic *sebaceous glands***Q *on* ***lips and oral mucosa***Q – *normal* condition.

Also Know

– ***Fox-Fordyce disease***Q: ***Apocrine miliaria****; itchy follicular papules* in **axillae *MC*** and groin; MC in ***women aged 13–35 years.***
– ***Miliaria***Q: Due to disruption of ***eccrine***Q ***sweat gland*** ductal integrity; ***miliaria rubra (prickly heat)***; miliaria crystallina (***sudamina***).
– ***Hidradenitis suppurativa***Q: Chronic suppurative condition of ***apocrine*** sweat glands.
– Apocrine: B***romhidrosis***: Offensive body odor.

29. Answer is d (Primary lymphatic malignancy).
Ref: The 5 Minute Pediatric Consult, edited by M William Schwartz, 2012 edition Pg 516.

Causes of lymphedema

Primary lymphedema	Secondary lymphedema
Developmental abnormality of lymphatic flow; has 3 forms but all may not be clinically evident at birth	Acquired abnormality of lymphatic flow
• ***Congenital*** lymphedema: Present at birth; MC in females; MC in lower limb; 2/3 cases are bilateral; may improve with age • ***Lymphedema praecox*** (***MC form*** of primary lymphedema): appears at puberty; MC in females; affects unilateral lower limb (L>R)	• Neoplasms • Postsurgical obstruction • Burns • Insect bites • Infection

• *Lymphedema tarda*: Presents at age 35 or older	• Surgery • Trauma

30. Answer is a (3 weeks).

Ref: Bailey and Love, 26th edition Pg 21; Transfusion and Transplantation Science, By Robin Knight. Pg 50.

➢ ***Shelf life of whole blood*** stored in ACD (Acid citrate dextrose) is approximately 3 ***weeks***. Whole blood is rarely used now.

Blood product	Shelf Life
Whole blood (in ACD)	3 weeks
Packed red cells (in CPD only)	3 weeks
Packed red cells (in SAG-M or CPD-A)	5 weeks
Fresh frozen plasma (FFP)	2 years at minus 40–50°C
Cryoprecipitate	2 years at minus 20°C
Platelets	5 days at 20–24°C (room temperature)
Granulocytes	24 hours

31. Answer is a (Innate immunity).

Ref: Harrison's, 19th edition Pg 950.

➢ ***Toll-like receptors*** have a crucial role in the detection of microbial infection in mammals and insects.

➢ In mammals, these receptors have evolved to recognize conserved products unique to microbial metabolism. This specificity allows the Toll proteins to detect the presence of infection and to induce activation of inflammatory and antimicrobial ***innate immune responses***.

➢ Recognition of microbial products by Toll-like receptors expressed ***on dendritic cells*** trigger functional maturation of dendritic cells and leads to initiation of antigen-specific adaptive immune responses.

32. Answer is b (*Cladosporium carrionii*).

Ref: CMDT 2013, Pg 1540.

- Chromoblastomycosis is a chronic, tropical cutaneous infection usually affecting young men, who are agricultural workers
- It is caused most commonly by two closely related black molds; ***Cladophialophora carrionii*** and ***Fonsecaea pedrosoi***.
- Lesions usually follow puncture wounds; develops into a a papule or ulcer—ultimately verrucous elevated nodules occur.
- ***Satellite lesions*** may appear along the lymphatics. ***Elephantiasis*** may result.
- The fungus is seen as brown, thick-walled, spherical, sometimes septate cells in potassium hydroxide preparations of pus or skin scrapings, which are quite sensitive for diagnosis (***medlar/sclerotic bodies***).
- Itraconazole or Terbinafine orally is used.

33. Answer is b (*Diphyllobothrium latum*).

Ref: Harrison's, 19th edition Pg 645.

- The ***fish tapeworm*** (***Diphyllobothrium latum***) lives in the small intestine of humans and accumulates cobalamin (B_{12}) from food, rendering the cobalamin unavailable for absorption.
- Because ***D. latum*** absorbs large quantities of vitamin B_{12} and ***interferes with ileal B_{12} absorption***, vitamin B_{12} deficiency can develop,
- Individuals acquire the worm by ***eating raw or partly cooked fish***.
- Infestation is common in ***Scandinavia***.
- ***Megaloblastic anemia*** or cobalamin neuropathy occurs only in those with a heavy infestation.

34. Answer is b (Interference microscope).
Ref: Ananthanarayan and Paniker's Textbook of Microbiology, Pg 8.

- ***Interference microscope***: *Reveals cell organelle* and also enables ***quantitative measurement of chemical constituents*** of cells such as *lipids, proteins and nucleic acids.*
- ***Polarization microscope***: Enables the study of intracellular structures using ***differences in birefringence.***
- ***Phase contract microscope***: Improves contrast and makes evident the structures within the cells that differ in thickness or refractive index.
- ***Dark field/Dark ground microscope***: ***Reflected light*** is used instead of transmitted light using a '***condenser***'.

35. Answer is a (*Staphylococcus aureus*).
Ref: Harrison's, 19th edition Pg 956.

- Virulence factors of *Staphylococcus aureus:*
  - ***Enterotoxin***[Q]: ***Preformed exotoxin***[Q] secreted in the intestines, heat resistant. Causes ***food poisoning*** typified by ***vomiting and diarrhea within 8 hours***[Q] of food consumption.
  - ***Toxic shock syndrome toxin 1 (TSST 1)*** – A ***superantigen***[Q] causing ***unregulated inflammation***; acquired from ***contaminated tampons***[Q] in ***menstruating women*** or from infected wounds; leads to ***Toxic shock syndrome***— signs are ***systemic hypotension***[Q], ***tachycardia***[Q], high fever, vomiting/diarrhea, ***headache***, sunburn such as ***rash***, muscle aches; redness of eyes and throat.
  - ***Exfoliatin:*** Another ***superantigen***[Q] causes ***Staphylococcal Scalded Skin Syndrome (SSSS)*** in children under 4 years; SSSS in neonates is called ***Ritter's disease***[Q] and in older individuals is called ***toxic epidermal necrolysis***[Q]. Diffuse tender erythema often with bullae and desquamation. ***Nikolksy sign***[Q] is present (sloughing of the epidermis can be provoked by gentle stroking of the skin). Milder and more common forms of SSSS include ***pemphigus neonatorum***[Q] *and* ***bullous impetigo***[Q].
  - ***Protein A***[Q] *(basis of* ***coagglutination reaction***[Q]*).*
  - *Beta hemolysin (exhibits* ***hot-cold*** *phenomenon)*
  - ***Synergohymenotropic***[Q] *toxin (biocomponent toxin such as gamma hemolysin + leucocidins).*
  - *Leukocidin:* ***Panton-Valentine***[Q]; important in ***MRSA infection.***
  - Others are, *Alpha and gamma hemolysin,;* ***clumping factor*** (responsible for *slide coagulase test).*
- ***Enzymes*** *produced: Coagulase, deoxyribonuclease, lipase, hyaluronidase, protease, fibrinolysin.*

36. Answer is d (12).
Ref: Donald School Basic Textbook of Ultrasound in Obstetrics & Gynecology, By V D'Addario, Pg 41.

- In ***ultrasonography***, the accuracy rate of sex determination increased with gestation from 70.3% at 11 weeks to ***98.7% at 12 weeks*** and 100% at 13 weeks.

37. Answer is a (1–1.5).
Ref: Gynaecological Oncology for the MRCOG and Beyond, By Nigel Acheson, David Luesley, Pg 137.

- The ***average woman*** has about a ***1.5% lifetime chance of developing ovarian cancer*** (with no family h/o ovarian cancer); in those with one first degree relative affected it is 5% and two first degree relatives affected it is 7%.
- She has about a ***12% chance of developing breast cancer*** at some point in her lifetime.

38. Answer is a (15).
Ref: Handbook of Diagnostic Endocrinology, edited by Janet E Hall, Lynnette K Niema, Pg 68.

- As ***endometrial cancer is responsible for*** 15% of all cases of ***postmenopausal bleeding (PMB)***, any such bleeding should be considered cancerous in origin until proven otherwise.
- ***MC cause of PMB*** in developing countries (like India) is ***Ca cervix.***
- ***MC cause of PMB*** in ***developed countries*** is ***endometrial and vaginal atrophy*** (30%).

39. Answer is d (Numerous acrochordons).
Ref: Harrison's, 16th (old) edition Pg 1733.

Clinical markers of insulin resistance:

- ***Acanthosis*** nigricans
- Multiple skin tags (***acrochordons***)
- ***Acromegaloid*** features
- ***Hyperandrogenism*** (acne, hirsutism, oligomenorrhea)
- Central obesity and ***high waist: hip*** ratio.
- ***High*** Body mass Index (BMI) > 30 kg/sq m

40. Answer is b (Renal imaging is not necessary in CBAVD).
Ref: Principles of Molecular Medicine, edited by J Larry Jameson, Pg 606.

- Congenital bilateral ***absence of the vas deferens*** (CBAVD) is responsible for 1–2% cases of male infertility;
- It is a/w ***CFTR gene*** mutation (80% cases) and cystic fibrosis;
- It is a/w ***seminal vesicle agenesis, low semen volume, low pH (acidic semen)*** with ***low fructose*** and ***azoospermia***.
- CFTR mutation negative CBAVD is a/w renal anomalies (horseshoe kidney, aplasia, renal ectopy) – abdominal U/S necessary

41. Answer is d (Concurrent use of combination of chemotherapy and brain irradiation).
Ref: Comprehensive Gynecology, By Gretchen M Lentz, Pg 788.

- ***Whole brain radiotherapy*** with to achieve hemostasis and tumor shrinkage has been used in ***conjunction with chemotherapy*** for patients with brain metastases, BUT chemotherapy is the preferred option.
- Given the vascular nature of these tumors and the fact that they are not protected by the blood brain barrier, intrathecal chemotherapy is unnecessary.
- Chemotherapy regimen used is EMA-CO: Etoposide, Methotrexate, Adriamycin- Cyclophosphamide, Oncovin (vincristine).

42. Answer is a (Germ cell tumor).
Ref: Dutta's gynecology, Pg 371.

- Malignant epithelial ovarian tumors constitute about 90% of all ovarian carcinomas (MC in women > 30 years of age).
- ***Germ cell tumors*** are the ***most common*** ovarian tumors of the ***first decade of life***.

43. Answer is c (*Corynebacterium*).
Ref: Textbook of Ophthalmology, By Sunita Agarwal, Pg 1002.

- ***Staphylococcus aureus, Streptococcus pneumoniae*** and ***Staphylococcus epidermidis*** are the ***most commonly*** encountered ***gram positive pathogens*** causing ***bacterial keratitis***.
- *Organisms less frequently* reported from bacterial keratitis include *Corynebacterium* species, *Propionibacterium* acnes, *Bacillus* species and *Neisseria* gonorrheae.

44. Answer is b (Vernal keratoconjunctivitis).
Ref: Parsons' diseases of the eye, 21st edition Pg 178-179.

Vernal Keratoconjunctivitis (VKC)

- A.k.a Spring Catarrh
- Affects ***children/young adults***[Q]; ***type I hypersensitivity***[Q] ***reaction*** due to external allergens
- A/w atopy (asthma, eczema, allergic rhinitis) OR a family h/o atopy
- Intense ***itching***[Q], *mucoid '****stringy/ropy***[Q]*' discharge:* ***Maxwell Lyon sign***[Q]
- ***Cobblestone***[Q] *papillae* on undersurface of upper eyelid
- ***Horner Trantas spots***[Q] at limbus
- Corneal ***'shield ulcer***[Q]***'*** may be seen
- ***Pseudogerontoxon***[Q] *(also called 'cupid's bow', peripheral corneal scar resembling arcus senilis)*; ***alkaline tears***[Q]

- Treatment: ***Mast cell stabilizers*** (sodium cromoglycate, ***olopatadine***Q); limited topical corticosteroids; topical ***cyclosporine***Q; cool compress
- Note: VKC patients have ↑ incidence of ***keratoconus***Q

45. Answer is b (Bone spicule pigmentary change).

Ref: Parsons' diseases of the eye, 21st edition Pg 320-321.

- The findings given are those of retinitis pigmentosa. See below for more details.

RETINITIS PIGMENTOSA (RP)

- Typical RP is a diffuse ***bilaterally symmetrical*** retinal ***dystrophy*** *predominantly affecting* ***rods***Q.
- Inheritance: Sporadic; ***AD*** (*MC, best prognosis*Q); AR; XLR (*least common, worst prognosis*, female carriers have normal fundi or show *'golden-metallic*Q*' tapetal reflex* temporal to the macula).
- **Clinical features:**
  - ***Defective dark adaptation (night blindness***Q***, nyctalopia)***, progressive visual field defect.
  - Classic triad of RP: (1) ***arteriolar attenuation***Q (2) ***bone-spicule pigmentation***Q that is perivascular and more in equatorial region (3) ***Waxy pallor of optic disk***Q that is *least reliable sign* of the triad.
  - Unmasking of larger choroidal vessels (due to pigment migration) gives the fundus a ***tessellated appearance***Q.
  - Three types of ***maculopathy***Q that may be seen are—atrophic, cellophane, cystoid macular edema.
  - *Associated ocular features*: optic disk drusen, open-angle glaucoma, *posterior subcapsular cataracts*Q, keratoconus, myopia, posterior vitreous detachment.

> - **RP** like **fundus picture is seen in**Q**:**
>   - End stage chloroquine retinopathy
>   - End stage syphilitic retinopathy
>   - Cancer related retinopathy

- **Investigations:**
  - ***ERG:*** *Reduced amplitude of scoptopic and photopic b-wave*Q, delay in time between the flash of light and peak of b-wave (*delayed implicit time*Q).
  - EOG: Absence of light rise.
  - Visual field: Initially annular/*ring* scotoma, later progressive constriction of visual field.
- **Atypical RP**
  - *Retinitis punctata albescens.*
  - *Sector RP:* Involves of only one quadrant (usually nasal) or one half (usually inferior); many cases remain stationary.
  - *Pericentric RP.*
  - *RP with exudative vasculopathy* (Coats disease such as telangiectasias).

Note: *Epiretinal and subretinal microchip implants*Q have been used with modest success in RP—still in research.

Syndromes A/W Retinitis Pigmentosa

Bassen-Kornzweig syn. (***Abetalipoproteinemia***Q): ***Acanthocytosis***, fat malabsorption, ataxia; ***jejunal biopsy is diagnostic***
Refsum'sQ **syn.:** Due to defective metabolism of ***phytanic acid***Q *that accumulates*. Peripheral neuropathyQ, cerebellar ataxia, elevated CSF proteins, deafness, icthyosis, cardiac arrhythmias
Bardet-Biedl synQ**.:** *Mental retardation, polydactyly, obesity, hypogonadism*; (coned rod dystrophy causing Bull's eye maculopathy is typically a/w Bardet Biedl syndrome)
Usher'sQ **syn.:** Sensorineural deafness.
Kearns-SayreQ **syn.:** Chronic progressive external ophthalmoplegia, heart block.
Cockayne'sQ **syn.:** *Bird-like facies*, dwarfism, flexion contracture of limbs, mental retardation, ataxia and premature aging.

Cohen syn.: Facial dysmorphism, prominent incisors, mental deficit, muscle hypotonia, truncal obsesity
Friedrich[Q] ataxia : Ataxia, nystagmus
HARP[Q] syn. - a.k.a. Hallervorden-Spatz disease : Hypoprebetalipoproteinemia, acanthocytosis, RP, Pallidal degeneration (Progressive extrapyramidal dysfunction and dementia)
NARP[Q] syn.: Neuropathy, ataxia, RP

Note: All are autosomal recessive.

46. Answer is d (i, ii and iii).

Ref: Parsons' diseases of the eye, 21st edition Pg. 281.

- The parameters to be assessed when evaluating a patient's optic disk for glaucoma are: *CDR* (cup-to-disk ratio); ***NRR area/thinning*** (neuroretinal rim) and ***RNFL defects*** (retinal nerve fiber layer).
- ***RNFL defects*** are best seen by ***red free (green) light***.
- In modern day glaucoma practice, size of optic disk also is to be assessed since larger disks will have larger cups and may not be necessarily glaucomatous. However, since option does not contain all of the above 'D' can be taken as the answer.

47. Answer is a (Myopia).

Ref: Ophthalmology, By Myron Yanoff, Jay S Duker, 3rd edition Pg 107.

- ***Myopia*** is the ***most common*** visually significant ***refractive error.***

48. Answer is a (Microvascular ischemia).

Ref: Parsons' diseases of the eye, 21st edition Pg 424-425.

- The ***most common cause*** of ***isolated cranial nerve palsies (III, IV or VI)*** is ***microvascular ischemia*** due to ***diabetes mellitus*** or ***hypertension***.

49. Answer is c (Fracture involves an abnormal bone)

Ref: Maheswari orthopedics textbook, 5th edition Pg 167.

- A ***stress fracture*** is common in ***the second metatarsal (March fracture)*** and has high occurrence rate in the military during training and marching.
- The fracture ***heals spontaneously***; treatment is ***usually symptomatic***.
- It occurs in a ***previously normal bone*** and is due to *accumulution of* ***microtrauma***.

50. Answer is e (Wrong stem/options as per revised answer key).

Ref: A short note given below.

Spondylolisthesis

- A forward slip of vertebra ***L5 on S1***.
- In a ***normal vertebra*** (in oblique view of spine), the interpeduncular region gives a ***'Scottish dog'*** appearance.
- In ***spondylolisthesis***, (in oblique view of spine), ***'Beheaded Scottish dog'*** appearance is seen
- ***AP view X-ray is least useful[Q] except*** in cases of ***Inverted Napoleon Hat*** sign (appearance of the L5 vertebra on an *AP X-ray in severe spondylolisthesis*).
- MRI shows spinal cord compression, CT scan shows bony slippage.

51. Answer is b (Medial tibial epiphysis).

Ref: Paediatric Orthopaedics: A system of decision-making, By Benjamin Joseph, Pg 455.

- **Blount's[Q] disease:** ***Tibia vara***[Q]; MC in West Indies; growth of the ***medial half of the proximal tibial epiphysis*** is retarded

COMED-K 2015 ANSWERS

52. Answer is d (Peginterferon with ribavarin).
Ref: CMDT 2013, Pg 676; Harrison's, 19th edition Pg 2042.

- Two formulations of ***pegylated interferon*** are approved for HCV infection: peginterferon alfa-2b and ***peginterferon alfa-2a*** (more efective). Both are given SC once per week
- ***Addition of the nucleoside analog ribavirin***, orally, results in ***higher sustained response rates*** than peginterferon alone in previously untreated patients with chronic hepatitis C and in patients, who have had a relapse after an initial response to interferon alfa and ribavirin.
- ***Still higher rates of response*** are achieved in persons infected with HCV ***genotype 1*** when a direct acting antiviral agent—***telaprevir or boceprevir*** (protease inhibitors) *is added to peginterferon and ribavirin.*

53. Answer is c (Right main bronchus).
Ref: An Illustrated Textbook: Ear, Nose & Throat and Head & Neck Surgery, By Rakesh Prasad Shrivastav, Pg 265.

- Over 80% of patients presenting with inhaled foreign bodies (FBs) are children under 4 years.
- The ***right main bronchus*** is *wider, shorter and more vertically placed* as compared to the left main bronchus which is more angled.
- Hence, ***FBs*** are more likely to be lodged in the ***right main bronchus.***

54. Answer is b (Herpes simplex encephalitis).
Ref: Harrison's, 19th edition Pg 1179.

- The clinical hallmark of HSV encephalitis has been the ***acute onset of fever*** and focal neurologic symptoms and signs, especially in the ***temporal lobe.***
- HSV encephalitis: ***Elevated cerebrospinal fluid (CSF) protein levels, leukocytosis (predominantly lymphocytes) and red blood cell counts*** due to hemorrhagic necrosis are common.
- While brain biopsy has been the gold standard for defining HSV encephalitis, a highly sensitive and specific PCR for detection of HSV DNA in CSF has largely replaced biopsy for defining CNS infection.

55. Answer is a (Antiepileptic therapy, continuous or intermittent is generally not recommended).
Ref: Pediatric Emergency Medicine Secrets, By Steven M Selbst, Pg 226

- Although it ***does not prevent simple febrile seizures, antipyretic therapy is desirable*** for other reasons.
- On the basis of risk/benefit analysis, ***neither long term nor intermittent anticonvulsant therapy is indicated for children,*** who have experienced one or more simple febrile seizures.
- The AAP recommends that an ***EEG should not be obtained in a neurologically healthy child with a first simple febrile seizure.***
- ***Lumbar puncture is no longer*** routinely recommended for well appearing, fully immunized children, who present with a simple febrile seizure
- ***If preventing subsequent febrile seizures is essential, oral diazepam would be the treatment of choice.*** It can reduce the risk of febrile seizure recurrence and because it is intermittent, probably has the fewest adverse effects.

More About Febrile Convulsions

Simple benign febrile convulsions

- Fits occur ***within 24 hours of onset of fever***[Q]
- Last < ***10 minutes***[Q] and are usually single per febrile episode
- Convulsions are ***generalized***[Q]
- ***NO***[Q] ***postictal*** neurological deficit
- ***Family history***[Q] may be present.

Atypical complex febrile convulsions

- Anything different from features of simple febrile convulsions are atypical fits. Presence of family h/o epilepsy, neurodevelopmental retardation and atypical episodes increase risk of febrile episodes and subsequent epilepsy.

Treatment

- Antipyretics[Q] (paracetamol, ibuprofen; *AVOID aspirin due to risk of Reye's syndrome*[Q])
- Hydrotherapy, tepid sponging, oxygen.
- IV diazepam or phenobarbitone for control of seizures

Prophylaxis

- Intermitent diazepam, clabazam, midazolam—most desirable.
- ***Continuous prophylaxis***[Q]***:*** In the form of antiepileptic drug therapy is advocated in event of failure of intermittent therapy, ***especially in recurrent atypical seizures*** or family h/o epilepsy (valproate or ***phenobarbitone***).

56. Answer is b (T cell lymphoma).

Ref: Harrison's, 19th edition Pg 1942.

- The most important complication of celiac disease is the development of cancer: Gastrointestinal and non-gastrointestinal neoplasms as well as ***intestinal lymphoma***.
- The frequency of ***lymphoma*** in patients with celiac disease is higher in ***Ireland and the United Kingdom***
- The possibility of lymphoma must be considered whenever a patient with celiac disease, who has previously done well on a gluten-free diet is *no longer responsive to gluten restriction or* a patient who presents with clinical and histologic features consistent with celiac disease *does not respond to a gluten-free diet.*
- Other complications of celiac disease:
  - Intestinal ulceration
  - Refractory sprue
  - Collagenous sprue (here a layer of collagen-like material is present beneath the basement membrane; patients with collagenous sprue generally do not respond to a gluten-free diet and often have a poor prognosis).

All about Celiac sprue (Gluten Sensitive Enteropathy)

- ❑ *Genetic* disorder (A/w ***HLA-DQ2***[Q] MC) of ***gluten***[Q] (e.g., ***wheat, barley, rye***[Q]) *intolerance*
- ❑ ***IgA antiendomysial***[Q]; ***Anti-tissue transglutaminase***[Q] *(tTGA) and* ***antigliadin***[Q] *(gliadin=wheat)* ***antibodies*** cause ***jejunal mucosal damage***[Q]
- ❑ Occurs ***within the 1st year***[Q] or in ***third decade***[Q] of life; MC in ***northern Europe***[Q].
- ❑ Proximal small bowel - jejunum affected - jejunal biopsy demonstrates loss of duodenal and jejunal villi, ***lymphocytes in lamina propria***[Q]
- ❑ Serum levels of ***tissue transglutaminase***[Q] are used for screening.
- ❑ A/w ***dermatitis herpetiformis***[Q]. Moderarely ↑ risk of malignancy (***T cell lymphoma***[Q]).
- ❑ Treatment: A ***gluten-free diet***[Q] (histology reverts to normal!).

57. Answer is d (Meckel's diverticulum).

Ref: Bailey and Love, 26th edition Pg 1169.

Meckel's Diverticulum

- ***Meckel's diverticulum***[Q] is the ***MC congenital abnormality***[Q] of the small intestine and GIT.
- Caused by an ***incomplete obliteration of the vitelline duct***[Q] (i.e., ***omphalomesenteric duct***[Q])—i.e., it represents the patent intestinal end of the vitellointestinal duct.

Rule of 2's - Meckel's diverticulum

- It is present in about 2% of subjects[Q]
- Its length is about *2 inches*[Q]
- Usually *2 feet*[Q] *(60 cm)* proximal to the ileocecal valve and occurs on the antimesenteric border of the ileum.
- *Present in 2%*[Q] of the population

- It is typically lined by ileal mucosa, but other *tissue types are also found* with varying frequency, ***ectopic gastric mucosa***[Q] in about 50%.
- A Meckel's diverticulum ***possesses all three coats of the intestinal wall***[Q] and ***has its own blood supply***[Q]. It is therefore *vulnerable to infection* and *obstruction* in the same way as the appendix
- Can also cause *intussusception, bleeding and volvulus*[Q].

58. Answer is a (Acute mastitis).
Ref: Bailey and Love, 26th edition Pg 1169.

- ***Bacterial mastitis*** is the ***most common*** variety of mastitis and is ***associated with lactation*** in the majority of cases.
- Most cases are caused by ***S. aureus*** and, if hospital acquired are likely to be penicillin resistant.
- The affected breast or more usually a segment of it, presents the classical signs of acute inflammation.
- Treatment: During the cellulitic stage: Flucloxacillin or coamoxi- clav. ***Feeding from the affected side may continue*** if the patient can manage.
- It used to be recommended that the breast should be incised and drained if the infection did not resolve within 48 hours. This advice has been replaced with the recommendation that ***repeated aspirations under antibiotic cover*** (if necessary using ultrasound for localization) be *performed*.
- For ***drainage***: The usual incision is sited in a ***radial direction*** over the affected segment, although if a ***circumareolar incision*** will allow adequate access to the affected area this is ***preferred, because it gives a better cosmetic result***.

59. Answer is e (Wrong question stem/options as per the revised answer key).
Ref: Harrison's, 19th edition Pg 2255.

ETIOLOGY OF HYPOPITUITARISM

- Development/Structural
  - Transcription factor defect
  - Pituitary dysplasia/aplasia
  - Congenital central nervous system mass, encephalocele primary empty sella
  - Congenital hypothalamic disorders (septo-optic dysplasia, Prader-Willi syndrome, Laurence-Moon-Biedl syndrome, Kallmann syndrome).
- Traumatic
  - Surgical resection radiation damage head injuries.
- Neoplastic
  - Pituitary ***adenoma***
  - Parasellar mass (germinoma, ependymoma, glioma) Rathke's cyst
  - Craniopharyngioma
  - Hypothalamic hamartoma, gangliocytoma
  - Pituitary metastases (breast, lung, colon carcinoma) lymphoma and leukemia
  - Meningioma.
- Infiltrative/Inflammatory
  - Lymphocytic hypophysitis
  - Hemochromatosis
  - Sarcoidosis

- Histiocytosis X
- Granulomatous hypophysitis
- Transcription factor antibodies.
- Vascular
  - Pituitary apoplexy (***Sheehan's*** syndrome)
  - Pregnancy related (infarction with diabetes; postpartum necrosis)
  - Sickle cell disease
  - Arteritis.
- Infections
  - Fungal (histoplasmosis)
  - Parasitic (toxoplasmosis)
  - Tuberculosis
  - *Pneumocystis carinii.*

- Note: Trophic hormone failure associated with pituitary compression/destruction occurs sequentially: ***GH first*** > FSH > LH > TSH> ACTH.
- During childhood, ***growth retardation is the presenting feature*** and in adults, ***hypogonadism*** is the ***earliest symptom.***

60. Answer is c (Increased bone resorption, fibrosis and cystic brown tumors).
Ref: Essential Revision Notes in Medicine for Students, Volume 1, By Philip A Kalra. Pg 200.

- von Recklinghausen's disease of bone also called ***Osteitis fibrosa cystica*** is seen in ***hyperparathyroidism*** and is characterized by ***parathyroid adenoma, pathological fracture*** and ***recurrent renal calculi.***
- ***Increased osteoclastic bone resorption*** releases minerals, including calcium from the bone into the bloodstream.
- In addition to elevated blood calcium levels, overactivity of this process results in a loss of bone mass, a weakening of the bones as their calcified supporting structures are replaced with fibrous tissue (peritrabecular fibrosis) and the formation of ***cyst-like brown tumors*** in and around the bone.

61. Answer is d (Duffy glycoproteins).
Ref: Harrison's, 19th edition Table 145e-1.

Microorganism	Microbial Ligand	Host receptor
Plasmodium Vivax	Merozoite form	Duffy Fy antigen
Plasmodium falciparum	Erythrocyte binding protein (EBA 175)	Glycophorin A

- The Duffy antigens are codominant alleles, ***Fya and Fyb***, that also serve as receptors for *Plasmodium vivax.*
- More than 70% of persons in malaria endemic areas lack these antigens.
- For unknown reasons, the lack of the Duffy antigen receptor for cytokines (DARC) is associ- ated with mild neutropenia.
- ***Duffy Negative*** blood group ***protects against Plasmodium*** infection.

62. Answer is d (Insulin resistance in peripheral tissue).
Ref: CMDT 2013, Pg 1192.

- Type 1 diabetes is due to pancreatic islet B cell destruction predominantly by an ***autoimmune process*** and these patients are ***prone to ketoacidosis.***
- This process occurs in ***genetically susceptible subjects,*** is probably triggered by one or more environmental agents (***MC is a viral infection***), and usually progresses over many months or years .
- ***Polymorphisms*** of ***multiple genes*** are reported to influence the risk of type 1A diabetes (including, HLA-DQalpha, HLA-DQbeta, HLA-DR, preproinsulin, the PTPN22 gene, CTLA-4, interferon-induced helicase, IL2 receptor (CD25), a lectin-like gene (KIA0035), ERBB3e and undefined gene at 12q)
- Note: ***Type 2 diabetes*** is the ***more prevalent form*** and ***results from insulin resistance*** with a *defect in compensatory insulin secretion.*

63. Answer is c (Sickle cell disease).
Ref: Harrison's, 19th edition Pg 634.

- Approximately half the individuals with homozygous Hb S disease experience vaso-occlusive crisis.
- Pain crises begin suddenly. The crisis may last several hours to several days and terminate as abruptly as it began.
- The pain can affect any body part. It often involves the ***abdomen***, bones, joints and soft tissue, and it may present as dactylitis (***bilateral painful and swollen hands and/or feet in children***), acute joint necrosis or avascular necrosis, or acute abdomen.
- In the classic picture of sickle cell anemia, the peripheral blood smear shows sickle cells and severe ***poikilocytosis.***

64. Answer is d [Intramascular (IM) injection preferred].
Ref: KD Tripathi, 7th edition Pg 415.

- Phenytoin is ***80–90% protein bound***.
- The kinetics of metabolism of phenytoin is capacity limited; changes from first order to zero order over the therapeutic range.
- When given by ***intramuscular injection***, phenytoin precipitates out at the injection site and is absorbed slowly and erratically. This route is NOT, therefore, recommended.
- ***Side effects: Gingival hyperplasia***[Q], ***hirsutism***[Q], ***lymphadenopathy***[Q], ***SJS***[Q], confusion, blurred vision, ***nystagmus***[Q], ***ataxia***[Q], diplopia, ***megaloblastic anemia***[Q], induction of cytochrome P-450, teratogenic.

65. Answer is d (Change to sodium valproate 500 mg/day).
Ref: CMDT 2013, Pg 1067.

- ***Anticholinergic*** effects of imipramine: ***dry mouth***, tachycardia, blurred vision, ***urinary retention*** (careful in BPH), sexual dysfunction.
- Hence the ***drug will have to be changed*** to a novel antidepressant like ***escitalopram*** which is a Selective Serotonin Reuptake Inhibitor (SSRI) and does not have significant anticholinergic side effects.

66. Answer is d (Lactic acidosis).
Ref: KD Tripathi, 7th edition Pg 275.

- ***Lactic acidosis*** is a rare ***side effect with metformin***. When, tissue hypoxia occurs, the metformin-treated patient is at higher risk for lactic acidosis due to compromised lactate removal.
- Almost all reported cases have involved subjects with associated risk factors that should have contraindicated its use (kidney, liver or cardiorespiratory insufficiency, ***alcoholism***, advanced age).
- Acute kidney failure can occur rarely in certain patients receiving ***radiocontrast agents***. Metformin therapy should therefore be temporarily halted on the day of radiocontrast administration and restarted a day or two later after confirmation that renal function has not deteriorated.

67. Answer is d (Piperacillin).
Ref: KD Tripathi, 7th edition Pg 724.

- It is an extended-spectrum β-lactam of the ***ureidopenicillin*** class
- Piperacillin is an ***antipseudomonal*** penicillin that is 8 times more active than carbenicillin.
- Piperacillin has been ***combined with tazobactam*** for use in severe infections such as peritonitis, UTI, respiratory infections caused by β-lactamase producing bacilli.
- When ***used alone, piperacillin lacks strong activity*** against the Gram-(+) pathogen *Staphylococcus aureus*, as it piperacillin is broken down by the Gram-(+) β-lactamases.

68. Answer is a (Alemtuzumab).
Ref: Parsons' diseases of the eye, 21st edition Pg 319, 320.

Anti VEGFS in Ophthalmology

- Vascular endothelial Grwoth Factor (VEGF) ***promotes angiogenesis***, increases vascular permeability and has proinflammatory action.
- In the human eye, *increased levels of VEGF correlate with retinal ischemia associated neovascularization* in diabetic retinopathy, retinal venous occlusion and retinopathy of pematurity; also VEGF levels are elevated in wet AMD.
- Hence, anti-VEGF agents are developed to use in these conditions; all are used ***intravitreally***.

Currently available anti-VEGFs are

Pegaptanib sodium[Q] (Macugen)	First FDA approved anti-VEGF; it is a pegylated ***aptamer***, which binds with high affinity to the major pathologic VEGF isoform, VEGF 165 thereby inhibiting it from binding to its receptor;
Bevacizumab (Avastin[Q])	Humanized ***monoclonal antibody*** against VEGF; currently ***FDA approved for IV treatment of colorectal cancer[Q]***; ***ocular uses are off-label***, but found safe and effective worldwide.
Ranibizumab[Q] (Lucentis)	Second FDA approved anti-VEGF; Humanized monoclonal antibody against VEGF
Aflibercept[Q]	Anti-VEGF fusion protein that binds all isoforms of VEGF-A and placental growth factor

Indications of anti-VEGFs

- ***Wet ARMD***[Q] (choroidal neovascular membrane, CNVM)
- ***Diabetic retinopathy***[Q] (for macular edema)
- ***Retinal venous***[Q] ***occlusive*** disease (for macular edema).

69. Answer is d (CYP2C9).
Ref: Pharmacogenomics in Psychiatry, edited by M Schwab, WP, Pg 60.

- Antidepressants are highly lipophilic agents subject to extensive biotransformation in the liver.
- In general their metabolism includes phase 1 oxidative reactions catalyzed by cytochrome P 450 (CYP) enzymes followed by phase 2 glucuronide conjugation.
- The human CYP system consists of a superfamily of more than 50 heme containing enzymes located in the membranes of the smooth endoplasmic reticulum in the liver and in many extrahepatic tissues that are responsible for the phase 1 oxidative reactions of many drugs and endogenous substances.
- Enzymes inolved in the biotransformation of ***mirtazapine*** are ***CYP2D6, CYP3A4, CYP1A2***.

70. Answer is b (Reduced time for calcium reuptake into sarcoplasmic reticulum).
Ref: Medical Physiology for Undergraduate Students, By Indu Khurana, Pg 77-79.

- Reduced time for calcium reuptake into sarcoplasmic reticulum leads to the plateau.

71. Answer is d (Leads to neurodegenerative diseases and cancer).
Ref: Medical Physiology for Undergraduate Students, By Indu Khurana, Pg 38.

Examples of Apoptosis

Apoptosis for proper development of tissues

- During formation of the fingers and toes of the fetus, the apoptosis plays an important role of removing the web tissue between the fingers and toes.
- During sexual development in fetal life, apoptosis is responsible for regression of duct systems.

Apoptosis for normal functioning of adult tissues

- Cyclic breakdown of endometrium that leads to start of menstruation caused by apoptosis.
- Epithelial cells that lose their connection to the basal lamina and surrounding cells undergo apoptosis.
- Enterocytes sloughed off the tips of intestinal villi undergo apoptosis.

Apoptosis that destroy cells that pose a threat to the integrity of the organism

- Apoptosis of virus infected cells, cancer cells, cells with DNA damage, autoreactive immunocytes.

72. Answer is c (Activating soluble guanylate cyclases to increase cGMP causing relaxation of smooth muscle enhancing blood).

Ref: Essentials of medical physiology, Sembulingam. 6th edition Pg 790.

- Nitric oxide activates the enzyme ***guanylyl cyclase,*** which in turn causes formation of cyclic guanosine monophosphate (*cGMP*) from GMP.
- The ***cGMP is a smooth muscle relaxant*** and it causes ***dilatation of arterioles.***
- Thus, nitric oxide indirectly causes dilatation of arterioles and ***helps in erection.***

73. Answer is d (Ganglion cells).

Ref: http://courses.washington.edu/psych333/handouts/coursepack/ch13-Information_processing_in_retina.pdf

- Remember: Rods and cones (photoreceptors) are the back of the retina (outer side) and NOT in front.
- Light passes through four other types of cells in the retina (ganglion cells, amacrine, bipolar and horizontal cells) before it reaches the photoreceptors.
- Once the photoreceptors are activated, they stimulate bipolar cells, which in turn stimulate ganglion cells.
- ***Ganglion cells*** are the ***ONLY cells*** in the retina that ***produce action potentials.***
- A ganglion cell only produces action potentials, however, when the release of glutamate by the bipolar cell(s) that contact it is sufficient to depolarize it to threshold. These action potentials are ***transmitted to the brain via the fibers of the optic nerve.***

74. Answer is c (DNA synthesis in the bone marrow).

Ref: Essentials of Medical Physiology, Sembulingam, 6th edition Pg 75.

- ***Erythropoiesis*** is the process in which new erythrocytes are produced.
- These new erythrocytes replace the oldest erythrocytes (normally about one percent) that are phagocytosed and destroyed each day.
- ***Folate, vitamin B_{12} and iron*** have crucial roles in erythropoiesis. Erythroblasts require folate and vitamin B12 for proliferation during their differentiation.
- Deficiency of folate or vitamin B_{12} *inhibits purine and thymidylate syntheses, impairs DNA synthesis and causes erythroblast apoptosis,* resulting in anemia from ineffective erythropoiesis.
- Vitamin B_{12}, Folic acid and intrinsic factor of castle are necessary for ***synthesis of DNA in the RBCs*** and ***maturation of RBCs.***

75. Answer is a (EEG shows low-voltage, high frequency waves).

Ref: Ref: Essentials of Medical Physiology, Sembulingam, 6th edition Pg 933.

- Sleep consists of two distinct states as shown by electroencephalographic studies:
  (1) ***REM (rapid eye movement) sleep,*** also called dream sleep, D state sleep, paradoxic sleep. Rapid conjugate movements of the eyeballs occur frequently BUT the sleep is deep—hence called ***paradoxical sleep.*** The eye movements are recorded by EOG - electro-oculogram. ***Low amplitude, Low voltage high frequency waves*** are seen on EEG like in awake state. ***EMG activity*** is ***absent.***
  (2) ***NREM (non-REM) sleep,*** also called S stage sleep, which is divided into stages 1, 2, 3 and 4 and is recognizable by different electroencephalographic patterns.
- Stages 3 and 4 are ***'delta'*** sleep.
- ***Dreaming occurs mostly in REM*** and to a lesser extent in NREM sleep.

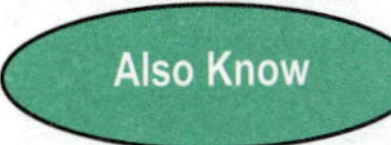

SLEEP DISORDERS

Dyssomnias	Parasomnias
• Dyssomnias are characterized by problems in the timing, quality or amount of sleep. • They include ***insomnia, hypersomnia, narcolepsy, sleep apnea and circadian rhythm sleep disorder.***	• Parasomnias are characterized by abnormalities in physiology or in behaviour associated with sleep. • They include the below mentioned ***non-REM sleep disorders and nightmare disorders.***

STAGES OF SLEEP AND THE EEG[Q]

Sleep stage and EEG waves	Features
Awake ➢ Beta ➢ Alpha	Active mental concentration Relaxed with eyes closed
Stage 1 ➢ Theta (4-6 Hz); low voltage alpha; vertex sharp waves	5% of sleep time Lightest stage of sleep characterized by peacefulness, slowed pulse and respiration, decreased BP and episodic body movements
Stage 2 ➢ Sleep spindles[Q] (12-14 Hz) and high amplitude 'K' complexes[Q]	Largest percentage of sleep time (45%)
Stages 3,4 ; Slow Wave Sleep, SWS ➢ High amplitude low frequency, 2 Hz, delta waves ➢ Stage 3 = < 50% delta waves with sleep spindles ➢ Stage 4 = > 50% delta waves but NO sleep spindles	25% of sleep time (decreases with age) Deepest, most relaxed stages of sleep' a/w sleep disorders mentioned below; SWS is most prominent in childhood (growth hormone secretion occurs) and in the healthy elderly male, SWS maybe completely absent
Rapid Eye Movement (REM) sleep ➢ 'Sawtooth' beta, alpha and theta waves; low amplitude high frequency waves on EEG.	***25%*** of sleep time (decreases with age) Dreaming[Q]; penile and clitoral erection[Q]; increased pulse, respiration, BP and gastric motility; ***low skeletal muscle tone***[Q] and paralysis

Note: NREM sleep = 75%; REM sleep = 25% of sleep time

Stages 3 And 4 (Slow Wave) Sleep Disorders

- **Night terrors (*Pavor nocturnu*[Q]*s*)=** The repetitive experience of ***fright in which a person (usually a child) screams in fear***. The child cannot be awakened and ***cannot remember the dream***. Sleep terrors that begin in adolescence may indicate *temporal lobe epilepsy*.
- **Sleep walking (*Somnambulism*[Q])=** Begins in childhood (4–8 years); the person walks around without being conscious and *DOES NOT REMEMBER* the episode.
- Sleep talking = ***Somniloquy***[Q]
- Nocturnal enuresis = ***Bedwetting***[Q]
- *Bruxism* = ***Teeth grinding***[Q]***.***

REM (Desynchronized or Paradoxical) Sleep Disorders

- **Nightmare[Q] disorder:** Repetitive frightening dreams that cause nighttime awakenings and the person can usually recall the nightmare.
- Narcolepsy
- Insomnia
- Sleep apnea.

76. Answer is b (De Clerambault's syndrome).

Ref: Kaplan & Sadock's Concise Textbook of Clinical Psychiatry, By Benjamin J Sadock, 3rd edition Pg 185.

- A woman believes that a man, who is inaccessible of a higher social status and to whom she has never spoken, loves her; a prominent feature of ***erotomania, de Clerambult's syndrome***[Q]
- When the content of delusion is mainly jealousy (infidelity) involving the spouse, it is called ***Othello's syndrome*** (conjugal paranoia, morbid jealousy). Morbid jealousy is more common among alcoholics.
- ***Ekbom's syndrome*** is restless legs syndrome.
- A ***querulant*** (from the Latin querulous—'*complaining*') is a person who obsessively feels wronged, particularly about minor causes of action. In particular, the term is used for those, who repeatedly petition authorities or pursue legal actions based on manifestly unfounded grounds. These applications include in particular complaints about petty offenses. In psychiatry, the terms ***querulous paranoia*** (Kraepelin) has been used to describe a paranoid condition, which manifested itself in querulant behavior (ICD-10, Paranoia querulans, section F22.8).

77. Answer is a (Genetic predisposition is significant).
Ref: Kaplan and Sadock's Synopsis of Psychiatry: Behavioral Sciences/Clinical Sciences, By Benjamin J Sadock. 10th edition Pg 1270.

- Bipolar disorders consist of episodic mood shifts into mania, major depression, hypomania and ***mixed mood states***.
- Some people alternate between extreme episodes of mania and depression, but most are ***depressed more often than they are manic***.
- ***Age of onset*** of bipolar disorder has classically been viewed as occurring commonly in ***late teens and young adulthood***.
- It is also thought ***bipolar disorder is linked to genetics***, as the condition seems to run in families. The ***family members*** of a person with the condition have an ***increased risk of*** developing it themselves. However, no single gene is responsible for bipolar disorder. Instead, a number of genetic and environmental factors are thought to act as triggers.

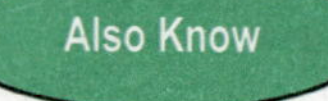

BIPOLAR DISORDERS

Patient Example: *A 29-year-old journalist is referred to a psychiatrist by his physician. He has become grandiose in his manner during the previous 2 months challenging the decisions of senior editorial staff and voicing his intention to take over the editorial chair. When seen he was in an elated mood, he had an inflated opinion of his abilities, was continuously talking and jumped from one subject to another. His manner was overfamiliar and he kept pacing up and down the room.*

Bipolar I **disorder**	***Bipolar II*** **disorder**
➢ Episodes of **both mania** (very elevated mood) and **major depression**.	➢ Episodes of both **hypomania** (elevated mood but not as sever as in mania) and **major depression**.

Cardinal features

- General criteria for a manic episode require a clear period of ***persistently elevated, expansive or irritable mood*** (3 or 4 of the below criteria) ***lasting 1 week***[Q] or severe enough to require hospitalization.
- *Criteria for a manic episode* are:
  1. ***Self-esteem***: ***Highly inflated***, grandiosity.
  2. ***Sleep***: ***Decreased need for sleep***, rested after only a few hours.
  3. ***Speech***: Pressure of speech, ***more talkative*** than usual.
  4. ***Thoughts***: Racing thoughts in the mind, ***flight of ideas*** (rapidly produced speech with abrupt shifts from topic to topic, the connections between shifts are apparent). When flight becomes severe, incoherence occurs.
  5. *Attention*: Easy distractibility.
  6. ***Activity***: ***Increased goal-directed activity***. In hypomania, there is a marked increase in productivity and creativity. Many artists and writers have contributed significantly in such periods.
  7. ***Hedonism***[Q]: High excess involvement in pleasurable activities (sex, spending, travel).
- The depressed phase of bipolar disorder resembles depression in major depressive disorder, but the first episode may differ.
- Untreated manic episodes last approximately 3 months; there is no unipolar manic disorder since depressive symptoms eventually occur. Therefore, one episode of mania or hypomania defines bipolar disorder.

☼ *'Rapid cycling[Q]'* = *4 or more episodes* of either depression or mania in a given year; maybe a/w *hypothyroidism*.

Treatment

➤ ***Mood stabilizers*** in conjunction with benzodiazepines (for rapid tranquilization) and antipsychotics; ***DOC*** for treating mania is ***lithium***[Q].
Anticonvulsants such as ***carbamazepine and valproic acid*** are also used to treat mania, particularly *rapid cycling bipolar disorder* and mixed episodes (mixed manic and depressive features).

78. Answer is d (Absence of activity on electro-oculogram).
Ref: Essentials of Medical Physiology, Sembulingam, 6th edition Pg 933.

➤ Please see explanation to ***answer no.*** 75 above.

79. Answer is c (Electromagnetic waves and particles).
Ref: Nanotechnology: Principles and Practices, By Sulabha K Kulkarni, Pg 1.1.

- Short ***electromagnetic waves*** such as ***X-rays*** behave ***like waves as well as particles*** when interacting with matter.
- These particles are discrete bundles of energy and are called ***photons***.
- The behavior of electromagnetic waves sometimes as waves and sometimes as particles is called ***'wave-particle' duality***.

80. Answer is d (Computed tomography).
Ref: Harrison's, 19th edition Pg 1695.

- Chest ***computed tomography (CT) is more specific for bronchiectasis*** and is the ***imaging modality of choice*** *for confirming the diagnosis.*
- CT findings include:
  - Airway dilation (detected as parallel ***'tram tracks'*** or as the ***'signet-ring sign'***)
  - Lack of bronchial tapering
  - Bronchial wall thickening in dilated airways
  - Inspissated secretions (e.g. the ***'tree-in-bud'*** pattern), or
  - Cysts emanating from the bronchial wall (especially pronounced in cystic bronchiectasis).

81. Answer is b (May show overinflation of the involved lung).
Ref: Encyclopedia of Imaging, Volume 2, By Albert L Baert, Pg 729.

- When foreign body aspiration is suspected in a patient, screening radiographic studies employed include anteroposterior (AP) and lateral imaging of the soft tissues of the neck, inspiratory and expiratory posteroanterior (PA) chest radiographs (CXRs) and lateral CXRs.
- ***Radiopaque foreign bodies are easy*** to diagnose by using radiographs obtaining two views of the foreign body helps in determining its location and excludes the presence of superimposed multiple foreign bodies
- With ***radiolucent foreign bodies***, *secondary radiographic signs*, such as *obstructive emphysema, atelectasis, pneumonia, and a mediastinal shift*, help in diagnosing foreign body aspiration.
- Patients with ***bronchial foreign bodies*** may have ***normal findings on CXRs***; however, the ***affected lung may show hyperaeration (obstructive*** emphysema—FB can partially obstruct the airway by acting like a ball valve, allowing air into the lung but not out—air trapping) and *shifting of the mediastinum away from the affected lung on expiratory CXRs*, because of the *ball-valve effect of the tracheal foreign body*. In such cases, the patients can inspire air past the foreign body but have difficulty exhaling.
- Inspiratory and expiratory films comparing the relative deflation of the two lungs may demonstrate unilateral air trapping indicative of a foreign body.
- Plain radiographic results cannot exclude foreign body aspiration. If the clinical suspicion is high for foreign body aspiration, ***endoscopy should be performed for definitive diagnosis and treatment***.

82. Answer is d (Respiratory acidosis with hypoxemia).
Ref: http://www.rnceus.com/abgs/abgmethod.html

- Please see the above link for an explanation of interpretation of arterial blood gases.
- For a more detailed review look at this link - http://www.medscape.com/viewarticle/763010_4

83. Answer is a or c (Nevirapine or Ritonavir).
Ref: CMDT 2013, Pg 1342.

- Taking nevirapine-based antiretroviral therapy together with tuberculosis treatment is complicated both by pharmacokinetic interactions related to ***rifampin*** and by overlapping toxicities of ***nevirapine*** and the first-line antituberculosis drugs, notably ***skin rash and hepatotoxicity***.
- Several studies have found that ***rifampin reduces serum concentrations of nevirapine*** by 20–55%.
- Combining increased doses of ***lopinavir/ritonavir*** tablets with the anti-tuberculosis drug ***rifampicin*** *increases the level of key liver enzymes and causes nausea and vomiting*.

84. Answer is c (Pleural effusion).
Ref: Harrison's, 19th edition Pg 1663.

- ***Ultrasonography*** is of limited value in disorders of the respiratory system.
- Because US energy is rapidly dissipated in air, it is ***NOT useful for evaluation of the pulmonary parenchyma*** and cannot be used if there is any aerated lung between the US probe and the abnormality of interest.
- However, ***ultrasound can detect and localize pleural abnormalities*** and is a quick and effective way of guiding percutaneous needle biopsy of peripheral lung, pleural or chest wall lesions.
- US is also ***helpful in identifying septations within loculated collections*** and ***can facilitate placement of a needle for sampling of pleural liquid*** (i.e. for thoracentesis), improving the yield and safety of the procedure.
- Bedside availability makes it valuable in the ICU.
- Real-time imaging can be used to assess the movement of the diaphragm.
- Endobronchial US is a valuable adjunct to bronchoscopy, allowing identification and localization of pathology adjacent to airway walls or within the mediastinum.

85. Answer is b (Membranous atresia is common than bony atresia).
Ref: Diseases of ENT, PL Dhingra, 6th edition Pg 163.

- Choanal atresia occurs due to ***persistence of the primitive bucconasal*** membrane.
- ***Bony atresia is more common*** (90%) than membranous atresia; ***Unilateral atresia is more common*** than bilateral.
- Symptoms of severe airway obstruction and cyclical cyanosis are the classic signs of neonatal ***bilateral atresia***—a ***life-threatening condition***.
- ***Unilateral*** choanal atresia presents with *unilateral nasal obstruction and mucoid rhinorrhea*.
- Diagnosis is by:
  - Presence of *mucoid discharge in the nose*
  - ***Absence of air bubbles*** in the ***nasal discharge***
  - ***Inability to pass a nasogastric tube into the nose*** of a newborn with *presence of air in the lower respiratory tree*
  - ***CT scan*** is investigation of choice.

86. Answer is c (Narrow interarytenoid cleft).
Ref: Diseases of ENT, PL Dhingra, 6th edition Pg 295.

- ***MC congenital abnormality***[Q] of larynx;
- ***MC*** cause of ***congenital laryngeal stridor/stridor in infants and children***[Q].
- ***Excessive flaccidity of supraglottic larynx***, which is sucked in during inspiration and child presents with ***inspiratory stridor***[Q] within 2 ***weeks***[Q] of birth; ***cry*** is normal.
- *Stridor is* ***relieved***[Q] *in* ***prone***[Q] position and *disappears spontaneously*[Q] by 2 years of age.
- Direct laryngoscopy: Elongated epiglottis curled on itself (***omega shaped***[Q] epiglottis); *floppy aryepiglotic folds and prominent arytenoids*.
- A/w ***gastroesophageal reflux***[Q] disease.

87. **Answer is e (Wrong stem/options as per revised answer key).**
Ref: Multiple sources.

- ***Fibrous dysplasia*** is a ***sporadic*** disorder characterized by the presence of ***one (monostotic)*** or ***more (polyostotic)*** expanding fibrous skeletal lesions composed of bone-forming mesenchyme.
- McCune-Albright syndrome (MAS) = polyostotic fibrous dysplasia + café au lait spots + pseudoprecocious puberty of ovarian origin; MC in girls (10:1).
- The monostotic form is the MC and is usually diagnosed in patients between 20 and 30 years of age
- The polyostotic form typically manifests in children of < 10 years old and may progress with age
- Fibrous dysplasia occurs with equal frequency in both sexes.
- In polyostotic fibrous dysplasia, the lesions MC involve the ***maxilla and other craniofacial bones***, ribs and metaphyseal or diaphyseal portions of the proximal femur or tibia.
- Sarcomatous degeneration involving the facial bones or femur is infrequent
- In ***long bones***, the fibrous dysplastic lesions are typically ***well defined, radiolucent areas*** with ***thin cortices*** and a ***ground-glass*** appearance.
- Involvement of ***facial bones*** usually presents as ***radiodense lesions***, which may create a ***leonine appearance (leontiasis osea)***.

88. **Answer is d (Near range of shotguns).**
Ref: Simpson's forensic medicine, 12th edition Pg 82.

- At ***intermediate ranges between 20 cm and 1m*** (of ***smooth bore firearms***), there will be diminishing smoke soiling and burning of the skin, but powder tattooing may persist.
- The spread of shot will begin, first causing an irregular margin to the wound.
- Often called a ***'rat hole'*** in USA, because of the nibbled edges, the same is called ***'scalloping'*** in the UK.

89. **Answer is b (Glycine).**
Ref: CMDT 2013, Pg 1429.

- See ***answer no. 13*** above.

90. **Answer is b (Torture).**
Ref: Textbook of Forensic Medicine and Toxicology, Krishan Vij, 4th edition Pg 729, Annexure 3.

- ***Declaration of Tokyo***: Guidelines for medical doctors ***concerning torture*** and other cruel, inhuman and degrading treatment or punishment in relation to detention or imprisonment. Adopted by the World Medical Assembly, Tokyo, Japan, 1975.
- ***Declaration of Helsinki***: The World Medical Association (WMA) has developed the Declaration of Helsinki as a statement of ***ethical principles for medical research involving human subjects***, including research on identifiable human material and data (1964).
- This is a repeat from ***COMEDK 2011, Q 93.***

91. **Answer is c (Shotgun).**
Ref: Narayan Reddy's FMT, 23rd edition Pg 109.

- Constriction of the barrel near the distal/muzzle end of the shotgun is called ***choking of shotgun***[Q] ***— reduces dispersion of pellets***.

92. **Answer is b (Takayasu's arteritis).**
Ref: Harrison's, 19th edition Pg 2190.

- The diagnosis of ***Takayasu arteritis*** should be ***suspected strongly in a young woman***, who develops a ***decrease or absence of peripheral pulses, discrepancies in BP*** and ***arterial bruits***.
- Takayasu arteritis is a systemic disease with generalized and vascular symptoms.

- Generalized symptoms: Malaise, fever, night sweats, ***arthralgias***, anorexia and weight loss.
- ***Pulses are commonly absent*** in the involved vessels, particularly the ***subclavian artery*** (MC vessel involved).
- ***Hypertension*** occurs in 35–90% of patients and contributes to renal, cardiac and cerebral injury.
- Characteristic laboratory findings include ***an elevated ESR, mild anemia*** and ***elevated immunoglobulin*** level.

93. Answer is b (Acute respiratory distress syndrome).
Ref: CMDT 2013, Pg 322.

ARDS

- Acute onset of ***respiratory failure***.
- Absence of elevated left atrial pressure (if measured, pulmonary capillary wedge pressure 18 mm Hg).
- Chest radiography shows diffuse or ***patchy bilateral infiltrates*** that rapidly become confluent; these *characteristically spare the costophrenic angles*.
- *Marked hypoxemia* occurs that is *refractory to treatment with supplemental oxygen*.

94. Answer is a (Constrictive pericarditis).
Ref: Harrison's, 19th edition Pg 1506.

- In chornic constrictive pericarditis, the apical pulse is reduced and may retract in systole (***Broadbent's*** sign).
- ***Constrictive pericarditis*** produces a ***square root sign*** in the *jugulars, right atrium and RV pressure tracings*.

95. Answer is a (Cor pulmonale).
Ref: Harrison's, 19th edition Pg 1506.

- *TAPSE:* Tricuspid Annular Plane Systolic Excursion (also called the ***Tei index***).
- In ***cor pulmonale***, two-dimensional echocardiography is useful for measuring RV thickness and chamber dimensions.
- Location of the RV behind the sternum and its crescent shape challenge assessment of RV function by echocardiography, especially when parenchymal lung disease is present.
- Calculated measures of RV function (TAPSE or the Tei Index) supplement more subjective assessments of RV function.

96. Answer is c (Turbulent blood flow).
Ref: Ultrasound in Obstetrics and Gynecology, Volume 1, By Eberhard Merz. Pg 449.

Doppler Ultrasonography

- Sound reflected from a mobile structure shows a variable frequency that corresponds to the speed of movement of the structure. The difference in frequency between the sound transmitted and received is known as the ***Doppler frequency shift***.
- ***Doppler angle***: Angle between the vessel and the transmitted sound wave.
- In Color Doppler imaging, the *different colors indicate the* ***direction of blood flow***[Q]: ***Red Toward***[Q] transducer; ***Blue Away***[Q] from the transducer; GREEN indicates turbulent flow *(Red Tower Blows Away !!)*.
- Shades (*intensity of color*[Q]) represent ***velocity***[Q] of flow.

Uses of Doppler

- Detect *venous thrombosis, arterial stenosis* and occlusion, particularly in *carotid arteries*.
- To assess *blood flow through the umbilical artery*; also estimate *tumor blood flow*.

97. Answer is c (Atrial septal defect).
Ref: Harrison's, 19th edition Pg 1850, 1855.

- ***Nephronophthisis:*** Autosomal ***recessive***; ***juvenile form is MC*** and usually caused by mutations in the ***NPHP2 gene***, it is the MC *inherited childhood form of kidney failure requiring kidney replacement therapy*.
- ***Small fibrotic*** kidneys; ***medullary cysts, Growth retardation, anemia***, visual loss, liver fibrosis, ***cerebellar ataxia, situs inversus.***

- ***Senior-Løken syndrome:*** NPHP + *retinitis pigmentosa.*
- Other associated syndromes are ***Joubert's syndrome*** and ***Bardet-Biedl*** syndrome.

98. Answer is c (It is characterized by brief period of thyrotoxicosis).
Ref: Harrison's, 19th edition Pg 2299.

- ***Painless thyroiditis***, or '***silent***' thyroiditis occurs in patients with underlying autoimmune thyroid disease and has a clinical course similar to that of subacute thyroiditis.
- It is more common in women with type 1 diabetes mellitus.
- The condition occurs in up to 5% of women 3–6 months after pregnancy and is then termed as ***postpartum thyroiditis***.
- Typically, patients have a ***brief phase of thyrotoxicosis*** lasting 2–4 weeks, followed by hypothyroidism for 4–12 weeks and then resolution.
- As in subacute thyroiditis, the uptake of 99mTc pertechnetate or radioactive iodine is initially suppressed.
- In addition to the painless goiter, silent thyroiditis can be distinguished from subacute thyroiditis by a ***normal ESR*** and the ***presence of TPO antibodies***.
- ***Glucocorticoid*** treatment is ***not indicated*** for silent thyroiditis.
- Severe thyrotoxic symptoms can be managed with a brief course of propranolol.

99. Answer is d (Anticoagulation).
Ref: Harrison's, 19th edition Pg 1565.

- LV apical ballooning (***takotsubo syndrome***; stress-induced cardiomyopathy; broken heart syndrome!) can follow a high catecholamine stress. The resulting shape of the LV suggests a rounded ampulla form similar to a Japanese octopus pot (tako-tsubo pot).
- Acute chest pain or shortness of breath.
- Predominately affects postmenopausal women.
- Presents as an acute anterior myocardial infarction, but coronaries normal at cardiac catheterization.
- Imaging reveals apical left ventricular ballooning due to anteroapical stunning of the myocardium.
- Most patients recover completely.
- Treatment: Include ***nitrates for pulmonary edema, intraaortic balloon pump*** if needed for low output, ***combined alpha and beta blockers*** rather than selective beta blockade if hemodynamically stable and ***magnesium for arrhythmias*** related to QT prolongation.
- ***Anticoagulation is generally withheld*** due to the occasional occurrence of ***ventricular rupture***.

100. Answer is a (Uncal herniation).
Ref: Harrison's, 19th edition Pg 1772.

- ***Herniation:*** Displacement of brain tissue by an overlying or adjacent mass into a contiguous compartment that it normally does not occupy.
- Coma and many of its associated signs can be attributed to these tissue shifts, and certain clinical features are characteristic of specific configurations of herniation.
- They are in essence 'false localizing' signs, because they derive from compression of brain structures at a distance from the mass.
- ***Transtentorial herniation***: Is the ***most common form of herniation***, here brain tissue is displaced from the supratentorial to the infratentorial compartment through the tentorial opening
- ***Uncal transtentorial herniation*** refers to impaction of the anterior medial temporal gyrus (the uncus) into the tentorial opening just anterior to and adjacent to the midbrain. The uncus compresses the third nerve as the nerve traverses the subarachnoid space, causing enlargement of the ipsilateral pupil (the fibers subserving parasympathetic pupillary function are located peripherally in the nerve).
- The coma that follows is due to compression of the midbrain against the opposite tentorial edge by the displaced parahippocampal gyrus.
- Lateral displacement of the midbrain may compress the opposite cerebral peduncle against the tentorial edge, producing a ***Babinski sign and hemiparesis contralateral to the hemiparesis*** that resulted from the mass (the ***Kernohan-Woltman sign***).

101. Answer is c (High-molecular-weight proteinuria).
Ref: Harrison's, 19th edition Pg 2459.

- ***Dent's disease*** and X-linked recessive nephrolithiasis (XRN) are two disorders, which represent unusual forms of the ***renal Fanconi syndrome*** are characterized by a ***low-molecular-weight proteinuria, hypercalciuria, nephrocalcinosis, nephrolithiasis*** and ***renal failure***.
- Repeated topic: Also please refer explanation under ***answer no. 165*** below.

102. Answer is b (60 mL/min).
Ref: http://www2.kidney.org/professionals/KDOQI/guidelines_ckd/p6_comp_g10.htm

- Bone disease and disorders of calcium and phosphorus metabolism develop during the course of ***chronic kidney disease*** and are associated with adverse outcomes.
- ***Patients with GFR < 60 mL/min/1.73 m***^{2} should be ***evaluated for bone disease*** and disorders of calcium and phosphorus metabolism.
- Bone disease associated with chronic kidney disease is composed of a number of abnormalities of bone mineralization. The major disorders can be classified into those associated with high bone turnover and high PTH levels (including osteitis fibrosa, the hallmark lesion of secondary hyperparathyroidism and mixed lesion) and low bone turnover and low or normal PTH levels (osteomalacia and adynamic bone disease).
- Altough I usually avoid giving internet refrences: This is an excellent article at the internet link above.

103. Answer is d (14 days).
Ref: Critical Care Nursing: Diagnosis and Management, By Linda D Urden, Pg 533.

- The administration of fibrinolytics in pulmonary embolism has had limited success.
- Currently fibrinolytic therapy is rserved for the patient with a massive pulmonary embolism and concomitant hemodynamic instability.
- Either ***rt-TPA or streptokinase*** may be used.
- The ***therapeutic window for using fibrinolytic therapy is up to 14 days*** although maximum benefit is usually obtained when given within 48 hours.

104. Answer is c (Amlodipine).
Ref: Harrison's, 17th edition Pg 1594.

Treatment of MI—'BeMOAN':

- **Be**ta blockers (metoprolol, atenolol—mortality, sudden death and infarct size are reduced in patients with Q-wave myocardial infarction when beta blockers are given early. Patients with unstable angina also benefit through a reduction in the incidence or severity of myocardial infarction).
- **M**orphine
- **O**xygen
- **A**spirin and ACE inhibitor
- **N**itroglycerine
- Thrombolytic therapy and streptokinase
- Antiplatelets and aspirin
- Antithrombotics
- Statins (early administration of high-dose statin therapy (pravastatin or atorvastatin) has been shown to reduce the risk of recurrent ischemic events during the 4-month period following hospital discharge).

Note:
- Unlike beta blockers, ***calcium antagonists are of little value in the acute setting***, and there is evidence that ***short-acting dihydropyridines (nifedipine, amlodepine)*** may be ***a/w an increased mortality risk!***.

105. Answer is c *(Campylobacter jejuni).*
Ref: Mayo Clinic Internal Medicine Board Review, edited by Robert D Ficalor, 2013 edition Pg 302.

- *Vibriocholerae,* Enterotoxigenic *Escherichia coli* and *Bacillus cereus* cause toxigenic diarrhea.
- Causes of invasive diarrhea are:
  - *Shigella*
  - EHEC, *E. coli* 0157:H7
  - *Camplylobacter jejuni*
  - *Yersinia*
  - *Vibrio parahemolyticus*

106. Answer is c or d (Often fatal in early middle age or Triad of loin pain, mass and attacks of renal colic).
Ref: Bailey and Love's, 26th edition Pg 1284.

- A direct pick from summary box 75.2 from the above page in Bailey and Love's textbook of surgery.
- ***Infantile polcystic kidney*** disease is ***autosomal recessive.***

Features of adult polycystic kidney disease:
- Inherited as an autosomal dominant trait
- An important cause of end-stage renal failure
- Pain, hematuria, infection and hypertension are common
- Often fatal in early middle age.

Autosomal Recessive (Childhood) Polycystic Kidney	Autosomal Dominant (ADult) Polycystic kidney
Genetics:	
– *ARPKD gene– chromosome* ***6p.*** – *Gene defect – PKHD1* which produces fibrocystin (polyductin) – (*PKHD*1 = **P**olycystic **K**idney **H**epatic **D**isease 1)	– ***APKD-1 gene***[Q] on chromosome ***16p***[Q] – *('Polycytsic kidney' =* ***16*** *letters =* ***16p!)*** – *Gene defect – PKD1 and PKD2, which code for polycystin 1 and 2* – Phenotypic heterogeneity is a hallmark of ADPKD, as evidenced by family members, who share the same mutation, but have a different clinical course
Clinically	
– Diagnosed in ***first year of life***[Q] presenting as *bilateral abdominal masses* – Enlarged with ***small cysts, < 5 mm, limited to the collecting tubules***[Q] – ***Death*** *in neonatal* period is MC due to ***pulmonary hypoplasia***[Q] – ***HTN***[Q] ***occurs in first few years of life*** – Longer-term survivors frequently develop ***portal hypertension, esophageal varices and hypersplenism from periportal fibrosis***	– *<u>DOES NOT</u> manifest before 30 years.* – Manifests disease as ***renomegaly***[Q]***, flank pain***[Q]***, haematuria***[Q]***, infection***[Q]***, hypertension***[Q]***, uremia***
Associated abnormalities	
– ***Congenital hepatic fibrosis***[Q]. – Maternal oligohydramnios – Potter's syndrome	– ***Hepatic cysts***[Q] (***MC extrarenal*** *anomaly*) – Also cysts in spleen, pancreas, ovaries – *Intracranial berry*[Q] *aneurysms* – *Mitral valve prolapse, colonic diverticula*

Imaging:	
– U/s shows large, echogenic kidneys – The diagnosis can be made *in utero after 24 weeks of gestation in severe cases*, but cysts generally become visible ONLY AFTER birth – The absence of renal cysts in either parent on ultrasonography helps to distinguish ARPKD from ADPKD in older patients	– IVU –'***spider-leg***[Q]' deformity – The sensitivity of ***renal ultrasonography***[Q] for the detection of ADPKD is 100% for subjects 30 years or older with a positive family history – ***Before the age of 30*** years, ***CT scan or T2-weighted MRI***[Q] is more sensitive for detecting presymptomatic disease
Treatment	
–	– ***Rovsing***[Q] operation

107. Answer is a (Isotonic formula).

Ref: Critical Care Medicine: The Essentials, By John J Marin. Pg 678.

- The principle of fluid resuscitation is that the intravascular volume must be maintained following a burn in order to provide sufficient circulation to perfuse not only the essential visceral organs such as the brain, kidneys and gut but also the peripheral tissues, especially the damaged skin.

Fluids for resuscitation:

- In children with burns over 10% TBSA and adults with burns over 15% TBSA, consider the need for intravenous fluid resuscitation
- If oral fluids are to be used, salt must be added
- Fluids needed can be calculated from a standard formula
- The key is to monitor urine output.

Parkland formula:

- Most widely used formula; this formula uses ***isotonic crystalloid solutions***.
- This calculates the fluid to be replaced in the first 24 hours by the following formula: total percentage body surface area × weight (kg) × 4 = volume (mL). Half this volume is given in the first 8 hours and the second half is given in the subsequent 16 hours.

There are three types of fluid used:

1. The most common is Ringer's lactate or Hartmann's solution.
2. Some centers use human albumin solution or fresh-frozen plasma.
3. Some centers use hypertonic saline.

- ***Ringer's lactate*** is the ***most commonly used crystalloid***. Crystalloids are said to be as effective as colloids for maintaining intravascular volume. They are also significantly less expensive. Another reason for the use of crystalloids is that even large protein molecules leak out of capillaries following burn injury; however, non-burnt capillaries continue to sieve proteins virtually normally.
- In children, maintenance fluid must also be given. This is normally dextrose saline.
- Human albumin solution (HAS) is a commonly used colloid.

108. Answer is b (Gastric arterial venous malformation).

Ref: Bailey and Love, 26th edition Pg 1043.

- ***Dieulafoy's*** disease: This is essentially a ***gastric arterial venous malformation*** that has a characteristic histological appearance.
- Bleeding due to this malformation is one of the most difficult causes of upper gastrointestinal bleeding to treat. The lesion itself is covered by normal mucosa and when not bleeding, it may be invisible.

109. Answer is c (Inferior surface of the liver).

Ref: Bailey and Love, 26th edition Pg 1098.

- ❑ **Calot's triangle:** 'Triangle' formed by the
  - *Cystic artery* superiorly
  - *Cystic duct* inferiorly
  - ***Hepatic duct*** and ***common hepatic artery*** medially.
- This was described in 1891 by Jean-Franc□ois Calot. It is an important surgical landmark and should be identified by surgeons performing cholecystectomy to avoid damage to the extrahepatic biliary system.

110. Answer is a (Hernias through the foramen of Morgagni are common at any age).
Ref: General Thoracic Surgery, By Thomas W Shields. Pg 719.

Congenital Diaphragmatic Hernia

(POsteroLAteRal hernia) **BochdaLek's Hernia (POLAR Bear!)**	**MoRgagni Hernia (retrosternal anterior hernia)**
– Due to ***persistence of the pleuroperitoneal canal***[Q]. – *MC diaphragmatic hernia*[Q] in children, MC on ***Left***[Q] *side*. – *Classic triad of* ***respiratory distress***[Q], ***apparent dextrocardia***[Q] *and a* ***scaphoid abdomen***[Q]	– Defect is between the sternal and costal attachments of the diaphragm. – Usually occurs on ***Right side***[Q], in ***adults***, particularly females. – ***MC*** involved viscus is the ***transverse colon***[Q]

- ***Pulmonary hypoplasia***[Q] is the ***MC*** *cause of morbidity and mortality. Hence,* medical therapy is directed toward ***optimizing oxygenation*** while ***avoiding barotrauma***.
- In the delivery room, if the infant is known or suspected to have ***congenital diaphragmatic hernia***, immediately place a vented ***orogastric tube and connect it to continuous suction***[Q] to prevent bowel distension and further lung compression.
- For the same reason, ***avoid bag and mask ventilation***[Q] and ***immediately intubate the trachea***[Q].
- ***Surgical repair***[Q] after stabilization is ***the treatment of choice***[Q].

111. Answer is c (2003).
Ref: http://www.genome.gov/10001772

- The ***Human Genome Project (HGP)*** was one of the great feats of exploration in history—an inward voyage of discovery rather than an outward exploration of the planet or the cosmos; an international research effort to sequence and map all of the genes together known as the genome of members of our species, Homo sapiens.
- ***Completed in April 2003***, the HGP gave us the ability for the first time to read nature's complete genetic blueprint for building a human being.

112. Answer is b [Adhesions (40%), Obstructed hernia (12%), Inflammatory (15%), Fecal impaction (8%)].
Ref: Bailey and Love's, 26th edition Pg 1181, Fig 70.1.

- This is a ***direct pick*** from the pie'chart figure on the above mentioned page from ***Bailey and Love*** textbook.
- Common causes of dynamic intestinal obstruction and their relative frequencies are as below:
  - Adhesions (40%)
  - Obstructed hernia (12%)
  - Inflammatory (15%)
  - Carcinoma (15%)
  - Fecal impaction (8%)
  - Pseudo-obstruction (5%)
  - Miscellaneous (5%).

113. Answer is a (Upper lateral quadrant).
Ref: Last's Anatomy, 9th edition Pg 166.

- In ***adults, the upper outer quadrant of the gluteus maximus*** is the most frequently used site for IM injection.

114. Answer is c (Product of digestibility coefficient and biological value divided by 100).
Ref: Essentials of Biochemistry (for Medical Students), By Pankaja Naik, Pg 148.

- The Net Protein Utilization (NPU) of a food is the percentage of protein contained in that food, which is retained by the body after the food has been eaten.
- NPU is used to describe the value or usefulness of certain proteins in a diet.
- ***NPU = Biological Value (BV) × Digestibility/100***
- Also, NPU = Nitrogen retained/Nitrogen intake × 100.

115. Answer is b (Periosteum is much thinner).
Ref: Nelson Textbook of Pediatric. 20th edition Ch 683.1.

- Growing bone is less dense and ***more malleable*** than mature bone due to fewer lamellar components and greater.
- The ***periosteum enveloping growing bones is stronger and thicke***r than mature periosteum and contributes to the lower
- The immature periosteum possesses increased osteogenic capability and new subperiosteal bone is rapidly laid down.
- ***Non-union is rare*** in children's fractures.
- Plane of deformity with respect to adjacent joint: ***Remodeling occurs more readily in the plane of a joint*** than with deformity not in the plane of the joint; also remodeling is better when fracture occurs close to the physis.

116. Answer is c (Coagulase negative *Staphylococcus*).
Ref: Oxford Handbook Clinical Medicine, Pg 264.

- Catheter-related infection is one of the most common clinical problems associated with the administration of parenteral nutrition.
- In addition to bloodstream infection, infection can occur at the exit site and in the subcutaneous tissue through which the catheter is placed.
- When a catheter related infection is identified, treatment may require catheter removal in addition to an appropriate systemic antimicrobial regimen.
- The use of antimicrobial lock solutions may reduce the risk of infection in high-risk patients. If catheter salvage is considered, systemic antimicrobials may be supplemented with antimicrobial lock solutions.
- ***Coagulase-negative staphylococci S. epidermidis*** is the MC cause.

117. Answer is d (Haloperidol).
Ref: Rang & Dale's Pharmacology. 8th edition Pg 564.

- ***Depot preparation*** is a special preparation of the medication, which is given by injection. The medication is ***slowly released into the body over a number of weeks.***
- Antipsychotic drugs available as depot preparations are ***haloperidol; fluphenazine, flupenthixol; sisperidone, aripiprazole,.***
- ***Note: Olanzapine*** and ***ziprasidone*** are also recently available as depot!.
- If same question gets repeated, the answer could be challenged with the above reference and other 2015 textbook references and this internet link also http://www.rcpsych.ac.uk/healthadvice/treatmentswellbeing/depotmedication.aspx.

118. Answer is b (Submandibular gland).
Ref: Bailey and Love, 26th edition Pg 726.

- ***80% of all salivary stones*** occur in the ***submandibular glands*** because their *secretions are highly viscous.*
- ***80% of submandibular stones*** are ***radio-opaque*** and can be *identified on plain radiography.*

119. Answer is b (Patient's in sinus Rhythm with an EF < 35% and a QRS > 120 ms).
Ref: CMDT 2013, Pg 406, Harrison's, 19th edition Pg 1514.

- Nonsynchronous contraction (***Mechanical dyssynchrony***) between the walls of the left ventricle (intraventricular) or between the ventricular chambers (interventricular) impairs systolic function, decreases mechanical efficiency of contraction and adversely affects ventricular filling.
- The single most important association of extent of dyssynchrony is a ***widened QRS interval*** particularly in the presence of a LBBB pattern.
- With placement of a pacing lead via the coronary sinus to the lateral wall of the ventricle, cardiac resynchronization therapy (CRT) enables a more synchronous ventricular contraction by aligning the timing of activation of the opposing walls.
- The COMPANION trial included 1,520 patients with NYHA class III or IV heart failure, ***EF of </= 35% and QRS duration >/= 120 milliseconds***. In addition to optimal medical therapy, resynchronization therapy with biventricular pacing with or without implantable defibrillator capability ***reduced death and hospitalization*** from any cause by about 20%.

120. Answer is d (Gastrinoma triangle).

Ref: Bailey and Love, 26th edition Pg 790, Fig 52.17.

Zollinger-Ellison Syndrome (ZES)

- ***ZES*** consists of ***severe peptic ulcers***Q secondary to ***gastric acid hypersecretion***Q due to ***unregulated gastrin release***Q from a ***non-β cell endocrine tumor (gastrinoma).***
- ***Age affected*** = 30–50 yearsQ
- ***Etiology***: Gastrinomas are classified into ***sporadic tumors (MC)*** and those ***a/w multiple endocrine neoplasia (MEN) type I***Q.
- ***Location***: Over 80% of these tumors are found within the hypothetical ***gastrinoma triangle***Q (confluence of the cystic and common bile ducts superiorly, junction of the second and third portions of the duodenum inferiorly, and junction of the neck and body of the pancreas medially).
- Around 90% of tumors occur in the *pancreatic head* or ***proximal duodenal wall***Q, the latter site being more common.

Clinically
- ***Peptic ulcers***, usually solitary and located in the duodenal bulb.
- ***Gastric acid hypersecretion*** can cause direct intestinal mucosal injury and pancreatic enzyme inactivation, resulting in *diarrhea, steatorrhea and weight loss;* nasogastric aspiration of stomach acid stops the diarrhea.
- ***Suspect ZES***Q when:
  - Increased fasting gastrin levels are a/w ulcers refractory to standard therapiesQ
  - ***Giant*** ulcersQ (> 2 cm)
  - Ulcers located distal to the duodenal bulb (***postbulbar*** ulcerQ), multiple duodenal ulcers
  - Frequent ulcer recurrences
  - Ulcers associated with *diarrhea*Q
  - Ulcers occurring after ulcer surgery
  - Patients with ulcer complications
  - Patients with hypercalcemia or family histories of ulcers (suggesting MEN 1)
  - Ulcers occurring in absence of *H. pylori* and NSAIDs usageQ.

Laboratory findings:
- ***Most sensitive and specific*** test: ***Increased fasting serum gastrin concentration***Q (> 150 pg/mL).
- *Gastric acid hypersecretion*Q is present (pH < 3.0)
- ***IV secretin***Q *produces a rise in serum gastrin* of over 200 pg/mL within 2–30 minutes.

Imaging:
- ***Somatostatin Receptor Scintigraphy***Q has a sensitivity (> 80%) for tumor detection that exceeds all other imaging studies combined.
- In patients with negative SRS, endoscopic ultrasonographyQ (EUS) may be useful to detect small gastrinomas in the duodenal wall, pancreas or peripancreatic lymph nodes.

Treatment:
- ***Proton pump inhibitors***Q are the *treatment of choice.*

Note:
- *Gastrinoma triangle* (*Psaros triangle*[Q]): 90% of gastrinomas are found here.

For questions 121-124

Ref: "Adverse reactions to iodinate contrast media". http://www.ncbi.nlm.nih.gov/pmc/articles/PMC3770975/

Explanation:
"Contrast media in radiology is an important topic for any PG medical entrance examination".

121. Answer is a (Iodine).
122. Answer is d (Non-ionic dimers).
123. Answer is d (Hypovolemia).
124. Answer is b (Water soluble non-ionic monomers).

- The frequency of allergic-like and physiologic adverse events related to the intravascular administration of ***iodinated contrast media (ICM) is low*** and has decreased considerably with changes in usage from ionic high-osmolality contrast media (HOCM) to nonionic low-osmolality contrast media (LOCM).
- The majority of adverse side effects to LOCM are mild non-life-threatening events that usually require only observation, reassurance and/or supportive measures.
- ***Ionic monomers*** has the ***lowest iodine-to-particle ratio*** of 1.5:1; it also has the highest osmolality ranging from five to eight times that of blood.
- ***Non-ionic monomeric and ionic dimeric*** ICM have the same iodine-to-particle ratio of 3:1. The osmolality of these preparations are approximately twice that of blood.
- ***Non-ionic dimeric contrast has the highest iodine-to-particle ratio*** of ***6:1***. It also has the most physiologic osmolality, approximately equal to that of blood.
- In general, as osmolality decreases, viscosity increases.
- The hyperosmolar contrast media have an osmolality that is 5 times greater than physiologic osmolality of body cells. Intravascular administration of hyperosmolar contrast medium may result in migration of fluid from extravascular soft tissues into blood vessels, consequently expanding blood volume. The ***hyperosmolar agents*** are associated with ***erythrocyte damage, endothelial damage, vasodilation, hypervolemia, interruption of blood brain barrier and cardiac depression.***
- ***Non-ionic low osmolality contrast media*** is recommended for intrathecal and vascular radiological procedures.

For questions 125-128

In a radiology department that uses conventional film and dark room techniques

Ref: *The Physics of Radiology and Imaging, By K Thayalan, Pg 178.*

125. Answer is c (Silver).
126. Answer is a (Red).
127. Answer is c (Reduces image contrast).
128. Answer is c (Electromagnetic waves and particles).

- Dark areas on any X-ray that you see are due to ***metallic silver*** (Comedk 2011 repeat).
- ***Safelights*** are ***special light*** fixtures ***(deep cherry-red[Q] color)*** fitted with filters used in the *X-ray darkroom, so that it will not affect the X-ray films and photographic paper* (Comedk 2013 repeat).
- Short ***electromagnetic waves*** such as ***X-rays*** behave ***like waves as well as particles*** when interacting with matter (refer answer 79 in the same paper above !!).
- When an X-ray beam enters a patient's body, a large portion of the photons engage in Compton interactions and produce scattered radiation. Some of this scattered radiation leaves the body in the same general direction as the

primary beam and exposes the image receptor. This ***scattered radiation reduces image contrast***. The degree of contrast loss depends on the scatter content of the radiation emerging from the patient's body. In most radiographic and fluoroscopic procedures, the major portion of the x-ray beam leaving the patient's body is scattered radiation. This, in turn, significantly reduces contrast.

For questions 129-132

Ref: Bailey and Love, 26th edition Pg 177-179.

Explanation:

" This is a set of questions based on MRI imaging – if you have read the below extract from Sure Success MAGIC, you should be easily able to answer the set".

129. Answer is d (Hydrogen).
130. Answer is b (High signal intensity on T2-weighted images).
131. Answer is a (Shortening of T1 and T2 relaxation times).
132. Answer is b (Gadolinium).

All About MRI (Magnetic Resonance Imaging)

- MRI was invented by ***Lauterbur***[Q] in **1973**[Q].
- MRI depends on the ***rearrangement of hydrogen nuclei***[Q] ***(protons***[Q]***)*** in water molecule and lipids when a tissue is *exposed to a short electromagnetic pulse.*
- When the pulse subsides, the nuclei return to their normal position, re-radiating some of the energy they have absorbed. Sensitive receivers pick up this electromagnetic echo.
- *Clinical MRI machines operate between* ***0.5 and 2.0 tesla;*** 3T–8T magnets are now available.

T1 and T2 images

- In MRI, the rate of return to equilibrium of perturbed protons is called ***relaxation rate***. The relaxation rate varies among normal and pathologic tissues.
- Two relaxation rates, T1 and T2 influence the signal intensity of the image.
- The T1 and T2 signals are analysed by the computer and reconstructed mathematically by a method called ***Fourier transformation***[Q].
- ***T1 relaxation time*** is the time, measured in milliseconds, for 63% of the hydrogen protons to return to their normal equilibrium state
- ***T2 relaxation*** is the time for 63% of the protons to become dephased owing to interactions among nearby protons.
- Various body tissues have different relaxation times, so that a given tissue may be ***T1 weighted or T2 weighted*** (i.e. best visualized on that particular type of image). In practice both types of scans are usually performed.
- ***Paramagnetic***[Q] ***substances*** such as *Fe, Mg and Gadolinium* cause a ***decrease in T1 and T2 times***[Q] (i.e., they increase the rate of relaxation of T1 and T2.).

	T1-weighted images	**T2-weighted images**
Best for	Normal anatomy, Subacute hemorrhage	Viewing pathological changes, Chronic hemorrhage
Hypointense (Dark/Black) structures	CSF, vitreous, edema	Blood vessels
Hyperintense (Bright/White) structures	Fat, blood and contrast agents	Water, CSF, vitreous, edema, inflammation (all have ***high water content***[Q]). 'waTer is whiTe on ***T2***'

Enhancement in MRI

- *Gadolinium*[Q] is a ***contrast agent given IV***, remains intravascular unless there is a breakdown of the BBB. It is ***only visualized***[Q] ***on T1-weighted images*** and ***enhancing lesion such as tumors and inflammation will appear bright on these images***. It DOES NOT show up on T2-weighted studies.
- **Fat suppression techniques**: Eliminate the brighter signal of fat and better delineates normal structures as well as tumors, inflammatory lesions and vascular malformations, e.g. T1 fat saturation with gadolinium; ***STIR***[Q] (Short T1 Inversion Recovery, *best for* ***optic neuritis***[Q]).
- **FLAIR[Q] (Fluid Attenuation Inversion Recovery)** *suppress the bright CSF on T2-weighted images* to allow *better visualization of adjacent pathological tissue such as periventricular plaques of demyelination*; FLAIR is more sensitive for ***edema***[Q].

Advantages of MRI

- NO ionizing radiation; images can be easily produced in any plane, e.g. sagittal and coronal (good for spinal cord, ,aorta, vena cava)
- Visualization of posterior fossa and other areas prone to bony artefact on CT is better (e.g. craniocervical junction).
- Shows vasculature without contrast
- High inherent soft tissue contrast, precise staging of malignancy possible.

Contraindications to MRI

- Patients with metallic FB[Q], e.g. pacemakers, cochlear implants, some types of aneurysmal clips, metallic intraocular FB,
- McGee stapedectomy piston[Q] prosthesis,
- Duraphase penile implant[Q],
- Swan-Ganz catheter[Q],
- Magnetic[Q] stoma plugs, magnetic dental implants, magnetic sphincters,
- Tattooed[Q] eyeliner (contains ferromagnetic material and may irritate eyes),
- Ferromagnetic[Q] IVC filters, coils, stents (safe 6 weeks after implantation).

Disadvantages of MRI

- High cost; ***Claustrophobic***; motion artifacts due to longer imaging time; ***Nephrogenic systemic fibrosis*** (in renal insufficiency patients due to gadolinium)
- Does ***NOT image bone/calcification*** (which appears black); although not always a disadvantage since bone marrow can be visualized (e.g. tumors extension into bone marrow).
- Does NOT detect acute hemorrhage.

- Echo-planar MRI (EPI): *Extremely rapid MRI of the* ***brain in 1-2 mins***. *Perfusion and diffusion imaging are EPI techniques* that are useful in early detection of ischemic injury of the brain and may be useful together to demonstrate infarcted tissue as well as, ischemic, but potentially viable tissue at risk of infarction (e.g. the ***ischemic penumbra***).
- ***Diffusion-weighted MRI:*** Is the *most sensitive technique for detection of* ***acute cerebral infarction of <7 days' duration***[Q] and is also sensitive to encephalitis and abscess formation.
- ***Perfusion MRI*** involves the acquisition of EPI images during a rapid intravenous bolus of gadolinium contrast material. It can also be used in the ***assessment of brain tumors*** to differentiate intra-axial primary tumors from extra-axial tumors or metastasis.
- ***Diffusion tensor imaging*** is a diffusion MRI technique that has great potential in the ***assessment of brain maturation***[Q]; valuable in *preoperative assessment of subcortical white matter tract anatomy prior to brain tumor surgery*.
- ***Functional MRI*** of the brain is an EPI technique that ***localizes regions of activity in the brain*** following task activation; useful in research. Currently ***preoperative somatosensory*** and ***auditory cortex localization***[Q] is possible.

- *Magnetic Resonance Neurography*[Q] is a T2-weighted MR technique that shows promise in detecting increased signal in irritated, inflamed or infiltrated peripheral nerves.
- ***Time-of-flight*[Q] *(TOF) imaging***, MC used method for MR angiogram (MRA).
- "When any motion of body produces disturbance and motion related artifact in images in radiology or during radiotherapy, then ***gating***[Q] is done to ***reduce the motion*** *related* ***artifacts***".

For questions 133-136

A 55-year-old male came for a routine medical health check up and his chest radiograph demonstrated a solitary calcific focus in the left upper lobe.

Ref: Computed Tomography and Magnetic Resonance of the Thorax, edited by David P Naidich, Pg 363; "The calcified lung nodule: What does it mean?" http://www.ncbi.nlm.nih.gov/pmc/articles/PMC2883201/

Explanation:
"This is a set of questions about solitary pulmonary nodule and lung calcification which are high yield topics for any PG medical entrance examination".

133. Answer is c (Varicella pneumonia).
134. Answer is c (Chondrosarcoma and osteogenic sarcoma).
135. Answer is a (Popcorn calcification and do not undergo malignant transformation).
136. Answer is b or c (Tuberculosis and silicosis or sarcoidosis and blastomycosis).

Causes of solitary calcified pulmonary nodule

- Granulomas:
  - Tuberculosis
  - Fungal infections
  - Vasculitides.
- Neoplasms:
  - Primary ***bronchogenic Ca***
  - ***Metastases.***
- ***Hamartoma***: MC benign tumor of the lung and shows popcorn calcification.

Note:
- Healed ***Varicella pneumonia*** is a/w ***multiple*** calcified nodules.
- Secondaries from Osteosarcoma and chondrosarcoma show diffuse clacification.

Egg shell calcification of lymph nodes

- **Sil**icosis[Q]
- **Sar**coidosis[Q]
- **Lymp**homa following radiotherapy[Q]
- **Coal mine**r's pneumoconiosis[Q]

"SILly **SAR**ah **LYMP**ed to the **COAL MINE"**

Note: Rare causes include TB, histoplasmosis, ***blastomycosis***, amyloidosis, scleroderma and Castleman's disease.

For questions 137-140

A child aged 3 years is brought to the pediatrician with a history of cough for 3 weeks treated at a local clinic conservatively. Serial radiographs of the chest revealed a large persistent right lower zone opacity with crowding of the ribs and a slight shift of the mediastinum to the same side.

Ref: Encyclopedia of Imaging, Volume 2, By Albert L Baert, Pg 729.

137. Answer is a (Collapse of right lower lobe).
138. Answer is b (May show overinflation of the involved lung).
139. Answer is b (Bronchiectasis).
140. Answer is a (Inspiratory and expiratory radiographs).

- Also see ***answer 81 above*** for explanation of question 138 which is a repeat question in the same paper and also for explanation for ***question 140 above***.
- Aspirated foreign material can result in focal ***bronchiectasis***. Persistence of a non-calcified foreign body, such as a vegetable fiber, within a bronchus for a prolonged period of time can serve as a nidus for calcium deposition.
- Chest X-ray signs of ***right lower lobe collapse:***
  - Increased opacity (triangular in shape) at the medial base of the right lung
  - Usually the medial aspect of the dome of right hemidiaphragm is lost
  - The right hilum is depressed
  - Descending right lower lobe pulmonary artery is not visualized
- Non-specific signs indicating right-sided atelectasis may also be present (although due to the small size of the right middle lobe they may well be subtle). They include:
  - Elevation of the hemidiaphragm
  - Crowding of the right sided ribs
  - Shift of the mediastinum to the right

For questions 141-144

A 58-year-old male visited a dermatologist with complaints of multiple eruptions on the skin all over the body. On examination, round to oval vesicles and bullae were seen on the scalp, face, chest, axilla and groin. Some of the vesicles had ruptured leaving erosions. A biopsy was performed and direct immunofluorescence showed fishnet-like pattern of IgG deposition in the squamous intercellular spaces in the lower epidermis.

Ref: Harrison's, 19th edition Pg 370.

Explanation:
" The case history given is that of a blistering skin disease – clues to daignosis are the 'fishnet pattern' in the 'lower epidermis' this rules out the other options which have a sub-peidermal blister".

141. Answer is c (Pemphigus vulgaris).
142. Answer is a (Subepidermal non-acantholytic blister).
143. Answer is d (Dermatitis herpetiformis).
144. Answer is c (Pemphigus vulgaris).

Summary of Immunologically Mediated Blistering Skin Diseases

Clinical features	Histology
Pemphigus vulgaris (PV)	
Flaccid blistersQ which rupture easily; ***Nikolsky's sign+***Q; ***Mouth***Q (~90% have oromucosal involvement), scalp, face, neck, axilla, trunk affected; lesions usually *heal* ***without scarring***Q; ***Anti-desmoglein***Q antibodies seen: anti-***Dsg3*** (plus anti-***Dsg1*** in patients with *skin involvement*)	Blisters formed in ***suprabasal***Q ***layer*** of epidermis. IgG and C3 on surface of keratinocytes in a ***fishnet pattern***Q; '***tombstones***Q'— *basal keratinocytes remaining attached to basemet membrane zone*
Pemphigus foliaceus (PF)	
Crusts and ***shallow erosions***Q on ***scalp, central face***Q, neck, upper chest and back. *Mucous membrane lesions are rare*. A/w thymoma/myasthenia.	Blister formed in ***superficial layers*** of epidermis (***subcorneal***Q)

Drug-induced pemphigus *resembles PF* (**penicillamine**[Q] **MC**, captopril, rifampin, piroxicam, penicillin, phenobarbital); ***Fogo selvagem*** = endemic form of PF in Brazil	
Paraneoplastic pemphigus (PNP)	
A/w ***Non-Hodgkin's lymphoma***[Q] ***(MC)***, CLL, thymoma, spindle cell tumors, Waldenstrom's macroglobulinemia, and *Castleman's disease*. PNP maybe a/w ***bronchiolitis obliterans***[Q]. Painful stomatitis and blisters; anti-***plakin***[Q] autoantibodies (desmoplakins I and II, bullous pemphigoid antigen 1, envoplakin, periplakin, and plectin) and anti-***cadherin*** autoantibodies (e.g. Dsg1 and Dsg3).	***Acantholysis, keratinocyte necrosis*** and ***vacuolar interface dermatitis***[Q]
Bullous pemphigoid(BP)	
Tense blisters[Q] on ***flexor surfaces***[Q], oromucosal lesions (RARE)*; anti* ***BPAG1 and BPAG2***[Q] *antibodies*	***Subepidermal*** blister ; (**B**ul**LO**us: **B**e**LO**w epidermis);
Pemphigoid (herpes) gestationis	
Variant of pemphigoid in ***pregnancy***[Q]; Pruritic, urticarial plaques, rimmed by vesicles and bullae on the ***trunk (periumbilical***[Q]***)*** and extremities; anti-BPAG2 antibodies; ***spontaneous remission***[Q] may occur.	Teardrop-shaped, ***subepidermal blisters***[Q]; ***eosinophil***-rich infiltrate;
Cicatricial pemphigoid	
Blistering lesions of mucous membranes and skin; scarring at some sites; ***anti-BPAG2***[Q] ***and laminin 332***[Q] ***antibodies***	***Subepidermal blister***
Dermatitis herpetiformis	
Extremely itchy[Q] small papules and vesicles on ***elbows, knees***, buttocks, and posterior nuchal area (***extensor surfaces***[Q]). A/ w ***subclinical, gluten sensitive***[Q] ***enteropathy*** (***celiac sprue***[Q]) A/w ***HLA B8/DRW3*** and HLA DQW2. Treatment is ***dapsone***[Q]. Strictly *exclude gluten* from the diet; ↑ risk of ***GI lymphoma***[Q]	***Subepidermal blister***[Q]; antibodies against ***epidermal transglutaminase 3***[Q] ***and anti-endomysial antibodies***[Q]***; Granular IgA deposits in dermal papillae***[Q] of perilesional skin observed by direct IF is the ***gold standard***[Q] of diagnosis
Linear IgA disease	
Itchy small papules on ***extensor surfaces***, ***anti-BPAG2*** antibodies	***Subepidermal blister***

For questions 145-148

A 5-year-old girl presents with recurrent itchy lesions on her face and limbs since the age of 6 months. The itching is worse in winter and there is a history of occasional oozing. It is temporarily relieved with topical steroids and emollient application. On examination, flexural areas are found to have lichenified skin, and there is erythema and scaling in the face.

Ref: CMDT 2013, Pg 103.

Explanation:

" The case history given is that of a child with atopic dermatitis—itching worse in winter, flexural areas affected are all catchwords here".

145. Answer is d (Wheal formation on stroking).
146. Answer is a (Pruritus).
147. Answer is c (House dust).
148. Answer is d (Isotretinoin).

- ***Diagnostic criteria*** for ***atopic dermatitis must include pruritus***, typical morphology and distribution (***flexural lichenification***, hand eczema, nipple eczema and eyelid eczema in adults), onset in childhood and chronicity

All About ATOPIC DERMATITIS

- ***Infancy:*** *Face, neck and extensor surfaces* involved. The *napkin area is frequently spared.*
- ***Childhood: Cubital***[Q] ***and popliteal fossae*** *involved*
- ***Adults:*** The face, trunk and ***flexures*** involved.
- Cardinal feature of AD is ***pruritus***[Q] and scratching account for most of the signs.
- Family history of atopic triad: *Dermatitis, Asthma and Allergic rhinitis.*
- ***Hanifin and Rajka Diagnostic Criteria***[Q] are used for atopic dermatitis.

Clinical Features of Atopic Dermatitis

- ***Lichenification***[Q]: Thick, leathery skin due to constant scratching and rubbing with exaggeration of normal skin lines and hyperpigmentation
- ***Pityriasis alba***[Q]: Hypopigmented poorly demarcated areas on cheeks and extremities
- ***Ichthyosis***: Dry, scaly skin
- ***Keratosis pilaris***[Q]: Follicular openings are filled with horny plugs; small, rough bumps seen on the face, posterolateral arms and anterior thighs
- ***Hyperlinear palms***[Q]: Increased number of skin creases on the palms
- ***Urticaria***: Hives (red, raised bumps), after exposure to allergen, or after exercise or a hot bath
- ***Cheilitis*** (perioral pallor[Q]): Inflammation of the skin on and around the lips
- ***Atopic pleat (Dennie-Morgan fold)*** [Q]: An extra fold of skin that develops under the eye
- ***Hertoghe's sign***[Q]: Thinning of the lateral half of the eyebrows
- ***Hyperpigmented lower eyelids***[Q]
- Firm rubbing of the skin elicits ***'white dermographism***[Q]***'*** with no erythema.

Treatment

- ***Emollients***[Q] for dry skin; bathe only once daily.
- Corticosteroid ointments sparingly with tapering.
- ***Tacrolimus*** and ***pimecrolimus*** ointment (*risk of T cell lymphoma*, not useful in acute weeping lesions)
- In 50% cases, disease ***remits spontaneously***[Q] ***between 2 and 5 years;*** in adults it is milder.
- Systemic therapy: Oral prednisone, antihistamines, antistaphylococcal antibiotics.
- Cyclosporine, mycophenolate mofetil or azathioprine in recalcitrant cases.

Special Concerns in Atopic Dermatitis

- *Associations*: ***shield cataract***[Q] ***(anterior subcapsular***[Q]***)*** and ***keratoconus***[Q], *food intolerance and food allergy*
- ***Genetic*** predisposition (both parents affected > 80% chances; one parent affected, 50% chance of child getting affected)
- Serum levels of ***IgE***[Q] ***are Elevated***
- Increased susceptibility to *papilloma virus* (warts) and *molluscum contagiosum* and superinfection with *S. aureus*
- *Susceptibility to severe* ***HSV 1 infection***[Q]: ***Eczema herpeticum***[Q] or ***Kaposi's varicelliform eruption***[Q]
- A/w positive skin reaction/aggravation to ***house dust mite allergens***.

For questions 149-152

A 40-year-old well-nourished female working as a top level executive at a law firm presented to the surgical clinic with complaints of well-localized midepigastric abdominal pain. The pain was usually tolerable and frequently relieved by food. The pain was episodic, seasonal in the spring and fall, and relapsed during periods of emotional stress. Upon further

enquiry she revealed that she had noticed that her stools were black tarry and foul smelling. She had undergone an upper GI endoscopy for the above complaints and was given medical management, which did provide her only symptomatic relief.

Ref: Harrison's, 19th edition Pg 1920.

Explanation:
"Pain relieved by food indicated duodenal ulcer; all other clinical signs mentioned point towards peptic ulceration.".

149. **Answer is b (Duodenal ulcer).**
150. **Answer is d (Rapid urease assay).**
151. **Answer is c (Somatostatin).**
152. **Answer is e (None of the above).**

Gastric versus Duodenal Ulcers

Characteristic	Gastric Ulcer	Duodenal Ulcer
Patients, Cause	Age > 50 years *NSAID[Q] users* H. pylori infection (*minor*) Blood type A (gAstric)	Younger **H. pylori**[Q] infection (almost 100%) Blood type O (duOdenal)
Frequency	25% cases	75% cases (*more common*[Q])
Timing of pain	*Soon after*[Q] eating	*2-4 hours after*[Q] eating, *night pain*[Q]
Vomiting	Considerable vomiting	*No vomiting*[Q]
Hemorrhage	Hemetemesis more frequent than melena	*Melena*[Q] more frequent
Gastric acid level	Normal/Low	High[Q]
Gastrin level	High	Normal
Effect of eating	Pain increases with meals—*afraid to eat—weight loss*[Q].	(*"Pain Decreases with meals in Duodenal ulcer!"*)—*good appetite—weight gain*[Q]
Dict	Lives on milk and fish	Eats almost anything
Sex	Equal in both sexes	MC in males

Tests for Diagnosis of *H. pylori*

Invasive (Endoscopic biopsy[Q] required)	
Rapid urease[Q]	Simple, rapid, false negative with recent use of PPIs, antibiotics or bismuth compounds, cannot be used for early follow-up. Some commercial kits inaccurate before 24 hour
Histology[Q]	May give additional histologic information, sensitivity dependent on experience and use of special stains
Culture[Q]	Allows determination of antibiotic susceptibility, time consuming
Noninvasive	
C13 of C14 urea breath test[Q]	Simple, useful for follow-up after treatment, low dose radiation exposure with C14 test
Stool antigen test[Q]	Simple, useful for follow-up after treatment, maybe useful in children
Serology	Cannot be used for early follow-up

- **Gastric acid secretion**: There are three regulatory molecules that ***stimulate acid secretion*** (***acetylcholine, histamine, gastrin***) and one regulatory molecule that ***inhibits acid secretion (somatostatin)***.

For questions 153 - 156

A 60-year-old male, presented to the surgical clinic with complaints of passing blood in stool for about 2 months. He had not sought medical intervention as the symptoms did not alarm him. He jokingly mentioned that he consumes red meat regularly. He said he was often fatigued, but could carry on his normal chores. He however, did not complain of abdominal pain. He mentioned that his trousers were loose and needed to wear a tight belt. He had undergone colonoscopy as advised by his physician and it revealed grade 1 hemorrhoids and an ulcer in the ascending colon. A diagnosis of colonic cancer was written on the pathology report.

153. Answer is b (Adenocarcinoma).
154. Answer is c (Proximal SMA with proximal IMA).
155. Answer is b (Contrast enhanced CT).
156. Answer is d (Right hemicolectomy).

Ref: Bailey and Love, 26th edition Pg 1163.

Explanation:

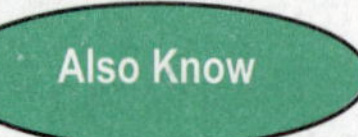

- Worldwide, the prevalence of colorectal cancer is closely associated with intake of red meat. There is ample evidence to suggest effects of red meat components (heme and N-nitroso compounds) on the DNA in the colorectal mucosa.

Risk factors

Age	Personal history	Family history	
		Colorectal cancer or adenomatous polyps	Hereditary syndromes (AD)
– > 50 years	– Previous colorectal cancer – ***Adenomatous polyps*** – IBD (particularly ***ulcerative colitis***Q) – ***Streptococcus bovis***Q bacteremia – Ureterosigmoidostomy – Decreased dietary fibre, increased ***red meat***Q consumption	– One first degree relative < 60 years of age or 2 first degree relatives of any age	– ***Familial Adenomatous Polyposis*** coli (responsible for 85% of colon cancers) – ***Non-polyposis coli syndrome (Lynch***Q syndrome – also a/w *endometrial, ovarian, stomach and small intestinal tumors,* ***AD***; a/w cancer of ***proximal colon***Q) – Cowden, Peutz- Jegher; Ruvalcaba-Smith-Myhre syndrome

- To prevent ischemic injury to the intestines, extensive collateralization occurs between major mesenteric trunks and branches of the mesenteric arcades.
- Collateral vessels within the colon meet at the splenic flexure and descending/sigmoid colon. These areas, which are inherently at risk for decreased blood flow, are known as ***Griffiths' point and Sudeck's point***, respectively, and are the most common locations for colonic ischemia
- *MC* colon cancer is ***adenocarcinoma***.
- ***Arc of Riolan*** = It is an inconstant artery that connects the ***proximal superior mesenteric artery (SMA)*** to the ***proximal inferior mesenteric artery (IMA)***. It is ***classically*** described as connecting the ***middle colic branch of the SMA with the left colic branch of the IMA***; also known as the ***mesenteric meandering artery (of Moskowitz)*** or *central anastomotic mesenteric artery*.
- Use of ***spiral CT of the chest and abdomen*** is now standard to ***stage colonic cancer by assessing T stage and detecting metastases.*** *Although chest X-ray and liver ultrasound are an alternative if CT is not readily available.*

Treatment

- *Carcinoma of the cecum or ascending colon* is treated when resectable by ***right hemicolectomy.***
- ***Carcinomas of the transverse colon and splenic flexure*** are most commonly treated by an ***extended right hemicolectomy.***
- For ***descending colon and sigmoid*** cancers: ***Left hemicolectomy*** is the operation of choice.

For questions 157 – 160

In a patient with gout

157. Answer is c (5–10 years after the onset of clinical symptoms).
158. Answer is b (1st MTP joint).
159. Answer is d (All of the above).
160. Answer is c (Punched out periarticular erosion).

Ref: Gout & Other Crystal Arthropathies, By Robert Terkeltaub. Pg 294.

Gout

- ***Asymmetric***[Q] joint distribution; joint is *swollen, red and painful.*
- Classically, painful ***MTP joint of big toe (podagra***[Q]***).***
- ***Tophus***[Q] ***formation*** (often on *external ear or Achilles tendon*). Acute attack[Q] tends to occur ***after alcohol consumption*** or a ***large meal.***
- Precipitation of ***monosodium urate***[Q] ***crystals*** into joints due to ***hyperuricemia***[Q], which can be caused by *Lesch-Nyhan syndrome, PRPP excess, ↓excretion of uric acid (e.g. thiazide diuretics), ↑cell turnover (cancer chemotherapy) or von Gierke's disease.* Crystals are *needle shaped*[Q] *negatively birefringent*[Q]. More common in *men*[Q].
- Treatment: ***Allopurinol, probenecid, colchicine,*** NSAIDs.
- Secondary gout, which may have a heritable component, is related to acquired causes of hyperuricemia, e.g. medication use (especially diuretics, low- dose aspirin, cyclosporine and niacin), myeloproliferative disorders, multiple myeloma, hemoglobinopathies, chronic kidney disease, hypothyroidism, psoriasis, sarcoidosis and lead poisoning
- Radiography is the main imaging modality for detecting the progression of gout, but there is a ***5-10 year latent period*** between first clinical symptoms and appearance of specific radiographic findings.
- Chronic gout shows '***punched out***' lesions on X-rays.

For questions 161 – 164

An adolescent male present with hypertension, hyperkalemia and metabolic acidosis with normal renal function

161. Answer is b (Gordon's syndrome).
162. Answer is a (DCT).
163. Answer is c (Thiazide diuretic).
164. Answer is c (WNK Kinase 1 and 4).

Ref: Harrison's, 19th edition Pg 301.

Explanation:
The clinical picture is of hereditary hypertension with kyperkalemia syndrome.

- Mutations in genes encoding ***WNK kinases, WNK-1 and WNK-4*** cause *pseudohypoaldosteronism type II* or ***Gordon syndrome*** characterized by hereditary hypertension with hyperkalemia.
- The clinical phenotype includes ***hypertension, hyperkalemia, hyperchloremic metabolic acidosis,*** suppressed PRA and aldosterone, hypercalciuria and reduced bone density.
- Treatment with ***thiazides*** results in resolution of the entire clinical phenotype.
- Gordon's syndrome, Liddle's syndrome and Gitelman's syndrome involve the ***distal tubule and collecting duct.***

For questions 165 - 168

A child present with low molecular proteinuria, hypercalciuria, nephrocalcinosis and nephrolithiasis. Later he progresses to renal failure from interstitial fibrosis, tubular atrophy and glomerulosclerosis.

165. Answer is d (Dent's disease).
166. Answer is c (X-linked recessive).
167. Answer is d (CLC-5).
168. Answer is a (PCT).

Ref: Harrison's, 19th edition Pg 2459.

Explanation: The case history given is that of Dent's disease. Although not a commonly encountered question OR condition that we see/read about—all the given clinical features do NOT fit into any of the other options and they can be ruled out.

- ***Dent's disease*** is an ***X-linked recessive*** disorder
- It is caused by inactivating mutations in ***CLCN5, a chloride transporter*** expressed in ***endosomes of the proximal tubule***. Impaired acidification of endocytic vesicles causes ***low-molecular-weight proteinuria***.
- Clinical features: ***Hypercalciuria, hypophosphatemia*** and ***recurrent nephrolithiasis*** *(kidney stones)*.
- Renal phosphate wasting is common among poorly controlled diabetic patients and alcoholics, who therefore are at risk for iatrogenic hypophosphatemia when treated with insulin or IV glucose, respectively.
- Diuretics and certain other drugs/toxins can cause defective renal tubular phosphate reabsorption.

For questions 169 – 172

A 50-year-old lady presented with chronic sinusitis. She was also having cough with hemoptysis. Her chest X-ray shows multiple cavities involving lower lobes. Her urine examination shows numerous RCB and proteinuria.

169. Answer is b [Granulomatosis with polyangitis (Wegener's)].
170. Answer is b (c-ANCA).
171. Answer is d (Large vessel vasculitis).
172. Answer is d (Plasmapheresis).

Ref: Harrison's, 19th edition Pg 2182.

Explanation:
The case history given is that of Wegener's granulomatosis—clues pointing to diagnosis are chronic sinusitis and lung and kindey involvement and c-ANCA positive—classic of Wegener's.

- ***Granulomatosis with polyangiitis*** *(formerly called* ***Wegener's****)* is characterized by granulomatous vasculitis of the ***upper and lower respiratory tracts*** together with ***glomerulonephritis***.
- ***Lung*** involvement typically appears as *multiple, bilateral, nodular* ***cavitary*** *infiltrates.*
- In its earliest form, ***renal*** involvement is characterized by a focal and segmental glomerulitis that may evolve into a rapidly progressive ***crescentic glomerulonephritis***.
- Involvement of the ***upper airway occurs in 95%*** of patients; severe upper respiratory tract findings such as ***chronic sinusitis***, paranasal sinus pain and drainage and purulent or bloody nasal discharge, with or without nasal mucosal ulceration.
- The ***histopathologic*** hallmarks: ***Necrotizing vasculitis of small arteries*** and veins together with ***granuloma formation***, which may be either intravascular or extravascular
- Approximately, 90% of patients with active disease have a positive antiproteinase-3 ANCA (*c-ANCA*).

Treatment

- For patients with severe disease, the combination of ***cyclophosphamide*** and ***prednisone*** is the standard of care
- ***Azathioprine*** has been shown to be as effective as cyclophosphamide in maintaining disease remissions
- Because of its superior side-effect profile, ***methotrexate*** is viewed as an appropriate substitute for cyclophosphamide

- *Rituximab*, a B-cell-depleting monoclonal antibody, has been shown to be as effective as cyclophosphamide for patients who have never been treated and may be more effective than cyclophosphamide for treating relapses.

For questions 173 -176

A 50 year old lady who was suffering from hypertension presented with sudden onset of severe headache and projectile vomiting. On examination she was drowsy with Glasgow coma scale of 7/14. Neck stiffness was present. There was no fever. Her CSF examination shows presence of xanthochromia.

173. Answer is b (Subarachnoid hemorrhage).
174. Answer is a (Hunt and Hess scale).
175. Answer is c (Nimodipine).
176. Answer is c (Hyponatremia).

Ref: *Harrison's, 19th edition Pg .*

Explanation:
The case history given is that of subarachnoid hemorrhage. The clues pointing to the diagnosis are hypertension, sudden severe headache and xanthochromia

All About Subarachnoid hemorrhage

- Bleeding into ***subarachnoid space***
- Overall *MC cause* is ***trauma***Q
- *MC* cause of ***spontaneous SAH***Q is rupture of ***Berry aneurysm***Q *(seen in Marfan's, Ehlers Danlos and ADPKD)*,
- Sudden onset, classically ***'worst headache in life' / thunderclap***Q headache; often a/w neck stiffness and vomiting.
- ***Bloody or xanthochromic CSF***Q on LP;
- Treat with ***nimodipine***Q
- ***Hunt and Hess scale***Q and *WFNS* (World federation of Neurological Societies scale) is for the severity of ***non-traumatic SAH***
- ***Fischer grading***Q is the severity of SAH by size (in mm).
- ***Non-contrast CT scan***Q confirms diagnosis
- Profound ***hyponatremia*** may develop quickly following ***SAH***. There is both natriuresis and volume depletion with SAH, so that patients become both hyponatremic and hypovolemic. Both atrial natriuretic peptide and brain natriuretic peptide have a role in producing this 'cerebral salt-wasting syndrome.'

For questions 177 - 180

A 15-year-old boy presented with a history of jaundice and pain in the knee joints after an episode of fever in the winter. On examination, no hepatosplenomegaly was seen. His hemoglobin was 8 g/dL and the anemia was normocytic and normochromic. His father too was anemic.

177. Answer is c (Sickle cell anemia).
178. Answer is d (Rouleaux formation).
179. Answer is b (*Salmonella*).
180. Answer is d (Parvovirus B19 infection).

Ref: *Harrison's, 19th edition Pg 634-635.*

Explanation:
The case history is that of sickle cell anemia. The clues pointing to the diagnosis are absence of hepatosplenomegaly and acute painful symptoms after and episode of fever.

- Painful crises are the most common clinical manifestation of sickle cell anemia.
- Provocative factors include infection, fever, excessive exercise, anxiety, abrupt changes in temperature, hypoxia or hypertonic dyes.
- Refer full details below.

All About Sickle Cell Disease

- *AR* disease; ***point mutation***[Q] in the ***β-globin***[Q] chain of Hb (***glutamic acid replaced by valine at position 6***[Q]) leads to the production of HbS, a form of Hb that is poorly soluble when deoxygenated.
- ***Heterozygotes*** are relatively ***malaria resistant***[Q].
  - ✈ Also know: *Duffy negativity, newborns (high HbF), thalassemia and G-6PD deficiency* have ***high resistance to P falciparum.***
- ***Acidosis, hypoxia*** and ***dehydration***[Q] → polymerization of HbS → distortion of RBCs into a ***sickle***[Q] ***shape*** that is susceptible to hemolysis and vascular clumping
- *Risk factors: African or Latin American*[Q] heritage
- Clinically:
  - Patients may be *asymptomatic between crises* or may note bone pain
  - Stressful events (e.g., infection, illness, trauma) incite sickle cell crises characterized by ***severe bone pain***[Q], ***chest pain***[Q], ***'hand foot syndrome' (dactylitis***[Q]***), dyspnea***[Q] and ***priapism***[Q].
  - Physical examination: Decreased growth velocity, jaundice or pallor, ***splenomegaly (in early stages***[Q]***)***, fever, possible leg ulcers.
- *Tests*:
  - ↓ Hb and ↑ reticulocytes; ↑ WBCs.
  - ↓ serum haptoglobin; ↑ indirect bilirubin
  - No HbA, ↑ HbF and presence of HbS (normally not present) on electrophoresis
  - Solubility tests (e.g. SICKLEDEX, Streck, Omaha, Nebraska) can detect Hgb abnormalities, but cannot differentiate between the carrier trait and homozygous disease states
  - Blood smear shows ***target cells, sickle cells and nucleated RBCs***[Q]
  - X-rays may show
    - ❑ *'**Fish-mouth**[Q]' vertebrae* OR *'**H shaped**[Q]' vertebrae*
    - ❑ ***Bone infarction = avascular necrosis***[Q] of bony regions with a tenuous blood supply (e.g. femoral head)
    - ❑ ***Periosteal reaction ('bone within bone***[Q]***').***
- *Treatment*:
  - Sickle cell crises are treated with hydration, supplemental oxygen and narcotic pain control
  - *Transfusions, exchange transfusions and hydroxyurea* (to shorten crises or to decrease the number of crises)
  - *Bone marrow transplantation:* Currently reserved for patients with severe disease and multiple complications.
- ***Complications***
  - Chronic anemia, pulmonary HTN, heart failure due to cardiac stresses, vascular insufficiency, renal failure and infections; ***Salmonella***[Q] ***osteomyelitis*** (***MC cause of osteomyelitis*** *in sickle cell patients*)
  - An ***aplastic crisis***[Q] may follow ***parvovirus B19***[Q] infection
  - Acute chest syndrome is severe chest pain due to pneumonia, embolization or pulmonary infarction and requires pain control and respiratory support
  - ***Autosplenectomy***[Q], stroke, osteonecrosis of the femoral or humeral head and multiorgan ischemia may result from vascular occlusion
  - Increased risk of infection by encapsulated organisms (e.g. *Streptococcus pneumoniae, Haemophilus influenzae, Neisseria meningitides, Klebsiella*) – keep *pneumococcal vaccinaction up to date.*
  - *Renal papillary necrosis*[Q] ***(Focal Segmental Glomerulosclerosis***[Q]***)*** occurs.
- Prognosis: Despite the multiple potential complications, survival at 18 years of age is 86%.

COMED-K 2014

COMED-K 2014 QUESTIONS

1. **Surgically used suture material—polydioxanone (PDS)**
   (a) Is nonabsorbable and remains encapsulated
   (b) Undergoes hydrolysis and complete absorption
   (c) Undergoes phagocytosis and enzymatic degradation
   (d) Is specifically used for heart valves or synthetic grafts

2. **Most common cause of abortion is**
   (a) Infection
   (b) Luteal phase defect
   (c) Immunological cause
   (d) Defective embryo

3. **Crackles are frequently heard in which of the following conditions?**
   (a) Pneumothorax
   (b) Pleural effusion
   (c) Bronchial asthma
   (d) Bronchiolitis

4. **Subepidermal blisters with granular deposits of Ig A selectively localized to the tips of dermal papillae is a feature of**
   (a) Dermatitis herpetiformis
   (b) Pemphigus vulgaris
   (c) Lichen planus
   (d) Psoriasis vulgaris

5. **Which of the following drugs causes an uncontrollable tendency to fall asleep at inappropriate time?**
   (a) Pramipexole
   (b) Methylphenidate
   (c) Dipyridamole
   (d) Memantine

6. **The following nerves invaginate the lateral dural wall of the cavernous sinus *EXCEPT***
   (a) Oculomotor nerve
   (b) Trochlear nerve
   (c) Abducens nerve
   (d) Ophthalmic nerve

7. **Inherited defect in the extracellular glycoprotein called fibrillin-1 results in which disease?**
   (a) Hereditary spherocytosis
   (b) Marfan syndrome
   (c) Cystic fibrosis
   (d) Duchenne muscular dystrophy

8. **'Tyre' sign is seen in**
   (a) Anal abuse
   (b) Bite mark
   (c) Buccal coitus
   (d) Vulvovaginal abuse

9. **The action of superior oblique muscle is**
   (a) Depressing the globe when the eye is abducted
   (b) Elevating the globe when the eye is adducted
   (c) Depressing the globe when the eye is adducted
   (d) Elevating the globe when the eye is abducted

10. **WHO definition of anemia complicating pregnancy is when the hemoglobin level is less than**
    (a) 10 g/dL
    (b) 11 g/dL
    (c) 12 g/dL
    (d) 14 g/dL

11. **Which of the following beta adrenergic agonists is a drug of abuse in sports as it has effects similar to anabolic steroids in muscles?**
    (a) Clenbuterol
    (b) Prenalterol
    (c) Colterol
    (d) Albuterol

12. **Which of the following drugs results in thrombocytopenia due to drug-antibody reaction?**
    (a) Aspirin
    (b) Quinine
    (c) Metronidazole
    (d) Artesunate

13. **Bone infarcts are seen in**
    (a) Iron deficiency anemia
    (b) Thalassemia
    (c) Sickle cell anemia
    (d) Hereditary spherocytosis

14. **Parafollicular cells (C-cells) in the thyroid are derived from**
    (a) Neural crest
    (b) Ultimobranchial body
    (c) Median bud of pharynx
    (d) Pharyngeal pouch

15. Mesangial deposits of IgA in renal glomeruli is a feature of
(a) Henoch-Schönlein purpura
(b) Membranoproliferative glomerulonephritis
(c) Lipoid nephrosis
(d) Alport syndrome

16. Horner's syndrome is characterized by all *EXCEPT*
(a) Ptosis
(b) Marcus Gunn pupil
(c) Anhydrosis
(d) Sympathetic lesion

17. The widest transverse diameter of the fetal skull is
(a) Biparietal diameter
(b) Bitemporal diameter
(c) Suboccipitobregmatic diameter
(d) Occipitofrontal diameter

18. Which of the following prosthesis is usually used without bone cement?
(a) Charnley's prosthesis
(b) Muller's total hip prosthesis
(c) Total knee prosthesis
(d) Austin Moore's prosthesis

19. Glaucoma should be suspected if the asymmetry in the cup-disk ratio between the two eyes is more than
(a) 0.1
(b) 0.2
(c) 0.3
(d) 0.4

20. Peritoneal dissemination of gastric cancer is best detected by
(a) Abdominal ultrasound
(b) Laparoscopy
(c) Computerized tomography
(d) Magnetic resonance imaging

21. Commonest cause of chest pain in pregnancy is
(a) Angina pectoris
(b) Musculoskeletal pain
(c) Gastritis
(d) Pleurisy

22. Which of the following is NOT increased during isometric exercise?
(a) Respiratory rate
(b) Heart rate
(c) Stroke volume
(d) Total peripheral resistance

23. Which of the following marker would be positive in both pre-B and pre-T lymphoblastic lymphomas?
(a) Terminal deoxynucleotidyl transferase
(b) CD 20
(c) Cyclin Dl
(d) Non-specific esterase

24. Characteristic endoscopic appearance of aphthous ulcer, skip lesions and anal sparing occurs in
(a) Ulcerative colitis
(b) Crohn's disease
(c) Tuberculous colitis
(d) Irritable bowel syndrome

25. Darling's disease is
(a) Chromoblastomycosis
(b) Sporotrichosis
(c) Cryptococcosis
(d) Histoplasmosis

26. Which one of the following is not a measure of dispersion?
(a) Range
(b) Mean deviation
(c) Median
(d) Standard deviation

27. A 60-year-old male, a known case of ischemic heart disease with chronic atrial fibrillation, complains of pain in the right foot since 1 day. The pain began suddenly, is continuous and made worse by lying down or elevation of the foot. The patient says that since the last few hours, he has been getting a tingling and numbness sensation in the foot. The most likely diagnosis in this patient is
(a) Deep vein thrombosis
(b) Acute nerve root compression
(c) Acute arterial occlusion
(d) Raynaud's syndrome

28. Argon laser trabeculoplasty is done in
(a) Open angle glaucoma
(b) Secondary glaucoma
(c) Angle-recession glaucoma
(d) Angle-closure glaucoma

29. In the 'Dugas' clinical test the patient is unable to
(a) Touch the opposite shoulder
(b) Abduct the shoulder
(c) Flex his elbow
(d) Supinate his forearm

30. As per the National Immunization Program, recommended diluent used for reconstitution of Japanese encephalitis vaccine is
(a) Normal saline
(b) Double distilled water
(c) Phosphate buffer solution
(d) Sucrose solution

31. Laser iridotomy is done in
(a) Open angle glaucoma
(b) Angle-closure glaucoma
(c) Iridocyclitis
(d) Posterior capsular opacification

32. Which one of the following is used as an irrigation solution during transurethral resection of the prostate?
(a) 1.5% glycine
(b) Physiological saline
(c) Ringer's lactate
(d) 5% dextrose

33. Erythromelalgia is associated with all of the following *EXCEPT*
(a) Gout
(b) Diabetes
(c) Amyloidosis
(d) Hypertension

34. A 32-year-old man with pelvic fracture is in urinary retention with blood at the external urinary meatus. Retrograde urethrogram shows prostatomembranous disruption. The most appropriate immediate treatment is
(a) Urethral catheterization
(b) Exploration and repair of urethra
(c) Suprapubic cystostomy
(d) Perineal urethrostomy

35. As per National Immunization Program, route of administration of BCG vaccine is
(a) Subcutaneous
(b) Intramuscular
(c) Oral
(d) Intradermal

36. National Rural Health Mission was launched in the year
(a) 2003
(b) 2005
(c) 2007
(d) 2010

37. Expressed breast milk can be stored at room temperature for
(a) Less than 2 hours
(b) 2–3 hours
(c) 4–5 hours
(d) 6–8 hours

38. In magnetic resonance imaging, paramagnetic substances cause
(a) Shortening of both T1 and T2 relaxation times
(b) Shortening of T2 relaxation times only
(c) Shortening of T1 relaxation times only
(d) No effect on both T1 and T2 relaxation times

39. Definition of critical limb ischemia includes
(a) Rest/Night pain
(b) Ankle blood pressure > 50 mm Hg
(c) Intermittent claudication
(d) Well-preserved tissues

40. Bovine cough is characteristic of
(a) Acute epiglottitis
(b) Tracheitis
(c) Laryngeal paralysis
(d) Chronic laryngitis

41. In normal pregnancy, amniotic fluid volume is maximum at
(a) 28 weeks
(b) 32 weeks
(c) 36 weeks
(d) 38 weeks

42. In an act of tribadism, the active partner is known as
(a) Bugger
(b) Butch
(c) Catamite
(d) Femme

43. Concentration of the dissolved gas in solution is given by
(a) Henry's law
(b) Dalton's law
(c) Boyle's law
(d) Ideal gas equation

44. Which of the following predisposes for adenocarcinoma of esophagus?
(a) Tylosispalmaris
(b) Plummer-Vinson syndrome
(c) Barrett's esophagus
(d) Alcohol

45. How long will *Treponema pallidum* survive in blood stored under ordinary refrigeration?
(a) Few hours
(b) 1 week
(c) 3 days
(d) Several years

46. Iliac 'horns' are seen in which of the following disorder?
(a) Achondroplasia
(b) Mucopolysaccharidosis
(c) Nail-Patella syndrome
(d) Down syndrome

47. What is the alveolar ventilation for person with vital capacity 500 mL, respiratory rate 14/min, tidal volume 500 mL and dead space 150 mL?
(a) 2,500 mL
(b) 3,500 mL
(c) 4,900 mL
(d) 6,000 mL

48. Unfavorable prognostic findings in a patient with non-small cell carcinoma include all of the following *EXCEPT*
(a) Pulmonary osteoarthropathy
(b) Chest wall invasion
(c) Adenocarcinoma cell type
(d) Hoarseness

49. Function of Golgi apparatus is
(a) Synthesis of protein
(b) Maturation of protein
(c) Degradation of protein
(d) Sequencing of protein

50. Which of the following vitamins contain sulfur in its structure?
(a) Thiamine
(b) Riboflavin
(c) Folic acid
(d) Niacin

51. Immunoglobulin acting as opsonin belong to the class
(a) IgG
(b) IgM
(c) IgD
(d) IgE

52. All of the following statements regarding niacin-induced flushing and pruritus are true *EXCEPT*
(a) Occurs due to release of prostaglandins by niacin
(b) More likely to occur if taken with ethanol containing beverages
(c) Warrants stoppage of niacin immediately
(d) Aspirin alleviates flushing in most patients

53. The microscopic feature that differentiates a follicular carcinoma from a follicular adenoma of thyroid is
(a) Nuclear pleomorphism
(b) Hurthle cell change
(c) Capsular invasion
(d) Absence of colloid

54. In which of the following conditions does the liver biopsy show presence of pigments composed of polymers of epinephrine?
(a) Crigler-Najjar syndrome
(b) Dubin-Johnson syndrome
(c) Alpha-1 antitrypsin deficiency
(d) Hemochromatosis

55. Executive magistrate are appointed by
(a) Central Government
(b) High Court
(c) State Government
(d) Supreme Court

56. Pott's puffy tumor refers to
(a) Osteomyelitis of the frontal bone
(b) Tuberculosis of the spine
(c) Actinomycosis of maxilla
(d) Odontogenic tumor of the jaw

57. The investigation of choice to detect gastrinoma less than 5 mm size is
(a) Endoscopic ultrasound
(b) Octreotide scan
(c) CT scan
(d) Portal venous sampling

58. Depression of consciousness level in hypothermia starts when the core body temperature falls below
(a) 35ºC
(b) 34ºC
(c) 33ºC
(d) 32ºC

59. The triad of diabetes, gallstones and steatorrhea is associated with
(a) Gastrinoma
(b) Somatostatinoma
(c) VIPoma
(d) Glucagonoma

60. **Picket fence type of fever with otalgia and ear discharge is seen in**
   (a) Suppurative labyrinthitis
   (b) Gradenigo's syndrome
   (c) Subdural abscess
   (d) Lateral sinus thrombophlebitis

61. **Renal papillary necrosis is seen in**
   (a) Sickle cell disease
   (b) Gouty nephropathy
   (c) Chronic glomerulonephritis
   (d) Tumor necrosis syndrome

62. **Local anesthetic agent with vasodilation property is**
   (a) Cocaine
   (b) Lidocaine
   (c) Mepivacaine
   (d) Prilocaine

63. **'Soiling index' is used to monitor**
   (a) Water pollution
   (b) Air pollution
   (c) Noise pollution
   (d) Chlorine levels in drinking water

64. **In India, legal blindness is defined as**
   (a) Best corrected visual acuity less than 3/60 in the better eye
   (b) Best corrected visual acuity less than 4/60 in the better eye
   (c) Best corrected visual acuity less than 5/60 in the better eye
   (d) Best corrected visual acuity less than 6/60 in the better eye

65. **Albright's syndrome includes all *EXCEPT***
   (a) Polyostotic fibrous dysplasia
   (b) Precocious puberty in girls
   (c) Patchy pigmentation
   (d) Pseudohypoparathyroidism

66. **Estimated HIV prevalence among adult population in India is**
   (a) 0.97%
   (b) 0.27%
   (c) 2.7%
   (d) 4.5%

67. **A bone bruise or contusion is best identified in the acute stage using**
   (a) Conventional X-rays
   (b) CT scans
   (c) MRI scans
   (d) PET scans

68. **Which dermatophyte affects skin and nails but not hair?**
   (a) *Epidermophyton floccosum*
   (b) *Trichophyton rubrum*
   (c) *Microsporum audouinii*
   (d) *Malassezia furfur*

69. **Which of the following nerves innervate a dermatome that does NOT lie superficial to its myotome?**
   (a) Musculocutaneous nerve
   (b) Axillary nerve
   (c) Radial nerve
   (d) Ulnar nerve

70. **Most common ligament injured around the ankle joint is**
   (a) Anterior talofibular
   (b) Posterior talofibular
   (c) Deltoid ligament
   (d) Spring ligament

71. **Grid laser photocoagulation is indicated in**
   (a) Ischemic maculopathy
   (b) Clinically significant macular edema
   (c) Macular hole
   (d) Proliferative diabetic retinopathy

72. **Gastrointestinal stromal tumor (GIST) occur from mutation of**
   (a) c-KIT oncogene
   (b) c-MYC oncogene
   (c) c-RAS oncogene
   (d) c-RET oncogene

73. **de Quervain's thyroiditis is characterized by**
   (a) Mononuclear cell infiltration
   (b) Histiocytic reaction
   (c) Giant cell infiltration
   (d) Eosinophilia

74. **The narrowest part of the ureter is at the**
   (a) Pelviureteric junction
   (b) Pelvic brim
   (c) Site it crosses common iliac artery
   (d) Vesicoureteric junction

75. **Selective medium used to isolate *Campylobacter jejuni* is**
   (a) Fletcher's medium
   (b) Skirrow's medium
   (c) Buffered charcoal yeast extract agar (BCYE)
   (d) Stuart's medium

76. Which of the following joint findings is most suggestive of an inflammatory rather than an osteo cause of joint pain?
(a) Painful range of motion
(b) Crepitus
(c) Bony articular enlargement
(d) Morning stiffness

77. Waldenstrom's macroglobulinemia is characterized by all *EXCEPT*
(a) IgE-secreting clone of plasma cells
(b) Hyperviscosity symptoms
(c) Hepatosplenomegaly
(d) Lymphadenopathy

78. In long-treated lepromatous patients, site from where bacilli are most frequently detected is
(a) Nasal mucosa
(b) Ear lobe
(c) Dorsum of fingers
(d) Skin lesion

79. Most common manifestation of cardiac lupus is
(a) Pericarditis
(b) Myocarditis
(c) Libman-Sacks endocarditis
(d) Aortic regurgitation

80. Mainstay of treatment for primary dysmenorrhea is
(a) Non-steroidal anti-inflammatory drugs
(b) Dicyclomine
(c) Hyoscine
(d) Paracetamol

81. The most common type of tracheoesophageal anomaly is
(a) Esophageal atresia with fistula to the distal esophagus
(b) Esophageal atresia without fistula
(c) Esophageal atresia with fistula to the proximal esophagus
(d) H-type fistula without esophageal atresia

82. Which of the following is an indication for renal biopsy in a child with nephrotic syndrome?
(a) Age at onset 2–6 years
(b) Low blood C3 levels
(c) High selective proteinuria
(d) Serum albumin less than 1 g/dL

83. Tennis elbow is caused due to inflammation of
(a) Common extensor origin
(b) Common flexor origin
(c) Brachioradialis
(d) Biceps muscle

84. In South India, important vector implicated in transmission of Japanese encephalitis is
(a) *Anopheles stephensi*
(b) *Culex vishnui*
(c) *Aedes aegypti*
(d) *Mansonia uniformis*

85. The millet rich in calcium is
(a) Rice
(b) Ragi
(c) Jowar
(d) Bajra

86. Posterior staphyloma occurs in
(a) Absolute glaucoma
(b) Perforated corneal ulcer
(c) Scleritis
(d) High myopia

87. Activation of which receptor causes pulmonary vasoconstriction?
(a) Alpha-2 adrenergic
(b) H2 histaminic
(c) M3 cholinergic
(d) ETA epithelial receptor

88. The ideal age of treatment of undescended testis is
(a) At birth
(b) From 1½ to 2 years of age
(c) From 5 to 10 years of age
(d) Above 15 years of age

89. 'Aortic nipple' in chest radiograph is formed by
(a) Arch of aorta
(b) Pulmonary trunk
(c) Left atrium
(d) Superior intercostal vein

90. In conditions of iron deficiency, which one of these parameters is increased?
(a) Serum iron
(b) Plasma transferrin
(c) Serum ferritin
(d) Blood hemoglobin

91. Which of the following antibiotics inhibit the action of antidiuretic hormone and used in the treatment of inappropriate secretion of antidiuretic hormone?
(a) Erythromycin
(b) Demeclocycline
(c) Tigecycline
(d) Doxycycline

92. The species of nontuberculous mycobacteria known to produce a toxin is
(a) *Mycobacterium vaccae*
(b) *Mycobacterium haemophilum*
(c) *Mycobacterium marinum*
(d) *Mycobacterium ulcerans*

93. With reference to neoplasia, the term 'tumor progression' means
(a) Spread of cancer to distant sites
(b) Rate of growth of tumors
(c) Ability of cancer cells to resemble their normal counterpart
(d) Sequential appearance of features of increasing malignancy

94. To term it as chronic rhinosinusitis, the symptoms should last for more than
(a) 4 weeks
(b) 6 weeks
(c) 12 weeks
(d) 24 weeks

95. HLA-B27 histocompatibility is correlated with
(a) Ankylosing spondylitis
(b) Scleroderma
(c) Felty's syndrome
(d) Sjögren's syndrome

96. The hallmarks of type Ia glycogen storage disease are all of the following *EXCEPT*
(a) Hypoglycemia
(b) Metabolic alkalosis
(c) Hyperuricemia
(d) Hyperlipidemia

97. All of the following skeletal muscle relaxants are metabolized by plasma cholinesterase *EXCEPT*
(a) Succinylcholine
(b) Atracurium
(c) Mivacurium
(d) Doxacurium

98. Absolute contraindications to pertussis vaccine includes all of the following *EXCEPT*
(a) Static neurological disease
(b) Progressive neurological disease
(c) Anaphylaxis after previous dose
(d) Encephalopathy within 7 days of previous dose

99. Which one of the following is not a high-risk group regarding transmission of HIV in India?
(a) Female sex workers
(b) Men who lives with men
(c) Injection drug users
(d) Pregnant women

100. First cell to migrate into a wound due to chemotaxis to start the process of wound healing is
(a) Lymphocyte
(b) Macrophage
(c) Platelet
(d) Neutrophil

101. The following are the therapeutic use of carbon dioxide gas *EXCEPT*
(a) For insufflation during abdominal laparoscopic surgeries
(b) To debubble cardiopulmonary bypass circuits
(c) To treat hypocarbia with respiratory alkalosis
(d) To flood the surgical field during cardiac surgeries

102. Anterior fontanel of neonate ossifies
(a) At birth
(b) At 6 months of age
(c) At 1 year of age
(d) At 18 months of age

103. Which of the following tests is most useful in the diagnosis of allergic rhinitis?
(a) Peripheral blood smear
(b) Measurement of specific serum anti-IgE
(c) Absolute eosinophil count in blood
(d) Eosinophil count in nasal secretions

104. All of the following diseases are transmitted by mosquito vectors *EXCEPT*
(a) West Nile fever
(b) Brugian filariasis
(c) Babesiosis
(d) Rift valley fever

105. Zymogen activation by partial proteolysis is an example of
(a) Allosteric modification
(b) Enzyme induction
(c) Enzyme repression
(d) Covalent modification

106. The method of choice for termination of pregnancy between 7 and 12 weeks is
(a) Mifepristone and misoprostol
(b) Dilatation and curettage
(c) Suction evacuation
(d) Menstrual regulation

107. All of the following are negative symptoms of schizophrenia *EXCEPT*
(a) Apathy
(b) Alogia
(c) Affective flattening
(d) Akathisia

108. Occupational disease caused by inhalation of sugarcane dust is
(a) Byssinosis
(b) Anthracosis
(c) Bagassosis
(d) Farmer's lung

109. The most sensitive among the following tests for diagnosis of malaria is
(a) Thin peripheral blood smear
(b) Quantitative buffy coat test
(c) PfHRP2 antigen
(d) Pan plasmodial LDH

110. Total electrical alternans in ECG along with sinus tachycardia is a specific sign of
(a) Left ventricular failure
(b) Cardiac tamponade
(c) Wet beriberi
(d) Hypertrophic cardiomyopathy

111. A 15-year-old girl with history of epistaxis has normal platelet count, but prolonged bleeding Ti prolonged activated partial thromboplastin time (APTT). She is likely to be suffering from
(a) Idiopathic thrombocytopenic purpura
(b) Hemophilia A
(c) von Willebrand disease
(d) Glanzmann thrombasthenia

112. Under Revised National Tuberculosis Control Program, drug used for chemoprophylaxis childhood contacts is
(a) Rifampicin
(b) Isoniazid
(c) Ethambutol
(d) Ciprofloxacin

113. Which of the following is considered as a marker for epididymal function?
(a) Fructose
(b) Testosterone
(c) Acid phosphatase
(d) Carnitine

114. Which of the following drugs inhibit the entry of human immunodeficiency virus (HIV)
(a) Enfuvirtide
(b) Efavirenz
(c) Etravirine
(d) Emtricitabine

115. Which one of the following statements about Km value is TRUE?
(a) Km is substrate concentration at maximal velocity
(b) Numerical value of Km is proportional to affinity of enzyme for substrate
(c) Km is independent of enzyme concentration
(d) Km denotes that 100% of enzyme molecules are bound with substrate molecules at that concentration

116. A child whose BMI lies in the 84th percentile for age is considered to be
(a) Overweight
(b) Obese
(c) Normal
(d) Undernourished

117. Which of the following is the criterion used for defining early gastric cancer?
(a) Size of the lesion
(b) Nodal involvement
(c) Depth of invasion
(d) Location in the stomach

118. A person falsely perceives that his close friend has been replaced by an exact double. This phenomenon is referred to as
(a) Cotard's syndrome
(b) Fregoli syndrome
(c) Capgras syndrome
(d) Delusional percept

119. In death due to criminal abortion with clostridial septicemia, the characteristic color of the skin is
(a) Bluish black
(b) Bronze
(c) Greenish
(d) Pinkish

120. The earliest antibody marker to appear in the serum in hepatitis B virus infection is
(a) Anti-HBs
(b) Anti-HBe
(c) Anti-HBc
(d) Anti-HBx

121. When the plasma glucose concentration falls to low levels, a number of difference hormones help combat the hypoglycemia. After intravenous administration

of a large dose of insulin, the return from hypoglycemia to normal glucose level is delayed in
(a) Adrenal medullary insufficiency
(b) Glucagon deficiency
(c) Combined adrenal medullary insufficiency and glucagon deficiency
(d) Thyrotoxicosis

122. All of the following are derivatives of neural crest *EXCEPT*
(a) Melanocytes
(b) Astrocytes
(c) Schwann cells
(d) Meninges

123. During childbirth, a woman suffers a serious hemorrhage and goes into shock. After she recovers, she displays symptoms of hypopituitarism. Which of the following will not be expected in this patient?
(a) Cachexia
(b) Infertility
(c) Pallor
(d) Low basal metabolic rate

124. Which of the following stains is used to demonstrate yeast forms of cryptococci in tissue sections?
(a) Mucicarmine
(b) Perl's
(c) Sudan black
(d) Fontana-Masson

125. All *EXCEPT* one characterizes focal segmental glomerulosclerosis
(a) Represents up to one third of cases of nephritic syndrome in adults
(b) The pathological features are most prominent in the renal cortex
(c) ACE inhibitors are useful to control proteinuria
(d) Overall prognosis worse than minimal change nephropathy

126. The hypothesis 'greater is the lipid solubility of the compound in olive oil, the greater is its anesthetic potency' is referred to as
(a) Meyer-Overton rule
(b) Pressure reversal rule
(c) Critical volume hypothesis
(d) Lipid bilayer expansion hypothesis

127. Which of the following is NOT an example of serotonin noradrenaline reuptake inhibitor?
(a) Sertraline
(b) Venlafaxine
(c) Duloxetine
(d) Milnacipran

128. Which one of the following is a cohort study?
(a) North Karelia project
(b) Stanford three community study
(c) MRFIT study
(d) Framingham Heart Study

129. Patient with 1.2 cm breast lump with three lymph nodes in the axilla with no metastasis is in which stage as per AJCC?
(a) T1N0M0
(b) T1bN1bM0
(c) T1cN1bM0
(d) T2N1cM0

130. Factors that increase risk of recurrence of febrile seizures include all *EXCEPT*
(a) Initial seizure at less than 12 months of age
(b) Positive family history
(c) Temperature more than 40°C
(d) Complex seizures

131. A 60-year-old male complains of tremors in his hands for the past 6 months. He does not smoke cigarettes, but drinks 6 beers daily. Physical examination reveals normal vital signs, diminished facial expression, a stooped posture, shuffling gait with short rapid steps and a 'pill rolling' tremor in both hands. Morphological changes in his brain will include
(a) Pallor and atrophy of the substantia nigra
(b) Marked atrophy of the caudate and putamen
(c) Frontotemporal atrophy of the cerebral cortex with enlarged ventricles
(d) Butterfly-shaped hemorrhagic mass extending across the corpus callosum

For questions 132 to 135

Q. A 33-year-old woman presented with a 4-day history of fever and abdominal pain, 7 days after undergoing a cesarean section. She had diffuse erythroderma and the blood pressure was 85/48 mm Hg. A workup revealed elevated creatinine and liver-enzyme levels. Her condition worsened over the next day, with acute respiratory distress; subsequently, desquamation of her hands occurred.

132. The patient is diagnosed to have
(a) Kwashiorkor
(b) Pseudoporphyria
(c) Toxic epidermal necrolysis
(d) Toxic shock syndrome

133. The condition is due to
(a) *Staphylococcus aureus*
(b) *Streptococcus pyogenes*
(c) Human papilloma virus
(d) Severe fungal infection

134. The treatment of the above condition
(a) Floxacillin
(b) Tetracycline
(c) Amphotericin B
(d) Antiviral acyclovir

135. A specimen of _______________ culture would be informative
(a) Vaginal swab
(b) From desquamated area
(c) Blood
(d) Wound of LSCS

From questions 136 and 137

Q. An 85-year-old male cigar smoker with no notable medical history presented with black discoloration and hairy appearance of the tongue, which had lasted several years. He said he did not use bismuth-containing compounds.

136. Cause for this lesion in the tongue is due to
(a) Aspergillosis
(b) Adrenal insufficiency
(c) Pellagra
(d) Lingua villosa nigra

137. This condition could be treated with all of the following *EXCEPT*
(a) Topical antibiotics
(b) Discounting smoking
(c) Application of 40% urea
(d) Applying topical retinoids

For questions 138 to 140

Q. A 55-year-old man presented with a two-day history of headache, fever and generalized weakness. He had received a cadaveric kidney transplant 5 years earlier. His medications included 5 mg of tacrolimus twice a day and 10 mg of prednisone daily. On neurologic examination, he was confused and incoherent. Cranial nerves were normal, but he had a hazy left retina. Magnetic resonance imaging of the brain with the administration of gadolinium showed multiple-enhancing lesion in both cerebral hemispheres.

138. The most probable diagnosis is
(a) Cerebral toxoplasmosis
(b) *Listeria monocytogenes* infection
(c) *Nocardia asteroides* infection
(d) Miliary tuberculosis

139. Patient had subretinal abscess, the aspirate was stained, the findings are likely to be
(a) Weakly positive acid-fast bacilli
(b) Gram-positive cocci
(c) Gram-negative cocci
(d) Coccobacillus

140. The treatment of choice in this condition is
(a) Trimethoprim-sulfamethoxazole
(b) Penicillin long acting
(c) Antitubercular therapy
(d) Steroids

For questions 141 to 143

Q. A 47-year-old woman was referred for bone pain and abnormal findings on radiography. The patient reported that for the past 17 years, she has habitually consumed water from that area. She reported a 5-year history of pain in the lower back, arms, legs and hips. Because of brittleness, all her teeth had been extracted. Radiography of the forearm revealed interosseous membrane calcification and radiography of the spine revealed a rugger-jersey appearance (striated pattern of increased density in the upper and lower zones of the vertebrae).

141. The probable diagnosis is
(a) Silicosis
(b) Fluorosis
(c) Vitamin D toxicity
(d) Hypercalcinosis

142. The condition can be treated with
(a) Supplementation of vitamin D
(b) Change in source of water
(c) Good-balanced diet
(d) Calcium chelation

143. This patient is likely to have
(a) Vitamin B deficiency
(b) Vitamin D toxicity
(c) Associated cardiac problems
(d) Renal damage

For questions 144 and 145

Q. A 65-year-old man presented with skin lesions on his chest and left arm and shoulder 6 weeks after returning from a vacation in Belize at the beach in

the rain forest. The lesions occasionally stung, drained a dark exudates, and enlarged despite 2 weeks of treatment with cephalexin. The patient had no constitutional symptoms. Physical examination revealed five nodules of varying sizes with surrounding erythema and a central pore through which a single, moving larva was observed.

144. This condition is caused by
(a) Bot fly
(b) Cutaneous leishmaniasis
(c) Tungiasis
(d) Onchocerciasis

145. The larvae coming out of the pores are
(a) *Dermatobia hominis*
(b) *Diphyllobothrium latum*
(c) *Loa loa*
(d) *Dracunculus medinensis*

For Questions 146 and 147

Q. A 40-year-old male complains of a vague dragging sensation in his abdomen for the last 6 months. There was no history of fever, renal colic or dysuria. Physical examination reveals a blood pressure at 150/96 mm Hg.

Renal ultrasound: Bilaterally enlarged kidneys with multiple cysts
Urine analysis: Protein +
WBCs 4/HPF (normal: < 5/HPF)
RBCs 10/HPF (normal: < 5/HPF)

146. He should be mentioned for the existence/development of
(a) Intracranial aneurysms
(b) Hyperthyroidism
(c) Hemolytic uremic syndrome
(d) Abdominal aortic aneurysm

147. The renal pathology was a result of
(a) Nephrolithiasis
(b) Enlarged prostate
(c) Ischemia to the renal medulla
(d) Deposition of immune complexes in the glomeruli

148. A 30-year-old homosexual male presented with a 1 week history of painful vesicular perianal lesions. There was an associated history of body aches, fever and joint pains. He claimed that his partner had similar lesion on his penis about 1 month ago with associated dysuria, which has resolved now. The microscopy of the lesion revealed multinucleated syncytial cells with intranuclear inclusion bodies and perinuclear halo. The most likely causative agent for these lesions is
(a) Herpes simplex virus
(b) Cytomegalovirus
(c) Epstein-barr virus
(d) Human immunodeficiency virus

149. A 45-year-old male is brought to the ER in an unconscious state. The wife informs the attending physician that he had complained of palpitations, tremors and dizziness prior to his recent presentation. Physical examination reveals excessive sweating of the extremities, RR-28/min and PR-110/min, rapid and bounding pulse. He made a significant improvement with administration of dextrose infusion. His condition is most likely related to a pathology in the
(a) Adrenal medulla
(b) Adrenal cortex
(c) Thyroid gland
(d) Pancreas

150. A 75-year-old man presented with complaints of progressive difficulty initiating urination, burning sensation while passing urine and terminal dribbling over the past 2 months. There was no history of weight loss. Digital rectal examination revealed a smooth and enlarged prostate, which was firm in consistency. Based on the pathogenesis of his condition, the likely target for therapy would be
(a) 14 hydroxylase
(b) Prostate specific antigen (PSA)
(c) 5-alpha-reductase
(d) Acid phosphatase

151. A 60-year-old female presented to the clinic with a history of vague lower abdominal pain and irregular vaginal bleeding for the past 3 months. She had an episode of hemoptysis 2 days ago. Physical examination revealed a thin female with a pulse rate of 140 beats per minute. Abdominal sonography showed an irregular mass in the left ovary. The uterus was normal. A chest X-ray showed multiple cannon ball-shaped lesions in both lung fields. Laboratory investigations were as follows:
Hb: 10 mg/dL (12–15 mg/dL)
Beta-hCG: Very high
The diagnosis is most likely
(a) Gestational choriocarcinoma
(b) Ovarian choriocarcinoma
(c) Partial mole
(d) Complete mole

152. A 31-year-old pregnant women at 29 weeks of gestation presents at the ER with complaints of headache and swelling of the legs of 2 days duration. Her last 3 antenatal visits had been uneventful. Physical examination reveals pitting edema of the

lower extremities, BP – 150/90 mm Hg and PR – 90/min. Which of the following investigations will be most helpful in the diagnosis of her condition?
(a) Blood culture
(b) Urinalysis
(c) Fasting blood sugar
(d) Bone marrow aspirate

For questions 153 and 154

Q. A 35-year-old male with a history of severe bronchial asthma for several months now complains of weight gain and the development of purple stretch marks. Physical examination showed BP – 149/95 mm Hg, supraclavicular fullness. The skin was thinned out with areas of bruising. Neurological examination revealed decreased strength in the proximal muscles. Laboratory investigation showed reduced serum cortisol and reduced plasma ACTH.

153. An electrolyte workup in this patient will most likely reveal
(a) Hyponatremia
(b) Hypomagnesemia
(c) Hypokalemia
(d) Hypercalcemia

154. His condition is most likely due to a/an
(a) Pituitary tumor
(b) Tumor of the adrenal cortex
(c) Iatrogenic cause
(d) Lung cancer

155. A 30-year-old female who underwent surgery for follicular carcinoma of the thyroid 4 months earlier now presents with muscle twitching, which began 2 weeks ago. Physical examination reveals no lymphadenopathy or palpable mass in the previous location of her thyroid. Tapping the facial nerve produces spasm of the facial muscles, laboratory studies show:
Serum Ca^{2+}: 7.3 mg /dL (N: 8.4–10.2 mg/dL)
Phosphate: 2.2 mmol/L (N: 0.8–1.4 mmol/L)
These features are best explained by
(a) Vitamin D deficiency
(b) Absence of parathyroid glands
(c) Gastrointestinal loss of calcium
(d) Autoimmune disease

156. A 32-year-old male with suspected neurofibromatosis was found to have a blood pressure of 178/110 mm Hg at a recent health fair. He complained of palpitations and excessive sweating. Today he presents to the clinic for a checkup because he has developed abdominal discomfort. His blood pressure is now recorded to be 130/80 mm Hg. Physical examination reveals multiple tumors of the oral mucosa and skin. Laboratory investigations reveal:
Serum K^+: 3.8 mEq/L (N: 3.5–5.0 mEq/L)
Serum Na^{++}: 136 mEq/L (N: 135–145 mEq/L)
Serum Ca^{2+}: 9.4 mg/dL (N: 8.4–10.2 mg /dL)
Genetic studies in this patient will most likely show
(a) N-myc amplification
(b) Overexpression of C-kit
(c) K-ras mutation
(d) RET oncogene

157. A 32-year-old African-American male presents with recurrent edema of the feet and periorbital swelling. He has a history of high-risk sexual behavior. The blood pressure was 110/85 mm Hg. Results of the laboratory investigations are as follows:
HBsAg: Negative
Blood glucose: Normal
HIV ELISA: Positive
24-hour urine protein: 3.9 g
Urine microscopy: Fatty casts, oval fat bodies
An H and E stain of the renal biopsy is most likely to show
(a) Segmental sclerosis of some of the glomeruli
(b) Diffuse thickening of the glomerular basement membrane
(c) Hypercellular glomeruli with thickening of the GBM
(d) Proliferation of the parietal cells filling of the Bowman's space

158. A 63-year-old male from the Middle East presented with hematuria. The urine showed RBCs, but no RBC casts. BUN level was normal. Cystoscopy revealed an irregular growth on the mucosa of the bladder. A biopsy from this growth revealed features of squamous cell carcinoma. The etiology of this condition is most likely linked to
(a) Cigarette smoking
(b) Infection by human papillomavirus (HPV)
(c) Parasitic infection
(d) Chronic alcohol abuse

159. A 60-year-old male presents to the clinic with complaints of abdominal pain, constipation and loin pain radiating to the groin of over a week duration. He has a 25-pack year smoking history and is currently being evaluated for a hilar mass picked up on chest radiography. As part of this laboratory work up, the serum calcium was found to be elevated. The elevated serum calcium level is most likely linked to
(a) Parathyroid adenoma
(b) Parathyroid hyperplasia
(c) Vitamin D intoxication
(d) Secretion of PTH-related peptide

160. A 45-year-old female had sought medical attention for her recent increase in weight and proximal limb weakness. She was diagnosed with rheumatoid arthritis. 1 week ago has been started on prednisolone tablets. Physical examination revealed truncal obesity; BP – 145/90 mm Hg and PR – 90/min. High levels of cortisol were found in her blood and 24-hour urine sample. A high dose dexamethasone suppression test was performed and the plasma cortisol level was suppressed. Serum ACTH level was high. The etiology of this condition can be confirmed by
(a) CT scan of the chest
(b) MRI of the brain
(c) CT scan of the abdomen
(d) Plasma metanephrine level

For questions 161 to 163

Q. An 87-year-old woman with severe retrosternal pain and intermittent dysphagia was referred to the clinic for further evaluation. She described paroxysms of crampy pain almost exclusively during the intake of solid foods. In the past several months, she noted a weight loss of 5 kg. Endoscopy revealed a pronounced helical configuration of the esophageal lumen. High-resolution manometry of the esophagus showed high-amplitude pressure waves, this patient had normal relaxation of the esophagogastric junction.

161. The most probable diagnosis in this lady would be
(a) Achalasia cardia
(b) Esophageal cancer
(c) Gastroesophageal reflux disease
(d) Nutcracker esophagus

162. The barium meal examination reveals
(a) Parrot beaking of the distal esophagus with proximal dilation
(b) Rat tail deformity of the esophagus
(c) Reflux of the barium
(d) Corkscrew appearance

163. The treatment of this condition
(a) High-dose proton-pump inhibitors
(b) Radical resection with continuity
(c) Treatment with long-acting diltiazem
(d) Balloon dilatation

For questions 164 to 166

Q. A 6-hour-old term male baby was observed to have yellowish discoloration of the skin up to the knee joints. He was born to a 30-year-old woman who had an abortion 2 years ago. The woman said she had an uneventful pregnancy and went for antenatal checkup only once. She came in advanced labor to the emergency ward where the baby was delivered. There was no prolonged rupture of membranes and the baby cried immediately after birth and accepted breast feeds soon after.

164. The most likely cause for jaundice in this baby is likely to be
(a) Physiological jaundice
(b) Rh hemolytic disease
(c) Neonatal sepsis
(d) Torch infection

165. What is the bilirubin value expected from the distribution of jaundice
(a) 6–9 mg/dL
(b) 9–12 mg/dL
(c) 12–15 mg/dL
(d) > 15 mg/dL

166. What should be the immediate treatment?
(a) Start phototherapy
(b) Start IV antibiotics
(c) Give phenobarbital
(d) Keep under warmer

For questions 167 and 168

Q. A 3-year-old female child sleeping in a thatched hut woke up in the middle of the night screaming. Her mother thought the child had a nightmare and tried to pacify her. After sometime she noticed that the child was sweating profusely and the hands were becoming cold. Child also vomited a couple of times. The mother immediately rushed the child to the emergency services. Her pulse was 150/minute and her BP 90/60 mm Hg.

167. This child is likely to have
(a) Snake bite
(b) Septic shock
(c) Food poisoning
(d) Scorpion envenomation

168. The first line of treatment for this condition is
(a) Corticosteroids
(b) Prazosin
(c) Anti-snake venom
(d) IV bolus of normal saline

For questions 169 to 171

Q. An 8-year-old girl was brought to the hospital for puffiness of eyes and swelling of legs of 2 days

duration. Mother said she was passing only small quantities of urine. Her urine was high colored and microscopic examination showed RBC and granular casts.

169. The likely diagnosis of her condition is
(a) Nephrotic syndrome
(b) Acute glomerulonephritis
(c) Hemolytic uremic syndrome
(d) Urinary tract infection

170. If this child develops headache and generalized convulsions the next day what complication she is most likely to have?
(a) Uremic encephalopathy
(b) Hypertensive encephalopathy
(c) Electrolyte imbalance
(d) Meningitis

171. What biochemical abnormality is not a feature of this condition?
(a) Raised ASLO titers
(b) Normal C3 levels
(c) Raised blood urea
(d) Dilutional hyponatremia

For questions 172 to 174

Q. A 3-year-old girl is brought for diarrhea of 2 weeks duration. She weighs 8 kg and her height is 93 cm.

172. Her nutritional status can be described as
(a) Mild malnutrition
(b) Moderate malnutrition
(c) Severe malnutrition
(d) Very severe malnutrition

173. She is lethargic and has cold extremities. Her pulse is 120/m, small volume and BP 70/40 mm Hg. Her axillary temperature is 36°C. Mother says she has no vomiting, but is not eating anything and had passed stools only once from morning. She has also voided urine. What is the most likely cause of her symptoms?
(a) Hypoglycemia
(b) Dehydration
(c) Hypothermia
(d) Hyponatremia

174. What IV fluids should she be given?
(a) Ringer lactate
(b) 10% dextrose
(c) Normal saline
(d) Isolyte P

For questions 175 to 177

Q. A 5-year-old boy was found to have a pansystolic murmur in the left lower sternal border during routine school health checkup. He is asymptomatic and has normal development. His ECHO showed a small muscular ventricular septal defect.

175. What should be the line of management in this child?
(a) Open closure of the defect
(b) Closure of VSD with a patch
(c) No intervention
(d) Indomethacin

176. What type of defect is most likely to undergo spontaneous closure?
(a) Perimembranous
(b) Muscular
(c) Subpulmonic
(d) Supracristal

177. Which cardiac chamber enlarges first in a VSD?
(a) Left ventricle
(b) Left atrium
(c) Right ventricle
(d) Right atrium

For questions 178 to 180

Q. A 3-day-old female baby was brought got oozing of blood from umbilical stump. The mother said she noticed blood-stained discharge from the nose when the baby sneeze. Baby did not have bleeding earlier. She was feeding and passing urine and stools normally. Her sleep was adequate.

178. The most probable diagnosis in this baby is
(a) Hemophilia A
(b) Early hemorrhagic disease of the newborn
(c) Classical hemorrhagic disease of the newborn
(d) Sepsis with disseminated intravascular coagulation

179. How should the baby be managed?
(a) Start IV antibiotics
(b) Give factor VIII concentrates
(c) Give vitamin K
(d) Give plasma transfusion

180. Bleeding in this child is due to deficiency of
(a) Factors II, VII, IX and X
(b) Fibrinogen, platelets and factor V
(c) Factor VIII
(d) Platelets, factors V and VII

COMED-K 2014

ANSWERS AND EXPLANATIONS

AUTHOR'S COMMENTS: The answers for this paper have been verified from the revised answer key from the Comed-website (last accessed on 1st September 2014).

1. **Answer is b (Undergoes hydrolysis and complete absorption).**
   Ref: Bailey and Love, 25th edition Pg 236-239, Table 18.2.

- Author's Comments: "This is a repeat question from *Comed-K 2005*".
- Suture materials absorb in one of two ways:
  - ***Catgut and collagen*** gets absorbed by ***enzymatic digestion***.
  - The other method is one of ***preliminary hydrolysis,*** which is the effect of water on suture materials. Once a suture has been broken up by hydrolysis, *polymorphonuclear cells and other macrophage (giant cells)* ***digest***. This type of suture degradation is seen in ***polydiaxonone*** (PDS).
- PDS is ***NOT*** used *a/w heart valves or synthetic grafts,* or in situations in which prolonged tissue approximation under stress is required.

Also Know

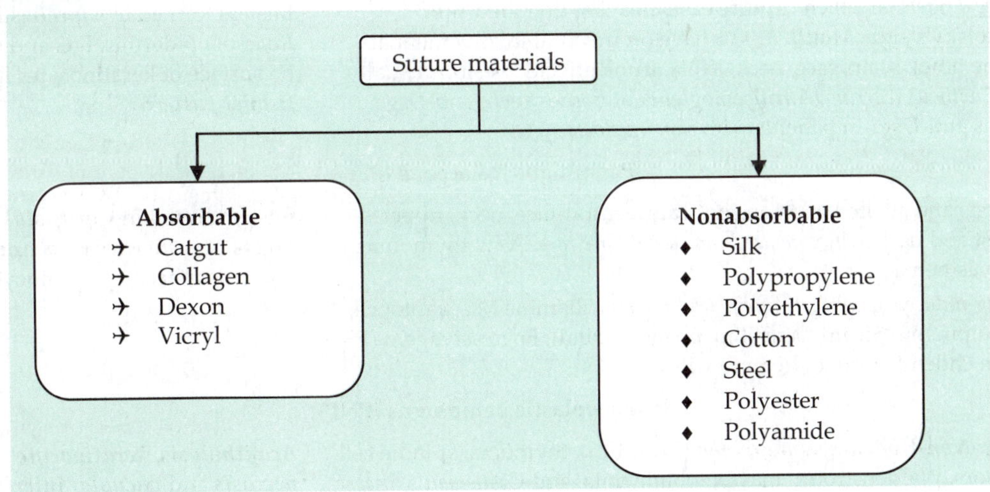

2. **Answer is d (Defective embryo).**
   Ref: Dutta's Obstetrics, 6th edition Pg 160.

- ***Chromosomal abnormalities*** are the ***MC cause of spontaneous abortion*** in the first trimester.
- ***MC chromosmal abnormality*** in spontaneous abortion is ***45,X***.

3. **Answer is d (Bronchiolitis).**
   Ref: MacLeod's Clinical Examination, 12th edition Pg 174.

- Interrupted ***non-musical sounds*** are called *crackles*. Crackles result from peripheral airway collapse on expiration.
- Air rapidly enters these distal airways on inspiration and small bronchi abruptly open producing the crackling noise.

- *Early inspiratory* crackles: Small airway disease such as ***bronchiolitis***
- ***Mid-inspiratory*** crackles: ***Pulmonary edema***
- ***Late inspiratory*** crackles: ***Pulmonary fibrosis*** *(fine)*
- Crackles ***throughout inspiration and expiration*: *Bronchiectasis*.**

4. Answer is a (Dermatitis herpetiformis).
Ref: CMDT 2013, Pg 122.

- **Author's Comments**: "Location of blisters in the blistering skin diseases is an important question in any PG entrance examination, so also the others details of all these diseases; be pucca with the table below".

Clinical features	Histology
Dermatitis herpetiformis	
Extremely itchy small papules and vesicles on ***elbows, knees,*** buttocks and posterior nuchal area (***extensor surfaces***). Almost all patients have an associated, usually ***subclinical, gluten sensitive enteropathy*** (celiac sprue). More than 90% express the ***HLA B8/DRW3*** and HLA DQW2. Treatment is **dapsone**. Strictly *exclude gluten* from the diet; ↑ risk of GI lymphoma	***Subepidermal blister*** with neutrophils in the dermal papillae; antibodies against ***epidermal transglutaminase 3*** *and* ***anti-endomysial antibodies; Granular IgA deposits in dermal papillae*** of perilesional skin observed by direct IF is the ***gold standard*** of diagnosis
Pemphigus vulgaris (PV)	
Flaccid blisters, which rupture easily leaving denuded skin; Nikolsky's sign; ***Mouth*** (~90% have oromucosal involvement at some time), scalp, face, neck, axilla, trunk affected; lesions usually *heal without scarring;* ***Antidesmoglein*** antibodies seen: anti-***Dsg3*** (plus anti-***Dsg1*** in patients with *skin involvement*)	Blisters formed in ***suprabasal layer*** of epidermis. IgG and C3 on surface of keratinocytes in a ***fishnet pattern***
Pemphigus foliaceous (PF)	
Crusts and shallow erosions on scalp, central-face, neck, upper chest and back. *Mucous membrane lesions are rare.* A/w thymoma /myasthenia. *Drug-induced pemphigus resembles PF* (penicillamine MC, captopril, rifampin, piroxicam, penicillin, phenobarbital); Fogo selvagem (FS) is an endemic form of PF in Brazil	Blister formed in ***superficial layers*** of epidermis (***subcorneal***); IgG on surface of keratinocytes
Paraneoplastic pemphigus (PNP)	
A/w ***Non-Hodgkin's lymphoma (MC)***, CLL, thymoma, spindle cell tumors, Waldenstrom's macroglobulinemia, and *Castleman's disease (more common among children)*. PNP maybe a/w ***bronchiolitis obliterans.*** Painful stomatitis and blisters; autoantibodies against cytoplasmic proteins of the ***plakin*** family (e.g. desmoplakins I and II, bullous pemphigoid antigen 1, envoplakin, periplakin, and plectin) and cell-surface proteins of the ***cadherin*** family (e.g. Dsg1 and Dsg3).	***Acantholysis, keratinocyte necrosis*** and ***vacuolar interface dermatitis;*** IgG and C3 on surface of keratinocytes
Bullous pemphigoid (BP)	
Large *tense blisters* on *flexor surfaces*, oromucosal lesions; *linear deposits of IgG and/or C3 in the epidermal BMZ; anti-**BPAG1** and **BPAG2** antibodies*	***Subepidermal*** eosinophil-rich blister; (**BulLOus: BeLOw** epidermis)

Pemphigoid (herpes) gestation	
Pruritic, urticarial plaques, rimmed by vesicles and bullae on the trunk and extremities; anti-BPAG2 antibodies	Teardrop shaped, ***subepidermal blisters*** in dermal papillae; ***eosinophil***-rich infiltrate; linear band of C3 in epidermal BMZ
Cicatricial pemphigoid	
Erosive and/or blistering lesions of mucous membranes and possibly the skin; scarring at some sites; *linear deposits of IgG and/or C3 in the epidermal BMZ; anti-BPAG2 and laminin 332 antibodies*	***Subepidermal blister*** and may or may not be a/w a mononuclear cell-rich infiltrate
Linear IgA disease	
Itchy small papules on extensor surfaces, occasionally larger arciform blisters. Linear band of IgA at BMZ; ***anti-BPAG2*** antibodies	***Subepidermal blister*** with ***neutrophils*** in the dermal papillae.

5. **Answer is a (Pramipexole).**
   Ref: CMDT 2013, Pg 1000.

- ***Pramipexole and ropinirole*** are two newer ***dopamine agonists*** that are not ergot derivatives.
- Adverse effects = *fatigue, somnolence, nausea, peripheral edema, dyskinesias, confusion, and postural hypotension*.
- Rarely, an ***irresistible urge to sleep*** may occur, sometimes ***in inappropriate and hazardous circumstances*** (driving).
- ***Impulse control disorders*** involving ***gambling, shopping, or sexual activity*** have also been reported.

6. **Answer is c (Abducens nerve).**
   Ref: Gray's Basic Anatomy: with STUDENT CONSULT Online Access, 2012 edition, Pg 439.

- Cavernous sinus is a collection of venous sinuses on either side of the pituitary
- Blood from eye and superficial cortex → cavernous sinus → internal jugular vein
- ***CN III, IV, V-1 (ophthalmic N), V-2 (Maxillary N)*** and ***postganglionic sympathetic fibers*** en route to orbit all pass through the ***wall of cavernous sinus***
- ***CN VI is 'free floating'*** in cavernous sinus
- Cavernous portion of ***internal carotid artery*** is also here.

7. **Answer is b (Marfan syndrome).**
   Ref: CMDT 2013, Pg 1670.

- Mutations in the ***fibrillin gene (FBN1)*** on ***chromosome 15*** cause ***Marfan syndrome***
- The nature of the FBN1 mutation has very little predictive value for prognosis.
- The pathogenesis of Marfan syndrome involves *aberrant regulation of* transforming growth factor ***(TGF)*** activity

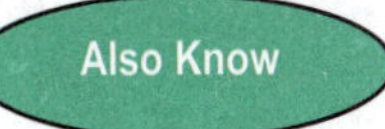

- **Marfan syndrome:**
  - ***AD***; mutation in ***fibrillin gene*** on chromosome ***15q***.
  - Ocular features: Lens subluxation that is ***upward and temporally, bilateral***, symmetrical. Angle anomaly (secondary glaucoma); ***retinal detachment*** (due to lattice degeneration); flat cornea, pupil difficult to dilate; blue sclera; axial ***myopia***.
  - Systemic features: ***Arachnodactyly; hyperextensible joints; pectus excavatum; high-arched palate; scoliosis and kyphosis; muscular underdevelopment (hernias); aortic dilation with dissecting aortic aneurysm; aortic regurgitation; mitral valve prolapse, dural ectasia.***

8. **Answer is a (Anal abuse).**
   Ref: http://www.dundee.ac.uk/forensicmedicine/Crimes_against_Women_and_Children/D12-Paediatrics.pdf; Paediatric Forensic Medicine and Pathology, 2nd edition Pg 40; http://www.biomedcentral.com/content/pdf/1471-2431-14-128.pdf

- Perianal venous congestion maybe found in about 25% of children following ***anal abuse***.
- The anus appears blue and there maybe some ***edema around the anus,*** which may last up to 2 days after the assault (‘***tire sign***’) – this maybe mistaken for hemorrhoids.

9. Answer is c (Depressing the globe when the eye is adducted).

Ref: Clinical Anatomy: a Problem Solving Approach, By Neeta V Kulkarni, 2nd edition Pg 403.

Muscle	Primary action	Subsidiary action	Nerve supply
Medial rectus	Adduction		Oculomotor N (III)
Lateral rectus	Abduction		Abducent N (VI)
Superior rectus	Elevation	Intorsion and adduction	Oculomotor N (III)
Inferior rectus	Depression	Extorsion and adduction	Oculomotor N (III)
Superior oblique	Intorsion (medial rotation)	Depression and abduction	Trochlear N (IV)
Inferior oblique	Extorsion (lateral rotation)	Elevation and abduction	Oculomotor N (III)

Insertions of recti from limbus
Superior = 7.7 mm
Lateral = 6.9 mm
Inferior = 6.6 mm
Medial = 5.5 mm
(‘*SLIM*’)

<u>Note</u>: III N. inferior division supplies MR, IR and IO; superior division supplies SR.

<u>Easy method to remember extraocular muscle (EOM) actions</u>

The actions of EOM is a straightforward question and should be answered correctly.

<u>Basic concepts</u>

- Primary action: It is the action when the eye is in the primary position.
- Subsidiary action: It is the additional effects on the position of the eye.

<u>Read and remember the below statements</u>

Horizontal recti have only one action (i.e. primary action only)

- ♦ Medical rectus: Adduction
- ♦ Lateral rectus: Abduction

AND

- *All other muscles have one primary and two subsidiary actions.*

AND

- *Primary action of oblique muscles is torsion (intorsion or extorsion).*

AND

- *Primary action of superior rectus is elevation and inferior rectus is depression.*

<u>After going through the above statements</u>

- JUST remember the ***mnemonic*** **‘SINRAD’,** which means: All **S**uperiors are **IN**tortors; all **R**ecti (obviously I am talking about only the 2 <u>*vertical*</u> recti) are **AD**ductors.
- The mnemonic also implies (inferiors are extortors and obliques are abductors) – but you do not need to remember this.
- ***Superior oblique:*** ‘Copying (in examination) muscle’; ALSO called 'tramp's muscle' – moves the eye 'down and out'. Superior oblique produces depression of the eye when the eye is adducted. Superior oblique paralysis causes NO obvious squint but ***diplopia on looking down***—typically ***while climbing down stairs***.
- ***Inferior oblique:*** ‘Stargazer’s muscle’ produces elevation of the eye when the eye is adducted.
- With the above knowledge read the below table once. Now take a paper and write down the actions once without looking. IT WORKS. And you won’t forget even if you want to!

- *Pure elevation* of eyeball is by the superior rectus with opposite named (i.e. inferior) oblique
- *Pure depression* of eyeball is by the inferior rectus with opposite named (i.e. superior) oblique

Mnemonic for EOM Nerve Supply

- $LR6(SO4)_3$ = Lateral **R**ectus by **VI** cranial nerve (abducent); Superior **O**blique by **IV** cranial nerve (trochlear) and the rest by **III** cranial nerve (Oculomotor).

More Important Points about Extraocular Muscles

- ***Inferior oblique*** is the ONLY muscle that does NOT arise from the apex of the orbit.
- ***Superior oblique*** muscle is usually NOT paralyzed in retrobulbar block, since the fourth cranial nerve is outside the muscle cone.
- ***Levator palpebrae superioris (LPS)*** is *considered by some to be an extraocular muscle.*
- LPS is supplied by a branch of superior division of oculomotor nerve.
- LPS acts as an elevator of upper eyelid—its action is anatgonized by palpebral portion of orbicularis oculi muscle.
- ***Müller's muscle*** consist of smooth muscle fibers; supplied by sympathetic nerve fibers; sympathetic irritation leads to retraction of lids and paralysis leads to Horner's syndrome.
- ***Orbicularis oculi*** consist of orbital and palpebral parts—supplied by facial nerve.
- The ***vertical recti*** form an angle of **23 *degrees with the visual axis***.
- The ***oblique muscles*** are inserted behind the equator and form an angle of **51 *degrees with the visual axis***.
- ***Spiral of Tillaux*** is an imaginary line joining the *insertions of the four recti* and is an important landmark when performing squint surgery.

10. Answer is b (11 g/dL).

Ref: deSwiet's Medical Disorders in Obstetric Practice, 5th edition Pg 48.

- ***WHO definition of anemia complicating pregnancy*** is when the ***hemoglobin level is less than 11 g/dL***.

11. Answer is a (Clenbuterol).

Ref: Sports Medicine; edited by Anthony A Schepsis, Brian D Busconi, LWW publishers, Pg 38.

- ***Clenbuterol is a potent, long-lasting bronchodilator*** that is prescribed for treating chronic asthma. Clenbuterol is a β-2 ***adrenergic agonist—bronchodilation***.
- However, clenbuterol like other β-adrenergic agonists can produce adverse cardiovascular and neurological effects, such as heart ***palpitations, muscle tremors and nervousness***.
- Activation of β receptors accounts for clenbuterol's ability to ***increase lean muscle mass and reduce body fat***.
- Clenbuterol is ***abused by athletes*** for its ability to alter body composition by reducing body fat and increasing skeletal muscle mass.
- ***Female athletes abuse*** this due to ***absence of typical androgenic side effects*** (hirsutism, deepening of voice).

12. Answer is b (Quinine).

Ref: Harrison's, 18th edition Pg 965-967.

- ***Drug-induced thrombocytopenia*** is ***more common with quinine and sulfonamides***—the thrombocytopenia typically occurs ***after*** a period of initial exposure (median length 21 days), or upon ***reexposure***, and usually resolves in 7–10 days after drug withdrawal.
- ***Quinine- and quinidine-induced thrombocytopenia***: ***Antibody-drug-antigen complexes*** may be passively absorbed by a bystander cell, which is then destroyed by activation of complement.
- The thrombocytopenia caused by the platelet ***GpIIbIIIa inhibitory drugs, such as abciximab***, *differs in that it may occur* ***within 24 h*** of initial exposure.

Also Know

- Drug stimulation of antibody production may mediate tissue injury by several mechanisms.
- ***Penicillin-induced hemolytic anemia***: The antibody may attack the drug when the drug is covalently attached to a cell and thereby destroy the cell.
- ***Heparin-induced thrombocytopenia***: Arises when ***antibodies against complexes of platelet factor 4 peptide*** and heparin generate ***immune complexes*** that activate platelets; thus, the thrombocytopenia is accompanied by ***'paradoxical' thrombosis*** and is treated with thrombin inhibitors.
- ***Procainamide and hydralazine***-induced ***lupus***: These drugs (or their reactive metabolites) can chemically alter nuclear material, stimulating the formation of antinuclear ***autoantibodies*** and occasionally causing ***lupus erythematosus.***
- ***Drug-induced pure red cell aplasia*** is due to an immune-based drug reaction.

13. Answer is c (Sickle cell anemia).
Ref: CMDT 2013, Pg 503.

X-ray findings in sickle cell disease include:

- ***Bone infarction = avascular necrosis*** of bony regions with a tenuous blood supply (e.g. femoral head)
- *'Fish-mouth' vertebrae* OR ***'H-shaped'*** vertebrae
- ***Periosteal reaction ('bone within bone')***

Also Know

- ***AR*** disease; point mutation in the β-globin chain of Hb (***glutamic acid replaced by valine at position 6***) leads to the production of HbS, a form of Hb that is poorly soluble when deoxygenated.
- ***Heterozygotes*** are relatively ***malaria resistant.***
  - ✈ ***Also know***: Duffy negativity, newborns (high HbF), thalassemia and G-6-PD deficiency have *high resistance to P. falciparum.*
- ***Acidosis, hypoxia and dehydration*** → polymerization of HbS → distortion of RBCs into a sickle shape that is susceptible to hemolysis and vascular clumping
- *Risk factors*: African or Latin American heritage
- Clinically:
  - Patients may be *asymptomatic between crises* or may note bone pain
  - Stressful events (e.g. infection, illness, trauma) incite sickle cell crises characterized by ***severe bone pain, chest pain, 'hand foot syndrome' (dactylitis), dyspnea and priapism.***
  - Physical examination: Decreased growth velocity, jaundice or pallor, ***splenomegaly (in early stages)***, fever, possible leg ulcers
- *Tests*:
  - ↓ Hb and ↑ reticulocytes; ↑ WBCs.
  - ↓ serum haptoglobin; ↑ indirect bilirubin
  - No HbA, ↑ HbF, and presence of HbS (normally not present) on electrophoresis
  - Solubility tests (e.g. SICKLEDEX, Streck, Omaha, Nebraska) can detect hemoglobin abnormalities, but cannot differentiate between the carrier trait and homozygous disease states
  - Blood smear shows target cells, sickle cells, and nucleated RBCs
- *Treatment*:
  - ***Sickle cell crises*** are treated with *hydration, supplemental oxygen, and narcotic pain control.*
  - ***Transfusions, exchange transfusions, and hydroxyurea*** are frequently useful to shorten crises or to decrease the number of crises in patients with frequent recurrences.
  - ***Bone marrow transplantation*** has demonstrated success as a ***curative therapy,*** but due to the appreciable mortality and morbidity rates it is currently reserved for patients with severe disease and multiple complications.

- *Complications*
  - Chronic anemia, pulmonary HTN, heart failure due to cardiac stresses, vascular insufficiency, renal failure, and infections; **Salmonella osteomyelitis** (however even in sickle cells patients also *S. aureus* is the MC cause).
  - An ***aplastic crisis*** may follow ***parvovirus B19*** infection.
  - Acute chest syndrome is severe chest pain due to pneumonia, embolization or pulmonary infarction and requires pain control and respiratory support.
  - *Autosplenectomy*, stroke, osteonecrosis of the femoral or humeral head and multiorgan ischemia may result from vascular occlusion.
  - Increased risk of infection by encapsulated organisms (e.g. *Streptococcus pneumoniae, Haemophilus influenzae, Neisseria meningitides, Klebsiella)*—keep pneumococcal vaccination up to date.
  - Renal papillary necrosis ***(focal segmental glomerulosclerosis)*** occurs.
  - Despite the multiple potential complications, survival at 18 years of age is 86%.

14. Answer is a (Neural crest).
Ref: Lippincott's Illustrated Embryology, Pg 264.

1. ***Neural crest cells*** *migrate into the ultimobranchial body to form* ***parafollicular C-cells*** of thyroid, which secrete calcitonin.
2. The ultimobranchial body ultimately fuses with the primordium of the thyroid gland and the neural crest cells are dispersed among the developing thyroid follicles.

Also Know

Branchial pouch derivatives
- ***1st pouch*** (***ventral*** part): ***Tongue***
- ***1st and 2nd pouch*** (***dorsal*** part): *Tubotympanic recess*, which forms the ***eustachian tube*** and ***middle ear cavity***.
- ***2nd pouch*** (***ventral*** part): ***Tonsil***
- 3rd pouch: ***Th***ymus, ***I***nferior parathyroid gland (***ThI***rd pouch)
- ***4th pouch***: Superior parathyroid gland, ***ultimobranchial body***.

Aberrant development of ***3rd and 4th pouches*** → ***DiGeorge syndrome*** → leads to T cell deficiency (*thymic aplasia*) and *hypocalcemia* (failure of parathyroid development).

15. Answer is a (Henoch-Schönlein purpura).
Ref: Comprehensive Clinical Nephrology, By Richard J Johnson, John Feehally, 2014 edition Pg 276.

- ***IgA nephropathy*** is very closely related to ***Henoch-Schönlein nephritis***.
- ***Diffuse mesangial IgA deposition*** is the hallmark of IgA nephropathy and Henoch-Schönlein nephritis.

16. Answer is b (Marcus Gunn pupil).
Ref: Parson's diseses of the eye, 21st edition Pg 124.

Horner's syndrome

Clinical features of Horner's syndrome	Causes of Horner's syndrome
Horner's syndrome (oculosympathetic paralysis) consists of ☐ ***Miosis*** (due to unopposed action of sphincter pupillae—parasympathetic) ☐ ***Ptosis*** and ***enophthalmos*** (due to loss of tone of Müller's muscle) ☐ ***Anhidrosis*** (unilateral)—only if lesion is below the superior cervical ganglion	– **Central (first-order neuron)** – Brainstem disease (tumor, vascular, demyelination) – Syringemyelia – Lateral medullary syndrome (Wallenberg) – Spinal cord tumor – Diabetic autonomic neuropathy – **Preganglionic (second-order neuron)** • Pancoast tumor (apical lung tumor)

❑ *Loss of ciliospinal reflex* ❑ In *congenital Horner's*, iris is ***hypochromic***	• Carotid and aortic aneurysm and dissection • Neck lesions (glands, trauma, postsurgical) – **Postganglionic (third-order neuron)** ✈ Cluster headache ✈ Internal carotid artery dissection ✈ Nasopharyngeal tumor ✈ Otitis media ✈ Cavernous sinus mass

- ***Cocaine confirms*** diagnosis of Horner's syndrome
- ***Hydroxyamphetamine*** (Paredrine) ***differentiates between a preganglionic and postganglionic*** lesions.

17. Answer is a (Biparietal diameter).
Ref: Dutta's, 6th edition Pg 85.

- ***Biparietal diameter (9.5 cm):*** Extends between the two parietal eminences—***widest transverse diameter*** of the ***fetal skull.***
- ***Engagement of the head*** has taken place when the ***widest transverse diameter (biparietal)*** has passed through the brim of the pelvis.

18. Answer is d (Austin Moore's prosthesis).
Ref: Total Hip Replacement, By Marye, 2009 edition Pg 24.

- The ***Austin Moore's prosthesis*** was designed for use ***without bone cement;*** using a fenestrated stem to allow ***'self-locking'*** of the prosthesis in the proximal femur.

19. Answer is b (0.2).
Ref: Parson's diseases of the eye, 21st edition Pg 281.

- The changes seen in the optic nerve head in glaucoma include:
  - ***Asymmetry of the cup-disk ratio (> 0.2)*** between the two eyes
  - A localized notch or thinning of the neuroretinal rim (NRR)
  - An enlarged cup-disk ratio (> 0.5) especially, if in the vertical axis
  - Pallor of the NRR
  - Superficial disk hemorrhages
  - 'Baring of circumlinear vessels' and 'overpass' of central vessels
  - Parapapillary atrophy.

20. Answer is b (Laparoscopy).
Ref: Radiology of the Stomach and Duodenum,By Alan H Freeman, Pg 154; Gastric Cancer, edited by Dongfeng Tan, Pg 275.

- ***Peritoneal carcinomatosis*** is common in gastric cancer and indicates ***advanced disease.***
- Diagnosis of early peritoneal involvement is difficult with CT and therefore ***diagnostic laparoscopy is commonly used*** to detect surgical resectability. Diagnostic laparoscopy ***detects < 0.5 cm of metastases*** on the peritoneum.
- ***MRI is most sensitive method to diagnose liver metastases*** BUT peritoneal carcinomatosis is <u>NOT</u> revealed, since the lesions are too small and maybe masked by ascites.
- Laparoscope is ***also superior*** to abdominal ultrasound.

21. Answer is b (Musculoskeletal pain).
Ref: Searching....

Sorry guys BUT couldn't find a reference here......anyway the revised answer key gives 'musculoskeletal pain' as the correct answer. If u find anything - message me on FB or email me; will update it for the benefit of all.

22. Answer is c (Stroke volume).

Ref: A Comprehensive Approach to Congenital Heart Diseases; edited by IB Vijayalakshmi, Pg 57.

	Isotonic	Isometric
Effect on heart	Volume load	Pressure load
BP	Increase in systolic and decrease in diastolic BP	Sudden increase in systolic BP
Heart rate	+++	+
Stroke volume	+++	***Unchanged***
Cardiac output	+++	+
Oxygen consumption	+++	+
Respiratory rate	+++	+++

Key: *+++ - significant increase; + - limited increase*

23. Answer is a (Terminal deoxynucleotidyl transferase).

Ref: Essentials of Anatomic Pathology; By Liang Cheng, David G. Bostwick; 3rd edition Pg 2-92; http://ajcp.ascpjournals.org/content/118/2/248.full.pdf

- ***Terminal deoxynucleotidyl transferase (TdT)*** is a nuclear enzyme whose expression is restricted, in normal tissues, to lymphoid precursors of B- and T-cell lineage.
- TdT is expressed in malignant tumors of lymphoblastic lineage (including ***precursor-B and T lymphoblastic leukemia/lymphoma*** and lymphoid blast crisis of chronic myeloid leukemia) and in a subset of acute myeloid leukemias.

24. Answer is b (Crohn's disease).

Ref: Harrison's, 18th edition Pg 2482-85.

Crohn's Disease and Ulcerative Colitis Compared

	Crohn's disease (CD)	Ulcerative colitis (UC)
■ Site of involvement	***Entire GI tract*** may be involved (mouth to anus) with 'skip' areas Distal ileum MC involved All layers of bowel wall involved (transmural); *Granulomas; creeping fat*	Continuous disease beginning at rectum and extending possibly as far as distal ileum Only mucosa and submucosa affected (mucosal) ***Crypt abscesses***
■ Symptoms	Watery diarrhea Abdominal pain, weight loss	***Bloody diarrhea*** Abdominal pain, urgency, tenesmus, weight loss, nausea, vomiting
■ Clinically	Palpable right lower quadrant ***abdominal mass*** *Perianal fissures and fistula* ***Oral (aphthous) ulcers*** Fever	Fever, abdominal tenderness, orthostatic hypotension, tachycardia, ***gross rectal bleeding***
■ Labs	ASCA frequently positive, pANCA rarely positive *Hemoccult positive stool* Biopsy diagnostic	ASCA rarely positive, pANCA frequently positive Biopsy diagnostic
■ Radiology	***Skip*** *lesions,* *Colonic ulcers* *Cobblestoning mucosa* *Strictures* *'String sign' on Ba swallow*	*Continuous involvement* *Fine mucosal ulcers (double contour)* *Pseudopolyps, friable mucosa* *'Lead pipe' colon without haustra and colon shortening*

■ Complications	Abscess formation ***Fistula*** and fissure common ***Malabsorption*** (since ileal disease)	Increased risk of colon cancer Hemorrhage Bowel obstruction ***Toxic megacolon***
■ Treatment	Mesalamine, broad-spectrum antibiotics, corticosteroids, immunosuppressives, surgical resection of severely affected areas, flares and remissions, recurrence after colectomy	***5-aminosalicylic acid*** compounds (***sulfasalazine is DOC,*** *mesalamine, balsalazide*), supplemental iron, corticosteroids, immunosuppressives, total colectomy is curative

To remember features of Crohn's disease you could imagine:

- ***"2 obsessed** (abscesses) **fish** (fissures and fistulas) **skipping** (skip lesions) on a **cobblestoned** (cobblestones) path **fully penetrated** (transmural) **fat** (creeping fat) **grandma's** (granuloma) house wall. She caught them with a **string** (strictures, String sign) and ate them and got **ulcers at both ends** (mouth and perianal), and screamed **'AMMA'!** (Abdominal Mass and MAlabsorption)"*

ASCA= Antiyeast saccharomyces cereveciae antibodies.

25. Answer is d (Histoplasmosis).

Ref: http://www.antimicrobe.org/history/Discovery%20of%20Histoplasmosis-Darling.asp

- ***Histoplasmosis is called Darling disease—*** named after ***Samuel Taylor Darling,*** a general knowledge question hence an interesting internet link for the explanation – go through if interested.
- Histoplasmosis is also known as ***Cave disease, Darling's disease, Ohio valley disease, Reticuloendotheliosis, Spelunker's Lung and Caver's disease.***

26. Answer is c (Median).

Ref: Epidemiology, Biostatistics, and Preventive Medicine,Elsevier Health Sciences, 2007, Pg 147.

Measures of Dispersion

Range	– The difference between the highest and lowest values
Percentile	– The level of measurement below which a specified proportion of the distribution falls, e.g. the 5th and 95th percentile are the values of a particular measurement below which 5% and 95% of people fall. A quartile is the division of the distribution using cutpoints at 25%, 50%, and 75%. The 'interquartile' range is the difference between the values of the 25th and 75th percentile
Standard deviation (SD)	– Measure of spread of observations about the mean. – SD = √Sum of individual observations - mean²/Number of observations
Coefficient of variation	– Ratio of the standard deviation of a series of observations to the mean of the observations. It is without units and is expressed as a percentage. – Coefficient of variation (%) = SD/Mean × 100 – Used to make comparisons of spread when the means are dissimilar, i.e. standard deviation of 10 around a mean of 40 indicates a greater degree of scatter than a standard deviation of 10 around a mean of 400
Mean deviation	Measure of dispersion
Variance	Measure of dispersion

27. Answer is c (Acute arterial occlusion).

Ref: Harrison's, 18th edition Pg 2069-70.

- The case history given is that of IHD patient with a trial fibrillation (AF) - *AF is the commonest cause of embolic acute arterial occlusion in the flower limb.*
- To diagnose acute ischemic foot, you need to check the initial critical cardinal signs, which are referred as "six Ps": ***pain, pallor, poikilothermia, pulselessness, paresthesia and paralysis***. The affected leg and foot will have ***no pulse and look pale initially***.
- *DVT* however, presents with ***leg swelling and leg is usually warmer to touch.***

28. Answer is a (Open angle glaucoma).
Ref: Kanski's clinical ophthalmology, 4th edition Pg 421.

- ***Laser Trabeculoplasty*** for ***POAG***: It involves laser application to the trabecular meshwork to enhance outflow of aqueous humor.
- It is NOT useful in angle closure/narrow angle glaucoma since the trabecular meshwork is not visible in these cases.

Argon laser trabeculoplasty	Selective laser trabeculoplasty
➢ Causes scarring of trabecular meshwork ➢ Not repeatable	➢ Uses 532 nm, frequency doubled, Q switched Nd: YAG laser ➢ NO scarring of trabecular meshwork ➢ Repeatable

29. Answer is a (Touch the opposite shoulder).
Ref: Orthopedics Ready Reckoner; By RM Shenoy, Pg 56.

Clinical signs of shoulder dislocation

- Patient enters casualty with ***shoulder abducted and elbow supported with opposite hand***
- ***Dugas test:*** Inability to touch opposite shoulder
- ***Hamilton ruler test:*** It is possible to place a ruler on the lateral side of the arm touching the acromion and lateral condyle of humerus simultaneously due to flattening of shoulder
- ***Callway's test:*** Increased vertical circumference of axilla compared to normal side
- ***Positive apprehension test***: With forced abduction and external rotation, patients experiences apprehension (a sense of impending doom).

30. Answer is c (Phosphate buffer solution).
Ref: http://www.who.int/immunization_standards/vaccine_quality/pq270_vpsar_jevlive_chengdu_12nov13.pdf.

- ➢ The ***Japanese encephalitis vaccine***, live is a preparation of Japanese encephalitis ***live attenuated virus strain (SA 14-4-2)***.
- ➢ It is a lyophilized vaccine that looks like a ***light yellow powder***.
- ➢ It should be *reconstituted with* ***phosphate-buffered saline.***
- ➢ ***Four new vaccines*** have been introduced into ***India's Universal Immunization Program (UIP)***, including injectable polio vaccine and an adult vaccine against Japanese encephalitis; vaccines against rotavirus, rubella.

31. Answer is b (Angle-closure glaucoma).
Ref: Parsons Disease of the Eye, 21st edition Pg 291.

- ➢ The ***MC mechanism of angle-closure*** glaucoma is ***pupillary block.***
- ➢ ***YAG laser peripheral iridotomy*** is indicated in ***angle-closure glaucoma***.
- ➢ ***Prophylactic laser iridotomy*** is indicated in stages of intermittent angle-closure glaucoma and as a definitive treatment in acute angle-closure glaucoma.
- ➢ ***Abram's lens*** is used for YAG PI.

32. **Answer is a (1.5% glycine).**
Ref: TURP syndrome – current concepts in the pathophysiology and management; Indian Journal of Urology; http://www.indianjurol.com/text.asp?2001/17/2/97/20247

- Irrigating fluids are used during endourological procedures for better vision. Ideally the irrigation solution should be isotonic, nonhemolytic, electrically inert (so that diathermy can be used), nontoxic, transparent, easy to sterilize and inexpensive.
- ***1.5% glycine is the MC irrigating solution used in TURP***. The osmolality of 1.5% glycine is 230 mosm/1 compared to serum osmolality of 290 mosm/L and hence cardiovascular and renal toxicities can occur at this concentration also. Further lowering of the concentration of glycine can lead to more complications due to hypotonicity and hence cannot be used for irrigation purposes. The ***distinct advantage of 1.5% glycine*** over sterile water is its tendency to cause less hemolysis and renal failure.
- Electrolyte solutions such as ***normal saline or Ringer's lactate*** do least harm when absorbed into the circulation. However they cause ***dispersion of high frequency current from the resectoscope and hence abandoned***.
- *Glucose* 2.5– 4%: This is not a widely used irrigating fluid since glucose produces ***tissue charring at the site of resection and associated hyperglycemia*** produced when glucose is absorbed into the circulation. It also causes ***stickiness of surgeons' gloves and instruments.***
- ***Urea 1%:*** This produces urea ***crystallization on the instruments*** during resection and hence NOT preferred.
- ***Mannitol*** 3%: Mannitol, though does not have the toxicities of glycine, drives water out of cells and may enhance ***circulatory overloading***. The ***cost of mannitol is also higher*** compared to glycine. The elimination of mannitol through kidney will be decreased in patients with impaired renal function.
- ***Cytal***: It is a mixture of sorbitol 2.7% and mannitol 0.54% widely used in USA as an irrigating fluid, has not gained popularity in India due to its ***high cost and nonavailability***. In the body, sorbitol is metabolized to fructose, which may present problems in a patient with ***hypersensitivity to fructose.***

33. **Answer is e (wrong options? as per revised answer key).**
Ref: Harrison's, 18th edition Pg 2073.

Erythromelalgia

- A disorder characterized by burning pain and erythema of the extremities.
- Affects ***Feet > hands*** and affects ***males > females***; MC in middle age.
- Causes:
  - ***Primary*** (also termed erythermalgia)
  - ***Secondary***: ***MC cause is myeloproliferative disorders*** (polycythemia vera and essential thrombocytosis)
  - Other causes: ***Drugs*** (calcium channel blockers, desmopressin, bromocriptine, and pergolide); ***neuropathies***; ***connective tissue diseases*** such as SLE and ***paraneoplastic*** syndromes.
- Clinically: Patients complain of ***burning in the extremities*** that is *precipitated by exposure to a warm environment and aggravated by a dependent position*. The symptoms are *relieved by exposing the affected area to cool air or water or by elevation*.
- REMEMBER: Peripheral pulses are present and the neurologic examination is normal.
- No specific treatment; ***aspirin*** may help in erythromelalgia secondary to myeloproliferative disease.
- I have gone through large number of reference books but found no a/w the options mentioned in the question – hence 'E' has been given as the answer I feel.

34. **Answer is c (Suprapubic cystostomy).**
Ref: Penn Clinical Manual of Urology; By Philip M Hanno, Pg 300.

- ***Suprapubic cystostomy*** remains ***standard management of prostomembraneous urethral disruption*** and straddle injuries to the bulbar urethra.

35. **Answer is d (Intradermal).**
Ref: OP Ghai, 7th edition Pg 166.

- ***Intradermal (ID) injection*** administers the vaccine in the topmost layer of the skin.
- ***BCG*** is the ***only vaccine*** with this route of administration.
- Intradermal injection of BCG vaccine ***reduces the risk of neurovascular injury***.
- A short narrow needle (15 mm, 26 gauge) is needed for BCG vaccine. All other vaccines are given with a longer, wider needle (commonly 25 mm, 23 gauge), either SC or IM.

36. Answer is b (2005).
Ref: http://nrhm.gov.in/nhm/nrhm.html

- The ***National Rural Health Mission (NRHM)*** was launched by the Hon'ble Prime Minister on ***12th April 2005***, to provide accessible, affordable and quality health care to the rural population, especially the vulnerable groups.
- The Union Cabinet vide its decision dated ***1st May 2013***, has approved the launch of ***National Urban Health Mission (NUHM)*** as a submission of an over-arching ***National Health Mission (NHM)***, with National Rural Health Mission (NRHM) being the other submission of National Health Mission.

37. Answer is d (6–8 hours).
Ref: OP Ghai, 7th edition Pg 127.

- ***Expressed breast milk*** can be stored:
  - At ***room temperature*** for 6–8 hours
  - In ***refrigerato*** for 24 hours
  - In ***freezer*** at –20°C for 3 months.

38. Answer is a (Shortening of both T1 and T2 relaxation times).
Ref: MR Imaging of the Body, edited by Ernst Rummeny, Peter Reime, Pg 26.

➢ ***Paramagnetic materials*** include oxygen and ions of various metals like ***Fe, Mg, and Gd***.
➢ These ions have unpaired electrons, resulting in a positive magnetic susceptibility. The magnitude of this susceptibility is less than 1,000 of that of ferromagnetic materials.
➢ The *effect on MRI is an increase in the T1 and T2 relaxation rates* (***decrease in the T1 and T2 times***).

39. Answer is a (Rest/Night pain).
Ref: Bailey and Love's, 25th edition Pg 902; Davidson's, 21st edition Pg 599; ABC of arterial and venous disease, 2nd edition Pg 3.

Critical Limb Ischemia (CLI) is defined as
➢ ***Rest (night) pain*** requiring opiate analgesia and/or tissue loss (***ulceration or gangrene***) present for more than 2 weeks in the presence of an ankle blood pressure of less than 50 mm Hg
➢ ABPI is < 0.5
Intermittent Claudication
❑ A *cramp-like pain* felt in the muscles that is
❑ Brought on/*precipitated by walking*
❑ NOT present on taking the first step (unlike osteoarthrosis)
❑ *Relieved by standing still* (unlike pseudoclaudication in lumbar intervertebral disk nerve compression)
Rest pain (night pain)
❖ Occurs with the leg at rest. Pain is worse in horizontal position (sleeping) and relieved by hanging the foot out of bed or sleeping in a chair.

Author's comment: "***Critical limb ischemia***" *IS* ***ABPI < 0.5****; (Davidson's, 21st/599 (specifically mentions "CLI"; Harrison's, 18th/2067 – mentions "< 0.5 is consistent with severe ischemia"; Bailey 25th/902 says < 0.3 suggests imminent necrosis). This has been a favorite question for both KCET and COMED-K many times earlier".*

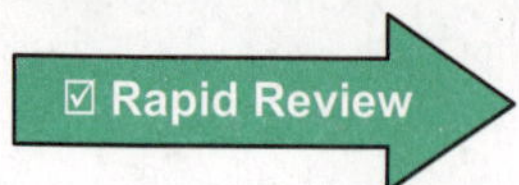

- *Ankle-brachial Pressure Index (ABPI)* = Ratio between the (highest systolic) ankle and brachial blood pressures.

In health	ABPI is >/= 1.0
In intermittent claudication	ABPI is 0.5–0.9
In critical limb ischemia	ABPI is < 0.5
Imminent necrosis suggested by	ABPI < 0.3

40. Answer is c (Laryngeal paralysis).

Ref: API Textbook of Medicine, 2012 edition Pg 26.

- The completely paralyzed vocal cord lies immobile midway between abduction and adduction (cadaveric position). Abductor paralysis is always organic in nature and it may be uni- or bi-lateral. On the other hand, pure adductor paralysis is always bilateral and it is functional in nature. This is frequently seen in hysteria.
- *Bovine cough*: A characteristic feature of organic laryngeal paralysis is a ***cow-like cough,*** which results from the ***loss of the explosive phase of normal coughing*** consequent upon the failure of the cords to close the glottis. Difficulty in bringing up sputum, which some patients experience is also explained on the same basis.
- A normal cough in patients with partial loss of voice or aphonia virtually excludes laryngeal paralysis.

41. Answer is c (36 weeks).

Ref: Dutta's, 6th edition Pg 30.

Amniotic Fluid

Volume	– 50 mL at 12 weeks – 400 mL at 20 weeks – ***1,000 mL at 36–38 weeks (maximum)*** – 600–800 mL at term – 100–400 mL at 43 weeks
Physical Features	– Fluid is faintly alkaline (pH 7.2) with a low specific gravity of 1.010 – It is hypotonic. An osmolarity of 250 mOsm/L is suggestive of fetal maturity – It is colorless, but becomes pale straw colored at term
Abnormal Color	– ***Meconium stained (green)***: Is suggestive of ***fetal distress*** in presentations *other than* transverse or breech – ***Golden color***: In ***Rh incompatibility*** due to excessive hemolysis – ***Greenish yellow (saffron)***: In ***postmaturity*** – ***Dark brown (tobacco juice)***: Found in ***intrauterine death***. The dark color is due to frequent presence of old ***HbA*** – Dark colored: In concealed accidental hemorrhage due to contamination of blood

- **Clarification**: Dutta's obstetrics and other standard books of India and UK give that maximum volume of amniotic fluid is at 34–36 weeks; BUT Williams obstetrics gives this as 20 weeks; SINCE in 2014 COMED-K paper also – 36 weeks was accepted as the 'correct' answer, if this question is repeated 36 weeks maybe marked as the answer.

42. Answer is b (Butch).

Ref: Textbook of FMT, By Krishnan Vij, Jaypee Brothers Medical Publishers (P) Ltd, Pg 322.

- Active lesbian: ***Butch or Dyke***
- Passive agent: ***Femme***
- Oral genital contact to female gentials: ***Cunnilingus***
- Tribaidsm: ***Lesbianism***

- *Sodomy:* Anal intercourse
- Oral genital contact to male genitals: ***Fellatio; buccal coitus or sin of Gomorrah.***

43. Answer is a (Henry's law).

Ref: Stoelting's Clinical Anesthesia, 2012 edition Pg 416.

- According to ***Henry's law***: At a constant temperature, the amount of a given gas that dissolves in a given type and volume of liquid is directly proportional to the partial pressure of that gas in equilibrium with that liquid.
- ***Carbonated beverages*** are an example of Henry's law in everyday life. The dissolved CO_2 stays in solution in a closed pop bottle or can where the partial pressure of CO_2 was set at a high value during bottling. When the can or bottle is opened the partial pressure of CO_2 is much lower and the dissolved carbon dioxide will gradually escape from the pop. When the new low partial pressure equilibrium is established the soda will be "flat" . This loss of dissolved CO_2 will happen faster for warm soda than for cold.
- Another example of Henry's law is in the ***decompression and decompression sickness of underwater divers.***

Also Know

Gas Laws	
• **Charles' law**	The volume of a gas changes in proportion to the change in temperature.
• **Boyle's law**	At constant temperature, the volume of a given weight of gas varies inversely as pressure, i.e. PXV = constant.
• **Gay-Lussac's law**	At constant volume, the absolute pressure of a given mass of gas varies directly with the absolute pressure.
• **Graham's law**	Rate of diffusion $\propto$ 1/molecular weight.
• **Henry's law**	Amount of gas dissolved $\propto$ partial pressure of the gas.
• **Fick's law**	Rate of diffusion across a membrane $\propto$ concentration gradient.
• **Adiabatic change**	A change in pressure, volume or temperature without change in energy of a gas (i.e. heat is lost or added).
• **Avogadro's hypothesis**	Equal volumes of 'ideal' gases at the same temperature and pressure contain the same number of molecules (Avogadro's number 6.022×10^{23} molecules occupying 22.4l at STP).
Pressure	
• **Dalton's law of partial pressures**	The pressure exerted by a mixture of gases is equal to the sum of the pressures, which each gas would exert on its own.
Solubility	
• **Ostwald solubility coefficient**	The amount of gas that dissolves in a unit volume of liquid under the stated temperature and pressure.
• **Bunsen solubility coefficient**	The amount of gas that dissolves in unit volume of a liquid at standard temperature (273K) and pressure (101.3 kPa).
Temperature	
• **Critical temperature**	Temperature above which a gas cannot be liquefied.
• **Critical pressure**	Pressure above which a gas at its critical temperature cannot be liquefied.
• **Pseudocritical temperature**	Temperature at which a mixture of gases separate out into their separate components, e.g. N_2O and O_2 in Entonox at –5.5°C.
• **Specific heat capacity**	Amount of heat required to increase the temperature of a substance by 1°C/kg.
Gas flow	
• **Bernoulli effect**	Fall of pressure at a constriction in a tube. Increased gas/fluid velocity results in increased kinetic energy with a reduction in potential energy and thus a decrease in pressure.

• **Coanda effect**	Streaming of a gas at a division in tubing along only one of the divisions. Used as logic valve in some ventilators.
• **Poynting effect**	A mixture of gases (e.g. Entonox) remains in a gaseous state, even though one component (N_2O) would normally be liquid at high storage pressures.
Humidification	
• **Absolute humidity**	Is the mass of water vapor present in a given volume of air.
• **Relative humidity**	Is the ratio of the mass of water vapor to the mass of water vapor when fully saturated, expressed as a percentage.

44. Answer is c (Barret's esophagus).
Ref: CMDT 2013, Pg 595.

CARCINOMA ESOPHAGUS

- ***MC malignant tumor** of esophagus* worldwide is still S***quamous cell carcinoma***. Adenocarcinoma is MC in Western countries; both cannot be distinguished radiographically or endoscopically; AdenoCa- MC in lower 1/3; squamous cells carcinoma inupper 2/3.
- *MC* in l***ower one third (H'son-18th)***, more common in ***men around 60*** years.

> - **Risk factors:**
>   - Excess ***alcohol*** consumption, cigarette ***smoking***, ingested ***carcinogens*** (*nitrates, smoked opiates, fungal toxins*), mucosal damage (from ingestion of *hot* ***tea*** *or* ***lye, radiation-induced*** strictures), ***tylosis*** (palmoplantar hyperkeratosis)
>   - Intrinsic esophageal disease like *chronic* ***achalasia***, B̲arret's esophagus (lead to *A̲D̲*enoCa), *P̲L̲U̲*mmer-Vinson syndrome (leads to S̲quamous cell Ca). "**BAD PLUS**"
>   - Dietary deficiencies of *selenium, molybdenum, zinc and vitamin A*

- Presents with ***dysphagia*** *(for solid foods)*, ***regurgitation*** (esophageal ***pseudovomiting***).
- **Therapy for non-operable disease:** Radiation therapy, chemotherapy (cisplatin, paclitaxel and 5-FU), and combined therapy.
- **For 'curable' disease:** Surgery (***transhiatal esophagectomy***); e***sophageal reconstruction: MC used is stomach*** (*practically feasible*), next choice is colon.
- *Prognosis is poor.*

45. Answer is c (3 days).
Ref: CP Baveja's Microbiology, 3rd edition Pg 45.

- ***Treponema pallidum*** may survive in ***refrigerated blood for 3 days***.
- May remain viable for ***several years, if frozen below –78°C***.

46. Answer is c (Nail-patella syndrome).
Ref: Harrison's, 18th edition Pg 2351.

- Patients with ***nail-patella syndrome*** develop ***iliac horns on the pelvis*** and dysplasia of the dorsal limbs involving the patella, elbows and nails; also associated are ***sensorineural hearing impairment, glaucoma***, and abnormalities of the GBM and podocytes, leading to ***hematuria, proteinuria, and FSGS***.
- ***Autosomal dominant***; mutations in the ***LIM domain region of LMX1B.***
- Histopath: ***Damage to the lamina densa*** of the GBM, an increase in collagen III fibrils along glomerular capillaries and in the mesangium, and damage to the slit-pore membrane, producing ***heavy proteinuria***—renal failure in 30% patients.
- Patients with renal failure do well with transplantation.

47. Answer is c (4,900 mL).
Ref: Ganong, 659, Table 34.4.

- ***Alveolar ventilation*** = Va = (Vt- Vd) × f—this means (tidal volume – dead space) × breath/min = (500 – 150) × 14 = 4,900 mL.

48. Answer is a (Pulmonary osteoarthropathy).
Ref: Various books.

- Hypertrophic osteoarthropathy does NOT add significantly to the mortality or morbidity of NSCLC.
- ***Hoarseness*** occurs due to tumor encroachment on the recurrent laryngeal nerve.
- Non-small cell lung cancer invading the chest wall represents an advanced stage of the disease.
- *SCC* has ***better prognosis*** than adenocarcinoma.

49. Answer is b (Maturation of protein).
Ref: Ganong, 24th edition Pg 46.

➢ The ***Golgi complex is a maturation site*** where newly synthesized proteins are glycosylated, concentrated and packaged into granules.

- Functions of Golgi complex include:
  - ***Post-translational modification of proteins***: Completion of N-linked glycosylation that began in the rER; O-linked glycosylation (addition of sugars to serine by the enzyme glycosyltransferase); sulfation and phosphorylation.
  - ***Protein sorting and packaging***: *Secretory proteins* (e.g. insulin) are packaged into *clathrin-coated vesicles; cell-membrane proteins* (e.g. hormone receptors) are packaged into *nonclathrin-coated vesicles;* and lysosomal enzymes are packaged into clathrin-coated vesicles after phosphorylation of mannose to form mannose-6-phosphatase.
  - ***Membrane recycling***.

50. Answer is a (Thiamine).
Ref: Nutrition & Dietetics, By Joshi, 3rd edition Pg 126.

- ***Sulfur*** is a constituent of two ***vitamins: Thiamine (B1)*** and ***Biotin***.
- ***Sulfur***-containing ***amino acids***: ***Methionine, Cysteine, Cystine.***

51. Answer is a (IgG).
Ref: Gujlun. Rapid review pathology, Pg 40.

- Antibodies of the ***IgG isotype*** coat (opsonize) microbes and promote their phagocytosis by binding to Fc receptors on phagocytes.
- The process of coating particles to promote phagocytosis is called ***opsonization***.
- ***C3b*** is another example of ***opsonin***.

52. Answer is c (Warrants stoppage of niacin immediately).
Ref: CMDT 2013, Pg 1253.

- ***Niacin*** causes a ***prostaglandin-mediated flushing*** that patients may describe as 'hot flashes' or pruritus and that ***can be decreased with aspirin*** or other non-steroidal anti-inflammatory agents taken during the same day.
- Flushing may also be decreased by initiating niacin therapy with a ***very small dose***, and ***later the dose is increased*** and divided over meals.
- Extended release niacin is tolerated better by patients.
- ***Spicy food, alcohol, hot baths*** can ***exacerbate the flushing***.

53. Answer is c (Capsular invasion).
Ref: Oncology: An Evidence-based Approach, By Alfred E Chang et al, Pg 988.

- The ***important feature that distinguishes follicular thyroid carcinoma from follicular adenoma*** is ***capsular*** and ***vascular invasion***.

54. Answer is b (Dubin-Johnson syndrome).
Ref: Harrison's, 18th edition Pg 2535-36.

- A cardinal feature of ***Dubin-Johnson syndrome*** is the accumulation in the lysosomes of centrilobular hepatocytes of ***dark, coarsely granular pigment***—the liver may be ***grossly black*** in appearance!!
- This pigment is thought to be derived from ***epinephrine metabolites*** that are not excreted normally.

55. Answer is c (State Government).
Ref: Textbook of FMT, NageshKumar G Rao, Pg 14.

- The ***magistrates*** are appointed by ***High Court***.
- ***Executive magistrates*** are appointed by ***state government—Cr PC 20***.

56. Answer is a (Osteomyelitis of the frontal bone).
Ref: Dhingra's EN, 5th edition Pg 213.

- ***Pott's puffy tumor:*** *Osteomyelitis of the frontal bone as a complication of* ***frontal sinusitis.***

57. Answer is a (Endoscopic ultrasound).
Ref: Harrison's, 18th edition Pg 3065.

- ***Endoscopic ultrasound (EUS)*** permits imaging of the pancreas with a high degree of ***resolution (< 5 mm)***.
- This modality is particularly helpful in excluding small ***gastrinomas*** within the pancreas and in assessing the presence of surrounding lymph nodes and vascular involvement.

58. Answer is d (32°C).
Ref: Harrison's, 18th edition Pg 165-67.

Author's comments: *"Repeat question from Comedk 2005! Even "OLD" papers questions get repeated in Comed-K – another example is the first question in this paper from Comed-K 2005!"*

Severity	Body Temperature	CNS	CVS	Respiratory	Renal and endocrine	Neuro-muscular
Mild	35°C (95°F)–32.2°C (90°F)	Depression of cerebral metabolism; *amnesia; apathy; dysarthria; impaired judgment*	Tachycardia, then progressive bradycardia; cardiac cycle prolongation; vasoconstriction; ***increase*** in cardiac output and BP	Tachypnea, then progressive decrease in respiratory minute volume; declining oxygen consumption; bronchorrhea; bronchospasm	Diuresis; increase in catecholamines, adrenal steroids, triiodothyronine and thyroxine; increase in metabolism with shivering	Increased preshivering muscle tone, then fatiguing
Moderate	< 32.2°C (90°F)–28°C (82.4°F)	EEG abnormalities; progressive ***depression of level of consciousness; pupillary dilation; paradoxical undressing;*** hallucinations	Progressive ***decrease*** in pulse and cardiac output; atrial and ventricular arrhythmias; ***suggestive (Osborne J-wave) ECG changes***	***Hypoventilation***; 50% decrease in carbon dioxide production per 8°C drop in temperature; absence of protective airway reflexes	50% increase in renal blood flow; renal autoregulation ***intact***; impaired insulin action	Hyporeflexia; reduced shivering-induced thermogenesis; rigidity

Severe	< 28°C (82.4°F)	Loss of cerebrovascular autoregulation; decline in cerebral blood flow; *coma*; loss of ocular reflexes; progressive decrease in EEG	Progressive decrease in BP, heart rate, and cardiac output; re-entrant dysrhythmias; maximum risk of ***ventricular fibrillation***; asystole	Pulmonic congestion and edema; 75% decrease in oxygen consumption; apnea	Decrease in renal blood flow parallels decrease in cardiac output; extreme oliguria; poikilothermia; 80% decrease in basal metabolism	No motion; decreased nerve-conduction velocity; peripheral areflexia; no corneal or oculocephalic reflexes

59. Answer is b (Somatostatinoma).
Ref: CMDT 2013, Pg 1188.

- ***Somatostatinomas*** can cause ***diabetes mellitus, steatorrhea and cholelithiasis***—they are a component of ***MEN-1 syndrome (Wermer syndrome)***.

Also Know

- ***Insulinomas*** cause hyperinsulinism and fasting hypoglycemia.
- ***Glucagonomas*** secrete glucagon and cause ***diabetes and migratory necrolytic erythema***.
- ***VIPomas*** secrete VIP (vasoactive intestinal polypeptide) and cause ***profuse watery diarrhea, hypokalemia, and achlorhydria*** (*WDHA, Verner-Morrison syndrome*).

60. Answer is d (Lateral sinus thrombophlebitis).
Ref: Pediatric Otolaryngology for the Clinician; By Ron B Mitchell, Kevin D Pereira, Pg 234.

- In children, the MC signs and symptoms of ***lateral sinus thrombosis*** include:
  - Intermittent spiking ***'picket fence' fever*** (due to periodic release of hemolytic streptococci) causing intermittent bacteremia in the blood.
  - Headache, vomiting, ***otalgia***, vertigo, diplopia and neck pain.

Also Know

"Named Fevers"

Break bone fever	Dengue
Gaol fever (epidemic typhus)	*R. prowazekii*
Haverhill fever	*Streptobacillus moniliformis*
Monkey fever	Kyasanur forest disease
Oraya fever (Carrion's disease)	*Bartonella baciliformis*
Oriental spotted fever	*R. japonica*
Q fever	*Coxiella burnetii*
Relapsing fever	*Borrelia recurrentis*
Rocky mountain spotted fever	*R. rickettsiae*
Trench fever	*R. quintana*
Undulant fever, Malta fever	*Brucella melitensis*

61. Answer is a (Sickle cell disease).
Ref: Harrison's, 18th edition Pg 854, 2381.

- In ***sickle cell nephropathy, renal papillary necrosis*** may result from ischemia due to ***sickling of red cells in the relatively hypoxemic and hypertonic medullary vasculature*** and ***present with gross hematuria*** and ureteric obstruction by sloughed ischemic papillae.

Major causes of renal papillary necrosis
– Analgesic nephropathy
– Sickle cell nephropathy
– Diabetes with urinary tract infection
– Prolonged NSAID use (rare)

62. Answer is e (wrong options – as per revised answer key).
Ref: Acute Pain Management; edited by Raymond S Sinatr, Pg 76.

- All local anesthetics except cocaine both ***constrict and dilate vascular smooth muscle*** depending on the concentration.
- At reduced concentrations local anesthetics ***inhibit nitric oxide release and cause vasoconstriction***.
- At ***higher concentrations used for regional anesthesia*** these agents cause ***vasodilation***.

63. Answer is b (Air pollution).
Ref: Textbook of Medical Biochemistry, By MN Chatterje, Pg 783.

- ***Soiling index*** is used for ***monitoring air pollution***.
- Smoke concentration is estimated and expressed as microgram per cubic meter of air as an average over a period of time.
- A known volume of air is filtered through a white filter paper under specified conditions and the stain is measured by photoelectric meter.

64. Answer is a (Best corrected visual acuity less than 3/60 in the better eye).
Ref: Parson's, 21st edition Pg 540.

– Parson's says < 1/60 os 'legal blindness' in some countries; and < 3/60 as 'social blindness'; could not find a reference for 3/60 as legal blindness in India – message me/mail me if you find a "PROPER reference" and I will update on my FB page for the benefit of all.

65. Answer is c (Patchy pigmentation).
Ref: Harrison's, 18th edition Pg 3142; CMDT 2013, Pg 1137.

Author's comments: "*The question asks about 'Albright's syndrome'; BUT the options have features of McCune Albright syndrome and Albrights hereditary osteodystrophy also; the answer given as 'pathcy pigmentation' – caf au;lait spots are actually patchy pigmented spots itself – do not know whether this question was challenged OR whether the challenge was not accepted; however the final answer key gave (C) as the answer; BUT I feel (D) maybe a better answer – it would be better if this question would have been scrapped itself*"

McCune Albright syndrome
• ***Gonadotropin-independent precocious puberty*** in females
• ***Polyostotic fibrous dysplasia***
• ***Cafe au lait spots*** (hyperpigmented skin lesions) that are undilateral and respect the midline
• Others: Growth hormone–secreting pituitary adenomas (***acromegaly***), and hypersecreting autonomous ***thyroid nodules*** and adrenal hypersecretion (***Cushing*** syndrome)

- In *pseudohypoparathyroidism type 1a (Albright hereditary osteodystrophy)*: Hypocalcemia and hyperphosphatemia with mental retardation, short stature, obesity, round face, short fourth metacarpals, ectopic bone formation, hypothyroidism, and hypogonadism.

66. Answer is b (0.27%).
Ref: NACO website (National AIDS Control organisation).

- The ***adult HIV prevalence in India is estimated to be 0.27%*** translating into 2.1 million people living with HIV/AIDS in 2011.
- This is ***third highest burden in the world***.
- On the other hand, ***India is highest tuberculosis (TB) burden country in the world*** with an estimated 2.2 million new TB cases occurring annually.

67. Answer is c (MRI scans).
Ref: Musculoskeletal Diseases: Diagnostic Imaging and Interventional Techniques, By Gustav K von Schulthess, et al, 2005 edition Pg 28.

- The term '***bone bruis***' or 'bone contusion' refers to trabecular microfractures due to impaction of bone.
- May occur due to blunt force from outside the body OR more commonly from two bones striking each other after ligament injuries.
- Conventional X-rays cannot detect bone bruises accurately and ***MRI is needed in acute stages***.
- It appears as ill-defined reticulated pattern, isointense to muscle on T1-weighted images and hyperintense on fat-suppressed T2 weighted images called '***bone marrow edema pattern***'.

68. Answer is a *(Epidermophyton floccosum)*.
Ref: Textbook of Microbiology,By CP Baveja, 2nd edition Pg 451.

Dermatophytes
• *Epidermophyton* (affects skin and nails). • *Microsporum* (affects hair and skin) • *Trichophyton* (affects skin, hair, nails) ("TRI= all Three!")

69. Answer is a (Musculocutaneous nerve).
Ref: Gray's Clinical Neuroanatomy; 2011 edition Pg 319.

- ***Dermatome***: The region of skin innervated by sensory afferent fibers from an individual spinal nerve.
- ***Myotomes*** are a group of muscles innervated by a spinal nerve.
- The ***musculocutaneous nerve (C5-C7)*** is formed as a continuation of the ***lateral cord*** of the brachial plexus. It pierces the ***coracobrachialis, supplies it, the biceps and brachialis***; then continues into the ***forearm as the lateral cutaneous nerve of the forearm***.

70. Answer is a (Anterior talofibular).
Ref: Postgraduate Orthopaedics; Paul A Banaszkiewicz, Pg 55.

- ***Anterior talofibular*** is the ***most commonly injured ligament*** around the ankle; ***posterior talofibular*** is the *least commonly injured*.

71. Answer is b (Clinically significant macular edema).
Ref: Parson's, 21st edition Pg 308.

Diabetic Maculopathy:
• Focal, diffuse, ischemic or mixed • ***Clinically significant macular edema (CSME)*** – Retinal edema within 500 μ of center of fovea

– Hard exudates within 500 μ of center of fovea + adjacent area of retinal thickening
– Retinal edema > 1 disk diameter, any part of which lies within 1 DD of center of fovea

Treatment of Diabetic Maculopathy

- *Focal maculopathy*: ***Focal*** argon laser photocoagulation required around the microaneurysms or leaking vessels.
- *Diffuse maculopathy*: ***'Macular-grid' photocoagulation*** required, but avoid the fovea.
- *Ischemic maculopathy*: Photocoagulation will not improve vision; follow-up is necessary as about 30% will develop PDR within 2 years.

72. Answer is a (c-KIT oncogene).
Ref: CMDT 2013; Pg 1620.

Oncogenes

- *Oncogenes* are mutated forms of genes that cause normal cells to grow out of control and become cancer cells. They are mutations of certain normal genes of the cell called **proto-oncogenes**.
- *Proto-oncogenes* are the genes that normally control how often a cell divides and the degree to which it differentiates (or specializes). When a proto-oncogene mutates (changes) into an oncogene, it becomes permanently 'turned on' or activated when it is not supposed to be. When this occurs, the cell divides too quickly, which can lead to cancer.

Common oncogenes

Gene	Associated cancer
c-kit	Gastrointestinal stromal tumor (GIST)
abl	CML
bcl-2	Follicular and undifferentiated lymphomas *(inhibits apoptosis)*
erb-b2	Breast, ovarian and gastric carcinomas
ras	Colon cancer
c-myc	Burkitt's lymphoma
L-myc	Lung cancer
N-myc	Neuroblastoma
ret	MEN types I and II

73. Answer is c (Giant cell infiltration).
Ref: Essentials of Rubin's Pathology, Howard Reisner, 6th edition Pg 600.

– ***Subacute thyroiditis*** - ***DeQeurvain's*** thyroiditis - ***Giant cell thyroiditis*** - are ***synonyms***.
– Numerous foreign body type multinucleated giant cells often containing colloid are present.
– Also Know—***Riedel's thyroiditis*** is a ***fibrosing thyroiditis***.

74. Answer is d (Vesicoureteric junction).
Ref: Smith's Textbook of Endourology, edited by Arthur D. Smith, 2nd edition Pg 216.

- Along the course of the ureter there are three constrictions:
  – At the pelviureteric junction
  – Here the ureter crosses the pelvic brim in the region of the bifurcation of the common iliac artery
  – The ***vesicoureteric junction—narrowest part.***

75. Answer is b (Skirrow's medium).
Ref: Textbook of Diagnostic Microbiology, By Connie R Mahon, Pg 477.

Selective Media

Organism	Medium
Campylobacter jejuni	CAMPY BAP, Skirrow's or Butzler's media; CCD agar
Bacillus anthracis	PLET medium
Bordetella	Bordet gengou medium
Brucella	Casteneda method of blood culture
Chlamydiae	Tissue culture (irradiated McCoy cells, HeLa cells treated with DEAE dextran)
Clostridia (anaerobic organisms)	Robertson's cooked meat broth
Corynebacterium diphtheriae	Loeffler's serum slope Tellurite blood agar
Mycobacterium tuberculosis	Lowenstein Jensen (LJ) medium
Neisseria gonorrheae	Thayer Martin medium Chacko nair medium
Pseudomonas	Cetrimide agar
Rickettsiae	Yolk sac of developing chick embryo
Shigella	Deoxycholate citrate agar (DCA)
Spirochaetes	Noguchi's medium
Staphylococcus	Ludlam's medium
Trypanosomes	Novy, McNeal, Nicole medium
Vibrio (holding or transport media)	Cary Blair medium Venkatraman Ramakrishnan (VR) medium
Transport of streptococci	Pike's medium
To differentiate lactose and non-lactose fermenters	MacConkey's medium

76. Answer is d (Morning stiffness).
Ref: Hutchinson's Clinical Methods, 23rd edition Pg 254.

- ***Early morning joint stiffness*** that persists for ***more than 30 minutes*** is an important sign of ***active inflammatory joint disease.***
- ***Painful range of motion, crepitus*** (clicking in osteoarthritis), and ***bony articular enlargement*** occur in both inflammatory and non-inflammatory joint disease.

77. Answer is a (IgE-secreting clone of plasma cells).
Ref: CMDT 2013, Pg 529.

- Waldenstrom macroglobulinemia is a syndrome of ***IgM hypergammaglobulinemia*** that occurs in the setting of a low-grade non-Hodgkin lymphoma characterized by B cells that are morphologically a hybrid of lymphocytes and ***plasma cells***—these cells characteristically secrete the ***IgM paraprotein.***

Clinical features of Waldenstrom

- Fatigue related to ***anemia***
- ***Hyperviscosity*** of serum: Mucosal and ***gastrointestinal bleeding*** (related to engorged blood vessels and platelet dysfunction)

- Nausea, vertigo and visual disturbances
- Alterations in consciousness vary from mild lethargy to ***stupor and coma***
- Cold agglutinin disease (***hemolysis***) or chronic demyelinating ***peripheral neuropathy*** (due to IgM paraprotein)
- ***Hepatosplenomegaly*** or ***lymphadenopathy***; retinal veins are engorged; purpura may be present
- NO bone tenderness and NO lytic bone lesions

78. Answer is c (Dorsum of fingers).
Ref: Looking for textbook reference; journal reference here – http://ila.ilsl.br/pdfs/v50n1a05.pdf.

➢ ***Ridley and Jopling*** found that in ***long-treated lepromatous patients***, bacilli were more frequently detected in the *fingers*.

79. Answer is a (Pericarditis).
Ref: Harrison's, 18th edition Pg 2729-30.

- MC *cardiac* manif of SLE = ***Pericarditis***
- MC ***respiratory*** manif of SLE = Pleurisy with/without effusion
- MC ***hematologic*** manif of SLE = Anemia
- Most ***SERIOUS*** manif of SLE = Nephritis.

80. Answer is a (Non-steroidal anti-inflammatory drugs).
Ref: CMDT 2013, Pg 750.

- ***Primary dysmenorrhea*** is ***menstrual pain*** a/w menstrual cycles in the ***absence of pathologic findings***.
- ***NSAIDs*** (ibuprofen, ketoprofen, mefenamic acid, naproxen) and the COX-2 inhibitor ***celecoxib*** are generally helpful. The medication should be started 1–2 days before expected menses. Symptoms can also be suppressed with the use of oral contraceptive pills.
- <u>**Note**</u>: ***Secondary dysmenorrhea*** is menstrual pain for which an ***organic cause exists***, often a/w ***endometriosis or uterine fibroids***.

81. Answer is a (Esophageal atresia with fistula to the distal esophagus).
Ref: OP Ghai's, 7th edition Pg 151.

- ***MC type*** of ***esophageal atresia*** is ***distal pouch communicating (fistula) with the trachea***.
- There may be ***maternal h/o polyhydramnios***.
- ***Saliva pours continuously*** from the mouth, ***regurgitation of first feeds*** occurs.
- ***VATER*** – Vertebral defects imperforate Anus, TracheoEsophageal fistula, Radial and Renal dysplasia.
- ***Immediate surgical correction*** is required.

82. Answer is b (Low blood C3 levels).
Ref: Nephrology Secrets; By Edgar V Lerma, Allen R Nissenson, Pg 116.

Criteria for performing renal biopsy in a child with nephrotic syndrome prior to treatment are:

- Age < 6 months
- Onset in adolescence
- Low C3 level
- Any unusual clinical feature.

<u>Note</u>: Most pediatricians defer a renal biopsy since minimal change disease is the MC cause of nephrotic syndrome in children and responds to steroid treatment.

83. Answer is a (Common extensor origin).
Ref: Maheswari, 4th edition Pg 293.

TEnnis Elbow (LaTEral epicondylitis)	– Inflammation where the ***common extensor tendon arises*** from ***lateral epicondyle*** of humerus. – ***Cozen's test:*** Pain at the lateral epicondyle when the patient extends his clenched fist against resistance. – ***Mill's Maneuver:*** Pain at the lateral epicondyle when patient's wrist is passively flexed with forearm is pronated. This gives rise to severe pain at attachment of common extensor tendons.
Golfer's elbow	– ***Medial*** humeral epicondylitis.
Student's elbow	– ***Olecranon bursitis*** (goose egg swelling at the tip of the elbow).
Pulled elbow / Nursemaid's elbow	– ***Subluxation of the head of radius*** from its encirclement by annular ligament in ***young children (< 6 years)***; occurs from sudden pull on upper limb by adult as to prevent from falling or trying to carry with one hand.
Little leaguers elbow	– *Avulsion of* ***medial epicondyle of humerus.***

84. Answer is b *(Culex vishnui).*
Ref: Park's textbook of PSM, 22nd edition Pg 261.

- In S***outh India***, the main vectors of ***Japanese encephalitis*** are ***Culex tritaeniorhynchus and Culex vishnui.***
- The ***rice fields*** are the *most important breeding places.*

85. Answer is b (Ragi).
Ref: Park, 22nd edition Pg 581.

- ***Ragi*** is one of the ***cheapest millets***; used ***widely in AP and Karnataka***; it is ***richest in calcium***.

86. Answer is d (High myopia).
Ref: Parson's diseases of the eye, 21st edition Pg 223.

Staphyloma

Staphyloma refers to a ***localized bulging (ectasia)*** of weak and thin outer tunic of the eyeball (cornea or sclera) lined by uveal tissue, which shines through the thinned out fibrous scar coat.

Staphyloma	Definition
• Anterior	A protrusion of the cornea with incarceration of the iris
• Intercalary	Ectasia of the sclera with incarceration of the root of the iris
• Ciliary	Ectasia of the sclera with incarceration of the ciliary body
• Equatorial	Ectasia of the sclera with incraceration of the choroids
• Posterior	Bulge of the weak sclera lined by choroid behind the equator, seen MC in ***high myopia***

87. Answer is d (ETA epithelial receptor).
Ref: Textbook of Pulmonary Vascular Diseases, Jason X et al, Springer publication, Pg 120.

- Endothelin-1 (ET-1) has been reported to induce pulmonary artery vasoconstriction via ETA receptor.
- Bosentan is an endothelin receptor antagonist approved for treating pulmonary artery hypertension.

88. Answer is b (From 1½ to 2 years age).
Ref: CMDT 2013, Pg 1177.

- ***Cryptorchism (undescended testes)***: One or both testes may be absent from the scrotum.
- ***Cryptorchism should be corrected before age 12–24 months*** in an attempt to ***reduce the risk of infertility.***

Also Note

- If the testes are not palpable, ***ultrasound or MRI*** can be used to locate them.
- Alternatively, ***hCG, 1500 units intramuscularly*** daily for 3 days, causes a *significant rise in testosterone, if the testes are present.*
- ***Therapy with hCG*** results in a ***testicular descent rate of about*** 25%.
- Cryptorchid testes increase the lifetime risk of ***testicular neoplasia*** (0.06%) and intra-abdominal testes have a much higher risk (5%). Orchiopexy decreases the risk of neoplasia when performed before 10 years of age.
- Retractile testes is different from cryptorchism and requires no treatment.

89. Answer is d (Superior intercostal vein).
Ref: http://radiopaedia.org/articles/aortic-nipple

- ***Aortic nippLE*** is seen as a small soft-tissue density adjacent to the lateral border of the aortic knob on a ***PA chest radiograph*** in up to ***10% of normal patients.***
- It represents the ***LEft superior intercostal vein.***

90. Answer is b (Plasma transferrin).
Ref: CMDT 2013, Pg 492.

Differential Diagnosis of Anemias

Tests	Iron deficiency	Thalassemia	Chronic disease	Sideroblastic
Serum iron	↓	N or ↑	↓	↑
Serum ferritin	↓	N	N or ↑	↑
TIBC (transferrin)	↑	N	↓	↓
Morphology	Microcytic, hypochromic	Microcytic, hypochromic with target cells	Normocytic	Variable, ringed sideroblasts

Also Know

- ***Mentzer index*** = MCV/RBC count; < 13 in thalassemia; > 13 in the rest of above.
- ***Zieve's syndrome:*** During withdrawal from prolonged alcohol abuse; defined by *hemolytic anemia, hyperlipoproteinaemia (excessive blood lipoprotein), jaundice and abdominal pain.*

91. Answer is b (Demeclocycline).
Ref: Harrison's, 18th edition Pg 349, 743, 828.

- ***Demeclocycline inhibits the effect of ADH*** on the ***distal tubule.***
- Onset of action may require 1 week, and urinary concentrating ability may be ***permanently impaired,*** resulting in ***nephrogenic diabetes insipidus*** and even ***hypernatremia.***
- Cirrhosis may increase the nephrotoxicity of demeclocycline.

92. Answer is d (*Mycobacterium ulcerans*).
Ref: Harrison's, 18th edition Pg 1067, 1369.

- ***M. ulcerans*** is a ***waterborne skin pathogen,*** found mainly in the tropical areas of ***Africa.***
- Infection follows ***skin trauma or insect bites*** that allow admission to ***contaminated water.***
- The skin lesions are ***typically painless, clean ulcers*** (***Buruli ulcer***) that slough and can cause osteomyelitis.
- The ***toxin mycolactone*** accounts for the modest host inflammatory response and the painless ulcerations.

93. **Answer is d (Sequential appearance of features of increasing malignancy).**
Ref: Robbins pathology, 7th edition Pg 288.

- The term ***tumor progression*** refers to "***sequential appearance of features of increasing malignancy***".

94. **Answer is c (12 weeks).**
Ref: Harrison's, 18th edition Pg 256-57.

- ***Acute rhinosinusitis defined as sinusitis of < 4 weeks' duration***—constitutes the vast majority of sinusitis cases.
- ***Chronic sinusitis*** is characterized by symptoms of ***sinus inflammation lasting > 12 weeks***. This illness is most commonly associated with either bacteria or fungi and clinical cure in most cases is very difficult.
- Also see question ***number 75 in Comed-K 2013*** paper.

95. **Answer is a (Ankylosing spondylitis).**
Ref: CMDT 2013, Pg 854.

Spondyloarthropathies

These disorders are noted for
- Striking a/w ***HLA-B27***
- ***Male*** predominance
- Onset usually ***before age 40***
- Inflammatory arthritis of the spine or the large peripheral joints (or both)
- ***Enthesopathy*** (inflammation of where ligaments, tendons, and joint capsule insert into bone)
- ***Uveitis*** in a significant minority
- **Absence of rheumatoid factor** in the serum (*hence 'seronegative'*).

Seronegative spondyloarthropathie[Q]***s*** are:
- Ankylosing spondylitis
- Psoriatic arthritis
- Reactive arthritis (***Reiter syndrome***)
- Arthritis a/w inflammatory bowel disease
- Undifferentiated spondyloarthropathy

96. **Answer is b (Metabolic alkalosis).**
Ref: Mayo Clinic Internal Medicine Concise Textbook, edited by Thomas M Habermann, Pg 313.

- ***Type I*** glycogen storage disease (AR): ***Glucose-6-phosphatase deficiency*** in liver, kidney, and intestinal mucosa.
- ***Type Ia***: Glucose-6-phosphatase enzyme is defective.
- ***Type Ib***: ***Translocase*** that transports glucose-6-phosphate across the microsomal membrane is defective.

Clinical features:
- ***Hypoglycemia and lactic acidosis*** during the neonatal period.
- Children usually have ***doll-like faces*** with fat cheeks, relatively thin extremities, short stature, and a protuberant abdomen that is due to ***massive hepatomegaly***.
- The ***kidneys are enlarged***, but the spleen and heart are of normal size.
- ***Easy bruising and epistaxis*** are associated with a prolonged bleeding time as a result of ***impaired platelet aggregation/adhesion***; ***menorrhagia*** occurs later in life.
- ***Hyperuricemia*** is present—leads to ***gout***.
- ***Hyperlipidemia*** includes elevation of triglycerides, cholesterol and phospholipids—leads to ***pancreatitis***; increased risk of ***CVS disease***.
- Type Ib patients have additional findings of ***neutropenia*** and impaired neutrophil function, resulting in recurrent bacterial ***infections***, oral and intestinal mucosal ulceration.
- GSD I patients may experience ***intermittent diarrhea***, which can worsen with age. In GSD Ib, it is largely due to loss of mucosal barrier function caused by inflammation.
- ***Puberty*** is often ***delayed***. Nearly all females have ultrasound findings consistent with ***polycystic ovaries***.

Glycogen Storage Disease

Disease	Enzyme deficient	Comments
Disorders with hepatomegaly and hypoglycemia		
Von Gierke's (type 1)	Glucose-6-phosphatase	Hepatomegaly and severe fasting hypoglycemia
Cori's, Forbe's - Limit dextrinosis (type 3)	Amyloglucosidase (debranching enzyme)	Hepatomegaly and hypoglycemia
Her's (type 6)	Liver phosphorylase	
Disorders with muscle-energy impairment		
McArdle's (type 5) *M*'s	*M*uscle glycogen phosphorylase	*M*uscle cramps, *M*yoglobinuria, *M*ale preponderance, exercise intolerance; compensated hemolysis in Tarui's
Tarui's (type 7)	Phosphofructokinase	
Disorders with skeletal and cardiac muscle impairment		
Pompe's (type 2) (Pumpe's = "*pump*" failure)	Acid a glucosidase (acid maltase)	Skeletal muscle weakness, severe cardiomegaly and failure
Disorders with liver cirrhosis		
Anderson's amylopectinosis	Amylotransglucosidase	Failure to thrive, hepatomegaly, progressive liver cirrhosis and failure (usually death before 5th year)

97. Answer is d (Doxacurium).

Ref: Miller's Basics of Anesthesia, Pg 154.

- ***Mivacurium*** is one of the shortest acting neuromuscular blocking agents available; it is unique among non-depolarizing agents in that it is metabolized by ***plasma cholinesterase*** similar to ***succinylcholine***.
- ***Doxacurium*** is ***NOT*** *metabolized by plasma cholinesterase.*
- ***Atracurium*** is metabolized by ***non-specific plasma esterases*** and also by ***Hoffman elimination***.

98. Answer is a (Static neurological disease).

Ref: Cleveland Clinic Intensive Review of Pediatrics, 4th edition Pg 29.

Absolute contraindications to pertussis vaccine are:

a. Immediate ***anaphylactic*** reaction to previous dose of vaccine
b. ***Progressive*** neurologic disorder
c. ***Encephalopathy*** occurring within 7 days of the vaccine.

99. Answer is d (Pregnant women).

Ref: Park, 22nd edition Pg 318.

- The primary drivers and risk groups of HIV infection in India are:
  - Unprotected paid sex/commercial female sex workers
  - Unprotected sex between men
  - Injecting drug use.

100. Answer is d (Neutrophil).
Ref: Essentials of Rubin's Pathology, By Howard Reisne, Pg 49.

- ***Polymorphonuclear leukocytes*** are ***rapidly recruited*** from the bone marrow, localize at the wound site by binding to activated endothelium and invade the wound site within the 1st day.

101. Answer is c (To treat hypocarbia with respiratory alkalosis).
Ref: various textbooks combined

Therapeutic uses of CO_2

- ***Laparoscopic surgery*** involves insufflation of a gas (***usually carbon dioxide***) into the peritoneal cavity producing a pneumoperitoneum.
- A very effective way to ***minimize air embolism during cardiac surgery*** is to ***flood the operative field with*** CO_2.
- ***Debubbling***: Generally, a 100% CO_2 flush of the arterial line filter, membrane oxygenator, and tubing for several minutes is used to remove all room air from the bypass circuit.
- ***Carbogen***, also called ***Meduna's mixture*** after its inventor Ladislas Meduna, is a mixture of carbon dioxide and oxygen gas. A ***carbogen mixture of 95% oxygen and 5% carbon dioxide*** can be used as part of the early treatment of ***central retinal artery occlusion and in radiotherapy to overcome radioresistance***.
- To ***facilitate vasodilation*** and thus lessen the degree of metabolic acidosis during the induction of ***hypothermia.***
- To ***prevent hypocapnia during hyperventilation.***
- For clinical and physiological investigations.
- In ***gynecological investigation*** for ***insufflation into fallopian tubes and abdominal cavities.***
- As ***solid carbon dioxide (dry ice) in tissue freezing techniques*** and for the ***destruction of warts by freezing***.
- To ***increase cerebral blood flow*** in arteriosclerotic patients undergoing surgery.
- To stimulate respiration after a period of apnea.
- In chronic respiratory obstruction after it has been relieved.
- To increase depth of anesthesia rapidly when volatile agents are being administered. It increases depth of respiration and helps to overcome breathholding and bronchial spasm.
- To facilitate blind intubation in anesthetic practice.

102. Answer is d (At 18 months of age).
Ref: Hutchison's Paediatrics, By Gupta Goel, Pg 7.

- The ***anterior fontanel*** close by ***18 months of age***.
- ***Posterior fontanel*** are fused by ***3 months of age***.

103. Answer is e (none—as per revised answer key).
Ref: Dhingra's ENT textbook, 5th edition Pg 182.

- Various test for allergic rhinitis are total and differential count, absolute eosinophil count, eosinophils in nasal smears, RAST, etc.

104. Answer is c (Babesiosis).
Ref: CMDT 2013, Pg 1499.

- ***Babesiosis*** is an ***intraerythrocytic infection*** caused mainly by two *Babesia* species (*B.microti and B.divergens*) and ***transmitted by Ixodes ticks.***

Also Know

Mosquito Borne Diseases

Type of mosquito	Disease
Anopheles	Malaria
Culex	Bancroftian filariasis Japanese encephalitis West Nile fever Viral arthritis (epidemic polyarthritis)
Aedes	Yellow fever (not in India) Dengue Dengue hemorrhagic fever Chikungunya fever Chikungunya hemorrhagic fever Rift valley fever Filaria (not in India)
Mansonoides	Malayan (Brugian) filariasis Chikungunya fever

105. Answer is d (Covalent modification).
Ref: Vasudevan's biochemistry, 7th edition Pg 64.

- ***Zymogen activation*** by partial proteolysis is an example of ***covalent modification***.
- The ***MC type of covalent modification*** is the ***reversible protein phosphorylation***.

106. Answer is c (Suction evacuation).
Ref: Dutta's, 6th edition Pg 175, 561.

- MTP method up to **42 *days***: ***Manual vacuum aspiration***.
- ***Menstrual regulation*** can be done for < 42 days gestation.
- ***Medical methods*** like mifepristone and misoprostol—within 50 days of gestation.
- ***Dilatation and evacuation*** is more commonly used for incomplete abortion.
- ***Suction evacuation*** is used more commonly for ***first trimester MTP***.

107. Answer is d (Akathisia).
Ref: Kaplan & Sadock's Concise Textbook of Clinical Psychiatry, 3rd edition Pg 158-60.

Positive symptoms	Negative symptoms
• Characterized by excessive function; positive symptoms include delusions, hallucinations, strange behavior and talkativeness. • These symptoms ***respond well*** to treatment with ***antipsychotic agents***.	• Characterized by decreased function; negative symptoms include: – ***Affective flattening*** – Attention impairment – ***Avolition apathy*** (lack of initiative) – Anhedonia (inability to experience pleasure) – Asociality (social withdrawal) – ***Alogia*** (lack of speech output). • Negative symptoms ***respond better to atypical antipsychotics*** like clozapine, olanzapine, quetiapine and risperidone.

- **Note**: Akathisia is characterized by a subjective desire to be in constant motion followed by an inability to sit or stand still and consequent pacing—motor restlessness. It is seen as a side effect of antipsychotics and SSRIs.

108. Answer is c (Bagassosis).
Ref: CMDT 2013, Pg 310.

Pneumoconiosis

- Particles > 5μ are filtered in upper airways and < 1μ can remain suspended, and are exhaled.
- Particles ***1-5μ settle in the alveoli as the most potentially dangerous*** particles.

Inorganic dusts	
Coal dust	Anthracosis
Silica	Silicosis
Asbestos	Asbestosis
Iron	Siderosis
Organic dusts	
Sugarcane fiber (bagasse)	Bagassosis (a/w *Thermoactinomyces sacchari and T. vulgaris)*
Cotton dust	Byssinosis ('Monday chest tightness')
Tobacco	Tobaccosis
Hay or grain dust	Farmer's lung (a/w *thermophilic actinomycetes and Micropolyspora faeni*)

109. Answer is b (Quantitative buffy coat test).
Ref: Panicker's textbook of medical parasitology, 7th edition Pg 80.

- The ***quantitative buffy coat test*** developed by Bectin Dickinson USA, is a new simplified method for diagnosing malaria.
- It is ***faster and more sensitive*** than peripheral blood smear.
- In this test, the centrifuged buffy coat is stained with a fluorochrome (e.g acridine orange), which lights up malarial parasites when viewed under UV light.
- *P. falciparum* specific, histidine-rich protein 2 (*PfHRP2*) or ***lactate dehydrogenase*** antigens in finger-prick blood samples—***sensitivity is similar to or lower*** than that of thick films.

110. Answer is b (Cardiac tamponade).
Ref:CMDT 2013, Pg 421.

- In ***cardiac tamponade***, the ECG often reveals non-specific T wave changes and low QRS voltage.
- ***Electrical alternans*** is present uncommonly, but is ***pathognomonic*** due to the heart swinging within the large effusion.
- Repeat question from Comed-K 2013.

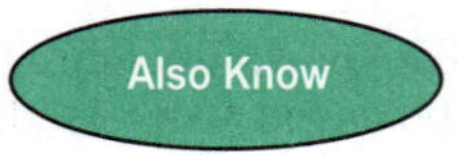

ECG Abnormalities

HyPERKalemia	***Tall, tented T-wave,*** decreased P-wave amplitude, widening of QRS, ***"sine wave pattern"*** (severe hyperkalemia causing cardiac arrest) (**"***Cadbury's* **PERK** with **T**ea**"**)

Hypokalemia	Prominent ***U-waves***, small T-waves, ventricular bigemini
*Hyper***calcemia**	***Shortens*** Q-T interval
*Hypo***calcemia**	***Lengthens*** Q-T interval
Subarachnoid hemorrhage	Marked QT prolongation with deep, wide T-wave inversions (***"CVA T-wave"***)
Hypothermia	Convex elevation of ***J point*** (J waves or Osborn waves)
Pericardial effusion	Total ***electrical alternans*** (often with tamponade)
TCA overdose	Sinus tachycardia with QRS and QT prolongation
Digoxin effect	Shortened QT interval with a characteristic "scooping" of the ST-T wave complex ST depression PR prolongation Inverted T-wave (***inverted check mark sign***) in V5-6 *QT (cutie!) Chhoti, depressed ST, PRolonged PR, ulta T)*
Pulmonary embolism	***MC: Sinus tachycardia with an otherwise normal ECG*** There may be deep S-waves in I, pathological Q-waves in III, inverted T-waves in III ('SIQIIITIII'), strain pattern V1-V3, right axis deviation, RBBB, atrial fibrillation
Syn. a/w prolonged QT interval	***Romano ward syn.*** (AD) and ***Jervell Lange Neilsen syn.*** (AR, congenital deafness)
Lev's disease and Lenegre's disease	Degenerative diseases commonly responsible for damage to the specialized conducting system and produce AV block usually associated with bundle branch block
Right bundle branch block (RBBB)	More common than LBBB; RBBB occurs with heart disease, both congenital (e.g. atrial septal defect) and acquired (e.g. valvular, ischemic)
Left bundle branch block (LBBB)	LBBB is often a marker of one of four underlying conditions: Ischemic heart disease, long-standing hypertension, severe aortic valve disease and cardiomyopathy

111. Answer is c (von Willebrand disease).
Ref: CMDT 2013, Pg 551.

- ***Platelet adhesion*** is mediated primarily by ***von Willebrand factor (vWF)***, a large multimeric protein present in both plasma and the extracellular matrix of the subendothelial vessel wall, which serves as the primary ***"molecular glue"***.
- ***vWD*** is the ***MC inherited bleeding disorder***; MC type of vWD is ***type 1 disease***.
- Patients have predominantly ***mucosal bleeding symptoms***. Bleeding symptoms are very uncommon in infancy and usually manifest ***later in childhood with excessive bruising and epistaxis***.
- Individuals with vWD will usually have ***normal PT, platelet count, thrombin time and fibrinogen level***. Some individuals may have ***prolonged aPTT*** that corrects in a mixing study. While a prolonged aPTT is consistent with vWD, the aPTT may be normal in untreated mild or moderate disease and alone cannot exclude vWD.

112. Answer is b (Isoniazid).
Ref:New pediatric guidelines - tbcindia.nic.in/Paediatric%20guidelines_New.pdf

- Under RNTCP, the currently recommended dose of ***INH for chemoprophylaxis is 10 mg/kg*** (instead of currently recommended dosage of 5 mg/kg) administered daily for 6 months. TB preventive therapy should be provided to:
  1. All asymptomatic contacts (under 6 years of age) of a smear positive case, after ruling out active disease and irrespective of their BCG, TST or nutritional status.
  2. Chemoprophylaxis is also recommended for all HIV-infected children who either had a known exposure to an infectious TB case or are tuberculin skin test (TST) positive (> = 5 mm induration) but have no active TB disease.
  3. All TST positive children who are receiving immunosuppressive therapy (e.g. children with nephritic syndrome, acute leukemia, etc.).
  4. A child born to mother who was diagnosed to have TB in pregnancy should receive prophylaxis for 6 months, provided congenital TB has been ruled out. BCG vaccination can be given at birth even if INH chemoprophylaxis is planned.

113. Answer is d (Carnitine).
Ref: Clinical Infertility and In Vitro Fertilization; edited by Botros RMB Rizk, Hassan N Sallam, Pg 87.

Structure	Marker
Prostatic function	Acid phosphatase, zinc, citric acid
Seminal vesicle function	Fructose, prostaglandins
Epididymal function	free L carnitine; glycerophosphocholine, neutral alpha glucosidase

114. Answer is a (Enfuvirtide).
Ref: CMDT 2013, Pg 1346.

ANTIRETROVIRAL DRUGS (ANTI-HIV AGENTS)

1. **Nucleoside Reverse Transcriptase Inhibitors (NRTIs)**	– Drugs: Abacavir Didanosine Emtricitabine Lamivudine, , Stavudine, Tenofovir Zalcitabine, Zidovudine – Mechanism: NNRTIs inhibit the reverse transcriptase enzyme; prevent incorporation of viral genome into host DNA
2. **Nonnucleoside Reverse Transcriptase Inhibitors (NNRTIs)**	– Drugs: Etravirine, Delavirdine, Efavirenz, Nevirapine, Rilpivirine – Mechanism: NNRTIs inhibit the reverse transcriptase enzyme; prevent incorporation of viral genome into host DNA
3. **Protease Inhibitors (PIs)**	– Drugs: Saquinavir, Ritonavir, Indinavir, Nelfinavir, Amprenavir, Tipranavir, Lopinavir, Fosamprenavir, Darunavir, Atazanavir – Mechanism: Inhibit assembly of new virus by blocking protease in progeny virions
4. **Entry Inhibitors - Fusion Inhibitors**	– Drug: ***Enfuvirtide*** – Mechanism: Bind viral gp41 subunit; inhibit conformational change required for fusion with CD4 cells, therefore block entry and subsequent replication – Clinical use: IN patients with persistent viral replication in spite of antiretroviral therapy; used in combination with other drugs
5. **Entry Inhibitors - CCR5 antagonists**	– Drug: ***Maraviroc*** – Mechanism: Specifically, maraviroc blocks the chemokine receptor CCR5, which HIV uses as a coreceptor to bind and enter a human helper T cell
6. **Integrase inhibitors**	– Drug: ***Raltegravir, dolutegravir*** – Mechanism: Raltegravir inhibits integrase, and prevents the integration of viral genetic material into human chromosomes also called strand transfer inhibitors (this refers to the process of DNA strand transfer from the viral genome to the host genome); the drug is metabolized away via glucuronidation

115. Answer is c (Km is independent of enzyme concentration).
Ref: Food Chemistry, By HD Belitz, Werner Grosch, Pg 119.

- In Michaelis Menton equation, the rate of reaction when the enzyme is saturated with substrate is the maximum rate of reaction, **Vmax**.
- The relationship between rate of reaction and concentration of substrate depends on the affinity of the enzyme for its substrate. This is usually expressed as the **Km** (Michaelis constant) of the enzyme, an inverse measure of affinity.
- For practical purposes, Km is the concentration of substrate, which permits the enzyme to achieve ***half Vmax.***
- ***Km is independent*** of ***enzyme concentration***.
- An enzyme with a ***high Km has a low affinity for its substrate***, and requires a greater concentration of substrate to achieve Vmax.

- The Km of an enzyme, relative to the concentration of its substrate under normal conditions permits prediction of whether or not the rate of formation of product will be affected by the availability of substrate.
- *An enzyme with a low Km* relative to the physiological concentration of substrate is normally saturated with substrate, and will act at a more or less constant rate, regardless of variations in the concentration of substrate within the physiological range.
- *An enzyme with a high Km* relative to the physiological concentration of substrate is not normally saturated with substrate, and its activity will vary as the concentration of substrate varies, so that the rate of formation of product will depend on the availability of substrate.
-

116. Answer is c (Normal).

Ref: http://www.cdc.gov/healthyweight/assessing/bmi/childrens_bmi/about_childrens_bmi.html

– BMI-for-age weight status categories and the corresponding percentiles are shown in the following table.

Weight Status Category	Percentile Range
Underweight	Less than the 5th percentile
Healthy weight	5th percentile to less than the 85th percentile
Overweight	85th to less than the 95th percentile
Obese	Equal to or greater than the 95th percentile

117. Answer is c (Depth of invasion).

Ref: Rubin's pathology, 6th edition Pg 629.

- The term '***early gastric cancer***' is strictly a ***pathologic diagnosis*** based on the ***depth of invasion***.
- The term does NOT refer to the duration of the disease, its size, presence of symptoms, absence of metastases or curability.
- Up to 20% of early gastric cancers have ***already metastasized*** to the regional lymph nodes by the time of diagnosis.
- The term ***'superficial spreading carcinoma'*** is a synonym.

118. Answer is c (Capgras syndrome).

Ref: Textbook of Postgraduate Psychiatry (2 Vols), By Vyas, Ahuj, Pg 226.

Capgras syndrome: Delusion of doubles

- MC in ***women***, MC in ***paranoid schizophrenia***, also seen in delusional disorders, Lewy body dementia, Alzheimer's dementia.
- ***Illusion des sosies:*** The person sees a familiar person (caregiver) as a stranger who is imposing as the caregiver.
- ***Illusion de Fregoli:*** The person falsely identifies strangers as familiar persons.

119. Answer is b (Bronze).

Ref: Knight's Forensic Pathology, 3rd edition Pg 12.

- Patients with ***clostridial sepsis*** are often *jaundiced (due to hemolysis) and that in combination with cutaneous vasodilation and pallor* produces a ***peculiar bronze skin discoloration***.

Also Know

Color of hypostasis	Poisoning
Cherry red	Carbon monoxide
Bright red/Brick red	Hydrocyanic acid; potassium cyanide; cyanide
Dark brown (chocolate)	Phosphorus
Red brown	Aniline, nitrates, potassium chloride/bicarbonate, nitrobenzene

Deep blue	CO_2 (aniline also as per some books)
Bluish green	Hydrogen sulfide (H_2S)
Black	Opium
Clostridial sepsis	Bronze

Note: Aniline and chlorate can cause various colors of hypoastasis !

120. Answer is c (Anti-HBc).
Ref: CMDT 2013, Pg 668.

HEPATITIS B SEROLOGY

■ HBsAg	*First virologic marker detectable in serum* after infection with HBV (even before elevation of serum aminotransferase and clinical symptoms appear) Indicates ***active hepatitis B infection***, either acute or chronic (> 6 months)
■ Anti-HBs	Antibody to HbsAg. Provides ***immunity to hepatitis B***. *Persists for years*
■ HBcAg	*Not routinely detectable* in blood
■ Anti-HBc	***First antibody*** to appear; ***Positive during the window period*** ***IgM anti-HBc*** is an indicator of ***recent disease***, IgG anti-HBc signifies chronic disease
■ HBeAg	Indicates ***active viral replication and high infectivity*** (**Be**ware!)
■ Anti-HBe	When present in HBsAg carrier, blood is potentially less infectious
■ ***PrEcorE mutants***	In hepatitis B are characterized by notable ***absence*** of HbEAg[Q]

121. Answer is c (Combined adrenal medullary insufficiency and glucagon deficiency).
Ref: Harrison's, 18th edition Pg 3006.

- ***Hypoglycemia-associated autonomic failure*** (HAAF) in diabetes: Recent antecedent iatrogenic hypoglycemia (by ***large dose insulin*** or sleep or prior exercise) causes both ***defective glucose counterregulation*** (by ***reducing the epinephrine response*** to a given level of subsequent hypoglycemia in the setting of ***absent insulin and glucagon responses***) and ***hypoglycemia unawareness*** (by reducing the sympathoadrenal response to a given level of subsequent hypoglycemia).
- These impaired responses create a vicious cycle of recurrent iatrogenic hypoglycemia.
- Also refer Fig 345-2 in Harrison's 18th edition for an excellent flowchart explanation.

122. Answer is b (Astrocytes).
Ref: Lippincott's Illustrated Q&A Review of Anatomy and Embryology, Pg 22.

GERM LAYER DERIVATIVES

ECTODERM	
Surface ectoderm	Epidermis, hair, nails, inner and external ear, tooth enamel, lens of the eye, anterior pituitary (from Rathke's pouch), parotid gland
Neurectoderm	Neural tube: CNS, retina and optic nerve, pineal gland, neurohypophysis, ***astrocytes***, oligodendrocytes
Neural crest	Adrenal medulla, ganglia (autonomic and sensory), melanocytes, Schwann cells, meninges (pia, arachnoid), pharyngeal arch cartilage, odontoblasts, parafollicular C cells, aorticopulmonary septum, endocardial cushions, chromaffin cells of adrenal medulla

MESODERM	Muscle (smooth, cardiac, skeletal), connective tissue, serous membranes, bone and cartilage, blood, lymph, cardiovascular organs, adrenal cortex, gonads and internal repoductive organs, spleen, kidney and ureter, dura mater
ENDODERM	Epithelial parts: GI tract, thymuc, tonsils, pharynx, larynx, trachea, bronchi, lungs, urinary bladder, urethra, tympanic cavity, auditory tube and other pharyngeal pouches Parenchyma: Liver, pancreas, thyroid, parathyroid, tonsils, glands of GI tract, submandibular an sublingual glands

123. Answer is a (Cachexia).
Ref: Jeffocoate, 6th edition Pg 644-45.

- ***Pituitary apoplexy***, either as a consequence of an infarcted pituitary adenoma or transient reduction in the blood supply of the pituitary during surgery or after ***rapid blood loss associated with parturition*** is termed Sheehan's syndrome.
- So symptoms of ***hypopituitarism*** will be there – ***low BMR*** (due to decreased TSH); ***infertility*** due to decreased gonadotropins; ***pallor*** (due to ACTH deficiency and blood loss-related anemia).
- Cachexia is not a part of this syndrome.

124. Answer is a (Mucicarmine).
Ref: Textbook of Microbiology & Immunology, By Parija, Pg 635.

- ***Mucicarmine stain*** is used to stain the mucinous capsule of ***Cryptoccoccus neoformans*** especially in tissues.
- ***India ink*** negative staining is used to detect ***budding yeast cells in the CSF***.

125. Answer is b (The pathological features are most prominent in the renal cortex).
Ref: CMDT 2013, Pg 930.

- ***FSGS*** accounts for ***35% cases of nephritic syndrome*** in adults.
- ***Angiotensin-converting enzyme inhibitors (ACEIs)*** and ***angiotensin receptor blockers (ARBs)*** are agents that ***reduce proteinuria*** because of their antihypertensive and intrarenal hemodynamic effects of reducing glomerular capillary pressure and resistance.
- ***Minimal change disease*** patients typically respond to corticosteroids, with ***excellent long-term prognosis***.
- Untreated FSGS has a progressive course leading to end-stage renal disease.
- The ***'tip' variant of FSGS*** has better prognosis compared to other variants of FSGS.

126. Answer is a (Meyer-Overton rule).
Ref: Stoelting's Clinical anesthesia, 7th edition Pg 109.

- More than 100 years ago, ***Meyer and Overton*** independently observed that the potency of gases as anesthetics was strongly correlated with their solubility in ***olive oil***.
- The ***Meyer-Overton rule*** states that the potency of anesthetic gases is ***proportional to their lipid solubility***.

127. Answer is a (Sertraline).
Ref: KD Tripathi, 7th edition Pg 461-63.

Classification of Antidepressants

Selective serotonin reuptake inhibitors (**SSRIs**)	Fluoxetine, Fluvoxamine, Paroxetine, Sertraline, Citalopram, Escitalopram
Tricyclic antidepressants : *NA and Serotonin reuptake inhibitors*	Imipramine, Nortriptyline (best tolerated), Amitriptyline, Desipramine, Protriptyline, Trimipramine, Clomipramine, Doxepine
Tetracyclic antidepressants	Amoxapine, Maprotiline, Mianserin
Selective serotonin noradrenaline	Duloxetine, Venlafaxine, Milnacipran

Reuptake inhibitors (**snris**)	
Noradrenaline reuptake inhibitors (**NARI**)	Reboxetine
5-HT2 antagonist	Nefazodone, Trazodone
Dopamine and NA reuptake inhibitors	Bupropion
Melatonin receptor ***agonist*** and 5-HT2c antagonist	Agomelatin

128. Answer is d (Framingham Heart Study).
Ref: Park's, 22nd edition 72, 77, 342.

- The ***Framingham heart study*** is a ***classic example of a cohort study***.
- The cohort design is always a ***follow-up study with forward directionality.***
- The cohort study can be *prospective or retrospective.*
- The Framingham heart study is a ***prospective cohort study*** because the study began before the health outcome occurred.
- It gave us knowledge of the ***risk factors for cardiovascular disease***.

129. Answer is c (T1cN1bM0).
Ref: AJCC TNM staging for Breast Cancer.

Primary Tumor

TX	Primary tumor cannot be assessed
T0	No evidence of primary tumor
Tis	Carcinoma *in situ*
Tis (DCIS)	DCIS
Tis (LCIS)	LCIS
Tis (Paget)	Paget disease of the nipple NOT associated with invasive carcinoma and/or carcinoma *in situ* (DCIS and/or LCIS) in the underlying breast parenchyma. Carcinomas in the breast parenchyma associated with Paget disease are categorized based on the size and characteristics of the parenchymal disease, although the presence of Paget disease should still be noted
T1	Tumor ≤ 20 mm in greatest dimension
T1mi	Tumor ≤ 1 mm in greatest dimension
T1a	Tumor > 1 mm but ≤ 5 mm in greatest dimension
T1b	Tumor > 5 mm but ≤ 10 mm in greatest dimension
T1c	Tumor > 10 mm but ≤ 20 mm in greatest dimension
T2	Tumor > 20 mm but ≤ 50 mm in greatest dimension
T3	Tumor > 50 mm in greatest dimension
T4	Tumor of any size with direct extension to the chest wall and/or to the skin (ulceration or skin nodules)[c]
T4a	Extension to the chest wall, not including only pectoralis muscle adherence/invasion
T4b	Ulceration and/or ipsilateral satellite nodules and/or edema (including peau d'orange) of the skin, which do not meet the criteria for inflammatory carcinoma
T4c	Both T4a and T4b
T4d	Inflammatory carcinoma

Regional Lymph Nodes

Clinical	
NX	Regional lymph nodes cannot be assessed (e.g. previously removed)
N0	No regional lymph node metastases
N1	Metastases to movable ipsilateral level I, II axillary lymph node(s)
N2	Metastases in ipsilateral level I, II axillary lymph nodes that are clinically fixed or matted
	OR
	Metastases in clinically detected[b] ipsilateral internal mammary nodes in the *absence* of clinically evident axillary lymph node metastases
N2a	Metastases in ipsilateral level I, II axillary lymph nodes fixed to one another (matted) or to other structures
N2b	Metastases only in clinically detected[b] ipsilateral internal mammary nodes and in the *absence* of clinically evident level I, II axillary lymph node metastases
N3	Metastases in ipsilateral infraclavicular (level III axillary) lymph node(s) with or without level I, II axillary lymph node involvement
	OR
	Metastases in clinically detected[b] ipsilateral internal mammary lymph node(s) with clinically evident level I, II axillary lymph node metastases
	OR
	Metastases in ipsilateral supraclavicular lymph node(s) with or without axillary or internal mammary lymph node involvement
N3a	Metastases in ipsilateral infraclavicular lymph node(s)
N3b	Metastases in ipsilateral internal mammary lymph node(s) and axillary lymph node(s)
N3c	Metastases in ipsilateral supraclavicular lymph node(s)

Regional Lymph Nodes (Pathologic)

pNx	Regional lymph nodes cannot be assessed (e.g. previously removed or not removed for pathologic study)
pN0	No regional lymph node metastasis identified histologically
pN1	Micrometastases
	OR
	Metastases in 1–3 axillary lymph nodes
	AND/OR
	Metastases in internal mammary nodes with metastases detected by sentinel lymph node biopsy, but not clinically detected
pN1mi	Micrometastases (> 0.2 mm and/or > 200 cells but none > 2.0 mm)
pN1a	Metastases in 1–3 axillary lymph nodes, at least one metastasis > 2.0 mm
pN1b	Metastases in internal mammary nodes with micrometastases or macrometastases detected by sentinel lymph node biopsy, but not clinically detected
pN1c	Metastases in 1–3 axillary lymph nodes and in internal mammary lymph nodes with micrometastases or macrometastases detected by sentinel lymph node biopsy, but not clinically detected
pN2a	Metastases in 4–9 axillary lymph nodes (at least 1 tumor deposit > 2 mm)

pN2b	Metastases in clinically detected[d] internal mammary lymph nodes in the *absence* of axillary lymph node metastases
pN3a	Metastases in ≥ 10 axillary lymph nodes (at least 1 tumor deposit > 2.0 mm)
	OR
	Metastases to the infraclavicular (level III axillary lymph) nodes
pN3b	Metastases in clinically detected[d] ipsilateral internal mammary lymph nodes in the *presence* of one or more positive axillary lymph nodes
	OR
	Metastases in > 3 axillary lymph nodes and in internal mammary lymph nodes with micrometastases or macrometastases detected by sentinel lymph node biopsy but not clinically detected[c]
pN3c	Metastases in ipsilateral supraclavicular lymph nodes

Distant metastases

M0	No clinical or radiographic evidence of distant metastases
cM0(i+)	No clinical or radiographic evidence of distant metastases, but deposits of molecularly or microscopically detected tumor cells in circulating blood, bone marrow, or other non-regional nodal tissue that are ≤ 0.2 mm in a patient without symptoms or signs of metastases
M1	Distant detectable metastases as determined by classic clinical and radiographic means and/or histologically proven > 0.2 mm

130. Answer is c (Temperature more than 40°C).
Ref: Current Management in Child Neurology; edited by Bernard L Maria; Pg 101, Epilepsy in Children, 2nd edition By Sheila J Wallace; Pg 127.

RISK OF RECURRENCE OF FEBRILE SEIZURES

- Family h/o febrile seizures
- First seizure before 1 year of age
- Brief duration (< 1 h) between onset of recognized fever and seizure
- Temperature (the lower the fever, the higher the risk of recurrence)
- Complex seizure.

Note: Initial temperature > 40°C is a/w a DECREASED risk of recurrence.

131. Answer is a (Pallor and atrophy of the substantia nigra).
Ref: CMDT 2013, Pg 998.

- In Parkinson disease there is a ***degeneration of the dopaminergic nigrostriatal*** system
- Given in the case history are the signs and symptoms of Parkinson disease:
  - ***Bradykinesia*** (slow dressing, feeding, writing, walking)
  - ***Mask-like*** face
  - Rigidity (***cogwheel***)
  - ***Tremor*** (*pill rolling, resting*)
  - ***Shuffling gait*** (small steps and involuntary gait acceleration after starting)
  - Postural instability and stooping
  - *Depression*
  - ***Micrographia*** (smaller handwriting compared to earlier)
  - ***Myerson sign***: Repetitive *tapping over the bridge of the nose* produces a *sustained blink response*.

For questions 132–135

A 33-year-old woman presented with a 4-day history of fever and abdominal pain, 7 days after undergoing a cesarean section. She had diffuse erythroderma, and the blood pressure was 85/48 mm Hg. A workup revealed elevated creatinine and liver-enzyme levels. Her condition worsened over the next day, with acute respiratory distress; subsequently, desquamation of her hands occurred.

132. Answer is d (Toxic shock syndrome).
133. Answer is a (*Staphylocccus aureus*).
134. Answer is a (Floxacillin).
135. Answer is a (Vaginal swab).

Ref: http://www.nejm.org/doi/pdf/10.1056/NEJMicm1213758 - DIRECT PICK.

Explanation:
The case history given is that of staphylococcal toxic shock syndrome. As seen by the explanation below, all the clinical features fit into the picture. However I feel a "vaginal swab" would not be of benefit in "non-menstrual TSS".

Case definition of *Staphylococcus aureus* toxic shock syndrome (TSS)

1. ***Fever***: Temperature of >/= 38.9°C (>/= 102°F).
2. ***Hypotension***: Systolic BP of 90 mm Hg, ororthostatic hypotension (orthostatic drop in diastolic blood pressure by 15 mm Hg, orthostatic syncope, or orthostatic dizziness).
3. ***Diffuse macular rash***, with ***desquamation*** 1–2 weeks after onset (including the palms and soles).
4. Multisystem involvement:
    a. Hepatic: Bilirubin or aminotransferase levels 2 times normal.
    b. Hematologic: Platelet count 100,000/L.
    c. Renal: Blood urea nitrogen or serum creatinine level 2 times the normal upper limit.
    d. Mucous membranes: Vaginal, oropharyngeal, or conjunctival hyperemia.
    e. Gastrointestinal: Vomiting or diarrhea at onset of illness.
    f. Muscular: Severe myalgias or serum creatine phosphokinase level 2 times the upper limit.

- More than 90% of menstrual cases are caused by ***TSST-1***, whereas a high percentage of non-menstrual cases are caused by enterotoxins.
- Although originally associated with tampon use, any focus (e.g. nasopharynx, bone, vagina, rectum, abscess or wound) harboring a toxin-producing *S. aureus* strain can cause toxic shock syndrome.
- Classically, ***blood cultures are negative*** because symptoms are due to the effects of the toxin and not systemic infection.
- ***Floxacillin*** is also called flucloxacillin and is used for treating staphylococcus infections.

For questions 136 – 137

An 85-year-old male cigar smoker with no notable medical history presented with black discoloration and hairy appearance of the tongue, which had lasted several years. He said he did not use bismuth-containing compounds.

136. Answer is d (Lingua villosa nigra).
137. Answer is a (Topical antibiotics).

Ref: http://www.nejm.org/doi/full/10.1056/NEJMicm050117.

Explanation:
The case history given is that of "Lingua villosa nigra !". Another direct pick from NEJM website - link above. NOT a routinely asked topic/queston !

- ***Black hairy tongue***, also known as ***lingua villosa nigra***, is a painless, benign disorder caused by defective desquamation and reactive hypertrophy of the filiform papillae of the tongue.

- Clinically: Abnormal ***brownish-black*** coating of the dorsal surface of the tongue.
- Etiology: Use of topical or systemic antibiotics as well as psychotropic agents, dehydration, hyposalivation, trigeminal neuralgia, poor oral hygiene, smoking, ingestion of alcohol and infections.
- Symptoms: Nausea, halitosis, dysgeusia and unattractive appearance of the tongue.
- Treatment options: *Increasing hydration and salivation,* ***discontinuing smoking****, brushing the tongue with a soft toothbrush enhanced by previous application of* ***40% urea****, applying* ***topical retinoids or salicylic acid****, or undergoing surgical excision.*

For questions 138 – 140

A 55-year-old man presented with a two-day history of headache, fever and generalized weakness. He had received a cadaveric kidney transplant 5 years earlier. His medications included 5 mg of tacrolimus twice a day and 10 mg of prednisone daily. On neurologic examination, he was confused and incoherent. Cranial nerves were normal, but he had a hazy left retina. Magnetic resonance imaging of the brain with the administration of gadolinium showed multiple-enhancing lesion in both cerebral hemispheres.

138. Answer is c (*Nocardia asteroides* infection).
139. Answer is a (Weakly positive acid-fast bacilli).
140. Answer is a (Trimethoprim-sulfamethoxazole).

Ref: http://www.nejm.org/doi/full/10.1056/NEJMicm990952 and HPIM - multiple pages - I have consolidated the info below for you.

Explanation:
The case history given is that of a late infection in a renal transplant recipient and its subsequent manifestations. Another direct pick from NEJM. The case history/clinical vignette given is that of ***cerebral nocardiosis***. This can be confused with cerebral toxoplasmosis due to the setting of immunosuppression and enhancing lesions on MRI. However, the quote from Harrison's given below states that toxoplasmosis typically occurs early after transplantation (here the infection is occurring after 5 years); also the second question under this case talks about subretinal abscesses whereas in toxoplasmosis subretinal abscess is very rare (chorioretinitis and vitritis may be seen). Other features in favor of nocardiosis are given below. Refer explanation below.

Harrison's, 17th/848 = 'Toxoplasmosis can occur in seropositive patients, but is ***less common than in other transplant settings, usually developing in the first few months after kidney transplantation***'.

Opportunistic infection in renal transplant recipients

Early (1–6 months)	Late (> 6 months)
• *Pneumocystis carinii*	• *Aspergillus*
• Cytomegalovirus	• ***Nocardia***
• *Legionella*	• BK virus (polyoma)
• *Listeria*	• Herpes zoster
• Hepatitis B	• Hepatitis B
• Hepatitis C	• Hepatitis C

- In ***immunocompromised hosts*** with underlying HIV infection, ***organ transplantation***, cancer or immunosuppressive therapy, most brain abscesses are caused by ***Nocardia* species**, *Toxoplasma gondii, Aspergillus* species, *Candida* species and *C. neoformans.*
- On contrast- enhanced T1-weighted MRI, a mature ***brain abscess*** has a ***capsule that enhances surrounding a hypodense center*** and surrounded by a hypodense area of edema. On T2-weighted MRI, there is a hyperintense central area of pus surrounded by a well-defined hypointense capsule and a hyperintense surrounding area of edema.
- The ***hazy left retina*** suggest ***endophthalmitis—Nocardia*** can cause ***subretinal abscess and ednophthalmitis***.

- The first step in diagnosis is examination of sputum or pus for crooked, branching, beaded, gram-positive filaments; most nocardiae are ***acid fast in direct smears, if a weak acid is used*** for decolorization (e.g. in the modified Kinyoun, Ziehl-Neelsen, and Fite- Faraco methods).
- *Sulfonamides:* Combination of ***sulfamethoxazole (SMX) and trimethoprim (TMP) is the drug of choice***.

For questions 141–143

A 47-year-old woman was referred for bone pain and abnormal findings on radiography. The patient reported that for the past 17 years, she has habitually consumed water from that area. She reported a 5-year history of pain in the lower back, arms, legs and hips. Because of brittleness, all her teeth had been extracted. Radiography of the forearm revealed interosseous membrane calcification and radiography of the spine revealed a rugger-jersey appearance (striated pattern of increased density in the upper and lower zones of the vertebrae).

141. Answer is b (Fluorosis).
142. Answer is b (Change in source of water).
143. Answer is d (Renal damage).

Ref: Manson's Tropical Diseases: Expert Consult - Online; By Jeremy Farrar, 204 edition Pg 1034; Textbook Of Orthopaedics By Kotwal; Pg 108.

Explanation:
The case history given is that of a patient with bone and teeth findings associated with water consumption – straightforward question especially with looking at the questions and options below.

- Ingestion of excess fluoride, most commonly in drinking water can cause fluorosis, which affects the teeth and bones. Moderate amounts lead to dental effects, but long-term ingestion of large amounts can lead to potentially severe skeletal problems. Paradoxically, low levels of fluoride intake help to prevent dental caries. The control of drinking water quality is therefore critical in preventing fluorosis.
- ***Dental fluorosis*** is caused by taking in too much fluoride over a long period when the teeth are forming under the gums. Only children aged 8 years and younger are at risk because this is when permanent teeth are developing under the gums.
- Adult fluorosis results in mottled and pitted defects in tooth enamel as well as brittle bone (skeletal fluorosis).
- Early skeletal fluorosis—***discomfort and parasthesiae in the limbs and trunk***; restriction of spine movements is the earliest clinical sign.
- ***Renal tubular damage and chronic kidney disease*** have been attributed to fluorosis.
- Radiological signs include increased bone density – osteosclerosis; osteopenia/osteoporosis; trabecular blurring or haziness; compact bone thickening; periosteal bone formation and ossification of the attachments of tendons, ligaments, and muscles; ***interosseous membrane calcification***; ossification of the posterior longitudinal ligament
- There is no specific drug treatment; changing source of water is necessary.

For questions 144 - 145

A 65-year-old man presented with skin lesions on his chest, left arm and shoulder 6 weeks after returning from a vacation in Belize at the beach in the rain forest. The lesions occasionally stung, drained a dark exudates, and enlarged despite 2 weeks of treatment with cephalexin. The patient had no constitutional symptoms. Physical examination revealed five nodules of varying sizes with surrounding erythema and a central pore through which a single, moving larva was observed.

144. Answer is a (Bot fly).
145. Answer is a *(Dermatobia hominis).*

Ref: Harrison's 18th edition Pg 3578.

Explanation:
The case history given is that of an insect bite. Although you will have to wonder where is Belize located! Refer the explanation from Harrison's below; for such cases the options should help you find the answer.

- *Myiasis* refers to infestations by diverse kinds of fly larvae (maggots) that invade living or necrotic tissue or body cavities.
- In forested parts of ***Central and South America (Belize is IN Central America)*** , ***larvae of the human botfly Dermatobia hominis*** produce ***boil-like subcutaneous nodules*** 3 cm in diameter.
- A sensation of ***movement under the patient's skin*** may lead to severe emotional distress. Botfly larvae may be induced to emerge if the ***air pore*** is coated with petrolatum or another occlusive substance.
- Removal may be facilitated by injection of a local anesthetic into the surrounding tissue, but surgical excision is often necessary because upward-pointing spines of some species hold the larva firmly in place.

<u>For questions 146 – 147</u>

A 40-year-old male complains of a vague dragging sensation in his abdomen for the last 6 months. There was no history of fever, renal colic or dysuria. Physical examination reveals a blood pressure at 150/96 mm Hg.

Renal ultrasound: Bilaterally enlarged kidneys with multiple cysts.

Urine analysis: Protein +; WBCs 4/HPF (Normal: < 5/HPF); RBCs 10/HPF (Normal: < 5/HPE).

146. Answer is a (Intracranial aneurysms).
147. Answer is c (Ischemia to renal medulla).

Ref: CMDT 2013, Pg 599.

<u>Explanation</u>:
The case history given is that of a young patient with hypertension, hematuria and proteinuria with cystic enlarged kidneys – polycystic kidney disease. Refer explanation below.

Autosomal Recessive (Childhood) Polycystic Kidney	<u>A</u>utosomal <u>D</u>ominant (<u>AD</u>ult) polycystic kidney
Genetics	
– *ARPKD gene – chromosome* ***6p***. – *Gene defect – PKHD1,* which produces fibrocystin (polyductin) – (***PKHD***1 = **P**olycystic **K**idney **H**epatic **D**isease 1)	– ***APKD-1 gene*** on chromosome ***16p*** – *"'Polycystic kidney' =* ***16*** *letters* = ***16p"*** – *Gene defect – PKD1 and PKD2, which code for polycystin 1 and 2* – Phenotypic heterogeneity is a hallmark of ADPKD, as evidenced by family members who share the same mutation, but have a different clinical course
Clinically	
– Diagnosed in ***first year of life*** presenting as *bilateral abdominal masses* – Enlarged, with ***small cysts, < 5 mm, limited to the collecting tubules*** – ***Death*** *in neonatal* period is MC due to ***pulmonary hypoplasia*** – ***HTN occurs in first few years of life*** – Longer-term survivors frequently develop ***portal hypertension, esophageal varices, and hypersplenism from periportal fibrosis***	– *<u>DOES NOT</u> manifest before 30 years.* – Manifests disease as ***renomegaly, flank pain. Hematuria, infection, hypertension, uremia***
Associated abnormalities	
– ***Congenital hepatic fibrosis*** – Maternal oligohydramnios – Potter's syndrome	– *Hepatic cysts* (also cysts in spleen, pancreas, ovaries) – (*MC extrarenal anomaly*) – *Intracranial* ***berry aneurysms*** – *Mitral valve prolapse* – *Colonic diverticula*

Imaging	
– U/s shows large, echogenic kidneys – The diagnosis can be made *in utero after 24 weeks of gestation in severe cases*, but cysts generally become visible ONLY AFTER birth – The absence of renal cysts in either parent on ultrasonography helps to distinguish ARPKD from ADPKD in older patients	– IVU – *"spider-leg"* deformity – The sensitivity of renal ultrasonography for the detection of ADPKD is 100% for subjects 30 years or older with a positive family history – Before the age of 30 years, CT scan or T2-weighted MRI is more sensitive for detecting presymptomatic disease

148. Answer is a (Herpes simplex virus).
Ref: CMDT 2013, Pg 1350-52.

- The case history is that of an ***STD in a homosexual man***—explanation below.
- ***HSV-2 lesions*** largely involve the genital tract, with the virus remaining latent in the presacral ganglia.
- The lesions consist of small, ***grouped vesicles*** that can occur anywhere but which most often occur on the vermilion border of the lips (Figure 6–15), the ***penile shaft, the labia, the perianal skin,*** and the buttocks.
- ***Intranuclear inclusion bodies and multinucleated giant cells*** on a Tzanck preparation or Calcofluor stain are indicative of herpetic infection.

149. Answer is d (Pancreas).
Ref: CMDT 2013, Pg 1350-52.

- ***Hypoglycemic symptoms***—frequently neuroglycopenic (confusion, blurred vision, diplopia, anxiety, convulsions).
- Common signs of hypoglycemia include ***diaphoresis and pallor. Heart rate and systolic blood pressure are typically increased,*** but may not be raised in an individual who has experienced repeated, recent episodes of hypoglycemia. Neuroglycopenic manifestations are often observable. Transient focal neurologic deficits occur occasionally.
- Neurogenic (or autonomic) symptoms of hypoglycemia:
  – Adrenergic symptoms: ***Palpitations, tremor, and anxiety***
  – Cholinergic symptoms: ***Sweating, hunger and paresthesias***.
- Clearly, these are non-specific symptoms. Their attribution to hypoglycemia requires a ***corresponding low plasma glucose concentration*** and their resolution after the glucose level is raised (***Whipple's tria***d).
- Immediate recovery occurs upon administration of glucose.

150. Answer is c (5-alpha-reductase).
Ref: CMDT 2013, Pg 959.

- ***Finasteride*** is a ***5 alpha-reductase inhibitor*** that blocks the conversion of testosterone to dihydrotestosterone.
- This drug acts upon the epithelial component of the prostate, resulting in ***reduction in size of the gland and improvement in symptoms***.
- ***6 months of therapy is required*** for maximum effects on prostate size (20% reduction) and symptomatic improvement.

151. Answer is b (Ovarian choriocarcinoma).
Ref: Shaw's gynecology, 15th edition Chapter 19.

- A ***60-year-old lady*** in the question is not in favor of gestational choriocarcinoma.
- A ***gestational ovarian choriocarcinoma*** may represent a metastasis from a uterine choriocarcinoma or much rarely arise from an ovarian ectopic pregnancy.
- ***Primary ovarian choriocarcinoma*** (non-gestational ovarian choriocarcinoma) arises presumably from a germ cell and is extremely rare. These may be mixed with other germ cell tumors such as immature teratoma, dysgerminoma or rarely occur in a pure form—pure primary choriocarcinoma of the ovary.
- The tumors are formed from placental trophoblastic elements—***serum β-HCG levels are often elevated.***
- The disease may present by way of its metastasis.

- *Neurological symptoms* such as hemiplegia, epilepsy, headache and visual disturbances suggests brain metastasis.
- *Pulmonary symptoms* may resemble pulmonary tuberculosis (*dyspnea and hemoptysis*). The *'cannon ball'* metastasis is typical of a malignant lesion.

152. Answer is b (Urinalysis).
Ref: Dutta, 6th edition Pg 221-223.

- The case history is that of *hypertension in pregnancy*.
- Mild *preeclampsia* is classically defined as *third trimester BP of > 140 systolic or > 90 diastolic* on two occassions at least 6 hours apart accompanied by *proteinuria > 300 mg/24 h* and *non-dependent edema* (face and/or hands).
- *Headache* can be a symptom of sever preeclampsia.

<u>For questions 153–154</u>

A 35-year-old male with a history of severe bronchial asthma for several months now complains of weight gain and the development of purple stretch marks. Physical examination showed BP – 149/95 mm Hg, supraclavicular fullness. The skin was thinned out with areas of bruising. Neurological examination revealed decreased strength in the proximal muscles. Laboratory investigation showed reduced serum cortisol and reduced plasma ACTH.

153. Answer is c (Hypokalemia).
154. Answer is c (Iatrogenic cause).

Ref: Harrison's, 17th edition Pg 2212.

<u>Explanation</u>:
The case history given is that of chronic asthmatic and symptoms and signs of Cushing's syndrome likely due to steroid dependance.

Cushing's Syndrome

- ↑ glucocorticoids due to various causes such as

↓ ACTH	↑ ACTH
• *<u>Iatrogenic</u>* (chronic steroid use); <u>MC cause of Cushing's syndrome</u> • Primary adrenal (hyperplasia/neoplasia)	• *<u>Cushing's disease</u>* (primary pituitary adenoma) • Ectopic ACTH production (small cell lung Ca)

- **Clinically**
  - HTN, weight gain, moon facies, truncal obesity, supraclavicular fats pads, buffalo hump, purple skin striae, hyperglycemia (insulin resistance), osteoporosis, amenorrhea, proximal myopathy, muscle wasting, posterior subcapsular cataracts, hypokalemic alkalosis and immune suppression.

155. Answer is b (Absence of parathyroid glands).
Ref: CMDT 2013, Pg 1137.

- *Acquired hypoparathyroidism* is *MC seen following thyroidectomy*. when it is usually transient, but may be permanent.

- Manifestations of *hypocalcemia* include ***tetany, muscle cramps, carpopedal spasm, irritability, altered mental status, convulsions, and stridor; tingling of the circumoral area, hands and feet*** is almost always present.
- ***Chvostek sign*** (***facial muscle contraction on tapping the facial nerve in front of the ear***) is positive.
- ***Trousseau phenomenon*** (carpal spasm after application of a sphygmomanometer cuff) is present.
- ***Serum calcium is low, serum phosphate high, urinary calcium low and alkaline phosphatase normal.***

156. Answer is d (RET oncogene).
Ref: CMDT 2013, Pg 1189.

- The case history gives ***episodic hypertension*** characteristic of ***pheochromocytoma, mucosal neuromas*** on oral mucosa and ***intestinal symptoms***.
- ***MEN 2B*** is a ***familial, autosomal dominant multiglandular syndrome*** that is caused by a mutation of the ***ret protooncogene (RET) on chromosome 10***.
- ***MEN 2B*** is characterized by ***mucosal neuromas with bumpy and enlarged lips and tongue, Marfan-like habitus***, adrenal ***pheochromocytomas*** and ***medullary thyroid carcinoma.***
- Patients also have ***intestinal abnormalities*** such as intestinal ganglioneuromas, skeletal abnormalities and delayed puberty.
- Medullary thyroid carcinoma is aggressive and presents early in life. Therefore, infants having a parent with MEN 2B receive genetic screening; those carrying the ***RET mutation*** undergo a prophylactic total thyroidectomy by age of 6 months.

157. Answer is a (Segmental sclerosis of some of the glomeruli).
Ref: Harrison's, 18th edition, Pg 1553.

- The case history given is that of a ***HIV-positive patient*** with ***signs of nephritis (edema, proteinuria***—normal 24-hour urine protein is about 80 mg/24 h).
- The MC type of glomerular affection in HIV is ***focal segmental glomerulosclerosis (HIV-associated nephropathy***—HIVAN, FSGS). ***Proteinuria*** is the hallmark of HIVAN.
- Here the kidney would show ***segmental sclerosis of some of the glomeruli***.

158. Answer is c (Parasitic infection).
Ref: CMDT 2013, Pg 1638.

Three types of bladder cancer and risk factors are:

- ***Transitional cell carcinoma*** is MC; a/w ***cigarette smoking***, exposure to ***industrial dyes***; chronic ***cyclophosphamide*** exposure.
- ***Pure squamous cell carcinoma***: Tend to be solid and nearly always associated with muscle invasion. A/w chronic ***Schistosoma hematobium*** exposure, chronic irritation by ***vesical calculi, leukoplakia*** of bladder and chronic ***catheter*** use.
- ***Pure adenocarcinoma*** usually arises in the fundus of the bladder at the site of *urachal remnant*.

159. Answer is d (Secretion of PTH-related peptide).
Ref: Harrison's, 18th edition Pg 742-43.

- ***Chronic smoker*** with ***hilar mass*** points towards ***lung cancer***.
- Signs and symptoms are those of ***hypercalcemia*** due to hyperparathyroidism, which is usually as a paraneoplastic syndrome a/w lung cancer.
- Classic mnemonic for clinical features of hyperparathyroidism is mnemonic "***stones*** (kidney stones , loin pain), ***bones*** (bone changes), ***abdominal groans*** (constipation, nausea, vomiting, pancreatitis), and ***psychiatric moans*** (CNS symptoms of psychosis, delirium, confusion)".

- Hence the answer here is secretion of PTH-related peptide, which is the mechanism of paraneoplastic syndrome in lung cancer.

160. Answer is b (MRI of the brain).
Ref: CMDT 2013, Pg 1159.

- The case history is that of ***Cushing's syndrome*** (*actually Cushing's disease by definition*). The signs fit into cortisol excess—truncal obesity, proximal muscle weakness, etc.
- For clinical features of Cushing's refer answer number 154 above.
- The diagnosis is ***ACTH-producing pituitary adenoma,*** hence can be detected ***by MRI of the brain***.

Dexamethasone suppression test
– *Healthy*: ↓ cortisol after low dose
– *ACTH-producing pituitary adenoma*: ↑ cotisol after low dose, ↓ cortisol after high dose
– *Ectopic ACTH-producing tumor* (small cell lung Ca): ↑ cortisol after low and high dose
– *Cortisol-producing adrenal tumor*: ↑ cortisol after low and high dose

<u>For questions 161–163</u>

An 87-year-old woman with severe retrosternal pain and intermittent dysphagia was referred to the clinic for further evaluation. She described paroxysms of crampy pain almost exclusively during the intake of solid foods. In the past several months, she noted a weight loss of 5 kg. Endoscopy revealed a pronounced helical configuration of the esophageal lumen. High-resolution manometry of the esophagus showed high-amplitude pressure waves, this patient had normal relaxation of the esophagogastric junction.

161. Answer is d (Nutcracker esophagus).
162. Answer is d (Corkscrew appearance).
163. Answer is c (Treatment with long-acting diltiazem).

Ref: http://www.nejm.org/doi/full/10.1056/NEJMicm1210209

<u>**Explanation**</u>:
"This is a direct pick from the above New England Journal of Medicine website link above. Pls refer that; anyway I have given the explanation below also".

- Nutcracker esophagus presents similar to diffuse esophageal spasms and is a manometric diagnosis.
- The ***pathognomonic feature on esophageal motility study*** is ***prolonged (> 7 seconds) high amplitude pressure waves (> 180 mm Hg)***.
- The lower esophageal sphincter shows normal resting pressure.
- The tertiray esophageal contractions are seen radiologically as ***corkscrew*** esophagus and ***helical configuration on endoscopy*** (NOTE: Classically corkscrew appearance on barium swallow is a/w diffuse esophageal spasm).
- Symptomatically, chest pain and dysphagia to solids and liquids is present.

<u>For questions 164–166</u>

A 6-hour-old term male baby was observed to have yellowish discoloration of the skin up to the knee joints. He was born to a 30-year-old woman who had an abortion 2 years ago. The woman said she had an uneventful pregnancy and went for antenatal check up only once. She came in advanced labor to the emergency ward where the baby was delivered. There was no prolonged rupture of membranes and the baby cried immediately after birth and accepted breast feeds soon after.

164. Answer is b (Rh hemolytic disease).
165. Answer is b (9–12 mg/dL).
166. Answer is a (Start phototherapy).

Ref: OP Ghai, 5th edition Pg 123.

Explanation:
A classic case of erythroblastosis fetalis.

Erythroblastosis Fetalis

- ***Hemolytic disease of the newborn*** (erythroblastosis fetalis) is caused by blood group incompatibility between the mother and fetus.
- ***Maternal IgG crosses the placenta*** and *destroys fetal erythrocytes.*
- An **Rh negative mother** carrying an **Rh positive fetus** is at highest risk.
- Risk increases when fetal blood crosses into the maternal circulation as in ***abortion, ectopic pregnancy, amniocentesis and motor vehicle accidents.***
- Affected neonates present with anemia, hyperbilirubinemia, hepatosplenomegaly, pulmonary edema and ascites.
- The **direct Coombs'** test is positive.
- Treat with exchange transfusions *(refer indications below).*
- Prevent disease with **anti-Rh IgG injections** for high-risk mothers at 28 weeks of delivery, *and at any other time of exposure to fetal blood.*
- Management of ABO HDN is usually successful with phototherapy alone provided by modern equipment.

Also Know

- Level of jaundice correlates with bilirubin level
- Visual jaundice indicates total bilirubin > 4 mg/dL
- Jaundice above nipple line: Bilirubin < 12 mg/dL
- Head and neck jaundice: 6 mg/dL bilirubin
- Trunk to umbilicus: 9 mg/dL bilirubin
- Trunk to knees: 12 mg/dL bilirubin
- Wrists and ankles: 15 mg/dL bilirubin
- Hands and feet: > 15 mg/dL bilirubin.

For questions 167 – 168

A 3-year-old female child sleeping in a thatched hut woke up in the middle of the night screaming. Her mother thought the child had a nightmare and tried to pacify her. After sometime she noticed that the child was sweating profusely and the hands were becoming cold. Child also vomited a couple of times. The mother immediately rushed the child to the emergency services. Her pulse was 150/minute and her BP 90/60 mm Hg.

167. Answer is d (Scorpion envenomation).
168. Answer is b (Prazosin).

Ref: CMDT 2013, Pg 1590.

Explanation:
The case history given is that of an envenomation—cannot be septic shock or food poisoning as per the history. Snake venom - maybe hemotoxic or neurotoxic and symptoms are slightly different—ptosis, dysphagis diplopia OR coagulopathy with local bleeding/redness. Hence scorpion sting would fit as the answer here".

- Scorpion venom is ***neurotoxic.***
- Such envenomations usually are a/w ***little swelling, but prominent pain, paresthesia,*** and hyperesthesia can be accentuated by tapping on the affected area (the tap test).
- Dysfunction of ***cranial nerves and hyperexcitability of skeletal muscles*** develop within hours.
- Patients present with restlessness, blurred vision, abnormal eye movements, profuse salivation, lacrimation, rhinorrhea, slurred speech, difficulty in handling secretions, diaphoresis, nausea and vomiting. Muscle twitching, jerking, and shaking may be mistaken for a seizure.
- Complications: ***Tachycardia, hypertension,*** arrhythmias, hyperthermia, rhabdomyolysis and acidosis.

- Fetal *respiratory arrest* is most common among young children and the elderly.
- Hypertension and pulmonary edema respond to ***nifedipine, nitroprusside, hydralazine or prazosin***, and bradyarrhythmias can be controlled with atropine.

For questions 169 – 171

An 8-year-old girl was brought to the hospital for puffiness of eyes and swelling of legs of 2 days duration. Mother said she was passing only small quantities of urine. Her urine was high colored and microscopic examination showed RBC and granular casts.

169. Answer is b (Acute glomerulonephritis).
170. Answer is b (Hypertensive encephalopathy).
171. Answer is b (Normal C3 levels).

Ref: Partha's Fundamentals of Pediatrics, By K Parthasarathy, Pg 336-37.

Explanation: Classical example of acute glomerulonephritis.

- ***Hematuria*** with RBC casts (smoky urine).
- ***Edema*** usually appears abruptly and first involves the periorbital area, but it may be generalized.
- ***Oliguria***: Azotemia (Rise in serum creatinine and blood urea nitrogen a/w a reduction in GFR).
- ***Proteinuria*** (1–2 g/24 h).
- ***Hypertension: Hypertensive encephalopathy*** can be the presenting feature of postinfectious glomerulonephritis; the most serious early complication of this disease. In these patients, hypertension is usually severe and is accompanied by signs of CNS dysfunction such as headache, vomiting, depressed sensorium, confusion, visual disturbances, aphasia, memory loss, coma, and convulsions.
- The mechanism of hypertension is most likely retention of sodium and water with resulting expansion of the extracellular space—***dilutional hyponatremia.***
- Laboratory features: ***Raised ASLO titer; low complement C3 levels.***

For questions 172 – 174

A 3-year-old girl is brought for diarrhea of 2 weeks duration. She weighs 8 kg and her height is 93 cm.

172. Answer is c (Severe malnutrition).
173. Answer is a (Hypoglycemia).
174. Answer is b (10% dextrose).

Ref: OP Ghai, 7th edition Pg 69; http://www.indianpediatrics.net/pdf/severe_acute_malnutrition.pdf

- As per the WHO weight for height charts, this falls under ***acute severe malnutrition***.
- All severely malnourished children are at risk for ***hypoglycemia***.
- Symptomatic hypoglycemia manifests as ***lethargy, seizures and unconsciousness; pallor and sweating*** are rare, but may occur; ***peripheral circulatory failure*** and hypothermia (normal body temperature is 37°C) may occur.
- Hypoglycemia, infection and ***hypothermia*** generally occur as a triad.
- Treat with ***10% glucose solution***.

For questions 175–177

A 5-year-old boy was found to have a pansystolic murmur in the left lower sternal border during routine school health checkup. He is asymptomatic and has normal development. His ECHO showed a small muscular ventricular septal defect.

175. Answer is c (No intervention).
176. Answer is b (Muscular).
177. Answer is a, b (Left ventricle, left atrium).

Ref: Partha's fundamentals of pediatrics, K. Parthasarathy, Pg 208-09.

Explanation:
The case history given is that of a VSD, which is already mentioned.

- VSDs can be small or large:
  - *Small VSDs* do not cause problems and often may close on their own. Because small VSDs allow only a small amount of blood to flow between the ventricles, they are sometimes called restrictive VSDs. Small VSDs do not cause any symptoms.
  - *Medium VSDs* are less likely to close on their own. They may require surgery to close and may cause symptoms during infancy and childhood.
  - *Large VSDs* allow a large amount of blood to flow from the left ventricle to the right ventricle. They are sometimes called non-restrictive VSDs. A large VSD is less likely to close completely on its own, but it may get smaller over time. Large VSDs often cause symptoms in infants and children, and surgery usually is needed to close them.
- *Small muscular VSDs* have the *greatest likelihood of spontaneous closure*, with closure rates approaching 80–90% by age 2 years.
- *Enlargement* of both *left atrium and left ventricle* occurs.
- **Modified Soto's classification:**
  - Perimembranous (infracristal or subaortic): 80%
  - Muscular: 10%
  - Outlet (supracristal or subpulmonic): 5%
  - Inlet: 5%

For questions 178 – 180

A 3-day-old female baby was brought got oozing of blood from umbilical stump. The mother said she noticed blood stained discharge from the nose when the baby sneeze. Baby did not have bleeding earlier. She was feeding and passing urine and stools normally. Her sleep was adequate.

178. Answer is c (Classical hemorrhagic disease of the newborn).
179. Answer is c (Give vitamin K).
180. Answer is a (Factors II, VII, IX and X).

Ref: Partha's fundamentals of pediatrics, K. Parthasarathy, Pg 40.

Explanation:
The case history is that of newborn bleeding. A 3-day-old female baby with symptoms mentioned falls into classical hemorrhagic disease of the newborn HDN.

Early-onset hemorrhagic disease of the newborn (HDN)
- This usually occurs *during first 24 hours* after birth; seen in infants born to mothers taking *warfarin, anticonvulsant or antituberculosis* medication.
- Vitamin K supplementation given after the birth for early-onset vitamin K deficiency bleeding may *be too late to prevent this disease.*

Classic HDN
- This usually occurs *after 24 hours and as late as the 1st week* of life; this is observed in infants who have not received prophylactic vitamin K at birth.
- Usually the *disease occurs from the second day of life to the end of the 1st week.*
- Bleeding *commonly occurs in the umbilicus, GI tract (i.e. melena), skin, nose, surgical sites (i.e. circumcision)* and, uncommonly, in the brain.

Late-onset HDN
- This usually occurs *between age 2–12 weeks*; however, late-onset vitamin K deficiency bleeding can be seen as long as *6 months after birth.*

- This disease is most common in ***breastfed infants who did not receive vitamin K prophylaxis at birth***.
- Vitamin K content is low in mature human milk and ranges from 1 to 4 µg/L.
- More than half of these infants present with ***acute intracranial hemorrhages.***

– ***Vitamin K prophylaxis at birth prevents classical and late HDN***.
– Coagulation factors ***II, VII, IX, and X*** and other Gla-proteins (e.g. protein C, protein S, protein Z) also depend on the presence of vitamin K for their activity.

NOTES

COMED-K 2013

COMED-K 2013 QUESTIONS

1. Energy requirement in most postsurgical adult patients can be met by administration of
(a) 30 kcal/kg/day
(b) 40 kcal/kg/day
(c) 50 kcal/kg/day
(d) 60 kcal/kg/day

2. Object constancy is a major cognitive milestone that is usually achieved at
(a) 6 months
(b) 9 months
(c) 12 months
(d) 15 months

3. A 54-year-old chronic smoker (smoking index—50 pack years) presents with lesions suggestive of oral leukoplakia. Which of the following intervention can cause regression of the lesion?
(a) α-tocopherol
(b) Isotretinoin
(c) β-carotene
(d) Selenium

4. Cystatin C is a novel marker of
(a) Fatty liver
(b) Glomerular filtration
(c) Vitamin K status
(d) Cholestasis

5. The following statements regarding phenytoin are true *EXCEPT*
(a) It is highly bound to plasma proteins
(b) It is a prodrug and requires activation in the liver
(c) It induces drug metabolizing enzymes
(d) At high concentrations, it follows zero order kinetics

6. Universal antidote contains the following *EXCEPT*
(a) Powdered charcoal
(b) Tannic acid
(c) Ground mustard
(d) Magnesium oxide

7. Comparing economic benefits of a program with the cost of that program, it is called
(a) Cost-accounting analysis
(b) Input-output analysis
(c) Cost-effective analysis
(d) Cost-benefit analysis

8. Following statements are true in leptospirosis *EXCEPT*
(a) It is a zoonosis
(b) Presents with fever, petechiae, jaundice and renal failure
(c) Doxycycline, penicillin and macrolides are used in treatment
(d) Demonstrated by phase contrast microscopy

9. Risk of ureteric injury during abdominal hysterectomy is increased in the following conditions *EXCEPT*
(a) Endometriosis
(b) Pelvic inflammatory disease
(c) Adenomyosis
(d) Broad ligament fibroid

10. Serum albumin level is a component of which of the following scoring systems?
(a) Ranson's criteria
(b) APACHE II score
(c) Child's scoring
(d) ASA physical status

11. Oxytocin
(a) Originates in the supraoptic nucleus of the hypothalamus
(b) Is essential for the onset of labor
(c) Stimulates the growth of uterine musculature
(d) Is synthesized by paraventricular nucleus of hypothalamus

12. Which of the following is an important feature of herpes simplex keratitis?
(a) Ciliary congestion
(b) Congestion haze
(c) Pannus
(d) Reduced corneal sensation

13. Association of sexual precocity, multiple cystic bone lesions and endocrinopathies is seen in
(a) McCune-Albright syndrome
(b) Granulose cell tumor
(c) Arrhenoblastoma
(d) Prolactinoma

14. Moth eaten alopecia is seen in
(a) Black dot tinea
(b) Telogen effluvium
(c) Alopecia areata
(d) Secondary syphilis

15. A 12-year-old child, a known case of rheumatic heart disease, presents with low grade fever of 1 month duration. She has pallor, splenomegaly, clubbing and microscopic hematuria. The most important diagnostic test, you would like to do is
(a) Antistreptolysin O titer
(b) C-reactive protein
(c) Urine culture
(d) Blood culture

16. Mallory bodies are derived from
(a) Cytokeratin
(b) Desmin
(c) Laminin
(d) Vimentin

17. All of the following drugs inhibit microbial cell wall synthesis *EXCEPT*
(a) Neomycin
(b) Vancomycin
(c) Meropenem
(d) Bacitracin

18. Fish tank granuloma is caused by
(a) *Mycobacterium ulcerans*
(b) *Mycobacterium marinum*
(c) *Mycobacterium kansasii*
(d) *Mycobacterium szulgai*

19. Which of the following is NOT TRUE of spasmodic croup?
(a) History of fever is present
(b) Cough is metallic
(c) Larynx is pale and edematous
(d) Occurs mostly at night

20. The most common cause of bronchopulmonary aspergillosis is
(a) *Aspergillus fumigatus*
(b) *Aspergillus clavatus*
(c) *Aspergillus flavus*
(d) *Aspergillus niger*

21. All of the following are indicators of physical quality of life index *EXCEPT*
(a) Infant mortality rate
(b) Life expectancy at 1 year
(c) Level of living
(d) Literacy

22. 'Le facies sympathique' may be seen in
(a) Hanging
(b) Strangulation
(c) Drowning
(d) Suffocation

23. Antigens presented along with HLA class II stimulate
(a) CD8 cells
(b) CD4 cells
(c) CD2 cells
(d) CD19 cells

24. Cell shape and physical structure is provided by
(a) Cell membrane
(b) Microtubules
(c) Microfilaments
(d) Golgi apparatus

25. The cavity of mesencephalic brain vesicle is
(a) Lateral ventricle
(b) Third ventricle
(c) Fourth ventricle
(d) Cerebral aqueduct

26. Stiffening of the body muscles after death due to the breakdown of ATP is known as
(a) Cadaveric rigidity
(b) Cadaveric spasm
(c) Postmortem hypostasis
(d) Postmortem lividity

27. Commonly, 'one dietary cycle' refers to
(a) 1 day
(b) 7 days
(c) 14 days
(d) 21 months

28. 'Shrinking lung' is a feature of
(a) Rheumatoid arthritis
(b) SLE
(c) Systemic sclerosis
(d) Polymyositis

29. Wolffian duct remnant may present in the female as
(a) Gartner's cyst
(b) Bartholin's cyst
(c) Endometriotic cyst
(d) Fimbrial cyst

30. 'Rodent ulcer' is the other name for
(a) Squamous cell carcinoma
(b) Malignant melanoma
(c) Basal cell carcinoma
(d) Actinic keratosis

31. The first step in conducting an epidemic investigation is to
(a) Determine the case count
(b) Calculate the incubation period
(c) Determine the population at risk
(d) Verify the diagnosis

32. The following syndrome is associated with bronchiectasis
(a) Kallmann's syndrome
(b) Kartagener's syndrome
(c) Kostmann's syndrome
(d) Klinefelter syndrome

33. In exocrine pancreatic cancer, the commonest tumor marker to be elevated is
(a) CA-125
(b) CEA
(c) CA 15–3
(d) CA 19–9

34. Recurrences of herpes genitalis
(a) More the HSV-2 than HSV-1
(b) Same in both HSV-1 and HSV-2
(c) More in HSV-1 than HSV-2
(d) Variable and insignificant with either type of HSV

35. Which of the following drugs is useful in the long-term treatment of alcohol dependence?
(a) Acamprosate
(b) Chlordiazepoxide
(c) Flumazenil
(d) Imipramine

36. March fracture is
(a) Stress fracture of neck of 2nd metatarsal
(b) Stress fracture of neck of talus
(c) Compression fracture of calcaneus
(d) Fracture lower end of fibula

37. Most frequent association of cryptorchidism is with
(a) Epididymo-orchitis
(b) Hernia
(c) Infertility
(d) Malignant transformation

38. All of the following are adverse effects of long-term corticosteroids *EXCEPT*
(a) Hypoglycemia
(b) Psychosis
(c) Peptic ulcers
(d) Osteoporosis

39. Laser iridotomy is done in
(a) Open angle glaucoma
(b) Angle-closure glaucoma
(c) Iridocylitis
(d) Posterior capsular opacification

40. An emerging viral pathogen causing pyelonephritis in kidney allografts is
(a) Rotavirus
(b) Herpes simplex virus
(c) Polyomavirus
(d) Influenza virus

41. Epidemic outbreak in birds is called
(a) Enzootic
(b) Ornithic
(c) Zoonotic
(d) Amphixenoses

42. The narrowest portion of fallopian tube in
(a) Interstitial part
(b) Isthmus
(c) Ampullary
(d) Infundibulum

43. The commonest variety of urinary bladder cancer is
(a) Squamous cell carcinoma
(b) Basal cell carcinoma
(c) Transitional cell carcinoma
(d) Adenocarcinoma

44. The commonest systemic abnormality associated with renal cell carcinoma is
(a) Hypertension
(b) Polycythemia
(c) Elevated ESR
(d) Pyrexia

45. Which of the following conditions cause congestive heart failure in neonates?
(a) Bicuspid aortic valve
(b) Tetralogy of Fallot
(c) ASD
(d) Total anomalous pulmonary venous return

46. The cause of gunstock deformity is
(a) Supracondylar fracture
(b) Fracture of both bones of the forearm
(c) Fracture of surgical head of humerus
(d) Fracture of fibula

47. Which of these statements about ulcerative colitis (UC) and colon carcinoma is FALSE?
(a) The risk of carcinoma increases with duration of UC
(b) Overall risk is less than 5%
(c) Cancer of rectum is more common than that of colon
(d) Surgery is indicated, if biopsy shows severe epithelial dysplasia

48. A hypertensive patient who is a chronic smoker presented with recurrent hemoptysis. On examination he had cushingoid features. Investigations revealed raised ACTH levels not suppressed by dexamethasone. The single diagnosis, which can account for all his symptoms is
(a) Multiple endocrine neoplasia I
(b) Pituitary adenoma
(c) Adrenocortical adenoma
(d) Ectopic ACTH-producing tumor

49. All of the following are skin antiseptics *EXCEPT*
(a) Chlorhexidine
(b) Ethylguaiacol
(c) Isopropyl alcohol
(d) Povidone-iodine

50. Cyclin B is required for cell cycle progression from
(a) G0 to G1
(b) G1 to S
(c) S to G2
(d) G2 to M

51. Which among the following drugs is LEAST likely to cause neutropenia?
(a) Chlorambucil
(b) Methotrexate
(c) Cyclophosphamide
(d) Vincristine

52. Which virus is NOT a teratogenic virus?
(a) Rubella
(b) Cytomegalovirus
(c) Herpes simplex
(d) Measles

53. The commonest valvular lesion in SLE-related cardiac disease is
(a) Tricuspid regurgitation
(b) Mitral regurgitation
(c) Mitral stenosis
(d) Aortic regurgitation

54. Safe lights in a radiographic darkroom are ideally light of which color?
(a) Red
(b) Blue
(c) White
(d) Yellow

55. Which joint is not fused in triple arthrodesis?
(a) Tibiotalar
(b) Calcaneocuboid
(c) Talonavicular
(d) Talocalcaneal

56. Tramline calcifications of the cerebral cortex is seen in
(a) Tuberous sclerosis
(b) Sturge-Weber syndrome
(c) von Hippel-Lindau disease
(d) von Recklinghausen's disease

57. Which of these is a sign of left atrial enlargement on a PA chest radiograph?
(a) Elevation of the right main bronchus
(b) Double density on the left side of the heart shadow
(c) Discrete bulge in the left cardiac margin below the pulmonary bay
(d) Displacement of the trachea to the right

58. District Mental Health Program was first implemented in
(a) Bellary district, Karnataka
(b) Trichy, Tamil Nadu
(c) Agra, Uttar Pradesh
(d) Mumbai, Maharashtra

59. The disease, which are imported into country in which they do not otherwise occur is termed as
(a) Endemic
(b) Exotic
(c) Epidemic
(d) Pandemic

60. 'Gandy-gamma' nodules are typically seen in chronic venous congestion of
(a) Lung
(b) Kidney
(c) Liver
(d) Spleen

61. Which of the morphological form of *Leishmania donovani* is seen in man?
(a) Promastigote
(b) Trypomastigote
(c) Amastigote
(d) Epimastigote

62. The primary visual area is located in the walls of
(a) Parieto-occipital sulcus
(b) Superior temporal sulcus
(c) Posterior part of calcarine sulcus
(d) Central sulcus

63. Thumb print sign in neck radiograph is characteristically seen in
(a) Ludwig's angina
(b) Croup
(c) Epiglottitis
(d) Lemierre's syndrome

64. **One of the most commonly used drugs worldwide is**
(a) Cannabis
(b) Alcohol
(c) Caffeine
(d) Cocaine

65. **The following may be found in the cortex of the ovary *EXCEPT***
(a) Primordial follicles
(b) Granulosa cells
(c) Hilus cells
(d) Corpus luteum

66. **A 30-year-old female patient underwent total thyroidectomy. After surgery, patient complained of inability to raise her voice pitch, the most likely cause is injury to**
(a) Internal branch of superior laryngeal nerve
(b) External branch of superior laryngeal nerve
(c) Recurrent laryngeal nerve
(d) Ansa cervicalis

67. **Lung compliance is increased in**
(a) The presence of intra-alveolar fluid
(b) Acute respiratory distress syndrome
(c) Idiopathic pulmonary fibrosis
(d) Emphysema

68. **A 2-year-old male child has a head circumference of 55 cm. Which one of the following intrauterine infection he might have acquired?**
(a) Rubella
(b) Toxoplasmosis
(c) Herpes
(d) Hepatitis

69. **Which one of the following is a life-threatening complication of talc pleurodesis?**
(a) Empyema
(b) Re-expansion pulmonary edema
(c) Hemothorax
(d) ARDS

70. **Haab striae are seen in**
(a) Congenital glaucoma
(b) Birth trauma
(c) Keratoconus
(d) Pseudoexfoliation glaucoma

71. **Hepatocellular carcinoma is associated with infection caused by**
(a) Hepatitis C virus
(b) Hepatitis E virus
(c) Hepatitis G virus
(d) Hepatitis A virus

72. **In thyroid gland, iodide is transported into the lumen of the follicles by**
(a) Endocytosis
(b) Pendrin protein
(c) Antiport
(d) Primary active transport

73. **The vitamin present in the fatty acid synthase complex is**
(a) Thiamine
(b) Folate
(c) Pantothenate
(d) Pyridoxine

74. **All of the following are antipseudomonal cephalosporins *EXCEPT***
(a) Ceftazidime
(b) Cefoperazone
(c) Cefpodoxime
(d) Cefpirome

75. **All of the following are true about acute rhinosinusitis *EXCEPT***
(a) It is less than 2 weeks of duration
(b) Can arise from infectious and non-infectious cause
(c) Most patients improve without antibiotics
(d) Fungal variety is called mucormycosis

76. **The art of winning friends and influencing people is called**
(a) Counseling
(b) Persuasion
(c) Education
(d) Motivation

77. **Pseudomembranous colitis is caused by**
(a) *Clostridium botulinum*
(b) *Clostridium perfringens*
(c) *Clostridium difficile*
(d) *Clostridium tetani*

78. **Which of the following carcinomas has a better prognosis?**
(a) Supraglottis
(b) Glottis
(c) Subglottis
(d) Epiglottis

79. **Which of the following organism in pus is acid fast with 1% sulfuric acid?**
(a) *Actinomyces israelii*
(b) *Nocardia brasiliensis*
(c) *Streptomyces somaliensis*
(d) *Blastomyces dermatitidis*

80. **The dartos muscle is innervated by**
(a) Ilioinguinal nerve
(b) Iliohypogastric nerve
(c) Sympathetic nerve
(d) Pudendal nerve

81. **REM sleep**
(a) Is associated with dreamless sleep
(b) Occupies 80% of the total sleep time in full-term infants
(c) Is associated with sleep walking
(d) Is associated with depressed muscle tone

82. **Otomycosis is caused by**
(a) *Aspergillus niger*
(b) *Histoplasma capsulatum*
(c) *Rhinosporidium seeberi*
(d) *Cryptococcus neoformans*

83. **Type of anemia developing commonly in a patient with carcinoma stomach is**
(a) Aplastic anemia
(b) Megaloblastic anemia
(c) Hemolytic anemia
(d) Iron deficiency anemia

84. **The commonest valvular lesion in SLE-related cardiac disease is**
(a) Tricuspid regurgitation
(b) Mitral regurgitation
(c) Mitral stenosis
(d) Aortic regurgitation

85. **The following drug is predominantly a dual serotonin and norepinephrine reuptake inhibitor**
(a) Fluvoxamine
(b) Duloxetine
(c) Fluoxetine
(d) Paroxetine

86. **In triage, green color indicates**
(a) Ambulatory patients
(b) Moribund patients
(c) High priority treatment or transfer
(d) Medium priority or transfer

87. **Bexarotene, an oral retinoid is indicated in**
(a) Severe acute vulgaris
(b) Pustular psoriasis
(c) Mycosis fungoides
(d) Lichen planus

88. **Which of the following is the most common cause of sensorineural hearing loss in adults?**
(a) Meniere's disease
(b) Presbycusis
(c) Cerebellopontine angle tumor
(d) Trauma

89. **Drugs that may increase the anticoagulant effect of warfarin include all of the following *EXCEPT***
(a) Fluconazole
(b) Aspirin
(c) Rifampicin
(d) Metronidazole

90. **Gastrointestinal stromal tumor originates from**
(a) Interstitial cells of Cajal
(b) Parietal cells
(c) Neuroendocrine cells
(d) Chief cells

91. **Retina develops from**
(a) Neural ectoderm
(b) Endoderm
(c) Surface ectoderm
(d) Mesoderm

92. **Consumption of even a moderate amount of alcohol during pregnancy is associated with**
(a) Goiter-like symptoms in the fetus
(b) Mental retardation in the newborn
(c) Increased risk of spontaneous abortion
(d) Fetal alcohol syndrome

93. **Hamman's sign is seen in**
(a) Pneumomediastinum
(b) Pericardial effusion
(c) SVC obstruction
(d) Thyrotoxicosis

94. **Which one of the following is a contraindication for liver transplantation?**
(a) Ongoing substance abuse
(b) Hepatorenal syndrome
(c) Portal hypertension
(d) Acute liver failure

95. **Amongst the following, the LEAST risk of malignant disease of bone or cartilage is seen with**
(a) Chondroblastoma
(b) Maffucci's syndrome
(c) Ollier's disease
(d) Familial retinoblastoma syndrome

96. **A 13-year-old male is injected with 5TU of tuberculin antigen. After 72 hours, the reading recorded is 15 mm × 10 mm. Which of the following statements is true regarding the test result?**
(a) Positive test—type I reaction
(b) Positive test—type IV reaction
(c) Negative test—type I reaction
(d) Negative test—type IV reaction

97. **Oral hairy leukoplakia occurs in**
(a) Carcinoma tongue
(b) Oral candidiasis
(c) HIV-AIDS
(d) Infectious mononucleosis

98. **Blackwater fever is seen in**
(a) Leishmaniasis
(b) Falciparum malaria
(c) Trypanosomiasis
(d) Leptospirosis

99. **The gap in time between the onset of primary case and the secondary case is called**
(a) Serial interval
(b) Generation time
(c) Communicable period
(d) Median incubation period

100. **The cell, which forms blood-testis barrier is**
(a) Spermatogonia
(b) Primary spermatocyte
(c) Leydig cell
(d) Sertoli cell

101. **Which among the following is NOT an adverse effect of furosemide?**
(a) Hypokalemia
(b) Ototoxicity
(c) Hypercalcemia
(d) Hyperuricemia

102. **In giant cell tumor of bone, the tumor cells are**
(a) Sinusoidal lining cells
(b) Osteoclastic giant cells
(c) Fibroblastic cells
(d) Mononuclear stromal cells

103. **'Germ theory of diseases' as advanced by**
(a) Louis Pasteur
(b) Lemuel Shattuck
(c) William Budd
(d) Antonie van Leeuwenhoek

104. **Copper sulfate poisoning manifests with**
(a) Acute hemolysis
(b) High anion gap acidosis
(c) Peripheral neuropathy
(d) Rhabdomyolysis

105. **The sensory nerve supply of the fallopian tube and ovary is from which nerve roots?**
(a) D6 to D8
(b) D8 to D10
(c) D10 to D12
(d) L1 to L2

106. **The most common benign lesion of the liver is**
(a) Hemangioma
(b) Hepatic adenoma
(c) Focal nodular hyperplasia
(d) Hepatoblastoma

107. **Celiac plexus block**
(a) Can be used to relieve pain from intra-abdominal malignancy
(b) May cause constipation
(c) May cause hypertension
(d) Causes constriction of the sphincter of Oddi

108. **A child whose weight for height is > 80% and height for age is < 90% is said to be**
(a) Normal
(b) Stunted
(c) Wasted
(d) Wasted and stunted

109. **The ratio between the uterine corpus and the cervix at birth is**
(a) 1:1
(b) 1:2
(c) 2:1
(d) 3:1

110. **The typical 'Orphan-Annie eye' nucleus is described in**
(a) Serous cystadenocarcinoma of ovary
(b) Renal cell carcinoma
(c) Papillary carcinoma of thyroid
(d) Seminoma

111. **The major cause of low birth weight in countries with high proportion of low birth weight is**
(a) Maternal anemia
(b) Preterm
(c) Maternal malnutrition
(d) Intrauterine growth retardation

112. Planned end-point of all activities is
(a) Objectives
(b) Goals
(c) Targets
(d) Results

113. Chronic zinc deficiency causes
(a) Hirsutism
(b) Gynecomastia
(c) Stunted growth
(d) Hypergeusia

114. Enteroclysis is
(a) Contrast study of small bowel fluoroscopically
(b) Double contrast study of colon fluoroscopically
(c) Laparoscopic lysis of adhesions
(d) Enema with a chemical substance

115. Regarding spinal anesthesia
(a) The spinal cord terminates at L4
(b) Aqueous 0.5% bupivacaine hyperbaric
(c) Bradycardia may be treated with IV ephedrine
(d) High block impairs the ability to cough

116. Which is TRUE of panic disorder?
(a) It is characterized by recurrent and unpredictable panic attacks
(b) The panic attacks always occur in specific situation
(c) Autonomic symptoms are rare in panic disorder
(d) The panic attacks evolve very slowly

117. The veins of the pericardium drain into
(a) Superior vena cava
(b) Inferior vena cava
(c) Azygos vein
(d) Left brachiocephalic vein

118. Blood flow of resting skeletal muscle is
(a) 1–1.5 mL/100 g/min
(b) 2–4 mL/100 g/min
(c) 5–7 mL/100 g/min
(d) 8–10 mL/100 g/min

119. Tension pneumothorax is associated with
(a) Mediastinal displacement away from the lesion
(b) Decreased percussion note on the side of the lesion
(c) Increased blood pressure
(d) Stridor

120. Carriers of avirulent organisms are called
(a) Healthy carriers
(b) Temporary carriers
(c) Inapparent carriers
(d) Pseudocarriers

121. An adenofibroma of ovary in which the epithelial component consists of nests of transitional cells is called
(a) Thecoma
(b) Granulosa cell tumor
(c) Brenner's tumor
(d) Serous cystadenofibroma

122. All of the following drugs can be used for the prophylaxis of migraine *EXCEPT*
(a) Propranolol
(b) Sumatriptan
(c) Amitriptyline
(d) Flunarizine

123. The biosynthesis of the enzyme pyruvate carboxylase is repressed by
(a) Insulin
(b) Glucagon
(c) Cortisol
(d) Epinephrine

124. Test used to find fixed flexion deformity of hip is
(a) Levin punch test
(b) Thomas test
(c) Telescopy test
(d) Laségue's test

125. Which of the following radionuclides is used to identify ectopic gastric mucosa?
(a) 99mTc-pertechnetate
(b) 99mTc-sulfur colloid
(c) 99mTc-labeled red cells
(d) 99mTc-albumen macroaggregates

126. The highest risk of malignant transformation in the oral cavity is seen in
(a) Oral submucous fibrosis
(b) Erythroplakia
(c) Oral lichen planus
(d) Discoid lupus erythematosus

127. Left ovarian vein drains into
(a) Left renal vein
(b) Internal iliac vein
(c) Inferior vena cava
(d) Azygos vein

128. Sjögren's syndrome affects
(a) Exocrine glands
(b) Paracrine glands
(c) Endocrine glands
(d) Autocrine glands

129. Treatment of choice for septate uterus with a high pregnancy success rate is
(a) Strassman operation
(b) Jones and Jones operation
(c) Tomkins operation
(d) Hysteroscopic metroplasty

130. A 62-year-old man with carcinoma lung presented to emergency department with respiratory distress. ECG showed electrical alternans. Most likely diagnosis is
(a) Pneumothorax
(b) Pleural effusion
(c) Cardiac tamponade
(d) Constrictive pericarditis

For questions 131–134

Q. A 4-year-old male child is brought to the pediatric outpatient department with sore throat and fever for 2 days and noisy breathing with inability to swallow for the past 4 hours. Examination showed a toxic, tachypneic child with inspiratory stridor and drooling of saliva. There is suprasternal, supraclavicular and intercostal recession during inspiration. No stridor heard during expiration.

131. The child's clinical presentation suggests
(a) Intrathoracic airway obstruction
(b) Extrathoracic airway obstruction
(c) Belladonna poisoning
(d) Bronchopneumonia

132. The appropriate next course of action is
(a) Arrange things for securing airway
(b) Give urgent stomach wash
(c) Immediate throat examination for a foreign body
(d) Sedate the child

133. Lateral view X-ray of the neck in this child is likely to reveal
(a) Steeple sign
(b) Thumb sign
(c) Scabbard trachea
(d) Normal airway

134. The child needs to be treated with
(a) Neostigmine
(b) Chelating agents
(c) Urgent adenoidectomy
(d) Antibiotics

For questions 135–138

Q. A 75-year-old woman with chronic atrial fibrillation presented to the hospital with a 2-day history of colicky abdominal pain. The physical examination revealed hypoactive bowel sounds and diffuse abdominal tenderness. Laboratory tests showed a white cell count of 19,400 per cubic millimeter with 92% neutrophils, a blood urea nitrogen level of 42 mg/dL (15 mmol/L) and a serum creatinine level of 3.0 mg/dL (267 µmol/L).

135. The plain skiagram in this patient would have revealed
(a) Gas under the diaphragm
(b) Dilated sigmoid colon
(c) Dilated gas-filled small bowel with thickening of the wall
(d) Colon cut off sign

136. The investigation of choice would be
(a) Contrast-enhanced CT abdomen
(b) Duplex Doppler of the abdomen
(c) MRI scan of the abdomen
(d) Ultrasonography of abdomen

137. The most probable diagnosis in this patient would be
(a) Portal view thrombosis
(b) Mesenteric ischemia
(c) Intestinal perforation
(d) Lynch syndrome

138. The common cause for this problem would be
(a) Occlusion of the portal vein
(b) Occlusion of the superior mesenteric vessel
(c) Occlusion of the inferior mesenteric vessel
(d) Perforation of the duodenum

For questions 139–141

Q. A 20-year-old female patient was stabbed with an ice pick in the xiphisternum, brought to the casualty in stupot, very pale, tachycardia, feeble pulse, prominent neck vein and muffled heart sounds on auscultation.

139. The investigation of choice in this patient would be
(a) Bedside ultrasound of chest
(b) Electrocardiogram
(c) CT chest
(d) Plain chest skiagram

140. The most likely problem in this patient is
(a) Tension pneumothorax
(b) Hemothorax
(c) Pericardial tamponade
(d) Diaphragmatic hernia

141. Immediate treatment of this condition is
(a) Massive infusion through wide bore needle
(b) Immediate ICD placement (intercostal drain)
(c) Immediate thoracotomy
(d) Pericardiocentesis

For questions 142–144

Q. A 60-year-old male has a long-standing history of breathlessness. He has been a heavy smoker since the age of 20 years. Physical examination reveals an anxious male who is emaciated, puffing for breath but is not cyanosed. The chest is barrel shaped.

142. An additional clinical finding would be
(a) Elevated domes of the diaphragm
(b) Left ventricular hypertrophy
(c) Muffled heart sounds
(d) Gynecomastia

143. The primary pathology of the lung in this patient is associated with which of the following pathogenetic mechanisms?
(a) Type I hypersensitivity
(b) Unabashed action of proteases
(c) Deposition of immune complexes
(d) Deficiency of a protein produced by the liver

144. The investigation of choice in this patient would be
(a) High resolution CT
(b) Contrast-enhanced CT
(c) Plain skiagram chest
(d) Ultrasound chest

For questions 145–146

Q. A 45-year-old multiparous perimenopausal women comes with a 6 cm lump in the right upper quadrant with puckering of the overlying skin and a small area of ulceration, on further examination she has three axillary firm palpable lymph node in the same side, she also has lymph node in the supraclavicular area, rest of the systems are clinically normal.

145. The most appropriate investigation, which was ordered from the outpatient department was
(a) Estimation of *BRCA I/II*
(b) Core needle biopsy
(c) Mammogram
(d) Ultrasonography

146. The clinical staging of this case would be
(a) T3 N2 M1
(b) T4 N2 M0
(c) T4 N3 M0
(d) T4 N3 M0

For questions 147–149

Q. A 38-year-old homeless male develops sudden onset hematemesis following a bout of severe vomiting and retching. He had no complaints prior to the onset of his symptoms. On examination, he is pale and looks anxious. The vital signs are normal. Laboratory investigations show normal liver function tests, a low Hb and high MCV, chest X-ray is normal.

147. The probable diagnosis in this patient is
(a) Variceal veins
(b) Mallory-Weiss syndrome
(c) Barrett's esophagus
(d) Boerhaave's disease

148. He should have an immediate
(a) Barium swallow
(b) Upper GI scopy
(c) Chest X-ray
(d) Ultrasound of abdomen

149. The above problem on endoscopy would appear as
(a) Dilated veins in lower esophagus
(b) Growth in the lower esophagus
(c) Linear tear in the OG junction
(d) Whitish plaques in esophagus

For questions 150-153

Q. A 58-year-old healthy man was evaluated for a toothache of 2 days duration. He was treated with oral penicillin and an opiate analgesic and advised to have the affected teeth pulled. He returned less than 24 hours later reporting severe swelling in the neck, sore throat, chills and chest pain. On examination, the floor of his oral cavity was indurated and woody, and he had marked tenderness and adenopathy throughout his neck. He had erythema spreading from his neck down over his anterior chest wall where his chest pain was localized.

150. The patient is suffering from
(a) Quinsy
(b) Ludwig's angina
(c) Acute parotitis
(d) Angioneurotic edema

151. This condition is an surgical emergency as it can lead to
(a) Airway obstruction
(b) Difficulty in swallowing
(c) Aspiration pneumonia
(d) CSOM

152. The infection spreads to the
(a) Submental, sublingual and submandibular space
(b) Parapharyngeal spaces
(c) Nasopharyngeal area
(d) Sinuses

153. The treatment of choice in such an acute condition would be
(a) Surgical decompression, antibiotic and intensive care
(b) Antifungal therapy
(c) Removal of the offending tooth
(d) Continue the penicillin in larger doses

For questions 154-157

Q. A 40-year-old veterinarian presented with complaints of abdominal pain. On examination he was found to be icteric, the liver was palpable, ultrasonography revealed the presence of cyst in the right lobe of liver.

154. The clinical picture is suggestive of infection caused by
(a) *Enteromonas hominis*
(b) *Echinococcus granulosus*
(c) *Endolimax nana*
(d) *Enterobius vermicularis*

155. The definitive hosts of the agent causing this infection are
(a) Humans
(b) Dogs
(c) Reptiles
(d) Deer

156. The skin hypersensitivity test is performed in this infection in the
(a) Patch test
(b) Napier's aldehyde test
(c) Casoni's test
(d) Sabin-Feldman dye test

157. The antigen used to perform the skin test is sterilized using the
(a) Hot air oven
(b) Gamma radiation
(c) Autoclaving
(d) Seitz filter

For questions 158-160

Q. A healthy 10-year-old girl presented to her physician with nontender, well circumscribed, mobile, slightly hyperneurotic erythematous plaques on the dorsal aspect of the interphalanged joints of both thumbs. The plaques had developed over several months.

158. These bilaterally symmetrical lesions are known as
(a) Garrod's pads
(b) Heberden's nodules
(c) Erythema nodosum
(d) Erythema marginatum

159. The diagnosis in this healthy young girl would be
(a) Bulimia nervosa
(b) Rheumatic fever
(c) Rheumatoid arthritis
(d) Scarlet fever

160. This kind of knuckle pads are also associated with all of the following *EXCEPT*
(a) Dupuytren's contracture
(b) Ledderhose's syndrome
(c) Bart-Pumphrey syndrome
(d) Rheumatic carditis

For questions 161–165

Q. A 45-year-old man presented with a 3-year-history of a painless soft and slow growing swelling of the neck, upper trunk, upper back and shoulders. The patient had a history of heavy alcohol consumption and was a non-smoker. Laboratory blood analysis showed minor elevations in aspartate aminotransferase (71 U/L), alanine aminotransferase (49 U/L), and total cholesterol [235 mg/dL (6.08 mmol/L)]. Triglycerides were elevated at 1,020 mg per deciliter (11.52 mmol/L). Magnetic resonance imaging revealed diffuse, non-encapsulated fatty deposits in the mediastinum and in the subcutaneous and deeper fascial compartments of the neck, upper trunk and back.

161. The probable diagnosis of the patient is
(a) Tuberculosis
(b) Rheumatoid arthritis
(c) Madelung's disease
(d) Hodgkin's lymphoma

162. This condition is seen in
(a) Renal insufficiency
(b) Hypercalcemia
(c) Tuberculosis
(d) Alcohol dependency

163. This condition is more common in
(a) Males
(b) Females

(c) Indians
(d) Children

164. The treatment for this patient would be
(a) Statins
(b) Aspirin
(c) B complex
(d) Anticoagulants

165. Which enzyme is specific indicator for alcohol-induced liver damage?
(a) SGOT
(b) SGPT
(c) GGTP
(d) All of the above

For questions 166–169

Q. A 25-year-old female patient presented with a history of bilateral hearing loss and tinnitus during pregnancy. She can hear better in a noisy environment. She speaks in a low volume monotonously. Otoscopy showed normal looking eardrums bilaterally and Rinne test negative bilaterally. Pure tone audiogram showed air bone gap with dip in bone conduction at 2 kHz.

166. What is the most probable diagnosis?
(a) Meniere's disease
(b) Acoustic neuroma
(c) Presbycusis
(d) Otosclerosis

167. Rinne test negative bilaterally means
(a) Bilateral conductive hearing loss
(b) Bilateral sensorineural hearing loss
(c) Bilateral normal middle ear function
(d) Bilateral acoustic nerve tumors

168. In the above patient, dip in bone conduction at 2 kHz is called
(a) Moore's sign
(b) Carhart's notch
(c) Schwartze's sign
(d) Thumb sign

169. The treatment of this patient is
(a) Endolymphatic sac decompression
(b) Myringotomy and grommet insertion
(c) Stapedotomy and piston insertion
(d) Retrosigmoid approach and excision

For questions 170–173

Q. A 6-year-old child who presented with perianal pruritus, excoriation of skin and nocturnal enuresis was found to be infected with a parasite causing autoinfection.

170. The causative agent is
(a) *Trichinella spiralis*
(b) *Giardia lamblia*
(c) *Enterobius vermicularis*
(d) *Wuchereria bancrofti*

171. The adult forms of the parasite are known to inhabit the
(a) Cecum, appendix and ascending colon
(b) Subcutaneous tissues
(c) Subcutaneous and lymphatic tissues
(d) Proximal small intestine

172. The infective form of parasite for humans is the
(a) Filariform larvae
(b) Embryonated egg
(c) Adult female
(d) Adult male

173. The causative agent is diagnosed by the
(a) NIH swab method
(b) String test
(c) Hetrazan test
(d) Encysted larvae on muscle biopsy.

For questions 174–177

Q. A 60-year-old male presents with progressive difficulty in swallowing, vomiting and occasional regurgitation for the past 3 months. Barium studies showed marked dilatation of the upper esophagus with narrowing of the lower segment. Manometry showed absent esophageal peristalsis.

174. The pathogenesis of this condition is most likely related to
(a) Reflux of gastric acid into the lower esophagus
(b) Abnormal dilatation of lower esophageal veins
(c) Incompetence of the lower esophageal sphincter
(d) Absence of ganglion cells in the myenteric plexus of the esophagus

175. Which of the following conditions is he most likely at risk of developing?
(a) Mallory-Weiss syndrome
(b) Peptic ulcer disease
(c) Squamous cell carcinoma of the esophagus
(d) Rupture of esophageal varies

176. He would also present to clinician with
(a) Recurrent chest infection
(b) Recurrent bleeding upper GI
(c) Recurrent colicky abdominal pain
(d) Esophageal perforation

177. This patient needs to have
(a) Balloon dilatation
(b) Endoscopic banding
(c) Sclerotherapy
(d) Proton pump inhibitor

For questions 178–180

Q. A 69-year-old female is being evaluated for constipation and an episode of blood-stained stools. Laboratory investigations show normal CBC and barium studies showed out-pouching of the sigmoid colon in multiple areas.

178. This patient has most likely developed the complication of
(a) Pseudomyxoma peritonei
(b) Herniation of the colonic wall at the sites of focal defects
(c) Absence of ganglion cells in the meissner plexus within the colon
(d) Atherosclerotic narrowing of the mesenteric arteries

179. 3 weeks later she develops fever left-sided abdominal pain and diarrhea. Vital signs are T-102°F (38.8°C), with tenderness in the left iliac fossa. Probable cause is
(a) Metastasis to the liver
(b) Acute ischemic colitis
(c) Perforation of the colon
(d) Crohn's disease

180. The investigation of choice in this patient with the above complication would be
(a) Computed tomography
(b) Ultrasound abdomen
(c) Colonoscopy with biopsy
(d) Barium enema

COMED-K 2013

ANSWERS AND EXPLANATIONS

1. **Answer is a (30 kcal/kg/day).**
   Ref: General Surgery: Principles and International Practice, edited by Kirby I Bland, Pg 31.

   – ***Postoperative energy*** and protein requirements depend upon body composition, clinical status and mobility.
   – An estimation of requirements is ***30 kcal/kg/day and a protein intake of 1 g/kg/day for the average adult*** patient.

2. **Answer is b (9 months).**
   Ref: Keeping Children Healthy in Body and Mind: Birth Through 10, By Farooq Mirza, 2001 edition, Pg 4.

   – A major milestone is the ***achievement*** of ***object constancy at about 9 months***—understanding the objects continue to exist even when not seen.
   – At 4–7 months infants look for an object that has been dropped, but quickly give up if it is not seen (***out of sight is out of mind***).
   – With object permanence infants persist in searching for the object even if hidden under a cloth.
   – ***Object permanence*** is ***firmly established*** at ***18 months*** of age.

3. **Answer is b (Isotretinoin).**
   Ref: Harrison's, 18th edition Pg 657.

   - ***Oral leukoplakia*** was a/w upregulation of retinoic acid receptor (RAR-beta)
   - Therapy with ***high, relatively toxic doses of isotretinoin (13-cis-retinoic acid) causes regression of oral leukoplakia***. However, the lesions recur when the therapy is withdrawn, suggesting the need for long-term administration.

4. **Answer is b (Glomerular filtration).**
   Ref: Nephrology and Clinical Chemistry: The Essential Link, edited by Pierre Delanaye, Pg 52.

   - ***Cystatin C*** is a *cysteine protease inhibitor* synthesized by all ***nucleated cells*** freely filtered by the glomerulus and not secreted by tubules.
   - It is ***reabsorbed in PCT*** and levels are ***not*** affected by age, sex, gender or muscle mass as seen with serum creatinine.
   - Due to these properties it is considered to be ***equal to if not superior than serum creatinine as a marker of GFR***.

5. **Answer is b (It is a prodrug and requires activation in the liver).**
   Ref: KD Tripathi, 7th edition Pg 413.

   - Phenytoin is widely distributed in the body and is ***80–90% bound to plasma proteins***.
   - ***Phenytoin is a potent inducer*** of CYP2C8/9, CYP3A4/5 and some other CYPs.
   - The kinetics of phenytoin metabolism is capacity limited; changes from first order to zero order over the therapeutic range.
   - ***Phenytoin is metabolized in the liver*** by hydroxylation involving CYP2C9 and 2C19 as well as glucuronide conjugation.
   - ***Fosphenytoin is a water-soluble prodrug*** of phenytoin that has been introduced to overcome the difficulties in IV administration of phenytoin, which it has replaced for use in status epilepticus.

6. **Answer is c (Ground mustard).**
   Ref: Narayan Reddy's synopsis of FMT, 23rd edition Pg.

   - The ***universal antidote*** is a mixture that contains ***activated charcoal, magnesium oxide and tannic acid***.
   - The ***mixture is ineffective*** and no longer used; ***activated charcoal*** is useful.

7. Answer is d (Cost-benefit analysis).
Ref: Park, 22nd edition Pg 814.

Cost-benefit analysis	• This has received the widest attention for application in health field • The economic benefits of any program are compared with the costs of that program
Cost-effectiveness analysis	• This is a more promising tool; it is similar to cost-benefit analysis except that, benefit instead of being expressed in monetary terms is expressed in terms of results achieved (e.g. number of lives saved)
Cost accounting	• Provides basic data on cost structure of any program • Financial records are kept in a manner permitting costs to be associated with the purpose for which they are incurred
Input-output analysis	• This is an economic technique, in the health field 'input' refers to all health service activities, which consume resources (manpower, money, materials and time) and 'output' refers to such useful outcomes as cases treated or lives saved

8. Answer is d (Demonstrated by phase contrast microscopy).
Ref: CMDT 2013, Pg 1477.

- ***Leptospirosis*** is caused by the multiple serovars of ***Leptospira interrogans***.
- It is among the ***most common zoonotic diseases***.
- The leptospires are often transmitted to humans by the ***ingestion of food and drink contaminated by the urine of the reservoir animal (rat's urine!)***—occupational cases occur among ***sewer workers, rice planters, abattoir workers, farmers***.
- Incubation period = ***2–20 days***.

Anicteric leptospirosis	Icteric leptospirosis (Weil syndrome)
➢ *MC and milder form of the disease*; often ***biphasic***. ➢ ***Initial "septicemic" phase***: Abrupt high fever, chills, abdominal pain, severe headache and myalgias, (calf muscles); marked conjunctival congestion; leptospires can be isolated from blood, CSF and tissues ➢ ***Second or "immune" phase***: Occurs following a 1- to 3-day period of improvement in symptoms and absence of fever; leptospires are absent from blood and CSF, but are still present in the kidney and specific antibodies appear; recurrence of symptoms is seen as in the first phase of disease with the onset of meningitis, panuveitis, rash and adenopathy may occur	➢ Impaired ***kidney and liver function (jaundice), abnormal mental status and hemorrhagic pneumonia*** and has a ***high*** (5–40%) ***mortality rate***

- Treatment: ***Penicillin*** or ***ceftriaxone*** is the ***DOC in severe leptospirosis***; ***Doxycycline*** is also effective as therapy if started early (most often used in mild-to-moderate disease); ***Azithromycin*** (macrolide) is also active, but clinical experience is limited.

Diagnosis:
➢ ***Neutrophilic leukocytosis*** ➢ Urine: May contain bile, protein, casts and red cells; oliguria is common ➢ *Elevated bilirubin and aminotransferases* ➢ *Elevated serum creatinine* ➢ Microscopy: Early in the disease, the organism may be identified by ***dark field examination*** of the patient's blood ➢ ***Culture*** on a semisolid medium (e.g. Fletcher EMJH): Take 1–6 weeks to become positive (the organism may also be grown from the urine from the 10th day to the 6th week) ➢ Diagnosis is usually made by means ***of serologic tests*** (ELISA, PCR)

9. Answer is a, d (Endometriosis, broad ligament fibroid).

Ref: Bonney's Gynaecological Surgery; By Tito Lopes, Nick Spirtos, Raj Naik, John M Monaghan, 11th edition Pg 235; http://www.ncbi.nlm.nih.gov/pmc/articles/PMC3285707/

Author's comments: *"The answer in the revised answer key gives a and d, BUT the above reference and many other books include a and d as seen below; however adenomyosis is not included in the reference – so is the revised key wrong? ....if anyone has any better reference - please message me on FB and I shall update.*

Predisposing factors for iatrogenic urologic injury:

- Uterus size larger than 12 weeks' gestation
- Large ovarian cysts 4 cm or larger
- ***Endometriosis***
- ***Pelvic inflammatory disease***
- Prior intra-abdominal operation
- Radiation therapy
- ***Broad ligament fibroid***
- Advanced state of malignancy
- Anatomical anomalies of the urinary tract (ectopic ureter, duplex ureter, etc.).

The six most common mechanisms of operative ureteral injury are as follows:

- Crushing from misapplication of a clamp
- Ligation with a suture
- Transection (partial or complete)
- Angulation of the ureter with secondary obstruction
- Ischemia from ureteral stripping or electrocoagulation
- Resection of a segment of ureter.

10. Answer is c (Child's scoring).

Ref: CMDT 2013, Pg 672, 692.

Components of Child-Pugh-Turcotte's scoring for staging cirrhosis	Total numerical score and corresponding Child class
• Ascites • Serum bilirubin • Serum albumin • Encephalopathy • Prothrombin time	• Class A = 5–6 • Class B = 7–9 • Class C = 10–15

Also Know

- Model for end-stage liver disease (MELD) scoring for cirrhosis includes INR, serum bilirubin and serum creatinine.
- A MELD score of > 14 is required for liver transplantation listing.

About Other Options

- ***APACHE II:*** Acute Physiology Assessment and Chronic Health Evaluation system
- ***Ranson's score:*** For acute pancreatitis

- *ASA*: American Society of Anesthesiologists score for assessing fitness for anesthesia based on coexisting systemic disease.

11. Answer is d (Is synthesized by paraventricular nucleus of hypothalamus).
Ref: KD Tripathi, 7th edition Pg 329.

Author's comments: "Although option a also may be correct, option d gives the word 'synthesized' and the revised answer key also give the same answer".

- ***Oxytocin and Vasopressin (ADH)*** are ***non-apeptides*** synthesized within the ***supraoptic and paraventricular nuclei*** of the hypothalamus and are transported down the axon and stored in the nerve endings within the neurohypophysis (posterior pituitary).
- Oxytocin ***increases the force of uterine contraction***.
- Oxytocin is released during labor and the uterus is highly sensitive to it at this time. However it ***does NOT appear to be obligatory for initiating parturition***—delivery occurs even in hypophysectomized animals and humans. It is only ***facilitatory in action***.
- Stimuli for oxytocin secretion—coitus, parturition, suckling, etc.
- Stimuli for vasopressin secretion—water deprivation, hemorrhage, hypertonic saline infusion, etc.

12. Answer is d (Reduced corneal sensation).
Ref: Parson's Diseases of the Eye, 21st edition Pg 201-202.

Herpes simplex keratitis

Epithelial keratitis
– Caused by ***actively replicating virus*** on corneal surface
– ***Dendritic ulcer***: Dichotomously branching lesion with ***terminal bulbs***; borders staining with Rose Bengal, epithelial defect stains with fluorescein – ***Geographic ulcer*** – ***Marginal keratitis*** – ***Metaherpetic/Trophic ulcer***: NOT a/w live virus and is due to inability of epithelium to heal
– ***Resolves spontaneously*** in 50% cases – ***Topical antivirals*** are mainstay of treatment
Stromal/Endothelial keratitis
– ***Immune-mediated response*** to non-replicating virus particles
– ***Endotheliitis*** ➢ Localized endotheliitis: Disciform keratitis ➢ Diffuse and linear endotheliitis – ***Necrotizing keratitis (uncommon)*** – ***Immune stromal keratitis (disciform keratitis)*** – ***Keratouveitis*** (a/w ***secondary glaucoma***)
– ***Topical steroids are mainstay*** (especially for stromal keratouveitis) with topical and oral antiviral cover is necessary; topical steroids may need slow tapering over months

13. Answer is a (McCune-Albright syndrome).
Ref: Harrison's, 18th edition Pg 3142.

McCune-Albright syndrome

- ➢ Gonadotropin-independent precocious puberty
- ➢ Polyostotic fibrous dysplasia

- Endocrine dysfunction: Acromegaly, adrenal adenomas and autonomous ovarian function
- Cafe-au-Lait spots

14. Answer is d (Secondary syphilis).
Ref: CMDT, 2013, Pg 1469.

- ***Moth eaten alopecia*** is a ***classic feature of secondary syphilis***—nonscarring, patterned hair loss in which many foci of hair loss are scattered throughout the scalp.

Also Know

SLE	Frontal alopecia with lupus hairs
Anagen effluvium	Arrow end hairs
Alopecia areata	Diffuse alopecia, exclamation mark hairs
Male pattern (androgenetic)	Frontoparietal thinning or diffuse thinning over crown
Lateral eyebrow alopecia	Queen Anne's sign in hypothyroidism

15. Answer is d (Blood culture).
Ref: CMDT 2013, Pg 1435.

- The case history given is that of ***infective endocarditis***. The keywords are *pallor, splenomegaly, clubbing and microscopic hematuria in a case of rheumatic heart disease (pre-existing heart disease)*.
- ***Blood culture*** confirms the ***diagnosis***.
- ***Hematuria and proteinuria*** may result from emboli or ***immunologically mediated glomerulonephritis***, which can cause ***kidney dysfunction***.
- Other lesions in infective endocarditis—petechiae (on the palate or conjunctiva, or beneath the fingernails), subungual ('splinter') hemorrhages, ***Osler nodes*** (painful, violaceous raised lesions of the fingers, toes or feet), ***Janeway lesions*** (painless erythematous lesions of the palms or soles) and ***Roth spots*** (exudative lesions in the retina)—occur in about 25% of patients. Strokes and major systemic embolic events are present in about 25% of patients and tend to occur before or within the 1st week of antimicrobial therapy.

16. Answer is a (Cytokeratin).
Ref: Fundamentals of Surgical Pathology, Shameem Shariff, 2010 edition Pg 129.

Mallory Hyaline

- These are aggregates of ***intermediate cytokeratin prekeratin filaments*** in the cytoplasm of hepatocytes *resulting from hepatocyte injury*.
- Also called ***alcoholic hyaline*** since ***MC seen in alcoholic hepatitis***.

Also seen in:
- Primary biliary cirrhosis
- Hepatocellular Ca
- Chronic cholestatic syndrome
- Focal nodular hyperplasia
- Indian childhood cirrhosis
- Wilson's disease
- Diabetes mellitus
- Morbid obesity, Jejunoileal bypass

17. Answer is a (Neomycin).
Ref: KD Tripathi, 7th edition Pg 689.

- ***Neomycin*** as a topical aminoglycoside antibiotic that acts by causing misreading of mRNA code by binding to 30S–50S ribosomes.

Mechanism of action	Drugs
Inhibit cell wall synthesis	Penicillins (all beta-lactam antibiotics including aztreonam and meropenem, cephalosporins, cycloserine, vancomycin, bacitracin
Cause leakage from cell membranes	Polypeptides: Polymyxin, Colistin, bacitracin; Polyenes: Amphotericin B, Nystatin, Hamycin
Block protein synthesis	Chloramphenicol, tetracyclines, macrolides, clindamycin, streptogramins (quinupristin, dalfopristin), linezolid
Cause misreading of mRNA code and affect permeability	Aminoglycosides
Interfere with DNA synthesis	Acyclovir, zidovudine
Block nucleotide synthesis by inhibiting folate metabolism	Sulfonamides, trimethoprim
Inhibitors DNA gyrase	FluoroQuinolones
Interfere with DNA function	Rifampicin
Block mycolic acid synthesis	Isoniazid
Interfere with intermediary metabolism	Sulfonamides, sulfones, PAS, pyrimethamine, metronidazole

18. Answer is b *(Mycobacterium marinum).*
Ref: CP Baveja's Textbook of Microbiology, 3rd edition Pg 343.

- ***Mycobacterium marinum*** is a ***photochromogen non-tuberculous Mycobacterium***.
- Causes a ***superficial granulomatous skin disease*** of man—***swimming pool granuloma or fish tank granuloma***.
- ***Buruli ulcer*** is caused by ***M. ulcerans***.

19. Answer is a (History of fever is present).
Ref: Practical Pediatrics. Don Roberton, 2007 edition Pg 486.

- ***Croup*** is ***acute laryngotracheobronchitis*** usually caused by ***viral illness (parainfluenza virus)***.
- ***Larynx is pale and edematous, barking/metallic cough*** maybe present; usually low grade or no fever; stridor; hoarseness—all ***worsen at night; short course of steroids*** may be required.
- ***Steeple sign*** is seen in ***frontal X-ray; Westley score*** is used for ***croup severity***.

20. Answer is a *(Aspergillus fumigatus).*
Ref: Harrison's, 18th edition Pg 1658, 2119.

➢ ***A. fumigatus*** is the ***MC cause of ABPA***.

Diagnostic features of ABPA

Main diagnostic criteria	Other diagnostic features
➢ Bronchial asthma ➢ Pulmonary infiltrates ➢ Peripheral eosinophilia (> 1,000/L) ➢ Immediate wheal-and-flare response to *A. fumigatus* ➢ Serum precipitins to *A. fumigatus* ➢ Elevated serum IgE ➢ Central bronchiectasis	➢ History of brownish plugs in sputum ➢ Culture of *A. fumigatus* from sputum ➢ Elevated IgE and IgG class antibodies specific for *A. fumigatus*

21. Answer is c (Level of living).
Ref: Park, 22nd edition Pg 16.

'Life' Indicators

Physical quality of life index (PQLI)	– **Infant mortality rate** – Life expectancy at age 1 – Literacy ('***ILL***') – PQLI in India is 45 (1999); ***Kerala*** *has high PQLI*
Human development index (HDI)	– Longevity (life expectancy at birth) – Income (real GDP per capita or purchasing power) – Knowledge/Education (adult literacy rate and mean years of schooling); **('*LIKE*')** – High HDI > 0.8; Medium HDI 0.7–0.799; Low HDI 0.50–0.41 – ***HDI for India is 0.547*** (medium HDI category)
Sullivan's index	– Expectation of life ***free of disability*** – Computed by subtracting from the life expectancy, the probable duration of bed disability and inability to perform major activities – One of the most advanced indicators currently available
Disability adjusted life year (DALY)	– *It expresses* years of life lost to premature death *and* years lived with disability *adjusted for the severity of the disability, one DALY is 1 lost year of healthy life* – ***Measure used to express global burden of disease***
Health-adjusted life expectancy (HALE)	– It is based on life expectancy at birth, but *includes an adjustment for time spent in poor health*. It means equivalent number of years in full health that a newborn can expect to live based on current rates of ill health and mortality
Life expectancy at birth	– As of 2009, for India it is ***63 for males and 66 for females***

22. Answer is a (Hanging).
Ref: Narayan Reddy's FMT, 23rd edition.

➢ **'Le facies sympathique:** A condition seen in hanging. If the ligature knot presses on ***cervical sympathetic chain***, *the eye on the same side may remain open and its pupil dilated*. It indicates ***antemortem hanging***.

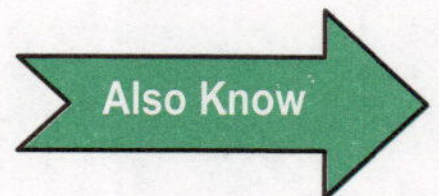

- **Ligature mark:** Most ***important and specific sign of death from hanging***. The mark *encircles the neck except for the place where the knot was located*: The mark is situated ***above the level of thyroid cartilage in 80%*** of cases.

- Antemortem hanging: *Saliva dribbling* **at angle of mouth is a sure sign (this is due to increased salivation just before death due to the stimulation of the salivary glands by the ligature); seminal emission is also a sign.**
- ***Amussat sign***: *Intima of carotid arteries* **show transverse split.**
- **Lynching:** Homicidal hanging in which the suspect/enemy is hanged by a ***rope from a tree by the mob***.

23. Answer is b (CD4 cells).
Ref: Harrison's, 18th edition, Pg 2686.

- There are structural contact sites for T cell molecules known as CD8 and CD4, expressed on the class I or class II membrane-proximal domains, respectively.
- This ensures that when peptide antigens are presented by ***class I molecules, the responding T cells are predominantly of the CD8 class***, and similarly, that ***T cells responding to class II pMHC complexes are predominantly CD4***.
- <u>Note</u>: ***"Rule of 8"***: "CD8 = 8 × 1 (class 1) = 8"; "CD4 = 4 × 2 (class 2) = 8"

24. Answer is b, c (Microtubules, Microfilaments).
Ref: Concepts in Biology, Enger Ross and Bailey, Pg 81.

- A complex array of ***microtubules, microfilaments and intermediate filaments*** provides the internal framework for the ***cell structure and shape***.

25. Answer is d (Cerebral aqueduct).
Ref: Color Atlas of Neuroscience: Neuroanatomy and Neurophysiology, By Ben Greenstein, Pg 66.

Parts of Developing Brain

The cavity of the developing brain shows three dilatations, craniocaudally these are given in the table below.

Developing Brain		Adult Derivatives
Prosencephalon (Forebrain)	→ ***Telencephalon*** (endbrain)	→ Cerebral hemispheres and lateral ventricle
	→ ***Diencephalon***	→ Thalamus, hypothalamus, optic stalk, retina, posterior pituitary and 3rd ventricle
Mesencephalon	→ ***Midbrain***	→ Aqueduct
Rhombencephalon (Hindbrain)	→ ***Metencephalon***	→ Pons and cerebellum and 4th ventricle
	→ ***Myelencephalon***	→ Medulla oblongata

26. Answer is a (Cadaveric rigidity).
Ref: Narayan Reddy's FMT, 23rd edition.

Rigor Mortis (RM)

- Occurs due to ***ATP depletion***.
- ***Appears first in*** **involuntary muscles of heart**; then it begins in the <u>*eyelids*</u> >> neck >> lower jaw >> muscle of face >> muscle of chest and UL >> abdomen >> LL muscle.
- Time of onset of RM: In India it *begins in 1–2 hours after death* and takes further 1–2 hours to develop.
- Duration of RM: In India it *lasts usually 24–48 hours in winter* and 18–36 hours in summer. It last for 2–3 days in temperate regions.
- RM does NOT OCCUR in a *fetus of less than 7 months*.

Early RM	Delayed RM
Occurs in death due to: ➢ Strychnine poisoning ➢ Cholera	Occurs in death due to: ➢ Arsenic poisoning ➢ Apoplexy

➢ Cancers ➢ TB ➢ Typhoid ➢ Fatigue/Exhaustion before death (due to rapid ATP depletion)	➢ Pneumonia ➢ Asphyxia

27. Answer is b (7 days).
Ref: Searching.

- One dietary cycle = 7 days.

28. Answer is b (SLE).
Ref: Harrison's, 18th edition Pg 2729.

Pulmonary Manifestations of SLE

- The ***MC pulmonary manifestation of SLE is pleuritis*** with or without pleural effusion; may respond to treatment with NSAIDs or a brief course of glucocorticoid therapy.
- Pulmonary infiltrates also occur.
- ***Life-threatening pulmonary manifestations*** include ***interstitial inflammation leading to fibrosis, shrinking lung syndrome and intra-alveolar hemorrhage***; all of these probably require early aggressive immunosuppressive therapy as well as supportive care.

29. Answer is a (Gartner's cyst).
Ref: Shaw, 13th edition Pg 13.

- Gartner's cyst is a cyst formed in Gartner's duct.
- ***Gartner's duct*** is a remnant of ***Wolffian duct***.

30. Answer is c (Basal cell carcinoma).
Ref: Bailey and Love's, 26th edition Pg 609-10.

Basal cell carcinoma

- BCC is MC skin cancer.
- It is *locally invasive*, but *rarely metastasizing* malignant epithelioid tumor of basal cells.
- Risk factors: Short wavelength *UV* radiation (290–320 nm, *sunburn* rays), X-rays and arsenic; immunosuppression, xeroderma pigmentosum, Gorlin syndrome, Bazex syndrome.
- ***Histologically:*** Dermis contains irregular masses of basaloid cells having characteristic peripheral ***palisaded*** appearance of the nuclei.

Clinical Types
• ***Noduloulcerative***: ***MC type***, begins as a small pearly nodule with telangiectatic vessels on its surface, may undergo ulceration, crusting, bleeding with a *rolled* border (***rodent ulcer***) • Pigmented, superficial (a/w *arsenic* exposure) and morphoeic (*scar like*)

- ***Treatment:*** Methods used are ***Mohs micrographic surgery (MMS)***, curettage and electrodessication and radiotherapy and cryotherapy.
- *MMS*—removal of the tumor followed by immediate frozen section histopathologic examination of margins with subsequent re-excision of tumor-positive areas and final closure of the defect—gives the ***highest cure rates (98%)*** and results in ***least tissue loss***.

31. Answer is d (Verify the diagnosis).
Ref: Park's, 22nd edition Pg 123.

Steps in investigation of epidemic

1. ***Verification of diagnosis.***
2. Confirmation of existence of epidemic.
3. Defining the population at risk.
4. Rapid search for all cases and their characteristics.
5. Data analysis.
6. Formulation of hypothesis.
7. Testing of hypothesis.
8. Evaluation of ecological factors.
9. Further investigation of population at risk.
10. Writing the report.

32. Answer is b (Kartagener's syndrome).
Ref: BIG Robbins, Pg 692, 750.

Kartagener's syndrome
- Bronchiectasis
- Sinusitis
- Situs inversus
- (A/w poor motility of cilia—***immotile cilia syndrome***)

33. Answer is d (CA 19-9).
Ref: CMDT 2013, Pg 1608.

- ***CA 19–9*** is raised in ***pancreatic cancer.***
- CA 19–9 with a sensitivity of 70% and a specificity of 87%, has *not proved sensitive enough for early detection of pancreatic cancer;* increased values are also found in ***acute and chronic pancreatitis and cholangitis***.

Tumor marker	Cancer
Hormones	
Human chorionic gonadotropin (hCG)	***Gestational trophoblastic disease, Gonadal germ cell tumor***
Calcitonin	***Medullary*** thyroid Ca
Catecholamines (epinephrine, norepinephrine)	***Pheochromocytoma***
Oncofetal antigens	
Alpha-fetoprotein (AFP)	***Hepatocellular Ca, gonadal germ cell tumor*** (NOT pure seminoma)
Carcinoembryonic antigen (CEA)	***Colon cancer*** Others (pancreas, lung, breast, ovary)
Enzymes	
Neuron-specific enolase	Small cell Ca of the lung, neuroblastoma
Prostatic acid phosphatase	Ca prostate
Lactate dehydrogenase	Lymphoma, Ewing's sarcoma
Alkaline phosphatase	***Osteosarcoma***
Placental alkaline phosphatase	Ca ovary, seminoma
Tumor-associated proteins	
Prostate-specific antigen (PSA)	***Prostate cancer***
Monoclonal immunoglobulin	Multiple myeloma

Bladder tumor antigen (BTA)	Bladder cancer
CA-15-3	Breast cancer
CA 27.29	Breast
CA-125 (a glycoprotein)	Ovarian cancer Other cancers (breast, hepatoma, lymphomas)
CA-19-9 (a carbohydrate)	***Pancreatic***, colon, cancer
CD30	Hodgkin's disease, anaplastic large cell lymphoma
CD25	Hairy cell leukemia, adult T-cell leukemia/lymphoma
S-100	***Melanoma***, CNS and nerve tumors
Intermediate filaments	
Keratins	Carcinomas, mesotheliomas
Desmin	Muscle tumors
Vimentin	Sarcomas
Others	
Factor VIII	Kaposi's sarcoma, angiosarcoma
Serum ferritin	Hepatoma
Thyroglobulin	Thyroid cancer and thyroid disorders

34. Answer is a (More the HSV-2 than HSV-1).
Ref: Manual of Clinical Problems in Infectious Disease; edited by Nelson Murray Gantz, 5th edition Pg 148.

- After the first episode of genital herpes infection, the major morbidity of the disease consists of frequent recurrences.
- Most patients with symptomatic genital herpes have generally 5–8 recurrences.
- *Only 14% of patients with genital HSV-1 note a recurrence* after their first episode compared with ***60% of patients with HSV-2***.

35. Answer is a (Acamprosate).
Ref: CMDT 2013, Pg 1082.

• Drugs helping in abstinence (by decreasing pleasurable effects of alcohol): Naltrexone and Acamprosate.
• Alcohol withdrawal symptoms: Detoxification – DOC benzodiazepines (chlordiazepoxide and diazepam); Clonidine suppresses cardiovascular signs of withdrawal and has some anxiolytic effect and may be used.
• Deterrent agents (alcohol sensitizing drugs) used are: – Disulfiram (aldehyde dehydrogenase inhibitor). – Citrated calcium carbide, Metronidazole, Nitrafezole, Methyltetrazolethiol, Animal charcoal, a fungus (coprinus atramentarius), sulfonylureas and certain cephalosporins also cause a disulfiram-like reaction.

36. Answer is a (Stress fracture of neck of 2nd metatarsal).
Ref: Essential Orthopedics, Maheshwari, Pg 87.

- ***Fatigue fracture*** of the ***shaft of the second or third metatarsal = March fracture*** – results from ***prolonged walking or running*** in those not accustomed to it – may occurs in ***fresh army recruits***.
- ***Repeat question*** *from KCET 2012 and 2009 papers.*

37. Answer is b (Hernia).
Ref: Bailey and Love's, 26th edition Pg 1378-79.

- ***Incompletely descended testes (cryptorchidism)*** is a/w ***patent processus vaginalis in 90% of cases***, although incidence of hernia is much lower.

- ***Infertility*** is another known association with paternity rates 2/3 of normal for unilateral and 1/3 of normal for bilateral undescended testis.
- ***Cancer risk*** for adults after cryptorchidism in childhood is 5–10 times greater than normal (***MC seminoma***).
- Undescended testis is more prone to ***testicular torsion***.

38. Answer is a (Hypoglycemia).
Ref: KD Tripathi, 7th edition Pg 293.

Adverse effects of glucocorticoids

- Cushing's habitus: Round face (moon face), narrow mouth, supraclavicular hump, obesity of trunk, with thin limbs
- Fragile skin, purple striae
- Hyperglycemia
- Proximal myopathy
- Susceptibility to infections
- Delayed healing of wounds
- Peptic ulceration
- Osteoporosis
- Avascular necrosis
- Posterior subcapsular cataract
- Steroid-induced glaucoma
- Growth retardation
- Fetal abnormalities: Cleft palate

39. Answer is b (Angle-closure glaucoma).
Ref: Parsons Disease of the Eye, 21st edition Pg 291.

- The ***MC mechanism of angle-closure*** glaucoma is ***pupillary block***.
- ***YAG laser peripheral iridotomy*** is indicated in ***angle-closure glaucoma***.
- ***Prophylactic laser iridotomy*** is indicated in stages of intermittent angle-closure glaucoma and as a definitive treatment in acute angle-closure glaucoma.

40. Answer is c (Polyomavirus).
Ref: BIG Robbins, 8th edition Pg 942-43.

- An emerging ***viral pathogen causing pyelonephritis in kidney allografts is polyomavirus***—direct pick from **Robbins textbook**.
- A distinct form of pyelonephritis called ***polyoma nephropathy***—viral infection of the tubular epithelial cell nuclei leading to nuclear enlargement and intranuclear inclusions visible by light microscopy—***cytopathic effect***.
- Interstitial inflammatory response is invariably present.

41. Answer is b (Ornithic).
Ref: Park, 22nd edition Pg 90.

Exotic	Disease imported into a country in which they do not otherwise occur, e.g. rabies in UK
Epornithic	An outbreak of disease in a ***bird population***
Enzootic	An endemic occurring in animals

42. Answer is a (Interstitial part).
Ref: A Comprehensive Textbook of OBG, Sadhana Gupta, Pg 8.

Uterine (fallopian) tube

- ***Fallopian tube*** is 10 cm long; blood supply = from ovarian A and uterine A; lymphatics = drain to para-aortic nodes.
- There are 4 parts:

Intramural or interstitial	Lies in uterine wall, narrowest part
Isthmus	MC site of ligation during tubal ligation
Ampulla	***Fertilization*** of ova takes place here, MC site of ***ectopic*** pregnancy
Infundibulum	Widest part

43. Answer is c (Transitional cell carcinoma).
Ref: Bailey and Love's, 26th edition Pg 1329.

- In total 95% of ***primary bladder tumors*** originate from ***transitional epithelium***.
- Over 90% of bladder cancers are ***urothelial (transitional cell)*** in origin.

44. Answer is c (Elevated ESR).
Ref: Harrison's, 17th edition Pg 592, Table 90.4.

- ***Increased ESR*** is present in almost ***55% patients*** of ***renal cell Ca***.
- The ***classic triad*** of ***hematuria, flank pain and flank mass*** is present in only 10–20%.
- **Author's comments**: This reference table has been deleted in 18th edition of Harrisons.

45. Answer is d (Total anomalous pulmonary venous return).
Ref: Pediatric Emergency Medicine, By Steven G Rothrock, Pg 70.

Causes of CHF in neonates

- ***Non-cardiac disorders*** (MC cause ion first 24 hours): Sepsis, severe anemia, metabolic causes acidosis, hypothermia, hypoglycemia, hypocalcemia.
- ***Left to right*** intracardiac shunt: Large VSD, complete AV canal, large PDA, AV malformation.
- ***Right to left*** intracardiac shunts: TGA, ***TAPVR***, truncus arteriosus.

46. Answer is a (Supracondylar fracture).
Ref: Essential Orthopedics, Maheshwari, 4th edition Pg 98.

- ***MC complication*** of ***supracondylar fracture of humerus*** due to ***malunion = cubitus <u>VAR</u>us (<u>GUN</u>stock) deformity*** occurs—treat with ***French osteotomy***, "Be<u>*VAR*</u>e of the <u>*GUN*</u>!".

47. Answer is b, c (Overall risk is less than 5%, cancer of rectum is more common than that of colon).
Ref: CMDT 2013, Pg 649.

- The risk of ***neoplasia in chronic UC increases with duration*** and extent of disease.
- A large meta-analysis of observational studies reported a cumulative incidence of 2% at 10 years, 8% at 20 years and 18% after 30 years of disease.
- Because of the relatively high incidence of concomitant carcinoma in patients with ***dysplasia*** (either low or high grade) in flat mucosa or non-endoscopically resectable mass lesions, ***colectomy*** is recommended.
- Chronic treatment with 5-ASA agents and folate is associated with a lower risk of cancer in patients with ulcerative colitis.

48. Answer is d (Ectopic ACTH-producing tumor).
Ref: Harrison's, 18th edition Pg 383, 627.

- Glucocorticoid excess is diagnosed by employing a dexamethasone suppression test—this test is useful to establish the diagnosis of Cushing's syndrome and to assist with the differential diagnosis of cortisol excess.
- Dexamethasone, a potent glucocorticoid, suppresses CRH/ACTH and, therefore, endogenous cortisol.

- **If cortisol production is autonomous** (e.g. adrenal nodule), ACTH is already suppressed and dexamethasone has little additional effect.
- **If cortisol production is driven by an ACTH-producing pituitary adenoma**, dexamethasone suppression is ineffective at low doses, but usually induces suppression at high doses.
- **If cortisol production is driven by an ectopic source of ACTH**, the tumors are usually resistant to dexamethasone suppression.

Note: Also the case history of chronic smoker with hemoptysis is given to suggest Ca lung—which could be the source ***of ectopic ACTH-MC is small cell lung*** cancers.

49. Answer is b (Ethylguaiacol).
Ref: KDT Tripathi, 7th edition Pg 898.

- ***Chlorhexidine, isopropyl alcohol and povidone-iodine*** are commonly used skin antiseptics.
- *Povidone-iodine* is used for routinely painting the parts preoperatively.
- *Chlorhexidine* and *alcohol* are components of many commercially available handwashes and sanitizers used in almost all hospitals these days.
- ***Ethyl guaiacol***: 4-ethylguaiacol, often abbreviated to 4-EG, is a phenolic compound not routinely used as skin antiseptic; a/w wine culturing.

50. Answer is d (G2 to M).
Ref: Genetics, By Patricia A Hoffee, 1999 edition Pg 11.

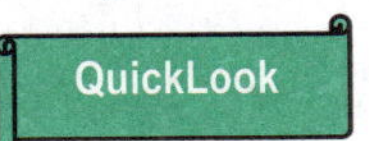

- The ***G2/M DNA damage checkpoint*** serves to prevent the cell from entering mitosis (M-phase) with genomic DNA damage. Specifically, the activity of the ***Cyclin B-cdc2 (CDK1) complex is pivotal in regulating the G2-phase transition*** wherein cdc2 is maintained in an inactive state by the tyrosine kinases Wee1 and Myt1.

51. Answer is d (Vincristine).
Ref: Still searching for accurate reference; KD Tripathi, 7th edition.

- Vincristine causes more of peripheral neuropathy, neurotoxicity and alopecia; SIADH and bone marrow suppression can occur.

52. Answer is d (Measles).
Ref: Nelson's Essentials of Pediatrics, 6th edition Chapter 66.

Known teratogenic viruses

- Cytomegalovirus: ***Petechial rash, periventricular calcifications, microcephaly, chorioretinitis***
- Herpes simplex virus (HSV-1 and 2): *Skin, eye and mouth vesicles*; can progress to severe systemic/CNS infection
- Rubella virus: ***Deafness (MC) 'blueberry muffin' rash, cataracts and 'salt and pepper'*** *chorioretinitis*, ***microcephaly; PDA*** and multiple pulmonary stenoses; encephalitis (*periventricular calcification*)
- Parvovirus B_{19}
- Varicella-zoster virus
- Venezuelan equine encephalitis virus

53. Answer is b (Mitral regurgitation).
Ref: CMDT 2013, Pg 833.

- In SLE; ***pericarditis*** is the ***most frequent cardiac*** manifestation.
- The endocardial involvement can lead to ***valvular insufficiencies, most commonly mitral regurgitation***.

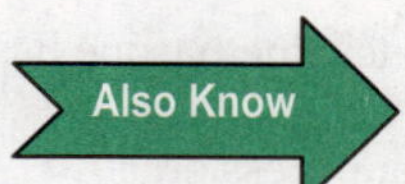

- The MC pulmonary manifestation of SLE is pleuritis with or without pleural effusion.
- The MC hematologic manifestation of SLE is anemia, usually normochromic normocytic, reflecting chronic illness.

54. Answer is a (Red).
Ref: Radiography Essentials for Limited Practice, By Bruce W Long, Eugene D Frank, Ruth Ann Ehrlich, Pg 590.

- ***Safelights*** are special ***light fixtures fitted with filters used in the X-ray darkroom.***
- The safelight filter should permit the passage of frequencies to which the X-ray film is least sensitive.
- ***GBX filters*** should be used in the darkroom.
- They are a ***deep cherry-red*** and are safe for use with blu-sensitive, green sensitive and X-ray sensitive films.
- A ***radiographic film*** can be ***left for 40 seconds*** in the safelight ***without getting fogged.***
- A ***distance of 4 feet*** should be maintained between the safe light and the processing tray.
- ***Wattage of safelight*** should be between ***7 and 15 W.***
- Inside of darkroom should be painted with light color to ensure that safelight is reflected throughout the room.

55. Answer is a (Tibiotalar).
Ref: Essential Orthopedics, Maheshwari, 4th edition Pg 209.

- ***In surgical treatment of CTEV; Triple arthrodesis*** involves fusion of the three joints of foot:
  - Subtalar (talocalcaneal)
  - Calcaneocuboid and
  - Talonavicular joints.

56. Answer is b (Sturge-Weber syndrome).
Ref: CMDT 2013, Pg 997.

- In ***Sturge-Weber syndrome, skull radiographs*** taken ***after the first 2 years of life*** usually reveal ***gyriform ("tramline") intracranial calcification,*** especially in the ***parieto-occipital region,*** due to mineral deposition in the cortex beneath the intracranial angioma.

Abnormal intracranial calcification
– Lipoma of corpus callosum (*bracket like*) – Oligodendroglioma (*serpentine*) – Meningioma (*ball like*) – Dermoid (*arc calcification*) – Craniopharyngioma (*punctate/curvilinear*) – Neurocysticercosis (*rice grain*) – CMV (*periventricular*) – Toxoplasmosis (*scattered flakey*)

57. Answer is c (Discrete bulge in the left cardiac margin below the pulmonary bay).
Ref: Hutchison's pediatrics, Gupta Goel, 2012 edition Pg 670.

Chest X-ray signs of left atrial enlargement
– *Displaced left main and lower lobe bronchi*
– ***Double density*** (double atrial shadow) right side of the left atrium projecting through the right atrium into the adjacent lung—a sign of left atrial enlargement
– ***Fourth mogul***
– *Posterior bulge of upper posterior cardiac outline*
– *Displaced barium filled esophagus*
– *Discrete bulge of left heart border below pulmonary bay*

58. Answer is a (Bellary district, Karnataka).
Ref: http://www.nimhans.kar.nic.in/dmhp/default.htm

- ***District Mental Health Program (DMHP)*** is an approach to decentralize mental health care in the community using the public health infrastructure and other resources.
- This model has been ***pilot tested in Bellary District of Karnataka State*** and found to be very useful to address the basic mental health needs of the population.
- This model has been implemented in all the states and currently there are ***125 DMHP sites in India***.

59. Answer is b (Exotic).
Ref: Park, 22nd edition Pg 90.

Exotic	Disease imported into a country in which they do not otherwise occur, e.g. rabies in UK
Epornithic	An outbreak of disease in a bird population
Enzootic	An endemic occurring in animals

60. Answer is d (Spleen).
Ref: BIG Robbins, 7th edition Pg 705.

- ***Gandy-gamna*** **bodies:** Seen in ***congestive splenomegaly***—areas of fibrosis containing deposits of iron and calcium salts encrusted on connective tissue and elastic fibers.

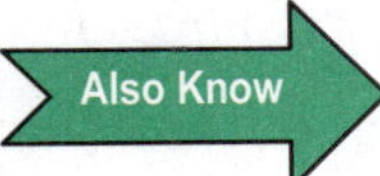

Chronic Venous Congestion of the liver	CVC of Lungs
♦ Seen in ***right ventricular failure***—leads to ***'Nutmeg'*** liver ♦ With severe CVC of liver, fibrous thickening of the walls of the veins and central sinusoids leads to ***'cardiac sclerosis' ('cardiac cirrhosis')***	♦ Seen in ***Left ventricular failure***; if chronic leads to—edematous hemosiderin laden septa become fibrotic—***'brown induration of lungs'*** ♦ ***'Heart failure cells'*** hemosiderin laden intra-alveolar macrophages

61. Answer is c (Amastigote).
Ref: Harrison's, 18th edition Pg 1714.

- ***Demonstration of amastigotes*** in smears of tissue aspirates (usually within macrophages) is the ***gold standard for the diagnosis*** of visceral and cutaneous leishmaniasis.
- Caused by ***Leishmania donovani in India.***
- Transmitted by ***sandfly bite***.
- ***Visceral leishmaniasis***: Irregular fever, progressive hepatosplenomegaly, pancytopenia, wasting.
- ***Cutaneous leishmaniasis***: Chronic, painless, moist ulcers or dry nodules.
- ***Mucocutaneous leishmaniasis***: Destructive nasopharyngeal lesions.

62. Answer is c (Posterior part of calcarine sulcus).
Ref: Atlas of Neurosurgical Techniques: Brain; edited by Laligam N Sekhar, Richard G Fessler, Pg 525.

- The ***posterior calcarine sulcus*** represents the ***primary visual (striate) cortex (Brodmann area 17)*** on its upper and lower lip whereas the anterior calcarine sulcus only on its lower lip—in the ***occipital lobe***.

63. Answer is c (Epiglottitis).
Ref: Textbook of ENT, Dhingra, 5th edition Pg 331.

Acute epiglottitis

- Caused by ***Haemophilus influenzae type B***.
- Marked *swelling of epiglottis,* which may extend to the supraglottic tissues.
- ***Dysphagia occurs early*** and a ***change in cry or voice*** is characteristic.
- ***Inspiratory stridor*** develops rapidly and may progress, if untreated, to fatal respiratory obstruction within a few hours.
- X-ray shows ***'thumb sign'*** *on lateral radiographs*—***enlarged epiglottis.***
- ***Tracheostomy*** should be done to relieve respiratory difficulty.
- Antibiotics (*ampicillin, cefotaxime, ceftriaxone, chloramphenicol*) are needed.

64. Answer is c (Caffeine).
Ref: Lowinson and Ruiz's Substance Abuse: A Comprehensive Textbook, edited by Pedro Ruiz, Eric C Strain, Pg 335.

- ***Caffeine is the most widely used mood altering drug*** in the ***world***.
- ***90% of people in the world*** use caffeine in one form or the other.

65. Answer is c (Hilus cells).
Ref: Fundamentals of Histology, GP Verma, Pg 380.

- In ***primordial follicles,*** the oocyte is arrested in the last stage of prophase (known as dictyotene). At this stage, it is surrounded by a single layer of flattened ovarian follicular epithelial cells (these cells are also known as ***granulosa cells***). They are small and usually found close to the ***outer edge of the cortex***.
- After ovulation, the ruptured follicle collapses and fills with a blood clot (corpus hemorrhagicum), which then forms the ***corpus luteum***. If pregnancy does not occur, then the corpus luteum degenerates into the ***corpus albicans***.
- ***Hilus cells*** are located within the ovarian hilum.

66. Answer is b (External branch of superior laryngeal nerve).
Ref: Textbook of ENT, Dhingra, 5th edition Pg 320.

- ***Paralysis of superior laryngeal nerve*** causes paralysis of cricothyroid muscle an ipsilateral anesthesia of the larynx above the vocal cord.
- ***Voice is weak and pitch cannot be raised***.
- Isolated paralysis of superior laryngeal nerve is uncommon—may occur due to thyroid surgery, tumors, neuritis or diphtheria.
- However thyroid surgery MC causes combined (complete) paralysis (recurrent and superior laryngeal nerve paralysis).

67. Answer is d (Emphysema).
Ref: CMDT 2013, Pg 260-61.

- ***Emphysema*** causes ***increased static lung compliance***.
- See answer for **Q no. 142–144** below.

68. Answer is b (Toxoplasmosis).
Ref: Washington Manual Pediatrics, 2012 edition Pg 314.

The rule of 3's and 9's for HEAD circumference

- Birth: 35 cm
- 3 months: 40 cm
- 3 years: 50 cm
- 9 years to adult: 55 cm

- Hence answer for above question is ***increased head circumference at 2 years***; ***toxoplasmosis*** can cause ***hydrocephalus leading to macrocephaly***.

69. Answer is d (ARDS).
Ref: 2010-Jun: Safety of talc pleurodesis, Nam et al, Journal of Hong Kong Respiratory Medicine.

- Talc is an effective agent for pleurodesis. ARDS is a potential life-threatening condition, which may be related to the dose and particle size of the talc.
- Current evidence suggests that calibrated large particle size talc may be a/w a lower risk of systemic complications.

70. Answer is a (Congenital glaucoma).
Ref: Parson's Diseases of the Eye, 2nd edition Pg 296.

- Haab's ***striae*** (Horizontal breaks in Descemet's membrane), increased IOP.
- Also remember: Vogt's striae are Vertical striae in keratoconus.

71. Answer is a (Hepatitis C virus).
Ref: CMDT 2013, Pg 1604-1607.

- Hepatocellular carcinomas are a/w cirrhosis in 80% of cases.
- Incidence rates are rising rapidly in Western countries, presumably because of the ***increasing prevalence of cirrhosis*** caused by ***chronic hepatitis C infection*** and *non-alcoholic fatty liver disease*.

Risk Factors for Hepatocellular Carcinoma

Common	Uncommon
– Chronic hepatitis B and hepatitis C – Cirrhosis (from any cause) – Chronic alcohol, hemochromatosis – Aflatoxin – Non-alcoholic fatty liver; non-alcoholic steatohepatitis	– Exposure to long-term estrogens in the form of contraceptives or androgens – Alpha-1-antitrypsin deficiency – Tyrosinemia, citrullinemia – Porphyria, cutanea, tarda, Wilson's disease

72. Answer is b (Pendrin protein).
Ref: Thyroid and Parathyroid Diseases: Medical and Surgical Management, edited by David Terris, Christine Gourin, 2009 edition Pg 19.

- ***Iodine*** is a crucial constituent of thyroid hormone and the first step in thyroid hormone synthesis is active transport of iodide against a large concentration and electrical gradient from the serum into the thyroid follicular cell.
- This is mediated by the sodium iodide transporter located in the basolateral membrane.
- ***Intracellular iodide*** is ***transported across the apical membrane into the follicular lumen by Pendrin*** an iodide-chloride transporter.
- ***Pendrin gene*** is on ***chromosome*** 7: Mutations give rise to ***Pendred's syndrome*** characterized by ***familial goiter, congenital sensorineural deafness*** and ***autosomal recessive***.

73. Answer is c (Pantothenate).
Ref: Lippincott's illustrated biochemistry, Pg 130.

COMED-K 2013 ANSWERS

Vitamin B_5 (pantothenic acid)

- ***Deficiency***: Dermatitis, alopecia, enteritis, adrenal insufficiency
- ***Function***: Constituent of ***CoA*** and component of ***fatty acid synthase.***

74. Answer is c (Cefpodoxime).
Ref: Katzung Basic and Clinical Pharmacology, 12th edition Pg 799, 800.

- ***First- and second-generation cephalosporins*** have limited or no activity against *Pseudomonas aeruginosa.*
- Even though ***cefpodoxime*** is a third-generation cephalosporin, it is ***inactive*** against *Pseudomonas.*

Cephalosporins with antipseudomonal activity

Third generation	Fourth generation
Ceftazidime and Cefoperazone	Cefpirome and Cefepime (due to zwitterion character)

75. Answer is a (It is less than 2 weeks of duration).
Ref: Harrison's, 18th edition Pg 256-57.

- ***Acute rhinosinusitis—defined as sinusitis of < 4 weeks' duration***—constitutes the vast majority of sinusitis cases.
- The ostial obstruction that results in rhinosinusitis can arise from both ***infectious and non-infectious causes***.
- ***Fungi are also*** established causes of sinusitis although most acute cases are in immunocompromised patients—rhinocerebral mucormycosis caused by fungi of the order ***Mucorales***, which includes Rhizopus, Rhizomucor, Mucor, Mycocladus.
- Most patients with a clinical diagnosis of acute rhinosinusitis ***improve without antibiotic therapy***.

76. Answer is b (Persuasion).
Ref: The Power of Persuasion: How We're Bought and Sold; By Robert Levine, Pg 241.

- ***Persuasion*** was seen as an essential skill of living—"the art of winning friends and influencing people" as the famous ***Dale Carnegie*** put it.

77. Answer is c (*Clostridium difficile*).
Ref: CMDT 2013, Pg 637.

- ***Clostridium difficile infection (CDI)*** is a unique colonic disease that is acquired almost ***exclusively in association with antimicrobial use*** and the consequent disruption of the normal colonic flora.
- CDI results from the ingestion of spores of *C. difficile* that vegetate, multiply and secrete toxins, causing ***diarrhea and pseudomembranous colitis (PMC)***.

78. Answer is b (Glottis).
Ref: Clinical Pathology; By James Carton, Pg 46.

- The two most important determinants of prognosis are the stage of the disease and the presence or absence of lymph node metastases.
- ***Glottic carcinomas have the best prognosis*** with a ***5 year survival rate of up to 85%,*** probably because they present early with hoarseness and tend to remain localized for longer.

79. Answer is b (*Nocardia brasiliensis*).
Ref: Medical Microbiology, edited by David Greenwood, 2012 edition Pg 235.

- Some species of ***Nocardia are partially acid fast*** (meaning that a less concentrated solution of sulfuric or hydrochloric acid should be used during the staining procedure) due to the presence of intermediate-length *mycolic acids in their cell wall.*
- With the ***modified Kinyoun acid-fast stain using weak acid (1% sulfuric acid) for decolorization,*** the nocardiae are often seen as partially acid-fast filamentous bacilli (showing both acid-fast and non-acid-fast organisms).

80. Answer is c (Sympathetic nerve).
Ref: SRB's Manual of Surgery SR Bhat.

- Layers of the ***scrotum*** from within outwards:
  - Skin
  - Dartos muscle
  - External spermatic fascia
  - Cremasteric fascia
  - Internal spermatic fascia.
- ***Dartos*** is supplied by ***sympathetic nerve***.

81. Answer is d (Is associated with depressed muscle tone).
Ref: Sleep Medicine, edited by Harold R Smith, Pg 11.

Sleep stage and EEG waves	Features
Awake ➢ Beta ➢ Alpha	 Active mental concentration Relaxed with eyes closed
Stage 1 ➢ Theta (4–6 Hz); low voltage alpha; vertex sharp waves	5% of sleep time Lightest stage of sleep characterized by peacefulness, slowed pulse and respiration, decreased BP and episodic body movements
Stage 2 ➢ Sleep spindles (12–14 Hz) and high amplitude 'K' complexes	Largest percentage of sleep time (45%)
Stages 3, 4: Slow wave sleep, SWS ➢ High amplitude low frequency, 2 Hz, delta waves ➢ Stage 3 = < 50% delta waves with sleep spindles ➢ Stage 4 = > 50% delta waves, but NO sleep spindles	25% of sleep time (decreases with age) Deepest, most relaxed stages of sleep a/w sleep disorders mentioned below; SWS is most prominent in childhood (growth hormone secretion occurs) and in the healthy elderly male, SWS maybe completely absent
Rapid eye movement (REM) sleep ➢ "Sawtooth" beta, alpha and theta waves	25% of sleep time (decreases with age) Dreaming; penile and clitoral erection; increased pulse, respiration, BP and gastric motility; low skeletal muscle tone and paralysis

82. Answer is a *(Aspergillus niger)*.
Ref: Textbook of ENT, Dhingra, 5th edition Pg 58.

- ***Otomycosis*** is a ***fungal infection of the ear canal*** that occurs often due to *Aspergillus niger, A. fumigatus or Candida albicans.*
- External canal is filled with ***wet debris or flakes resembling wet newspaper/blotting paper***; musty odor.
- Keep ear ***clean and dry***; suction clearance; ***antifungal*** ear drops.

83. Answer is d (Iron deficiency anemia).
Ref: CMDT 2013, Pg 1616.

- ***Iron deficiency anemia*** due to ***chronic blood loss or anemia of chronic disease*** is common in ***gastric cancers***.

84. Answer is b (Mitral regurgitation).
Ref: CMDT 2013, Pg 833.

- See ***answer no. 53 above*** since this a ***repeat topic*** in the same question paper.

85. Answer is b (Duloxetine).
Ref: KD Tripathi, 7th edition Pg 458.

Classification of Antidepressants

Selective serotonin reuptake inhibitors (**SSRIs**)	Fluoxetine, Fluvoxamine, Paroxetine, Sertraline, Citalopram, Escitalopram
Tricyclic antidepressants: *NA and serotonin reuptake inhibitors*	Imipramine, Nortriptyline (best tolerated), Amitriptyline, Desipramine, Protriptyline, Trimipramine, Clomipramine, Doxepine
Tetracyclic antidepressants	Amoxapine, Maprotiline, Mianserin
selective serotonin noradrenaline reuptake inhibitors (**SNRIs**)	Duloxetine, Venlafaxine, Milnacipran
Noradrenaline reuptake inhibitors (**NARI**)	Reboxetine
5-HT2 antagonists	Nefazodone, Trazodone
Dopamine and NA reuptake inhibitors	Bupropion
Melatonin receptor ***agonist*** and 5-HT2c antagonist	Agomelatin

86. Answer is a (Ambulatory patients).
Ref: Bailey and Love's, 25th edition Pg 286.

Triage Four Color Codes

Red: High priority treatment or transfer
Yellow: Medium priority
Green: Ambulatory patients
Black: Dead or moribund patients

87. Answer is c (Mycosis fungoides).
Ref: CMDT Pg 115-116.

- ***Bexarotene*** is a *synthetic retinoid X receptor ligand*, which has activity in ***cutaneous T cell lymphoma (Mycoses fungoides).***

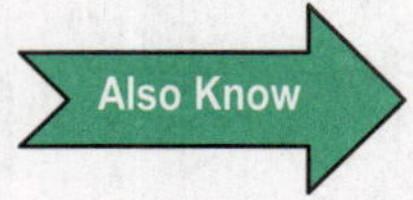

- Patients with ***localized early-stage mycosis fungoides*** can be cured with radiotherapy, often ***total-skin electron beam irradiation***.
- More advanced disease has been treated with *topical glucocorticoids, topical nitrogen mustard, phototherapy, psoralen with ultraviolet A (PUVA), extracorporeal photopheresis, retinoids (bexarotene), electron beam radiation, interferon, antibodies, fusion toxins, histone deacetylase inhibitors (vorinostat and romidepsin) and systemic cytotoxic therapy.*

88. Answer is b (Presbycusis).
Ref: Textbook of ENT, Dhingra, 5th edition Pg 206.

- ***Presbycusis*** or ***age-related hearing loss*** is the ***most frequent cause of sensory hearing loss*** and is progressive, predominantly high-frequency and symmetrical.

89. Answer is c (Rifampicin).
Ref: Katzung Basic and Clinical Pharmacology, 12th edition Pg 610; KD Tripathi, 7th edition Pg 623.

Factors Increasing Effect of Warfarin	Factors Decreasing Effects of Warfarin
Aspirin	Barbiturates
Fluconazole	Rifampicin
Metronidazole	Carbamazepine
Amiodarone	Griseofulvin
Cimetidine	OCPs
Disulfiram	Cholestyramine
Phenylbutazone	Diuretics
Sulfinpyrazone	Vitamin K
TMP-SMX	Hypothyroidism
III gen cephalosporins	
Heparin	
Hepatic disease	
Hyperthyroidism	

90. Answer is a (Interstitial cells of Cajal).
Ref: CMDT 2013, Pg 1619.

GASTROINTESTINAL MESENCHYMAL (STROMAL) TUMORS

- These occur throughout the GIT, but MC ***in the stomach (66%)***; a/w neurofibromatosis.
- MC stromal tumors are ***gastrointestinal stromal tumors ('GIST')***, originate from ***interstitial cells of Cajal***.
- GIST are a/w mutations in ***KIT, a receptor tyrosine kinase***; most GIST stain positively for ***CD117*** (part of the KIT protein); high CD117 = high malignant potential.
- Usually asymptomatic; GIST may be discovered incidentally; may cause hematemesis, melena, pain.
- ***Endoscopic US*** (possibly with guided FNA biopsy) is the optimal study
- ***Surgery*** is recommended for all patients with tumors that are symptomatic; or for risk of malignancy.
- Treatment: ***Tyrosine kinase inhibitor imatinib mesylate***; if resistant may respond to ***sunitinib***.
- ***Carney's triad***: GIST, pulmonary chondroma and/or functioning extra-adrenal paraganglioma.

91. Answer is a (Neural ectoderm).
Ref: Parson's diseases of the eye, 22nd edition Pg 5.

– ***Retina and retinal pigment epithelium develops from the neural ectoderm*** and in fact is considered a 'nerve' itself due to the nature of its functions.

EMBRYOLOGY OF EYE STRUCTURES

Surface ectoderm	Neural ectoderm	Neural crest
◆ Conjunctival epithelium ◆ Corneal epithelium ◆ Lens ◆ Lacrimal glands ◆ Tarsal glands (Meibomian, Zeis, Moll) ◆ Skin of eyelids and eyelashes	◆ Smooth muscles of iris (sphincter and dilator pupillae) ◆ Optic vesicle and cup ◆ Iris epithelium ◆ Ciliary epithelium ◆ Part of vitreous ◆ Retina and retinal pigment epithelium	◆ Corneal stroma, keratocytes and endothelium ◆ Sclera (maximally) ◆ Trabecular meshwork endothelium ◆ Iris stroma ◆ Ciliary muscles ◆ Choroidal stroma ◆ Part of the vitreous ◆ Uveal and conjunctival melanocytes
Mesoderm		

• Extraocular muscles • Corneal stroma • Sclera (temporal small portion) • Iris • Choroid • Vascular endothelium of eye and orbit • Part of vitreous	• Optic nerve	• Meningeal sheaths of the optic nerve • Ciliary ganglion • Schwann cells of the ciliary nerves • Orbital bones • Orbital connective tissue • Connective tissue sheath and muscular layer of ocular, and orbital blood vessels • Melanocytes (uveal and conjunctival)

92. Answer is d (Fetal alcohol syndrome).
Ref: KD Tripathi, 7th edition Pg 392.

- Even ***moderate drinking of alcohol during pregnancy*** can result in ***fetal alcohol syndrome*** resulting an ***intrauterine and postnatal growth retardation, low IQ, microcephaly, craniofacial*** *and other abnormalities and immunological impairment.*
- ***Heavy drinking*** of alcohol during pregnancy = ***increased miscarriages, stillbirths and low-birth-weight babies***.

93. Answer is a (Pneumomediastinum).
Ref: Harrison's, 18th edition Pg 2182.

- ***Hamman's sign,*** which is a crunching or clicking noise synchronous with the heartbeat and is best heard in the left lateral decubitus position—in pneumomediastinum.
- In pneumomediastinum, there is ***gas in the interstices of the mediastinum***.
- Typically, there is ***severe substernal chest pain*** with or without radiation into the neck and arms. The physical examination usually reveals ***subcutaneous emphysema in the suprasternal notch***.
- The diagnosis is confirmed with the ***chest radiograph***.
- Usually no treatment is required, but the mediastinal air will be absorbed faster, if the patient ***inspires high concentrations of oxygen.***

94. Answer is a (Ongoing substance abuse).
Ref: Harrison's, 18th edition Pg 2608.

For Liver Transplantation

Absolute contraindications	Relative contraindications
• ***Sepsis*** • ***Active alcohol or drug abuse (should be abstinent for 6 months)*** • ***Malignancy*** to liver • Advanced ***cardiopulmonary disease*** • Cholangiocarcinoma • AIDS	• Age > 70 years • Morbid obesity • Portal and mesenteric vein thrombosis • Severe malnutrition • Lack of patient understanding

<u>Note</u>: *MC indication of liver transplantation* ***in children = biliary atresia; in adults = end-stage cirrhosis*** of all causes.

95. Answer is a (Chondroblastoma).
Ref: Orthopedic secrets, David E Brown, 3rd edition Pg 78.

- ***Chondroblastomas*** are typically ***benign tumors***; histology shows "***chicken wire***" appearance; risk of malignancy is only 2%.

<u>Bone diseases with high risk of malignancy</u>

- Multiple hereditary exostoses: 10%
- ***Ollier's*** disease (enchondromatosis): 30%

- *Maffucci* syndrome: 100%
- ***Familial retinoblastoma*** syndrome patients are at high risk for developing ***osteosarcoma.***

96. Answer is b (Positive test—type IV reaction).
Ref: CMDT 2013, Pg 283.

- Tuberculin test is a ***type IV*** hypersensitivity reaction.
- AND 15 mm × 10 mm is certainly a positive test.

97. Answer is c (HIV-AIDS).
Ref: CMDT 2013, Pg 224, 225, Fig 8.4.

- ***Oral hairy leukoplakia*** occurs on the ***lateral border of the tongue*** and is a ***common early finding in HIV infection***.
- It often develops quickly and appears as slightly raised leukoplakic areas with a corrugated or 'hairy' surface.
- Clinical regression following administration of ***zidovudine or acyclovir*** has been reported and *treatment is under active investigation*.

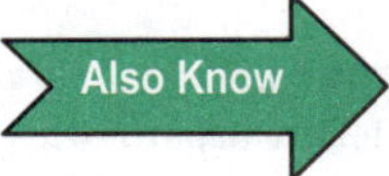

Premalignant lesions of oral cavity
- Oral leukoplakia
- Oral submucus fibrosis
- Oral lichen planus
- Syphilis: Syphilitic interstitial glossitis with endarteritis
- Carcinogenic irritants
- Chronic hyperplastic candidiasis
- Discoid lupus erythematosus
- Dyskeratosis congenita (a/w oral leukoplakia)
- Plummer vinson syndrome (Paterson-Kelly syndrome or sideropenic dysphagia): Achlorhydria, iron deficiency anemia, esophageal ***(hypopharyngeal, postcricoid)*** *webs, atrophy of mucosa of mouth, pharynx; a/w SCC*

98. Answer is b (Falciparum malaria).
Ref: CMDT 2013, Pg 1495.

- ***Blackwater fever*** is a rare severe illness, probably due to hypersensitivity that includes marked hemolysis and hemoglobinuria (DIC and renal failure) in the setting of ***quinine therapy for falciparum malaria***.

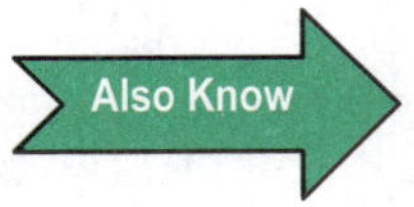

Clinical features of malaria

- ***Fever with rigors; anemia, splenomegaly*** (early with *P. vivax* and *P. falciparum,* late in *P. malariae).*
- Complications
  - *P. falciparum* = Malignant tertian malaria; ***Cerebral malaria, Blackwater fever*** (*DIC and renal failure*); ***Algid malaria*** (*peripheral circulatory failure*)
  - ***P. vivax*** = **splen**ic rupture. "**Why wax** (vivax) spleen?!"
  - ***P. malariae*** = **Neph**rotic syndrome. **"Malariae** is **Neph**arious"!

99. Answer is a (Serial interval).
Ref: Park, 22nd edition Pg 96.

Author's comments: "An often repeated question in all PG entrance examinations including KCET 2002 and 2009 in the same form and in almost every year paper in a different form".

- ***Serial interval***: The ***gap in time between the onset of the primary case and the secondary case is called serial interval***.
- In actual practice we seldom know the incubation period of a disease. But we know when an outbreak of disease occurs say in a family, which is the smallest group and also a closed group, there is an initial primary case.
- The primary case is followed by 2 or 3 secondary cases within short time. By collecting information about a series of such onsets, we get a distribution of secondary cases from which we can guess the incubation period of the disease.

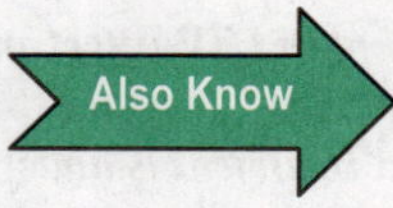

- ***Latent period*** is *equivalent of incubation period* in infectious diseases. It is used in non-communicable disease and is defined as the period from disease initiation to disease detection.
- ***Generation time*** is defined as *"the interval of time between receipt of infection by a host and maximal infectivity of the host"*. In general, generation time is roughly equal to the incubation period. However, these two terms are not the same. Incubation period can be applied to infections that result in manifest disease, whereas generation time refers to transmissions of infection, whether subclinical or clinical.
- ***Communicable period*** is defined as *"the time during which an infectious agent may be transmitted directly or indirectly from an infected person to another person, from an infected animal to a man or from an infected person to an animal including arthropods"*.

100. Answer is d (Sertoli cell).
Ref: Essentials of Medical Physiology, Indu Khurana, Pg 493.

- ***Sertoli cells*** (supporting or sustentacular cell) are present in the epithelial layer of the seminiferous tubules.
- The ***tight junctions between the Sertoli cells*** creates a barrier between the seminiferous tubules and the bloodstream called ***blood testis barrier***.

101. Answer is c (Hypercalcemia).
Ref: Harrison's, 18th edition Pg 445, 967.

Adverse effects of Loop (high ceiling) and thiazide type diuretics include

- *Hypo*kalemia
- *Hypo*calcemia
- *Hypo*magnesemia
- Dilutional *hypo*natremia
- Hyper<u>G</u>lycemia, Hyper<u>U</u>ricemia and Hyper<u>L</u>ipidemia (***Hyper- <u>GU</u>r<u>L</u>!***)
- Acute saline depletion
- Hearing loss/ototoxicity.

102. Answer is d (Mononuclear stromal cells).
Ref: MRI of Bone and Soft Tissue Tumors and Tumor-like Lesions: Differential; By Steven P Meyers, Pg 462.

- Giant cell tumors are composed of neoplastic, ovoid and/or spindle-shaped mononuclear stromal cells, CD68 positive monocytes and multinucleated osteoclast-like giant cells.

103. Answer is a (Louis Pasteur).
Ref: Textbook of Immunology and Microbiology, Parija, 2012 edition Pg 4.

Contributions of Louis Pasteur "Father of Microbiology" include

- He proposed the "*germ theory of disease*".
- Coined the term *vaccine* and pioneered vaccination against anthrax and rabies.
- ***Pasteruization.***
- Control of ***pebrine disease of silkworms***.

104. Answer is a (Acute hemolysis).

Ref: Harrison's, 18th edition Pg 595.

- ***Copper sulfate poisoning*** is usually accidental and manifests with nausea and vomiting, diarrhea, hepatic failure, mental deterioration, ***hemolytic anemia*** and renal dysfunction.

105. Answer is c (D10 to D12).

Ref: Essential Obstetrics and Gynaecology, edited by E Malcolm Symonds et al; Pg

- ***Sympathetic fibers*** arise from *preganglionic fibers at the* ***T10/T11 level*** and supply the ***ovaries and fallopian tubes*** through sympathetic fibers that follow the ovarian vessels.

106. Answer is a (Hemangioma).

Ref: CMDT 2013. Pg 701.

- The ***MC benign neoplasm of the liver is the cavernous hemangioma***, often an *incidental finding on ultrasonography or CT.*

About the Other Options

- ***Focal nodular hyperplasia*** occurs at all ages and in both sexes and is probably ***not caused by the oral contraceptives***. It is often ***asymptomatic*** and appears as a ***hypervascular mass***, often with a ***central hypodense 'stellate' scar on CT or MRI***. It is not a true neoplasm, but a non-specific reaction to altered blood flow.
- ***Hepatocellular adenoma*** occurs ***MC in women in their 30s–40s*** usually caused by ***oral contraceptives***; acute *abdominal pain may occur, if the tumor undergoes necrosis or hemorrhage.*
- ***Hepatoblastoma***: It is an uncommon malignant liver neoplasm occurring in infants and children; usually present with an abdominal mass; most commonly diagnosed during a child's first 3 years of life; α-fetoprotein (AFP) commonly is elevated.

107. Answer is a (Can be used to relieve pain from intra-abdominal malignancy).

Ref: Miller's Basic of Anesthesia, 6th edition Pg 711.

- The ***MC application of neurolytic celiac plexus block*** is to ***treat pain a/w intra-abdominal malignancy***; particularly pain a/w ***pancreatic cancer***.
- ***Physiologic effects*** following celiac plexus block include: ***Orthostatic hypotension; sudden diarrhea and abdominal camping, hiccups.***
- ***Complications*** include: ***Retroperitoneal hematoma, abdominal aortic dissection, paraplegia, interscapular back pain, reactive pleurisy, hematuria, pneumothorax.***

108. Answer is b (Stunted).

Ref: Achar's Textbook of Pediatrics, 4th edition Pg 46.

Interpretation of nutritional status (waterflow classification)

Code	Height for age	Weight for height	Interpretation of nutritional status
A	Normal	Low	Wasted
B	Low	Low	Stunted + wasted
C	Low	Normal	Stunted
D	Low	High	Stunted + obese
E	Normal	High	Obese
F	High	Low	Wasted

109. Answer is c (2:1).
Ref: Doubtful....

- Most books including ***Shaw's Textbook of Gynaecology (15th edition, page 8)*** mentions that ***before puberty the body: cervix ratio is 1:2, at puberty 2:1*** and during the ***reproductive years it may be 3:1 or 4:1*** and then the organ atrophies even though, the revised answer key still maintained this as the reverse (2:1), if u have a good reference this can be challenged, in case this question repeats (thanks many of u).

110. Answer is c (Papillary carcinoma of thyroid).
Ref: Bailey and Love's 26th edition Pg 765, Fig 51.40.

Thyroid cancers

Type	Cells affected	Characteristics	Prognosis
Papillary	Columnar cells of gland	**Most common form** (80% cases); more common in **younger** patients begins as slow-growing nodule; eventually metastasis to local **cervical lymph nodes**; *Orphan annie* (ground glass) nuclei; ***Psammoma bodies;*** ↑ risk with childhood irradiation ("Remember As Papiral**LY** - **LY**mph nodes")	**Excellent**; few recurrences
Follicular	Cuboid cells in follicles	10% of thyroid cancers; MC in older patients; may function like normal thyroid tissue; metastasizes to liver, lung, bone and brain	Good, but worse than papillary cancer; 50% 10-year survival
Medullary	*Parafollicular C cells*	**Produces calcitonin;** may present with other endocrine tumors (e.g. ***MEN2a and MEN2b, a/w ret oncogene***)	Worse in older patients; metastases common at diagnosis
Anaplastic	Poorly differentiated	**Very aggressive**; local extension causes hoarseness, dysphagia	***Very poor***

111. Answer is d (Intrauterine growth retardation).
Ref: Park, 22nd edition Pg 495.

- ***Low-birth-weight (LBW) infant*** is any infant with ***birth weight less than 2.5 kg regardless of gestational age***.
- Two main groups of LBW babies:
  - *In countries where the population of LBW infants is less—**short gestation period*** is major cause.
  - *In countries where the proportion of LBW babies is high (India),* the majority of cases can be attributed to ***fetal growth retardation***.

112. Answer is a (Objectives).
Ref: Park, 22nd edition Pg 811.

- ***An objective (point)*** is precise; it is either achieved or not achieved; it is ***the planned end point of all activities***.
- ***Target*** often refers to a ***discrete activity*** such as the number of blood films collected, etc.
- *Goals*: Is the ***ultimate desired state*** toward, which *objectives and resources are directed*.

113. Answer is c (Stunted growth).
Ref: Harrison's, 18th edition Pg 595.

Zinc	
Deficiency	**Toxicity**
Growth retardation, ↓ taste and smell, alopecia, dermatitis and diarrhea (***acrodermatitis enteropathica***), immune dysfunction, failure to thrive, ***gonadal atrophy***, congenital malformations	General: Reduced copper absorption, gastritis, sweating, fever, nausea, vomiting Occupational: Respiratory distress, ***pulmonary fibrosis***

114. Answer is a (Contrast study of small bowel fluoroscopically).
Ref: S Das Textbook of Surgery, Pg 617.

- Author's Comments: "This is a repeat question from ***KCET 2007***".
- ***'Entero'*** is Greek for intestine. ***'Clysis'*** is Greek for washing out. Thus, enteroclysis is ***washing out of the intestine***.
- With this in mind, an enteroclysis study of the small bowel is a minimally invasive radiographic procedure of the small intestine, which requires the introduction of a catheter into the small intestine followed by the injection of barium and methylcellulose. The barium coats the intestine and the methylcellulose distends the lumen to give a double contrast examination that allows for fluoroscopic visualization of the entire small bowel.

115. Answer is d (High block impairs the ability to cough).
Ref: Concise Anatomy for Anaesthesia; By Andreas G Erdmann, 2nd edition Pg 167.

Spinal Anesthesia

- Site: *L3-L4* **space in** *adults; L4-L5* **space in *children*.**

Structures that the needle will pierce

1. Skin/Subcutaneous fat, fascia
2. Supraspinous ligament
3. Interspinous ligament
4. Ligamentum flavum
5. Epidural space
6. Dura mater
7. Arachnoid mater
8. Subarachnoid space—CSF

Baricity

- Local anesthetic agents are either **heavier (*hyperbaric*)**, **lighter (*hypobaric*)** or have the same specific gravity **(*isobaric*)** as the CSF.
- Hyperbaric solutions tend to spread below the level of the injection, while isobaric solutions are not influenced in this way.
- It is ***easier to predict*** the spread of spinal anesthesia when using a hyperbaric agent.

Drugs

- ***Bupivacaine***: 0.5% ***hyperbaric*** (heavy) ***is the best agent to use***; it *lasts longer than most other spinal anesthetics*: usually 2–3 hours.
- ***Lignocaine***: 5% hyperbaric (heavy) lignocaine gives best results, which lasts 45–90 minutes. 2% lignocaine can also be used, but it has a much shorter duration of action. If 0.2 mL of adrenaline 1:1,000 is added to the lignocaine, it will usefully prolong its duration of action. Lignocaine from multidose vials should *NOT* be used for intrathecal injection as it contains potentially harmful preservatives.

Factors affecting height or level of block

- Volume of drug—m*ore* ***volume, more the height*** of block
- Height of patient—in ***tall patients more drug is required***
- Obesity, ascites, pregnancy.

Complications of spinal anesthesia

1. ***Hypotension (MC complication):***
   - Prophylactic Rx: Treat by ***preloading with 1.5 L Ringer lactate solution***
   - Curative Rx: *Head low position, fluids, vasopressors (ephedrine, mephentermine), inotropes (dopamine) and oxygen inhalation*
2. **Postspinal headache:**
   - Usually ***occipital***, relieved on lying down, lasting for ***7–10 days***
   - Prophylactic: Use small bore needle, adequate hydration, avoid sitting position postoperatively
   - Curative: Lie supine, analgesia, abdominal binder, epidural blood patch
3. **Total spinal anesthesia ('high block'):**
   - Sensory block that rises *above the cervical region;* it is unintentional and may occur due to patient movement, inappropriate positioning or inappropriate dose of local anesthetic
   - Manifests as ***bradycardia, hypotension, dyspnea, inability to speak and cough, difficulty in swallowing*** and ***loss of consciousness***; *Ephedrine is used for hypotension*
   - Treat supportively with oxygenation, ventilation and maintain circulation until the block wears off (*usually wears off rapidly*)

Note: The ***spinal cord terminates*** the ***lower border of L1 in adults***.

116. Answer is a (It is characterized by recurrent and unpredictable panic attacks).
Ref: CMDT 2013, Pg 1041.

- ***Panic disorder*** is characterized by ***sudden, short lived, recurrent, unpredictable episodes of intense anxiety*** accompanied by marked ***physiologic manifestations***.
- *Etiology*: Mean age of onset is *25 years;* MC in ***women***; often accompanied by ***agoraphobia***.
- Panic disorder is a/w ***separation anxiety disorder*** of childhood; a/w ***mitral valve prolapse;*** *a/w* ***depression*** in approximately *50%* patients.
- *Characteristics:* Panic attacks, defined as episodic periods of anxiety symptoms that have a sudden onset and increase in intensity over a period of approximately 10 minutes—*palpitations, sweating, tremors, dyspnea, chest pain, nausea, fear of losing control;* ***autonomic symptoms***.
- Panic attacks occur approximately ***twice weekly*** and last approximately ***30 minutes***. Between attacks the patient fears having another attack (***anticipatory anxiety***). For diagnosis at least 1 ***month of worry about attacks*** should be present.
- Conditions mimicking panic disorder: *Myocardial infarction, pheochromocytoma, hyperthyroidism and various recreational drug reactions.*
- Panic attack can be evoked by: *IV infusion of* ***sodium lactate***; *α-2 adrenergic antagonist* ***yohimbine, CCK-4*** *and* ***CO_2 inhalation***.

Treatment

- ***For immediate relief*** or anticipatory anxiety, benzodiazepines, particularly ***alprazolam*** with gradual withdrawal over 8–12 months.
- ***For maintenance***, antidepressant medication: SSRIs, tricyclics, MAOIs.
- Psychological treatment: ***Systematic desensitization and cognitive therapy*** are useful.

117. Answer is a, c, d (Superior vena cava, Azygos vein, Left brachiocephalic vein).
Ref: Clinically Oriented Anatomy, Keith L Moore, 7th edition Pg 131.

The ***venous drainage of the pericardium*** is from the:

- Pericardiophrenic veins: Tributaries of the ***brachiocephalic or internal thoracic veins***.
- Variable tributaries of the ***azygous veins,*** which inturn drains into the *SVC*.

118. Answer is b (2–4 mL/100 g/min).
Ref: Essentials of Medical Physiology, Khurana, Pg 378.

- ***Blood flow in resting skeletal muscle (white type) is 2–4 mL/min/ 100 g,*** which may increase to 50–80 mL/min/100 g during maximal exercise.
- In red muscle fibers, which employ aerobic metabolism and contract all the time, this is 30 mL/min/100 g.

119. Answer is a (Mediastinal displacement away from the lesion).
Ref: Bailey and Love, 26th edition Pg 354.

- A ***tension pneumothorax*** develops when a ***one-way valve air leak*** occurs either from the lung or through the chest wall.
- Air is sucked into the thoracic cavity without any means of escape, completely collapsing and compressing the affected lung.
- The ***mediastinum is displaced to the opposite side,*** decreasing venous return and ***compressing the opposite lung.***
- Patient is panicky with ***tachypnea, dyspnea and distended neck veins; tracheal deviation*** may be seen; ***hyper-resonance and absent breath sounds*** *over the affected hemithorax.*
- Treat with ***immediate decompression by rapidly inserting a large bore needle into the second intercostal space*** in *the midclavicular line* of the affected hemithorax followed by ***insertion of chest tube in the fifth intercostal space in mid-axillary line.***

120. Answer is d (Pseudocarriers).
Ref: Park, 22nd edition Pg 92.

- ***Carriers of avirulent organisms*** are called ***pseudocarriers***; they are ***not important epidemiologically.***
- ***Temporary carriers*** are those who shed the infectious agent for short periods of time.
- ***Healthy carriers*** emerge from subclinical cases; they have developed carrier state without suffering from overt disease.

121. Answer is c (Brenner's tumor).
Ref: BIG Robbins, 8th edition Pg 1046.

- ***Brenner's tumors*** are classified as adenofibromas in which the epithelial cell component consist of nests of transitional-type epithelial cells resembling those lining the urinary bladder.
- They are usually ***unilateral and benign.***

122. Answer is b (Sumatriptan).
Ref: KD Tripathi, 7th edition Pg 176-180.

Drugs for migraine

Treatment	Prophylaxis
– ***Analgesic*** (e.g. *aspirin, PCT, ibuprofen or naproxen*) – ***Cafergot***, a combination of ***ergotamine tartrate*** and ***caffeine*** (avoid ergot in pregnancy and CVS disease) – ***Prochlorperazine*** – ***Triptans*** (sumatriptan, zolmitriptan, etc.)—oral, nasal or SC – ***Lasmiditan*** (5HT1F receptor agonist) is in clinical trials	– ***Topiramate*** (SE: nystagmus, diplopia, glaucoma, renal calculi, weight loss, hypohidrosis, hyperthermia) – ***Valproic*** acid – ***Candesartan*** (ARB) – ***Beta blockers*** (propranolol; timolol) – ***Verapamil*** (CCB) – ***Amitriptyline*** – ***Botulinum toxin*** A

123. Answer is a (Insulin).
Ref: Vasudevan's Biochemistry, 6th edition Pg 283.

- ***Gluconeogenesis*** is ***inhibited by insulin by repressing the key enzymes pyruvate carboxylase,*** *phosphoenolpyruvate kinase and glucose-6-phosphatase.*

124. Answer is b (Thomas test).
Ref: Essential Orthopedics, Maheshwari, 4th edition Pg 349.

- ***Thomas test***: Place your hand under the patient's lumbar spine to stop any lumbar movements and fully flex one of the hips. Observe the other hip; if it lifts off the couch then it suggests a ***fixed flexion deformity*** of that hip.

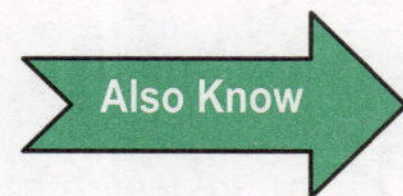

- ***Lewin punch test*** is used for evaluating low back pain—may indicate protruded intervertebral disk; done by punching the buttocks.

125. Answer is a (99mTc-pertechnetate).
Ref: Case-Based Nuclear Medicine, edited by Kevin Donohoe, 2011 edition Pg 123.

- A ***Meckels' diverticulum*** may be demonstrated by IV injection of ***99mTc pertechnetate,*** which localizes in the *ectopic gastric mucosa*—***Meckel scan.***

126. Answer is b (Erythroplakia).
Ref: Textbook of ENT, Dhingra, 238.

- ***Erythroplakia*** has ***17 times higher malignant potential*** than leukoplakia. It is a red plaque or patch on the mucosal surface.

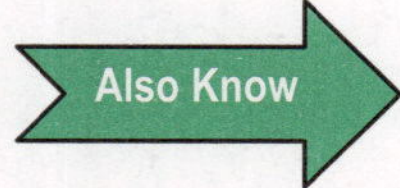

- ***Leukoplakia*** is any white lesion that cannot be removed by simply rubbing the oral mucosal surface. It is the ***MC premalignant oral lesion***.

127. Answer is a (Left renal vein).
Ref: Essentials of Anatomy, By IB Singh, 2nd edition Pg 279.

- **Right** ovarian V. drains into IVC; **Left ovarian V.** drains into **left renal vein.** Similar to right and left adrenal veins.
- Also remember **Right** testicular V. drains into IVC; **Left testicular V.** drains into **left renal vein.** Similar to right and left adrenal veins.

128. Answer is a (Exocrine glands).
Ref: CMDT 2013, Pg 842.

- ***Sjögren syndrome*** is a ***systemic autoimmune disorder*** whose clinical presentation is usually ***dominated by dryness of the eyes and mouth*** due to ***immune-mediated dysfunction*** of the ***exocrine glands*** (***lacrimal and salivary glands***).

129. Answer is d (Hysteroscopic metroplasty).
Ref: Textbook of Hysteroscopy, By Nandita Palshetkar, Rishma Dhillon Pai, Hrishikesh D Pai, Jaypee Brothers Medical Publishers (P) Ltd, Pg 41.

- ***Division of uterine septum*** was one historically by laparotomy, but now is ***MC done by hysteroscopy***.
- ***Hysteroscopic metroplasty*** leads to significant improved rates of pregnancy.

- *Pregnancy rates* have been estimated to rise from 3% prior to surgery to ***80% postsurgery*** with hysteroscopic correction.
- Also hysteroscopic metroplasty has ***lesser complications*** compared to *Tomkin's, Jones and Strassman procedures.*

130. Answer is c (Cardiac tamponade).
Ref: CMDT 2013, Pg 421.

- ***Electrical alternans*** is present uncommonly, but is ***pathognomonic*** due to the heart swinging within the large effusion in cardiac tamponade.
- ***Spread of adjacent lung cancer*** as well as invasion by breast cancer, renal cell carcinoma, Hodgkin's disease and lymphomas are the ***most common neoplastic processes involving the pericardium*** and have become the most ***frequent causes of pericardial tamponade in many countries***.

For questions 131–134

A 4-year-old male child is brought to the pediatric outpatient department with sore throat and fever for 2 days, and noisy breathing with inability to swallow for the past 4 hours. Examination showed a toxic, tachypneic child with inspiratory stridor and drooling of saliva. There is suprasternal, supraclavicular and intercostal recession during inspiration. No stridor heard during expiration.

131. Answer is b (Extrathoracic airway obstruction).
132. Answer is a (Arrange things for securing airway).
133. Answer is b (Thumb sign).
134. Answer is d (Antibiotics).

Ref: Harrison's, 18th edition Pg 265-66.

Explanation:
The case history given is that of acute epiglottitis. The clinchers/keywords are 'fever, inspiratory stridor, salivary drooling and recession'. Also know that Croup and epiglottitis cause extrathoracic airway obstruction.

	Croup (laryngotracheobronchitis)	**Acute epiglottitis (emergency)**
Etiology	**MC** *parainfluenza virus 1*; **also by RSV**	MC by ***H. influenzae* type b**
Presenting age	3 months to 3 years	**3–7 years**
Clinically	*Prodrome* with URI symptoms for 1–7 days; ***low*** grade fever, ***inspiratory stridor*** that worsens with agitation; ***hoarseness of voice, barking cough,***	***Rapid onset (4–12 hours)***; high ***fever, dysphagia, drooling, muffled voice, inspiratory stridor;*** retractions of chest wall; patients may be in ***'sniffing' position*** with neck hyperextended and chin protruding
X-ray	***'Steeple sign'*** on A-P view neck film	***'Thumb sign'*** (enlarged epiglottis) on lateral neck film
Treatment	Mist therapy, oxygen, *aerosolized racemic epinephrine*, ***dexamethasone (steroids)***	***Call anesthesia***, transfer to ***operation theater***, ***endotracheal intubation*** and ***IV antibiotics for 7–10 days***

For questions 135–138

A 75-year-old woman with chronic atrial fibrillation presented to the hospital with a 2-day history of colicky abdominal pain. The physical examination revealed hypoactive bowel sounds and diffuse abdominal tenderness. Laboratory tests showed a white cell count of 19,400/mm^3 with 92% neutrophils, a blood urea nitrogen level of 42 mg/dL (15 mmol/L) and a serum creatinine level of 3.0 mg/dL (267 μmol/L).

135. Answer is c (Dilated gas-filled small bowel with thickening of the wall).
136. Answer is d (Ultrasonography of abdomen).
137. Answer is b (Mesenteric ischemia).
138. Answer is b (Occlusion of the superior mesenteric vessel).

Ref: *Harrison's, 18th edition Pg 2510-13; CMDT 2013, Pg 471.*

Explanation:
The case history given is that of 'acute mesenteric ischemia'. The keywords/clinchers are 'atrial fibrillation-indicating that embolus has occurred, hypoactive bowel sound and tender abdomen with leukocytosis'.

- ***Occlusive intestinal ischemia*** is a result of disruption of blood flow by an ***embolus or progressive thrombosis*** in a ***major artery supplying the intestine. Emboli originate from the heart in > 75% of cases*** and lodge preferentially just ***distal to the origin of the middle colic artery from the superior mesenteric artery.***
- ***Acute mesenteric ischemia*** presents with ***severe acute, non-remitting abdominal pain*** strikingly out of proportion to the physical findings (with the exception of ***minimal abdominal distention*** and ***hypoactive bowel sounds***). Nausea and vomiting, transient diarrhea and bloody stools may be present.
- Earlier features of intestinal ischemia seen on abdominal radiographs include ***bowel-wall edema, known as 'thumbprinting'.*** If the ischemia progresses, ***air can be seen within the bowel wall (pneumatosis intestinalis)*** and within the portal venous system.
- A ***mesenteric duplex scan (i.e. ultrasound scan) demonstrating a high-peak velocity of flow in the superior mesenteric artery (SMA)*** is associated with an ~80% positive predictive value of mesenteric ischemia. More significantly, a negative duplex scan virtually precludes the diagnosis of mesenteric ischemia.
- ***Gold*** standard test is laparotomy.
- A ***high white cell count***, *lactic acidosis, hypotension* may aid in the diagnosis.

For questions 139–141

A 20-year-old female patient was stabbed with an ice pick in the xiphisternum, brought to the casualty in stupor, very pale, tachycardia, feeble pulse, prominent neck vein and muffled heart sounds on auscultation.

139. Answer is c (CT chest).
140. Answer is c (Pericardial tamponade).
141. Answer is d (Pericardiocentesis).

Ref: *Harrison's, 18th edition Pg 1972-74; CMDT 2013, Pg 421.*

Explanation:
The case history given is that of cardiac tamponade. The clinchers/keywords are 'history of trauma to heart and Beck's triad (Distended neck veins; Distant or muffled heart sounds and Decreased BP)'.

- The accumulation of fluid in the pericardial space in a quantity sufficient to cause serious obstruction to the inflow of blood to the ventricles results in ***cardiac tamponade.***
- Common causes of tamponade are neoplastic disease, idiopathic pericarditis and renal failure; it may also result from ***bleeding into the pericardial space after cardiac operations, trauma and*** anticoagulants usage.
- The three principal features of ***tamponade (Beck's triad)*** are ***hypotension, soft or absent heart sounds and jugular venous distention*** with a prominent x descent, but an absent y descent.
- The quantity of fluid necessary to produce this critical state may be as small as 200 mL when the fluid develops rapidly or > 2,000 mL in slowly developing effusions when the pericardium has had the opportunity to stretch and adapt to an increasing volume.
- There may be reduction in amplitude of the QRS complexes and ***electrical alternans*** of the P, QRS or T waves should raise the suspicion of cardiac tamponade.
- When ***tamponade*** is present, ***urgent pericardiocentesis*** is required.

For questions 142–144

A 60-year-old male has a long-standing history of breathlessness. He has been a heavy smoker since the age of 20 years. Physical examination reveals an anxious male who is emaciated, puffing for breath, but is not cyanosed. The chest is barrel shaped.

142. Answer is c (Muffled heart sounds).
143. Answer is b (Unabated action of proteases).
144. Answer is a (High resolution CT).

Ref. CMDT 2013, Pg 260-61.

Explanation:
The case history given is that of COPD (emphysema). The clinchers/keywords are 'smoker for 40 years and a 'puffer' but not cyanosed'.

- ***Patient profile in emphysema predominant COPD (pink puffer):*** Severe ***dyspnea***, cough is rare with clear mucoid sputum; patients are thin with recent weight loss and appear ***uncomfortable***; Also evident is use of accessory muscles of respiration. ***Chest is very quiet without adventitious sounds***. No peripheral edema. ↓ FEV1 , ↓ FVC, ↑ TLC; ***barrel chest,*** respiratory acidosis, pulmonary hypertension, cor pulmonale.
- ***Plain radiographs are insensitive for the diagnosis of emphysema***.
- ***CT of the chest, particularly using a high-resolution*** reconstruction, is more sensitive and specific than plain radiographs for the diagnosis of emphysema.
- In smokers, ***unabated action of proteases*** is the common mechanism of asthma; as per the protease-antiprotease hypothesis; however this was NOT corrected in the revised answer key earlier in 2013—in case this question gets repeated you can mark 'b' as above as correct answer.

For questions 147–149

A 45-year-old multiparous perimenopausal women comes with a 6 cm lump in the right upper quadrant with puckering of the overlying skin and a small area of ulceration, on further examination she has three axillary firm palpable lymph node in the same side, she also has lymph node in the supraclavicular area, rest of the systems are clinically normal.

145. Answer is b (Core needle biopsy).
146. Answer is e (e indicates wrong question wording or wrong options).

Ref: CMDT 2013, Pg 728-29.

Explanation:
The case history given is that of breast cancer/lump with metastases. The clinchers/keywords are 'puckering, ulceration and metastases to lymph nodes'.

- The diagnosis of breast cancer depends ultimately on ***examination of tissue or cells removed by biopsy***.
- Treatment should never be undertaken without an unequivocal histologic or cytologic diagnosis of cancer.
- The ***simplest biopsy method is needle biopsy,*** either by aspiration of tumor cells (***FNA cytology***) or by obtaining a ***small core of tissue with a hollow needle (core biopsy).***
- Large needle (core needle) biopsy removes a core of tissue with a large cutting needle and is the ***diagnostic procedure of choice for both palpable and image-detected abnormalities***. Hand-held biopsy devices make large-core needle biopsy of a palpable mass easy and cost effective in the office with local anesthesia. As in the case of any needle biopsy, the main problem is sampling error due to improper positioning of the needle, giving rise to a false-negative test result can be overcome with image-guided biopsies. Core biopsy has the *advantage that tumor markers, such as estrogen receptor (ER), progesterone receptor (PR) and HER-2/neu overexpression can be performed on cores of tissue.*
- ***FNAC disadvantages are*** skilled pathologist required; core of lesion may be missed; tumor markers cannot be performed.

For questions 147–149

A 38-year-old homeless male develops sudden onset hematemesis following a bout of severe vomiting and retching. He had no complaints prior to the onset of his symptoms. On examination, he is pale and looks anxious. The vital signs are normal. Laboratory investigations show normal liver function tests, a low Hb and high MCV, chest X-ray is normal.

147. Answer is b (Mallory-Weiss syndrome).
148. Answer is b (Upper GI scopy).
149. Answer is c (Linear tear in the OG junction).

Ref: *CMDT 2013, Pg 599.*

Mallory-Weiss tear

- A vertical split in the gastric mucosa, immediately below the squamocolumnar junction at the cardia in 90% of cases (on lesser curvature).
- In only 10%, the tear is in the esophagus.
- Occurs following ***retching/vomiting after alcohol*** ingestion; causes ***upper GI bleeding/hematemesis***; diagnosed by ***endoscopy***; ***alcoholism*** is a strong-predisposing factor.
- In most patients, ***bleeding ceases spontaneously***; continued bleeding may respond to vasopressin therapy or *angiographic embolization*.

For questions 150–153

A 58-year-old healthy man was evaluated for a toothache of 2 days duration. He was treated with oral penicillin and an opiate analgesic and advised to have the affected teeth pulled. He returned less than 24 hours later reporting severe swelling in the neck, sore throat, chills and chest pain. On examination, the floor of his oral cavity was indurated and woody, and he had marked tenderness and adenopathy throughout his neck. He had erythema spreading from his neck down over his anterior chest wall where his chest pain was localized.

150. Answer is b (Ludwig's angina).
151. Answer is a (Airway obstruction).
152. Answer is a (Submental, sublingual and submandibular space).
153. Answer is a (Surgical decompression, antibiotic and intensive care).

Ref: *CMDT 2013, Pg 230.*

Explanation:
The case history given is that of Ludwig's angina. The clinchers/keywords are 'tooth extraction, neck swelling, woody indurated floor of mouth and neck adenopathy'.

- ***Ludwig's angina*** is caused by a virulent ***streptococcal*** infection a/w anaerobic organisms *(Bacteroides* and *Fusarium)* and sometimes with other lesions of the floor such as carcinoma.
- It is a ***cellulitis of the sublingual and submaxillary spaces***, often arising from ***infection of the mandibular dentition***.
- It is characterized by:
  - ➢ ***Brawny (board like)*** swelling of the submandibular region combined with inflammatory edema of the mouth; ***combined cervical and intraoral signs***.
  - ➢ Putrid ***halitosis***.
  - ➢ The infection encompasses both sides of the mylohyoid muscle causing edema and inflammation such that the tongue may be displaced upwards and backwards, giving rise to ***dysphagia***.
  - ➢ Unless treated cellulitis may extend below the deep fascial layers of the neck to involve the larynx (deep neck abscess), ***causing glottic edema and painful airway compromise***.
- Treatment: ***Immediate antibiotic therapy*** (cefuroxime with metronidazole); if not responding ***drain both submandibular triangles*** under local anesthesia.

For questions 154–157

A 40-year-old veterinarian presented with complaints of abdominal pain. On examination he was found to be icteric, the liver was palpable, ultrasonography revealed the presence of cyst in the right lobe of liver.

154. Answer is b *(Echinococcus granulosus).*
155. Answer is b (Dogs).
156. Answer is c (Casoni's test).
157. Answer is d (Seitz filter).

Ref: *Textbook of Medical Laboratory Technology, By Ramnik Sood, Pg 182.*

Explanation:
The case history given is that of hydatid cyst of liver. The clinchers/keywords are 'veterinarian, liver enlarged and cyst in liver'.

- *E. granulosus* is transmitted by ***domestic dogs (definitive host)*** in areas with livestock (***sheep, goats, camels and horses) as intermediate*** hosts.
- After humans ingest parasite eggs, the eggs hatch in the intestines to form oncospheres, which penetrate the mucosa, enter the circulation and encyst in specific organs as ***hydatid cysts***. *E. granulosus* forms cysts most commonly in the ***liver (65%)*** and lungs.
- Findings may include ***abdominal or chest pain, biliary obstruction (jaundice)***, cholangitis, portal hypertension, cirrhosis, bronchial obstruction leading to segmental lung collapse and abscesses.
- ***Casoni's test*** is an ***intradermal skin test for hydatidosis*** consisting of fresh sterile hydatid fluid (sterilized by ***Seitz filter***).

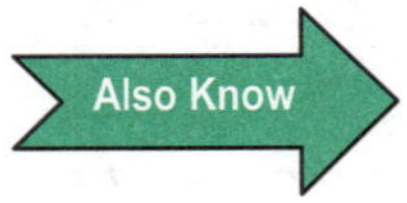

Sabin Feldman dye test	Toxoplasmosis
Frenkel's skin test	Toxoplasmosis
Casoni's test	Hydatid cyst
Montenegro test	Leishmaniasis
Scotch tape test	Enterobiasis (pinworm)
Fairley's test	Schistosomiasis
Skin snip test	Onchocerciasis

For questions 158–160

A healthy 10-year-old girl presented to her physician with nontender, well circumscribed. Mobile, slightly hyperneurotic erythematous plaques on the dorsal aspect of the interphalangeal joints of both thumbs. The plaques had developed over several months.

158. Answer is a (Garrod's pads).
159. Answer is a (Bulimia nervosa).
160. Answer is d (Rheumatic carditis).

Ref: http://www.nejm.org/doi/full/10.1056/NEJMicm1008915

Explanation:
"This is a direct pick from the above New England Journal of Medicine website link above. Please see that; anyway I have given the explanation below also".

- ***Knuckle pads*** are a type of benign fibroma that typically occurs over the small joints of the hands and feet.
- Also known as ***Garrod's pads***, these lesions have been associated with repetitive friction or pressure, as may occur with *habitual chewing or sucking of the fingers, with repetitive occupational activities, with athletic activities (e.g. boxing and surfing)* and with ***bulimia nervosa*** with self-induced vomiting.
- Knuckle pads have also been associated with a number of ***fibrosing disorders*** (such as ***Dupuytren's contracture, Ledderhose's syndrome and Peyronie's disease***), the autosomal dominant Bart–Pumphrey syndrome and a variety of other medical conditions.
- Knuckle pads in the ***pediatric population*** are often ***idiopathic***.

For questions 161–165

A 45-year-old man presented with a 3 year history of a painless soft and slow growing swelling of the neck, upper trunk, upper back and shoulders. The patient had a history of heavy alcohol consumption and was a non-smoker. Laboratory

blood analysis showed minor elevations in aspartate aminotransferase (71 U/L), alanine aminotransferase (49 U/L) and total cholesterol [235 mg /dL (6.08 mmol/L)]. Triglycerides are elevated at 1,020 mg /dL (11.52 mmol/L). Magnetic resonance imaging revealed diffuse, non-encapsulated fatty deposits in the mediastinum and in the subcutaneous and deeper fascial compartments of the neck, upper trunk and back.

161. Answer is c (Madelung's disease).
162. Answer is d (Alcohol dependence).
163. Answer is a (Males).
164. Answer is a (Statins).
165. Answer is c (GGTP).

Ref: http://www.nejm.org/doi/full/10.1056/NEJMicm1003531.

Explanation:
Another direct pick from NEJM. The case history given is most likely that of Madelung's disease. The clinchers/keywords are "alcoholism, nonsmoker, multiple fatty deposits". Quite a rare condition and question also!

- ***Madelung's disease (benign symmetric lipomatosis)*** is a rare condition characterized by presence of ***multiple and symmetric non-encapsulated masses of fatty tissue*** usually involving the neck and upper region of the trunk ***horse collar pattern of lipomas.***
- MC seen in ***Mediterranean population with M:F = 15:1***; in 30–50 year age group.
- Most patients have a history of ***moderate-to-severe alcoholism.***
- Fat is deposited in subcutaneous tissue of the neck deep under the sternocleidomastoid and trapezius muscles, posterior cervical triangle and around the salivary glands.
- Treatment consist of ***surgical resection or liposuction and medically—use of statins.***
- ***Gamma Glutamyl Transferase*** is not a specific indicator of ***alcohol-induced liver damage*** *(Harrison's, 19th/1992); BUt increased serum GGT levels are seen in alcoholic hepatitis. The same question about "specific" to alcoholic liver disease - can be found in 2007 Comed-K question no.1; BUT all recent textbooks say that GGT is NOT specific to alcoholic liver; BUT all sources DO say that GGT is increased in alcoholic liver disease, hence GGT may be chosen based on the wording of the question in future also.*

For questions 166–169

A 25-year-old female patient presented with a history of bilateral hearing loss and tinnitus during pregnancy. She can hear better in a noisy environment. She speaks in a low volume monotonously. Otoscopy showed normal looking eardrums bilaterally and Rinne test negative bilaterally. Pure tone audiogram showed air bone gap with dip in bone conduction at 2 KHz.

166. Answer is d (Otosclerosis).
167. Answer is a (Bilateral conductive hearing loss).
168. Answer is b (Carhart's notch).
169. Answer is c (Stapedotomy and piston insertion).

Ref: Textbook of ENT, Dhingra, 5th edition Pg 97.

Explanation:
The case history given is that of otosclerosis. The clinchers/keywords are "bilateral, female, worsened in pregnancy and Carhart's notch".

Otosclerosis

Etiopathogenesis

- AD, ***family H/o deafness*** ++ in 70% cases; ***common in South Indians and Whites***; M:F = 1:2 in ***15–35 year*** *age* group; ***pregnancy may initiate or aggravate*** otosclerosis.
- Normal temporal bone has embryonic cartilage rests called ***globuli interossei;*** *sites of predilection for otosclerosis.*

- This is a disease of the bony labyrinth in which ***vascular spongy bone formation*** near the ***oval window*** causes ***fixation or ankylosis of the footplate of the stapes***.
- ***MC site is fissula antefenestram*** in front of the oval window.

Clinically
- *MC cause of non-supportive conductive deafness in the adult.*
- Main symptom is ***progressive deafness usually bilateral. Tinnitus*** is present in *80%* cases.
- ***Paracusis Willisii (Lombard effect)*** is present. It is the ability to hear better in noisy surroundings as people talk louder in a noisy place.
- Otoscopy reveals normal intact and mobile tympanic membrane in most cases.
- In some *(2%)* cases ***flamingo pink tinge*** may be seen due to vascular otospongiotic mass and is called positive ***Schwartze's sign.***
- Systemic associations: ***Van der Hoeve's syndrome:*** Otosclerosis with blue sclera and pathologic bone fractures; ***Paget's disease.***

Investigations
- ***Rinne's test is negative*** and ***Weber is lateralized to the more affected ear*** (conductive deafness); *Gelle's test is negative;* ***Type A or type AS tympanogram.***
- ***In early cochlear otosclerosis, cookie-bite curve*** shows that there is greatest degree of hearing loss in mid-frequency range.
- ***Carhart's notch in BC at 2,000 Hz*** is present in some cases.
- Histologically, ***first sign*** is a change in the extracellular staining pattern—'***blue mantle***'; later 'otospongiosis' and finally 'otosclerosis'.

Treatment
- ***Stapedectomy with artificial prosthesis*** *is the surgery of choice*. Here the stapes including its footplate is removed.
- ***Indications*** for stapedectomy:
  - ➢ Firmly fixed staped as indicated by an air-bone gap of 30 dB.
  - ➢ Negative Rinne for 256 and 512 Hz magnesium tuning forks.
  - ➢ Speech discrimination score of 30% or more.
- ***Hearing aids*** that amplify the sound waves and this overcomes the resistance to sound transmission.
- ***Cochlear otosclerosis*** is treated by ***Fluoride therapy***.

For questions 170–173

A 6-year-old child who presented with perianal pruritus, excoriation of skin and nocturnal enuresis was found to be infected with a parasite causing autoinfection.

170. Answer is c *(Enterobius vermicularis).*
171. Answer is a (Cecum, appendix and ascending colon).
172. Answer is b (Embryonated egg).
173. Answer is a (NIH swab method).

Ref: *Harrison's 18th edition Pg 1740, 1743.*

Explanation:
The case history given is that of enterobius vermicularis. The clinchers/keyword are "perianal pruritus, autoinfection".

- ***Enterobius vermicularis,*** the ***pinworm,*** is a common cause of intestinal infections worldwide, with maximal prevalence in school-age children. Enterobiasis is transmitted ***person-to-person via ingestion of eggs*** after contact with the hands or perianal region of an infected individual. ***Autoinfection*** also occurs.
- ***Eggs hatch in the duodenum*** and larvae migrate to the ***cecum and appendix***. Females mature in about a month and remain viable for about another month. During this time they migrate through the anus to deposit large ***numbers of eggs on the perianal skin.***

- Most individuals with pinworm infection are ***asymptomatic***. The most common symptom is ***perianal pruritus***, particularly at night, due to the presence of the female worms or deposited eggs. Insomnia, restlessness and enuresis are common in children. Perianal scratching may result in excoriation and impetigo.
- *NIH swab/scotch tape/cellophane tape test*: Eggs are detected by the application of clear cellulose acetate tape to the perianal region in the morning. After the tape is transferred to a slide, microscopic examination will detect pinworm eggs.
- Treatment is with single oral doses of albendazole, mebendazole or pyrantel pamoate. The dose is repeated in 2 weeks due to frequent reinfection.
- Treatment is with single oral doses of albendazole (400 mg), mebendazole (100 mg) or pyrantel pamoate (11 mg/kg, to a maximum of 1 g). The dose is repeated in 2 weeks due to frequent reinfection.

<u>For questions 174–177</u>

A 60-year-old male presents with progressive difficulty in swallowing, vomiting and occasional regurgitation for the past 3 months. Barium studies showed marked dilatation of the upper esophagus with narrowing of the lower segment. Manometry showed absent esophageal peristalsis.

174. Answer is d (Absence of ganglion cells in the myenteric plexus of the esophagus).
175. Answer is c (Squamous cell carcinoma of the esophagus).
176. Answer is a (Recurrent chest infection).
177. Answer is a (Balloon dilation).

<u>*Ref*</u>*: Harrison's, 18th edition Pg 2430-31.*

<u>Explanation</u>:
The case history given is that of achalasia cardia. The clinchers/keywords are 'dilated esophagus with absent peristalsis and narrow lower segment'.

Achalasia (failure to relax)

- Achalasia is an idiopathic ***motility*** *disorder* characterized by loss of peristalsis in the distal two thirds (smooth muscle) of the esophagus and ***impaired relaxation of the lower esophageal sphincter***. There appears to be denervation of the esophagus resulting from ***loss of ganglion cells in Auerbach's*** plexus.
- Gradual, ***progressive dysphagia*** for solids and liquids.
- Radiologic findings are air-fluid level in the enlarged, fluid-filled esophagus, *smooth narrowing* of lower esophagus ***(bird's beak), lack of gas bubble in stomach, S-shaped (sigmoid) lower esophagus***, uncoordinated peristalsis.
- *Strategies to overcome dysphagia*: Arching the neck and shoulders, raising the arms, standing or sitting up straight during the meal and ***walking around after a meal***.
- Patients are also at risk for ***bronchitis, pneumonia and lung abscess*** due to ***chronic regurgitation***.
- ***Esophageal manometry*** **confirms** diagnosis.
- ***Pneumatic dilation***: Over two thirds of patients derive good to excellent relief of dysphagia after one or two sessions of ***pneumatic dilation*** of the lower esophageal sphincter.
- Endoscopically guided injection of botulinum toxin directly into the lower esophageal sphincter results in a marked reduction in lower esophageal sphincter pressure and sustained improvement in symptoms in two thirds of patients for 6–24 months.
- Surgical: ***Heller's cardiomyotomy*** in patients who fail to improve with the above two methods.
- ***Chronic achalasia*** is believed to be ***risk factor*** for ***Ca esophagus***.

<u>For questions 178–180</u>

A 69-year-old female is being evaluated for constipation and an episode of blood-stained stools. Laboratory investigations show normal CBC and barium studies showed out pouching of the sigmoid colon in multiple areas.

178. Answer is b (Herniation of the colonic wall at the sites of focal defects).
179. Answer is c (Perforation of the colon).
180. Answer is a (Computed tomography).

Ref: Bailey and Love, 25th edition Pg 1160-1162.

Explanation:
The case history given is that of sigmoid colonic diverticulosis. The clinchers/keywords in the question are "out pouching of the sigmoid colon and blood in stools".

- ***Diverticulosis*** is the ***MC cause of acute lower GI bleeding.***
- Acute uncomplicated diverticulitis characteristically presents with ***fever, anorexia, left lower quadrant abdominal pain and obstipation.***
- Perforation of a colonic diverticulum results in an intra-abdominal infection that may vary from microperforation (most common) with localized paracolic inflammation to macroperforation with either abscess or generalized peritonitis.
- The ***diagnosis of diverticulitis*** is ***best made on CT*** with the following findings: Sigmoid diverticula, thickened colonic wall > 4 mm and inflammation within the pericolic fat ± the collection of contrast material or fluid.

NOTES

COMED-K 2012

COMED-K 2012 QUESTIONS

1. **Superior colliculus is concerned with**
   (a) Olfaction
   (b) Hearing
   (c) Vision
   (d) Pain sensation

2. **A failure of synthesis of ceruloplasmin is seen in**
   (a) Hemochromatosis
   (b) Weil's disease
   (c) Wilson's disease
   (d) Wernicke's encephalopathy

3. ***Bacillus anthracis***
   (a) Produces an endotoxin
   (b) Produces terminal bulging spores
   (c) Is an anaerobic organism
   (d) Capsule is demonstrated by M'Fadyean's reaction

4. **A 45-year-old chronic alcoholic male with severe ascites, presented with the history of passing bright red blood in his stools, since 3 days. There was no pain or diarrhea. What would you suspect in this case?**
   (a) Intestinal infarction
   (b) Chronic ischemic colitis
   (c) Hemorrhoids
   (d) Angiodysplasia

5. **The quantity of water considered adequate in urban areas (in liters per day person) is**
   (a) 50–100
   (b) 100–150
   (c) 150–200
   (d) 200–250

6. **Which one of the following manifestations is more likely to be found in the diffuse form of systemic sclerosis than in the limited variant?**
   (a) Esophageal dysmotility
   (b) Pulmonary involvement
   (c) Distal skin thickening
   (d) Renal disease

7. **Radiofemoral delay is characteristic of**
   (a) Patent ductus arteriosus
   (b) Coarctation of aorta
   (c) Aortic dissection
   (d) Takayasu's disease

8. **Fetal middle cerebral artery Doppler is most useful in the evaluation of**
   (a) Intrauterine growth restriction
   (b) Preeclampsia
   (c) Fetal anemia
   (d) Fetal metabolic disorders

9. **Spine metastasis from all the following malignancies are 'radiosensitive' *EXCEPT***
   (a) Prostate
   (b) Breast
   (c) Lung
   (d) Kidney

10. **Which element is used safely as an intravascular radiological contrast agent?**
    (a) Iodine
    (b) Barium
    (c) Bromine
    (d) Fluorine

11. **Which of the following is true of infantile autism?**
    (a) Onset after 5 years of age
    (b) Normal language and communication
    (c) High intelligence scores
    (d) Impaired reciprocal interactions

12. **A 23-year-old female patient presents with 2 months history of low grade fever and moderate right-sided pleural effusion. Pleural fluid shows lymphocyte predominance with ADA levels of 120 IU/L. The patient is started on anti-tubercular therapy (WHO Category I). Two months later the patient presents with**

progressive breathlessness, generalized body swelling and raised JVP. Pleural fluid is now predominantly transudate. This patient is likely to have developed

(a) Hypoproteinemia
(b) Drug resistant TB
(c) Collagen vascular disease
(d) Constrictive pericarditis

13. Exfoliatin (exfoliative toxin) is implicated in

(a) Toxic epidermal necrolysis
(b) Staphylococcal scalded skin syndrome
(c) Septicemia due to gram-negative organisms
(d) Idiopathic exfoliative dermatitis

14. Ureteral tumor occurs MOST frequently in

(a) Upper 1/3 of ureter
(b) Middle 1/3 of ureter
(c) Lower 1/3 of ureter
(d) Equally along the length of ureter

15. Which of the following techniques is NOT a treatment option for vaginal atresia?

(a) McIndoe's operation
(b) Williams operation
(c) Strassman operation
(d) Frank procedure

16. The most readily detected clinical sign of hypermagnesemia is

(a) Drowsiness
(b) Hypotension
(c) Cerebellar ataxia
(d) Disappearance of deep tendon reflexes

17. Non-sampling errors may occur due to all of the following, *EXCEPT*

(a) Inadequately calibrated instruments
(b) Repeated sampling
(c) Observer variation
(d) Conceptual errors

18. Ludwig's angina is

(a) Infection of carotid sheath
(b) Infection of submandibular space
(c) Necrotizing ulcerative gingivitis
(d) Peritonsillar abscess

19. An important triggering event in acute pancreatitis is activation of

(a) Pepsinogen
(b) Prekallikrein
(c) Trypsinogen
(d) Lipase

20. Inhibitors of bacterial protein synthesis include all of the following *EXCEPT*

(a) Streptomycin
(b) Erythromycin
(c) Clindamycin
(d) Vancomycin

21. Posterior ethmoidal air sinus opens into

(a) Superior meatus
(b) Middle meatus
(c) Inferior meatus
(d) Sphenoethmoidal recess

22. Hemorrhagic meningitis is caused by

(a) Streptococcus pneumoniae
(b) Haemophilus influenzae
(c) Bacillus anthracis
(d) Neisseria meningitidis

23. The following documentary evidences are accepted by the court without confirmation by oral evidence *EXCEPT*

(a) Dying declaration
(b) Chemical examiner's report
(c) Medicolegal report
(d) Reports of Master of Mint

24. The pulse polio immunization (PPI) was first launched in India in

(a) 1995
(b) 1996
(c) 1999
(d) 2000

25. IgA nephropathy has all the following characteristics *EXCEPT*

(a) Hematuria
(b) Hypertension

(c) Nephritic syndrome
(d) Thin basement membrane on renal biopsy

26. Dosage of folate for the prevention of recurrence of neural tube defects is
(a) 50 ug
(b) 500 ug
(c) 5 mg
(d) 500 mg

27. Toxic megacolon is a complication of which following condition?
(a) Sigmoid volvulus
(b) Hirschsprung's disease
(c) Ulcerative colitis
(d) Diverticulitis

28. Normal plasma osmolality in mOsmol/kg H_2O
(a) 285
(b) 385
(c) 485
(d) 585

29. Which of the following cyanotic heart diseases is associated with left axis deviation and left ventricular hypertrophy?
(a) Transposition of great vessels
(b) Truncus arteriosus
(c) Tricuspid atresia
(d) Total anomalous pulmonary venous drainage

30. The following is an example of atypical antipsychotic
(a) Olanzapine
(b) Haloperidol
(c) Amitriptyline
(d) Zuclopenthixol

31. Which one of the following reactions has flavin mononucleotide (FMN) as a coenzyme?
(a) Amino acid oxidation reaction
(b) Conversion of xanthine to uric acid
(c) Conversion of succinate to fumarate
(d) Conversion of pyruvate to acetyl CoA

32. Cardiotoxicity of anthracyclines can be reduced by
(a) Mesna
(b) Dexrazoxane
(c) Leucovorin
(d) Erythropoietin

33. The following are attributes of hepatitis B infection *EXCEPT*
(a) Establishes chronic infections in those infected as infants
(b) HBcAg in serum indicates active infection
(c) Can cause hepatocellular carcinoma
(d) Alpha interferon is used for the treatment of chronic infection

34. A 35-year-old female, presents with chronic irritation in both eyes. On examination, there is mild papillary conjunctivitis, punctuate staining of the superior cornea and corneal filaments. Which of the following diagnostic tests would be most appropriate?
(a) Histamine level of tear film
(b) Thyroid function test
(c) Bacterial culture of eyelid margin
(d) Serum rheumatoid factor

35. *Thermoactinomyces sacchari* is the causative agent of
(a) Occupational asthma
(b) Bagassosis
(c) Byssinosis
(d) Farmer's lung

36. Fixed and wide splitting of second heart sound is characteristic of
(a) VSD
(b) ASD
(c) PDA
(d) Fallot's tetralogy

37. Thymoglobulin is a
(a) Polyclonal antibody
(b) Polyclonal antigen
(c) Thyroid antigen
(d) Monoclonal antibody

38. Infantile polycystic disease is
(a) Autosomal dominant
(b) Autosomal recessive
(c) X-linked
(d) Multifactorial genetic disease

39. The SI unit of radiation absorbed dose is
(a) Rad
(b) Becquerel
(c) Gray
(d) Sievert

40. The letter 'S' in DOTS stands for
(a) Strategy
(b) Scheme
(c) Short course
(d) System

41. Ectopic pheochromocytoma may be found in
(a) Organ of Zuckerkandl
(b) Bladder
(c) Filum terminale
(d) Meckel's diverticulum

42. The commonest cause of death in ARDS is
(a) Hypoxemia
(b) Hypotension
(c) Non-pulmonary organ failure
(d) Respiratory failure

43. The first step in planning cycle for health is
(a) Fixing priorities
(b) Establishment of objectives and goals
(c) Analysis of the health situation
(d) Assessment of resources

44. Marked diminution of vision is a feature of
(a) Papilledema
(b) Lattice degeneration
(c) Retinal hole
(d) Papillitis

45. Increased rouleaux formation in the peripheral blood is a characteristic feature of
(a) Multiple myeloma
(b) Non-Hodgkin's lymphoma
(c) Tuberculosis
(d) Malaria

46. The largest gene expressed in cardiac and smooth muscle is
(a) Dystrophin gene
(b) Semiphorin gene
(c) Tumor suppressor gene
(d) Huntington gene

47. Fertilization takes place in which part of the fallopian tube?
(a) Fimbriae
(b) Isthmus
(c) Ampulla
(d) Intramural part

48. Neurotransmitter implicated in pleasure seeking behavior
(a) Dopamine
(b) Serotonin
(c) Nor epinephrine
(d) GABA

49. Nodular scabies is found in
(a) Web space of fingers
(b) Chest
(c) Scrotum
(d) Abdomen

50. Which one of the following is a premalignant condition in stomach
(a) Ménétrier's disease
(b) Eosinophilic gastritis
(c) Erosive gastritis
(d) Type A gastritis

51. Therapy of choice for sleep-apnea syndrome is
(a) Invasive ventilation
(b) Non-invasive ventilation
(c) Oxygen inhalation
(d) Use of respiratory stimulants

52. Theory of contagion was first enunciated by
(a) Paracelsus
(b) Fracastorius
(c) Vesalius
(d) Pare

53. Normal anion-gap metabolic acidosis is seen in
(a) Addison's disease
(b) Diabetic ketoacidosis
(c) Renal failure
(d) Lactic acidosis

54. The sacrotuberous ligament is the degenerated tendon of
(a) Semitendinosus
(b) Semimembranosus
(c) Long head of biceps femoris
(d) Short head of biceps femoris

55. **The test which can be used for the detection of arsenic is**
(a) Reinsch test
(b) Marsh test
(c) Mc Ewan test
(d) Marquis test

56. **Phosphate test is used to check**
(a) Specific gravity of milk
(b) Bacteriological quality of milk
(c) Fat content of milk
(d) Pasteurization of milk

57. **Carotenes are converted into vitamin A in the**
(a) Liver
(b) Skin
(c) Small intestine
(d) Large intestine

58. **Bowen's disease is seen in the**
(a) Ovary
(b) Tube
(c) Vagina
(d) Vulva

59. **Prominent U waves on the ECG is a feature of**
(a) Hyponatremia
(b) Hypernatremia
(c) Hypokalemia
(d) Hyperkalemia

60. **Hallucination is**
(a) False perception in absence of a stimulus
(b) Misinterpretation of a stimulus
(c) Sensory distortion
(d) Thinking abnormality

61. **Ectopic gastric mucosa in Meckel's diverticulum is best identified by which of the following investigation**
(a) Technetium scan
(b) MIBG scan
(c) CT scan
(d) MRI scan

62. **'Xerostomia' is seen in all the following *EXCEPT***
(a) Postirradiation
(b) Anticholinergics therapy
(c) Sjögren's syndrome
(d) Oral sepsis

63. **The limiting amino acid in wheat is**
(a) Methionine
(b) Tryptophan
(c) Lysine
(d) Isoleucine

64. **Molluscum contagiosum is caused by**
(a) Human immunodeficiency virus
(b) Cytomegalovirus
(c) Poxvirus
(d) Epstein-Barr virus

65. **Salutatory conduction refers to all of the following *EXCEPT***
(a) It is a rapid process
(b) Jumping of depolarization from node to node
(c) Current flow through myelin is negligible
(d) Depolarization travels in opposite directions

66. **Bochdalek's foramen is a defect due to developmental failure of**
(a) Pleuroperitoneal membrane
(b) Cervical myotomes
(c) Septum transversum
(d) Dorsal mesentery of esophagus

67. **Hypertriglyceridemia is not a feature of**
(a) Alcoholism
(b) Diabetes mellitus
(c) Obesity
(d) Pregnancy

68. **The removal of surgical segments V,VI,VII and VIII is termed as**
(a) Right hepatectomy
(b) Extended right hepatectomy
(c) Trisegmentectomy
(d) Left hepatectomy

69. **Phocomelia due to thalidomide in the past has resulted from**
(a) Use in a large number of pregnant women with leprosy
(b) Use as a safe sleeping aid
(c) Immunosuppressive effects
(d) Use for leprosy in reactions

70. Nodular bronchiectasis is seen in
(a) Allergic bronchopulmonary aspergillosis
(b) Infection with *Mycobacterium tuberculosis*
(c) Infection with *Pseudomonas aeruginosa*
(d) Infection with *Mycobacterium avium* complex

71. Which one of the following drugs does NOT cause SIADH?
(a) Carbamazepine
(b) Chloramphenicol
(c) Cyclophosphamide
(d) Chlorpropamide

72. A cohort study is
(a) An analytical study
(b) A descriptive study
(c) A corelational trial
(d) An experimental study

73. Indian Evidence Act was enacted in
(a) 1861
(b) 1872
(c) 1880
(d) 1882

74. Major histocompatibility complex class I proteins are found in
(a) The surface of body cells
(b) Macrophages only
(c) All the body cells surface except erythrocytes
(d) B cells only

75. Which of the following is useful in differentiating the site of sensorineural hearing loss?
(a) Pure tone audiometry
(b) Brain stem auditory evoked response
(c) Speech reception threshold
(d) Tympanometry

76. Small for date baby is below
(a) 10 percentile for that gestational age
(b) 50 percentile for that gestational age
(c) 2,000 g
(d) 2,500 g

77. Which of the following is NOT a contraindication of combined oral contraceptive pills?
(a) Ischemic heart disease
(b) Focal migraine
(c) History of preeclampsia
(d) Acute liver disorders

78. The minimum systolic blood pressure in mm of mercury required to feel a carotid pulse is
(a) 40 mm Hg
(b) 60 mm Hg
(c) 80 mm Hg
(d) 100 mm Hg

79. What is the age of gestation when ovaries and testis are first distinguishable?
(a) 4 weeks
(b) 8 weeks
(c) 12 weeks
(d) 16 weeks

80. Bony ankylosis results from
(a) Pyogenic arthritis
(b) Tuberculosis arthritis
(c) Osteoarthritis
(d) Rheumatic arthritis

81. All these criteria are used for child's classification of hepatocellular function *EXCEPT*
(a) Serum bilirubin
(b) Serum albumin
(c) Ascites
(d) Prothrombin time

82. Wastes not to be incinerated are those
(a) With a low heating volume
(b) Whose content of combustible matter is above 60%
(c) Whose content of non-combustible solids is below 5%
(d) With a moisture content above 30%

83. All are predisposing causes of cerebral venous thrombosis *EXCEPT*
(a) Hypotension
(b) Oral contraceptives
(c) Aplastic anemia
(d) Pregnancy

84. Band-shaped keratopathy is seen in
(a) Hyperthyroidism
(b) Still's disease
(c) Absolute glaucoma
(d) Buphthalmos

85. Paget's disease of bone is also called
(a) Osteitis deformans
(b) Brittle bone disease
(c) Fibrous dysplasia
(d) Osteomalacia

86. All of the following are tumor necrosis factor blocking agents *EXCEPT*
(a) Adalimumab
(b) Etanercept
(c) Infliximab
(d) Abciximab

87. Trans fatty acids are known to form during
(a) Hydrogenation of oils
(b) Beta oxidation of palmitate
(c) Rancidity of fats
(d) Prostaglandin biosynthesis

88. Chondroblastoma arises from
(a) Epiphysis
(b) Metaphysis
(c) Diaphysis
(d) Flat bones

89. Pleural calcification is seen in
(a) Malignant mesothelioma
(b) Asbestosis inhalation
(c) Pleural fibroma
(d) Long standing bronchiectasis

90. Which of the following is an abnormal cystometry finding?
(a) Residual urine of less than 50 mL
(b) First desire to void is 150 mL
(c) Presence of systolic detrusor contractions
(d) Voiding detrusor pressure rise of less than 70 cm of H_2O for a volume of more than 150 mL

91. MRI is the investigation of choice in all of the following *EXCEPT*
(a) Syringomyelia
(b) Brain stem tumors
(c) Skull bone tumors
(d) Multiple sclerosis

92. Triage means classification of injuries based on
(a) Severity of injury
(b) Mode of injury
(c) Treatment protocol
(d) Supervision
(e) Required

93. Most common site for extranodal lymphoma
(a) Esophagus
(b) Stomach
(c) Intestine
(d) Skin

94. The following are attributes of endotoxin *EXCEPT*
(a) It is heart stable
(b) Protein-polysaccharide-lipid complex
(c) Action is often enzymatic
(d) Associated with gram-negative bacteria

95. Thyroid storm can be treated by all the following drugs *EXCEPT*
(a) Propylthiouracil
(b) Dexamethasone
(c) Propranolol
(d) Aspirin

96. The highest risk of developing malignancy is seen in association with this breast pathology
(a) Apocrine metaplasia
(b) Squamous metaplasia
(c) Florid adenosis
(d) Atypical hyperplasia

97. A specific heated vaporizer is required for the use of
(a) Sevoflurane
(b) Halothane
(c) Desflurane
(d) Isoflurane

98. In a crying infant presenting with blood in stools and mass in abdomen, the likely diagnosis is
(a) Intussusceptions
(b) Volvulus
(c) Abdominal lymphadenitis
(d) Hirschsprung's disease

99. In a classical radical neck dissection, all the following important structures are removed *EXCEPT*
(a) Accessory nerve
(b) Internal jugular vein
(c) Vagus nerve
(d) Sternocleidomastoid muscle

100. The systolic ejection murmur in hypertrophic obstructive cardiomyopathy is diminished when a patient
(a) Performs the Valsalva maneuver
(b) Lies down
(c) Inhales amyl nitrite
(d) Stands up

101. Endodermal sinus tumor is characterized by
(a) Schiller-Duval bodies
(b) Psammoma bodies
(c) Call-Exner bodies
(d) Homer-Wright rosettes

102. Which among the following is NOT a contraindication for combined oral contraceptives?
(a) Thromboembolic disorders
(b) Suspected breast cancer
(c) Vaginal bleeding of unknown cause
(d) Iron deficiency anemia

103. Lipoprotein X is most likely to be seen with
(a) Cholestasis
(b) Gilbert syndrome
(c) Increased intake of trans fatty acids
(d) Increased intake of PUFA

104. Pneumoconiosis is caused due to inhalation of dust within the size range of
(a) 0.5–3 microns
(b) 3.5–6 microns
(c) 6.5–8 microns
(d) 10–20 microns

105. Urogenital diaphragm consists of the following muscle
(a) Pubococcygeus
(b) Superficial transverse perineal muscle
(c) Deep transverse perineal muscle
(d) Iliococcygeus

106. Double bubble sign on antenatal ultrasonography is seen in
(a) Duodenal atresia
(b) Jejunal atresia
(c) Ileal atresia
(d) Colonic atresia

107. 'Card test' tests the function of
(a) Median nerve
(b) Ulnar nerve
(c) Ileal atresia
(d) Colonic atresia

108. The following immunoglobulin is not known to fix complement
(a) IgE
(b) IgM
(c) IgA
(d) IgG

109. Which one of the following decreases Na+ K+ ATPase activity?
(a) Thyroid hormone
(b) Aldosterone
(c) Dopamine
(d) Insulin

110. A 25-year-old male complaints of progressive loss of vision of 10 years duration. On examination, the cornea shows bifurcating criss-cross lines associated with punctuate opacities. Histology shows that the lesions are composed of amyloid. The most probable diagnosis is
(a) Schnyder dystrophy
(b) Lattice dystrophy
(c) Granular dystrophy
(d) Reis-Buckler's dystrophy

111. The commonest etiological agent in urinary tract infection is
(a) *Escherichia coli*
(b) *Staphylococcus*
(c) *Proteus mirabilis*
(d) *Klebsiella*

112. A patient with pneumonia for 5 days is admitted to the hospital. He suddenly ceases to recognize the doctor and staff, thinks that he is in jail and complains of scorpions attacking him. He is in altered sensorium, this condition is

(a) Acute delirium
(b) Acute dementia
(c) Acute schizophrenia
(d) Acute paranoia

113. The fetal effects caused by maternal alcohol consumption are all *EXCEPT*
(a) Low set ears
(b) Fetal growth restriction
(c) Small head
(d) Spina bifida

114. 'Auer rods' are seen in
(a) Lymphoblast
(b) Myeloblast
(c) Erythroblast
(d) Megakaryoblast

115. The drug of choice in paroxysmal supraventricular tachycardia is
(a) Digoxin
(b) Adenosine
(c) Nifedipine
(d) Esmolol

116. Galeazzi fracture is
(a) Fracture of upper ulna with disruption of superior radioulnar joint
(b) Fracture of lower ulna with disruption of inferior radioulnar joint
(c) Fracture of upper radius with disruption of superior radioulnar joint
(d) Fracture of lower radius with disruption of inferior radioulnar joint

117. The concentration of sodium ion is least in the
(a) Small intestinal juice
(b) Bile
(c) Gastric juice
(d) Pancreatic juice

118. Fitz-Hugh-Curtis syndrome is associated with
(a) Chlamydial infection
(b) Genital tuberculosis
(c) Syphilis
(d) Candidal infection

119. The following are indications for use of prostaglandin analogs *EXCEPT*
(a) Termination of pregnancy
(b) Prevention of NSAID-induced ulcers
(c) Closure of patent ductus arteriosus
(d) Reduction of intraocular pressure

120. The protein content in 100 g of cow's milk
(a) 1.2 g
(b) 2.2 g
(c) 3.2 g
(d) 4.2 g

121. The following are attributes of histoplasmosis *EXCEPT*
(a) Is an intracellular infection
(b) Is a superficial fungal infection
(c) Infection is acquired by inhalation
(d) Treated by IV amphotericin B

122. 'Knudson's two-hit' hypothesis is associated with
(a) Retinoblastoma
(b) Melanoma
(c) Ulcerative colitis
(d) Crohn's disease

123. A child has presented with a BP of 190/110, pedal edema++, facial edema, gross hematuria and absent ascites. The most probable diagnosis is
(a) Acute glomerulonephritis
(b) Minimal change nephritic syndrome
(c) Renal vein thrombosis
(d) Renal amyloidosis

124. A chronically draining ear that fails to respond to appropriate antibiotic therapy should raise the suspicion of
(a) Cholesteatoma
(b) Otosclerosis
(c) Presence of third window
(d) Stapes Gusher syndrome

125. Which among the following is NOT an adverse effect of lithium?
(a) Tremor
(b) Diabetes mellitus
(c) Hypothyroidism
(d) Edema

126. Muscle relaxant of choice in a patient with renal failure posted for surgery is
(a) Atracurium
(b) Vecuronium
(c) Pancuronium
(d) Pipecuronium

127. The most common cardiac defects seen in congenital rubella syndrome is
(a) Pulmonary artery stenosis and coarctation of aorta
(b) Ventricular septal defect (VSD) and patent ductus arteriosus (PDA)
(c) VSD and pulmonary artery stenosis
(d) Pulmonary artery stenosis and PDA

128. Lewy bodies are found in the substantia nigra neurons in
(a) Alzheimer disease
(b) Parkinson disease
(c) Huntington disease
(d) Pick disease

129. Which of the following is a lung fluke?
(a) Clonorchis sinensis
(b) Paragonimus westermani
(c) Fasciolopsis buski
(d) Gastrodiscoides hominis

130. Birbeck granules are present in
(a) Merkel cell
(b) Melanocytes
(c) Langerhans cells
(d) Keratinocytes

For questions 131–134

Q. A 50-year-old male smoker presents with history of hearing loss on the right ear for the past 6 weeks. Examination revealed dull tympanic membrane on right and normal left tympanic membrane. Rinne test was negative on the right and positive on the left. Weber was lateralized to the right ear. Absolute bone conduction is normal bilaterally.

131. What is the nature of his hearing loss?
(a) Right-sided conductive hearing loss
(b) Right-sided mixed hearing loss
(c) Left-sided sensorineural hearing loss
(d) Bilateral mixed hearing loss

132. What is the most appropriate next course of action?
(a) Prescribe neurovitamins and follow-up after 3 months
(b) Advise hearing aid
(c) Do urgent CT scan of brain
(d) Do posterior rhinoscopy

133. Tympanometry in this patient is most likely to reveal
(a) Bilateral type 'Ad' curve
(b) Right type 'Ad' curve and left type 'B' curve
(c) Right type 'B' curve and left type 'A' curve
(d) Right type 'A' curve and left type 'C' curve

134. Likely cause of this patient's clinical features is
(a) Demyelination of auditory nerve
(b) Presbycusis
(c) Cerebral infarct in the auditory area
(d) Nasopharyngeal carcinoma

For questions 135–137

Q. A 50-year-old male was met with motorcycle accident, the handle bar hit his left chest, patient is conscious, breathless, has tachycardia, feeble radial pulse, chest examination reveals a bruise in the left chest with a segment of chest moving up and down, it is tender to palpate and there is surgical emphysema, crepitus. Auscultation reveals decreased breath sounds on the left chest.

135. Management of this patient at the accident site would include
(a) Wide bore IV line, rapid Ringer's lactate infusion, oxygen by mask
(b) Wide bore IV line, rapid Ringer's lactate infusion and insertion of left chest tube
(c) Just shift the patient to the hospital
(d) Wide bore IV line, rapid Ringer's lactate infusion and insertion of right chest tube

136. The most probable diagnosis of this condition would be
(a) Open pneumothorax
(b) Flail chest
(c) Tension pneumothorax
(d) Hemothorax

137. **The least the patient would require is a**
   (a) Chest skiagram
   (b) CT chest
   (c) MRI chest
   (d) Pulmonary function test

For questions 138–141

Q. A 30-year-old female patient presented with difficulty in swallowing to both solids and liquids for 8 months duration following accidental ingestion of toilet cleaner, endoscopy was done and dilation done following which the patient had severe retrosternal pain, radiating to back with breathlessness.

138. **This patient is probably having**
   (a) Acute myocardial infarction
   (b) Dissecting aneurysm thoracic aorta
   (c) Iatrogenic perforation of esophagus
   (d) Severe aspiration pneumonia

139. **The classical sign on examination of this patient would reveal**
   (a) Crepitus at the suprasternal notch
   (b) Prominent enlarged neck veins
   (c) Gallop rhythm on auscultation
   (d) Bronchial breath sounds right base

140. **A chest skiagram of this patient should reveal**
   (a) Enlarged boot-shaped heart
   (b) Pneumomediastinum with pleural effusion
   (c) Consolidation right lower lobe
   (d) Widening of the anterior mediastinum

141. **The ideal treatment of this condition would be**
   (a) Conservative management
   (b) Thrombolytic therapy
   (c) Cardiac catheterization
   (d) Thoracotomy procedure

For questions 142–146

Q. A 50-year-old male, a chronic 'gutka' consumer has a 3 cm ulcerative lesion, with everted margin in the left cheek, skin not involved, it is non-tender, foul smelling, bad oral hygiene, one submandibular node felt firm, mobile, 2.5 cm in greatest diameter, with no other clinical evidence of metastasis.

142. **The TNM stage of the tumor is**
   (a) T2 N1 M0
   (b) T1 N1 M0
   (c) T3 N3 M0
   (d) T1 N2 M0

143. **A sample for histopathology of the primary is obtained by**
   (a) FNAC
   (b) Edge wedge biopsy
   (c) Core needle biopsy
   (d) Imprint biopsy

144. **The premalignant conditions of oral cancer include all *EXCEPT***
   (a) Leukoplakia
   (b) Erythroplakia
   (c) Submucosal fibrosis
   (d) Oral candidiasis

145. **The treatment consist of**
   (a) Surgery
   (b) Chemotherapy
   (c) Radiotherapy
   (d) Combined modality

146. **Predisposing factors for carcinoma cheek are all of the following *EXCEPT***
   (a) Smoking
   (b) Gutka
   (c) Khaini
   (d) Sweets

For questions 147–149

Q. A 65-year-old man died on arrival at the ER despite vigorous resuscitative measures. Histopathological sections of his lungs at autopsy reveal alveolar spaces filled with acellular granular pink fluid. The alveolar capillaries were engorged. There is no inflammatory infiltration.

147. **This patient most likely died from**
   (a) Viral pneumonia
   (b) Cardiac failure
   (c) Pulmonary embolism
   (d) Infection by *Pneumocystis jirovecii*

148. This patient could have had the all of the following conditions *EXCEPT*
(a) Mitral stenosis
(b) Hypertension
(c) Ischemic heart disease
(d) Cor pulmonale

149. The diagnosis could have been established antemortem by
(a) Blood analysis
(b) Echocardiography
(c) ECG
(d) EEG

For questions 150–153

Q. A 33-year-old male is violently stabbed in the supraclavicular region. He immediately develops shortness of breath and bloats like a balloon. Physical examination reveals puffiness of the face, swelling of the eye lids, neck and chest wall. Crepitus is felt over the chest wall. Widespread crepitations are heard on chest auscultation.

150. Which of the following features explains his present condition?
(a) Mediastinal emphysema
(b) Pneumothorax
(c) Hemothorax
(d) Aortic rupture

151. He should have an immediate
(a) Skiagram of chest
(b) MRI chest
(c) Echocardiogram
(d) FAST

152. This condition should be treated with
(a) Oxygen by mask and pleurocentesis
(b) Only by oxygen mask
(c) Intubation and controlled ventilation
(d) Thoracotomy and repair of the heart

153. This condition
(a) Is fatal
(b) Is progressive
(c) Has to be aggressively managed
(d) Has to be managed conservatively

For questions 154–157

Q. A 17-year-old male complains of recurrent episodes of cough, wheezing and shortness of breath particularly at night for the last 3 days. His sibling has a history of similar symptoms. A skin test with pollen produces immediate wheal and flare.

154. The laboratory finding most consistent with his clinical condition would be
(a) Neutrophilia
(b) Cold agglutinins
(c) Positive direct antiglobulin test
(d) Eosinophilia

155. He should be treated with
(a) Bronchodilators
(b) Steroids
(c) Antibiotics
(d) Cough sedative

156. The pulmonary function test done on this patient would be
(a) Noninformative
(b) Obstructive pattern
(c) Restrictive pattern
(d) Destructive pattern

157. Which of the following morphological changes in the lungs would be found in this patient?
(a) Destruction and dilation of the bronchi and bronchioles
(b) Free air in the interstitium
(c) Viscid mucus plugs in the small airways
(d) Peribronchiolar fibrosis

For questions 158–160

Q. A 60-year-old male has weight loss, bloody stools and constipation for the past 6 months. Colonoscopy showed an irregularly shaped ulcerative lesion in the descending colon.

158. A biopsy of the lesion on colonoscopy revealed
(a) Adenocarcinoma
(b) Amoedoma
(c) Squamous carcinoma
(d) Ulcerative colitis

159. **A barium enema in this patient would have revealed**
   (a) 'Apple core' stricture of the colon
   (b) A smooth narrowing
   (c) Lead pipe appearance
   (d) Bowel wall thickening

160. **This patient should have**
   (a) Left sigmoid colectomy
   (b) Left radical hemicolectomy
   (c) Abdominoperineal resection
   (d) Exenteration pelvic

For questions 161–163

Q. A 70-year-old male has been experiencing intermittent epistaxis, fatigue and pain in bones for the past 4 months. Laboratory investigations are as follows:
Serum Ca^{2+}: 11.2 mg/dL (Normal: 8.9–10.1 mg/dL)

161. **A bone marrow aspirate in this patient will most likely reveal**
   (a) Sheets of myeloid blast cells
   (b) Numerous plasma cells
   (c) A 'dry' tap
   (d) Abundance of lymphoid blast cells

162. **This patient is likely to develop a complication of**
   (a) Floppy mitral valve
   (b) Autoimmune hemolytic anemia
   (c) Amyloidosis
   (d) Calcific aortic valve disease

163. **The above condition is to be treated with**
   (a) Radiotherapy
   (b) Chemotherapy
   (c) Antibiotics
   (d) Antifungal therapy

For questions 164–166

Q. A 5-year-old female child develops reduced urine output, irritability, lethargy and restlessness over a period of 8 hours. She has several episodes of bloody diarrhea in the past 24 hours and has become very weak. Examination reveals mild pallor and dehydration. Laboratory investigation results are as follows:
Hb: 9 g/dL (normal: 12–16 g/dL)
Platelets: 90,000/mm^3 (Normal: 150,000–450,000)
Peripheral blood smear: Numerous schistocytes.
The BUN and creatinine were elevated.

164. **These features are suggestive of**
   (a) Parvovirus infection of the bone marrow
   (b) B cell lymphoma
   (c) Hemolytic uremic syndrome
   (d) Autoimmune hemolytic anemia

165. **A similar finding in the peripheral blood film can be seen in**
   (a) Disseminated intravascular coagulopathy
   (b) Hairy cell leukemia
   (c) Megaloblastic anemia
   (d) Thalassemia minor

166. **Her condition worsened and her BUN creatinine raised further, urine output nil, the treatment would then consist of**
   (a) Hemodialysis
   (b) Intravenous fluid
   (c) Antidiarrheal
   (d) Elective ventilation

For questions 167–170

Q. A 27-year-old male develops high grade fever with chills. A heart murmur is heard on cardiac auscultation. There is evidence of splenomegaly and splinter hemorrhages in the nails.

167. **The damage to the heart was predominantly a result of**
   (a) Ischemia to the myocardium
   (b) Abnormal coagulation process
   (c) Infection
   (d) Vasculitis

168. **This patient is likely to show**
   (a) Mycotic aneurysms
   (b) Arthritis
   (c) Leucopenia
   (d) Berry aneurysms

169. He should be treated with

(a) Anticoagulants
(b) Antibiotics
(c) Valve replacement
(d) Anti-inflammatory

170. The patient is suffering from

(a) Subacute bacterial endocarditis
(b) Malaria
(c) Kala-azar
(d) DIC

For questions 171–174

Q. A 60-year-old male with weight loss, epigastric pain radiating to the back, passage of pale bulky stools, jaundice and elevated levels of CA 19–9.

171. This clinical condition is likely to be associated with

(a) Hepatitis
(b) Diabetes
(c) Hypertension
(d) Vasculitis

172. The investigation of choice in this patient would be

(a) Plain CT scan
(b) Contrast-enhanced CT scan
(c) Ultrasound
(d) Plain X-ray abdomen

173. This patient is probably suffering from

(a) Chronic pancreatitis
(b) Choledochal cyst
(c) Carcinoma head of pancreas
(d) Hepatoma

174. This patient should under go

(a) Whipple's procedure
(b) Hepatectomy
(c) Puestow's procedure
(d) Excision of the cyst

For questions 175–177

Q. A newborn baby delivered at 38 weeks gestation, died a few days after developing severe pallor, jaundice and generalized body swelling. The mother who was Rh-negative had irregular antenatal visits and has a previous history of termination of pregnancy. Autopsy revealed hepatosplenomegaly and bile-stained organs.

175. The clinical features reflected a destruction of the red blood cells by

(a) IgE-mediated hypersensitivity
(b) Antibody-mediated reaction
(c) Immune complex-mediated injury
(d) Endotoxin-mediated injury

176. The deposition of the bile pigment in the brain is referred to as

(a) Kernicterus
(b) Jaundice
(c) Unconjugated hyperbilirubinemia
(d) Gliosis

177. This condition can be prevented to great extent by

(a) Immunizing the mother with anti-D
(b) Immunizing the unborn fetus with anti-D
(c) Administration of phenobarbitone to the mother
(d) Kasai's operation

For questions 178–180

Q. A 5-week-old male baby has developed progressively worsening projectile vomiting following breastfeeding. Physical examination showed dehydration, visible peristalsis in the abdomen and a firm oval mass in the epigastrium.

178. The pathogenesis of this condition is most likely related to

(a) *Helicobacter pylori* infection of the antrum
(b) Hypertrophy of the circular muscle layer in the pylorus

(c) Aspiration of the amniotic fluid
(d) Autoimmune destruction of the glands in the fundus of the stomach

179. This child is likely to have the following electrolyte imbalance
(a) Hypochloremic hypokalemic alkalosis
(b) Hypochloremic hypokalemic acidosis
(c) Hyperchloremic hypokalemic acidosis
(d) Hypochloremic hyperkalemic alkalosis

180. This child should have
(a) Ramstedt's operation
(b) Duhamel's operation
(c) Heller's myotomy
(d) Toupet procedure

COMED-K 2012
ANSWERS AND EXPLANATIONS

1. Answer is c (Vision).
Ref: Ganong's Physiology, 23rd edition Pg 199.

- The ***superior colliculi*** form the ***rostral two bumps*** (one on each side) on the ***dorsal aspect of the midbrain***.
- The ***caudal two bumps are the inferior colliculi*** and together they (inferior and superior colliculi) comprise the TECTUM or roof of the midbrain.
- In *contrast to the* ***inferior colliculus***, which is an ***AUDITORY*** structure, the ***superior colliculus*** is usually described as a **VISUAL *reflex center***. It is a highly laminated (layered) structure.
- The *top or dorsal-most three layers receive visual information primarily from two sources, i.e. the retina (retinocollicular) and the visual cortex (area 17; corticotectal).*
- The *intermediate and deep layers receive projections from many functionally different areas of* the brain. These inputs are both 'motor' and 'sensory' (visual, auditory and somatosensory inputs); hence you can see that the superior colliculus is *not exclusively related to visual function*. Instead, it ***plays a role in helping orient the head and eyes to all types of sensory stimuli***.

Note:

- The two superior and two inferior colliculi are collectively called '***corpora quadrigemina***'.
- How to remember easily: Superior = Vision; Inferior = Hearing—'***Eyes are above the ears***':) !!!
- Clinical syndrome that 'maybe' related to superior colliculus: ***Parinaud's dorsal midbrain syndrome***: ***paralysis of upward gaze***.

2. Answer is c (Wilson's disease).
Ref: Harrison's, 18th edition Pg 3188.

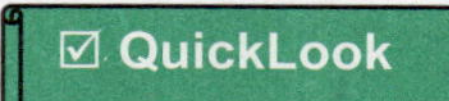

Wilson's Disease (Hepatolenticular Degeneration)

Etiology	Diagnosis
• ***AR***, inherited disorder of copper homeostasis; a/w ***mutation in ATP7B gene*** → results in ***excess accumulation of copper*** in ***liver*** and ***brain***.	• ↓ ***ceruloplasmin level.*** • ↑ ***urinary excretion of copper.*** • ↑ ***hepatic copper level.*** • Liver biopsy may show acute or chronic hepatitis or cirrhosis. • MRI of the brain may show evidence of increased basal ganglia, brainstem and cerebellar copper even early in the course of the disease.
Clinically	**Treatment**
• ***Liver related features***: ***Chronic hepatitis, hepatic steatosis and cirrhosis*** in ***adolescents and young adults***. • ***CNS features***: Indicates that liver disease is present and include ***speech disorders*** and various ***movement disorders***. • Eye: ***Kayser-Fleischer rings*** in the periphery of cornea and ***copper deposition in Descemet's membrane***; best seen by ***slit lamp examination***.	• Early in the treatment phase, ***restriction of dietary copper*** (shellfish, organ foods, nuts, mushrooms and chocolate) may be of value copper chelating medications such as ***D-penicillamine*** and ***trientine***. Oral ***zinc acetate*** competes with copper absorption in the gut and induces ***metallothionein*** in the intestine, which then sequesters copper and promotes fecal copper excretion.

3. **Answer is d (Capsule is demonstrated by M'Fadyean's reaction).**
Ref: CP Baveja's Textbook of Microbiology, 3rd edition Pg 220.

Bacillus anthracis

- ***Aerobic***, gram positive, spore (refractile, oval, central, ***NON-bulging*** spores) forming rod; only bacterium with a protein capsule.

– **First** pathogenic bacterium observed under microscope. – **First** communicable disease shown to be transmitted by inoculation of blood. – **First** bacillus to be isolated in pure culture and shown to possess spores. – **First** bacterium used for the preparation of an attenuated vaccine.	Culture appearances – ***Bamboo stick or boxcar*** appearance. – ***Medusa head*** appearance. – ***Inverted fir tree*** appearance. – ***String of pearls*** reaction.
– ***Pulmonary anthrax (Wool sorter's disease)***— following inhalation of spores flu-like symptoms that rapidly progresses to fever, pulmonary hemorrhage, shock. X-ray shows hemorrhagic mediastinitis with mediastinal widening. – ***Cutaneous anthrax (Hide porter's disease)***— MC in humans; contact leads to malignant pustule (painless ulcer) that can progress to bacteremia and death. – DOC for anthrax is penicillin G.	– *B. anthracis* is susceptible to gamma phage but *B. cereus* is not. – ***M'Fadyean's reaction (to demonstrate capsule)*** is characteristic of *B. anthracis*.
– ***Duckering***—destruction of anthrax spores in animal products imported into non-endemic countries. – ***Sterne and Mazucchi vaccine*** used to prevent anthrax in animals only. – *Obsolete treatment* used for humans was ***Sclavo's serum***.	
– ***Bioterrorism: Bacillus anthracis*** (anthrax) is the prototypic disease of bioterrorism. – ***Other agents*** studied for use in ***bioterrorism*** are ***Yersinia pestis (pneumonic plague), Francisella tularensis (tularemia), Variola major (small pox), Botulinum toxin.***	

4. **Answer is c (Hemorrhoids).**
Ref: Bailey and Love's 25th edition Pg 1253-59.

The case history given is that of alcoholic cirrhosis with portal hypertension and ascites—leading to hemorrhoids causing bright red blood in stool.

❖ Typically hemorrhoids present with bright red blood in stools or on toilet paper.

About the other options:
- ***Ischemic colitis*** and ***intestinal infarction*** is typically associated with abdominal pain (abdominal angina)
- ***Angiodysplasia*** can present with painless acute GI bleeding; more common in elderly and presents as melena.

COMED-K 2012 ANSWERS

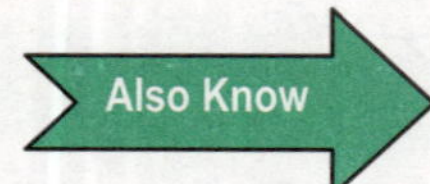

Sites of portal systemic anastomoses

Site of anastomosis	Clinical sign	Portal → systemic
➲ Lower end of esophagus	Esophageal varices	Left gastric → esophageal
➲ Umbilicus	Caput meduase	Paraumbilical → superficial and inferior epigastric
➲ Anal canal wall	Hemorrhoids	Superior rectal → middle and inferior rectal

5. Answer is c (150–200).
Ref: Park's 21st edition Pg 617.

- A ***daily supply of 150–200 liters per capita*** is considered as an adequate supply to meet the needs for all urban domestic purposes.
- In India, 40 liters of water supply per capita per day was the set target to be achieved in rural areas.
- The basic physiological requirements for drinking water have been estimated at about 2 liters/head/day.

6. Answer is b, d (Pulmonary involvement, Renal disease) — Answer verified with revised answer key!
Ref: Harrison's, 18th edition Pg 2757-58.

Systemic Sclerosis

- ***Diffuse cutaneous SSc (dcSSc)*** presents with progressive skin induration (scleroderma), starting in the fingers and ascending from distal to proximal extremities, the face and the trunk.
- ***dcSSc*** patients are at risk for ***early pulmonary fibrosis and acute renal involvement***.
- In ***limited cutaneous SSc (lcSSc),*** patients generally have long standing Raynaud's phenomenon before other manifestations of SSc appear. Skin induration is limited to the fingers (sclerodactyly), distal extremities and face and the trunk is not affected.
- A subset of patients with lcSSc have *CREST syndrome*:
  - ☐ Calcinosis cutis
  - ☐ Raynaud's phenomenon
  - ☐ Esophageal dysmotility
  - ☐ Sclerodactyly
  - ☐ Telangiectasia.
- ***Pulmonary involvement*** is the ***leading cause of death*** in systemic sclerosis.

Features	Limited cutaneous SSc	Diffuse cutaneous SSc
Skin involvement	Limited to fingers, distal to elbows, face; slow progression	Diffuse: fingers, extremities, face, trunk; rapid progression
Raynaud's phenomenon	Precedes skin involvement; associated with critical ischemia	Onset contemporaneous with skin involvement
Pulmonary fibrosis	May occur, moderate (35%)	***Frequent, early and severe (65%)***
Pulmonary arterial hypertension	Frequent, late, may be isolated	May occur, associated with pulmonary fibrosis
Scleroderma renal crisis	Very rare (2%)	Occurs in 15%; early
Calcinosis cutis	Frequent, prominent	May occur, mild
Autoantibodies	Anticentromere	Antitopoisomerase I (Scl-70)

7. Answer is b (Coarctation of aorta).
Ref: Harrison's, 18th edition Pg 1925.

- ***Radiofemoral delay*** is ***classically attributed to coarctation of the aorta***, usually due to narrowing of the aorta just ***distal to origin of the left subclavian artery***.
- It is ***more often seen in young men***. Sometimes a noticeably lower pulse volume in the femoral artery compared to radial artery is all that is appreciated rather than the classic delay in the femoral pulse.

Normal time delay for pulse wave propagation

Carotid	30 msec
Brachial	60 msec
Radial	80 msec
Femoral	75 msec

Note:

- The ***brachiofemoral delay*** rather than radiofemoral delay appears to be ***more sensitive*** in the diagnosis of coarctation, since there is already a delay of 15 msec from brachials to femorals in normals.
- Unless the ***delay is more than 20 msec***, it is NOT appreciable clinically.
- ***BP measurement (upper limb hypertension) is a more sensitive indicator*** of coarctation than radiofemoral delay.
- A ***radioradial delay*** (palpating radial arteries on both sides together) is suggestive of vascular obstruction anywhere from the *innominate artery on the right or subclavian artery on the left to the site of palpation*; also a sign of ***dissection of thoracic aorta***.
- In the elderly, ***advanced atherosclerosis/arteriosclerosis maybe a cause of radiofemoral delay*** (due to differences in peripheral artery calcification and stiffness between the lower limbs and upper limbs arteries).

Short synopsis of Coarctation of Aorta

- Infantile type: Aortic stenosis proximal to insertion of ductus (preductal).
- Adult type: **Postductal. MC coarctation is** ***just below origin of left subclavian A***.
- A/w ***HTN in upper extremities, weak pulses in lower extremities (radiofemoral delay).***
- A/w ***Turner syndrome***.
- Palpable arterial pulsations in interscapular region (***Suzzman's sign***).
- Aortic ***ejection systolic murmur.***
- Chest X-ray: ***3-sign, Dock sign*** (***rib notching*** due to collateral circulation).
- Treatment: Mainly surgical repair and stenting.

8. Answer is c (Fetal anemia).

Ref: Obstetrics: Normal and Problem Pregnancies; By Steven G Gabbe, Jennifer R Niebyl, Joe Leigh Simpson, Mark B Landon, MD, 6th edition Elsevier, Pg 749.

- The advent of non-invasive testing for ***fetal anemia through the use of middle cerebral artery (MCA) Doppler*** has ***replaced the serial amniocentesis*** for ΔOD450 except in rare circumstances:
  - Where MCA Doppler is not available or
  - In the management of alloimmunized pregnancy after 35 weeks of pregnancy.
- ***Serial MCA Doppler studies are now the mainstay of surveillance for fetal anemia*** in the red cell alloimmunized gestation.

9. Answer is d (Kidney).

Ref: Spinal Cord and Spinal Column Tumors: Principles and Practice; By Curtis A Dickman, Michael G Fehlings, Ziya L Gokasla; Pg 389; Table 24-4.

Radiosensitivity of various metastatic spinal tumors

Sensitivity	Tumor type
High	Lymphoma, multiple myeloma
Intermediate	Breast, prostate, small cell lung cancer
Low (relatively radioRESISTANT)	Sarcoma, Renal cell Ca, Non-small cell Lung cancer, colon, melanoma

10. Answer is a (Iodine).

Ref: Practical Atlas of Computed Tomography, By Hariqbal Singh, MD, Hariqbal Singh MD DMRD, Sushil Kachewar, MD, Pg 441; Textbook of Interventional Neurology, edited by Adnan I Qureshi, Pg 21, Table 2.5.

- ***Intravascular radiological contrast media*** are ***iodine containing chemicals,*** which add information to the details given from any CT scan and therefore aid in the diagnosis.
- Iodine (atomic weight 127) is an ideal choice element for X-ray absorption because the k-shell binding energy of iodine is (33.7) nearest to the mean energy used in diagnostic radiography and thus maximum photoelectric interactions can be obtained, which are a must for best image quality.

Classification of iodinated contrast media:

High osmolality (ionic)	*Low osmolality (nonionic)*
Iothalamate, Ioxaglate, Meglumine Diatrizoate, Metrizoate	Iohexol, Iopamidol, Iodixanol, Ioversol, Iopromide, Ioxilan, Metrizamide

Note:

– Barium sulfate preparations are used for **investigation of *alimentary tract*;** it is completely insoluble and is therefore neither acted on by the alimentary secretions nor absorbed through the intestine.

11. Answer is d (Impaired reciprocal interactions).

Ref: Niraj Ahuja's Psychiatry, 7th edition Pg 164.

Autistic Disorder

Patient Example: A 3-year-old boy shows no interest in or connection to his parents, other adults or children. He does not speak voluntarily and is fascinated with watching rotating objects. He screams fiercely when his environment is altered in any way, such as when his mother tries to dress him (Also see Dustin Hoffman in the movie, *Rain Man*).

Cardinal features and treatment

- Autism is the most important ***pervasive developmental disorder*** **(PDD)** of childhood.
- ***Leo Kanner*** described the condition and gave the name ***infantile autism.***
- MC in ***boys***; onset ***BEFORE*** *the age of 30 months;* Autism is a ***failure to make social contact; aloofness, lack of eye contact***, etc.
- Major ***defects in language*** development – babbling, echolalia, perseveration, poor articulation, pronominal reversal (I-you) are common.
- Resistance to change with associated ***ritualistic and/or manneristic behaviors – stereotyped behaviors like head-banging, body-spinning, hand-flicking,*** etc.
- ***Idiot-savant syndrome:*** Some autistic children have ***isolated well-developed skills (rote memory, computation, musical ability)***.
- *Etiology*: *Perinatal complications, genetic loading* (concordance rate is 35% in monozygotic twins, lower in dizygotic twins and have been implicated. Earlier theories of 'cold and aloof' refrigerator mothers have not been substantiated.
- Behavior therapy ***(operant conditioning)*** may reduce stereotypies.
- Prognosis is poor with persistent impairments in 60%. Most patients remain severely impaired in adulthood; only 2% approximately can work and live independently.

Differential diagnosis of autistic disorder

Asperger's syndrome	**Rett syndrome**
– It is a l***ess severe form of PDD*** with *later onset;* – MC in *boys;* – NORMAL *language development and intelligence;* schizoid personality.	– ***X-linked****;* affects girls only (*affected males die in utero*). – After an apparently normal early development and normal head circumference at birth, there is

– *Pedantic speech* and a *preoccupation with obscure facts* often occur.	*deceleration of head growth between the age of 5 and 30 months*. – Stereotyped movements develop with *hand clapping and head wringing*. Expressive and receptive *language is impaired with mental retardation*.

12. Answer is d (Constrictive pericarditis).
Ref: Harrison's, 18th edition Pg 1976, 1348-49.

- The case history given is that of ***tuberculosis with pleural effusion*** as evidenced by the following facts—2 months low grade fever; pleural fluid showing predominance of lymphocytes and increased ADA levels.
- Normally, TB results in exudative pleural effusion. Transudative pleural effusion results from systemic factors (due to either increased hydrostatic pressure or decreased osmotic pressure—MC due to cardiac failure—so cardiac failure may have developed).
- In ***developing nations a high percentage of cases of constrictive pericarditis is of tuberculosis origin***.
- ***Exertional dyspnea, generalized edema*** and ***raised JVP which fails to decline during inspiration*** **(*Kussmaul's sign*)** are all features of constrictive pericarditis.

13. Answer is b (Staphylococcal scalded skin syndrome).
Ref: CP Baveja's Microbiology textbook. 3rd edition Pg 176.

Virulence factors of *Staphylococcus aureus*

➢ ***Exfoliatin***—another superatigen causes *Staphylococcal Scalded Skin Syndrome (SSSS)* in children less than 4 years; SSSS in neonates is called ***Ritter's disease*** and in older individuals is called ***toxic epidermal necrolysis***. Diffuse tender erythema often with bullae and desquamation. ***Nikolsky sign*** is present (sloughing of the epidermis can be provoked by gentle stroking of the skin). Milder and more common forms of SSSS include pemphigus neonatorum and bullous impetigo.

➢ ***Enterotoxin***—preformed exotoxin secreted in the intestines, heat resistant. Causes food poisoning typified by vomiting and diarrhea within 8 hours of food consumption.

➢ ***Toxic shock syndrome toxin 1 (TSST 1)***—a superantigen binds to a constant region of the T cell receptor, non-specifically activating T lymphocytes resulting in unregulated inflammation; acquired from *contaminated tampons* in menstruating women or from infected wounds; leads to systemic hypotension, tachycardia.

➢ Others are *protein A, alpha-toxin (hemolysin), Panton-Valentine leukocidin.*

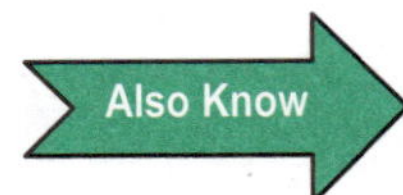

- Diseases caused by *Staphylococcus aureus*:
  - Skin infection: ***Furuncles, boils, abscesses, carbuncles, impetigo, acute paronychia, folliculitis.***
  - ***Pneumonia*** *classically seen during resolution phase of a prior viral pneumonia;* ***pneumatoceles*** *seen in children*; also *follows tracheal intubation of a hospitalized patient.*
  - Bacteremia commonly due to IV drug abuse, postsurgical via wounds or nosocomial via intravenous catheters.
  - Acute severe bacterial endocarditis of both native and prosthetic valves.
  - Osteomyelitis, sphenoid sinusitis, spinal epidural abscess; septic intracranial thrombophlebitis; septic bursitis, postoperative wound infections.
  - ***MRSA*** (methicillin-resistant *S. aureus*) infection: Important cause of serious nosocomial and community-acquired infections. Resistant to β-lactams due to altered penicillin-binding protein.
- DOC for *S. aureus*:
  - **For MSSA** (methicillin sensitive *S. aureus*): ***Penicillinase-resistant penicillin*** (oxacillin, nafcillin) with 1st generation cephalosporin as second line (Methicillin caused interstitial nephritis and no longer available).
  - **For MRSA:** Vancomycin, linezolid (bacteriostatic, oral, hematotoxicity) and daptomycin (bactericidal IV only), clindamycin and TMP-SMZ.

14. Answer is c (Lower 1/3 of ureter).
Ref: Radiological Imaging of the Kidney, edited by Emilio Quaia, Pg 606.

- ***Ureteral neoplasms*** are ***most commonly located in the distal third of the ureter*** and more rarely in the middle and proximal third.

15. Answer is c (Strassman operation).
Ref: Postgraduate Gynecology, By B Presannakumari, 2011 edition Pg 24.

Treatment of vaginal agenesis/atresia

- ***Frank and Ingram procedure***: ***Non-surgical procedure***: A vagina can be created using serial vaginal dilators pressed into the perineal body—this can take from 4 months to several years.
- ***William's*** vulvovaginoplasty.
- ***Abbe-Wharton-McIndoe*** operation: Most popular procedure.
- ***Bowel vaginoplasty.***

→ Note: ***Strassman operation*** is for abdominal repair of ***bicornuate uterus***.

16. Answer is d (Disappearance of deep tendon reflexes).
Ref: Neurology and General Medicine: Expert Consult - Online and Print, By Michael J Aminof, Pg 353; The 5-Minute ICU Consult, By Jose R Yunen, 2012, Pg 152.

- ***Loss of deep tendon reflexes*** is an ***early sign*** of ***hypermagnesemia*** and occurs at serum Mg levels of 5–6 mEq/L; at > 7.3 mEq/L, DTR are absent.
- Other manifestations are ***hypotension, bradycardia, lethargy and confusion***.

17. Answer is b (Repeated sampling).
Ref: Park's, 21st edition Pg 753.

- The sampling error is not the only error, which arises in a sample survey.
- ***Non-sampling errors*** given below are more important than sampling errors:
  - *Inadequately calibrated instruments*
  - *Observer variation*
  - *Incomplete coverage achieved in examining the subjects selected*
  - *Conceptual errors.*

18. Answer is b (Infection of submandibular space).
Ref: Bailey and Love, 25th edition Pg 731.

- ***Ludwig's angina*** is caused by a virulent ***streptococcal*** infection a/w anaerobic organisms and sometimes with other lesions of the floor such as carcinoma.
- It is characterized by:
  - ***Brawny (board like)*** swelling of the ***submandibular region*** combined with inflammatory edema of the mouth—***combined cervical and intraoral signs***.
  - Putrid ***halitosis***.
  - The infection encompasses both sides of the mylohyoid muscle causing edema and inflammation such that the tongue may be displaced upwards and backwards, giving rise to ***dysphagia***.
  - Unless treated cellulitis may extend below the deep fascial layers of the neck to involve the larynx, ***causing glottic edema and painful airway compromise***.
- Treatment: ***Immediate antibiotic therapy*** (cefuroxime with metronidazole); if not responding ***drain both submandibular triangles*** under local anesthesia.

19. Answer is c (Trypsinogen).
Ref: Harrison's, 18th edition Pg 2634.

- ***Autodigestion*** is a pathogenic theory of ***acute pancreatitis*** according to which pancreatitis results when ***proteolytic enzymes*** (e.g. ***trypsinogen, chymotrypsinogen, proelastase and phospholipase A***) are activated in the pancreas ***rather than*** in the intestinal lumen.
- A number of factors (e.g. *endotoxins, exotoxins, viral infections, ischemia, anoxia and direct trauma*) are believed to activate these proenzymes.
- Activated proteolytic enzymes, ***especially trypsin*** not only digest pancreatic and peripancreatic tissues but also can activate other enzymes, such as elastase and phospholipase.
- ***Pepsinogen***: It is an inactive zymogen is secreted into gastric juice from both mucous cells and chief cells. Once secreted, pepsinogen is activated by stomach acid into the active protease pepsin, which is largely responsible for the stomach's ability to initiate digestion of proteins.
- ***Prekallikrein***: It (or ***Fletcher factor***) is a proenzyme that circulates in plasma in a 1:1 complex with high-molecular weight kininogen (HWMK). Prekallikrein is converted to kallikrein by factor XIIa. Once formed, kallikrein enhances the activation of factor XII and (with factor XIIa) converts HWMK into bradykinin, which is an important mediator of vasodilation, inflammation and fibrinolysis (by stimulating the release of tissue plasminogen activator from endothelial cells).

20. Answer is d (Vancomycin).
Ref: KD Tripathi, 6th edition Pg 668-69.

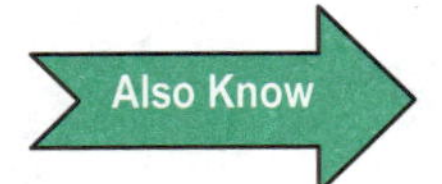

Mechanism of action	Drugs
Inhibit cell wall synthesis	Penicillins, cephalosporin's, Cycloserine, ***Vancomycin***, Bacitracin
Block protein synthesis at 30S ribosomal subunit	Aminoglycosides (***streptomycin*** etc..), tetracyclines S-I-M 'AmIno Tet 30? (Am I not yet 30?)'
Block protein synthesis at 50S ribosomal subunit	Chloramphenicol, macrolides (***erythromycin***, etc.), ***clindamycin***, streptogramins (quinupristin, dalfopristin), linezolid
Cause leakage from cell membranes	Polymyxin, Colistin, Bactitracin, Amphotericin B, Nystatin, Hamycin
Cause misreading of mRNA code and affect permeability	Aminoglycosides (streptomycin, gentamicin, etc.)
Inhibit DNA gyrase	Fluoroquinolones (ciprofloxacin, etc.)
Interfere with DNA function	Rifampin, Metronidazole
Interfere with DNA synthesis	Acyclovir, Zidovudine
Interfere with intermediary metabolism	Sulfonamides, sulfones, PAS, trimethoprim, pyrimethamine, ethambutol

21. Answer is a (Superior meatus).
Ref: Dhingra's ENT textbook, 5th edition Pg 150-153.

Meatus and openings into them

☼ **Inferior meatus**	Receives the **N**asolacrimal **D**uct S-I-M **(INDia)**
☼ **Middle meatus**	Receives **FR**ontal sinus, **A**nterior and **M**iddle **E**thmoid sinus. Hiatus semilunaris receives **M**axillary sinus S-I-M **(FRAME-M)**
☼ **SuPErior meatus**	Receives **P**osterior **E**thmoid sinus
☼ **Sphenoethmoidal recess**	Receives the sphenoid sinus.

22. Answer is c (*Bacillus anthracis*).

Ref: Medical Response to Terrorism: Preparedness and Clinical Practice, By Daniel C Keye, Pg 60, 2005 edition.

- ***Hemorrhagic meningitis*** occurs in approximately 50% of ***inhalational anthrax cases*** and is believed to develop as result of frank bacteremia.
- The ***CSF is hemorrhagic*** in most cases and polymorphs pleocytosis is present.
- Numerous large, encapsulated, gram-positive bacilli are seen under microscope.
- Anthrax meningitis is ***almost always fatal*** despite intensive antibiotic therapy, with death occurring 1–6 days after onset of illness.

23. Answer is c (Medicolegal report).

Ref: Principles of Forensic Medicine and Toxicology, By Rajesh Bardale, Pg 9; http://healthdrip.com/oral-evidence

- ***Medicolegal report*** is attached to the file relating to the case and the file is produced in the court—it will be open to scrutiny of the defense lawyer. It will NOT be admitted as evidence unless the doctor attends the court and testifies to the facts under oath.
- **Author's comments**: *'This question should be easy for any of us who have attended court for any reports we have given in MLC cases!'*

Exceptions to oral evidence are

- Dying declaration (Section 32 & 157, I.E.A)
- Chemical examiner's report
- Expert opinion expressed in a treatise may be proved in court by producing such book if the author is dead or cannot be found or cannot be called witness without unreasonable delay or expense (Section. 60, IEA)
- Oral Evidence of Mint officers or an officer of the India Security Press (Section. 292, CrPC)
- Deposition of medical witness in a lower court
- Evidence given by a witness in a lower court.

24. Answer is a (1995).

Ref: Park's, 21st edition Pg 183, 378.

Program	Year of launch
Universal immunization program	1974
National Program for Control of Blindness (NPCB)	1976
20-point program	1975
Pulse polio immunization	1995
National Rural Health Mission (NRHM)	2005

25. Answer is d (Thin basement membrane on renal biopsy).

Ref: Harrison's, 18th edition Pg 2342-2343.

IgA Nephropathy (Berger's disease)

- ***Mesangial IgA deposits***; ***CD71*** mesangial IgA1 receptor is expressed more
- ***Painless, recurrent hematuria*** in ***young males*** usually ***Asian*** origin; *24–48 hours* ***after pharyngeal/GI infection***
- Henoch-Schönlein purpura is distinguished clinically from IgA nephropathy by prominent systemic symptoms, a younger age (< 20 years old), preceding infection and abdominal complaints.

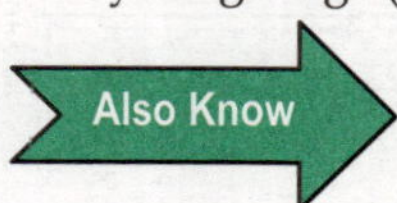

- **Thin basement membrane disease**: It is a ***variant of Alport's syndrome;*** thin basement membranes are found in 5–10% of the so-called normal population. These subclinical patients have ***normal blood pressure*** and ***little proteinuria*** and they ***rarely*** progress to renal failure.

26. Answer is c (5 mg).
Ref: Neurology of the Newborn, 5th edition, Volume 899, By Joseph J Volpe, Pg 19.

27. Answer is c (Ulcerative colitis).
Ref: Harrison's, 18th edition Pg 2482.

- ***Toxic megacolon*** is defined as a ***transverse colon*** with a ***diameter of > 5–6 cm***, with loss of haustration in patients with severe attacks of ulcerative colitis.
- It occurs in about 5% of attacks and can be triggered by electrolyte abnormalities and narcotics. About 50% of acute dilations will resolve with medical therapy alone, but urgent colectomy is required for those that do not improve.

Crohn's Disease and Ulcerative Colitis Compared

	Crohn's disease (CD)	Ulcerative colitis (UC)
■ Site of involvement	***Entire GI tract*** may be involved (mouth to anus) with 'skip' areas Distal ileum MC involved All layers of bowel wall involved (transmural); *Granulomas; creeping fat*	Continuous disease beginning at rectum and extending possibly as far as distal ileum Only mucosa and submucosa affected (mucosal) ***Crypt abscesses***
■ Symptoms	Watery diarrhea Abdominal pain, weight loss	***Bloody diarrhea*** Abdominal pain, urgency, tenesmus, weight loss, nausea, vomiting
■ Clinically	Palpable right lower quadrant ***abdominal mass*** *Perianal fissures and fistula* Oral ulcers Fever	Fever, abdominal tenderness, orthostatic hypotension, tachycardia, ***gross rectal bleeding***
■ Labs	ASCA frequently positive, pANCA rarely positive *Hemoccult positive stool* Biopsy diagnostic	ASCA rarely positive, pANCA frequently positive Biopsy diagnostic
■ Radiology	*Skip lesions,* *Colonic ulcers* *Cobblestoning mucosa* *Strictures* *'String sign' on Ba swallow*	*Continuous involvement* *Fine mucosal ulcers (double contour)* *Pseudopolyps, friable mucosa* *'Lead pipe' colon without haustra and colon shortening*
■ Complications	Abscess formation ***Fistula*** and fissure common ***Malabsorption*** (since ileal disease)	Increased risk of colon cancer Hemorrhage Bowel obstruction ***Toxic megacolon***
■ Treatment	Mesalamine, broad spectrum antibiotics, corticosteroids, immunosuppressives, surgical resection of severely affected areas, flares and remissions, recurrence after colectomy	Mesalamine, supplemental iron, corticosteroids, immunosuppressives, total colectomy is curative

To remember features of Crohn's disease you could imagine:

- *"2* ***obsessed*** *(abscesses)* ***fish*** *(fissures and fistulas)* ***skipping*** *(skip lesions) on a* ***cobblestoned*** *(cobblestones) path* ***fully penetrated*** *(transmural)* ***fat*** *(creeping fat)* ***grandma's*** *(granuloma) house wall. She caught them with a* ***string*** *(strictures, String sign) and ate them and got* ***ulcers at both ends*** *(mouth and perianal) and screamed* ***'AMMA'!*** *(Abdominal Mass and MAlabsorption)"*

ASCA= Anti-yeast *Saccharomyces cerevisiae* antibodies.

28. Answer is a (285).
Ref: Harrison's, 18th edition Pg 341.

- The ***solute or particle concentration of a fluid is known as its osmolality*** and is expressed as milliosmoles per kilogram of water (mOsmol/kg).
- Vasopressin secretion, water ingestion and renal water transport collaborate to ***maintain human body fluid osmolality between 280 and 295 mOsmol/kg***.
- *AVP secretion is stimulated* as systemic osmolality increases ***above a threshold level of 285 mOsmol/kg*** above which there is a linear relationship between osmolality and circulating AVP. Thirst and thus water ingestion also are activated at 285 mOsmol/kg beyond which there is an equivalent linear increase in the perceived intensity of thirst as a function of circulating osmolality.

29. Answer is c (Tricuspid atresia).
Ref: Harrison's, 18th edition Pg 1927.

- ***Tricuspid Atresia*** is characterized by atresia of the tricuspid valve, an interatrial communication and, frequently, hypoplasia of the right ventricle and pulmonary artery.
- Clinically, there is ***severe cyanosis*** due to obligatory admixture of systemic and pulmonary venous blood in the left ventricle.
- The ***ECG characteristically shows RA enlargement, left-axis deviation and LV hypertrophy***.

30. Answer is a (Olanzapine).
Ref: KD Tripathi, 6th edition Pg 429.

- ***Atypical antipsychotics*** are new/second generation antipsychotics that have ***weak D2 blocking, but potent 5-HT2 antagonistic activity***; extrapyramidal side effects are minimal and they may improve the impaired cognitive effect function in psychotics.

Atypical antipsychotic	Comments
Clozapine	0.8% risk of ***agranulocytosis*** (monitor ***leukocyte count*** weekly); ***epileptogenic***; myocarditis; used as a reserve drug in schizophrenia
Olanzapine	Broader spectrum than clozapine; NO agranulocytosis; causes weight gain, worsening of diabetes
Risperidone	Postural hypotension; increases prolactin levels; stroke in elderly
Quetiapine	Short acting; sedating; cataracts
Aripiprazole	Partial agonist at D2 and 5-HT1A receptor, but antagonist at 5HT2 receptor; minimally sedating (may cause insomnia)
Ziprasidone	Cardiac arrhythmias

31. Answer is a (Amino acid oxidation reaction).
Ref: Vasudevan's Biochemistry, 6th edition Pg 393.

- Enzymes containing ***riboflavin*** are called ***flavoproteins***.
- The two coenzymes are ***FMN (Flavin Mono Nucleotide)*** and ***FAD (Flavin Adenine Dinucleotide)***.

FMN-dependent enzymes	FAD-dependent enzymes
– During ***amino acid oxidation***, FMN is reduced. It is reoxidized by molecular O_2 to produce hydrogen peroxide – In ***respiratory chain***, NADH dehydrogenase contains FMN	– Succinate to fumarate by succinate dehydrogenase – Xanthine to uric acid by xanthine oxidase – Pyruvate to acetylCo-A by pyruvate dehydrogenase – Alpha-ketoglutarate to succinyl Co-A by AKG dehydrogenase – Acetyl Co-A to alpha beta unsaturated acylCo-A by acyl Co-A dehydrogenase

32. Answer is b (Dexrazoxane).
Ref: Physician's Cancer Chemo Drug Manual 2010, Pg 129.

- *Dexrazoxane* is classified as an iron chelating agent; chemoprotective drug; used IV.
- FDA approved to prevent/reduce anthracycline-induced cardiotoxicity.

SUPPORTIVE AGENTS IN ANTICANCER TREATMENT

- **Allopurinol** (Prevents *hyperuricemia from tumor lysis syndrome*).
- **Mesna** (Prevents *ifosfamide bladder toxicity*).
- **Leucovorin** (*Protects against methotrexate toxicity* to normal cells).
- **Amifostine** (*Prevents radiation toxicity*).
- **Palifermin** (*Prevents mucositis*).
- **Pilocarpine hydrochloride** (*Ameliorate dry mouth* from *radiation*).
- **Pamidronate** (Treat *hypercalcemia*, reduce effects of bone metastases).
- **Zoledronic acid** (Treat *hypercalcemia*, reduce effects of bone metastases).
- **Epoetin alfa** (erythropoietin) and **Darbepoetin alfa** (Long-acting erythropoietin): (Treat cancer or chemotherapy-related anemia).
- **Dexrazoxane**: is a *chelating agent*, a cyclic *derivative of EDTA* that may *prevent anthracycline-induced cardiomyopathy*.
- **Amifostine**: Cytoprotective agent, ***prevents radiation toxicity***. MOA: It is dephosphorylated by alkaline phosphatase in tissues to a pharmacologically active *free thiol metabolite*. The higher concentration of free thiol in normal tissues is available to bind to and thereby detoxify reactive metabolites of cisplatin. Free thiol may also act as a scavenger of free radicals that may be generated in tissues exposed to cisplatin.
- **Filgrastim**: G-CSF, *granulocyte colony stimulating factor; reduces severity and duration of chemotherapy-induced neutropenia.* SE: bone pain, hypoxia.
- **Sargramostim:** GM-CSF, *granulocyte-macrophage colony stimulating factor* SE: Fluid retention, dyspnea, capillary leak (rare), supraventricular tachycardia (rare), bone pain, irritation at injection sites.
- **Neumega, oprelvekin (IL-11):** Interleukin-11 used to *treat chemotherapy-induced thrombocytopenia*. SE: Fluid retention, headache, arrhythmias, arthralgias, myalgias.

33. Answer is b (HBcAg in serum indicates active infection).
Ref: Harrison's, 18th edition Pg 2539-40.

- *HBsAg* in serum indicates ***active infection***; ***HBcAg is NOT*** routinely detectable in blood: Hepatitis B can cause ***hepatocellular carcinoma***.
- ***Chronic hepatitis*** is an important ***late complication of acute hepatitis B*** occurring in a small proportion of patients with acute disease, but ***more common in those who present with chronic infection without having experienced acute illness, as occurs typically after neonatal infection*** or after infection in an immunosuppressed host.

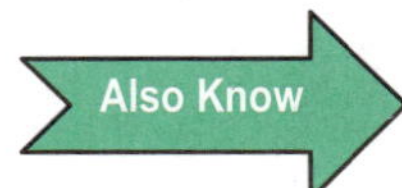

Hepatitis B Serology

■ HBsAg	*First virologic marker detectable in serum* after infection with HBV (even before elevation of serum aminotransferase and clinical symptoms appear) Indicates ***active hepatitis B infection***, either acute or chronic (> 6 month)
■ Anti-HBs	Antibody to HBsAg. Provides ***immunity to hepatitis B***. *Persists for years*
■ HBcAg	*Not routinely detectable* in blood
■ Anti-HBc	***Positive during the window period*** ***IgM anti-HBc*** is an indicator of ***recent disease***, IgG anti-HBc signifies chronic disease
■ HBeAg	Indicates ***active viral replication and high infectivity***. S-I-M (**Be**ware!)
■ Anti-HBe	When present in HBsAg carrier, blood is potentially less infectious

Summary of Hepatitis Viruses

Name	Viral characteristics	Transmission	Special features
❑ **Hepatitis A (infectious hepatitis)**	RNA picornavirus	Fecal-oral, food borne	Onset usually abrupt, disease mild, self-limiting, no chronic infection, NOT a/w cancer Vaccine: active immunization available
❑ **Hepatitis B (serum hepatitis)**	*DNA* hepaDNAvirus	Parenteral or sexual transmission	Insiduous onset common, disease may be severe with 1–2% mortality; a/w *primary hepatocellular carcinoma, cirrhosis* Vaccine available
❑ **Hepatitis C (post-transfusion hepatitis)**	RNA flavivirus	Parenteral or sexual transmission	Acute disease is usually subclinical with *high rate of chronicity* with ~4% mortality; A/w *primary hepatocellular carcinoma, cirrhosis* NO vaccine
❑ **Hepatitis D (delta hepatitis)**	Defective-enveloped RNA virus, requires hepatitis B as helper virus to replicate	Coinfection or superinfection	Coinfection (both acquired at same time) is occasionally severe; Superinfection (patient already infected with B, then acquires B and D) has high mortality; cirrhosis, fulminant hepatitis
❑ **Hepatitis E (enteric hepatitis)**	RNA calicicvirus	Fecal-oral, food borne	Severe and *high 20% mortality in pregnant patients*. No chronic infection, NOT a/w cancer

Mnemonics for hepatitis S-I-M

- **A** and **E** feco-oral: "The vowels hit your bowels!"
- Hepatitis **A**: **A**symptomatic (usually), **A**cute, **A**lone (no carriers)
- Hepatitis **B**: **B**lood borne
- Hepatitis **C**: **C**hronic, **C**irrhosis, **C**arcinoma, **C**arriers
- Hepatitis **D**: **D**efective, **D**ependent on HBV
- Hepatitis **E**: **E**xpectant mothers, **E**pidemics

34. Answer is b (Thyroid function test).
Ref: Kanski, 6th edition Pg 239.

The case history given is that of superior limbic keratoconjunctivitis, SLK (question says 'mild papillary conjunctivitis' 'punctate corneal staining superiorly' and corneal filaments—all point to SLK).

- SLK typically affects middle-aged women who have ***thyroid dysfunction***.
- Pain, redness, watering.
- ***Superior bulbar conjunctival*** congestion, ***papillary*** conjunctival hypertrophy.
- *Corneal pannus* and ***filamentary keratitis (stains with rose Bengal).***
- *Dry eyes (50% cases).*
- Treatment: ***Lubricant*** eyedrops, ***cyclosporine*** eyedrops; *silver nitrate* on cotton bud for 1-20 second followed by thorough irrigation and antibiotic ointment; bandage soft contact lenses.

35. Answer is b, d (Bagassosis, Farmer's lung)—verified from revised answer key.
Ref: Harrison's, 18th edition Table 2117.

- ***Thermophilic actinomycetes*** = *Micropolyspora faeni, Thermoactinomyces vulgaris,* ***T. saccharrii****, T. viridis and T. candidus.*
- ***Thermophilic actinomycetes*** are implicated in causing:
  - ***Bagassosis*** ('moldy' bagasse or sugarcane)
  - ***Farmer's lung*** ('moldy' hay)
  - Humidifier or air-conditioner lung
  - Mushroom worker's lung
  - Potato Riddler's lung.

36. Answer is b (ASD).
Ref: OP Ghai, 7th edition Pg 398, 399 and Fig 14.8; Harrison's, 17th edition Pg 1459.

Repeat Topic	Qn

- See ***answer no. 57 in COMEDK 2010 answers*** for detailed explanation.

37. Answer is a (Polyclonal antibody).
Ref: Pediatric Acute Care: Management for the Nurse Practitioner, By Karin Reuter-Rice, Beth Bolic, Pg 224, Table 22-14, 2012 edition.

- ***Thymoglobulin*** is the brand name for a polyclonal antithymocyte globulin preparation.
- Also please be aware of the brand name Herceptin—see table below (asked in APPG and AIPGE) earlier.

Immunosuppressive antibody preparations

Medication	Mechanism of action/features
Polyclonal antibody preparations	
Antithymocyte globulin ➢ Rabbit ATG (Thymoglobulin) ➢ Equine/Horse ATG (ATGAM)	Targets numerous B and T cell surface antigens; used to prevent acute transplant rejection
Monoclonal antilymphocytes preparations	
Muromonab (OKT3)	Targets CD3 receptors on T cells; used to prevent acute transplant rejection
Monoclonal anti-IL2R antibodies	
Basiliximab	Chimeric antibody that inhibits activation and clonal expansion
Daclizumab	Humanized antibody that inhibits activation and clonal expansion; used to prevent acute transplant rejection
Anti-TNF alpha antibodies	
Infliximab	Used in Crohn's disease, rheumatoid arthritis, psoriatic arthritis, ankylosing spondylitis
Adalimumab	Used in Crohn's disease, rheumatoid arthritis, psoriatic arthritis
Others	
Abciximab	Targets Glycoprotein IIb/IIIa; to prevent cardiac ischemia in unstable angina and in patients treated with percutaneous coronary intervention
Trastuzumab (Herceptin)	Targets erb-B2; used in HER-2-overexpressing breast cancer
Rituximab	CD20; B cell non-Hodgkin's lymphoma
Omalizumab	IgE; Additional line of treatment for severe asthma

38. Answer is b (Autosomal recessive).
Ref: Harrison's, 18th edition, Pg 2359.

Autosomal Recessive (Infantile) Polycystic Kidney	Autosomal Dominant (ADult) polycystic kidney
Genetics	
– *ARPKD gene—chromosome* ***6***	– ***APKD-1*** *gene* on chromosome ***16p***

– *Gene defect*—PKHD1, which produces fibrocystin (polyductin) – (***PKHD***1 = **P**olycystic **K**idney **H**epatic **D**isease 1)	– **S-I-M** *"Polycytsic kidney'* = **16** *letters* = ***16p'*** – *Gene defect – PKD1 and PKD2, which code for polycystin 1 and 2* – Phenotypic heterogeneity is a hallmark of ADPKD, as evidenced by family members who share the same mutation, but have a different clinical course
Clinically	
– Diagnosed in ***first year of life*** presenting as *bilateral abdominal masses* – Enlarged, with ***small cysts, < 5 mm, limited to the collecting tubules*** – ***Death*** *in neonatal* period is MC due to ***pulmonary hypoplasia*** – ***HTN occurs in first few years of life*** – Longer-term survivors frequently develop ***portal hypertension, esophageal varices and hypersplenism from periportal fibrosis***	– *DOES NOT manifest before 30 years* – Manifests disease as ***renomegaly, flank pain, hematuria, infection, hypertension, uremia***
Associated abnormalities	
– ***Congenital hepatic fibrosis*** – Maternal oligohydramnios – Potter's syndrome	– *Colonic diverticula (MC extrarenal anomaly),* – *Hepatic cysts* (also cysts in spleen, pancreas, ovaries) – *Intracranial berry aneurysms* – *Mitral valve prolapse*
Imaging	
– U/s shows large, echogenic kidneys – The diagnosis can be made *in utero after 24 weeks of gestation in severe cases*, but cysts generally become visible ONLY AFTER birth – The absence of renal cysts in either parent on ultrasonography helps to distinguish ARPKD from ADPKD in older patients	– IVU—***'spider-leg'*** deformity – The sensitivity of renal ultrasonography for the detection of ADPKD is 100% for subjects 30 years or older with a positive family history – Before the age of 30 years, CT scan or T2-weighted MRI is more sensitive for detecting presymptomatic disease

39. Answer is c (Gray).

Ref: International System of Units (SI) (rev, 2008 Ed.), edited by Barry N Taylor, Pg 67.

Radiation Derived Units

Quantity	Old unit	SI unit	Name for SI unit	*Mnemonic*
Radioactivity	**Curie (Ci)**	Disintegrations per second (dps)	Becquerel (Bq)	*"Becky and Curie are Active"*
Radiation Absorbed Dose	**RAD**	Joule per kilogram (J/kg)	Gray (Gy)	*Colors—"Red and Gray"*
Radiation Exposure	Roentgen (R)	Coulomb per kilogram (C/kg)	-	
Dose equivalent	rem	Joule per kilogram (J/kg)	Sievert (Sv)	

40. Answer is c (Short course).

Ref: Park's, 21st edition Pg 167.

- *DOTS* = *D*irectly *O*bserved *T*reatment, *S*hort course.
- ***DOTS Plus*** = Dots and use of second line anti-TB drugs to prevent MultiDrug Resistant (MDR TB).

41. Answer is a (Organ of Zuckerkandl).
Ref: Robbin's pathology, Big, 8th edition Pg 1159.

- The ***organ of Zuckerkandl*** is a ***chromaffin body*** derived from ***neural crest*** located at the ***bifurcation of the aorta or at the origin of the inferior mesenteric artery***. It can be the source of paraganglioma or extra-adrenal pheochromocytoma.
- The organ of Zuckerkandl is of pathological significance in the adult as a ***common extra-adrenal site of pheochromocytoma*** though the *most common extra-adrenal site is in the superior para-aortic region between the diaphragm and lower renal poles.*

42. Answer is c (Non-pulmonary organ failure).
Ref: Harrison's, 18th edition Pg 2209.

- ***Mortality in ARDS*** is largely attributable to ***non-pulmonary causes***, with ***sepsis and non-pulmonary organ failure accounting for > 80% of deaths***.
- Thus, improvement in survival is likely secondary to advances in the care of septic/ infected patients and those with multiple organ failure.

43. Answer is c (Analysis of the health situation).
Ref: Park's, 21st edition Pg 772-73.

Steps of planning cycle
1. Analysis of health situation
2. Establishment of objectives and goals
3. Assessment of resources
4. Fixing priorities
5. Write-up of formulated plan
6. Programming and implementation
7. Monitoring
8. Evaluation

44. Answer is d (Papillitis).
Ref: Parson's diseases of the eye, 21st edition Pg 346.

- About option B—***lattice degeneration*** predisposes to retinal detachment; by itself it is asymptomatic.
- About option C—***retinal hole***, by itself may be asymptomatic; maybe a/w lattice degeneration in which cases barrage laser is needed to prevent retinal detachment.
- About option A—***papilledema usually has preserved vision*** to begin with, in fact this differentiates it from ***papillitis***, which typically is a cause of sudden loss of vision.
- See detailed table below.

Differences between Papilledema and Papillitis (optic neuritis)

	Papilledema	Papillitis (Optic neuritis)
History	***Headache and vomiting***, initially NO visual symptom	***Sudden loss of vision***, h/o fever or URTI
Laterality	Usually ***bilateral***	Usually ***unilateral***
Visual acuity	Remains *normal until late stage*	*Severely reduced* (6/60 or less)
Pain or tenderness of the eyeball	***Absent***	May be present
Pupil	Normally reacting	Relative Afferent Pupillary Defect ***(RAPD)*** or Marcus Gunn Pupil
Disk swelling	More than +3D elevation in established case	Usually +2D to +3D elevation

Hemorrhage and exudates	More in established case	Relatively *less*
Visual fields	***Enlargement of blind spot*** and later constriction of peripheral fields	***Central or centrocecal*** scotoma
CT scan or MRI	Intracranial space-occupying lesion ***(ICSOL)*** can be detected	***Demyelinating disorder*** can be seen
Recovery of vision	Usually not complete after treatment	Usually complete with adequate and prompt treatment

45. Answer is a (Multiple myeloma).
Ref: Medical Laboratory Technology; By Sood, 5th edition Pg 202; Wintrobe's clinical hematology, 12th edition Pg 785.

- Rouleaux formation of RBC is demonstrated by 'stacking' of RBCs.
- Also see ***answer no. 161*** in the same Comedk 2012 answers for a detailed summary of multiple myeloma.

Increased Rouleaux formation	Decreased Rouleaux formation
Caused by increased fibrinogen or globulins in the blood—as in multiple myeloma, hyperfibrinogenemia, macroglobulinemia	Due to abnormally shaped RBCs as in hereditary spherocytosis.

46. Answer is a (Dystrophin gene).
Ref: Molecular Pathology in Clinical Practice, edited by Debra GB Leonard, Pg 87.

- The ***DMD gene*** is the ***largest human gene isolated*** spanning more than 2,000 kilobases of genomic DNA, which is translated into a protein named ***dystrophin***.
- Dystrophin is found in ***cardiac, smooth muscle, skeletal muscle and brain***.

47. Answer is c (Ampulla).
Ref: Dutta's, 6th edition Pg 21.

Fertilization

- Fertilization is the process of fusion of the spermatozoon with the mature ovum.
- It occurs in the ***ampulla*** of the fallopian tube.
- Out of hundreds of millions of sperm deposited in the vagina at a single ejaculation, ***only 300–500 reach the ovum***.
- It takes about *1 hour for the sperms to reach the site (at ~3 mm/min)*.

48. Answer is a, b (Dopamine, Serotonin).
Ref: The Encyclopedia of Positive Psychology, edited by Shane J Lopez. Pg 288.

- ***Dopamine*** is highly associated with the ***pleasure seeking system*** of the brain and is released by naturally rewarding experiences such as food, sex, some drugs (cocaine, nicotine and amphetamines).
- ***Serotonin and dopamine*** play an important role in ***pleasure seeking***.
- ***Nucleus accumbens*** is referred to as the ***brain's pleasure center***.

49. Answer is c (Scrotum)
Ref: Dermatalogical Diseases : A Practical Approach, By Venkataram Mysore, Pg 201, Table 35.3.

– ***Nodular scabies***: In some cases, itching nodules persist for several months. They are found most commonly on the scrotum.

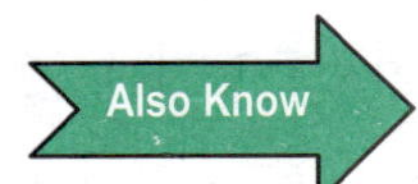

Scabies

Etiology and spread

- Caused by ***itch mite***[Q], ***Sarcoptes scabiei***[Q]; spread through ***contact***[Q] ***(sexual promiscuity, crowding, uncleanliness)*** with infected individuals, spread is common in families.

Presentation

- Intense **pruritus**[Q] **(itching) that *worsens* at *night* and *after a hot shower***[Q].
- Burrows[Q] appear as dark wavy lines in the epidermis that measure 3–15 mm and end in a small pearly bleb that contains the female mite.
- Lesions are seen on ***interdigital webs, flexor aspects of wrists***, the elbows, anterior axillary folds, around the nipples, umbilicus, lower abdomen, genitalia, buttocks, medial aspects of thighs, legs and feet.
- The ***face, scalp, neck, palms and soles* are *spared***[Q] *except in children.*

Varieties of scabies

- ***Scabies incognito***[Q]: Occurs in persons treated with steroids.
- ***Norwegian scabies***[Q]: Hyperinfestation with millions of mites may result from glucocorticoid use, immunodeficiency[Q] or AIDS.
- ***Sarcoptic mange***[Q]: Animal scabies.

Treatment

- All the family members should be treated at the *same time.*
- ***5% permethrin cream***[Q] applied from the neck down after bathing and removed 8 h later with soap and water.
- Alternatives include *benzyl benzoate, sulfur ointments, topical crotamiton cream, ivermectin.*
- *Lindane solution* was used earlier, but it causes *neurotoxicity* (seizures) and *aplastic anemia.*
- Contraindicated in pregnant women and infants.

50. Answer is a, d (Menetrier's disease, Type A gastritis) — verified from answer key.

Ref: Harrison's, 18th edition Pg 765-66.

Risk factors

- *H. pylori* infection
- Chronic Atrophic gastritis (***type A*** gastritis)
- Blood group **A**
- Pernicious Anemia
- Adenomatous polyps
- Smoking and Alcohol
- Nitrosamines in smoked fish
- Menetrier's disease
- Postantrectomy — 15-20 years after Billroth II anastomosis

Also Know About Stomach Cancer

- **Morphologically**
  - MC site is proximal third of stomach (including the esophagogastric junction). ***Lauren classification*** below:
  - Polypoid — solid mass projecting into stomach lumen
  - Ulcerative — ulcer through all layers
  - Superficial spreading — most favorable prognosis
  - Leather-bottle type (*linitis plastica*) — poor prognosis.

- **Symptoms**: Dyspepsia lasting longer than a month in patients > 40 years. Weight loss and the 3 **A**s – **A**nemia (iron deficient), **A**norexia, **A**sthenia.
- **Signs**: *Epigastric mass*, obstructive jaundice and hepatomegaly (due to secondaries in liver), ***ascites*** (from peritoneal carcinomatosis), enlarged left supracalvicular **(*Virchow's*)** node, migratory thrombophlebitis **(*Trousseau's sign*)**, ***acanthosis nigricans***, microangiopathic hemolytic anemia.
- **Metastases:** To the ovary (***Krukenberg's tumor*** – classically from colloid Ca); periumbilical region (***'Sister Mary Joseph node'***), peritoneal cul-de-sac/pouch of Douglas (***Blumer's shelf*** palpable on rectal or vaginal exam); to supraclavicular node (*Virchow's node*). ***Liver*** is the MC site for hematogenous spread of tumor.
- Diagnosis – ***endocscopy with multiple biopsies*** (most accurate), barium upper GI series, abdominal CT scan also used.
- Classification systems for gastric adenocarcinomas are: ***Lauren system;*** WHO classification; ***Ming*** classification; ***Japanese*** classification; ***Borrmann's*** (macroscopic – polypoid/fungating, ulcerating with raised borders, ulcerative infiltrating and diffuse infiltrative)
- **Treatment**: Surgical removal of the complete tumor with resection of adjacent lymph nodes offers the only chance for cure, but this is possible in less than one third of patients. Metastasis is obvious in > 60% of patients and is a contraindication to surgery. Palliation involves use of drugs, surgery and radiotherapy.

51. Answer is b (Non-invasive ventilation).
Ref: Harrison's, 18th edition Pg 2189.

- ***Obstructive sleep apnea/hypopnea syndrome (OSAHS)*** is defined as the coexistence of unexplained excessive daytime sleepiness with at least five obstructed breathing events (apnea or hypopnea) per hour of sleep.
- ***Continuous Positive Airway Pressure (CPAP)*** is the ***treatment of choice***.
- ***CPAP*** is a type of ***non-invasive ventilation***.
- ***Invasive ventilation*** is ventilation with ***endotracheal intubation***.

52. Answer is b (Fracastorius).
Ref: Basic Epidemiological Method & Biostat: A Practical Guidebook; By Randy M Page, Galen E Cole, Thomas C Timmreck, Pg 6.

- The notion that disease could be caused by germs was largely popularized by an Italian poet and physician ***Heironymous Fracatsorius***.
- His belief that disease was transmitted from one person to another by particles too small to be seen was put forth in his book called *Des Res Contagiosa*.
- Calling this transmission process as '***contagion***' he hypothesized that minute germs could be spread by close personal contact and conveyed person to person by 'fomes' or inanimate objects.

53. Answer is a (Addison's disease).
Ref: Harrison's, 18th edition Pg 368-69.

Increased anion gap metabolic acidosis ('*MUDPILES*')	Normal anion gap metabolic acidosis ('*DURHAM*')
M – Methanol	D – Diarrhea
U – Uremia	U – Ureteral diversion
D – Diabetic ketoacidosis, alcoholic ketoacidosis, drugs	R – Renal tubular acidosis
P – Phosphate or paraldehyde	H – Hyperalimentation
I – Ischemia or Iron or INH	A – Addison's disease, Ammonium chloride, Acetazolamide
L – Lactate	M – Miscellaneous (amphotericin B)
E – Ethylene glycol	
S – Starvation or salicylates	

54. Answer is c (Long head of biceps femoris).
Ref: IB Singh, Anatomy, 2008 edition Pg 341.

- The *lower border of the sacrotuberous ligament* was found to be directly continuous with the ***tendon of origin of the long head of the Biceps femoris*** in approximately 50% of subjects.

55. Answer is a, b (Reinsch test, Marsh test)—*verified from answer key.*
Ref: Narayan Reddy's FMT, 23rd edition Pg 265-66.

Arsenic Poisoning

Chemical nature
- Metallic arsenic is ***not*** poisonous, as it is not absorbed from the alimentary canal.
- Arsenic or white arsenic is arsenious oxide or arsenic trioxide (Sankhya or Somalkhar).
- Copper arsenite is ***Scheele's green***; Copper acetoarsenite is ***Paris green.***
- Arsenic combines with ***sulfhydryl enzymes*** and interferes with cell metabolism.
- Most popular homicidal poison.

Acute poisoning
- Resembles cholera, gastroenteritic type; ***garlic*** odor.
- When acute arsenic poisoning is suspected, an X-ray of the abdomen may reveal ingested arsenic, which is ***radiopaque.***
- Arsenic is rapidly cleared from blood and distributed to various organs and tissues. Blood sample is useful only in acute poisoning.

Chronic poisoning
- Skin and nail changes, such as hyperkeratosis, ***'rain drop'*** hyperpigmentation , exfoliative dermatitis and ***Mee's*** lines (transverse white striae of the fingernails).
- Sensory and motor ***polyneuritis*** manifesting as numbness and tingling in a 'stocking-glove' distribution.
- ***Subendocardial hemorrhages*** of the left ventricle.
- ***Stomach*** mainly affected and shows red-velvety appearance.
- Chronic consumption of water containing arsenic at high concentration leads to vasospasm and peripheral vascular insufficiency culminating in ***'blackfoot disease,'*** a gangrenous condition affecting the extremities.
- Risk of ***skin cancer*** and possibly of ***cancers*** of the lung, liver (*angiosarcoma*), bladder, kidney and colon.

Tests
- **MAR**sh test and Reinsch tests are positive.
- Arsenic can be detected in completely decomposed bodies since it is present in hair, nails and bones.

Treatment
- Freshly prepared hydrated ferric oxide (Fe_2O_3) is ***arsenic antidote***; Dialyzed iron maybe used as substitute.
- Alkalis should NOT be given as they increase the solubility of arsenic.
- ***Lillys antidote kit*** is used.

56. Answer is d (Pasteurization of milk).
Ref: Park, 21st edition Pg 569.

- Tests of pasteurized milk are:
  - Phosphatase test
  - Standard plate count
  - Coliform count.

57. Answer is c (Small intestine).
Ref: Vitamins for natural healing, GC Goyal, Pg 21; Food, Jenny Ridgewell, Pg 35.

- There are two major forms of vitamin A—***retinol and beta-carotene.***
- ***Retinol*** is mainly found in ***animal foods***— milk, cheese, butter and oily fish.
- ***Beta-carotene*** is found in ***green vegetables, red and orange fruits*** (carrots, tomatoes and apricots).
- ***Beta-carotene is converted in the body to retinol in the small intestine.***

58. Answer is d (Vulva).
Ref: Robbins pathology, Big, 8th edition Pg 1012.

- ***Bowen disease*** is a form of ***intraepidermal carcinoma***, a malignant tumor of keratinocytes. Bowen disease may ultimately progress to an invasive ***squamous cell carcinoma***.
- MC on ***head and neck***; next is ***limbs***; ***vulva*** can be affected and so also ***glans penis*** (erythroplasia of Queyrat).

59. Answer is c (Hypokalemia).
Ref: Harrison's, 18th edition Pg 1838, 47.

ECG – Abnormalities – Must Know for any PG entrance examination

• **HyPERKalemia**	***Tall, tented T-wave***, decreased P-wave amplitude, widening of QRS, ***'sine wave pattern'*** (severe hyperkalemia causing cardiac arrest) **S-I-M** **'PERK with Tea'**
• **Hypokalemia**	Prominent ***U-waves***, small T-waves, ventricular bigeminy
• *Hyper***calcemia**	***Shortens*** Q-T interval
• *Hypo***calcemia**	***Lengthens*** Q-T interval
• **Subarachnoid hemorrhage**	Marked QT prolongation with deep, wide T-wave inversions (***'CVA T-wave'***)
• **Hypothermia**	Convex elevation of ***J point*** (J waves or Osborn waves)
• **Pericardial effusion**	Total ***electrical alternans*** (often with tamponade)
• **TCA overdose**	Sinus tachycardia with QRS and QT prolongation
• **Digoxin effect**	Shortened QT interval with a characteristic 'scooping' of the ST-T wave complex ST depression PR prolongation Inverted T-wave (***inverted check mark sign***) in V5-6 **S-I-M** *QT Choti, depressed ST, PRolonged PR, ulta T)*
• **Pulmonary embolism**	***MC: Sinus tachycardia with an otherwise normal ECG*** There may be deep S-waves in I, pathological Q-waves in III, inverted T-waves in III ('SIQIIITIII'), strain pattern V1-V3, right axis deviation, RBBB, atrial fibrillation
• **Syndrome a/w prolonged QT interval**	***Romano ward syndrome*** (AD) and ***Jervell and Lange-Neilsen syndrome*** (AR, congenital deafness)
• **Lev's disease and Lenegre's disease**	Degenerative diseases commonly responsible for damage to the specialized conducting system and produce AV block usually associated with bundle branch block
• **Right bundle branch block (RBBB)**	More common than LBBB; RBBB occurs with heart disease, both congenital (e.g. atrial septal defect) and acquired (e.g. valvular, ischemic)
• **Left bundle branch block (LBBB)**	LBBB is often a marker of one of four underlying conditions: Ischemic heart disease, long-standing hypertension, severe aortic valve disease and cardiomyopathy

60. Answer is a (False perception in absence of a stimulus).
Ref: Niraj Ahuja's Psychiatry, 7th edition Pg 13.

Illusions	Hallucinations
❑ Illusions are ***misconceptions*** of external stimuli, e.g. at dusk, a common illusion is to perceive the outline of a bush as that of a man.	❑ A ***perception experienced in the absence of external stimulus*** to the sense organs. ❑ A few normal people also experience them during transition between sleep and waking (when tired); they are called *hypnagogic* if experienced, while falling asleep and *hypnopompic* if experienced during awakening.

Types Of Hallucinations

According to Complexity

1. ***Elementary*** *hallucinations*—bangs, whistles, flashes of light.
2. ***Complex*** *hallucinations*—hearing voices or music, or seeing faces and scenes.

According to Sensory Modality

1. Auditory hallucinations:
- Voices, music or noises; common in non-organic psychiatric disorders.
- ***Voices addressing the patient*** (*second-person hallucinations* and voices talking to one another referring to the patient (***third person hallucinations***) seen commonly in ***schizophrenia***.
- Sometimes voices seem to anticipate what the patient thinks a few moments later or speak his own thoughts as he speaks them (*Gedankenlautwerden*), or repeat his thoughts immediately after he has thought of them (*echo de la pensee*).

2. Visual hallucinations:
- These may be elementary or complex; common in *organic mental disorders* also seen in hysteria, severe affective disorders.
- ***Extracampine:*** Visual hallucinations are experienced as located outside the field of vision, i.e. ***behind the head***.

3. **Olfactory and gustatory hallucinations** are frequently experienced together, often as unpleasant smell or tastes; may suggest severe depressive disorders, schizophrenia, ***temporal lobe epilepsy***, irritation of the olfactory bulb by a tumor.

4. ***Tactile (haptic) hallucinations***: Experienced as insects crawling on the body or under the skin; occurs with ***cocaine abuse (formication of Magnan's bugs), amphetamine abuse, delirium tremens, opioid withdrawal and*** occasionally in schizophrenics.

5. ***Autoscopic hallucination*** is the experience of seeing one's own body projected into space, usually in front of oneself for short periods. This experience may convince the person that he has a ***double (doppelganger)***; this is a rare phenomenon encountered mainly in a small minority of patients with ***temporal lobe epilepsy*** or other organic brain disorders.

61. Answer is a (Technetium scan).

Ref: Bailey and Love's, 25th edition Pg 1158-59.

- A ***technetium-99m (99mTc) pertechnetate scan, also called Meckel scan*** is the ***investigation of choice to diagnose Meckel's*** diverticula.
- This scan ***detects gastric mucosa***; since approximately 50% of symptomatic Meckel's diverticula have ectopic gastric or pancreatic cells contained within them [9] this is displayed as a spot on the scan distant from the stomach itself. This scan is highly accurate and noninvasive.

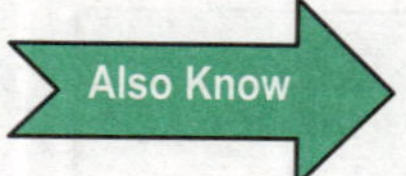

Commonly Used Scans in Medicine

1. Adrenal scan	– For localization of ***pheochromocytoma*** when CT or MRI findings are equivocal – *Labeled* ***MIBG*** is used; patients should return for imaging several days after MIBG administration
2. Bleeding scan	– Detection of source of GI bleeding – **Technetium-99m (^{99m}Tc)** sulfur colloid scan – **Technetium-99m (^{99m}Tc)** red cell scan—superior for localizing ***intermittent bleeding***
3. Bone scan	– ***Metastatic workups*** (Ca likely to go to bone—breast, prostate, kidney, thyroid, lung) – Evaluation of delayed union of fractures – Osteomyelitis – Avascular necrosis of femoral head – Evaluation for hip prosthesis – Differentiation of traumatic and pathologic fractures
4. Brain scan	– Metastatic workup – **Determination of** blood flow in brain death or atherosclerotic disease) – Evaluation of space-occupying lesions (tumor, hematoma, abscess, AV malformation) – Encephalitis
5. Cancer scan	– **Technetium-99m** (^{99m}Tc) + **arcitumomab, CEA-Scan**. For imaging of cancers with increased levels of CEA and has been found to be more sensitive and specific than CT scans in the detection of both resectable and non-resectable disease
6. Cardiac scans	– **Diagnosis of MI**, stress testing, measurement of ejection fraction and cardiac output, diagnosis of ventricular aneurysms – **Thallium-201** (^{201}Tl). Measurement of myocardial perfusion by uptake of ^{201}Tl by normal myocardium. Normal myocardium appears hot and ischemic or infarcted areas appear cold – Acute MI (< 12 h) seen as hotspot, old MI (scar) seen as cold on both resting and exercise scans – Ischemia is cold on exercise scan and returns to normal after rest – **Technetium-99m** (^{99m}Tc) **pyrophosphate**. Recently damaged myocardium concentrates 99mTc pyrophosphate producing a myocardial hotspot. Most sensitive 24–72 hours after AMI – **Technetium-99m** (^{99m}Tc) labeled **ventriculogram.** ^{99m}Tc labeled serum albumin or RBCs are used. Shows abnormal wall motion, cardiac shunt, size and function of heart chambers, cardiac output and ejection fraction. Another form of this study is **MUGA scan** in which data collected are synchronized to an ECG and used to provide a 'moving picture' of cardiac function. Performed with patient at rest or during exercise stress test
7. Gallium scan	– *Location of* ***abscesses*** (5–10d old) and chronic inflammatory lesions, lymphoma, staging and follow-up for disease detection, diagnosis of lung cancer, melanoma and other neoplasms
8. Hepatobiliary scan (HIDA or BIDA scan)	– Differential diagnosis of **biliary obstruction** (when bilirubin between 15 and 7 mg/dL), *acute cholecystitis*, biliary atresia; not good for stones unless cystic duct is completely occluded and cholecystitis is present

9. **Indium-111 (^{111}In) Octreotide scan**	– Imaging of *tumors with somatostatin receptors* (gastrinoma, insulinoma, pheochromocytoma, small cell lung cancer)
10. **Iodine-125 (^{125}I) Fibrinogen scanning**	– ***Detection of venous thrombosis*** in the lower extremities. Patient is scanned several hours and several days after injection of tracer. Identification of clots at or below knees. False positives with varicosities, cellulitis, incisions, arthritis and hematomas. Tracer availability problem
11. **Lungs scan (V/Q scan)**	– Evaluation of ***pulmonary embolism***
12. **Renal scans**	– **Iodine-131** (^{131}I) **Hippuran**. Evaluation of function in renal insufficiency; visualization is poor and radiation dose can be high – **Technetium-99m** (^{99m}Tc) **glucoheptonate**. Combination renal cortical imaging and renal function; evaluation of overall function, but can be used to determine vascular flow and visualize renal parenchyma and collecting system – **Technetium-99m** (^{99m}Tc) **DMSA** (dimercaptosuccinic acid). Renal cortical imaging only – **Technetium-99m** (^{99m}Tc) **DTPA** (diethylenetriaminepentaacetic acid). Renal function, renal blood flow studies, estimation of GFR, evaluation of collecting system – **Technetium-99m** (^{99m}Tc) mercaptoacetyltriglycine **(MAG3)**. Renal function. Imaging of the renal parenchyma within minutes of injection and with low radiation dose, *May eventually replace* all other agents
13. **Strontium-89 (^{89}Sr) Metastron**	– ***Palliative therapy*** for multiple **painful bony metastases** (prostate or breast cancer). Because agent is a pure beta emitter, radioactivity remains in the body, so no special precautions are needed
14. **Thyroid scan**	– **Technetium-99m** (^{99m}Tc) **pertechnetate**. Evaluation of nodules. Scan patterns in conjunction with laboratory test may help in diagnosing hyperfunctioning adenoma. Plummer and Grave's disease, multinodular goiter, localization of ectopic thyroid tissues (especially after thyroidectomy for cancer), identification of superior mediastinal masses

62. Answer is d (Oral sepsis).

Ref: Shafers Oral Pathology, 6th edition Pg 36.

Causes of xerostomia (DRY mouth)

Systemic causes	Local causes
– Autoimmune connective tissue disorders: Sjögren's syndrome, primary and secondary – Granulomatous diseases: Sarcoidosis, tuberculosis – Graft-versus-host disease – Cystic fibrosis Bell's palsy Diabetes (poorly controlled) – Amyloidosis – Human immunodeficiency virus infection – Thyroid disease: Hypo- and hyper-thyroidism – Late stage liver disease – Affective disorder Eating disorders and malnutrition • anorexia, bulimia, dehydration – Drugs: Anticholinergic	– Salivary duct calculi (especially submandibular duct) – Sialadenitis – Salivary gland aplasia – Postradiotherapy

63. Answer is c (Lysine).
Ref: Park, 21st edition Pg 342.

64. Answer is c (Poxvirus).
Ref: Textbook of Microbiology, CP Baveja, 3rd edition Pg 436.

- ***Molluscum contagiosum*** is a viral infection of the skin or occasionally of the mucous membranes, sometimes called water warts. It is caused by a ***DNA poxvirus*** called molluscum contagiosum virus (MCV). MCV has no non-human-animal reservoir (infecting only humans).
- Infection is ***most common in children*** aged 1–10 years old. MC can affect any area of the skin, but is most common on the trunk of the body, arms and legs. It is spread through direct contact or shared items such as clothing or towels.
- Histologically, molluscum contagiosum is characterized by ***molluscum bodies in the epidermis above the stratum basale***, which consist of large cells with abundant granular eosinophilic cytoplasm (accumulated virons) and a small peripheral nucleus.

65. Answer is d (Depolarization travels in opposite directions).
Ref: Ganong's physiology, 23rd edition Pg 87-88.

- Depolarization in myelinated axons ***jump from one node of Ranvier to the next***, with current sink at the active node serving to electronically depolarize the node ahead of the action potential to the firing level.
- Myelin is an effective insulator and current flow through it is ***negligible***.
- This jumping of depolarization from node to node is called ***saltatory conduction***.
- It is a ***rapid process*** that allows myelinated axons to conduct up to 50 times faster than unmyelinated fibers.

66. Answer is a (Pleuroperitoneal membrane).
Ref: Fundamentals of Diagnostic Radiology, By William E Brant, Clyde Helms, Pg 345.

- The ***foramina of Bochdalek*** are defects in the closure of the posterolateral diaphragm at the junction of the ***pleuroperitoneal membrane*** with the transverse septum.
- The ***foramina of Morgagni*** are triangular gaps in the muscles of the anteromedial diaphragm.
- Both are potential sites of ***diaphragmatic hernia***.

67. Answer is NONE – verified with revised answer key.
Ref: Harrison's, 18th edition Pg 3149.

- ***Familial hypertriglyceridemia*** is autosomal dominant; elevated VLDL levels.
- Secondary causes of hypertriglyceridemia:
  - ***Obesity***
  - ***Type 2 DM***
  - Glycogen storage disease
  - Hepatitis
  - ***Alcohol***
  - Renal failure
  - Sepsis
  - Stress
  - Cushing's syndrome
  - ***Pregnancy***
  - Acromegaly
  - Lipodystrophy
  - Drugs: Estrogen, beta blockers, glucocorticoids, bile acid binding resins, retinoic acid.

68. Answer is a (Right hepatectomy).
Ref: Mastery of Surgery, Vol 1, Josef Fischer, Pg 1014; Minimally Invasive Surgical Oncology: State-Of-The-Art Cancer Management, By Ronald Matteott, 2012 edition Pg 284.

- ***Right hepatectomy***: Removes four segments 5.6.7.8.
- ***Left hepatectomy***: Removes three segments 2, 3, 4.
- ***Trisegmentectomy***: Removal of any combination of three segments.
- ***Extended right hepatectomy***: Involves five segments; a right hepatectomy, which extends into segments 1 or 4.
- ***Extended left hepatectomy***: Involves four segments; a left hepatectomy, which extends into segments 1, 5 or 8.

69. Answer is b (Use as a safe sleeping aid).
Ref: http://en.wikipedia.org/wiki/Phocomelia.

- Pls go thru the above article..........from Wikipedia..........quite interesting too.
- I usually do not give Wikipedia/internet links........but then the thalidomide tragedy is something which no textbook gives in so much detail.......so the Wikipedia article.

70. Answer is d (Infection with *Mycobacterium avium* complex).
Ref: Bronchiectasis; By RA Floto, CS Haworth, Pg 119, June 2011 – European respiratory society clinical handbook.

<u>***Mycobacterium avium* complex (MAC) lung disease**</u>

- ***Traditional presentation***: ***Fibrocavitary disease*** of lung apex: similar to TB especially in males with h/o cigarette smoking and/or alcohol abuse.
- ***Nodular/bronchiectasis***: ***Nodular*** and ***interstitial infiltrates*** involving the right middle lobe or lingual predominantly in the *postmenopausal non-smoking Caucasian females: slower progression, detected on HRCT.*

71. Answer is b (Chloramphenicol).
Ref: Harrison's, 18th edition Pg 2908, Table 340-2.

Drugs causing SIADH

- Carbamazepine
- Chlorpropamide
- Cyclophosphamide
- Vasopressin or desmopressin
- Oxytocin, high doses
- Nicotine
- Vincristine
- Phenothiazines
- Tricyclics
- MAO inhibitors
- Serotonin reuptake inhibitors.

72. Answer is a (An analytical study).
Ref: Park's, 20th edition Pg 66, 71.

- ***Analytical studies*** are of two types of ***observational*** studies:

Case control study	Cohort study
A ***retrospective*** study; a common first approach to test causal hypothesis	Undertaken to obtain additional evidence to support or refute the existence of an association between suspected cause and disease; also called ***prospective study***, longitudinal study, incidence study and forward-looking study

73. Answer is b (1872).
Ref: Narayan Reddy's FMT, 23rd edition Pg 2.

- Indian Penal Code (IPC) = 1860
- Indian Evidence Act (IEA) = 1872
- Criminal Procedure Code (CrPC) = 1973.

74. Answer is c (All the body cells surface except erythrocytes).
Ref: Robbins Pathology, Big, 8th edition Pg 191.

Major Histocompatibility Complex (MHC)

- MHC encoded by **H**uman **L**eukocyte **A**ntigens (HLA) genes located on **<u>short arm of Chromosome 6 (6p)</u>**.

MHC 1	MHC 2
– MHC 1 (Class 1) = HLA-A, HLA-B and HLA-C – **MHC 1** antigens are expressed on **all nucleated cells and platelets *except mature RBCs*** – Antigen is loaded in RER of mostly intracellular peptides – Mediates viral immunity – Pairs with β2-microglobulin	– MHC 2 (Class 2) = HLA-DP, HLA-DQ, HLA-DR – MHC 2 antigens expressed only on **'antigen presenting cells' (APCs)**, including **dendritic** cells, **macrophages, B cells** and **activated T cells** – Antigen is loaded in an acidified endosome

75. Answer is b (Brain stem auditory evoked response).
Ref: Dhingra's ENT textbook, 5th edition Pg 32.

- Brain stem auditory evoked response is useful in differentiating the site of sensorineural hearing loss.
- The exact anatomic site of neural generation of various waves is disputed, but latest studies indicate following sites:
  - Wave 1—Distal part of CN VIII
  - Wave 2—Proximal part of CN VIII near brainstem
  - Wave 3—Cochelar nucleus
  - Wave 4—Superior olivary complex
  - Wave 5—Lateral lemniscus
  - Wave 6, 7—Inferior colliculus.

76. Answer is a (10 percentile for that gestational age).
Ref: Park, 20th edition Pg 460.

- ***Low-birth-weight (LBW) baby*** = birth weight measured within ***first hour of life* < 2,499 g (2.5 kg)** regardless of gestational age.
- So, LBW babies may be:
  - ***Small for date*** babies may be born at term or preterm; they weigh ***less than 10th percentile for the gestational age***—these babies are ***clearly the result of IUGR***.
  - Preterm babies: Born before 37 weeks (259 days); ***intrauterine growth may be normal***.

77. Answer is c (History of preeclampsia).
Ref: Park, 20th edition Pg 432.

Combined Pill

- Estrogen (ethinyl estradiol) + progestin (levonorgestrel, norethisterone or norgestrel).
- Mala-N contains Norethisterone 1.0 mg and ethinyl estradiol 0.03 mg.
- Mala-D contains D-norgestrel 0.30 mg and ethinyl estradiol 0.03 mg.
- Mode of action: They inhibit ovulation by preventing LH and FSH release from the pituitary; produce static endometrial hyperplasia; make the cervical mucus hostile to sperm entry and penetration; interfere with motility and secretion of the fallopian tubes.

Side effects	– Nausea, vomiting, headache and leg cramps; mastalgia; breakthrough bleeding (especially with progestin only preparations) – Weight gain; chloasma and acne; pruritus vulvae; carbohydrate intolerance, mood swings (due to alteration in tryptophan metabolism), abdominal distension – Leg vein and pulmonary thrombosis – Coronary and cerebral thrombosis – Hypertension – Gallstones, cholestatic jaundice, benign hepatomas
Beneficial effects	– Protection against at least six diseases: Benign breast disorders including fibrocystic breast disease and fibroadenoma, ovarian cysts and ovarian cancer, endometrial cancer ectopic pregnancy, pelvic inflammatory disease and iron deficiency anemia
Absolute contraindications	– Thromboembolic disease or a past history of it – Cardiac abnormalities – Suspected/overt malignancy of genitals, breast – Moderate-to-severe hypertension, hyperlipidemia – Active liver disease, hepatoma or h/o jaundice during past pregnancy – Undiagnosed abnormal uterine bleeding – Porphyria – Impending major surgery
Relative contraindications	– Migraine, Obesity, Varicosities, Epilepsy, Bronchial asthma, Age over 35, Diabetes, Nursing mothers in the first 6 months, Smoking, Gallbladder disease

78. Answer is b (60 mm Hg).

Ref: The Anesthesia Technician and Technologist's Manual: All You Need to Know; By Glenn Woodworth, Jeffrey R Kirsch, Shannon Sayers-Rana, 2012 edition Pg 292, Table 33-2.

Minimum systolic pressure required to palpate these pulses
- Carotid: 60 mm Hg
- Femoral: 70 mm Hg
- Radial: 80 mm Hg
- Dorsalis pedis: 90 mm Hg

79. Answer is b (8 weeks).

Ref: Gender Development; By Judith E Owen, 2009 edition Pg 44; Pediatric endocrinology, Mark A Sperling, 3rd edition Pg 532.

- The ***ovaries*** begin to become ***distinguishable from the testis*** by ***8 weeks*** of gestation.

80. Answer is a (Pyogenic arthritis).

Ref: Textbook of orthopedics, Maheswari, 4th edition Pg 177, Essential Handbook of Practical Orthopaedic Examinations. By K Banerjee, Pg 163-164.

- ***Immobility*** or stiffening of a joint often in an abnormal position due to surgery, injury or disease is called ankylosis.

Fibrous ankylosis (false ankylosis)	Bony ankylosis (true ankylosis)
• Due to proliferation of fibrous tissue • Common outcome of ***TB arthritis*** (except in spine)	• Due to total destruction of articular cartilage • Found in ***untreated septic arthritis classically***; in TB spine, ankylosing spondylitis, rheumatoid arthritis, etc.

81. Answer is d (Prothrombin time)—verified with revised answer key....BUT read on.

Ref: Diseases of Liver and biliary system, Sheila Sherlock, 2002 edition.

- *Child-Pugh classification* is a means of *assessing the severity of liver cirrhosis*.

Score	1	2	3
S. bilirubin (micromol/L)	< 34	34–50	> 50
S. albumin (g/L)	> 35	28–35	< 28
Prothrombin time (seconds prolonged) OR	< 4	4–6	> 6
Prothrombin time INR	< 1.7	1.7–2.3	> 2.3
Encephalopathy	None	Mild	Marked
Ascites	None	Mild	Marked

- If there is primary biliary cirrhosis or sclerosing cholangitis then bilirubin is classified as < 68 = 1; 68–170 = 2; > 170 = 3.
- The individual scores are summed and then grouped as:
  - < 7 = A
  - 7–9 = B
  - 9 = C
  - A C classification forecasts a survival of less than 12 month.

Note:
The original Child's classification had 'nutrition' instead of 'prothrombin time'; 'nutrition' being graded as 'excellent, good and poor'. The ORIGINAL Child's classification DOES NOT have prothrombin time, but Child-Pugh's HAS!!
Dr CG Child and Dr JG Turcotte of the University of Michigan first proposed the scoring system in 1964. It was modified by Pugh et al in 1972. They replaced Child's criterion of nutritional status with the prothrombin time or INR and thus eliminated the most subjective part of the score.

82. Answer is d (With a moisture content above 30%).
Ref: Parks', 20th edition Pg 696.

Wastes suitable for incineration	Wastes NOT to be incinerated are
Low heating volume – above 2,000 kcal/kg for single chamber incinerators and above 3,500 kcal/kg for double chamber incinerators	Pressurized gas containers
Content of combustible matter above 60%	Large amount of reactive chemical wastes
Content of non-combustible solids below 5%	Silver salts and photographic or radiographic wastes
Content of non-combustible fines below 20%	Halogenated plastic such as PVC
Moisture content below 30%	Wastes with high mercury/cadmium content such as broken thermometers, used batteries and lead-lined wooden panels
	Sealed ampules or ampules containing heavy metals

83. Answer is 'NONE' – verified with revised answer key!
Ref: Harrison's, 18th edition Pg 462.

- Hypercoagulable disorders primarily cause increased risk of venous thrombosis and therefore may cause venous sinus thrombosis.

Risk factors for venous thrombosis

Inherited	Acquired	Unknown
Factor V Leiden	Age	Elevated factor II, IX, XI
Prothrombin G20210A	Previous thrombosis	Elevated TAFI levels
Antithrombin deficiency	Immobilization	Low levels of TFPI
Protein C and S deficiency	Major surgery	
Elevated FVIII	Pregnancy and puerperium	

	Hospitalization Obesity Infection APC resistance, non-genetic Smoking	

84. Answer is b (Still's disease).

Ref: Parson's diseases of the eye, 21st edition Pg 209-10.

- ***Band keratopathy*** is characterized by deposition of ***calcium*** *in Bowman's membrane, epithelial basement membrane and anterior stroma.*
- Ocular causes: ***Chronic anterior uveitis*** (especially in ***children with Juvenile Rheumatoid Arthritis—Still's disease***); ***phthisis bulbi, silicone oil in AC, chronic corneal edema, severe chronic keratitis.***
- Others: Age related; metastatic calcification, increased serum calcium and phosphorus, chronic renal failure, hyperuricemia); familial and ichthyosis.
- Treatment: ***Chelation with EDTA.***

85. Answer is a (Osteitis deformans).

Ref: Harrison's, 18th edition Pg 3136.

Paget's Disease (Osteitis Deformans)

- Abnormal bone architecture caused by ↑ in both osteoblastic and osteoclastic activity. Possibly viral in origin.
- Serum calcium, phosphorus and PTH levels are **normal**. ↑ ***serum ALP***. Mosaic bone pattern; long bone chalk-stick fractures.
- *Age* > 40 y; M:F 2:1.
- ***Pain*** *is* the MC presenting symptom.

Skull:	**Spine:**
➲ ***Osteoporosis circumscripta*** (outer table destroyed only) ➲ ***'Cotton wool'*** areas of sclerotic bone ➲ ↑ ***Hat size***! (facial bones not commonly affected, cf. fibrous dysplasia) ➲ ***Hearing*** loss common due to auditory foramen narrowing	➲ Especially lumbar spine. Enlargement of vertebrae and coarsened trabeculae and cortical thickening produces the ***'picture frame' vertebral body***
Pelvis:	**Extremities:**
➲ Cortical thickening ➲ Enlargement of pubis/ischium ➲ Coarse trabecular pattern ➲ ***'Brim sign'***	➲ Leading edge of the lytic phase of the disease has a ***'Blade of grass'*** appearance ➲ ***'Banana fractures'*** (incomplete pathologic fractures)

☐ *Complications:*

- ***Pathological fractures*** (usually femur = 'Shepard's crook' deformity).
- Sarcomatous change in **1%** (usually ***osteosarcoma*** or less commonly fibrosarcoma).
- ↑ blood flow from ↑ arteriovenous shunts may cause high output ***CHF***.
- ***Calcific aortic stenosis*** and diffuse vascular calcifications.
- Osteoclast-rich ***benign giant cell tumors*** may arise in areas adjacent to pagetic bone and respond to glucocorticoid therapy.
- ***Hyperuricemia*** and ***urinary stones*** may occur.

☐ *Treatment*: ***Bisphosphonates*** are the drugs of choice.

86. Answer is d (Abciximab).

Ref: KD Tripathi, 6th edition Pg 204-05.

- ***TNF-alpha inhibitors*** suppress inflammation and are used in the treatment of autoimmune diseases such as RA, IBD, psoriasis, etc.
- Examples are:
  - ***Etanercept***: Recombinant fusion protein of TNF-receptor and Fc portion og human IgG.
  - ***Infliximab***: Chimeral monoclonal antibody.
  - ***Adalimumab***: Recombinant monoclonal anti-TNF antibody.

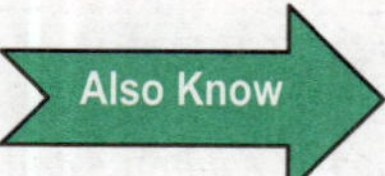

  - **Anakinra**: ***IL-1 receptor antagonist*** used in RA.
  - **Abciximab**: Monoclonal ***antibody against Glycoprotein GP IIb/IIIa receptor—platelet aggregation inhibitors***—used in unstable angina and as adjuvant to coronary thrombolysis/percutaneous coronary intervention with stent placement.

87. Answer is a (Hydrogenation of oils).
Ref: Vasudevan's biochemistry, 6th edition Pg 298.

- ***Trans Fatty Acids*** (TFA) are formed during the ***partial hydrogenation of vegetable oils***.
- TFA are more atherogenic than saturated fatty acids.
- Clinical studies have shown that ***DHA (Docosa Hexanoic acid)*** and ***EPA (Eicosa pentanoic acid)*** lower triglycerides slow the buildup of atherosclerotic plaques and reduce risk of heart attacks.

88. Answer is a (Epiphysis).
Ref: Maheswari's orthopedics textbook, 4th edition, Pg 229.

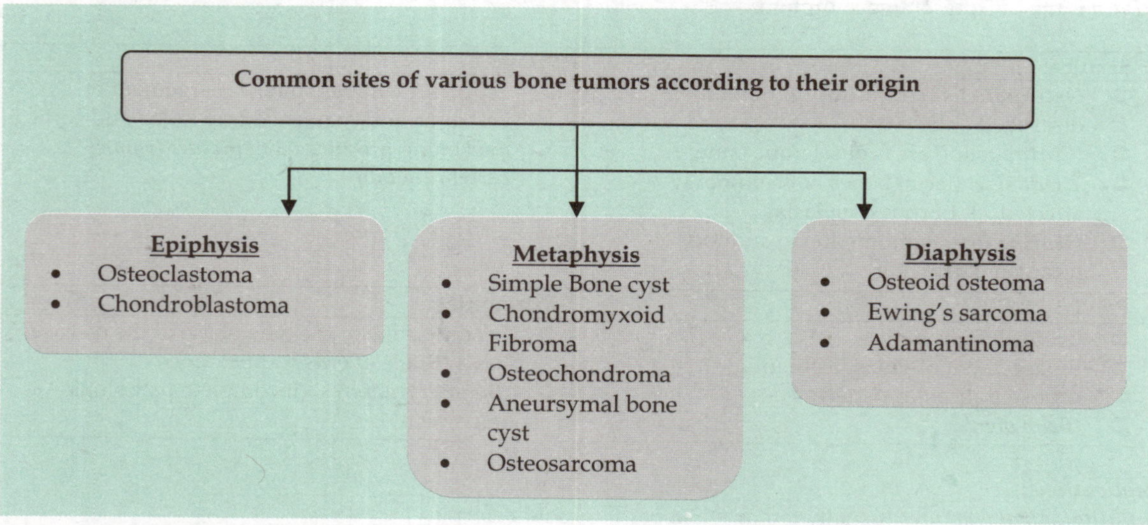

89. Answer is b, c (Asbestosis inhalation, Pleural fibroma).
Ref: Aids to radiological D/D, Stepehn Davies, Pg 122.

90. Answer is c (Presence of systolic detrusor contractions).
Ref: Berek & Novak's Gynecology: Edited by Jonathan S Berek, Issue 935, Volume 2007, Pg 867.

Normal cystometry findings/values

Residual urine < 50 mL
First desire to void occurs between 150–250 mL

Strong desire to void does not occur until after 250 mL Cystometric capacity between 400–600 mL No uninhibited detrusor contractions during filling, despite provocation No urge or stress incontinence despite provocation Voiding occurs as a result of voluntarily initiated and sustained detrusor contraction. Flow rate during voiding is greater than 15 mL/sec with a detrusor pressure of < 50 c H_2O

91. Answer is c (Skull bone tumors).
Ref: Harrison's, 18th edition Pg 3241-3243.

– For ***skull bone tumors, CT scan*** is more suitable.

92. Answer is a (Severity of injury).
Ref: Bailey and Love's, 25th edition Pg 286.

Triage 4 Color Codes

Red: High priority treatment or transfer

Yellow: Medium priority

Green: Ambulatory patients

Black: Dead or moribund patients

93. Answer is b (Stomach).
Ref: Harrison's, 18th edition Pg 646.

Gastric lymphoma

- Second MC gastric malignancy; usually **solitary**; 95% ARE **non-Hodgkin's lymphomas of B cell** origin; ***H. pylori*** infection increases the risk of gastric lymphoma.
- The **stomach** is the **MC extranodal location** for lymphoma.
- The treatment of gastric lymphoma is controversial and may involve surgical resection, radiotherapy or combination chemotherapy.

94. Answer is c (Action is often enzymatic).
Ref: CP Baveja's microbiology, 3rd edition Pg 82, Table 10.1.

Endotoxins	Exotoxins
Lipopolysaccharide in nature	Proteins (polypeptides)
Heat stable	Heat labile (> 60°C)
Form integral part of cell wall; released only on disruption of bacterial cell	Actively secreted by living cells into the medium
Weakly antigenic; antitoxin is not formed but antibodies against polysaccharide are raised	Highly antigenic; stimulates formation of antitoxin, which neutralizes toxin
Cannot be toxoided	Converted into toxoid by formaldehyde
No enzymic action	Enzymic in action
Non-specific action of all endotoxins	Specific pharmacological effect of each exotoxin
Low potency	Very high potency
Non-specific in action	Highly specific for particular tissue, e.g. tetanus toxin for CNS
Usually produce fever	Do not produce fever in host
Produced by Gram-negative bacteria	Produced mainly by Gram-positive bacteria and also by some Gram-negative bacteria

95. Answer is d (Aspirin).
Ref: Irwin and Ripe's Intensive Care medicine, 2008 edition Pg 1271.

Thyroid storm (thyrotoxic crisis)

- An acute, life-threatening, hypermetabolic state induced by excessive release of thyroid hormones (THs) in individuals with thyrotoxicosis.
- *Clinical*: Fever, tachycardia, hypertension and neurological and GI abnormalities. Hypertension may be followed by congestive heart failure that is associated with hypotension and shock.
- Because thyroid storm is almost invariably fatal if left untreated, rapid diagnosis and aggressive treatment are critical.
- Treatment:
  - Aggressively ***control hyperthermia*** by applying ice packs and cooling blankets and by administering acetaminophen (15 mg/kg orally or rectally every 4 h).
  - Promptly administer ***antiadrenergic drugs (e.g. propranolol)*** to minimize sympathomimetic symptoms.
  - Correct the hyperthyroid state. Administer antithyroid medications to block further synthesis of thyroid hormones (THs) - ***High-dose propylthiouracil (PTU)*** is preferred because of its early onset of action and capacity to inhibit peripheral conversion of T4 to T3.
  - Administer ***iodine compounds*** (Lugol iodine or potassium iodide) orally or via a nasogastric tube to block the release of THs (at least 1 h after starting antithyroid drug therapy). If available, intravenous radiocontrast dyes such as ipodate and iopanoate can be effective in this regard. These agents are particularly effective at preventing peripheral conversion of T4 to T3.
  - Administer ***glucocorticoids*** to decrease peripheral conversion of T4 to T3. This may also be useful in preventing relative adrenal insufficiency due to hyperthyroidism.

96. Answer is d (Atypical hyperplasia).
Ref: Breast Imaging, 3rd edition By Daniel B Kopan, Pg 82, Table 3.2.

Histologic subtypes of benign breast lesions and subsequent risk of developing invasive breast cancer

NO increased risk
Adenosis, Apocrine metaplasia, cysts, ductal ectasia, fibrosis, fibroadenoma, hyperplasia (mild), inflammation (mastitis, squamous metaplasia)
SLIGHTLY increased risk (1.5–2 times, baseline risk)
Hyperplasia (moderate or florid, solid or papillary) Papilloma with fibrovascular core Sclerosing adenosis
Moderately increase risk (4–5 times baseline risk)
Atypical hyperplasia (ductal or lobular)

97. Answer is c (Desflurane).
Ref: Stoelting's Clinical Anesthesia, 2009 edition Pg 665.

- An ***anesthetic vaporizer*** is a device generally attached to an anesthetic machine, which delivers a given concentration of a volatile anesthetic agent.
- A much more acceptable way is to convert the liquid inhalational agent into a form that can be delivered by the inhalational route to the patient. The most convenient way is to deliver the 'vapor' form of the liquid inhalational agent. A device which converts liquid to vapor is called vaporizer.
- ***Desflurane*** has a ***very low boiling point*** (about 23 degrees Centigrade) and even at room temperature, has an high vapor pressure. The solution chosen for the problem is to have a ***vaporizer that heats the Desflurane to a very precisely controlled temperature*** that is not affected by changes in room temperature. The heated vapor is then 'injected' into the fresh gas flow.

98. Answer is a (Intussusception).
Ref: Bailey and Love's, 25th edition Pg 80.

Name	Presenting age	Vomit description	Findings/Comments
Intussusception	4 month–2 year	Bilious	Currant-jelly stools (blood and mucus); Palpable sausage-shaped mass; sign de Dance; treat with barium enema (diagnostic and therapeutic)

99. Answer is c (Vagus nerve).
Ref: Dhingra's ENT textbook, 5th edition Pg 396.

- **Classical radical neck dissection**: ***Saves the following structures***: carotid artery; brachial plexus; phrenic nerve; ***vagus nerve***; cervical sympathetic chain, marginal mandibular branch of facial nerve, lingual and hypoglossal nerves.
- **Modified radical neck dissection**: Similar to above radical neck dissection and in addition also saves one or more of the following structures: ***Spinal accessory nerve; internal jugular vein and sternocleidomastoid muscle***.

100. Answer is b (Lies down).
Ref: Harrison's, 18th edition Pg 1828.

Effects of Various Interventions on Systolic Murmurs

Intervention	HOCM	Aortic stenosis	Mitral regurgitation	Mitral valve prolapse
Squatting or handgrip	↓	↓ or ↔	↑	↓
Standing	↑	↑ or ↔	↓ or ↔	↑
Valsalva	↑	↓	↓ or ↔	↑
Exercise	↑	↑ or ↔	↓	↑
Amyl nitrite	↑↑	↑	↓	↑

101. Answer is a (Schiller-Duval bodies).
Ref: Robbins pathology, Big, 8th edition Pg 1049.

- ***Schiller-Duval body*** is a structure seen in the ***endodermal sinus tumor***.
- It consists of a central vessel surrounded by tumor cells—the whole structure being contained in a cystic space often lined by flattened tumor cells.
- ***Call exner bodies*** are seen in ***granulosa cell tumor***.
- ***Psammoma bodies*** are seen in **P**apillary Ca thyroid, **S**erous cystadenoma of ovary, **M**eningioma, **M**alignant **M**esothelioma; S-I-M **PSaMMoma**.
- ***Homer Wright*** (pseudo) rosettes are seen in neuroblastoma.

102. Answer is d (Iron deficiency anemia).
Ref: Dutta's OBG, 6th edition Pg 544.

- See ***answer no. 77*** above in the same ***Comed-k 2012 answers***.

103. Answer is a (Cholestasis).
Ref: Clinical Biochemistry 2e: Metabolic and Clinical Aspects, By William J Marshall, Pg 777.

- ***Lipoprotein-X*** is an abnormal lipoprotein that appears in the sera of patients with obstructive jaundice and thus is a ***sensitive indicator of cholestasis***.

104. Answer is a (0.5–3 microns).
Ref: Park, 21st edition Pg 711.

105. Answer is c (Deep transverse perineal muscle).
Ref: Snell's Anatomy regional, Pg 314.

- The ***urogenital diaphragm is a triangular*** musculofacial diaphragm situated in the anterior part of the perineum filling in the gap of the pubic arch.
- It is formed by the ***sphincter urethrae*** and the ***deep transverse perineal muscles***.

106. Answer is a (Duodenal atresia).
Ref: Bailey and Love's, 25th edition Pg 85.

- ***Double bubble*** sign = Duodenal atresia.
- ***Triple bubble*** sign = Jejunal atresia.

107. Answer is b (Ulnar nerve).
Ref: Maheswari's orthopedics, 4th edition Pg 65, Fig 10.6.

Upper Limb Nerves and their tests

• **Radial N**	– Innervates **B**rachioradialis, **E**xtensors of wrist and fingers, **S**upinator, **T**riceps **S-I-M (BEST)**; also called ***'great extensor nerve'***. – Injury results in ***Wrist drop***, also involved in ***Crutch palsy/Saturday night palsy.***
• **Median N**	Palsy tested by: – ***Pointing index (Oschner's clasping test)*** – *Flexor digitorum superficialis and flexor digitorum profundus of the index finger* are paralyzed. – ***Pen test*** – tests the *abductor pollicis brevis*. – ***Ape thumb*** (simian deformity).
• **Ulnar N**	– ***Only Ulnar nerve Injury*** results in ***partial claw hand.*** – ***If both ulnar and median nerves are involved*** (low ulnar and low median; high ulnar and low median) the deformity of ***total or combined claw hand*** otherwise called 'simian hand' develops. Palsy tested by: – ***Froments sign/Book test***: when the adductor pollicis (Ulnar.N) is paralyzed patient tries to hold the book by using the flexor pollicis longus (Median.N) in place of adductor. – ***Egawa test (weak dorsal interossei)*** – unable to abduct middle finger/fingers against resistance. – ***Card test (weak palmar interossei)*** – unable to hold card between fingers **S-I-M** **PAD** = **P**almars **AD**duct; **DAB** = **D**orsals **Ab**duct. **Ulnar Paradox** ➢ High ulnar nerve palsy = injury proximal to the elbow. ➢ Low ulnar nerve palsy = injury in distal third of forearm. ❖ In ***high Ulnar nerve lesion***, the flexor carpi ulnaris is paralyzed and there is '***ulnar paradox***', i.e. higher the injury lesser the deformity as along with intrinsic muscles, extrinsic muscles are also paralyzed. Medial half of flexor digitorum profundus is paralyzed resulting in lesser amount of clawing than in lower ulnar nerve palsy.

108. Answer is a (IgE).
Ref: CP Baveja's microbiology textbook, 3rd edition Pg 104.

Ig	Features
1. IgG	– ***Most abundant*** Ig (80%), distributed in blood and interstitial fluids – Main Ig in ***secondary immune response*** – Only Ig that ***crosses placenta***, so the *major protective Ig in neonate* – ***Opsonized bacteria, neutralizes*** bacterial toxins and viruses, coats cells prior to killing by killer cells – ***Activates complement*** via ***classical*** pathway

2. **IgA**	– Principal ***Ig in secretions*** of respiratory and GI tract and in sweat, saliva, tears and colostrums – Key ***defense for mucosal surfaces***—prevents attachment of bacteria and viruses to mucosa – J (joining) chain is seen in dimeric forms of IgA, it is synthesized by epithelial cells – When aggregated binds polymorphs and ***activates complement via alternate*** pathway
3. **IgM**	– **M**acroglobulin made up of 5 monomeric Ig subunits linked by a J chain—**M**assive, **M**ax. mol. weight – Mainly ***intravascular*** – **M**ajor Ig of primary immune response (pri**M**ary = Ig**M)** – Does not cross placenta, fetal production of high levels of IgM may be of diagnostic significance (e.g. rubella) – ***Activates complement*** via ***classical*** pathway – ***Blood group*** antibodies are IgM
4. **IgD**	– Unclear function; resembles IgG structurally – Found on ***surface of many B cells*** and in serum
5. **IgE**	– Produced in linings of intestine and respiratory tract; mostly distributed extravascularly – Cannot cross placental barrier; cannot fix complement

109. Answer is c (Dopamine).
Ref: Sodium In Health And Disease, By Michel Burnie, Pg 8.

- ***Dopamine inhibits Na⁺K⁺ATPase activity in renal tubule cells.***
- This inhibition is associated with phosphorylation and internalization of the alpha subunit, both events being protein kinase C-dependent.

110. Answer is b (Lattice dystrophy).
Ref: Parson's diseases of the eye, 21st edition Pg 208.

The case history given is that of Lattice dystrophy - easy way of detecting the answers/guessing (even if u do not know) is by remembering that 'lattice' basically means 'criss cross'.

- See the detailed table and the mnemonic!

Corneal Stromal Dystrophies

Feature	**Granular**	**Lattice**	**Macular**
Inheritance	AD	AD	*AR*
Age of onset			
Deposits	1st decade	1st decade	1st decade
Symptoms	3rd decade of asymptomatic	2nd decade	1st decade
Diminished vision	By *4th or 5th decade*	By 2nd or 3rd decade	1st or 2nd decade
Corneal Erosions	Uncommon	Frequent	Common
Opacities	Discrete *sharp borders* Intervening stroma clear early, but becomes hazy Not to limbus	Early *Refractile* tiny lines and dots Subepithelial spots Diffuse central haze Limbal zone clear except in extreme cases	***Indistinct margins*** Hazy intervening stroma Extends to limbus *Endothelium affected* Central lesions more anterior; Peripheral lesions more posterior
Corneal thickness	Normal	Normal	Thinned
Material accumulated	<u>H</u>yaline	<u>A</u>myloid	<u>M</u>ucopolysaccharides /

			proteoglycans / glycosaminoglycans
Stains	**M**asson's trichrome	**C**ongo red	**A**lcian blue
Distinguishing clinical features	***Clear*** *limbal zone*	*Lattice lines*	***Opacities reach limbus*** Cornea thinned unless decompensated MOST SEVERE

Mnemonic for material accumulated and stains in corneal dystrophies (see bold and underlined letters in table above): "**M**arilyn **M**onroe **A**lways **G**ets **H**er **M**en in **L**.**A**. **C**ity"

- **MC Anterior Corneal Dystrophy** = *Epithelial Basement Membrane Dystrophy*
- **MC Stromal Corneal Dystrophy** = *Lattice dystrophy (Lattice type 1 MC)*
- **Least Common Stromal Corneal Dystrophy** = *Macular dystrophy*
- **MC Posterior/Endothelial Corneal Dystrophy** = *Fuch's endothelial dystrophy*

111. Answer is a (*Escherichia coli*).
Ref: Davidson's, 21st edition Pg 2388.

112. Answer is a (Acute delirium).
Ref: Niraj Ahuja's psychiatry, Pg 20-21.

Delirium (Acute Confusional State)

Cardinal features

- MC organic disorder seen in clinical practice; ***Impaired conscious level*** with ***acute onset*** (over hours or days); ***Disorientation in time (MC)*** and in place with a decreased attention span and distractibility; Fluctuation of symptoms, worse in the evening and night (***sun downing***); ***disturbance of sleep-wake cycle*** with insomnia at night and daytime drowsiness.
- Perceptual disturbances such as illusions, ***hallucinations*** (***MC visual***) are common; motor activity may be increased, but is usually purposeless—***asterixis, myoclonus, carphologia/floccillation (picking at bed clothes)***.
- ***Thinking*** is slow and muddled; ideas of reference and delusions (often persecutory) are common; ***Mood disturbances***—lability, apathy, depression irritability; ***Autonomic dysfunction***: sweating, tachycardia, pupillary dilatation; ***Memory—impaired registration***, retention and recall of recent memory with relatively intact remote memory; ***Insight is impaired***; EEG fast wave activity or generalized slowing.

Etiology

- CNS illness (meningitis, head trauma); systemic illness (e.g. liver, kidney, cardiovascular or lung disease); drug abuse (e.g. alcohol, sedatives, phencyclidine); drug withdrawal, particularly from sedatives (e.g. alcohol, benzodiazepines, barbiturates).

113. Answer is a, d (Low set ears, Spina bifida)—verified with revised answer key!!
Ref: Essentials of Pathophysiology: Concepts of Altered Health States, By Carol M Porth, Pg 125.

- ***Fetal alcohol syndrome***: Prenatal-onset growth deficiency, developmental delay, facial dysmorphism (short palpebral fissures, ptosis, strabismus, ear abnormality, long philtrum with a thin upper lip), multiple joint anomalies and cardiac defects (*ASD > VSD*); ***ADHD***; mental subnormality.

114. Answer is b (Myeloblast).
Ref: Robbins pathology, Big, 8th edition Pg 623.

- ***Myeloblasts*** have delicate nuclear chromatin, two or four nucleoli and more voluminous cytoplasm than lymphoblasts.
- ***Auer rods*** are distinctive needle-like azurophilic granules present in myeloblasts in ***AML with t(15:17) translocation***.

115. Answer is b (Adenosine).
Ref: KD Tripathi, 6th edition Pg 518.

- An attack of paroxysmal supraventricular tachycardia ***(PSVT)*** can be terminated by IV verapamil, diltiazem, esmolol or digoxin; BUT ***most cardiologists now prefer adenosine***.
- Administered by rapid IV injection over 1–3 seconds, adenosine terminates within 30 seconds more than 90% episodes of PSVT involving the AV node.

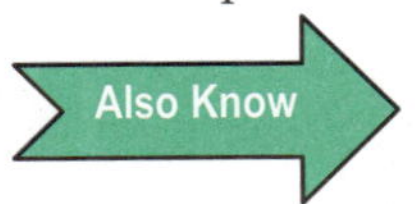

Other uses of adenosine
- Diagnosis of tachycardias.
- For inducing brief vasodilation.
- To produce controlled hypotension during surgery.

116. Answer is d (Fracture of lower radius with disruption of inferior radioulnar joint).
Ref: Maheswari's orthopedics, 4th edition Pg 107.

❑ **Monteggia # dislocation**	– Fracture of upper third of ulna with dislocation of head of radius; very unstable injury. S-I-M MonteggiA =ulnA.
❑ **Galeazzi # dislocation**	– Fracture of lower third of radius with dislocation or subluxation of radioulnar joint; ***Perfect reduction essential*** for complete restoration of all functions.

117. Answer is c (Gastric juice).
Ref: Fluid and Electrolyte Balance, By Norma Methen, Pg 193, Table 13-1.

Secretion	**Na^+**	**K^+**	**Cl^-**
Saliva	10	26	10
Gastric	60	10	130
Duodenal	140	5	80
Ileal	140	5	104
Colonic	60	30	40
Pancreatic	140	5	75
Bile	145	5	100

118. Answer is a (Chlamydial infection).
Ref: Harrison's, 18th edition Pg 1424-25.

- The ***Fitz-Hugh-Curtis syndrome*** is an ***extrapelvic manifestation of pelvic inflammatory disease***. The syndrome was first reported in 1920 and describes the development of inflammation of the liver capsule and diaphragm (***perihepatitis***).
- The disorder is largely restricted to women and seems likely to reflect intra-abdominal spread of infection from the pelvis to the subphrenic space via the right paracolic gutter.
- Typical symptoms include pain in the right upper quadrant of the abdomen, sometimes with pleuritic features and with radiation of pain into the right shoulder. Most patients also have symptoms of acute salpingitis.
- MC causative is ***Chlamydia trachomatis*** (at least 80% of cases).
- It is rare for the diagnosis to be established by imaging but, at laparoscopy, the liver capsule is inflamed with patchy exudate formation. The appearance has been described as '***looking like salt sprinkled on a moist surface***'. If the

infection becomes chronic, '***violin-string***' adhesions develop between the liver capsule and the anterior abdominal wall or diaphragm.

119. Answer is c (Closure of patent ductus arteriosus).
Ref: KD Tripathi, 6th edition Pg 181-82.

Clinical uses of prostaglandins and their analogues

- Abortion: During first trimester MTP.
- Induction/Augmentation of labor.
- Cervical priming.
- Postpartum hemorrhage control (carboprost).
- Peptic ulcer healing (misoprostol).
- Reduction of IOP in glaucoma (latanoprost, travoprost and bimatoprost).
- To maintain patency of PDA (alprostadil).
- To avoid platelet damage and prevent platelet aggregation.

Note:
For ***closure of PDA, aspirin and indomethacin*** inhibit prostaglandin production and bring about closure within a few hours.

120. Answer is c (3.2 g).
Ref: Park, 20th edition Pg 545.

Differences between human breast milk and cow's milk

Constituent	Breast milk (g/L)	Cow milk (g/L)
Proteins	11	32
Carbohydrates	**70**	50
Lactose	**62**	50
Minerals	2	8
Energy	640–720 kCal	650 kCal
Amino acids	Rich in cystine, taurine	Rich in methionine
Fats	Rich in **linoleic acid**	

121. Answer is b (Is a superficial fungal infection).
Ref: Harrison's, 18th edition Pg 1640.

Histoplasmosis - deep fungal infection

- ***Intracellular*** (tiny yeast inside macrophages); n capsule despite its name; Also called ***Darling's disease***.
- Acquired via ***inhalation*** of spores in ***bat guano*** **or** ***bird droppings***.
- Causes:
  - Pneumonia, chronic pulmonary histoplasmosis. Sputum culture is the preferred method for diagnosis.
  - Ocular histoplasmosis syndrome is a distinct clinical form of uveitis, although a positive histoplasmin skin test is a requisite for diagnosis, none of the patients involved has had active histoplasmosis.
- Treatment— itraconazole for pneumonia, ***amphotericin*** for disseminated disease.

122. Answer is a (Retinoblastoma).
Ref: Yanoff's ocular pathology, Pg 343.

- ***Knudston's 2-hit hypothesis***—both alleles must be knocked out for tumor to develop. Classically described in ***retinoblastoma***.

123. Answer is a (Acute glomerulonephritis).
Ref: Harrison's, 18th edition Pg 2340.

Common pediatric renal diseases

Acute Post Streptococcal Glomerulonephritis

- Following h/o **recent streptococcal** ***pyoderma or pharyngitis***.
- **Edema, Oliguria, hematuria, hypertension,** ***decreased C3 levels***
- Fluid restriction, furosemide, penicillin, antihypertensives
- ***> 95% have good prognosis***.

Nephrotic syndrome

- ❑ MC cause in children is ***minimal change disease*** *(normal histology on light microscopy)*.
- ❑ Clinically:
  - *Massive* ***edema***
  - *Massive* ***selective proteinuria*** *(> 2 g/day)*
  - ***Hypoalbuminemia*** *(< 2.5 g/dL)*
  - ***Hypercholesterolemia*** *(> 200 mg%)*.
- ❑ Gene mutation a/w **congenital NS *(Finnish)* type** = ***Nephrin*** (NPHS1). **S-I-M** **PH**innish = Ne**PH**rin.
- ❑ Gene mutation a/w steroid-resistant NS = *Podocin* (NPHS2).
- ❑ Treatment: Initial longer course of ***corticosteroids***; *relapses are common*. For steroid-resistant nephritic syndrome, cyclosporine A is used.

124. Answer is a (Cholesteatoma).
Ref: Dhingra's ENT textbook, 5th edition Pg 75-76.

125. Answer is b (Diabetes mellitus).
Ref: Niraj Ahuja's psychiatry, Pg 190; KD Tripathi, 6th edition Pg 434-36.

- Lithium (Li) is small ***monovalent cation***; Li is used as its ***carbonate salt*** because, it is less hygroscopic and less gastric irritant than LiCl or other salts. It is *converted into chloride in the stomach*.
- Mechanism of action is not known exactly. Probably because ***Li inhibit hydrolysis of inositol-1-phosphate***.
- **Pharmacokinetics:**
  - Lithium is *well-absorbed orally; hyponatremia and diuretics cause ↑plasma levels of Li*.
  - Steady state plasma concentrations are reached in *7 days*.
  - *Prophylactic* blood lithium levels (for maintenance therapy) = 0.5–0.8 mEq/L.
  - *Therapeutic* blood lithium levels (for treatment of acute mania) = 0.8–1.2 mEq/L.
  - *Serious toxic effects* occur with plasma concentrations above 2.0 mEq/L.
  - Renal excretion is increased by diuresis and urinary alkalinization and decreased by hypovolemia and hyponatremia.

- **Side effects:**
  - Acute *toxicity: Li causes* **tremors**; *treatment of choice* is ***hemodialysis***. Osmotic diuretics and sodium bicarbonate infusion promote Li excretion.
  - ***Renal diabetes insipidus*** (thirst and polyuria); ***hypothyroidism*** may occur.
  - Li is *contraindicated in pregnancy* (***Ebstein anomaly*** in neonate if Li ingested in first trimester).
  - *Neurological:* ***tremor*** *MC.*
  - *Pedal* ***edema.***
- **Uses of lithium are:**
  - In treatment of ***acute mania and prophylaxis of bipolar mood disorder***.
  - Other uses are in ***Cluster headache; Cancer chemotherapy-linked agranulocytosis*** **and** ***neutropenia*** **(Li increases leukocyte count);** ***SIADH; Cyclical vomiting; Huntington's chorea***.

126. Answer is a (Atracurium).
Ref: KD Tripathi, 6th edition Pg 345.

Atracurium
– At body temperature and pH, atracurium undergoes spontaneous degradation via ***'Hoffmann elimination'*** and is therefore stored at 4°C to reduce the rate of spontaneous degradation; major metabolite is ***laudanosine****, which is a CNS stimulant*.
– It is the *relaxant of choice* in patients with *hepatic or renal* (anephric) dysfunction.
– It is *suitable for patients with atypical cholinesterase; organophosphorus poisoning and in myasthenia gravis.*
– Its actions will be prolonged in hypothermic patients, e.g. during cardiac surgery.
– *Histamine release* occurs causing flushing of skin. Also contraindicated in asthmatics.

127. Answer is d (Pulmonary artery stenosis and PDA).
Ref: Harrison's, 18th edition Pg 1605-06.

Congenital Rubella

- ***Deafness (MC)***
- ***'Blueberry muffin' rash,***
- ***Cataracts and 'salt and pepper' chorioretinitis***
- *PDA* and multiple pulmonary stenoses
- Encephalitis (periventricular calcification)
- Maximum fetal transmission if infected between 6 and 8 weeks of pregnancy.

128. Answer is b (Parkinson disease).
Ref: Harrison's, 18th edition Pg 3312.

129. Answer is b (Paragonimus westermani).
Ref: Harrison's, 18th edition Pg 1757-58.

Trematodes (Flukes)

1. Schistosoma (Bladder fluke)	*Snails* are host; *cercariae* penetrate skin of humans; causes granulomas, fibrosis and inflammation of the spleen and liver; ***portal hypertension, bladder cancer, hematuria.***	*Praziquantel*
2. Clonorchis sinensis (Asian liver fluke)	***Undercooked fish****; causes inflammation of the* ***biliary tract - pigmented gallstones****. Also associated with* ***cholangiocarcinoma****.*	*Praziquantel*
3. Paragonimus westermani (Lung fluke)	Undercooked ***crab meat****;* causes inflammation and 2° bacterial infection of the lung.	*Praziquantel*

130. Answer is c (Langerhans cells).
Ref: Robbins pathology, Big, 8th edition Pg 631.

For questions 131–134

A 50-year-old male smoker presents with history of hearing loss on the right ear for the past six weeks. Examination revealed dull tympanic membrane on right and normal left tympanic membrane. Rinne test was negative on the right and positive on the left. Weber was lateralized to the right ear. Absolute bone conduction is normal bilaterally (ENT).

131. Answer is a (Right-sided conductive hearing loss).
132. Answer is d (Do posterior rhinoscopy).
133. Answer is c (Right type 'B' curve and left type 'A' curve).
134. Answer is d (Nasopharyngeal carcinoma).

Ref: Dhingra's ENT textbook, 5th edition Pg 265.

Explanation:
The case history given is that of nasopharyngeal cancer. The clinchers/keywords are "smoker, adult, dull tympanic membrane, conductive hearing loss".

- Presence of ***serous otitis media (dull tympanic membrane)*** in an adult, especially a ***smoker*** should raise the suspicion of ***nasopharyngeal growth***.
- Negative Rinne test on right indicates right conductive hearing loss.
- Posterior rhinoscopy should be done to look for the growth.

Types of tympanogram

1. **A** – Normal (normal middle ear pressure)
2. **As** – Reduced compliance at ambient pressure (***otosclerosis***)
3. **Ad** – Increased compliance at ambient pressure (***ossicular discontinuity***)
4. **B** – ***Flat or dome-shaped*** tympanogram (fluid in middle ear—***otitis media***)
5. **C** – ***Rounded tympanogram***; maximum compliance at pressures more than 100 mm H_2O (negative pressure in middle ear—***eustachian tube dysfunction***)

For questions 135–137

A 50-year-old male was met with motorcycle accident, the handle bar hit his left chest, patient is conscious, breathless, has tachycardia, feeble radial pulse, chest examination reveals a bruise in the left chest with a segment of chest moving up and down, it is tender to palpate and there is surgical emphysema, crepitus. Auscultation reveals decreased breath sounds on the left chest.

135. Answer is a (Wide bore IV line, rapid Ringer's lactate infusion, oxygen by mask).
136. Answer is b (Flail chest).
137. Answer is a (Chest skiagram).

Ref: Greenberg's Text-Atlas of Emergency Medicine, By Michael I Greenberg, 2005 edition Pg 20; http://www.trauma.org/archive/thoracic/CHESTflail.html

Explanation:
The case history given is that of flail chest. The keywords/clinchers are "handlebar hitting chest, bruise in that area and tenderness, segment of chest moving up and down". All these are features, which differentiate it from a tension pneumothorax also....as given below pneumothorax can be associated with flail chest in > 50% of cases.

- A ***flail chest*** occurs when a ***segment of the thoracic cage is separated from the rest of the chest wall***. This is usually defined as ***at least two fractures per rib*** (producing a free segment), in at least two ribs.
- A flail chest is identified as ***paradoxical movement of a segment of the chest wall*** – i.e. indrawing on inspiration and moving outwards on expiration. This is often better appreciated by palpation than by inspection. This may NOT be so evident in patients already on mechanical ventilation.
- H/O ***direct trauma to chest*** is present; since significant trauma is required to cause flail chest, intrathoracic or intra-abdominal injuries (or both) are also usually present.
- ***Pneumothorax*** is present in > 50% of cases as an association.
- The question talks of ***feeble pulse, which could indicate intra-abdominal bleeding*** and hence an ***IV line is mandatory***.
- The ***anteroposterior chest radiograph*** will identify most significant chest wall injuries, but will not identify all rib fractures (hence this is the ***'least; investigating*** the patient requires as asked in the above question). Lateral or

anterior rib fractures will often be missed on the initial plain film. However, since the management of rib fractures is determined by their clinical significance rather than by their number or position, dedicated rib views are never indicated.

- *CT chest is the 'gold standard'* for detection of flail chest.
- All patients should initially be placed on ***100% oxygen via a non-rebreathing facemask***.
- Patient controlled administration of an opioid infusion (PCA) is the best method for cooperative patients.

For questions 138–141

A 30-year-old female patient presented with difficulty in swallowing to both solids and liquids for 8 months duration following accidental ingestion of toilet cleaner. Endoscopy was done and dilation done following which the patient had severe retrosternal pain, radiating to back with breathlessness.

138. Answer is c (Iatrogenic perforation of esophagus).
139. Answer is a (Crepitus at the suprasternal notch).
140. Answer is b (Pneumomediastinum with pleural effusion).
141. Answer is d (Thoracotomy procedure).

Ref: The Washington Manual of Surgery, 2007 edition Pg 160-162.

Explanation:
The case history given is that of iatrogenic perforation of esophagus. The clinchers/keywords are "h/o toilet cleaner ingestion (leads to strictures), dilation of esophagus done and symptoms developing soon after that".

- The *MC cause* of ***perforation of esophagus is iatrogenic*** (75%).
- MC sites are anatomic sites of narrowing, i.e. cricopharyngeus and GE junction.
- ***Toilet cleaners*** contain ***caustics,*** which can lead to ***stricture*** of esophagus as a complication.
- Clinical signs: ***Dysphagia, pain,*** fever, leukocytosis, tachycardia, respiratory distress and shock.
- Cervical perforations may present with ***neck stiffness and subcutaneous emphysema.***
- Intrathoracic perforation: Chest pain, subcut emphysema, dyspnea and ***pleural effusion.***
- Definitive management requires ***operative repair***.

For questions 142–146

A 50-year-old male, a chronic 'gutka' consumer has a 3 cm ulcerative lesion, with everted margin in the left cheek, skin not involved, it is nontender, foul smelling, bad oral hygiene, one submandibular node felt firm, mobile, 2.5 cm in greatest diameter, with no other clinical evidence of metastasis.

142. Answer is a (T2 N1 M0).
143. Answer is b (Edge wedge biopsy).
144. Answer is d (Oral candidiasis).
145. Answer is d (Combined modality).
146. Answer is d (Sweets).

Ref: Comprehensive preventive dentistry, By Hardy limeback, Pg 64, Table 4-5; Oral Cancer, By Jatin P Shah, Newell W Johnson, Pg 27 Table 2.3; Surgical Diseases in Tropical Countries, By Sood, Table 3.1, Pg 29.

Explanation:
The case history given is that of oral, cheek cancer. The clinchers/keywords are "gutka, cheek ulcerative lesion".

Risk factors for oral cancer	Premalignant lesions and conditions
Strong associations Tobacco smoking Smokeless tobacco (gutka, paan, kahini, mischri, zarda, gadaku, mawa, nas, naswar, shammah, toombak)	**Lesions** Leukoplakia Homogenous Nonhomogenous (Verrucous, nodular,

Alcohol consumption Betel quid and areca nit chewing Sun exposure (cancer of lip) **Weak associations** HPV infections (strong a/w oropharyngeal cancer) Marijuana smoking Chronic periodontal disease Low intake of fruit and vegetable	erythroleukoplakia) Erythroplakia **Conditions** Oral submucous fibrosis Sideropenic dysphagia Lichen planus DLE Syphilis

TNM classification for oral cancer

Primary tumor (T)	TS	Primary tumor cannot be assessed
	T0	No e/o primary tumor
	T1s	Ca in situ
	T1	Tumor < or + 2 cm in greatest dimension
	T2	Tumor > 2 cm in greatest dimension, but < or = 4 cm
	T3	Tumor > 4 cm
	T4	Tumor invades deep or adjacent structures
Regional lymph nodes	Ns	Lymph nodes cannot be assessed
	N0	No lymph node mets
	N1	Metastases in a single ipsilateral lymph node measuring < or = 3 cm
	N2a	Metastases in single ipsilateral node measuring > 3 cm, but < or = 6 cm
	N2b	Metastases in multiple ispilateral nodes, none measuring > 6 cm
	N2c	Metastases in bilateral or contralateral nodes, none > 6 cm
	N3	Metastases in a node > 6 cm
Distant metastases	M1	Distant metastases cannot be assessed
	M2	No distant metastases
	M3	Distant metastases present

- ***Histopathology*** sample is obtained by ***edge wedge biopsy***.
- ***Orthopan tomogram*** = oblique and occlusion views of the mandible or CT scan oral cavity to demonstrate involvement of the bone.
- ***Treatment:*** Surgery, radiotherapy and chemotherapy—combined modality may be required.

For questions 147–149

A 65-year-old man died on arrival at the ER despite vigorous resuscitative measures. Histopathological sections of his lungs at autopsy reveal alveolar spaces filled with acellular granular pink fluid. The alveolar capillaries were engorged. There is no inflammatory infiltration.

147. Answer is b (Cardiac failure).
148. Answer is d (Cor pulmonale).
149. Answer is b (Echocardiography).

- The case history gives the pathology of ***Pulmonary Edema***: Intra-alveolar accumulation of fluid AND heavy wet lungs with engorged alveolar capillaries and intra-alveolar granular pink precipitate.
- Pulmonary edema is usually due to left heart failure from any cause; ***cor pulmonale*** indicates right heart failure.
- A bedside ***echocardiogram*** in a patient with decompensated CHF is an important diagnostic tool in determining the etiology of pulmonary edema. Echocardiography can be used to evaluate LV systolic and diastolic function, as well as valvular function.

For questions 150–153

A 33-year-old male is violently stabbed in the supraclavicular region. He immediately develops shortness of breath and bloats like a balloon. Physical examination reveals puffiness of the face, swelling of the eye lids, neck and chest wall. Crepitus is felt over the chest wall. Widespread crepitations are heard on chest auscultation.

150. Answer is a (Mediastinal emphysema).
151. Answer is a (Skiagram of chest).
152. Answer is b (Only by oxygen mask).
153. Answer is d (Has to be managed conservatively).

Ref: see FB page /website please – facebook.com/suresuccessramgopal.

Explanation:
The case history given is that of mediastinal emphysema (also called pneumomediastinum). The clinchers/keywords are "stabbing the lungs, subcut emphysema and crepitus".

- ***Penetrating or blunt injury*** to the thorax may cause air leak syndromes including ***pneumomediastinum.***
- The most common symptoms seen with pneumomediastinum (PM) were ***subcutaneous emphysema*** (76% of patients) and neck or chest pain (38% of patients)
- Although not pathognomic of pneumomediastinum, the presence of ***subcutaneous crepitations*** suggests free air is present within the thoracic cavity
- ***Hamman sign***: Is pathognomic of pneumomediastinum, consists of precordial systolic crepitations and diminution of heart sounds
- ***Chest radiography*** usually (although not invariably) reveals a pneumomediastinum. Chest radiography reveals air within the mediastinal space. Coexisting disease (e.g. pneumothorax, pneumoperitoneum, pneumoretroperitoneum of pneumopericardium) may also be evident.

For questions 154–155

A 17-year-old male complains of recurrent episodes of cough, wheezing and shortness of breath particularly at night for the last 3 days. His sibling has a history of similar symptoms. A skin test with pollen produces immediate wheal and flare.

154. Answer is d (Eosinophilia).
155. Answer is a (Bronchodilators).
156. Answer is b (Obstructive pattern).
157. Answer is c (Viscid mucus plugs in the small airways).

Ref: Harrison's, 18th edition Pg 2102.

Explanation:
The case history given is that of bronchial asthma. The clinchers/keywords are "wheezing at night, similar history in siblings and pollen allergy".

Asthma

Two types	–	***Extrinsic asthma***: ***Type 1 hypersensitivity*** reaction.
	–	***Intrinsic asthma***: Trigger is ***non-immune*** and may include ***aspirin, cold, exercise,*** psychogenic or ***infection.***
Pathology	–	Bronchial wall edema and development of inflammatory infiltrate with increased number of eosinophils, thickening of basement membrane, bronchial smooth muscle hypertrophy and hyperplasia and hypertrophy of submucosal mucus glands.
Microscopically	–	Whorled mucus plugs (***Curschmann's spirals***) and crystalloid debris of eosinophil membranes (***Charcot-Leyden crystals***) are seen within airways.

❖ ***Samter's triad*** = *bronchial asthma + nasal allergy/polyposis + hypersensitivity to aspirin.*

For questions 158–160

A 60-year-old male has weight loss, bloody stools and constipation for the past 6 months. Colonoscopy showed an irregularly shaped ulcerative lesion in the descending colon.

158. Answer is a (Adenocarcinoma).
159. Answer is a ('Apple core' stricture of the colon).
160. Answer is b (Left radical hemicolectomy).

Ref: Bailey and Love's surgery, 25th edition Pg 1179-1181.

Explanation:
The case history given is that of carcinoma colon. The clinchers/keywords are "colonoscopy, weight loss and bloody stools and ulcerative lesion in colon".

For detailed explanation: Please see website and FB page – facebook.com/suresuccessramgopal.

For questions 161–163

A 70-year-old male has been experiencing intermittent epistaxis, fatigue and pain in bones for the past 4 months. Laboratory investigations are as follows:
Serum Ca^{++}: 11.2 mg/dL (Normal: 8.9–10.1 mg/dL)

161. Answer is b (Numerous plasma cells).
162. Answer is c (Amyloidosis).
163. Answer is b (Chemotherapy).

Ref: Harrison's, 18th edition Pg 937.

Explanation:
The case history given is most likely that of ***multiple myeloma***. The clinchers/keywords are "bone pains, elderly male and hypercalcemia". Also the subsequent questions (161, 162, 163) reveal the answer.

Multiple Myeloma

- Monoclonal ***plasma cell*** cancer (fried egg appearance) that arises *within the bone marrow* and produces *large amounts of IgG* (55%) or IgA
- *MC primary bone tumor* on the elderly (> 40–50 years)
- Symptoms: *Back pain* (MC presenting symptom); ***hypercalcemic*** symptoms (*stones, bones, abdominal moans and psychiatric groans*), pathologic fractures, ***fatigue*** and frequent infections. Renal failure, anemia. A/w primary ***amyloidosis*** (AL)
- Testing:
  - Skeletal survey—to detect punched out osteolytic lesions. S-I-M 'MyeLoma = Lytic'
  - Serum protein electrophoresis (SPEP)—monoclonal immunoglobulin spike (*M spike*)
  - Urine protein electrophoresis—Ig light chains in urine (*Bence Jones proteins*)
  - Peripheral smear—***rouleaux formation*** of RBCs
  - ↑ serum calcium; ***beta-2 microglobulin*** level is a prognostic indicator
  - Most specific test is ***bone marrow biopsy***.
- Treatment: ***Melphalan and steroids***. Thalidomide (inhibitor of TNF) may be added
- ***International Staging System***: for ***multiple myeloma***Q relies on two factors, beta-2-microglobulin and albumin.

For questions 164–166

A 5-year-old female child develops reduced urine output, irritability, lethargy and restlessness over a period of 8 hours. She has several episodes of bloody diarrhea in the past 24 hours and has become very weak. Examination reveals mild pallor and dehydration. Laboratory investigation results are as follows:
Hb: 9 g/dL (Normal: 12–16 g/dL).

Platelets: 90,000/mm³ (normal: 150,000–450,000).
Peripheral blood smear: Numerous schistocytes.
The BUN and creatinine were elevated.

164. Answer is c (Hemolytic uremic syndrome).
165. Answer is a (Disseminated intravascular coagulopathy).
166. Answer is a (Hemodialysis).

Ref: Harrison's, 18th edition Pg 156, 970, 1283.

Explanation:
The case history given is that of Hemolytic Uremic syndrome. The clinchers/keywords are "bloody diarrhea – suggesting ? *Shigella;* and signs of renal dysfunction and uremia".

Common Pediatric Hematologic Disorders

	HUS	HSP	TTP	ITP
MC age	Children	Children	Young adults	Children or adults
Previous infection	Diarrhea (*EHEC, Shigella*)	URI	None	*Viral* (especially in children)
RBC count	↓	N	↓	N
Platelet count	↓	N	↓	↓
Peripheral smear	Hemolysis, schistocytes	N	Hemolysis	N
Kidney effects	ARF, hematuria	Hematuria	ARF, proteinuria	None
Treatment	Supportive*	Supportive*	Plasmapheresis, NSAIDs; NO platelets**	*Steroids****, *splenectomy* if drugs fail
Key differential points	*Age, diarrhea*	*Rash, abdominal pain, arthritis, melena*	*CNS changes, age*	*Antiplatelet antibodies*

Key:
HUS = Hemolytic uremic syndrome; HSP = Henoch-Schönlein purpura; TTP = Thrombotic thrombocytopenic purpura; ITP = Idiopathic thrombocytopenic purpura; ARF = Acute renal failure; EHEC = Enterohemorrhagic *E.coli*.
* In HUS and HSP, patients may need dialysis and transfusions.
** Do not give platelet transfusion to patients with TTP, clot may form.
*** Give steroids only if the patient is bleeding.

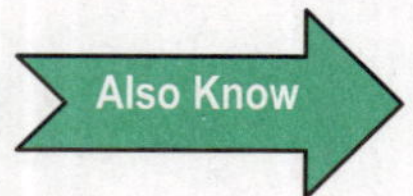

Common Red Cell Appearances and their Causes

Microcytosis (reduced average cell size, MCV< 76 fl)	– Iron deficiency anemia – Sideroblastic anemia – Thalassemia – Pyridoxine deficiency – Lead poisoning – Copper deficiency – *Also* Anemia of chronic inflammation (<u>BUT</u> more commonly presents as normocytic anemia)
Macrocytosis (increased average cell size, MCV > 100 fl)	– Megaloblastic anemia

Target cells (central area of Hb)	–	HbC disease
	–	Asplenia (Postsplenectomy)
	–	Liver disease
	–	Thalassemia
	–	S-I-M *"HALT and aim for the Target"*
Spherocytes (dense cells, no area of central pallor)	–	Hereditary spherocytosis
	–	Autoimmune hemolysis
	–	Postsplenectomy
	–	Disseminated intravascular coagulation (DIC)
Nucleated red blood cells (normoblasts)	–	Marrow infiltration
	–	Myelofibrosis
	–	Severe hemolysis
Howell-Jolly bodies (small round nuclear remnants)	–	Postsplenectomy
	–	Hyposplenism
	–	Dyshematopoiesis
Polychromasia (young red cells—reticulocytes present)	–	Hemolysis
	–	Increased red cell turnover
Basophilic stippling (abnormal ribosomes appear as blue dots)	–	Thalassemia
	–	Anemia of chronic disease
	–	Iron deficiency
	–	Lead poisoning
	–	S-I-M *'TAIL'*
Helmet cell, Schistocyte	–	DIC
	–	Hemolytic Uremic Syndrome (HUS)/Thrombotic Thrombocytopenic Purpura (TTP)
Burr cell	–	HUS/TTP
Poikilocytes	–	Non-uniform shapes in HUS/TTP, microvascular damage, DIC
Teardrop cell	–	Myeloid metaplasia with myelofibrosis
Bite cell	–	G6PD deficiency

For questions 167–170

A 27-year-old male develops high grade fever with chills. A heart murmur is heard on cardiac auscultation. There is evidence of splenomegaly and splinter hemorrhages in the nails.

167. Answer is c (Infection).
168. Answer is a (Mycotic aneurysms).
169. Answer is b (Antibiotics).
170. Answer is a (Subacute bacterial endocarditis).

Ref: Harrison's, 18th edition.

Explanation:
The case history given is that of infective endocarditis. The clinchers/keyword are "high grade fever, cardiac murmur, splenomegaly and splinter hemorrhages on nails".

Infective Endocarditis

Acute endocarditis	Subacute endocarditis
– *S. aureus* MC (high virulence)	– *S. viridans* (low virulence)
– Rapid onset	– Insidious onset
– ***Large vegetations*** on ***previously normal valves***	– ***Smaller vegetations*** in ***congenitally abnormal or diseased valves***
	– Sequel of dental procedures

Clinical features

- Mitral valve MC involved; **Tri**cuspid valve in IV **drug** abusers. S-I-M 'Never **Tri drugs**'.

  - ☐ ***Fever with chills***
  - ☐ ***Roth spots*** (round white spots on retina surrounded by hemorrhage)
  - ☐ ***Osler's nodes*** (tender raised lesions on finger or toe pads)
  - ☐ ***Janeway lesions*** (small erythematous lesions on palms and soles)
  - ☐ ***Splinter hemorrhages*** on nail beds
  - ☐ ***New murmur***

Management

- Multiple blood cultures (3) needed for diagnosis.
- If transthoracic ECHO is negative, do ***transesophageal*** *ECHO* (more sensitive).
- Duke criteria (clinical, biochemical and ECHO changes) are used for **D**iagnosis.
- Treat with prolonged antibiotic therapy for 4–6 weeks.

For questions 171–174

A 60-year-old male with weight loss, epigastric pain radiating to the back, passage of pale bulky stools, jaundice and elevated levels of CA 19-9.

171. Answer is b (Diabetes).
172. Answer is b (Contrast-enhanced CT scan).
173. Answer is c (Carcinoma head of pancreas).
174. Answer is a (Whipple's procedure).

Ref: Harrison's, 18th edition Pg 786-788.

Explanation:
The case history given is that of Ca pancreas. The clinchers/keywords are "epigastric pain radiating to the back – this you would associate with pancreatic pain especially if you have seen any pancreas case in surgical wards/clinics; weight oss and CA 19-9 is associated with Ca pancreas".

Pancreatic Cancer

- MC ductal ***adenocarcinomas***; MC in the ***head and neck*** of the pancreas.
- ***Risk factors***:
  - *Cigarette smoking; previous gastric resection, chronic pancreatitis and possibly* ***diabetes***.
  - Point mutations in ***codon 12 of the K-ras oncogene*** are found in 70–100%, inactivation of the tumor suppressor genes *INK4A, TP53, MADH4*, mutation of the ***palladin gene*** is reported to be common.
  - As part of several hereditary syndromes: Hereditary pancreatitis, familial atypical multiple mole melanoma, Peutz–Jeghers syndrome, ataxia-telangiectasia, familial breast cancer (*BRCA-2*) and hereditary non-polyposis colorectal cancer.
  - Polymorphisms of the genes for methylenetetrahydrofolate reductase and thymidylate synthase.
- ***Symptoms***: ***Epigastric pain*** that is intractable, severe, radiates to the back and may be *relieved by sitting/leaning forward*; ***dramatic weight loss***; dyspepsia, pruritus is uncommon.
- ***Signs***: Obstructive ***jaundice, cachexia***, fever, enlarged gallbladder.
- ***Rarer presentations***: Superficial thrombophlebitis migrans (***Trousseau's syndrome***); marantic endocarditis; gastric outlet obstruction; ***diabetes mellitus***; pancreatitis, hepatomegaly, splenomegaly.

- ***Contrast-enhanced CT scan is the preferred*** investigation over ERCp and MRI.
- The most widely used ***serum marker in pancreatic cancer is cancer-associated antigen 19-9 (CA 19-9)***. It has a reported sensitivity and specificity of about 80–90% and is suggestive, rather than confirmatory, of the diagnosis of pancreatic cancer.
- Only 13% are suitable for resection by ***Whipple's operation*** (***pancreaticoduodenectomy***—head and neck of the pancreas together with the duodenum is resected). Others may benefit from palliative surgery.
- Combined irradiation and chemotherapy (***gemcitabine***) may be used for palliation of unresectable cancer confined to the pancreas.

For questions 175–177

A newborn baby delivered at 38 weeks gestation died a few days after developing severe pallor, jaundice and generalized body swelling. The mother who was Rh-negative had irregular antenatal visits and has a previous history of termination of pregnancy. Autopsy revealed hepatosplenomegaly and bile-stained organs.

175. Answer is b (Antibody-mediated reaction).
176. Answer is a (Kernicterus).
177. Answer is a (Immunizing the mother with anti-D).

Ref: Dutta's obsetetrics, 6th edition Pg 331, 479.

Explanation:
The case history given is that of Rh isoimmunization. The clinchers/keywords are "Rh-negative mother; previous history of MTP; baby dying soon after born with jaundice and generalized edema".

- Isoimmunization is defined as production of immune antibodies in an individual in response to an antigen derived from another individual of the same species provided the first one lacks the antigen.
- In the given case history previous sensitization to the Rh antigen has occurred during the MTP.
- Kernicterus refers to the yellow staining of the brain by unconjugated bilirubin resulting in neuronal injury.
- To prevent active immunization of Rh-negative yet unimmunized mother, Rh anti-D immunoglobulin (IgG) is administered IM to the mother following childbirth and abortion.

For questions 178–180

A 5-week-old male baby has developed progressively worsening projectile vomiting following breastfeeding. Physical examination showed dehydration, visible peristalsis in the abdomen and a firm oval mass in the epigastrium.

178. Answer is b (Hypertrophy of the circular muscle layer in the pylorus).
179. Answer is a (Hypochloremic hypokalemic alkalosis).
180. Answer is a (Ramstedt's operation).

Ref: Bailey and Love's, 25th edition Pg 79.

Explanation:
The case history given is that of congenital hypertrophic pyloric stenosis. The clinchers/keywords in the question are "male baby, projectile vomiting, visible peristalsis and epigastric mass". This one should be easy for you to answer.

Congenital Hypertrophic Pyloric Stenosis (CHPS)

- Presents **MC between** ***3rd and 6th week*** of life.
- **M:F = 4:1;** classically seen in ***first born male babies***, one of the parents (mother in 50% of cases) has a **scar** of operation for CHPS.
- *Etiology*: Failure of the pylorus to relax (**achalasia**).

- *Clinically*: ***Projectile vomiting (bile is absent)***; ***visible peristalsis*** may be seen; ***palpation of hypertrophic pylorus ('olive'-shaped mass in epigastrium)***; ***constipation*** is usually present (***rabbit stools*** *or* ***starvation stools***); loss of weight; change from one type of feeding to another brings about a remission.
- In ***premature infants*** there may be ***paradoxical symptoms,*** anorexia instead of voracious appetite, vomiting is regurgitant, rather than projectile and peristalsis is normally visible. But the diagnostic rock is the palpation of hypertrophic pylorus.
- Leads to low Cl^-/low K^+ metabolic alkalosis (***Hypochloremic hypokalemic alkalosis***)
- U/S detects early, hard-to-feel pyloric tumors (~14% of cases).
- Surgery is ***Ramstedt's pyloromyotomy.***
- In the living, veins of Mayo are helpful landmarks in distinguishing the pyloric canal from the first part of the duodenum.

COMED-K 2011

COMED-K 2011 QUESTIONS

Section A (Q No. 1–150)

MEDICINE

1. **A 60-year-old patient with a past history of treated pulmonary TB presents with massive hemoptysis. What is the most likely cause for hemoptysis?**
   (a) Pulmonary amyloidosis
   (b) Aspergilloma
   (c) Broncholith
   (d) Relapse of TB

2. **King's College criteria for orthotopic liver transplantation in acute liver failure (paracetamol induced) include all of the following *EXCEPT***
   (a) pH < 7.30
   (b) PT > 100 s
   (c) Grade three encephalopathy
   (d) Serum bilirubin > 300 μmol/L

3. **Which one of the following clinical features is NOT seen in pheochromocytoma?**
   (a) Hypertension
   (b) Episodic palpitations
   (c) Weight loss
   (d) Diarrhea

4. **All of the following are causes of giant 'a' wave in JVP *EXCEPT***
   (a) Tricuspid stenosis
   (b) Pulmonary stenosis
   (c) Pulmonary hypertension
   (d) Aortic stenosis

5. **A 50-year-old male presents with severe refractory hypertension, weakness, muscle cramps and hypokalemia, the most likely diagnosis is**
   (a) Hypoaldosteronism
   (b) Hyperaldosteronism
   (c) Cushing's syndrome
   (d) Pheochromocytoma

6. **Mental retardation is NOT a feature of one of the Mucopolysaccharidosis**
   (a) Hurler MPS-I
   (b) Hunter MPS-II
   (c) Sanfilippo MPS-III
   (d) Morquio MPS-IV

7. **Wernicke's hemianopic pupillary response is seen in lesion of**
   (a) Optic tract
   (b) Optic chiasm
   (c) Optic radiation
   (d) Lateral geniculate body

8. **Dissociated sensory loss is seen in**
   (a) Syringomyelia
   (b) Vitamin B_{12} deficiency
   (c) Transverse myelitis
   (d) Pellagra

9. **Pulmonary mycetomas on radiographs most commonly show as**
   (a) Air fluid level
   (b) Lucent crescent
   (c) Eccentric nodule
   (d) Rim calcification

10. **All of the following immunosuppressives cause profound myelosuppression *EXCEPT***
    (a) Sirolimus
    (b) Cyclosporine
    (c) Azathioprine
    (d) Mercaptopurine

11. **Molecular pathogenesis of α thalassemia involves**
    (a) Mutation in transcription promoter sequence
    (b) Gene deletion
    (c) Codon termination mutation
    (d) mRNA splicing defect

12. **McArdle's syndrome is due to**
    (a) Deficiency of glucose-6-phosphatase
    (b) Absence of muscle phosphorylase
    (c) Deficiency of liver phosphorylase
    (d) Deficiency of liver phosphorylase kinase

13. **Which of the following illnesses increases the risk of developing tuberculosis?**
    (a) Anthracosis
    (b) Berylliosis
    (c) Sarcoidosis
    (d) Silicosis

14. **Cell of origin of hairy cell leukemia is**
    (a) B cell
    (b) T cell

(c) NK cell
(d) Dendritic reticulum cell

15. The commonest cause of chronic renal failure is
(a) Diabetes mellitus
(b) Hypertension
(c) Pyelonephritis
(d) Cystic disease of kidneys

16. Plasmapheresis is indicated in each of the following *EXCEPT*
(a) Hemolytic-uremic syndrome
(b) Goodpasture's syndrome
(c) Polycythemia vera
(d) Landry-Guillain-Barré syndrome

17. 'Square root' sign is characteristic of
(a) Dilated cardiomyopathy
(b) Restrictive cardiomyopathy
(c) Constrictive pericarditis
(d) Cardiac tamponade

18. A 40-year-old woman presented to the surgical OPD with features suggestive of colitis. She was on prolonged treatment with clindamycin. Fecal sample was positive for toxin produced by this agent. Her condition improved on treatment with metronidazole. The clinical condition is associated with
(a) *Bacillus anthracis*
(b) *Acinetobacter baumannii*
(c) *Clostridium difficile*
(d) *Listeria monocytogenes*

19. Prophylaxis for *Pneumocystis carinii* is indicated in HIV positive patients when CD4 count is
(a) < 300 cells/mm^3
(b) < 200 cells/mm^3
(c) < 100 cells/mm^3
(d) < 50 cells/mm^3

20. Following statements regarding ulcerative colitis is true
(a) Smoking has a protective effect
(b) Smoking does not have a protective effect
(c) There is no relation to smoking
(d) Smoking causes relapses

21. Localization in insulinoma is best with
(a) Contrast computerized tomography
(b) Magnetic resonance imaging
(c) Somatostatin receptor scintigraphy
(d) Selective arteriography

SURGERY

22. Benign prostatic hyperplasia first develops in the
(a) Periurethral transition zone
(b) Peripheral zone
(c) Central zone
(d) Anterior fibromuscular stroma

23. Zollinger-Ellison syndrome is NOT caused by tumors from
(a) Pancreas
(b) Ovary
(c) Colon
(d) Duodenum

24. The use of 5% dextrose as an intravenous resuscitation fluid can
(a) Improve cerebral perfusion
(b) Provide glucose substrate for cerebral metabolism
(c) Reduce intracranial pressure and cause laxity of brain
(d) Reduce serum osmolality and cause brain edema

25. A 40-year-old female presents with fever, fatigue, diffuse painful swelling in the midline of the neck, FNAC of the same reveals epithelioid cells and giant cells, the likely diagnosis is
(a) Acute thyroiditis
(b) Subacute thyroiditis
(c) Tubercular lymphadenitis
(d) Hashimotos thyroiditis

26. All are precancerous for carcinoma esophagus *EXCEPT*
(a) Achalasia
(b) Paterson-Brown-Kelly syndrome
(c) Zenker's diverticulum
(d) Ectodermal dysplasia

27. An ulceroproliferative lesion in the antrum of the stomach 6 cm in diameter, invading the serosa, with 10 enlarged lymph nodes around the pylorus with no distant metastasis, the TNM staging is
(a) T2N1M0
(b) T3N2M0
(c) T4N1M0
(d) T1N3M0

28. **A 10-year-old female presents with pain in the right hypochondrium, fever, jaundice and a palpable mass in the right hypochondrium the probable diagnosis is**
   (a) Hepatitis
   (b) Hepatoma
   (c) Choledochal cyst
   (d) Mucocele gallbladder

29. **A 50-year-old male presents with pain upper abdomen, pruritus, jaundice and weight loss, elevated ANA, the likely diagnosis is**
   (a) Primary sclerosing cholangitis
   (b) Klatskin tumor
   (c) Secondary sclerosing cholangitis
   (d) Choledocholithiasis

30. **Bilateral, multicentric type of carcinoma in breast is usually**
   (a) Mucoid carcinoma
   (b) Invasive lobular carcinoma
   (c) Infiltrating ductal carcinoma
   (d) Non-infiltrating ductal carcinoma

31. **Crohn's disease is associated with**
   (a) *NOD2/CARD15* gene
   (b) *P53* suppressor gene
   (c) Philadelphia chromosomes
   (d) *BRAC1* gene

32. **Investigation of choice to diagnose Hypertrophic Pyloric Stenosis in infants is**
   (a) Contrast radiology
   (b) Gastroscopy
   (c) Ultrasound abdomen
   (d) CT scan abdomen

OBG

33. **Delivery of head in normal labor is by the following movement**
   (a) Flexion
   (b) Extension
   (c) Rotation
   (d) Restitution

34. **The following conditions are associated with endometriosis *EXCEPT***
   (a) Anovulation
   (b) Luteinized unruptured follicle
   (c) Hyperprolactinemia
   (d) Hypothyroidism

35. **The karyotype of complete mole is**
   (a) 46XX
   (b) 46XY
   (c) 45XX or 46XY
   (d) Triploid

36. **Fitz-Hugh-Curtis syndrome is associated with**
   (a) Chlamydial infection
   (b) Genital tuberculosis
   (c) Syphilis
   (d) Candida infection

37. **Human Chorionic Gonadotropin levels are increased if the fetus is having**
   (a) Down syndrome
   (b) Anencephaly
   (c) Hydrocephalus
   (d) Spina bifida

38. **Most likely cause for amenorrhea in cases of vesicovaginal fistula is**
   (a) Asherman's syndrome
   (b) Hypothalamic suppression
   (c) Nutritional
   (d) Infection

39. **Mayer-Rokitansky-Kuster-Hauser syndrome is characterized by all *EXCEPT***
   (a) Urinary tract abnormality in 30%
   (b) Phenotypically male
   (c) Presence of ovaries
   (d) Absence of uterus

40. **All the following are primary solid ovarian tumors *EXCEPT***
   (a) Krukenberg's tumor
   (b) Dysgerminoma
   (c) Brenner's tumor
   (d) Carcinoid tumor

41. **A women presents with 10 weeks of amenorrhea, pain and bleeding. On examination the uterus is 10 weeks size, soft and internal os is open. The diagnosis is**
   (a) Threatened abortion
   (b) Missed abortion
   (c) Ectopic pregnancy
   (d) Inevitable abortion

42. **The lowest failure rate is seen with which of the following techniques of tubectomy**
   (a) Pomeroy's method
   (b) Laparoscopic ligation

(c) Madlener's technique
(d) Aldridge method

PEDIATRICS

43. Pharmacological closure of patent ductus arteriosus in a premature infant is by administration of
(a) Aspirin
(b) Estrogen
(c) Ibuprofen
(d) Prednisolone

44. The main infectious agent associated with recurrent pulmonary infections in patients with cystic fibrosis is
(a) *Mycoplasma*
(b) *Pseudomonas*
(c) *Pneumocystis*
(d) *Aspergillus*

45. The guidelines for immunization against infectious disease includes all of the following *EXCEPT*
(a) Live vaccines are contraindicated in pregnant women
(b) Live vaccines should not be administered within 3 months of giving human immunoglobulin
(c) Inactivated vaccines should not be given, if there has been significant reaction to previous dose
(d) Hay fever, sickle cell anemia and tuberculosis are contraindications for vaccination

46. Initial manifestation as an infection of the limbic regions of the brain is seen in children with the following infection
(a) Enterovirus
(b) Rabies
(c) Epstein-Barr virus
(d) Cytomegalovirus

47. Which of the following is the best indicator of long-term nutritional status?
(a) Mid arm circumference
(b) Height for age
(c) Weight for age
(d) Weight for height

48. Conjugated hyperbilirubinemia is seen in
(a) Dubin-Johnson syndrome
(b) Crigler-Najjar syndrome-I
(c) Crigler-Najjar syndrome-II
(d) Gilbert's syndrome

49. A reversal of shunt to right-to-left producing late cyanosis is called
(a) Lutembacher's syndrome
(b) Eisenmenger's syndrome
(c) Kartagener syndrome
(d) Corrected transposition

50. All the following diseases are associated with triplet and other repeat sequences *EXCEPT*
(a) Huntington's disease
(b) Friedreich's ataxia
(c) Myotonic dystrophy
(d) Hereditary motor – sensory neuropathy

51. Attention deficit hyperactivity disorder is seen in
(a) Insulin resistance
(b) Thyroid hormone resistance
(c) Testosterone deficiency
(d) Calmodulin deficiency

52. Which is the age limit for further developmental assessment in a child NOT reaching for objects?
(a) 3 months
(b) 5 months
(c) 9 months
(d) 12 months

53. Respiratory Syncytial Virus causes all of the following in children *EXCEPT*
(a) Bronchiolitis
(b) Croup
(c) Pneumonia
(d) Rhinosinusitis

ORTHOPEDICS

54. A 2-day-old child with bilateral idiopathic clubfeet is best managed by
(a) Manipulation by the mother
(b) Manipulation and Denis-Browne splint
(c) Manipulation and casts
(d) Surgical release

55. A 2-year-old male child has been limping ever since he has started walking. Examination reveals a short right lower limb with limited abduction at the hip. The Trendelenburg sign is positive however telescopy is absent. The most probable diagnosis is
(a) Kirner's deformity
(b) Congenital dislocation of the hip
(c) Congenital coxa vara
(d) Perthes' disease

56. **Peripheral nerves can withstand ischemia up to**
(a) 30 minutes
(b) 1 hour
(c) 3 hours
(d) 4 hours

57. **The primary site of infection in Pott's spine is**
(a) Vertebral body
(b) Intervertebral disk
(c) Transverse process
(d) Spinous process

OPHTHALMOLOGY AND ENT

58. **Shield cataract is seen in**
(a) Diabetes
(b) Atopic dermatitis
(c) Neurofibromatosis type-2
(d) Galactosemia

59. **The following bacteria can invade intact corneal epithelium *EXCEPT***
(a) *Neisseria gonorrhoeae*
(b) *Corynebacterium diphtheriae*
(c) *Staphylococcus aureus*
(d) *Listeria monocytogenes*

60. **Which is the most appropriate parameter for assessment of hearing in a 9-month-old child?**
(a) Shows some response to his/her own name
(b) Searches for quiet sounds made out of sight
(c) Turns the head when spoken to from side
(d) Pauses and listens to prolonged sound

61. **Progressive unilateral sensorineural deafness with tinnitus and disequilibrium is seen in**
(a) Secretory otitis media
(b) Benign paroxysmal positional vertigo
(c) Vestibular neuronitis
(d) Acoustic neuroma

62. **The most critical and constant finding of Retinitis pigmentosa is**
(a) Dense bone spicule in the retinal periphery
(b) A significantly reduced electroretinogram
(c) Tubular visual fields
(d) Attenuated retinal arteries

63. **Prominent or enlarged corneal nerves are seen in all of the following conditions *EXCEPT***
(a) Keratoconus
(b) Acanthameba keratitis
(c) Fuch's endothelial dystrophy
(d) Congenital hereditary endothelial dystrophy

64. **Fever, headache and nasal obstruction with bilateral bulging of nasal septum is due to**
(a) Septal hematoma
(b) Rhinoscleroma
(c) Septal abscess
(d) Tuberculosis of nasal septum

65. **Buphthalmos usually presents as**
(a) High intraocular pressure
(b) Optic cupping
(c) Field defects
(d) Enlarged cornea

66. **Down beat nystagmus can occur in each of the following *EXCEPT***
(a) Multiple sclerosis
(b) Craniocervical junction lesion
(c) Labyrinthine lesion
(d) Cerebellar stroke

67. **All the following develop from surface ectoderm, *EXCEPT***
(a) Corneal epithelium
(b) Conjunctival epithelium
(c) Iris epithelium
(d) Lens

68. **Massive retinal hemorrhages are seen in**
(a) Central retinal artery occlusion
(b) Central retinal vein occlusion
(c) Carotid artery occlusion
(d) Branch artery occlusion

69. **In electroretinogram, the A wave is generated by**
(a) Rods and cones
(b) Retinal pigment epithelial cells
(c) Anterior lens cells
(d) Amacrine cells

DERMATOLOGY, ANESTHESIOLOGY, RADIOLOGY AND PSYCHIATRY

70. **Erythema Nodosum Leprosum is seen in**
(a) Lepromatous leprosy
(b) Indeterminate leprosy
(c) Borderline tuberculoid leprosy
(d) Tuberculoid leprosy

71. **Ecthyma gangrenosum is typically due to**
(a) *Escherichia coli*
(b) *Pseudomonas aeruginosa*
(c) *Staphylococcus aureus*
(d) *Candida albicans*

72. Seborrheic dermatitis is frequently seen in
(a) Lipid storage disorders
(b) Psoriasis vulgaris
(c) Hypertension
(d) Parkinson disease

73. Apple jelly nodules are seen in
(a) Tuberculosis verrucosa cutis
(b) Tuberculous gumma
(c) Scrofuloderma
(d) Lupus vulgaris

74. In the context of inhalation anesthetics, MAC refers to
(a) Maximum anesthetic concentration
(b) Minimum anesthetic concentration
(c) Minimum alveolar concentration
(d) Maximum alveolar concentration

75. Which of the following stages is described as State of surgical anesthesia?
(a) 1
(b) 2
(c) 3
(d) 4

76. Postspinal headache is due to
(a) Injury to spinal cord
(b) CSF leak from dura
(c) Meningitis
(d) Raised intracranial pressure

77. Contraindication to nasotracheal intubation is
(a) Basilar skull fracture
(b) Severe otitis media
(c) Labyrinthitis
(d) Pituitary microadenoma

78. Diffusion into gas-containing spaces is a problem with
(a) Halothane
(b) Nitrous oxide
(c) Isoflurane
(d) Ether

79. Radiographic features of pulmonary embolism include all *EXCEPT*
(a) Westermark's sign
(b) Fleischner sign
(c) Hampton's hump
(d) Virchow's sign

80. 'Rugger jersey' spine is seen in
(a) Fluorosis
(b) Achondroplasia
(c) Renal osteodystrophy
(d) Marfan's syndrome

81. Which of these is a sign of left atrial enlargement on a PA chest radiograph?
(a) Elevation of the right main bronchus
(b) Double density on the left side of the heart shadow
(c) Discrete bulge of the left cardiac margin below the pulmonary bay
(d) Displacement of the trachea to the right

82. The dark areas in a conventional radiographic film are due to particulate deposits of
(a) Carbon
(b) Iron
(c) Silver
(d) Copper

83. The only atypical antipsychotic drug that is indicated to reduce the risk of suicide is
(a) Clozapine
(b) Ziprasidone
(c) Risperidone
(d) Asenapine

84. Restless leg syndrome is commonly caused by addiction to which of the following
(a) Caffeine
(b) Cocaine
(c) Cannabis
(d) Opium

85. Which of the following is a necessary criterion to diagnose a depressive episode?
(a) Past history of mania
(b) Suicidal attempt
(c) Presence of a stress
(d) Depressed mood for a minimum 2 weeks duration

86. Which is true of Anxiety disorders?
(a) They are the least prevalent psychiatric disorders in the general population
(b) They are present in 15–20% of patients attending medical clinics
(c) They are characterized by pervasive sadness
(d) They are primarily treated with antipsychotics

87. A 9-year-old boy complains of 'something crawling inside my head'. He was conscious with no eye blinking. The most likely diagnosis is

(a) Simple partial seizure
(b) Tics
(c) Migraine
(d) Dissociative disorder

88. **Which is true of schizophrenia?**
(a) It is characterized by pure negative symptoms
(b) Positive symptoms occur in the later part of the illness
(c) There is a pathognomonic feature for the diagnosis
(d) Marked variability in the 'course' of symptoms is common

89. **Dissociative fugue is disorder that refers to one of the following**
(a) Patient being dominated by two or more distinct personalities of which only one is being manifest at a time
(b) Loss of memory following a traumatic event
(c) Episodes of unexpected yet organized wandering away from home
(d) Absence of voluntary movements or speech

FORENSIC MEDICINE

90. **Study of lip prints is known as**
(a) Poroscopy
(b) Rugoscopy
(c) Cheiloscopy
(d) Oroscopy

91. **Strychnine acts by inhibiting**
(a) GABA
(b) Glycine
(c) Acetylcholine
(d) Dopamine

92. **The shape of the curve, which best describes the cooling of the body after death is**
(a) Parabola
(b) Hyperbola
(c) Sigmoid
(d) Linear

93. **'Declaration of Tokyo' deals with**
(a) Abortion
(b) Torture
(c) Human experimentation
(d) Consumerism

PREVENTIVE AND SOCIAL MEDICINE

94. **A night blood survey is done in**
(a) Malaria
(b) Filariasis
(c) Plague
(d) Dengue

95. **What percentage of the healthcare waste generated is infectious?**
(a) 10–15%
(b) 50%
(c) 75%
(d) 100%

96. **The vector for Dengue fever is**
(a) *Culex fatigans*
(b) *Anopheles culicifacies*
(c) *Aedes aegypti*
(d) *Aedes africanus*

97. **All of the following are techniques of quantitative management, *EXCEPT***
(a) Cost benefit analysis
(b) Network analysis
(c) Work sampling
(d) Management by objectives

98. **The Government of India launched National Mental Health Program in the year**
(a) 1982
(b) 1983
(c) 1984
(d) 1985

99. **The type of study that determines the norms and limits of the distribution of variables, including the characteristics of the events and population under study, is referred to as**
(a) Explanatory
(b) Cross-sectional
(c) Descriptive
(d) Analytical

100. **Claviceps fusiformis is responsible for**
(a) Neurolathyrism
(b) Ergotism
(c) Epidemic dropsy
(d) Endemic ascites

101. Experimental studies are meant to
(a) Test etiological hypothesis
(b) Find out prevalence rates
(c) Find out causes of epidemics
(d) To find out the history of disease

102. Amongst the following fats and oils, highest proportion of poly unsaturated fatty acids (PUFA) is found in
(a) Groundnut oil
(b) Coconut oil
(c) Safflower oil
(d) Butter

103. The permissible dose of radiation from man-made sources in terms of rads per year should NOT exceed
(a) 1
(b) 5
(c) 10
(d) 15

104. Tuberculosis control is achieved when
(a) Tuberculosis conversion index in infants is < 1%
(b) Prevalence of natural infection in age group 0–14 years is in order of 10%
(c) Annual infection rate < 5%
(d) Prevalence of natural infection in 0–14 years is < 1%

105. The disaster cycle progresses from
(a) Rehabilitation → Reconstruction
(b) Mitigation → Reconstruction
(c) Mitigation → Response
(d) Rehabilitation → Response

106. In the life cycle of malaria parasite, the definitive host is
(a) Mosquito
(b) Man
(c) Pig
(d) Sandfly

107. 'Sensitivity' of a test is
(a) True negative/(False positive + True negative)
(b) True positive/(True positive + False negative)
(c) False positive/(True positive + True negative)
(d) False negative/(True positive + False negative)

108. The validity period of 'valid certificate of yellow fever vaccination' is
(a) 7 days after date of vaccination up to 10 years
(b) 10 days after date of vaccination up to 7 years
(c) 10 days after date of vaccination up to 10 years
(d) 7 days after date of vaccination up to 7 years

109. According to concept of iceberg phenomenon of diseases, all of the following statements about the submerged portion of iceberg are true *EXCEPT*
(a) It includes subclinical cases
(b) It includes carriers
(c) It constitutes undiagnosed reservoir of infection
(d) Diagnosis can be made with available techniques

MICROBIOLOGY

110. Which of the following statements is NOT TRUE about *Trichomonas vaginalis*?
(a) Cyst is the infective form
(b) Possesses 3–4 anterior and 1 posterior flagella
(c) Trophozoite is pear shaped
(d) Vagina is the usual site of infection

111. The opportunistic fungi, which produces mycotoxins is
(a) *Aspergillus flavus*
(b) *Penicillium marneffei*
(c) *Allescheria boydii*
(d) *Phialophora jeanselmei*

112. Prions are infectious agents consisting of
(a) A single DNA chain
(b) A pair of DNA chains
(c) A single RNA chain
(d) Molecules

113. The rabies virus recovered from naturally occurring case of rabies is called
(a) Fixed virus
(b) Street virus
(c) Negri body
(d) None of the above

114. A kidney transplant between identical twins is an example of
(a) Isograft
(b) Allograft
(c) Autograft
(d) Xenograft

115. Lymphogranuloma venereum is caused by
(a) *Chlamydia trachomatis*
(b) *Haemophilus ducreyi*
(c) Human T-cell lymphoma virus type II
(d) Donovania granulomatis

116. Weil-Felix test is referred to as a 'Heterophile agglutination test' as the antigens used to detect infection is obtained from
(a) *Peptostreptococcus*
(b) *Proteus*
(c) *Pseudomonas*
(d) *Pasteurella*

PHARMACOLOGY

117. The following drug is predominantly a dual serotonin and norepinephrine reuptake inhibitor
(a) Fluvoxamine
(b) Duloxetine
(c) Fluoxetine
(d) Paroxetine

118. Which among the drugs given below, does NOT act by protease inhibition?
(a) Ritonavir
(b) Saquinavir
(c) Nelfinavir
(d) Zanamivir

119. Cardiomyopathy has the strongest association with the use of which of the following drugs?
(a) Didanosine
(b) Zidovudine
(c) Zalcitabine
(d) Lamivudine

120. A 160 mg dose of a drug was administered IV, and 80 mg was eliminated during the first 120 minutes. If the drug follows first order elimination kinetics, how much of the drug will remain 6 hours after its administration?
(a) None
(b) 20 mg
(c) 10 mg
(d) 40 mg

121. A 25-year-old male is brought to the emergency room with accidental ingestion of moth balls. He is found to have severe hemolysis. The most likely mechanism for hemolysis is
(a) G6PD deficiency
(b) Pyrimidine 5′-nucleotidase deficiency
(c) RBC glutathione deficiency
(d) Pyruvate kinase deficiency

122. Which is true of Lithium?
(a) It is extensively protein bound
(b) It is excreted unchanged by the kidneys
(c) It is exchanged for potassium by the kidneys
(d) It often causes hyperthyroidism

123. One of the following drugs is a weak, reversible monoamine oxidase inhibitor. There are case reports of serotonin syndrome occurring, when this drug is coadministered with selective serotonin reuptake inhibitors. Name the antibiotic
(a) Quinupristin-dalfopristin
(b) Clindamycin
(c) Linezolid
(d) Capreomycin

124. Which of the following is also known as Mickey Finn?
(a) Ethylene glycol
(b) Chloral hydrate
(c) Methyl alcohol
(d) Chloroform

125. The following chemical mediator is a product of arachidonic acid metabolism by cyclooxygenase pathway
(a) LXA4
(b) LXB4
(c) 5HETE
(d) PGH2

PATHOLOGY

126. Glycoprotein IIb – IIIa complex is deficient in
(a) Bernard-Soulier syndrome
(b) Glanzmann's disease
(c) Gray platelet syndrome
(d) von Willebrand's disease

127. Acute cellular rejection following solid Organ transplantation occurs
(a) Within minutes to hours of transplantation
(b) Within 48 hours of transplantation
(c) Between 5 and 30 days of transplantation
(d) Beyond 30 days after transplantation

128. Lipschutz inclusion bodies are seen in infections caused by
(a) Herpes virus
(b) Vaccinia virus
(c) Hepatitis A virus
(d) Hanta virus

129. Isolated deletion of which chromosome causes Myelodysplastic syndrome?
(a) 2q
(b) 5q
(c) 8q
(d) 11q

130. Middle meningeal vessel damage results in
(a) Subdural hemorrhage
(b) Subarachnoid hemorrhage
(c) Intracerebral hemorrhage
(d) Epidural hemorrhage

131. One of the statements regarding Hermansky-Pudlak syndrome is FALSE
(a) It is characterized by tyrosinase positive oculocutaneous albinism
(b) Bleeding tendencies are secondary to decreased platelets
(c) Restrictive lung disease is a rarity in the syndrome
(d) Cardiomyopathy is expected to occur in the 3rd or 4th decade of life

ANATOMY, PHYSIOLOGY AND BIOCHEMISTRY

132. Skin of dorsum of first web space of foot is supplied by
(a) Sural nerve
(b) Saphenous nerve
(c) Deep peroneal nerve
(d) Lateral plantar nerve

133. The ductus arteriosus is derived from the following aortic arch
(a) 3rd
(b) 4th
(c) 5th
(d) 6th

134. A 37-year-old male with a history of a penetrative trauma to the neck complains of pain and 'drooping' of the right shoulder with inability to hunch the shoulders and weakness of abduction. The nerve most likely to have been affected is the
(a) Axillary nerve
(b) Suprascapular nerve
(c) Spinal accessory nerve
(d) Long thoracic nerve

135. Cells present in the medulla of the ovary, which are homologous to interstitial cells of the testes
(a) Stromal cells
(b) Hilus cells
(c) Germinal epithelium
(d) Tunica albuginea

136. Structure passing through foramen Rotundum is
(a) Ophthalmic nerve
(b) Mandibular nerve
(c) Maxillary nerve
(d) Abducens nerve

137. The transpyloric plane passes through the
(a) Pylorus of the stomach
(b) Fundus of the stomach
(c) Fundus of the uterus
(d) Fundus of the gallbladder

138. All the following open into Right atrium *EXCEPT*
(a) Anterior cardiac vein
(b) Venae cordis minimi
(c) Coronary sinus
(d) Middle cardiac vein

139. The stria of Gennari is a histological feature of
(a) Motor speech area
(b) Auditory area
(c) Visual area
(d) Prefrontal area

140. The syndrome of growth failure, rash and hypogonadism is due to deficiency of
(a) Calcium
(b) Copper
(c) Zinc
(d) Magnesium

141. The receptors giving rise to signals that bring about Hering-Breuer inflation reflex are
(a) Proprioceptors
(b) J receptors
(c) Pain receptors
(d) Stretch receptors

142. Nasion lies at the junction of
(a) Frontonasal and internasal suture
(b) Frontonasal and interparietal suture
(c) Frontonasal and frontozygomatic suture
(d) Frontozygomatic and internasal suture

143. Salivary centers are located in
(a) Spinal cord
(b) Medulla
(c) Hypothalamus
(d) Cerebellum

144. **Ganglion of hay fever is**
(a) Otic ganglion
(b) Pterygopalatine ganglion
(c) Submandibular ganglion
(d) Geniculate ganglion

145. **The normal daily excretion of uric acid ranges from**
(a) 10 to 30 mg
(b) 50 to 70 mg
(c) 100 to 300 mg
(d) 500 to 700 mg

146. **Selenocysteine residues are present in**
(a) Pyruvate carboxylase
(b) Xanthine oxidase
(c) Deiodinase
(d) Lysyl oxidase

147. **The activities of all the following enzymes are increased in starvation *EXCEPT***
(a) Pyruvate kinase
(b) Pyruvate carboxylase
(c) Phosphoenolpyruvate carboxykinase
(d) Glucose-6-phosphatase

148. **Which of the following amino acids is purely ketogenic?**
(a) Phenylalanine
(b) Leucine
(c) Proline
(d) Tyrosine

149. **A mutation that results in premature termination of incorporation of amino acid into a peptide chain is a**
(a) Nonsense mutation
(b) Transversion
(c) Silent mutation
(d) Frameshift mutation

150. **Which of the following groups of contrast agents may be safely injected intrathecally?**
(a) Water-soluble ionic monomers
(b) Water-soluble non-ionic monomers
(c) Water-soluble ionic dimers
(d) Oil-based iodinated contrasts

Section B (Q No. 151–180)

(Question Number 151–153)
A 40-year-old male presents to the Accident and Emergency ward of the hospital with sudden onset of severe central abdominal pain of few hours duration, increasing in intensity with time, with severe abdominal distension, a skiagram of the abdomen revealed a 'coffee bean' appearance.

151. **The diagnosis of the above condition would be**
(a) Acute pancreatitis
(b) Duodenal ulcer perforation
(c) Sigmoid volvulus
(d) Ureteric calculus

152. **After optimization this patient should have**
(a) Exploratory laparotomy
(b) Urgent sigmoidoscopy
(c) Computed tomography
(d) Esophagogastroscopy

153. **This condition is more common in the**
(a) Africans
(b) Europeans
(c) Asians
(d) Chinese

(Question Number 154–157)
A 35-year-old female presented to the outpatient with a swelling in the neck for the past 2 months, she had treatment for Hodgkin's lymphoma when she was 22 years with irradiation. On examination, her vitals were normal, there was a single, firm, irregular nodule, moving with deglutition in the left side of midline. Clinical examination also revealed a single node in the left side of the neck.

154. **The most likely clinical diagnosis of this condition is**
(a) Recurrence of lymphoma
(b) Malignant goiter
(c) Benign multinodular goiter
(d) Toxic nodular goiter

155. **Most probable pathological diagnosis would be**
(a) Anaplastic carcinoma
(b) Follicular carcinoma
(c) Medullary carcinoma
(d) Papillary carcinoma

156. **The FNAC (FINE NEEDLE ASPIRATION CYTOLOGY) of the lesion should reveal**
(a) 'Orphan-Annie eye' nucleus cells
(b) Amyloid deposits
(c) Epithelioid cells and giant cells
(d) Follicular cells

157. **The ideal treatment of the above condition would be**
(a) Total thyroidectomy with lymph nodal dissection of the same side
(b) Radiotherapy

(c) Lobectomy
(d) Lobectomy with isthmusectomy

(Question Number 158–160)
A 55-year-old man presented with a two-day history of headache, fever and generalized weakness. He had received a cadaveric kidney transplant 5 years earlier. His medications included 5 mg of tacrolimus twice a day and 10 mg of prednisone daily. On neurologic examination, he was confused and incoherent. Cranial nerves were normal, but he had a hazy left retina. Magnetic resonance imaging of the brain with contrast showed multiple enhancing lesions in both cerebral hemispheres.

158. The most probable diagnosis is
(a) Cerebral toxoplasmosis
(b) *Listeria monocytogenes* infection
(c) *Nocardia asteroides* infection
(d) Miliary tuberculosis

159. Patient had subretinal abscess, the aspirate was stained, the findings are likely to be
(a) Weakly positive acid fast bacilli
(b) Gram positive cocci
(c) Gram negative cocci
(d) *Coccobacillus*

160. The treatment of choice in this condition is
(a) Trimethoprim – sulfamethoxazole
(b) Antitubercular therapy
(c) Steroids
(d) Long acting penicillin

(Question Number 161–163)
A 47-year-old man was brought to the AE because of altered mental status and acute renal failure. Previous evening after working on his car, later at 8 PM. his speech was slurred and he was lethargic. By 9 PM, the patient was vomiting and becoming increasingly lethargic. At 3:30 AM, his wife found him unresponsive. Approximately 30 minutes after his arrival at this hospital, the patient had a generalized tonic-clonic seizure. He had severe metabolic acidosis associated with an anion gap. Numerous needle-shaped crystals were seen in the urinary sediment.

161. The first investigation done on his arrival to the hospital is
(a) CT brain
(b) MRI brain
(c) Blood glucose
(d) Lumbar puncture

162. The probable cause for his condition
(a) Lesch-Nyhan syndrome
(b) Rhabdomyolysis
(c) Ethylene glycol poisoning
(d) Primary hyperparathyroidism

163. The drug of choice in this condition is
(a) Fomepizole
(b) Bisphosphonates
(c) 25% glucose
(d) Antibiotics

(Question Number 164–167)
A 30-year-old male presented to the clinic complaining of anorexia, nausea, vomiting and malaise since 1 week. He had not eaten anything for the last 3 days and had lost 10 kg weight. He had received a blood transfusion 2 months back. Physical examination revealed yellowish discoloration of his eyes. There was tender hepatomegaly, 3 cm below the costal margin. Total bilirubin 12.0 mg/dL, Direct bilirubin 8.0 mg/dL, Aspartate aminotransferase 1,240 U/L, Alanine aminotransferase 1,650 U/L, Alkaline phosphatase 198 U/L, HBsAg positive, Anti-HBc Total-positive; IgM fraction – positive, Anti-HIV negative. A liver biopsy was done.

164. What would be the most likely finding in the liver biopsy?
(a) Cholangitis
(b) Cirrhosis
(c) Bridging necrosis
(d) Fatty change

165. What would you expect to find in this patient's urine?
(a) Excess of urobilinogen
(b) Hemoglobin
(c) Fatty casts
(d) Bilirubin

166. A marker of active viral replication is
(a) HBsAg
(b) HBeAg
(c) IgM anti-HBc
(d) Anti-HBe

167. Chronic hepatitis is defined as the presence of continuing liver disease for more than
(a) 1 month
(b) 2 months
(c) 4 months
(d) 6 months

(Question Number 168–171)
A 60-year-old man presented with weight loss over a 4 month period and the recent onset of fever in the evenings with night sweats. He had enlarged cervical

lymph nodes. FNAC of the nodes showed epithelioid cells and giant cells. Chest X-ray revealed an irregular opacity of the right upper lung with pleural effusion. Thoracentesis was performed, and examination of the pleural fluid was done.

168. What findings would you expect in the pleural fluid?
(a) Increased proteins, decreased glucose and plenty of mesothelial cells
(b) Decreased proteins, increased glucose and plenty of neutrophils
(c) Increased proteins, decreased glucose and plenty of lymphocytes
(d) Decreased proteins, increased glucose and plenty of lymphocytes

169. The lesion of secondary pulmonary tuberculosis begins near the
(a) Interlobar fissure
(b) Hilum
(c) Apical region
(d) Blood vessels

170. Multidrug resistant tuberculosis is caused by *Mycobacterium tuberculosis* that is resistant to
(a) Rifampicin and Isoniazid
(b) Rifampicin, Isoniazid and Ethambutol
(c) Rifampicin, Isoniazid, Ethambutol and Pyrazinamide
(d) Any of the two first line antitubercular drugs

171. Which one of the following is FALSE about tuberculosis in the HIV infected patient?
(a) There is a 7–10% annual risk of reactivation of tuberculosis
(b) Disseminated tuberculosis is common
(c) The clinical presentation of tuberculosis is independent of the CD4 count
(d) Lower lobe pulmonary tuberculosis is common with low CD4 counts

(Question Number 172–174)
A 55-year-old man presented with a 1 month history of yellow discoloration of his palms and soles. Diabetes mellitus had been diagnosed 1 month before admission. His conjunctiva was not icteric. The fasting glucose level was 293 mg/dL (16.2 mmol/L) and the glycated hemoglobin value was 12.8%.

172. The cause for the yellow discoloration of the palms in this patient was due to
(a) Vitamin B_{12} deficiency
(b) Amiodarone exposure
(c) Diabetes mellitus
(d) Hyperlipidemia type III

173. Yellow discoloration of the skin is NOT a feature of
(a) Hypothyroidism
(b) Liver disease
(c) Diabetes mellitus
(d) Hyperlipidemia type III

174. The treatment for this patient is
(a) Good glycemic control
(b) Vitamin B_{12} injection
(c) Lower his cholesterol
(d) Thyroxine

(Question Number 175–177)
A 55-year-old man presented with intermittent, crampy pain in the right lower quadrant of the abdomen of 2 days duration. He reported perianal itching, otherwise no change in bowel movements, no nausea, vomiting, hematochezia, fever or other systemic symptoms. The physical examination revealed only for mild tenderness on deep palpation in the right lower quadrant.

175. The probable cause for this pain abdomen could be due to
(a) *Trichuris trichiura*
(b) *Ancylostoma duodenale*
(c) *Ancylostoma duodenale*
(d) *Enterobius vermicularis*

176. Non-bile stained ova seen on microscopy of the stools is due to
(a) *Trichuris trichiura*
(b) *Taenia solium*
(c) *Ascaris lumbricoides*
(d) *Enterobius vermicularis*

177. The treatment of choice for this patient is
(a) Albendazole
(b) Metrogyl
(c) Mebendazole
(d) Benzodiazepine

(Question Number 178–180)
A 2-year-old boy has a 1 week history of facial puffiness. His blood pressure is 100/160 mm Hg and there is generalized edema and ascites. Serum concentrations are: creatinine 0.4 mg/dL, albumin 1.4 g/dL and cholesterol 569 mg/dL. Urine analysis shows 4+ protein and no blood. The 24-hour urinary protein excretion is 3,865 mg/day.

178. The most likely diagnosis is
(a) Acute poststreptococcal glomerulonephritis
(b) Nephrotic syndrome due to minimal change disease

(c) Nephrotic syndrome due to focal segmental glomerulosclerosis
(d) Henoch purpura with nephritis

179. The above presentation in an adult patient with the presence of granular immunofluorescent deposits of immunoglobulins and complement along the glomerular basement membrane would suggest the diagnosis of

(a) Membranous glomerulonephritis
(b) Wegener granulomatosis
(c) Goodpasture's syndrome
(d) Postinfectious glomerulonephritis

180. A contraindication to renal biopsy is

(a) Lupus nephritis
(b) Polycystic kidney disease
(c) Chronic kidney disease
(d) Postoperative oliguria in a renal transplant

COMED-K 2011
ANSWERS AND EXPLANATIONS

Section A (Q No. 1–150)

MEDICINE

1. **Answer is b (Aspergilloma).**
   Ref: Textbook of pulmonary medicine, D Behera, Vol 1, 2nd edition Pg 508.

   - Infection of ***inactive tubercular cavities by Aspergillus fumigatus*** gives rise to solid mass like lesions inside the cavity (***aspergilloma***/ mycetoma or fungus ball).
   - They give rise to ***classic 'air-crescent' signs in the X-ray—Lucent crescent*** along the inner border of a cavity or between a dense parenchymal lesion and surrounding lung structures.
   - The position is changed when the patient is screened in different positions.
   - Most give rise to ***hemoptysis, which may be massive***.

2. **Answer is d (Serum bilirubin > 300 µmol/L).**
   Ref: Liver transplantation, Dilip Chakravarty et al, Jaypee, 2010 edition Pg 390.

King's College Hospital criteria for liver transplantation in acute liver failure

Patients with acetaminophen (paracetamol) **toxicity**
- pH < 7.3 (or irrespective of grade of encephalopathy)
- Prothrombin time > 100 seconds (or INR > 7.0)
- Serum creatinine level > 3.4 mg/dL (> 300 µmol/L), if in grade III or IV encephalopathy

Other patients
- Prothrombin time > 100 seconds or *Three of the following variables*:
  - Age < 10 years or > 40 years
  - Cause:
    - Non-A, non-B hepatitis
    - Halothane hepatitis
    - Idiosyncratic drug reaction
  - Duration of jaundice before encephalopathy > 7 days
  - Prothrombin time > 50 seconds (INR > 3.5)
  - Serum bilirubin level > 17.6 mg/dL (> 300 µmol/L)

3. **Answer is d (Diarrhea).**
   Ref: Davidson's, 21st edition Pg 779, Box 20.50.

Clinical Features of Pheochromocytoma

- Paroxysms of hyperadrenergic symptoms (***<u>5P's</u>):***
  - Pressure (elevated BP, often postural drop of BP)
  - Pain (headache)
  - Perspiration (sweating)
  - Palpitation (tachycardia)

– Pallor
- Anxiety (fear of death)
- Abdominal pain
- Vomiting
- Constipation
- Weight loss
- Glucose intolerance

More about pheochromocytoma

- **MC tumor of *adrenal medulla*** in adults.
- Derived from ***chromaffin* cells** (derived from neural crest).
- Tumors secrete epinephrine, NE and dopamine.
- ↑↑ Urinary *VMA*, ↑↑ plasma and urinary catecholamine levels.
- A/w ***MEN II* and *MEN III*.**
- ***CT scan*** of adrenal glands; ***MIBG scan*** is a nuclear isotope scan to detect occult collections of metastatic pheochromocytoma.
- Treat with ***phenoxybenzamine***, irreversible **α-blocker, to *first* control BP**. Without α-blockade BP can drop significantly postoperatively. Propranolol is used *after* the α-blocker.

✈ **Rule of 10s for pheochromocytoma: 10%** malignant; **10%** bilateral; **10%** extra-adrenal; **10%** calcify; **10%** in kids; **10%** familial.

4. Answer is d (Aortic stenosis).
Ref: Harrison's, 17th edition Pg 1384.

Abnormalities of JVP

⊕ **Large a wave**	Tricuspid stenosis, pulmonary stenosis/hypertension, some cases of left ventricular hypertrophy (Bernheim effect)
⊕ **Cannon a wave**	Complete heart block, junctional rhythm, atrioventricular dissociation with ventricular tachycardia
⊕ **Absent a wave**	Atrial fibrillation
⊕ **Raised JVP with normal waveform**	Fluid overload, right heart failure
⊕ **Raised JVP with absent pulsation**	SVC obstruction (edema of head and neck, collateral veins, and absent venous pulsation)
⊕ **Systolic *(cv)* waves**	Tricuspid regurgitation, look for earlobe movement
⊕ **Slow y descent**	Tricuspid stenosis
⊕ **Deep x and y descents**	Constrictive pericarditis and pericardial tamponade

Normal Jugular Venous Pulse (JVP)

The *right internal jugular vein* is the best vein for accurate estimation of the central venous pressure. The waves in the normal JVP are:

♦ *a wave*	atrial contraction
♦ *c wave*	bulging of tricuspid valve into right atrium during right ventricular isovolumetric systole
♦ *v wave*	increasing volume of blood in the right atrium during ventricular systole as the tricuspid valve is closed
♦ *x descent*	atrial relaxation and downward displacement of tricuspid valve during ventricular systole
♦ *y descent*	opening of tricuspid valve and rapid inflow of blood into right ventricle

5. Answer is b (Hyperaldosteronism).
Ref: Harrison's, 17th edition Pg 2260.

- The criteria for the diagnosis of ***primary hyperaldosteronism (Conn's syndrome)*** are:
  - ➢ Diastolic ***hypertension*** without edema.
  - ➢ Hyposecretion of renin (as judged by low plasma renin activity levels) that fails to increase appropriately during volume depletion (upright posture, sodium depletion).
  - ➢ Hypersecretion of aldosterone that does not suppress appropriately in response to volume expansion.
- ***Hypokalemia may be severe; Hypernatremia is infrequent.***
- Individuals with primary hyperaldosteronism are usually asymptomatic BUT:
  - ➢ Sodium retention may cause edema.
  - ➢ Hypokalemia may cause ***muscle weakness.***
  - ➢ Polyuria and occasionally tetany are seen.

Note:

- ♦ ***HYPOaldosteronism*** is characterized by HYPOnatremia, HYPOtension and HYPERkalemia.
- ♦ ***Cushing's syndrome*** is characterized by HYPERglycemia.

6. Answer is d (Morquio MPS-IV).
Ref: Harrison's, 17th edition Pg 2452, Table 355-1.

- ♦ ***Morquio's disease*** and MPS-1S ***Scheie*** are NOT a/w mental retardation.

Also Know

- ➢ Hunter's disease is the only MPS with X-linked recessive inheritance (all others are autosomal recessive)
  Clue: Hunter's aim for the 'X'!
- ➢ Also NO corneal opacity for Hunter (Clue" Hunter cannot hunt with a corneal opacity).

7. Answer is a (Optic tract).
Ref: Parson, 19th edition Pg 528, 120.

- Wernicke's hemianopic pupil is caused by division of the optic tract that results in a contralateral homonymous hemianopia.
- Though the direct and consensual responses still occur, the pupils fail to react when a narrow pencil of light is shone onto the non-seeing half of the retina, but they do react, if it falls onto the seeing retinal half.
- It is also characterized by ptosis on the same side as the hemianopia and anisocoria with the larger pupil also on the same side as the hemianopia.
- The macular area is often involved and optic atrophy may follow.
- Due to fact that the pupillary and visual fibers deviate in the posterior aspect of the optic tract, ***Wernicke's Hemianopic pupil occurs as a result of a lesion in the optic tract*** in an area that precedes the splitting of the two types of fibers.
- Not a very clinically useful test, since it is difficult to make the slit lamp light/torchlight to fall only on one half of the retina.

8. Answer is a (Syringomyelia).
Ref: Davidson's, 21st edition Pg 1157.

- ❖ *Lesions in the center of the spinal cord* (such as ***syringomyelia***) spare the dorsal columns, but affect the spinothalamic fibers crossing the cord from both sides over the length of the lesion.
- ❖ The ***sensory loss is therefore dissociated*** (in terms of the modalities affected) and suspended (in sense that segments above and below the lesions are spared), often with reflex loss, if afferent fibers of the reflex arc within the cord are affected.

9. **Answer is b (Lucent crescent).**
Ref: Textbook of pulmonary medicine, D Behera, Vol 1, 2nd edition Pg 508.

Answer no. 1 above for detailed explanation.

10. **Answer is b (Cyclosporine).**
Ref: KD Tripathi, 6th edition Pg 839.

- ***Cyclosporine*** is ***uniquely different*** from other immunosuppressives in that it does not hinder neutrophil function and is NOT *myelosuppressive.*
- Side effects of cyclosporine are:
  – ***Nephrotoxicity***
  – ***Tremor***
  – ***Hirsutism***
  – ***Hypertension***
  – ***Hypomagnesemia***
  – ***Gum hyperplasia***.

11. **Answer is b (Gene deletion).**
Ref: Harrison's, 17th edition Pg 641; Davidson's, 21st edition Pg 1030.

- In alpha thalassemia there is reduced or absent alpha chain synthesis.
- There are two alpha gene loci on chromosome 16 and therefore each individual carries 4 alpha gene alleles:
  - If 1 is ***deleted,*** there is no clinical effect
  - If 2 are deleted, there maybe a mild hypochromic anemia
  - If 3 are deleted the patient has hemoglobin H disease
  - If 4 are deleted the baby is stillborn (hydrops fetalis).

12. **Answer is b (Absence of muscle phosphorylase).**
Ref: Harrison's, 17th edition Pg 2458, Table 356-1.

Glycogen Storage Diseases

Disease	Enzyme deficient	Comments
Disorders with hepatomegaly and hypoglycemia		
Von Gierke's (Type 1)	Glucose-6-phosphatase	Hepatomegaly and severe fasting hypoglycemia
Cori's, Forbe-Limit dextrinosis (Type 3)	Amyloglucosidase (Debranching enzyme)	Hepatomegaly and hypoglycemia
Her's (Type 6)	Liver phosphorylase	
Disorders with muscle-energy impairment		
McArdle's (Type 5) M's	*M*uscle glycogen phosphorylase	*M*uscle cramps, *M*yoglobinuria, *M*ale preponderance, exercise intolerance; compensated hemolysis in Tarui's
Tarui's (Type 7)	Phosphofructokinase	
Disorders with skeletal and cardiac muscle impairment		
Pompe's (type 2) (Pumpe's = **'pump'** failure)	Acid a glucosidase (Acid maltase)	Skeletal muscle weakness, severe cardiomegaly and failure
Disorders with liver cirrhosis		
Anderson's amylopectinosis	Amylo-transglucosidase	Failure to thrive, hepatomegaly, progressive liver cirrhosis and failure (usually death before 5th year)

13. Answer is d (Silicosis).

Ref: Davidson's, 21st edition Pg 712; Harrison's, 17th edition Pg 1614.

- ***Silicosis*** results from the inhalation of free silica usually in the form of quartz by workers grinding and polishing stone.
- Silicosis is a/w egg shell calcification of lymph nodes; HRCT shows 'crazy paving' pattern.
- Silicosis is a/w an **increased risk of tuberculosis (silicotuberculosis)**, lung cancer and COPD; associations with renal, and connective tissue disease have been described.
- Because of the ***increased risk of active tuberculosis***, the recommended treatment of latent tuberculosis in these patients is longer.

14. Answer is a (B cell).

Ref: Davidson's, 21st edition Pg 1036.

- ***Hairy cell leukemia*** *is a* ***Mature B*** lymphocyte proliferative disorder.
- ***Affects M****iddle* aged (55 years) ***Men*** (M:F=5:1); *Massive* splenomegaly is present. **S-I-M** *"**Mature Middle aged Men** will **B** Massively Hairy".*
- Patients present with fatigue and frequent infections.
- Pancytopenia is the hallmark; hairy cells are present in blood smear and bone marrow biopsy. Bone marrow is usually inaspirable (***dry tap***). Hairy cells stain with tartrate resistant acid phosphatase (TRAP) and CD11c positive.
- The treatment of choice is ***cladribine*** (2-chlorodeoxyadenosine, 2-CDA). Treatment with *pentostatin* is somewhat similar, but this drug is *more cumbersome to administer*.

15. Answer is a (Diabetes mellitus).

Ref: Davidson's, 20th edition Pg 486, Box 17.29; Harrison's, 17th edition Pg 1762.

Common causes of chronic renal failure

Diabetes mellitus type-2	20–40%
Hypertension	5–25%
Glomerular diseases	10–20%
Interstitial disease	5–15%
Renal artery stenosis	5%
Systemic inflammatory diseases	5%
Congenital and inherited (e.g. polycystic kidneys, Alport's syndrome)	5%

16. Answer is c (Polycythemia vera).

Ref: Harrison's, 17th edition Pgs 1788, 2670, 1737

- ***Plasmapheresis*** is the removal, treatment and return of (components of) blood plasma from blood circulation.
- Plasmapheresis is used to remove antibodies from the bloodstream, thereby preventing them from attacking their targets. It does not directly affect the immune system's ability to make more antibodies and therefore may only offer temporary benefit.
- The basic procedure consists of removal of blood, separation of blood cells from plasma and return of these blood cells to the body's circulation, diluted with fresh plasma or a substitute. Because of concerns over viral infection, and allergic reaction, fresh plasma is not routinely used. Instead, the most common substitute is saline solution with sterilized human albumin protein. During the course of a single session, 2–3 L of plasma is removed and replaced.
- Plasmapheresis ***may offer benefit and is done in:***
  - Goodpasture's syndrome
  - Landry-Guillain-Barre syndrome
  - Hemolytic-uremic syndrome
  - ANCA small vessel vasculitis

- Antiphospholipid syndrome
- Essential mixed cryoglobulinemia
- IgA nephropathy
- Myasthenia gravis
- Pemphigus vulgaris
- Waldenstrom's macroglobulinemia.

✈ Note: Periodic phlebotomies are useful in polycythemia vera.

17. Answer is c (Constrictive pericarditis).
Ref: Harrison's, 17th edition Pg 1493.

- In ***constrictive pericarditis***, the ventricular pressure pulses in both ventricles exhibit characteristic ***'square root' signs*** during diastole.

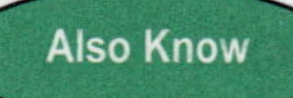

D/D of Constrictive Pericarditis

Feature	Cardiac Tamponade	Constrictive pericarditis	Restrictive cardiomyopathy	Right ventricular MI
Pulsus paradoxus	*Common*	Usually absent	Rare	Rare
Kussmaul's sign	Absent	*Present*	Absent	Absent
Third heart sound (S3)	Absent	Absent	Rare	*May be present*
Pericardial knock	Absent	*Often present*	Absent	Absent
Electrical alternans	*May be present*	Absent	Absent	Absent
Thickened pericardium, pericardial calcification	Absent	*Present*	Absent	Absent
JVP				
Prominent y descent	Absent	*Usually present*	Rare	Rare
Prominent x descent	*Present*	*Usually present*	Rare	Rare

❖ Note: ***Beck's triad*** in ***cardiac tamponade*** consists of distended neck veins, distant heart sound, hypotension

18. Answer is c (*Clostridium difficile*).
Ref: Davidson's, 21st edition Pg 338; Harrison's, 17th edition Pg 818.

- ***Clostridium difficile*** *associated* disease (CDAD) is a unique colon infection that is acquired almost exclusively in a/w antimicrobial use and the consequent disruption of the normal colonic flora.
- The most commonly diagnosed diarrheal illness acquired in the hospital, CDAD results from the ingestion of spores of *C. difficile* that vegetative, multiply and secrete toxins, causing diarrhea and ***Pseudomembranous colitis*** (PMC).
- PMC is a more advanced form of CDAD with ***abdominal pain and colitis*** and is visualized at endoscopy in only ~50% of patients with diarrhea who have a positive stool culture and toxin assay for *C. difficile*.
- ***Clindamycin***, ampicillin and cephalosporins were the first antibiotics associated with CDAD.
- The diagnosis of CDAD is based on a combination of clinical criteria: (1) diarrhea (≥ 3 unformed stools per 24 h for ≥ 2 days), with no other recognized cause; plus (2) ***toxin*** A or B detected in the stool, toxin-producing *C. difficile* detected by stool culture, or ***pseudomembranes*** seen in the colon.
- Treatment: Traditionally ***metronidazole*** was started and ***vancomycin*** used for relapses; however some authorities now recommend vancomycin as first line drug.

19. Answer is b (< 200 cells/mm^3).
Ref: Harrison's, 17th edition Pg 1172; Davidson's, 20th edition Pg 384, Box 14.7.

Repeat Topic

Indications for Prophylaxis for Pneumocystis Jiroveci Pneumonia (PCP)

For any HIV-infected individual
- Who has experienced a prior bout of PCP?
- Any patient with a ***CD4+ T cell count of < 200/μL*** or a CD4 percentage < 15
- Any patient with unexplained fever for > 2 weeks and
- Any patient with a history of oropharyngeal candidiasis

Agents for prophylaxis

- ***TMP/SMX***, one double-strength tablet daily (preferred regimen—*also provides protection against toxoplasmosis*)

For patients who cannot tolerate TMP/SMX, alternatives for prophylaxis include
- *Dapsone plus pyrimethamine plus leucovorin*
- *Aerosolized pentamidine* administered by the Respirgard II nebulizer and
- *Atovaquone*

- Also see ***answer no. 114 in Karnataka 2007 answers*** for detailed correlation between CD4 counts and HIV prophylaxis.

20. Answer is a (Smoking has a protective effect).
Ref: Davidson's, 21st edition Pg 896, Box 22.71; Harrison's, 17th edition Pg 1886, Table 289-1.

- Ulcerative colitis is more common in non-smokers and ex-smokers.
- ***Smoking may prevent ulcerative colitis.***

Note: Smoking is a/w a two-fold increased risk of Crohn's disease.

21. Answer is d (Selective arteriography).
Ref: See below with answer.

- "***Arteriography*** was previously considered to be **the gold standard for the diagnosis of insulinoma**. Now its use has declined to improvement in alternative imaging modalities." —*Clinical Endocrine Oncology By Ian D Hay, John AH Wass, 2nd edition Pg 458-59.*
- "The choice of imaging modality for insulinoma has been the subject of much debate. We believe that the choice is dependant on the expertise and technology (Ultrasound + CT/MRI) available at a particular center as well as the patient characteristics (previous abdominal surgery, obesity)." —*Clinical Endocrine Oncology By Ian D Hay, John AH Wass, 2nd edition Pg 458-59.*
- "In insulinomas, Somatostatin Receptor Scintigraphy (SRS) shows only a low sensitivity because many insulinomas do not express the respective somatostatin receptor subtypes binding octreotide. Hence, ***in insulinomas SRS plays only a minor role*** in comparison to other pancreatic neuroendocrine tumors." —*Methods of Cancer Diagnosis, Therapy and Prognosis: Gastrointestinal Carcinoma By MA Hayat, Pg 44-45. Vol 3, 2008 edition.*

SURGERY

22. Answer is a (Periurethral transition zone).
Ref: Bailey and Love's, 25th edition Pg 1343.

- Based on the work of ***McNeal***, classification of the prostate into two zones:
  - Peripheral zone—Carcinoma arises
  - Periurethral (central) zone—BPH arises.

Other high yield points about Ca Prostate

- MC malignant tumor in ***men > 65 years***.
- Over 95% of prostatic cancers are ***adenocarcinomas*** that arise in the *prostatic acini*, usually in the *'peripheral' zone* of the prostate.
- As ***axial skeleton is the MC site of metastases***, patients may present with back pain or *pathologic fractures*.
- ***Hematogenous metastases*** occur to ***bone***
- The **TNM staging** scheme has replaced the *Whitmore-Jewett system*. The route of lymphatic spread (in decreasing order) is to obturator, internal iliac, common iliac, presacral and para-aortic nodes.
- *Prostate Specific Antigen (PSA)*: The serum level is the ***most sensitive test*** for early detection of prostate cancer and is elevated in approximately 65% of cases. Normal upper limit is 4 ng/mL. Prostate confined cancers are associated with levels of less than 10 ng/mL; whereas metastatic disease may be associated with more than 30 ng/mL. This antigen is an imperfect tumor marker because of insensitivity (false negatives) and lack of specificity (elevations can occur with BPH, prostatitis and prostatic infarction). Earlier serum acid phosphatase was used as a tumor marker.
- *Ultrasound*: On transrectal sonography, carcinoma is revealed as hypoechoic densities within the peripheral zone.
- *Transrectal prostatic biopsy* with a rapid-fire spring loaded needle provides the most accurate sampling of the index lesion and the remainder of the gland and is the preferred technique.
- The ***Gleason score (2–10)*** remains the best predictor of tumor biology. It sums the scores of two most dysplastic biopsy samples on a scale of 1–5 (well differentiated to poorly differentiated).
- The ***CAPRA nomogram*** uses serum PSA, Gleason grade, clinical stage, percent positive biopsies and patient age in a point system to risk stratify, and predict the likelihood of PSA recurrence 3 and 5 years after radical prostatectomy. The CAPRA has been validated on large multicenter radical prostatectomy cohorts.
- For metastatic disease, androgen ablation is used either in the form of orchiectomy or by giving LHRH agonists (leuprolide, buserelin). Other drugs used are estrogen administration, aminoglutethimide, ketoconazole and antiandrogens (flutamide, cyproterone or bicalutamide).

23. Answer is c (Colon).

Ref: Harrison's, 17th edition Pg 1868.

Tumor Location of Gastrinomas in Zollinger-Ellison syndrome (ZES)

- ***Location:*** Over 80% of these tumors are found within the hypothetical ***gastrinoma triangle*** (confluence of the cystic and common bile ducts superiorly, junction of the second and third portions of the duodenum inferiorly and junction of the neck and body of the pancreas medially).
- ***Duodenal tumors constitute the MC non-pancreatic lesion***; between 50% and 75% of gastrinomas are found here. *(HPIM 17th, 1868)*. Primary gastrinomas may arise in the pancreas (25%), duodenal wall (45%), or lymph nodes (5–15%) and in other locations or of unknown primary in 20% *(CMDT, Chapter 15)*. Around 90% of tumors occur in the pancreatic head or proximal duodenal wall, the latter site being more common *(Davidsons, 20th edition Pg 890)*.
- Less-common extrapancreatic sites include ***stomach, bones, ovaries, heart, liver and lymph nodes***.

Simple Synopsis of Zollinger-Ellison Syndrome (ZES)

- ***ZES*** consists of ***severe peptic ulcer*** diathesis secondary to ***gastric acid hypersecretion*** due to ***unregulated gastrin release*** from a ***non-β cell endocrine tumor (gastrinoma)***.
- ***Age affected*** = 30–50 years.
- ***Etiology:*** Gastrinomas are classified into ***sporadic tumors (MC)*** and those ***a/w multiple endocrine neoplasia (MEN) type I***.

Clinically

- ***Peptic ulcers***, usually solitary and located in the duodenal bulb; isolated gastric ulcers do not occur.
- ***Gastric acid hypersecretion*** can cause direct intestinal mucosal injury and pancreatic enzyme inactivation, resulting in diarrhea, steatorrhea and weight loss; nasogastric aspiration of stomach acid stops the diarrhea.
- ***Suspect ZES*** when:
  - Increased fasting gastrin levels are a/w ulcers refractory to standard therapies
  - Giant ulcers (> 2 cm)

- ➢ Ulcers located distal to the duodenal bulb (postbulbar ulcer), multiple duodenal ulcers
- ➢ Frequent ulcer recurrences
- ➢ Ulcers associated with diarrhea
- ➢ Ulcers occurring after ulcer surgery
- ➢ Patients with ulcer complications
- ➢ Patients with hypercalcemia or family histories of ulcers (suggesting MEN 1); ulcers occurring in absence of *Hpylori* and NSAIDs usage.

Laboratory Findings

- ***Most sensitive and specific test: Increased fasting serum gastrin concentration*** (> 150 pg/mL)
- Gastric acid hypersecretion is present (pH < 3.0)
- ***IV secretin*** produces a rise in serum gastrin of over 200 pg/mL within 2–30 minutes in 85% of patients with gastrinoma

Imaging

- ***Somatostatin Receptor Scintigraphy*** has a sensitivity (> 80%) for tumor detection that exceeds all other imaging studies combined. If SRS is positive for tumor localization, further imaging studies are not necessary.
- In patients with negative SRS, endoscopic ultrasonography (EUS) may be useful to detect small gastrinomas in the duodenal wall, pancreas or peripancreatic lymph nodes

Treatment

- *Metastatic disease*: In patients with multiple hepatic metastases, initial therapy should be directed at controlling hypersecretion. Oral proton pump inhibitors
- *Localized Disease*: Cure can be achieved only, if the gastrinoma can be resected before hepatic metastatic spread has occurred.

Note:

- ✈ ***Gastrinoma triangle*** (Psaros triangle): 90% of gastrinomas are found here.

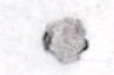

24. Answer is d (Reduce serum osmolality and cause brain edema).
Ref: http://www.trauma.org/archive/neuro/icpcontrol.html; http://www.nursingcenter.com/prodev/ce_article.asp?tid=1157503

- ❖ *5% Dextrose in water (D5W)* is unique in that it may be categorized as both an isotonic and a hypotonic solution.
- ❖ D5W should NOT be used in isolation to treat fluid volume deficit because it dilutes plasma electrolyte concentrations. It's also contraindicated in these clinical circumstances:
  - ***For resuscitation***, because the solution won't remain in the intravascular space.
  - In the ***early postoperative period***, because the body's reaction to the surgical stress may cause an increase in antidiuretic hormone secretion.
  - In ***patients with known or suspected increased intracranial pressure*** (ICP) due to its hypotonic properties following metabolism—it can ***increase cerebral edema***.

25. Answer is b (Subacute thyroiditis).
Ref: Harrison's, 17th edition Pg 2238.

SUBACUTE THYROIDITIS—also termed *de Quervain's thyroiditis, granulomatous thyroiditis* or *viral thyroiditis.*

- ♦ The diagnosis of subacute thyroiditis is often overlooked because the ***symptoms can mimic pharyngitis***.
- ♦ Peak incidence = 30–50 years, ***F:M = 3:1***.
- ♦ Pathology: Thyroid shows a characteristic patchy inflammatory infiltrate with disruption of the thyroid follicles and ***multinucleated giant cells*** within some follicles.
- ♦ The patient usually presents with a ***painful and enlarged thyroid***, sometimes accompanied by ***fever***.
- ♦ There may be features of thyrotoxicosis or hypothyroidism, depending on the phase of the illness.
- ♦ Malaise and symptoms of an upper respiratory tract infection may precede the thyroid-related features by several weeks.

- In other patients, examination reveals a small goiter that is exquisitely tender. Pain is often referred to the jaw or ear. Complete resolution is the usual outcome, but permanent hypothyroidism can occur.
- Relatively large doses of aspirin or NSAIDs are sufficient to control symptoms in many cases. If this treatment is inadequate, or if the patient has marked local or systemic symptoms, glucocorticoids should be give.

Quick summary

	Grave's disease	Subacute thyroiditis (de Quervain's)	Hashimoto's disease
Etiopathology	Antibody to TSH receptor, MC in females	Viral (possibly Coxsackie virus or Mumps)	Autoimmune
Clinically	Hyperthyroidism; diffuse painless goiter; ophthalmic (proptosis, lid lag, conjunctival injection); pretibial myxedema	Hyperthyroidism → hypothyroidism ***Painful tender thyroid gland***; jaw pain, ***granulomatous inflammation***	Hypothyroidism; painless thyroid enlargement; slow course, ***lymphocyte infiltrate*** with germinal centers, ***Hürthle cells*** on histology; may lead to ***lymphoma***
Diagnosis	**↑ RAIU**	↓ RAIU, ↑ ESR, thyroid antibodies are negative	Antimicrosomal and antithyroglobulin antibodies
Treatment	Propylthiouracil, methimazole, thyroid ablation with I 131	NSAIDs, steroids if pain severe	Levothyroxine

26. Answer is c (Zenker's diverticulum).
Ref: Harrison's, 17th edition Pg 570, Table 87-1.

- **Risk factors for Ca esophagus:**
  - Excess **alcohol** consumption, cigarette **smoking**, ingested **carcinogens** (nitrates, smoked opiates, fungal toxins, betel chewing), mucosal damage (from ingestion of hot **tea** or **lye**, **radiation induced** strictures, postcricoid web), tylosis (palmoplantar hyperkeratosis also called palmoplantar ectodermal dysplasia).
  - Intrinsic esophageal disease such as chronic **achalasia**, **B**arrett's esophagus (lead to **AD**enoCa), **PLU**mmer-Vinson syndrome (Paterson-Brown-Kelly syndrome)—leads to **S**quamous cell Ca (Mnemonic: **BAD PLUS)**.

- **Zenker's diverticulum**: Zenker's diverticulum, also pharyngoesophageal diverticulum, also pharyngeal pouch, is a diverticulum of the mucosa of the pharynx, just above the cricopharyngeal muscle (i.e. above the upper sphincter of the esophagus). It is a false diverticulum (not involving all layers of the esophageal wall).

27. Answer is b (T3N2M0).
Ref: TNM Staging Atlas By Philip Rubin, John T Hansen, 2007 edition Pg 216, Fig 25.2.

- The prognosis of ***gastric carcinoma*** is related to the stage of the disease at the time of diagnosis and to the histologic grade of the carcinoma. Staging is by TNM staging:
- The T stage, representing the extent of penetration through the gastric wall, is categorized are as follows:
  - T0: Carcinoma in situ, intraepithelial tumor
  - T1: Tumor extension to submucosa
  - T2: Tumor extension to the muscularis propria or subserosa
  - T3: Tumor penetration of the ***serosa***
  - T4: Tumor invasion of the adjacent organs.
- The N stage, representing the number and site of draining lymph nodes involved, is categorized are as follows:
  - N0: No lymph nodes involved
  - N1: Metastases in 1–6 regional lymph nodes
  - N2: Metastases in ***7–15*** regional lymph nodes
  - N3: Metastases in > 15 regional lymph nodes.

- The M stage, representing the presence of metastases, is categorized are as follows:
  - M0: No distant metastases
  - M1: Distant metastases.

28. Answer is c (Choledochal cyst).
Ref: Harrison's, 17th edition Pg 1998.

- Cystic dilatation involving the free portion of the CBD is a choledochal cyst.
- ~50% of patients present with onset of symptoms ***after age 10***.
- Only one-third of patients show the ***classic triad of abdominal pain, jaundice and an abdominal mass***.
- Ultrasonographic detection of a cyst separate from the gallbladder should suggest the diagnosis of choledochal cyst, which can be confirmed by demonstrating the entrance of extrahepatic bile ducts into the cyst.
- Surgical treatment involves excision of the 'cyst' and biliary-enteric anastomosis (hepaticojejunostomy).
- There is increased risk for cholangiocarcinoma.

29. Answer is a (Primary sclerosing cholangitis).
Ref: Davidson's, 21st edition Pg 966.

- ***Primary sclerosing cholangitis*** is a cholestatic disease characterized by diffuse inflammation and fibrosis; it can involve entire biliary tree and leads to gradual obliteration of the bile ducts, and ultimately biliary cirrhosis.
- M:F = 2:1; age peak = 25–40 years.
- 2/3 of patients have associated ***ulcerative colitis***.
- Common symptoms include ***fatigue, intermittent jaundice, weight loss, right upper quadrant abdominal pain and pruritus***.
- Elevated ***p-ANCA, serum alkaline phosphatase, ANA and anti-smooth muscle antibodies*** may be found.

30. Answer is b (Invasive lobular carcinoma).
Ref: Contemporary Issues in Breast Cancer: A Nursing Perspective By Karen Hassey Dow, Pg 67, 2nd edition AND also see with answer below.

- ***Invasive (infiltrating) lobular carcinoma*** arises from the lobular and terminal duct epithelium, and accounts for approximately 5–10% of all breast cancers.
- ***Among all types of breast cancers, it is the most often multicentric*** representing multiple quadrants of the breast and it ***can be bilateral***.
- "Pathologically, ***breast cancer can be a multicentric and bilateral disease***. Bilateral disease is somewhat ***more common in patients with infiltrating lobular carcinoma***"-
  http//www.cancer.gov/cancertopics/pdq/treatment/breast/healthprofessional/page 1

31. Answer is a (*NOD2/CARD15* gene).
Ref: Harrison's, 17th edition Pg 1886, 2117.

→ **Direct quote:** "Three alleles of the ***NOD2/CARD15* gene** on chromosome 16 have been found in approximately half of patients with Crohn's disease" (Harrison's, 17th edition Pg 2118).

- *CARD15* (caspase-associated recruitment domain containing protein 15) on chromosome 16 is a cytosolic molecule that senses bacterial muramyl dipeptide and regulates intracellular signaling.
- *CARD15* protein is expressed by intestinal epithelial cells, including Paneth cells, monocytes, macrophages and dendritic cells.
- Loss-of-function mutations in *CARD15* are highly associated with CD and may account for up to 10% of CD risk.
- Homozygosity for these mutant alleles confers up to a 40-fold increased risk for fibrostenosing Crohn's disease, esp. of the ileum.

32. Answer is c (Ultrasound abdomen).
Ref: Fundamentals of Pediatric Surgery By Peter Mattei, 2011 edition Pg 341.

- An ***ultrasound*** performed by a skilled technician has a sensitivity and specificity approaching 100%, and is the ***diagnostic procedure of choice*** in diagnosis of ***infantile hypertrophic pyloric stenosis*** (HPS).
- Ultrasound features confirming HPS include:
  - A *pyloric muscle thickness of 4 mm*
  - A *channel length of 16 mm* or greater.

Also Know

♦ **Pyloric stenosis**	– Hypertrophy of pylorus → gastric outlet obstruction – Affects ***first-born male infants*** at ***2 weeks of life*** (range 2 week–4 month); – ***Non-bilious projectile vomiting, palpable olive shaped mass in epigastrium; hypochloremic, hypokalemic metabolic alkalosis*** secondary to emesis – *U/S is gold standard* – Treat by first correcting dehydration and metabolic abnormalities, surgery is ***pyloromyotomy (Ramstedt's)***

OBSTETRICS AND GYNECOLOGY

33. Answer is b (Extension).
Ref: Dutta's, 6th edition Pg 127.

→ ***Delivery of the head*** takes place by ***extension*** through 'couple of force' theory.

- The principal movement in normal labor is:
  - Engagement
  - Descent
  - Flexion
  - Internal rotation
  - Crowning
  - Extension (delivery of the head)
  - Restitution
  - External rotation
  - Expulsion of the trunk

34. Answer is d (Hypothyroidism).
Ref: Endometriosis: Current Management and Future Trends, Juan Gracia et al, 2010 edition Pg 125, Table 16-2.

- **Ovulation disorders in patients with endometriosis:**
  - ***Anovulation*** (15–25%)
  - ***Hyperprolactinemia***
  - Abnormal follicular genesis
  - Premature follicular rupture
  - ***Luteinized unruptured follicles***
  - Luteal phase defect.

→ **Note**: *Hypothyroidism, chronic fatigue syndrome and fibromyalgia* are more common in endometriosis patients—however not a direct association.

35. Answer is NONE; wrong options given according to revised answer key.
Ref: Dutta's, 6th edition Pg 193-202.

Complete versus Partial Hydatidiform Mole

Feature	Complete mole	Partial mole
Karyotype	46XX (85%), 46XY	Triploid, 69XXY or 69XYY
Villous edema	All villi	Some villi
Trophoblast proliferation	Diffuse, circumferential	Focal, slight
Atypia	Often present	Absent
Serum hCG	Elevated	Less elevated
hCG in tissue	++++	+
Behavior	2% choriocarcinoma	Rare choriocarcinoma
Fetal parts	Rarely seen	More common

36. Answer is a (Chlamydial infection).
Ref: Harrison's, 17th edition Pg 1073, 830.

- ***Perihepatitis*** or the ***Fitz-Hugh-Curtis syndrome,*** was originally described as a complication of gonococcal PID. Most cases are now known to be due to chlamydial salpingitis.
- The syndrome should be suspected whenever a young, sexually active woman presents with an illness resembling cholecystitis (fever and right-upper-quadrant pain of subacute or acute onset). Symptoms and signs of salpingitis may be minimal.
- Cultural and/or serologic ***evidence of C. trachomatis infection is found in three-quarters of women*** with this syndrome.
- In patients with ***Chlamydial salpingitis,*** serum titers of microimmunofluorescent antibody to *C. trachomatis* are typically much higher when perihepatitis is present than when it is absent.

37. Answer is a (Down syndrome).
Ref: Dutta's, 6th edition Pg 59.

- ↑ ***hCG levels*** = multiple pregnancy, hydatidiform mole or choriocarcinoma, Down syndrome fetus.

Also Know

- HCG is synthesized by the ***syncytiotrophoblast*** of the placenta and secreted into the blood of the mother and fetus.

Functions of hCG	Levels of hCG
▪ hCG ***maintains the corpus luteum*** (and thus progesterone) for the 1st trimester by acting like LH (otherwise no luteal cell stimulation and abortion results). In the 2nd and 3rd trimester, the placenta synthesizes its own estriol and progesterone, and the corpus luteum degenerates. ▪ hCG ***stimulate Leydig cells of male fetus*** to produce testosterone in conjunction with fetal pituitary gonadotropin—thus indirectly involved in development of male external genitalia. ▪ hCG has got ***immunosuppressant*** activity. ▪ hCG ***stimulates both adrenal and placental steroidogenesis; stimulates maternal thyroid*** because of thyrotropic activity.	▪ *t½* = 24 hours; ***doubling time*** = 1.4–2 days. ▪ By RIA it can be detected in the maternal serum or urine ***as early as 8–9 days following ovulation***—used to detect pregnancy. ▪ ***Maximum blood and urine levels*** seen ***between 60 and 70 days of pregnancy*** (100–200 IU/mL). ▪ ***Low levels*** of between 10 and 20 IU/mL at 100–130 days. ▪ ***Slight secondary peak*** at ***32 weeks.*** ▪ hCG ***disappears from the circulation within*** 2 ***weeks following delivery.***

38. Answer is b (Hypothalamic suppression).
Ref: Shaw's gynecology (Big), 4th edition Pg 885.

- Most cases of amenorrhea in vesicovaginal fistula are ***secondary amenorrhea*** due to ***hypothalamic dysfunction***.

39. Answer is b (Phenotypically male).
Ref: Shaw's gynecology (Big), 4th edition Pg 192.

Mayer-Rokitansky-Kuster-Hauser syndrome

- 46XX genotype
- Normal female phenotype
- Spontaneous development of secondary sexual characters, since ovarian tissue is present and functions normally
- Vaginal agenesis and absent uterus
- A/w renal tract abnormalities (15–40%) and skeletal abnormalities (10–20%)
- Ovarian estrogen normal, ovulation normal
- Vaginoplasty is usually required

40. Answer is a (Krukenberg's tumor).
Ref: Robbins pathology, 8th edition Pg 1052.

- ***Krukenberg's tumor***: Stomach malignancy that metastasizes to ovaries causing a ***mucin-secreting signet cell adenocarcinoma.*** It is a metastases to the ovary and is NOT primary ovarian tumor.

41. Answer is d (Inevitable abortion).
Ref: Dutta's, 6th edition Pg 163.

- ***Inevitable abortion***: It is the clinical type where the changes of pregnancy have progressed to s state from where continuation of pregnancy is impossible.
- Clinical features:
  - Increased ***vaginal bleeding***
  - Lower abdominal ***pain***
  - ***Dilated internal os*** of cervix through which products of conception are felt.

42. Answer is a (Pomeroy's method).
Ref: Dutta's, 6th edition Pg 557.

Female sterilization

Methods	Comments
Pomeroy's tubectomy	Convention laparotomy; segment of loop is excised; lowest failure rate of 0.1–0.5%
Madlener's technique	Convention laparotomy; loop is not excised; abandones due to high failure rate of 3%
Minilaparotomy (Mini-lap, Uchida)	Main method in National Family Planning Program
Laparoscopic sterilization	Silastic ring (Falope) or Filshie clip is used

PEDIATRICS

43. Answer is c (Ibuprofen).
Ref: OP GHai, 7th edition Pg 407.

- ***Indomethacin or Ibuprofen*** is often tried for ***pharmacological closure of PDA***.

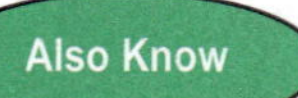

PGE (***alprostadil***) is used to keep PDA open, which is necessary in conditions mentioned below:

→ Patent Ductus Arteriosus ***(PDA) is beneficial*** (i.e. if closure is avoided) in:
  - Hypoplastic left heart
  - Pulmonary stenosis
  - Eisenmenger's physiology
  - TGA with intact ventricular septum
  - Interrupted aortic arch.

44. Answer is b *(Pseudomonas).*
Ref: Harrison's, 17th edition Pg 952.

- ***Pseudomonas aeruginosa*** is responsible for ***chronic infections of the airways*** associated with a number of underlying or predisposing conditions—most commonly ***Cystic Fibrosis*** in Caucasian populations.
- ***Burkholderia cepacia*** is also a common cause of respiratory infection in cystic fibrosis.

45. Answer is d (Hay fever, sickle cell anemia and tuberculosis are contraindications for vaccination).
Ref: Foundations of Community Medicine, Dhaar By 2nd edition Pg 374; Park, 20th edition Pg 98.

Contraindications/Precautions with/To immunization

- Live vaccines CI in pregnancy
- Live vaccines CI in immunodeficiency
- Vaccination after administration of immunoglobulin's is CI for atleast 3 months.
- Inactivated vaccines should not be given, if there has been significant reaction to previous dose-toxigenic reaction.
- Hay fever, sickle cell anemia and TB are relative contraindications sometimes.

46. Answer is b (Rabies).
Ref: Harrison's, 17th edition Pg 1222.

- The ***limbic system*** is a complex set of structures that lies on both sides of the thalamus, just under the cerebrum. It includes the ***hypothalamus, the hippocampus, the amygdala*** and several other nearby areas.
- ***Negri bodies*** are eosinophilic cytoplasmic inclusions in brain neurons and are composed of randomly oriented rabies virus nucleocapsids embedded in an amorphous substance or matrix. These inclusions occur in a minority of infected cells, are *most commonly present in Purkinje cells of the cerebellum and in pyramidal cells in the* ***hippocampus*** and are less frequently seen in cortical neurons and in the brainstem.
- For obscure reasons, Negri bodies are rarely produced in infections caused by laboratory variants of rabies virus, whereas wild, or 'street', rabies infection results in Negri bodies in ~80% of cases. Thus, the absence of Negri bodies does not exclude the diagnosis.

47. Answer is b (Height for age).
Ref: Park, 20th edition Pg Nutrition Assessment: A Comprehensive Guide for Planning Intervention By Margaret D Simko, Catherine Cowell, Judith A Gilbride, 1995 edition Pg 94.

Anthropometric indicators in children

Weight for height	▪ Acute undernutrition generally characterized by low weight for height has been termed *wasting*. ▪ Conversely, overnutrition or *obesity* is characterized by high weight for height. This is an indicator of present nutritional status.
Height for age	▪ This is a measure of linear growth. Frequent periods of acute food deprivation or infection or prolonged period of inadequate food intake—especially during the rapid growing years

	(esp, first 2 years of life) may cause measurable growth retardation—the result is a child who is low in height for age—called *stunting*. ▪ This is an ***indicator of long term nutritional adequacy***.
Weight for age	▪ Does NOT distinguish between present and long-term malnutrition. ▪ Useful in *children under 1 year of age* in whom length measurement may not be accurate.

48. Answer is a (Dubin-Johnson syndrome).
Ref: Davidson's, 21st edition Pg 932, Box 23.10.

Jaundice

Hyperbilirubinemia	Cause	Examples
Unconjugated (indirect)	↑ bilirubin production	Hemolytic anemia Disorders of erythropoiesis Internal hemorrhage resorption
	Impaired conjugation	Physiologic jaundice of newborn Deficiency of glucuronosyltransferase (e.g. ***Gilbert disease, Crigler-Najjar syndrome***) Hepatocellular disease (e.g. cirrhosis, hepatitis)
Conjugated (direct)	↓ hepatic bilirubin excretion	Impaired bilirubin transport (e.g. ***Dubin-Johnson syndrome, Rotor syndrome***) Hepatocellular disease (e.g. cirrhosis, hepatitis) Drug impairment
	Extrahepatic biliary obstruction	Intrahepatic bile duct disease (e.g. PBC, PSC) Gallstone obstruction of bile ducts (i.e. choledocholithiasis) Pancreatic or biliary cancer Biliary atresia

Key: PBC, primary biliary cirrhosis; PSC, primary sclerosing cholangitis.

49. Answer is b (Eisenmenger's syndrome).
Ref: Davidson's, 21st edition Pg 630.

- Persistently raised pulmonary blood flow (e.g. with left to right shunt) causes increased pulmonary resistance followed by pulmonary hypertension. Progressive changes including obliteration of distal vessels occur and are irreversible. Central cyanosis and digital clubbing occur.
- The CXR shows enlarged central pulmonary arteries and peripheral 'pruning' of pulmonary vessels. ECG shows RVH.
- If severe pulmonary hypertension develops, a left-to-right shunt may ***reverse resulting in right-to-left shunt*** and marked cyanosis (***Eisenmenger's syndrome***), which may be more apparent in the feet and toes than in upper part of the body: *differential cyanosis*. This is MC with large VSD or PDA than with ASD.
- Patients with Eisenmenger's syndrome are at particular risk from abrupt changes in afterload that exacerbate right-to-left shunting such as vasodilation, anesthesia and pregnancy.

50. Answer is d (Hereditary motor—sensory neuropathy).
Ref: Davidson's, 21st edition Pg 53.

Diseases a/w triplet and other repeat sequences	
Coding repeat expansion	**Non-coding repeat expansion**
– Huntington's disease	– Myotonic dystrophy
– Spinocerebellar ataxia types (1, 2, 3, 6, 7)	– Friedrich's ataxia
– Dentatorubral pallidoluysian atrophy	– Progressive myoclonic epilepsy
– Machado-Joseph disease	– Fragile X mental retardation (XLD)
– Spinobulbar muscular atrophy (XLR)	– Fragile site mental retardation 2 (XLR)

51. Answer is b (Thyroid hormone resistance).
Ref: Child and adolescent psychiatry, Sandra Sexon, 2nd edition Pg 97.

- Medical conditions associated with attention deficit hyperactivity disorder (ADHD) like conditions include:
  - Increased serum lead level
  - ***Thyroid hormone resistance*** and
  - Seizure disorder.

Note: "Earlier studies have found the prevalence of thyroid abnormalities to be higher in children with ADHD (Weiss et al, 1993) and that ADHD was strongly a/w generalized resistance to thyroid hormone (Hauser et al, 1993). Subsequent research failed to find evidence for generalized resistance to thyroid hormone (Spencer et al, 1995) or any strong correlation between thyroid hormone concentrations and symptoms of hyperactivity and inattention (Stein and Weiss, 2003). Clinically, routine estimation of thyroid functions are not warranted in individuals with ADHD" = However, the answer given in the revised key is b (Thyroid Hormone Resistance)—and that is selected.

All About

ATTENTION DEFICIT HYPERACTIVITY DISORDER (HYPERKINETIC SYNDROME)

Patient Example: A 7-year-old boy frequently gets into trouble at school because he interrupts the teacher, disturbs the other students and cannot seem to sit still in class

Cardinal Features and Treatment

- Described first by ***Heinrich Hoff***, also called ***Strauss syndrome***.
- Characterized by an **early onset** (***usually 3–8 years***) of ***short attention span, distractibility, overactivity, impulsivity, clumsiness and language delay, which lasts longer than 6 months***.
- MC in ***boys***, present in ***two or more settings (school, home, work)*** and is often ***a/w antisocial behavior/conduct disorder***; *50% continue to have ADHD into adulthood.*
- Etiology: Genetic loading, poverty, ***parental alcohol abuse***, dietary constituents (***lead, tartrazine***) and ***exposure to tranquilisers (barbiturates)***.
- **Treatment** (CNS stimulants) is given *only when severe* and includes the drug of choice ***methylphenidate***; others like pemoline and dextroamphetamine are also tried.
- ***Adverse effects*** of CNS stimulants in children include failure to gain weight and inhibition of growth. ***Barbiturates are contraindicated*** as they ***increase hyperactivity.***
- ***Pemoline and imipramine*** should *NOT be given before 6 years of age.*

52. Answer is c (9 months).
Ref: OP Ghai, 7th edition Pg 29, Table 2.2.

- ***Bidextrous*** reach: ***4 months***, reaching out for objects with both hands.
- ***Unidextrous*** reach: ***6 months***, reaching out for objects with one hand, transfers objects.

"Nearest answer in the options given is 9 months."

53. Answer is d (Rhinosinusitis).
Ref: Davidson's, 21st edition Pg 323, 680.

- ***Respiratory syncytial virus causes:***
  - Bronchiolitis
  - Pneumonia
  - Croup
  - Upper respiratory tract disease (coryza, common cold)

ORTHOPEDICS

54. Answer is a, c (Manipulation by the mother, Manipulation and casts) — verified with revised answer key — both a, c are given.

Ref: John Ebenezer's, 4th edition Pg 507; Maheshwari, 4th edition Pg 207.

- In a ***newborn***, the ***mother is taught to manipulate the foot*** after every feed. Minor deformities are corrected by this method alone — *Maheshwari, 4th edition Pg 207.*
- Conservative management is the treatment of choice in infants less than 6 months of age. For ***first 6 weeks of life*** — weekly ***serial manipulation of the deformities and above knee casting*** for the first 6 weeks of life. Later it is done every fortnight until correction is achieved. ***Manipulation by mother is NOT sufficient*** — *John Ebenezer's, 4th edition Pg 507.*

Comment: *"That explains why both options a and c are given in the revised answer key".*

55. Answer is c (Congenital coxa vara).

Ref: Maheshwari's, 4th edition Pg 313; (http://www.jbjs.org/article.aspx?Volume 31 and Pg 115 - Full text article about congenital coxa vara – from 1946! – but still good enough to answer this MCQ).

- Congenital coxa vara is a term used to describe a reduced angle between the neck and shaft of femur — resulting from some unknown growth anomaly at upper end of femoral epiphysis.
- Noticed as a ***painless limp*** in a child who has just started walking.
- O/E, ***abduction and internal rotation of the hip are limited*** and the ***leg is short***.
- Epiphyseal plate may be too vertical.
- There maybe a separate triangle of bone in the inferior portion of the metaphysis called ***Fairbank's triangle***.
- ***Trendelenburg sign is positive*** (in coxa valga also); ***NO*** telescoping
- Treatment is by ***subtrochanteric corrective osteotomy***.

56. Answer is c (3 hours).

Ref: Apley, 8th edition Pg 256; Trauma manual By Ernest Eugene Moore, David V Feliciano, Kenneth L Mattox, 4th edition Pg 356.

- ***Peripheral nerves*** can withstand ***ischemia up to 3 hours***.

57. Answer is b (Intervertebral disk).

Ref: Maheshwari's, 4th edition Pg 180.

- TB of spine is also called ***Pott's disease***
- ***Spine is MC site of skeletal TB***
- Bacilli reach spine through paravertebral (*Batson's*) plexus; ***Paradiscal type*** is MC (***Infection starts in the intervertebral disk***)
- MC symptom is ***back pain***; on X-ray reduction of disk space is ***earliest sign***
- Anterior type of vertebral TB may show erosion of anterior part of the body, much the same as that in aneurysm of aorta — ***aneurysmal sign***
- TB spine with neurological involvement is ***Pott's paraplegia*** — MC in ***thoracic spine***.

Also Know

Summary of Musculoskeletal TB

Tissue	Disease	Remarks
Bone		
1. Long bone	**TB osteomyelitis**	*Tibia* commonly affected; lots of lytic lesions, minimal newbone formation unlike pyogenic osteomyelitis; thin watery discharge; multiple sinuses

2. **Short bone (phalanges)**	**TB dactylitis**	Also called ***spina ventosa***
3. **Spine**	**TB spondylitis**	Also called ***Pott's disease—see above***
Joints		
1. **Arthritis**	**TB arthritis**	***Hip joint*** commonly affected; MC in children/adolescents; pain referred to knee severe at night (***night cries***); ***true shortening*** of lower limb present, ***Thomas test*** used to detect fixed flexion deformity of hip Shoulder joint TB may not produce any pus/cold abscess—***'Caries sicca'***
2. **Synovium**	**Synovial TB**	***Knee joint*** commonly affected; begins in synovium; long standing TB knee causes ***triple subluxation*** (flexion of knee, posterior subluxation and external rotation of tibia); ***X-ray*** essentially ***normal***
Others		
1. **Tendon (synovium)**	**TB tenosynovitis**	***Compound palmar ganglion*** (of flexor tendons at wrist, ***melon seed bodies*** may be seen)
2. **Bursae**	**TB bursitis**	Trochanteric bursitis

OPHTHALMOLOGY AND ENT

58. Answer is b (Atopic dermatitis).
Ref: Parson's diseases of the eye, 250, Table 18.2.

Some distinct cataracts

Type of cataract	Comment
❖ **Oil drop cataract**	*Galactosemia*
❖ **Diabetic cataract**	In diabetes mellitus, in the lens *glucose is converted to sorbitol by aldose reductase* → diabetic cataract; aldose reductase inhibitors are being studied to prevent diabetic cataract
❖ **Blue dot cataract**	*MC Congenital cataract*; no significant visual symptoms
❖ **Radiation cataract**	Posterior subcapsular cataract
❖ **Steroid induced cataract**	Posterior subcapsular cataract
❖ **Sunflower cataract**	*Chalcosis* (excess copper accumulation in lens)
❖ **Traumatic cataract**	*Rosette cataract*, *Vossius ring* (pigments on anterior lens capsule due to *constricted pupil* striking lens during blunt trauma)
❖ **After Cataract**	Posterior capsule opacification, *Elschnig's pearls*, *Soemmering's ring*
❖ **Anterior Lenticonus**	**AL**port's syndrome
❖ **Complicated cataract**	Due to any disease process in eye (e.g. Uveitis), Polychromatic luster, Bread crumb appearance
❖ **Christmas tree cataract**	Myotonic dystrophy
❖ **Glass blowers cataract**	Heat cataract, Infrared rays
❖ **Posterior subcapsular cataract**	Even in the early stages, vision is usually impaired owing to the position of the opacity near the *nodal point of the eye*; more blurring in bright sunlight and headlights of oncoming cars
❖ **Nuclear cataract**	*'Second sight'* due to induced myopia—person who was using glasses to read earlier will be able to read better without glasses
❖ **Posterior polar**	Early visual impairment, since located at nodal point of the eye; high risk of posterior capsule rupture during surgery

❖ **Zonular (lamellar) cataract**	*Hypocalcemia, Riders* are seen
❖ **Snowflake cataract**	*Diabetes mellitus*
❖ **Rubella cataract**	Congenital nuclear cataract with necrosis of lens nucleus

59. Answer is c (*Staphylococcus aureus*).
Ref: Parson's, 20th edition Pg 187; Kanski, 6th edition Pg 254; Cornea and External Eye Disease, Volume 2 By Thomas Reinhard, Frank Larkin, Vol 2, Pg 22; Infectious Diseases in 30 days By Frederick S Southwick, Pg 157.

Bacteria that ***invade intact corneal epithelium*** are:

- *Neisseria*
- *Corynebacterium*
- *Listeria, Shigella* and
- *H. influenzae*

60. Answer is b (Searches for quiet sounds made out of sight).
Ref: Dhingra's TB of ENT, 5th edition Pg 131.

- *Distraction techniques* are used in children 6–7 months of age.
- The child at this age turns the head to locate the source of sound.
- In this test, the child is seated on his mother's lap; an assistant distracts the child's attention, while the examiner produces a sound from behind or from one side to see if the child tries to locate it.

61. Answer is d (Acoustic neuroma).
Ref: Dhingra's TB of ENT, 5th edition Pg 123.

Acoustic Neuroma (Vestibular Schwannoma)

Origin
- Benign slow growing tumor that arises from the neurilemmal sheath of the ***superior Vestibular N.***
- ***MC (80%) of all CPA angle tumors***; age group 40–60 years.

Clinically
- Early symptom is ***unilateral sensorineural deafness with tinnitus.***
- In advanced cases CN5 is involved first (↓ corneal sensation and reflex, MC presenting sign), followed by CN7 and CN3.
- ***Hitzelberger's sign***: hypoesthesia of posterior meatal wall because of facial nerve (CN7) involvement.

Investigations
- X-ray of internal auditory meatus may show expansion and erosion of canal.
- Audiometry shows dip in audiogram at 4,000 Hz.
- *Speech discrimination is poor.*
- ***Roll over phenomenon*** is present.
- *Recruitment absent.*
- Threshold tone decay test shows retrocochlear type of lesion.
- ***BERA*** (Brainstem evoked response audiometry) is preferred investigation.
- ***MRI is gold standard*** for imaging the tumor.

Treatment
- ***Stereotactic radiosurgery or Gamma knife.***

About the other options

- Secretory otitis media causes conductive deafness.
- Vestibular neuronitis shows sudden severe vertigo with NO cochlear symptoms.
- BPPV is characterized by vertigo, when the head is placed in a certain critical position.

62. Answer is b (A significantly reduced electroretinogram).
Ref: Parson's diseases of the eye, 20th edition Pg 309.

- The classical features of ***retinitis pigmentosa*** (RP) are:
  - Waxy pallor of optic disk
  - Attenuated arterioles
  - Bone spicule pigmentation.
- The ***ERG in RP is markedly subnormal or completely extinguished early in the disease*** before subjective symptoms or objective signs appear, a point of great prognostic importance in assessing the future of a young child in an affected family.

63. Answer is d (Congenital hereditary endothelial dystrophy).
Ref: Parson's diseases of the eye, 20th edition Pg 185.

Prominent corneal nerves seen in

Systemic conditions	Ocular conditions
Leprosy	Acanthamoeba keratitis
MEN 2b	Keratoconus
Neurofibromatosis	Fuch's endothelial dystrophy
Refsum's disease	Congenital glaucoma
Riley-Day syndrome	Corneal edema

64. Answer is c (Septal abscess).
Ref: Dhingra's ENT textbook, 5th edition Pg 166.

- ***Septal abscess*** MC results from infection of septal hematoma.
- There is ***severe bilateral nasal obstruction with pain and tenderness*** over the bridge of the nose.
- ***Fever, chills and frontal headache*** may be present.
- Abscess should be ***drained*** as early as possible; systemic antibiotics for 10 days.

65. Answer is d (Enlarged cornea).
Ref: Parson's diseases of the eye, 20th edition Pg 284.

- ***Congenital glaucoma*** is usually detected by the parents ***when the affected eye is noted to enlarge or the cornea becomes hazy***.
- In ***buphthalmos*** deep cupping may be seen. But it is not the presenting feature.
- *Field defects* may not be made out in infants and young children, since they are unable to perform the visual fields test.
- *High IOP* is not the presenting feature of buphthalmos since the scleral stretching and enlarging globe may mask the increased IOP.

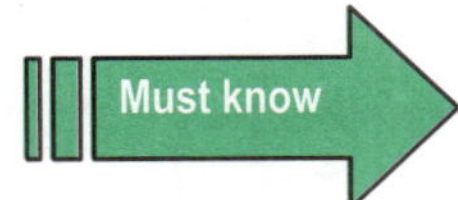

Congenital Glaucoma

Etiopathogenesis	– ***MC Boys, MC Bilateral***, AR, chromosome 2. – Corneal diameter more than ***12 mm*** within the 1st year is always pathological. – Pathology: ***Trabeculodysgenesis***? *Barkan's membrane* covering angle of eye.

Clinically	– Watering and photophobia; Hazy cornea, Large cornea – *Buphthalmos=Ox eye (occurs only if age < 3 years)* – **H**aab's striae (**H**orizontal breaks in Descemet's membrane), increased IOP – progressive myopia due to globe enlargement; subluxated lens.
Treatment	– Mainly surgical—Goniotomy; trabeculotomy +/- trabeculectomy (*Brimonidine* can cause *apnea in children* < *6 years*).

66. Answer is c (Labyrinthine lesion).
Ref: Harrison's, 17th edition Pg 195.

Downbeat nystagmus	Upbeat nystagmus
▪ Lesions near the craniocervical junction (Chiari malformation, basilar invagination) ▪ Brainstem or cerebellar stroke ▪ Lithium or anticonvulsant intoxication ▪ Alcoholism ▪ Multiple sclerosis	▪ Due to damage to the pontine tegmentum, from stroke, demyelination or tumor

Note: ***Vestibular nystagmus*** results from dysfunction of the labyrinth (Meniere's disease), vestibular nerve or vestibular nucleus in the brainstem.

67. Answer is c (Iris epithelium).
Ref: Parson's diseases of the eye, 20th edition Pg 5.

Embryology of Ocular Structures

Surface ectoderm	Mesoderm	Neural ectoderm
◆ Epithelium of ***Conjunctiva***, ***cornea***, crystalline ***lens*** and glands (Meibomian, lacrimal, Zeis, Moll) ◆ Skin of eyelids and eyelashes	◆ Corneal stroma and endothelium ◆ Iris stroma ◆ Ciliary muscles and choroids ◆ Extraocular muscles ◆ Sclera ◆ Bony orbit ◆ Vitreous	◆ Retina and retinal pigment epithelium ◆ ***Epithelium of Iris*** and Ciliary body ◆ Optic Nerve ◆ Sphincter and Dilator pupillae ◆ Melanocytes

- Eyelids and Zonules: Both from surface ectoderm and mesoderm
- Bruchs membrane: Neural ectoderm and mesoderm

68. Answer is b (Central retinal vein occlusion).
Ref: Parson's diseases of the eye, 20th edition Pg 303, Fig 20.18.

- In ***central retinal vein occlusion (CRVO)***, all the veins of the retina become enormously engorged with blood and extremely tortuous and the ***retina is covered with extensive hemorrhages***.
- Vision is very impaired—painless loss of vision.
- ***Neovascular glaucoma*** may ensue in 3 months' time (*'100 day glaucoma'*).

69. Answer is a (Rods and cones).
Ref: Parson's diseases of the eye, 21st edition Pg 107, 110.

Electroretinogram

- 'a' wave = photoreceptor (rods and cones) activity
- 'b' wave = response of bipolar cells
- 'c' wave = generated by retinal pigment epithelium and related to retinal metabolism

DERMATOLOGY, ANESTHESIOLOGY, RADIOLOGY AND PSYCHIATRY

70. Answer is a (Lepromatous leprosy).
Ref: Harrison's, 17th edition Pg 1023.

Direct quote: "Erythema nodosum leprosum (ENL) occurs exclusively in patients near the lepromatous end of the leprosy spectrum (BL-LL), affecting nearly 50% of this group."

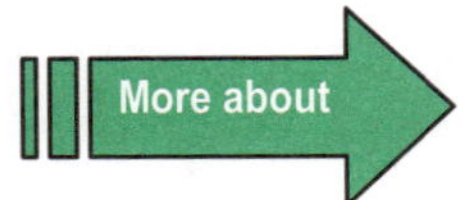

Lepra reactions

Lepra reaction	Type 1 (Reversal reaction)	Type 2 (Erythema nodosum leprosum)
Mechanism	***Cell mediated*** hypersensitivity	***Immune complexes*** Arthus phenomenon
Seen in	***BT*** (more common), BB, BL patients	***LL and BL*** patients, most often in the latter half of the initial year of treatment
Clinical features	***Painful tender nerves***, loss of function Swollen and erythematous skin lesions and new lesions may appear, rarely fever	Tender, inflamed ***subcutaneous nodules***, may ulcerate; *Fever, arthralgia, iritis, orchitis*
Management	Mild: Aspirin Severe: Glucocorticoids	Mild: Aspirin Severe: Glucocorticoids Severe and recurrent/unresponsive: Thalidomide

71. Answer is b *(Pseudomonas aeruginosa).*
Ref: Harrison's, 17th edition Pg 126, 764.

Ecthyma gangrenosum

- *Caused by P. aeruginosa.*
- Indurated plaque evolving into hemorrhagic bulla or pustule that sloughs, resulting in eschar formation; erythematous halo; most common in axillary, groin, perianal regions.
- Usually affects neutropenic patients; occurs in up to 28% of individuals with *Pseudomonas* bacteremia.

72. Answer is d (Parkinson disease).
Ref: Harrison's, 17th edition Pg 315.

- ***Seborrheic dermatitis*** is a common, chronic disorder, characterized by *greasy scales overlying erythematous patches* or plaques.
- Induration and scales are generally ***less prominent*** than in psoriasis.
- *Most common location is in the scalp,* where it may be recognized as severe dandruff; scaling of the external auditory canal is common; additionally, the postauricular areas often become macerated and tender.
- Seborrheic dermatitis may also develop in the central chest, axilla, groin, submammary folds and gluteal cleft. Rarely, it may cause a widespread generalized dermatitis. Pruritus is variable.
- Seborrheic dermatitis may be evident within the first few weeks of life and within this context it occurs in the scalp ('***cradle cap***'), face or groin.

- Although it is frequently seen in patients with ***Parkinson disease,*** in those who have had ***cerebrovascular accidents*** and in those with ***HIV infection,*** the vast majority of individuals with seborrheic dermatitis have no underlying disorder.

73. Answer is d (Lupus vulgaris).
Ref: Dermatology Terminology By Herbert B Allen, Pg 47, Fig 3.8.

Lupus vulgaris

- ***MC* form of skin TB**; seen in *previously infected/sensitized persons;* ***MC*** **in** ***females***; often a/w *underlying active TB* in the lung or lymph nodes.
- *MC* in ***head and neck*** and are red-brown plaques; ***'apple-jelly nodules'*** on diascopy; ***scarring and SCC*** can develop within the plaques.
- Cartilage (nose, ears) within the affected area is progressively destroyed **(*lupus vorax*)**; *bone usually is spared.*
- Culture or PCR analysis of the lesions should be done because it is rare for the acid-fast stain to show bacilli within the granulomas.

74. Answer is c (Minimum alveolar concentration).
Ref: KD Tripathi, 6th edition Pg 365.

Minimum Alveolar Concentration (MAC)

❖ **Definition**
– MAC is a measure of the ***minimum alveolar concentration*** of an inhalational agent that has to be achieved ***to prevent movement in 50% of subjects following a surgical stimulus***. A high alveolar concentration will need to be achieved for agents that have low potency (desflurane) compared with those that have a high potency (halothane). – The anesthetic effects of inhalational agents are additive and therefore two values of MAC are often quoted—the value in oxygen and the value when administered with a certain percentage of nitrous oxide, which will clearly be less. – An alternative method of expressing the potency of inhalational agents is as **the alveolar concentration, which prevents movement in response to surgery in 95% of patients—the** ***AD95***. This gives values approximately 1.5 times the MAC value and is probably a more relevant figure for clinical anesthesia.
❖ **↓ MAC due to**
– Increasing age, hypothermia, hypothyroidism and concurrent use of opioids.
❖ **↑ MAC due to**
– Infants, patients with pyrexia and in chronic drug abusers.

MAC of some inhaled anesthetics

- Nitrous oxide = 105% (least potent)
- Isoflurane = 1.2%
- Sevoflurane = 2%
- Desflurane = 6%
- Halothane = 0.7% (most potent)

75. Answer is c (3).
Ref: KD Tripathi, 6th edition Pg 367.

Stages of Anesthesia (Guedel)

Stage I: Stage of Analgesia	Preliminary excitement until voluntary control is lost. Because hearing is the last sense to be lost, the conversation of operating room staff should be guarded during this stage.

Stage II: Stage of Delirium	Loss of voluntary control.
Stage III: Stage of Surgical Anesthesia	Entire relaxation, no muscular rigidity and deep regular breathing.
Stage IV: Stage of Respiratory Paralysis	

76. Answer is b (CSF leak from dura).

Ref: Pocket Anesthesia By Richard D Urman, Jesse M Ehrenfel, Pg 6-3, 2009 edition LWW.

Postspinal headache

- Seen as a complication of spinal anesthesia (dural puncture).
- Cause: ***CSF leaking from a dural puncture*** would lead to a loss of CSF pressure in the spine and a loss of buoyancy supporting the brain. When the patient assumes an upright posture, the brain sags and tension on the meninges, and other intracranial structures creates the pain seen with postdural puncture (postspinal) headache.
- Usually ***occipital***, relieved on lying down, lasting for ***7–10 days***.
- Prophylactic: Use small bore needle, adequate hydration, avoid sitting position postoperatively.
- Curative: Lie supine, analgesia, abdominal binder, epidural blood patch, caffeine.

77. Answer is a (Basilar skull fracture).

Ref: Principles of airway management, Brendan TF et al, 4th edition Pg 318-19.

Contraindication to nasotracheal intubation are:

- Bleeding disturbances (coagulopathies or on anticoagulants)
- Nasal pathology (epistaxis, deviated septum, polyps, infections)
- Basal skull fractures
- Midfacial fractures including maxillofacial fractures
- In patients with apnea
- CFS leakage
- Chronic sinusitis
- Nasal stenosis

78. Answer is b (Nitrous oxide).

Ref: KD Tripathi, 6th edition Pg 371.

- ***Nitrous oxide diffuses more rapidly into air-filled cavities*** than any nitrogen can escape *causing either a rise in pressure (e.g. in the middle ear) or an increase in volume (e.g. within the gut of an air embolism).*
- ***Contraindicated in pneumothorax*** and in patients who have been scuba diving within the previous 24 hours due to the potential for decompression sickness.

Also Know

All About Nitrous Oxide

- ***Pharmacology***
  - First ***prepared by Priestley*** *in* 1772 and was called ***'laughing gas'***; first used as an anesthetic agent in **1845 by Horace Wells.**
  - It is a colorless, sweet-smelling, non-irritant gas; ***good analgesic*** *BUT* ***weak anesthetic*** with an *MAC of 105.*
  - Maximum safe concentration that can be administered without the risk of hypoxia is ***approximately 70%.***
  - ***Diffusion hypoxia or 'Fink effect'***: At the end of anesthesia, rapid excretion of nitrous oxide into the alveoli dilutes any oxygen present. This can be overcome by increasing the inspired oxygen concentration during recovery.
  - ***Poynting effect***: Certain mixtures of nitrous oxide and oxygen will remain in the gaseous phase at pressures, and temperatures, at which, nitrous oxide by itself would normally be liquid.

- *Second gas effect* is significant, when N_2O is given at 70–80% concentration. However this effect accounts for only a small increase in the concentration of accompanying volatile anesthetic.
- Nitrous oxide is premixed with oxygen as a 50%: 50% mixture called ***'Entonox'***, which is widely used analgesic in obstetrics.

◆ *Other Systemic Effects*
- ***Methemoglobinemia***, mainly due to its impurities (nitric oxide and nitrogen dioxide).
- ***Megaloblastic anemia*** because nitrous oxide inhibits methionine synthase; also it may cause bone marrow suppression.
- Reduces bowel motility, increases ICT, causes nausea and vomiting.

79. Answer is d (Virchow's sign).
Ref: Cardiopulmonary imaging By Ella A Kazerooni, Barry H Gross, Pg 583; Radiology of chest diseases By Sebastian Lange, Geraldine Walsh (FRCR), Pg 188.

Chest X-ray signs in pulmonary embolism

Embolism without Infarction (90%)	Embolism with Infarction (10%)
▪ ***Normal chest*** (most common!); Platelike atelectasis; Segmental/lobar consolidation; Pleural effusion	▪ ***Hampton hump*** (a peripheral, pleural-based, wedge-shaped density above the diaphragm)
▪ ***Westermark sign*** (focal oligemia in the embolized zone)	▪ Pleural effusion (50%)
▪ ***'Knuckle' sign*** (abrupt tapering off of an occluded vessel distally)	▪ ***'Melting' sign*** (regression of consolidation from periphery to center; appears within days to weeks)
▪ Enlarged right descending pulmonary artery (***Pall's sign***)	▪ ***Fleischner*** lines
▪ Local widening of artery by impacted embolus	▪ Platelike atelectasis; cardiomegaly/CHF; Elevated hemidiaphragm; no air bronchogram

80. Answer is c (Renal osteodystrophy).
Ref: Musculoskeletal imaging: a teaching file By Felix S Chew, Catherine C Roberts, Anand P Lalaji, 2nd edition Pg 177, Fig 3.26.

✈ 'Rugger jersey' spine = seen in **R**enal **O**steodystrophy, osteo**PET**rosis

Also Know

➤ **'Ivory' vertebrae** = **L**ymphoma (Hodgkin's), **I**nfection, **M**etastases, **P**aget's disease.
➤ **'Codfish' vertebrae** = **O**steoporosis, **O**steomalacia, **S**ickle cell disease.
➤ **'Bullet shaped' vertebrae** = **H**urler's disease, **A**chondroplasia, **M**orquio disease.

81. Answer is c (Discrete bulge of the left cardiac margin below the pulmonary bay).
Ref: Chest radiology: A resident's manual By J Kirchner, 2011 edition Pg 1-42.

Left atrial enlargement is characterized by following features on PA chest X-ray
✈ Visualization of an atrial double shadow
✈ ***Double 'right heart border' sign***
✈ Protrusion in the pulmonary bay (***enlarged left atrial appendage***)
✈ ***Splaying of the carina*** resulting from ***cranial displacement of left main bronchus***
✈ Protrusion of the right cardiac border
✈ Displacement of the esophagus (barium swallow).

82. Answer is c (Silver).
Ref: Understanding Radiography By Stephen H Hiss, 4th edition Pg 37.

- The ***silver bromide grain*** is the heart of the radiographic image.
- These grains when exposed to light/X-rays have the ability to change their composition during film processing and become tiny particles of ***black metallic silver***.
- In fact the final radiograph with all its details is an accumulation of specks of black metallic silver, which have been fused to the film's base.
- The clustering of these black metallic silver particles on the film's base as the film is hung on an illuminator produces patterns of ***clear and dark areas***, which in aggregate—reveal visual patterns, which recognize as various body tissues or structures.

83. Answer is a (Clozapine).

Ref: The American Psychiatric Publishing Board Review Guide for Psychiatry, 2009 edition Pg 630.

- ***Clozapine*** is the ***ONLY antipsychotic*** that has received ***FDA approval*** for the ***treatment of recurring suicidal behavior*** in patients with schizophrenia and schizoaffective disorder.

84. Answer is a (Caffeine).

Ref: Restless legs syndrome: coping with your sleepless nights, Mark JB et al, 2006 edition Pg 48.

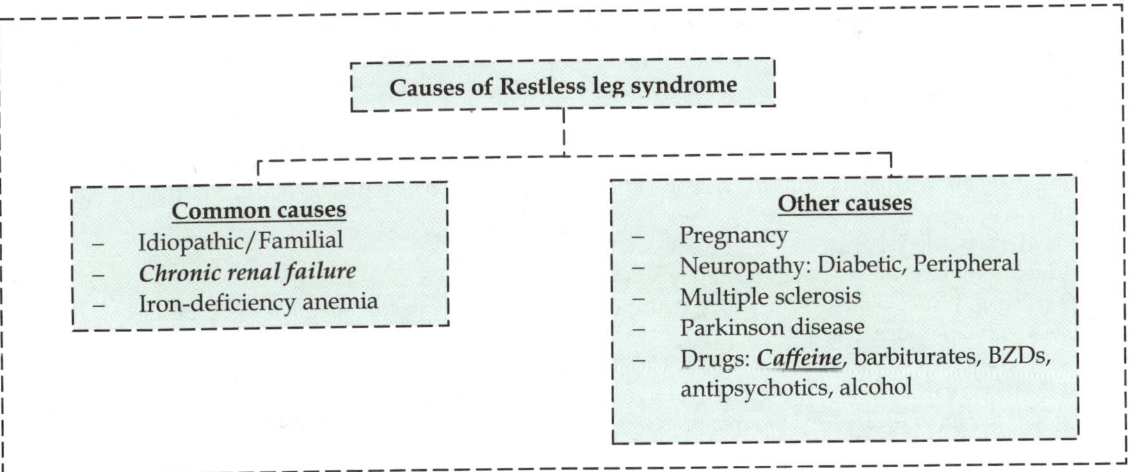

85. Answer is d (Depressed mood for a minimum 2 weeks duration).

Ref: Harrison's, 17th edition Pg 2716, Table 386-9.

Criteria for Major Depression

A. Five (or more) of the following symptoms have been present during the ***same 2-week period*** and represent a change from previous functioning; at least one of the symptoms is either (1) depressed mood or (2) loss of interest or pleasure. **Note:** Do not include symptoms that are clearly due to a general medical condition or mood-incongruent delusions, or hallucinations.

1. Depressed mood most of the day, nearly every day, as indicated by either subjective report (e.g. feels sad or empty) or observation made by others (e.g. appears tearfully sad).
2. Markedly diminished interest or pleasure in all, or almost all, activities most of the day, nearly every day (as indicated by either subjective account or observation made by others).
3. Significant weight loss when not dieting or weight gain (e.g. a change of > 5% of body weight in a month) or decrease, or increase in appetite nearly every day.
4. Insomnia or hypersomnia nearly every day.
5. Psychomotor agitation or retardation nearly every day (observable by others, not merely subjective feelings of restlessness or being slowed down).
6. Fatigue or loss of energy nearly every day.

7. Feelings of worthlessness or excessive or inappropriate guilt (which may be delusional) nearly every day (not merely self-reproach or guilt about being sick).
8. Diminished ability to think or concentrate or indecisiveness, nearly every day (either by subjective account or as observed by others).
9. Recurrent thoughts of death (not just fear of dying), recurrent suicidal ideation without a specific plan or a suicide attempt, or a specific plan for committing suicide.

B. The symptoms do NOT meet criteria for a mixed episode.
C. The symptoms cause clinically significant distress or impairment in social and occupational functioning.
D. The symptoms are NOT due to the direct physiologic effects of a substance (e.g. a drug of abuse, a medication) or a general medical condition (e.g. hypothyroidism).
E. The symptoms are NOT better accounted for by bereavement, i.e. after the loss of a loved one, the symptoms persist for > 2 months or are characterized by marked functional impairment, morbid preoccupation with worthlessness, suicidal ideation, psychotic symptoms or psychomotor retardation.

86. Answer is b (They are present in 15–20% of patients attending medical clinics).
Ref: Niraj Ahuja's psychiatry textbook, 20th edition Pg 89-91; Harrison's, 17th edition Pg 2710.

- Anxiety is the commonest psychiatric symptom in clinical practice and anxiety disorders are one of the ***commonest psychiatric disorders*** in general population. They are present in ***15–20% of patients*** attending medical clinics.
- ***Drugs of choice*** for treatment are ***antidepressants***; BZDs are also used in treatment.
- ***Pervasive sadness*** is usually associated with ***depression***.

87. Answer is a (Simple partial seizure).
Ref: Interpreting signs and symptoms, LWW, Pg 557.

- Resulting from an irritable focus in the cerebral cortex, simple partial seizures do NOT alter the patients consciousness.
- They may be classified as
- ***Motor*** (including Jacksonian march and epilepsia partialis continua)
- ***Somatosensory*** (visual, olfactory, auditory sensation—***'something crawling in my head'***; pins and needles feeling, numbness—all fall under this)

88. Answer is d (Marked variability in the 'course' of symptoms is common).
Ref: Harrison's, 17th edition Pg 2721.

- ***Schizophrenia*** is a heterogeneous syndrome characterized by perturbations of language, perception, thinking, social activity, affect and volition.
- There are NO ***pathognomonic features***.
- Schizophrenia commonly begins in late adolescence, has an insidious (and less commonly acute) onset and, often, a poor outcome, progressing from social withdrawal, and perceptual distortions to recurrent delusions and hallucinations.
- Patients may present with ***positive symptoms*** (such as conceptual disorganization, delusions or hallucinations) or ***negative symptoms*** (loss of function, anhedonia, decreased emotional expression, impaired concentration and diminished social engagement) and must have at least two of these for a 1-month period and continuous signs for at least 6 months to meet formal diagnostic criteria.
- ***As individuals age, positive psychotic symptoms tend to attenuate*** and some measure of social and occupational function may be regained.
- However, ***marked variability in the course and individual character of symptoms is typical***.
- 'Negative' symptoms predominantly occur in one-third of the schizophrenic population and are associated with a poor long-term outcome, and a poor response to drug treatment.

89. Answer is c (Episodes of unexpected yet organized wandering away from home).
Ref: Niraj Ahuja's TB of Psychiatry, 20th edition Pg 101.

- Dissociative fugue is characterized by ***sudden inability to remember pertinent personal information*** coupled with ***wandering away from home*** and taking on a new identity. The person usually is ***not aware*** that she has assumed a new identity.
- The onset is usually sudden in the presence of severe stress. The ***termination too is abrupt*** and is followed by amnesia for the episode, but with recovery of memories of earlier life.

FORENSIC MEDICINE

90. Answer is c (Cheiloscopy).
Ref: Narayan Reddy's FMT, 23rd edition Pg 51.

Cheiloscopy	Study of ***lip prints***
Poroscopy	Examination of impressions left by the sweat pores of fingers to check or support ***fingerprint evidence***
Rugoscopy	The observation and study of the patterns of the grooves, wrinkles and ridges ***(rugae) of the palate*** to identify individual patterns
Oroscopy	Examination of ***buccal cavity***

91. Answer is b (Glycine).
Ref: Narayan Reddy's FMT, 23rd edition Pg 308-09.

→ **Mechanism of strychnine poisoning:** ***Strychnine*** depresses the inhibitory postsynaptic potentials in the spinal cord and ***prevents the affects of glycine*** (the presumed inhibitory neurotransmitter). Widespread inhibition in the spinal cord results in 'release' excitation.

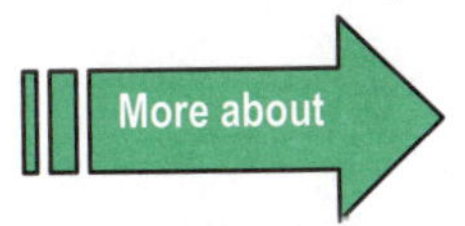

Strychnine Poisoning

- Caused by ***Strychnos nux vomica***—contains 2 alkaloids strychnine and brucine-neurotoxic.

Trait	Strychnine	Tetanus
Onset	Sudden	Gradual
History	No history of injury	H/o injury present
Convulsions	All muscles of body are affected at a time	All muscles are not affected at same time
Lower jaw	Does not start in or especially affect the jaw	Starts in and especially affects the jaw
Muscular condition	Between fits muscles are completely relaxed	Between fits muscles are slightly rigid
Fatal period	1–2 hours	More than 24 hours
Chemical analysis	Strychnine found	No poison found

92. Answer is c (Sigmoid).
Ref: Narayan Reddy's FMT, 23rd edition Pg 78.

- ***Algor mortis (chill of death)*** = Cooling of the body after death.
- Does not occur at same rate throughout the body.
- For about half to one hour after death the rectal temperature falls little or not at all.
- Then the cooling rate is relatively uniform in its slope.
- The ***curve of the cooling*** is '***sigmoid***' or inverted S-shape in pattern.

93. Answer is b (Torture).

Ref: Textbook of Forensic Medicine and Toxicology By Krishan Vij, 4th edition Pg 729, Annexure 3.

- ***Declaration of Tokyo***: Guidelines for medical doctors ***concerning torture*** and other cruel, inhuman, and degrading treatment or punishment in relation to detention or imprisonment. Adopted by the World Medical Assembly, Tokyo, Japan, 1975.

Also Know

- ***Declaration of Helsinki***: The World Medical Association (WMA) has developed the Declaration of Helsinki as a statement of ***ethical principles for medical research involving human subjects***, including research on identifiable human material and data (1964).

PREVENTIVE AND SOCIAL MEDICINE

94. Answer is b (Filariasis).

Ref: Park's, 20th edition Pg 234.

- In ***filariasis***, a considerable proportion of people are asymptomatic although their blood is positive for microfilaria.
- They may remain without any symptoms for months or years.
- They are an important source of infection in the community.
- These carriers are usually detected by ***night blood examination***.

95. Answer is a (10–15%).

Ref: Park's, 20th edition Pg 694-95.

- Between 75 and 90% of the waste produced by the healthcare providers is non-risk or 'general' healthcare waste comparable to domestic waste.
- It comes from administrative and housekeeping functions of the hospitals and may also include waste generated during maintenance of healthcare premises.
- The remaining ***10–25% healthcare waste is regarded as hazardous*** and may create a variety of health risk.

96. Answer is c (*Aedes aegypti*).

Ref: Harrison's, 17th edition Pg 1230; Park 20th edition Pg 675.

- All four distinct ***dengue*** viruses (dengue 1-4) have ***Aedes aegypti*** as their principal vector and all cause a similar clinical syndrome.

Also Know

Mosquito-borne diseases

Mosquito	Disease
□ *Anopheles*	– Malaria
□ *Culex*	– Bancroftian filariasis – Japanese encephalitis – West Nile fever – Viral arthritis (epidemic polyarthritis)

☐ *Aedes*	– Yellow fever (not in India) – Dengue – Dengue hemorrhagic fever – Chikungunya fever – Chikungunya hemorrhagic fever – Rift valley fever – Filaria (not in India)
☐ **Mansonoides**	– Malayan (Brugian) filariasis – Chikungunya fever

97. Answer is d (Management by objectives).
Ref: Park, 20th edition Pg 774-75.

Management methods and techniques

Methods based on behavioral sciences	Quantitative methods
– Organizational design – Personnel management – Communication – Information systems – Management by objectives	– Cost benefit analysis – Cost effectiveness analysis – Cost accounting – Input output analysis – Model – Systems analysis – Network analysis – Program evaluation and review technique (PERT) – Critical path method (CPM) – Planning programming budgeting system (PPBS) – Work sampling – Decision making

98. Answer is a (1982).
Ref: Park, 20th edition Pg 389.

Program	Launch date
National Mental Health Program	1982
National Cancer Control Program	1975–1976
National Program for Control and Treatment of Occupational Disease	1998–1999
Integrated Disease Surveillance Project	2004
National Guinea Worm Eradication Program	1984
National Rural Health Mission	2005 (up to–2012)
Pulse Polio Immunization	1995
National Program for Control of Blindness	1976
National AIDS Control Program	1987
Modified Plan of Operation (Malaria)	1977
National Leprosy Control Program	1955

99. Answer is c (Descriptive).
Ref: Park, 20th edition Pg 59.

❖ ***Descriptive studies*** are concerned with observing the distribution of disease or health related characteristics in human populations and identifying the characteristics with which the disease in question seems to be associated. Such studies basically ask the questions:
- When is the disease occurring (time distribution)?
- Where is it occurring (place distribution)?
- Who is getting the disease (person distribution)?

100. Answer is b (Ergotism).
Ref: Park, 20th edition Pg 571.

- ***Claviceps fusiformis*** is the ergot fungus responsible for ergotism.

Also Know

❖ ***Neurolathyrism*** caused by beta-N-oxalylamino-L-alanine (BOAA) found in seeds of the pulse *L. sativus* (kesari dal).
❖ ***Epidemic dropsy*** is due to contamination of mustard oil with argemone oil (toxin – sanguinarine).
❖ ***Endemic ascites*** is due to seeds of *Crotalaria* (Jhunjhunu), which contain pyrrolizidine alkaloids.
❖ ***Aflatoxins*** are produced by *Aspergillus fumigatus.*

101. Answer is a (Test etiological hypothesis).
Ref: Park, 20th edition Pg 76.

The aims of ***experimental studies*** are:
✈ To provide ***'scientific proof' of etiological (or risk) factors,*** which may permit the modification or control of these diseases.
✈ To provide a method of measuring the effectiveness and efficiency of health services for the prevention, control, and treatment of disease and improve the health of the community.

102. Answer is c (Safflower oil).
Ref: Park, 20th edition Pg 528, Table 2.

➢ ***Maximum content of PUFA*** is found in ***Safflower oil***.
➢ Maximum content of *saturated fatty acids* is found in *coconut oil*.

103. Answer is b (5).
Ref: Park, 20th edition Pg 651.

➢ The permissible dose of radiation from man-made sources ***should NOT exceed 5 rads/year***.106

104. Answer is d (Prevalence of natural infection in 0–14 years is < 1%).
Ref: Park, 20th edition Pg 164.

- ***Tuberculosis control*** means reduction in the prevalence and incidence of disease in the community.
- The WHO defines that tuberculosis control should be achieved when the ***prevalence of natural infection in the group of ages 0–14 years is of the order of 1%***.
- This is about 40% in India.

105. Answer is a (Rehabilitation → Reconstruction).
Ref: Park, 20th edition Pg 701.

- There are three fundamental aspects of disaster management:
  - Disaster response
  - Disaster preparedness
  - Disaster mitigation
- These three aspects of disaster management correspond to different phases in the so-called 'disaster cycle' shown below.
- ***Preparedness → Response → Rehabilitation → Reconstruction → Mitigation → Preparedness.***

106. Answer is a (Mosquito).
Ref: Park, 20th edition Pg 223.

- ***Malaria***:
  - *Definitive host*: Mosquito
  - *Intermediate host*: Man.

107. Answer is b [True positive/(True positive + False negative)].
Ref: Park, 20th edition Pg 126.

Analysis of Diagnostic Tests

Test result	Disease	
	⊕	–
⊕	a (true positive)	b (false positive)
–	**c (false negative)**	d (true negative)

☼ **Sensitivity**	– The test's ability to all people with disease, who truly have the disease (***true positives***) = $a / a + c \times 100 = 1 -$ false negative rate – Most acceptable screening tests are > 80% sensitive – A false negative is a negative test in a patient with the disease
☼ **Specificity**	– The test's ability to correctly identify all people without disease, i.e. those who do not have the disease (***true negatives***) = $d / b + d \times 100 = 1 -$ false positive rate – Used as confirmatory test after a positive screening test – Most acceptable confirmatory tests are > 85% specific – Example: HIV testing; screen with ELISA (sensitive, high false positive rate, low threshold); confirm with Western blot (specific, high false negative rate, high threshold)
Mnemonic	**SPIN** = **SP**ecificity rules **IN**; **SNOUT** = **S**e**N**sitivity rules **OUT**
☼ **Predictive value**	– Reflects the diagnostic power of the test
☼ **Positive Predictive value**	– Proportion of positive test results that are true positive, i.e. the probability that a person with a positive test actually has the disease = $a / a + b \times 100$
☼ **Negative Predictive value**	– Proportion of negative test results that are true negative, i.e. the probability that a person with a negative test actually is disease free = $d / c + d \times 100$

108. Answer is c (10 days after date of vaccination up to 10 years).
Ref: Park, 20th edition Pg 248.

All About Yellow Fever Vaccine

- Sensitivity of the lyophilized 17D vaccine to *heat is major drawback* to the use of this vaccine in mass campaigns in tropical countries.
- Vaccine is given *SC at the insertion of deltoid* in a single dose of 0.5 mL irrespective of age.
- Immunity appears to begin on the 7th day and lasts for more than 35 years and possibly for life.
- Revaccination after 10 years is recommended for international travel.
- Cholera and yellow fever vaccines together or within 3 weeks interfere with each other, so whenever possible they should be given 3 weeks or more apart.
- ***The validity of the certificate (international certificate of vaccination) begins 10 days after the date of vaccination and extends up to 10 years.***

109. Answer is d (Diagnosis can be made with available techniques).
Ref: Park, 20th edition Pg 123.

- The submerged portion of the iceberg ***represents the hidden mass of disease*** (e.g. ***subclinical cases, carriers, undiagnosed cases***).
- The *floating tip* represents what *the physician sees in practice.*
- The ***hidden part of the iceberg*** thus represents the mass of unrecognized disease in the community and its ***detection and control is a challenge*** to modern techniques in preventive medicine.

MICROBIOLOGY

110. Answer is a (Cyst is the infective form).
Ref: Harrison's, 17th edition Pg 1315; Review of medical microbiology and immunology By Warren Levinson, 9th edition Pg 356; Parasitology for Medical and Clinical Laboratory Professionals By Ridley, John W Ridley, Pg 43.

- ***Trichomonas vaginalis*** is a pear shaped organism with **4–5 *anterior flagella and one posterior flagella***; actively motile and anaerobic.
- It has **NO** cyst form and the ***trophozoite is the infective stage.***
- It is a major cause of ***vaginitis (see below).***

Also Know

Trichomonas Vaginitis

- ***Sexually transmissible***; its ingress into the vagina is favored when the ***pH is raised (5–6) as during a menstrual period.***
- It is characterized by ***copious, green, frothy discharge***, which may be associated with ***foul odor* and *vulvar pruritus***.
- On examination ***punctuation on the cervix, classically called 'strawberry cervix'*** is seen.
- Diagnosis may be made by saline wet mount of the vaginal discharge, which reveals highly *motile trichomonads.*
- Treatment is by ***metronidazole***.

111. Answer is a (*Aspergillus flavus*).
Ref: Textbook of Microbiology By CP Baveja, 3rd edition Pg 552.

Fungi and their mycotoxins

Fungus	Mycotoxin produced
Aspergillus fumigatus	Aflatoxin, fumigation
A. ochraceus	Ochratoxin
Fusarium graminearum	Mycotoxin
Mushrooms (toadstool)	Mycotoxin

Claviceps species	Ergot alkaloids
Penicillium rubrum	Rubratoxin
P. puberculum	Penicillic acid
Fusarium nivale	Sciepenols
Amanita muscaria	Muscarine

112. Answer is d (Molecules).
Ref: Harrison's, 17th edition Pg 2646.

❖ ***PRION = Proteinaceous infectious particle*** that ***lacks nucleic acid*** (NO DNA or RNA). Prions are composed largely, if not entirely, of ***PrPSc molecules***.

Also Know

Prion diseases

Human prion diseases	Animal prion diseases
➲ ***Creutzfeldt-Jakob disease (MC)*** ➲ Gerstmann-Straussler-Scheinker disease ➲ Fatal Familial insomnia ➲ Kuru	➲ Scrapie ➲ Bovine spongiform encephalopathy ➲ Chronic wasting disease

113. Answer is b (Street virus).
Ref: Park, 20th edition Pg 239.

- ***Rabies virus*** has been grouped into street virus and fixed virus.
- The ***street virus*** is derived from one that exists in nature in naturally occurring cases and the ***fixed virus*** denotes to strains of virus that has been adapted by serial intracranial passage in some animal (rabbit) in the laboratory, and this is used in vaccine production.

114. Answer is a (Isograft).
Ref: Textbook of Microbiology By Baveja, 3rd edition Pg 163.

Types of Grafts

☼ **Autograft**	: From ***self***
☼ **Syngeneic graft /Isograft**	: From ***identical twin*** or clone (i.e. genetically identical with recipient)
☼ **Allograft /Homograft**	: From non-identical member of ***same species***
☼ **Xenograft**	: From ***different species***

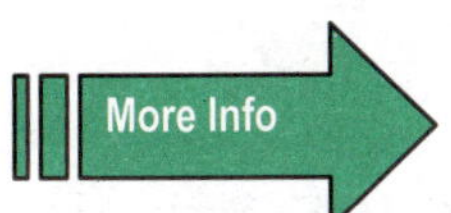

• **Heterotopic**	Graft placed in a ***different type of tissue***, e.g. thyroid tissue in subcutaneous pocket
• **Isotopic**	Graft placed in the ***same anatomical location*** of tissue from which the graft came
• **Orthotopic**	Graft placed in same type of tissue as graft origin, but a ***different anatomical position***, e.g. skin grafted from thigh to arm

115. Answer is a *(Chlamydia trachomatis)*.
Ref: Harrison's, 17th edition Pg 1071.

Etiology of common STDs

Lymphogranuloma venereum (LGV)	*C. trachomatis* strains of the *L1, L2 and L3* serotypes, *L2 is MC*
Granuloma inguinale (Donovanosis)	*Calymmatobacterium granulomatis*, a *pleomorphic, gram-negative rod*
Chancroid	*Gram-negative* bacillus *Haemophilus ducreyi*
Syphilis	*Treponema pallidum*

116. Answer is b *(Proteus).*
Ref: Textbook of Microbiology By CP Bavjea, 3rd edition Pg 391.

Weil Felix Test

- This test is used to identify the presence of R*ickettsiae* without specifying a particular species.
- A sample of patients blood is first obtained and the clean serum is separated from the red blood cells. A sample of serum is mixed with the cells of the bacterium, ***Proteus OX19***.
- The bacteria will clump together, if the serum contains antibodies against the *Rickettsiae,* indicating that a person has the disease or once had it.
- If no clumping takes place, Rickettsial antibodies are probably not present.
- The Weil-Felix test works because *Rickettsiae* possess antigens, also located in Proteus cells and therefore, both organisms stimulate the immune system to produce the same antibodies – hence an example of ***heterophile agglutination test***.

PHARMACOLOGY

117. Answer is b (Duloxetine).
Ref: KD Tripathi, 6th edition Pg 447.

- ***Duloxetine and venlafaxine*** are serotonin + noradrenaline reuptake inhibitors (SNRI's).

CLASSIFICATION OF ANTIDEPRESSANTS

• **Tricyclic antidepressants**	
– **Noradrenaline and Serotonin Reuptake Inhibitors (NA:5-HT)**	– Imipramine, Amitriptyline, Trimipramine, Clomipramine, Doxepin, Dothiepin
– **Selective Noradrenaline (NA > 5-HT) Reuptake Inhibitors**	– Nortriptyline, Desipramine, Amoxapine and Reboxetine
• **Selective Serotonin Reuptake Inhibitors (SSRIs)**	Fluoxetine (bicyclic), Femoxetine, Fluvoxamine, Paroxetine, Sertraline, Citalopram
• **Selective Dopamine Reuptake Inhibitors**	Bupropion, Nomifensine
• **Selective Serotonin Reuptake Enhancers (SSRE)**	Tianeptine, Amineptine
• **Atypical antidepressants**	Mianserin, Trazodone, Duloxetine, Venlafaxine, Mirtazapine

118. Answer is d (Zanamivir).
Ref: KD Tripathi, 6th edition Pg 778.

❖ ***Zanamivir, Oseltamivir*** and ***Amantadine*** are ***anti-influenza virus drugs***.

Also Know

Protease Inhibitors	– Drugs: Saquinavir, Ritonavir, Indinavir, Nelfinavir, Amprenavir, Tipranavir, Lopinavir, Fosamprenavir, Darunavir, Atazanavir. – Mechanism: Inhibit assembly of new virus by blocking protease in progeny virions.

119. Answer is b (Zidovudine).
Ref: Textbook of Cardiovascular Medicine By Eric Topol, Vol 355, Pg 1416.

❖ ***Zidovudine*** is associated with ***dilated cardiomyopathy*** rarely that appears to be related to ***mitochondrial dysfunction***.

120. Answer is b (20 mg).
Ref: KD Tripathi, 6th edition Pg 32.

- ***First order kinetics*** means, a constant fraction of the drug present in the body is eliminated in unit time.
- For a drug following first order kinetics, the t½ (plasma half-life) remains constant.
- In the given example, 160 mg becomes 80 mg (i.e. 50% eliminated) in 120 minutes (2 hours) → the t½ is 2 hours.
- So in 4 hours (½ of 80) = 40 mg will remain.
- ***In 6 hours (½ of 40) = 20 mg will remain.***

121. Answer is a (G6PD deficiency).
Ref: Harrison's, 17th edition Pg 657.

✈ Neonatal jaundice (NNJ) can be very severe in some G6PD-deficient babies, especially in association with prematurity, infection and/or environmental factors [such as ***naphthalene-camphor balls*** (these are ***Moth Balls***) used in babies' bedding and clothing]. In these cases, if inadequately managed, NNJ associated with G6PD deficiency can produce kernicterus and permanent neurologic damage.

✈ Similarly in adults (with G6PD deficiency) also, these moth balls if ingested can cause severe hemolytic anemia.

More about G6PD Deficiency

Maintenance of integrity of RBC membrane is as follows:

- HMP pathway—production of NADPH, which maintains glutathione in, reduced state—this in turn detoxifies free radicals and peroxides.
- Glycolysis—to produce 2ATP, which maintains Na^+ and K^+ distribution across the cell membrane.

In G6PD deficiency → ↓ NADPH → poor defense against oxidizing agents → RBC lysis → hemolytic anemia.

♦ Precipitating factors in G6PD deficiency: Infection (*MC cause*); oxidant drugs (antibiotics, antimalarials, antipyretics, antituberculous); favism (ingestion of fava beans); neonatal jaundice	♦ G6PD deficiency is more among ***Blacks*** ♦ **H**einz bodies—altered **H**b precipitates within RBCs ♦ ***Bite cells*** result from phagocytic removal of Heinz bodies from macrophages ♦ XLR; ↑ *resistance to falciparum malaria*

122. Answer is b (It is excreted unchanged by the kidneys).
Ref: KD Tripathi, 6th edition Pg 435.

- Lithium is slowly, but well absorbed orally and is NEITHER protein bound or metabolized and is excreted unchanged solely by the kidneys (Direct quote from Psychiatry: 1,200 questions to help you pass the boards By Maju Mathews, Kumar Budur, Biju Basil, 2004 edition Pg 274).
- Lithium is handled by the kidney in much the same way as sodium.
- Long term lithium use may cause ***HYPO***thyroidism.

Summary about Lithium

- Lithium (Li) is small ***monovalent cation***; Li is used as its ***carbonate salt*** because, it is less hygroscopic and less gastric irritant than LiCl or other salts. It is *converted into chloride in the stomach.*
- Mechanism of action is not known exactly. Probably because ***Li inhibit hydrolysis of inositol-1-phosphate.***
- Pharmacokinetics
  - Lithium is *well-absorbed orally; hyponatremia and diuretics cause ↑plasma levels of Li.*
  - Steady state plasma concentrations are reached in *7 days.*
  - *Prophylactic* blood lithium levels (for maintenance therapy) = 0.5–0.8 mEq/L.
  - *Therapeutic* blood lithium levels (for treatment of acute mania) = 0.8–1.2 mEq/L.
  - *Serious toxic effects* occur with plasma concentrations above 2.0 mEq/L.
  - Renal excretion is increased by diuresis and urinary alkalinization and decreased by hypovolemia, and hyponatremia.
- *Side effects*
  - Acute *toxicity: Li causes* ***tremors***; *treatment of choice* is ***hemodialysis***. Osmotic diuretics and sodium bicarbonate infusion promote Li excretion.
  - ***Renal diabetes insipidus*** (thirst and polyuria); ***hypothyroidism*** may occur.
  - Li is *contraindicated in pregnancy* (***Ebstein anomaly*** in neonate if Li ingested in first trimester).
- Uses of lithium
  - In treatment of ***acute mania and prophylaxis of bipolar mood disorder.***
  - Other uses are in ***Cluster headache; Cancer chemotherapy linked agranulocytosis*** **and** ***neutropenia*** **(Li increases leukocyte count);** ***SIADH; Cyclical vomiting; Huntington's chorea.***

123. Answer is c (Linezolid).

Ref: KD Tripathi, 6th edition Pg 732.

- ***Linezolid*** is an oxazolidinedione antibiotic useful for treatment of resistant gram-positive coccal and bacillary infections.
- Linezolid binds to the 50S ribosomal subunit and blocks the initiation of protein synthesis.
- Because ***linezolid is a MAO inhibitor, interaction with adrenergic/serotonergic drugs*** and excess dietary tyramine are expected.

124. Answer is b (Chloral hydrate).

Ref: Kaplan & Sadock's concise textbook of clinical psychiatry By Benjamin J Sadock, Virginia A Sadock, 2008 edition Pg 488.

- The concoction of ***chloral hydrate with alcohol*** is known as ***Mickey Finn***. This mixture was used to incapacitate customers and rob them.
- For more details on the story of Mickey Finn - see this wikipedia link: http://en.wikipedia.org/wiki/Mickey_Finn_(drugs)
- For more on slangs for drugs of abuse (quite and exhaustive list) go to http://www.drugrehab.co.uk/street-drug-names.htm.

125. Answer is d (PGH2).

Ref: KD Tripathi, 6th edition Pg 172, Fig 13.1.

- Arachidonic acid derivatives are called eicosanoids. Either cyclo-oxygenase (COX) or lipo-oxygenase (LOX) may act on arachidonic acid.

- ***COX pathway*** → prostaglandins and thromboxane.
- COX exists in two isoforms **COX-1** and **COX-2**.
- Eicosanoids produced by ***COX-1 participate in physiological (house-keeping) functions*** such as secretion of mucus for protection of gastric mucosa, hemostasis and maintenance of renal functions.
- Eicosanoids produced by ***COX-2 lead to inflammatory and pathological changes***. Hence **selective COX-2 inhibitors (celecoxib, rofecoxib)** are now available as NSAIDs to counter gastritis side effects.
- Aspirin, ibuprofen and naproxen, inhibit both COX-1 and COX-2.
- ***LOX pathway*** → leukotrienes.
- ***LOX*** pathway operates mainly in the ***lung, WBC and platelets***.

Arachidonic Acid Derivatives

Leukotrienes (LTC4, LTD4, LTD4)	↑ vascular tone ↑ bronchial tone ↑ vascular permeability; Components of SRS-A	Leukotrienes (**Leako** = ↑ vascular permeability)
Leukotriene A4, B4	Increased neutrophil chemotaxis Release of lysosomal enzymes	
Thromboxane A2	↑ vascular tone ↑ bronchial tone Produced by platelets, promotes platelet aggregation	Throm**BOX**ane = gathers platelets in **BOX**es
Prostacyclin (PGI)	↓ vascular tone ↓ bronchial tone ↓ uterine tone ↓ platelet aggregation Produced by vascular endothelium	**PGI** = Platelet-Gathering Inhibitor and Power-Gaining Inhibitor (all ↓ tone)
Prostaglandins (PGE and PGF)	↓ vascular tone ↓ bronchial tone ↑ uterine tone Produced by most tissues, especially kidney	Used to induce labor

PATHOLOGY

126. Answer is b (Glanzmann's disease).
Ref: Harrison's, 17th edition Pg 723.

Inherited Platelet Membrane Defects (AR)

- *Glanzmann thrombasthenia*: Defective platelet aGgregation from a deficiency of platelet membrane glycoproteins, GP IIb-IIIa.
- *BernarD-Soulier Syndrome*: Defective platelet aDhesion (↓ GP Ib).

Note:

- ***von Willebrand's disease*** = deficiency of von Willebrand's factor → defect of platelet adhesion and ↓ factor VIII survival.
- ***Gray platelet syndrome*** = Platelet alpha-granule deficiency – causes macrothrombocytopenia – thrombocytopenia with increased platelet size.

127. Answer is c (Between 5 and 30 days of transplantation).
Ref: Davidson's, 21st edition Pg 93, Table 4.24.

Classification of transplant rejection

Type	Time	Pathological findings	Mechanism	Treatment
Hyperacute rejection	Minutes to hours	Thrombosis, necrosis	Preformed antibody and complement activation (type II hypersensitivity)	None-rapid and irreversible graft loss
Acute vascular rejection	5–30 days	Vasculitis	Antibody and complement activation	Increase immunosuppression
Acute cellular rejection	5–30 days	Cellular infiltration	CD4+ and CD8+ T cells (type IV hypersensitivity)	Increase immunosuppression
Chronic allograft failure	> 30 days	Fibrosis, scarring	Immune and non-immune mechanisms	Minimize drug toxicity, control high BP and hyperlipidemia

128. Answer is a (Herpes virus).
Ref: TB of Microbiology By Ananthnarayan, 7th edition Pg 474.

Viral Inclusion Bodies

Intracytoplasmic	Fowl Pox	Bollinger, Borrel's body
	Molluscum contagiosum	Henderson-Peterson body
	Rabies	Negri bodies
	Smallpox	Guarnieri's bodies
Intranuclear	Cowdry type A	Herpes virus and Varicella (***Lipschutz body***), Yellow fever (Torres body)
	Cowdry type B	Adenovirus, poliovirus

129. Answer is b (5q).
Ref: Myelodysplastic syndromes: clinical and biological advance By Peter L Greenberg, Pg 43.

- The notable example of morphologic cytogenetic correlation in ***myelodysplastic syndrome*** is the ***5q del (5q) syndrome***.
- Predominantly occurs in middle aged females and is generally accompanied by favorable prognosis.

130. Answer is d (Epidural hemorrhage).
Ref: Harrison's, 17th edition Pg 2599, Fig 373-4.

Traumatic Vascular Injury

Epidural (Extradural) hematoma	**Subdural hematoma**
– Usually *arterial blood* accumulates between skull bone and dura	– *Venous blood* accumulates between dura and arachnoid
– Usually rupture of ***middle meningeal artery*** after trauma to temporal bone	– Rupture of torn superficial bridging veins between cerebral cortex and sinuses
– Brief unconsciousness followed by **LUC**id interval for several hours	– Occur in elderly and alcoholics after relatively minor trauma
– CT scan: conv**ex** mass *(lentiform)* **Mnemonic:** *"EXtradural = convEX; Always give LUCy EXtra attention!"*	– Concave (crescent-shaped) mass, which is less dense than epidural, since blood is diluted with CSF

131. Answer is c (Restrictive lung disease is a rarity in the syndrome).
Ref: Harrison's, 17th edition Pg 1650; Harley's pediatric Ophthalmology, Pg 371.

The Hermansky-Pudlak syndrome (autosomal recessive):

- Granulomatous colitis.
- Oculocutaneous albinism (tyrosinase positive, meaning can develop some pigmentation—partial albinism).
- Bleeding diathesis secondary to platelet dysfunction.
- Accumulation of a chromolipid, lipofuscin material in cells of the reticuloendothelial system.
- Interstitial lung disease: A restrictive fibrotic pattern; alveolar macrophages may contain cytoplasmic ceroid-like inclusions.
- Cardiomyopathy (due to accumulation of ceroid in heart).

ANATOMY, PHYSIOLOGY AND BIOCHEMISTRY

132. Answer is c (Deep peroneal nerve).
Ref: Surgical Exposures in Orthopaedics: The Anatomic Approach By Stanley Hoppenfeld, Piet DeBoer, Richard Buckley, Richard Eric Buckley, 4th edition Pg 9-249.

- The ***skin of the dorsum of the first web space*** is supplied by ***branches of the deep peroneal nerve***.
- Numbness in the first web space is the earliest sign of a deep peroneal nerve lesion in the anterior compartment of the leg.

133. Answer is d (6th).
Ref: Clinical anatomy for students: problem solving approach By Neeta V Kulkarni, Pg 205.

Aortic Arches and their derivatives

- The ***six pairs of aortic arches***, develop in a ***cephalocaudal direction*** and interconnect the ventral aortic roots, and the dorsal aorta.
- They are never all present in the developing human heart. Of the six pairs of aortic arches, most of the 1st, 2nd and 5th arches disappear. The fate of the remaining arches is listed below.

– ***3rd aortic arch***	→ Common carotid and proximal internal carotid artery
– ***4th aortic arch (Right)***	→ Proximal right subclavian A and brachiocephalic A
– ***4th aortic arch (Left)***	→ Arch of aorta and left subclavian A
– ***6th aortic arch***	→ Right and left pulmonary arteries, and ductus arteriosus (on left only)

134. Answer is c (Spinal accessory nerve).
Ref: Essentials of orthopedics, RM Shenoy, Pg 141.

- In ***spinal accessory nerve injury***, patients usually present with
  - A ***dull ache*** of the shoulder region
  - An ***inability to use the affected arm overhead*** (inability to lift shoulder > 90°)
  - Scapular winging and
  - Atrophy of the trapezius
  - Although a lower, ***drooping, shoulder*** is often present, many patients do not complain of this per se, being more concerned with the pain or weakness.

135. Answer is b (Hilus cells).
Ref: Krause's Essential Human Histology for Medical Students By Krause J William, 3rd edition Pg 242.

- ***Hilus cells*** are large epithelioid cells found a/w vascular spaces and unmyelinated nerves in the hilus of the ovary.
- The cells appear ***similar to the interstitial cells of the testis*** and contain lipid, lipochrome pigments, and cholesterol esters.
- Hilus cells are found most commonly at pregnancy and at menopause, but their function is unknown.
- Tumors arising from these cells cause ***masculinization***.

136. Answer is c (Maxillary nerve).
Ref: Clinical anatomy for students: problem solving approach By Neeta V Kulkarni, Pg 459.

Major Foramina of the Skull and Structures Transmitted

Foramen ovale	**Foramen spinosum**	**Foramen rotundum**
Mandibular N (CN V3) Accessory meningeal A Lesser petrosal N Emissary vein Ovale = *MALE*	Middle meningeal A Meningeal branch of mandibular N (nervus spinosus) Posterior trunk of middle meningeal V	*Maxillary Nerve* (CN V2)
Carotid canal	**Jugular foramen**	**Optic canal**
Internal carotid A Venous and sympathetic plexus around the artery	CN IX, CN X and CN XI Internal jugular V	Optic nerve (CN II) Ophthalmic A Central retinal V
Superior orbital fissure	**Inferior orbital fissure**	**Foramen lacerum**
CN III, CN IV, CN V1 (Ophthalmic) and CN VI Inferior ophthalmic V	Maxillary N Zygomatic N Orbital branches of the pterygopalatine ganglion Infraorbital vessels	Internal carotid A Lesser petrosal N (branch of IX) Greater petrosal N (branch of VII) Deep petrosal nerves (autonomic)

137. Answer is a, d (Pylorus of the stomach, Fundus of the gallbladder)—revised answer key gives both a, d as answers.
Ref: Clinical anatomy by regions By Richard S Snell, 8th edition Pg 192.

- The abdomen is divided into 9 regions by 4 imaginary planes, 2 horizontal and 2 vertical.

• **Transpyloric plane of Addison** (horizontal)	It is called '***trans-pyloric***', since it ***cuts across the pylorus of the stomach***; Passes midway between the suprasternal notch and the symphysis pubis. It lies about a hand's breadth below the xiphisternal joint. Anteriorly, it passes through the tips of the ninth costal cartilages and posteriorly through the body of L1 vertebra (near its lower border).
• **Transtubercular plane** (horizontal)	Passes through tubercles of iliac crest and the body of vertebra L5 near its upper border.
• Right and left lateral planes (vertical)	Correspond to midclavicular or mammary lines indicated by lines drawn on the surface through points halfway between the anterior superior iliac spine and symphysis pubis (mid-inguinal point).
• **Subcostal plane** (horizontal, sometimes used)	Passes through the lower borders of the 10th costal cartilage and body of vertebra L3 (near its upper border).

138. Answer is d (Middle cardiac vein).
Ref: Clinical anatomy by regions By Richard S Snell, 8th edition Pg 107: BD Chaurasia, 3rd edition Vol 1, Pg 219.

- **Openings into the right atrium**
  - Superior vena cava
  - Inferior vena cava

- Coronary sinus
- Venae cordis minimae (Thebesian vessels)
- Anterior cardiac veins
- Right atrioventricular orifice.

139. Answer is c (Visual area).
Ref: Textbook of Ophthalmology By Sunita Aggarwal, Vol 2, Pg 313.

- ***Band of Gennari (Stria occipitalis):*** Typical white stripe (geniculocalcarine fibers) visible with naked eye, which is the characteristic feature of the ***area 17 (striate cortex)*** of the ***primary visual cortex***.

140. Answer is c (Zinc).
Ref: Harrison's, 17th edition Pg 449.

Trace Elements—a Summary

Elements	Deficiency	Toxicity
Zinc	***Growth retardation***, ↓ taste and smell, alopecia, dermatitis (rash) and diarrhea (***acrodermatitis enteropathica***), immune dysfunction, failure to thrive, ***gonadal atrophy***, congenital malformations	General: Reduced copper absorption, gastritis, sweating, fever, nausea, vomiting Occupational: Respiratory distress, ***pulmonary fibrosis***
Selenium	***Cardiomyopathy*** (**Keshan disease** endemic in children. Young women in regions of China), Heart failure, Striated muscle degeneration	General: Alopecia, nausea, vomiting, abnormal nails, emotional lability, peripheral neuropathy, lassitude, garlic odor to breath, dermatitis Occupational: Lung and nasal carcinomas, liver necrosis, pulmonary inflammation
Calcium	Reduced bone mass, osteoporosis	Renal insufficiency (***milk-alkali syndrome***), nephrolithiasis, impaired iron absorption
Iodine	Thyroid enlargement, ↓ T4, cretinism	Thyroid dysfunction, ***acne-like eruptions***
Copper	***Anemia*** (***microcytic***), growth retardation, defective keratinization and pigmentation of hair, hypothermia, degenerative changes in aortic elastin, osteopenia, mental deterioration	Nausea, vomiting, diarrhea, ***hepatic failure***, tremor, mental deterioration, hemolytic anemia, renal dysfunction
Fluoride	↑ Dental caries	Dental and skeletal ***fluorosis, osteosclerosis***
Iron	Muscle abnormalities, ***koilonychia, pica, microcytic hypochromic anemia***, ↓ work performance, impaired cognitive development, premature labor, ↑ perinatal maternal mortality	Gastrointestinal effects (nausea, vomiting, diarrhea, constipation), iron overload with organ damage, acute systemic toxicity
Manganese	Impaired growth and skeletal development, reproduction, lipid, and carbohydrate metabolism; ***upper body rash***	General: Neurotoxicity, Parkinson-like symptoms Occupational: Encephalitis-like syndrome, ***Parkinson-like syndrome***, psychosis, pneumoconiosis

141. Answer is d (Stretch receptors).
Ref: Ganong's medical physiology, 23rd edition Pg 632.

- Pulmonary ***stretch receptors*** are located in the smooth muscle of the bronchial wall especially at points of bronchial branching.
- These are slow adapting mechanoreceptors responsible for the ***Hering-Breuer reflex***.

Reflexes Related to Respiration

- ***Hering-Breuer inflation reflex***: It is an increase in the duration of expiration produced by steady lung inflation and Hering-Breuer deflation reflex is a decrease in the duration of expiration produced by marked deflation of the lung.
- ***Pulmonary chemoreflex***: It is due to the stimulation of J (juxtacapillary) receptors, which are actually C fiber endings, by hyperinflation of the lung or intracardiac administration of capsaicin. The reflex response that is produced is apnea followed by rapid breathing, bradycardia and hypotension.
- ***Bezold-Jarisch reflex (coronary chemoreflex)***: The above response is also produced by receptors in the heart and is called coronary chemoreflex.

142. Answer is a (Frontonasal and internasal suture).

Ref: Color Atlas and Textbook of Human Anatomy: Locomotor system By Werner Platzer, Werner Kahle, 5th edition Pg 310.

- The ***nasion*** is the ***intersection of the frontal and two nasal bones of the human skull***.
- Its manifestation on the visible surface of the face is a distinctly depressed area directly between the eyes just superior to the bridge of the nose

143. Answer is b, c (Medulla, Hypothalamus).

Ref: Human physiology: from cells to systems By Lauralee Sherwood. 2011 edition Pg 598.

- The ***salivary center is located in the medulla*** as seen in the above reference and almost all anatomy, and physiology.
- Salivary reflex is mediated via the feeding center ion the lateral hypothalamus.
- I could not find a reference to explain why the revised answer key has both b, c as the answer. Will try to update it on my blog—*suresuccessinpg.blogspot.com*.

144. Answer is b (Pterygopalatine ganglion).

Ref: Clinical anatomy for students: problem solving approach By Neeta V Kulkarni, Pg 460.

- Pterygopalatine ganglion is the largest of the peripheral parasympathetic ganglia.
- Though topographically it is related to the maxillary nerve, functionally it is related to the facial nerve.
- Nerve of the pterygoid canal (Vidian nerve) is formed by the union of deep petrosal nerve and greater petrosal nerve in the foramen lacerum.
- Irritation of the nerve of pterygoid canal causes lacrimation and excessive secretion of nasal and palatine glands (typical features of allergic rhinitis or hay fever).
- Therefore this nerve is called the 'nerve of hay fever' and the ***pterygopalatine ganglion is called 'hay fever ganglion'***.

145. Answer is d (500 to 700 mg).

Ref: Clinical laboratory medicine, Volume 2001 By Kenneth D McClatchey, Pg 366.

- Only 6–12% of the original filtered uric acid is excreted in the urine, which amounts to ***400-800 mg excreted*** in the urine daily.

146. Answer is c (Deiodinase).

Ref: Harrison's, 17th edition Pg 449.

- Selenium, in the form of ***selenocysteine*** is found in the ***deiodinase*** enzymes, which mediate the deiodination of thyroxine to triiodothyronine.
- Selenocysteine is also found in ***glutathione peroxidase***, which serves to protect proteins, cell membranes, lipids and nucleic acids from oxidant molecules.
- Such as, selenium is being actively studied as a ***chemopreventive*** agent against certain cancers, such as prostate.
- Rich dietary sources of selenium include seafood, muscle meat and cereals, although the selenium content of cereal is determined by the soil concentration.

147. Answer is a (Pyruvate kinase).

Ref: Vasudevan's TB of Biochemistry, 6th edition Pg 102, 288.

- In starvation the dietary supply of glucose is decreased. Oxaloacetate is diverted for gluconeogenesis.
- The ***activity of key gluconeogenic enzymes is increased,*** viz.:
  - Pyruvate carboxylase
  - Phosphoenolpyruvate carboxykinase
  - Fructose-1,6-biphosphatase
  - Glucose-6-phosphatase.

Note: Pyruvate kinase activity decreases during starvation.

148. Answer is b (Leucine).
Ref: Vasudevan's TB of Biochemistry, 6th edition Pg 21.

• Essential amino acids (Aa's) **S-I-M (PVT, TIM, HALL)**	PVT—Phenylalanine (Phe); Valine (Val); Threonine (Thr) TIM—Tryptophan (Try); Isoleucine (Ile); Methionine (Met) HALL—Histidine (His); Arginine (Arg), Leucine (Leu); Lysine (Lys)
• ***Purely Ketogenic Aa's*** • Purely Glucogenic Aa's • Glucogenic/Ketogenic	Leu, Lys Met, Val, Arg, His Ile, Phe, Tyr, Thr
• Acidic Aa's • Basic Aa's	Asp, Glu (Monoamino-dicarboxylic acids) Arg (**most basic**), Lys, His
• Sulfur containing Aa's	**Methionine, Cysteine, Cystine** S-I-M (Sulfur is **MeCCy**)
• Aromatic Aa's	**His**tidine, **Phe**nylalanine, **T**yrosine, **T**ryptophan S-I-M (**His PheTT** have aroma)
• Aa's with **ALI**phatic side chains	**Alanine, Leucine, Isoleucine, Glycine, Valine** S-I-M **(ALI-GV)**
• Aa's with hydroxyl (OH) groups	Serine, Threonine, Tyrosine S-I-M **(OH! - STT)**
• Imino acids	Proline

149. Answer is A (Nonsense mutation).
Ref: Vasudevan's TB of Biochemistry.

Missense mutation	This type of mutation is a change in one DNA base pair that results in the substitution of one amino acid for another in the protein made by a gene (e.g. sickle cell anemia).
Nonsense mutations	A nonsense mutation is also a change in one DNA base pair. Instead of substituting one amino acid for another, however, the altered DNA sequence prematurely signals the cell to stop building a protein. This type of mutation results in a shortened protein that may function improperly or not at all (e.g. 15–30% of all inherited diseases including cystic fibrosis, hemophilia, retinitis pigmentosa and duchenne muscular dystrophy).
Frameshift mutation	This type of mutation occurs when the addition or loss of DNA bases changes a gene's reading frame. A reading frame consists of groups of 3 bases that each code for one amino acid. A frameshift mutation shifts the grouping of these bases and changes the code for amino acids. The resulting protein is usually nonfunctional ('garbled'). Insertions, deletions and duplications can all be frameshift mutations.
Silent mutation	A point mutation may change the codon for one amino acid to a synonym for the same amino acid. Then the mutation is silent and has no effect on the phenotype (e.g. CUA is mutated to CUC, both code for leucine and so the mutation has no effect).

150. Answer is b (Water-soluble non-ionic monomers).
Ref: Contrast Media: Safety Issues and ESUR Guidelines By Henrik S Thomsen, Judith AW Webb, Pg 4,45.

– ***Non-ionic water soluble monomers*** are the contrast agents of choice these days and ***can be safely used intrathecally also***.

Classification of iodinated contrast media

High osmolality (ionic)	*Low osmolality (non-ionic)*
Monomeric, Iothalamate, Oxalate, Diatrizoate, Metrizoate	Iohexol, Iopamidol, Iodixanol, Ioversol, Iopromide, Ioxilan, Metrizamide

Advantages of Non-ionic Over Ionic Contrast Agents

- ***Reduced tonicity***: Since most side effects are related to hypertonicity, the change to nearly isotonic has significantly decreased reactions in man.
- ***Myelography***: ***Cannot use ionic contrast media for myelography***. So discovery of non-ionic in 1974 (metrizamide) revolutionized this procedure. Newer agents (iopamidol and iohexol) have even lower neurotoxicity.
- ***Chemical toxicity***: Increased hydrophilic means fewer tendencies to cross cell membranes.

Note: ***Oil-based agents*** (e.g. iophendylate) were introduced many years ago for intrathecal use, but lack of fine image detail (due to cohesiveness) and the need to remove the dye (to prevent arachnoiditis and postspinal headaches) made these agents ***suboptimal***.

Section B (Q No. 151–180)

151. Answer is c (Sigmoid volvulus).
152. Answer is b (Urgent sigmoidoscopy).
153. Answer is a (Africans).

Explanation:
The clinical vignette given is that of an acute abdominal emergency. Abdominal distension and the classic coffee bean sign give away the diagnosis as ***sigmoid volvulus***. More given below.

Ref: The Ascrs Textbook of Colon and Rectal Surgery edited By David E Beck, Pg 396, 2011 edition.

- Twisting of loop of sigmoid intestine around its mesenteric attachment is called sigmoid volvulus
- Sigmoid volvulus most common form of GI tract volvulus
- Accounts for up to **8%** of all intestinal obstructions
- Most common in **elderly** persons (often neurologically impaired)
- More common in Africans using a high fiber diet
- Patients almost always have a history of chronic constipation
- **Clinical features:**
  - May present as abdominal emergency
  - Acute distension
  - Colicky pain (often LLQ)
  - Failure to pass flatus or stool (**constipation is prevailing feature**)
  - Vomiting is late sign.

Abdominal plain X-ray usually diagnostic

- **Inverted U-shaped** appearance of distended sigmoid loop
- Largest and most dilated loops of bowel are seen with volvulus
- **Loss of haustra**
- **Coffee-bean sign** – midline crease corresponding to mesenteric root in a greatly distended sigmoid

– **Sigmoid volvulus**—bowel loop points to RUQ
– **Bird's-beak or bird-of-prey sign**—seen on barium enema as it encounters the volvulated loop.

154. Answer is b (Malignant goiter).
155. Answer is d (Papillary carcinoma).
156. Answer is a ('Orphan-Annie eye' nucleus cells).
157. Answer is a (Total Thyroidectomy with lymph nodal dissection of the same side).

Explanation:
The given case history/clinical vignette is of **thyroid carcinoma** as evidenced by the prior exposure to radiation and midline swelling moving with deglutition (a basic fact, which u learn in the surgery clinics).

Ref: Davidson's, 21st edition Pg 751-52; Harrison's, 17th edition Pg 2243-45.

- ***Radiation exposure*** increases the risk of benign and malignant thyroid nodules, is associated with multicentric cancers, and shifts the incidence of thyroid cancer to an earlier age group.
- ***Papillary carcinoma*** accounts for 90% of radiation induced cancer.
- Papillary carcinoma spreads more commonly to ***regional lymph nodes***.
- Follicular carcinoma spread is usually hematogenous.
- Characteristic cytologic features of papillary carcinoma help make the diagnosis by FNA or after surgical resection; these include psammoma bodies, cleaved nuclei with an ***'orphan-Annie'*** appearance caused by large nucleoli and the formation of papillary structures.
- Treatment is usually by ***total thyroidectomy*** followed by large dose of I 131 irradiation. Lymph node removal can also be done. Lobectomy is NOT usually preferred.

158. Answer is c (*Nocardia asteroides* infection).
159. Answer is a (Weakly positive acid fast bacilli).
160. Answer is a (Trimethoprim—sulfamethoxazole).

Explanation: See answer no.138–140 in 2014 COMED-K paper, since this is a repeat question.

161. Answer is a (CT brain).
162. Answer is c (Ethylene glycol poisoning).
163. Answer is a (Fomepizole).

Explanation:
The case history/clinical vignette given is that of ***ethylene glycol poisoning***, Clues: working with car; CNS symptoms; high anion gap metabolic acidosis and specific antidotes asked in the third question.

Ref: Davidson's, 21st edition Pg 220-221; http://www.mnpoison.org/index.asp? Page ID=155

- ***Ethylene glycol (EG)*** is used as ***antifreeze and coolant***, it is also found in solvents, humectants, brake fluids, paints and lacquers. Ingestion of as little as one mouthful of a 99% EG antifreeze solution by either a child or adult may lead to toxic signs and symptoms.
- Ethylene glycol's major toxicities are a result of it is metabolites: ***glycolaldehyde, oxalic acid, glycolic acid and glyoxylate***. These metabolites cause (1) tissue destruction, primarily from calcium oxalate crystal deposition and (2) metabolic abnormalities, specifically a ***high anion-gap metabolic acidosis***, lactic acidosis and hypocalcemia.
- Oxalic acid combines with calcium to form ***calcium oxalate crystals, which deposit in the kidneys and seen in the urine***. This can result in hypokalemia, hematuria and proteinuria, increased creatinine, and ***renal failure***.
- The first enzyme in the metabolic pathway of EG is ***alcohol dehydrogenase***. By blocking the action of this enzyme, the production of toxic metabolites can be stopped.

Clinical Symptoms

- **Phase 1** (Minutes–12 hours): ***CNS toxicity*** predominates with inebriation (without odor of ethanol on the breath), coma, nystagmus, paralysis and ***seizures***. Nausea, vomiting and papilledema may also occur. An elevated serum osmolality is seen early in this phase. Calcium oxalate crystals may be present.

- **Phase 2** (12–24 hours): ***Cardiopulmonary symptoms*** predominate with mild tachycardia and hypertension. Other effects include anion gap metabolic acidosis (possibly severe) with compensatory hyperventilation, hypoxia, CHF and ARDS.
- **Phase 3** (> 24 hours): This ***renal phase*** is characterized by acute tubular necrosis and renal failure. Oliguria, anuria, hematuria and proteinuria are common.

Treatment: ***Fomepizole*** blocks alcohol dehydrogenase and delays the formation of toxic metabolites until parent drug is eliminated naturally or by hemodialysis. Metabolic acidosis should be treated with sodium bicarbonate.

❖ Why CT scan as first test upon arrival? – Here the revised answer key gives CT scan as the answer. Possibly because here we have an unresponsive patient arriving with h/o CNS symptoms for 6 and half hours followed by a generalized tonic clonic seizure. Most textbooks give that a CT scan should be done for all patients presenting with a first time seizure.

164. Answer is c (Bridging necrosis).
165. Answer is d (Bilirubin).
166. Answer is b (HBeAg).
167. Answer is d (6 months).

Ref: Harrison's, 17th edition Pg 1939.

Explanation:
The case history/clinical vignette given is that of ***acute viral hepatitis B*** as evidenced by HBsAg positivity, recent blood transfusion (parenteral transmission), jaundice and tender hepatomegaly.

Pathology:
– The typical morphologic lesions of all types of viral hepatitis are similar and consist of panlobular infiltration with mononuclear cells, hepatic cell necrosis, hyperplasia of Kupffer cells, and variable degrees of cholestasis.
– A more severe histologic lesion, ***bridging hepatic necrosis***, also termed ***subacute*** **or** ***confluent necrosis*** **or** ***interface hepatitis***, is occasionally observed in some patients with acute hepatitis.

Clinical Features
– The *prodromal symptoms* of acute viral hepatitis are systemic and quite variable. Constitutional symptoms of anorexia, nausea and vomiting, ***fatigue, malaise***, arthralgias, myalgias, headache, photophobia, pharyngitis, cough, and coryza may precede the onset of jaundice by 1–2 weeks.
– Dark urine and clay-colored stools may be noticed by the patient from 1–5 days before the onset of clinical jaundice.
– With the onset of ***clinical jaundice***, the constitutional prodromal symptoms usually diminish, but in some patients mild ***weight loss*** (2.5–5 kg) is common and may continue during the entire icteric phase.
– The ***liver becomes enlarged and tender***, and may be associated with ***right upper quadrant pain*** and discomfort.

Serology
– HBeAg, appears concurrently with or shortly after HBsAg. Its appearance coincides temporally with high levels of virus replication and reflects the presence of circulating intact virions, and detectable HBV DNA.

Hepatitis B Serology

■ HBsAg	*First virologic marker detectable in serum* after infection with HBV (even before elevation of serum aminotransferase and clinical symptoms appear). Indicates ***active hepatitis B infection***, either acute or chronic (> 6 months).
■ Anti-HBs	Antibody to HbsAg. Provides ***immunity to hepatitis B***. *Persists for years*.
■ HBcAg	*Not routinely detectable* in blood.
■ Anti-HBc	***Positive during the window period.*** ***IgM anti-HBc*** is an indicator of ***recent disease***, IgG anti-HBc signifies chronic disease.

■ HBeAg	Indicates ***active viral replication and high infectivity***. **S-I-M** (Beware!).
■ Anti-HBe	When present in HBsAg carrier, blood is potentially less infectious.

Laboratory Features

– The ***serum aminotransferases aspartate aminotransferase (AST) and ALT*** (previously designated SGOT and SGPT) show a ***variable increase*** during the prodromal phase of acute viral hepatitis, and precede the rise in bilirubin level

The ***serum bilirubin may continue to rise*** despite falling serum aminotransferase levels.

Chronic hepatitis

– This represents a series of liver disorders of varying causes and severity in which hepatic inflammation, and necrosis continue for atleast 6 months.

168. Answer is c (Increased proteins, decreased glucose and plenty of lymphocytes).
169. Answer is c (Apical region).
170. Answer is a (Rifampicin and Isoniazid).
171. Answer is c (The clinical presentation of tuberculosis is independent of the CD4 count).

Ref: Harrison's, 17th edition Pg 1010, 1011; 1171-72; Park, 20th edition Pg 173, 175.

Explanation:
The case history/clinical vignette given is that of ***pulmonary tuberculosis***. Evening rise of temperature with night sweats and pulmonary manifestations should clinch the diagnosis.

- ***TB lymphadenitis*** (cervical lymphadenopathy MC) is the most common manifestation of extrapulmonary TB. The diagnosis is established only by fine-needle aspiration (FNAC) or surgical biopsy—shows granulomatous lesion with epithelioid and giant cells.
- ***Postprimary disease also called adult-type, reactivation or secondary tuberculosis***, postprimary disease results from endogenous reactivation of latent infection and is usually localized to the ***apical, and posterior segments of the upper lobes***, where the substantially higher mean oxygen tension (compared with that in the lower zones) favors mycobacterial growth.
- **Primary disease:** Primary pulmonary tuberculosis occurs soon after the initial infection with tubercle bacilli. In areas of high tuberculosis transmission, this form of disease is often seen in ***children***. Because most inspired air is distributed to the ***middle and lower lung zones***, these areas of the lungs are most commonly involved in primary tuberculosis.
- ***Pleural fluid in TB pleural effusion*** = The fluid is straw-colored and at times hemorrhagic; it is an exudate with a ***protein concentration > 50%*** of that in serum (usually ~4–6 g/dL), a ***normal-to-low glucose concentration***, a pH of ~7.3 (occasionally < 7.2) and detectable white blood cells (usually 500–6,000/µL). Neutrophils may predominate in the early stage, while mononuclear cells (***lymphocytes***) are the typical finding later. Mesothelial cells are generally rare or absent.
- ***MDRT: WHO*** defines multidrug resistant TB strain as one that is at least resistant to ***isoniazid and rifampicin***.
- The estimated 10% activation of dormant TB over the life of an infected person is increased to ***10% activation in one year, if HIV infection is superimposed*** (Harrison's, 17th/1172 = For the patient with untreated HIV infection and a positive PPD skin test, the rate of reactivation TB is 7–10% per year).
- The clinical manifestations of TB in HIV-infected patients are quite varied and generally show different patterns as a function of the CD4+ T cell count.
- ***In patients with relatively high CD4+ T cell counts***, the typical pattern of pulmonary reactivation occurs in which patients present with fever, cough, dyspnea on exertion, weight loss, night sweats and a chest X-ray showing cavitary apical disease of the *upper lobes*.
- ***In patients with lower CD4+ T cell counts, disseminated disease*** is more common. In these patients the chest X-ray may show ***diffuse or lower lobe bilateral reticulonodular infiltrates*** consistent with miliary spread, pleural effusions, hilar and/or mediastinal adenopathy.

172. Answer is c (Diabetes mellitus).
173. Answer is d (Hyperlipidemia type III).
174. Answer is a (Good glycemic control).

Explanation:
The clinical vignette given is that of a patient with ***diabetes mellitus***—this question is a direct lift from the below given web page reference from New England Journal of Medicine. Even otherwise diabetes is the most likely answer.

Ref: http://www.nejm.org/doi/pdf/10.1056/NEJMicm050780

- Yellow discoloration of the skin may be associated with
  - Carotenemia (carrots, squash and green beans)
  - Hypothyroidism
  - Diabetes mellitus
  - Liver disease
  - Renal disease.
- ***Yellow skin*** is an *uncommon finding* in patients with diabetes. Traditionally, it is considered to be related to carotenemia, but it may also be associated with end products of advanced glycation.
- This patient needs to be treated with oral hypoglycemic medication, his glycated hemoglobin brought under control and the yellow discoloration of his palms and soles ***will improve***.

175. Answer is d (*Enterobius vermicularis*).
176. Answer is d (*Enterobius vermicularis*).
177. Answer is a (Albendazole).

Ref: Harrison's, 17th edition Pg 1320, 1322.

Explanation:
The case history/clinical vignette given is that of a case of ENTEROBIASIS (pinworm).

Clinical features:
- Most pinworm infections are ***asymptomatic***.
- Perianal pruritus is the cardinal symptom. The itching, which is often worse at night as a result of the nocturnal migration of the female worms, may lead to excoriation and bacterial superinfection.
- Heavy infections may cause abdominal pain and weight loss.
- Rarely, pinworms invade the female genital tract, causing vulvovaginitis and pelvic or peritoneal granulomas.
- Eosinophilia is uncommon.

Diagnosis
- Since pinworm eggs are not released in feces; eggs are detected by the application of clear cellulose acetate tape (***Scotch tape test***) to the perianal region in the morning. After the tape is transferred to a slide, microscopic examination will detect pinworm eggs, which are oval and are flattened along one side.

Treatment:
- Infected children and adults should be treated with mebendazole (100 mg once), albendazole (400 mg once) or pyrantel pamoate (11 mg/kg once; maximum, 1 g), with the same treatment repeated after 2 weeks.
- Treatment of household members is advocated to eliminate asymptomatic reservoirs of potential reinfection.

178. Answer is b (Nephrotic syndrome due to minimal change disease).
179. Answer is a (Membranous glomerulonephritis).
180. Answer is b (Polycystic kidney disease).

Ref: Harrison's, 17th edition Pg 1785, 1790, 1791; Davidson's, 21st edition Pg 469, Box 17.6.

Explanation:
The case history/clinical vignette given is that of NEPHROTIC SYNDROME.

- *Nephrotic syndrome* describes the onset of
  - Heavy proteinuria (> 3.0 g/24 h)
  - Hypertension
  - Hypercholesterolemia
  - Hypoalbuminemia
  - Edema/anasarca
  - Microscopic hematuria.
- Minimal change disease (MCD), sometimes known as nil lesion (since no changes on light microscopy), causes 70–90% of nephrotic syndrome in childhood but only 10–15% of nephrotic syndrome in adults.
- Most common cause of nephrotic syndrome in adults is membranous glomerulonephritis (A/w: lymphoma, Malaria, HBV, Syphilis and ***Drugs*** (gold, penicillamine, captopril).
- All patients are treated with ***corticosteroids.***
- Relapse possible, but ***most patients have good prognosis*** with eventual cessation of relapses.

Renal Biopsy

Indications	**Contraindications**
– ARF that is not adequately explained – CKD with normal sized kidneys – Nephrotic syndrome or glomerular proteinuria in adults – Nephrotic syndrome in children that has atypical features or is not responding to treatment – Isolated hematuria or proteinuria with renal characteristics or associated abnormalities	– Disordered coagulation/ thrombocytopenia/aspirin usage – Uncontrolled hypertension – Polycystic kidneys – Kidneys < 60% of predicted size – Solitary kidney (relative CI)
Complications	
– Pain, usually mild – Minor bleeding into urine, may produce clot colic/obstruction – Bleeding around the kidney – AV fistula	

NOTES

COMED-K 2010

COMED-K 2010 QUESTIONS

MEDICINE

1. **The diabetes control and complication trial (DCCT) provided definitive proof that reduction in chronic hyperglycemia helps to improve**
   (a) Microvascular complications of type 1 DM
   (b) Macrovascular complications of type 1 DM
   (c) Microvascular complications of type 2 DM
   (d) Macrovascular complications of type 2 DM

2. **The most common cause of severe hypercalcemia is**
   (a) Vitamin D toxicity
   (b) Sarcoidosis
   (c) Chronic renal failure
   (d) Malignancy

3. **Investigation of choice in bronchiectasis is**
   (a) Bronchoscopy
   (b) MRI thorax
   (c) HRCT lung
   (d) Chest X-ray

4. **The most strongly implicated premalignant condition of the oral cavity is**
   (a) Fordyce spots
   (b) Erythroplakia
   (c) Median rhomboid glossitis
   (d) Erythema multiforme

5. **Kyasanur forest disease (KFD) is transmitted by**
   (a) Fleas
   (b) Mosquitoes
   (c) Ticks
   (d) Mites

6. **All the following drugs are to be avoided in hypertrophic cardiomyopathy *EXCEPT***
   (a) Diuretics
   (b) Beta blockers
   (c) Digitalis
   (d) Nitrates

7. **The most common organ involved in MEN 1 is**
   (a) Parathyroid
   (b) Thyroid
   (c) Adrenal
   (d) Testis

8. **Which of the following conditions does NOT cause right axis deviation in ECG?**
   (a) Lying down posture
   (b) End of deep inspiration
   (c) Right ventricular hypertrophy
   (d) Right bundle branch block

9. **In primary immune deficiency, the following plasma protein fraction is reduced**
   (a) α-1-globulin
   (b) α-2-globulin
   (c) β-globulin
   (d) γ-globulin

10. **Niacin should be avoided in patients with**
   (a) Peptic ulcer
   (b) Hypertension
   (c) Alzheimer's disease
   (d) Parkinsonism

11. **A patient with pCO_2 80 mm Hg and plasma bicarbonate 33 mEq/L is having**
   (a) Metabolic acidosis
   (b) Respiratory acidosis
   (c) Respiratory alkalosis
   (d) Excessive renal bicarbonate loss

12. **Which of the following is TRUE regarding classical spontaneous bacterial peritonitis?**
   (a) Ascitic fluid neutrophil count is > $250/mm^3$
   (b) Bowel perforation should be present
   (c) Multiple organisms are isolated from ascitic fluid
   (d) Board-like rigidity is present in abdomen

13. **A 35-year-old lady presented with dysphagia, nocturnal asthma and weight loss for 6 years. The most probable diagnosis is**
   (a) Achalasia cardia
   (b) Lye stricture of esophagus
   (c) Gastroesophageal reflux disease
   (d) Cancer esophagus

14. **Fresh water swimming can lead to**
   (a) Brucellosis
   (b) Leptospirosis
   (c) Babesiosis
   (d) Lassa fever

15. **Waddling gait is seen in**
   (a) Muscular dystrophy
   (b) Traumatic paraplegia
   (c) Parkinsonism
   (d) Cerebellar infarct

16. Heyde's syndrome is
(a) Mitral stenosis, arthritis and biliary cirrhosis
(b) Mitral regurgitation, hiatus hernia and cirrhosis
(c) Aortic stenosis, gastrointestinal bleeding and angiodysplasia of colon
(d) Pulmonary arterial hypertension, tricuspid regurgitation and cirrhosis

17. Which muscle is relatively spared in facioscapulohumeral muscular dystrophy?
(a) Deltoid
(b) Biceps
(c) Triceps
(d) Orbicularis oris

18. All the following statements are TRUE regarding methyl alcohol poisoning *EXCEPT*
(a) It is characterized by high anion gap acidosis
(b) It causes ocular toxicity
(c) It causes high osmolal gap
(d) Concurrent ethanol ingestion worsens the clinical features

19. The most likely cause of fluctuating jaundice in a middle-aged or elderly man is
(a) Periampullary carcinoma
(b) Liver fluke infestation
(c) Choledochal cyst
(d) Carcinoma head of pancreas

20. Which vesiculobullous disease is associated with enteropathy?
(a) Pemphigus
(b) Linear IgA dermatosis
(c) Chronic bullous disease of childhood
(d) Dermatitis herpetiformis

21. Which of the following antibodies is involved in the tissue destructive process associated with hypothyroidism in Hashimoto's and atrophic thyroiditis?
(a) Thyroperoxidase antibody
(b) Thyroglobulin antibody
(c) TSH receptor antibody
(d) Thyroid-stimulating antibody

22. Which of the following is NOT used in post-exposure prophylaxis for HIV?
(a) Zidovudine + Lamivudine
(b) Nelfinavir
(c) Stavudine + Didanosine
(d) Acyclovir

23. Reversible airway obstruction is defined as _____ percentage increase in FEV1, 15 minutes after an inhaled short-acting β2-agonist therapy
(a) $\geq 5\%$
(b) $\geq 10\%$
(c) $\geq 15\%$
(d) $\geq 20\%$

24. The ideal tidal volume in a patient ventilated for ARDS is
(a) 6 mL/kg
(b) 10 mL/kg
(c) 14 mL/kg
(d) 20 mL/kg

25. En-coup-de sabre is a form of
(a) Scleroderma
(b) Syphilis
(c) Lupus erythematosus
(d) Alopecia

26. Which of the following is the agent of choice for treating thyrotoxicosis during pregnancy?
(a) Carbimazole
(b) Propylthiouracil
(c) Methimazole
(d) Radioactive I 131

27. Persistent priapism is rarely seen as a consequence of
(a) Sickle cell disease
(b) Leukemia
(c) Spinal cord disease
(d) Prolonged sexual activity

28. Diagnosis of colonic polyps is best done radiologically using
(a) Barium meal series
(b) Double-contrast barium enema
(c) Instant enema
(d) Water-soluble contrast enema

29. The most common location of ventricular septal defect is
(a) Perimembranous
(b) Muscular
(c) Doubly – committed subarterial
(d) Inlet septal

30. Hepatitis B virus is NOT present in
(a) Milk
(b) Sweat
(c) Stool
(d) Lymph

31. A 20-year-old male presents with fever, fatigue, posterior cervical lymphadenopathy, palatal petechiae and splenomegaly. Peripheral smear shows atypical lymphocytes and heterophile antibody is positive. The likely diagnosis is
(a) Acute leukemia
(b) Lymphocytic leukemia
(c) Infectious mononucleosis
(d) Chronic myeloid leukemia

32. The most common site of acute aortic dissection is
(a) Right lateral wall of ascending aorta
(b) Arch of aorta
(c) Suprarenal abdominal aorta
(d) Infrarenal abdominal aorta

SURGERY

33. Polycystic kidney disease is associated with all of the following *EXCEPT*
(a) Cerebral aneurysms
(b) Mitral valve prolapse
(c) Renal cell carcinoma
(d) Hepatic cysts

34. A 45-year-old postmenopausal lady presents with an 8 cm breast lump that is adherent to the skin, with one firm apical lymph node in the axilla and one more node in the ipsilateral supraclavicular area with no clinical evidence of distant metastasis. The staging is
(a) T3 N2 M1
(b) T4 N3c M0
(c) T4 N2c M1
(d) T3 N3 M0

35. In a head injury patient, Mannitol should NOT be used for control of increased intracranial pressure when
(a) Serum osmolality is more than 320 mOsmol/kg
(b) Arterial $PaCO_2$ is less than 35 mm Hg
(c) Arterial PaO_2 is more than 100 mm Hg
(d) Arterial pH is less than 7.35

36. In a healthy adult scheduled for an elective operation, solid food should be withheld for at least ________ hours before surgery
(a) 2
(b) 4
(c) 6
(d) 8

37. Struma ovarii is a
(a) Metastatic tumor
(b) Teratoma
(c) Sex cord tumor
(d) Surface epithelial tumor

38. The indications of colonoscopy in a patient with ulcerative colitis are all of the following *EXCEPT*
(a) Diagnosis of the extent of inflammation
(b) Differentiating it from Crohn's disease
(c) Diagnosis of toxic megacolon
(d) Monitoring the response to treatment

39. Stress-induced ulcers are most commonly found in the
(a) Fundus of stomach
(b) Antrum of stomach
(c) Pyloric channel
(d) First part of duodenum

40. The ideal replacement for the esophagus after esophagectomy is
(a) Stomach
(b) Jejunum
(c) Colon
(d) Synthetic stent

41. Which of the following is NOT a sign of pulmonary hydatidosis?
(a) Water lily sign
(b) Rising sun sign
(c) Meniscus sign
(d) Drooping lily sign

42. The most common cause of epididymitis is
(a) Gonococcal infection
(b) Chlamydia infection
(c) Proteus infection
(d) Tubercular infection

43. The most important prognostic factor of carcinoma breast is
(a) Tumor size
(b) DNA content of tumor
(c) Histologic subtype
(d) Tumor grade

44. A 40-year-old male driver had a car accident in which he got wedged in-between. He complained of severe abdominal pain with radiation to the back. The initial CT on admission was negative except for minimal retroperitoneal hematoma. The diagnosis is
(a) Liver injury
(b) Duodenal perforation

(c) Bowel rupture
(d) Pancreatic injury

45. Choledochotomy is indicated in all of the following *EXCEPT* in patients with
(a) Palpable CBD stones
(b) History of jaundice or cholangitis
(c) Abnormal alkaline phosphatase
(d) Abnormal gamma-glutamyl transferase

46. The most popular incision for open general thoracic surgical procedure is
(a) Anterior thoracotomy
(b) Median sternotomy
(c) Lateral thoracotomy
(d) Transverse thoracosternotomy

OBG

47. The class of antihypertensive drugs, which is contraindicated in pregnancy is
(a) Central sympatholytics
(b) Calcium channel antagonists
(c) Beta blockers
(d) Angiotensin-converting enzyme inhibitors

48. Vulvovaginitis in children could be due to any of the following *EXCEPT*
(a) Worm infestation
(b) Forgotten foreign body
(c) Estrogen deficiency
(d) Chlamydia infection

49. Risk of scar rupture in classical cesarean section is
(a) 0–1.5%
(b) 1.5–4%
(c) 4–9%
(d) 10–12%

50. Hematospermia is due to
(a) Damage of blood-testis barrier
(b) Testicular malignancy
(c) Infection of testis
(d) Infection of urethra

51. With regard to trichomonal vaginitis the following statements are true *EXCEPT*
(a) Discharge is greenish and frothy
(b) It is described as strawberry vagina
(c) Culture of discharge is not necessary for diagnosis
(d) It is treated with doxycycline

52. The composition of Mala-N is
(a) Norgestrel 0.30 mg and Ethinyl estradiol 0.30 µg
(b) Norgestrel 3.0 mg and Ethinyl estradiol 3.0 µg
(c) Norgestrel 0.30 mg and Ethinyl estradiol 30 µg
(d) Norgestrel 30 mg and Ethinyl estradiol 30 µg

53. The correct method to conduct the third stage of normal labor is
(a) Fundal pressure
(b) Bimanual massage
(c) Controlled cord traction
(d) Manual removal

54. In early pregnancy, the doubling time of the concentration of human chorionic gonadotropin in plasma is
(a) 1 day
(b) 2 days
(c) 3 days
(d) 4 days

55. Characteristic fetal anomaly in maternal diabetes is
(a) Sacral agenesis
(b) Anencephaly
(c) Transposition of great vessels
(d) Renal agenesis

56. Chronic treatment with Tamoxifen can cause
(a) Carcinoma ovary
(b) Carcinoma endometrium
(c) Carcinoma cervix
(d) Carcinoma vulva

PEDIATRICS

57. Widely split S1 is heard in
(a) Right bundle branch block (RBBB)
(b) Mitral regurgitation (MR)
(c) Atrial septal defect (ASD)
(d) Ventricular septal defect (VSD)

58. Chest radiographs of children with foreign body aspiration
(a) Are always abnormal
(b) May show overinflation of the involved lung
(c) Always show the foreign body
(d) Commonly show pneumothorax

59. Viral gastroenteritis may be caused by all of the following in infant and young children *EXCEPT*
(a) Enterovirus
(b) Coronavirus
(c) Calicivirus
(d) Adenovirus

60. Conjugated hyperbilirubinemia in neonates is a feature of
(a) Breast milk jaundice
(b) Gilbert's syndrome
(c) Hypothyroidism
(d) Rotor syndrome

61. 10-year-old male with poor growth, poor appetite, recurrent chest infection and steatorrhea is likely to have
(a) High sodium and chloride levels in the sweat
(b) Diabetes mellitus
(c) Recurrent skin allergy
(d) Mental retardation

62. Extraluminal abdominal calcifications in the newborn may be seen in
(a) Meconium aspiration
(b) Hirschsprung's disease
(c) Meconium peritonitis
(d) Meconium plug syndrome

63. Non-immune hydrops fetalis is caused by all *EXCEPT*
(a) Parvo B19 virus
(b) Chromosomal abnormalities
(c) α-thalassemia
(d) ABO incompatibility

64. The most common cause of short stature is
(a) Constitutional
(b) Systemic diseases
(c) Hypothyroidism
(d) Growth hormone deficiency

65. An infant has eczematous rash, rhythmic rocking, microcephaly and hypertonia. What is the likely diagnosis?
(a) Phenylketonuria
(b) Homocystinuria
(c) Tyrosinosis
(d) Autism

66. All of the following are accepted therapeutic measures initiated in hyperammonemic states in an infant *EXCEPT*
(a) Intravenous administration of 10% dextrose with lipids (l g/kg/24 h)
(b) Addition of a mixture of essential amino acids (0.25 g/kg/24 h)
(c) Intravenous infusion of sodium benzoate, sodium phenylacetate and arginine
(d) Exchange transfusion to remove ammonia

67. The most effective method of reduction of incidence of institutional pediatric *Staphylococcus aureus* infection is
(a) Mask and gown use with each suspected patient
(b) Meticulous handwashing before and after contact with patients
(c) Treatment of all culture positive patients with vancomycin
(d) Routine isolation of culture positive patients

ORTHOPEDICS

68. A 50-year-old patient presents with long-standing backache. Skiagram shows lesion in the midline involving the sacrum, which is lytic and expansile. What is the likely diagnosis?
(a) Chordoma
(b) Synovial sarcoma
(c) Osteoclastoma
(d) Fibrosarcoma

69. A 15-year-old with slipped capital femoral epiphysis develops increasing pain and stiffness in the affected hip. Serial X-rays showed progressive reduction in joint space. What complication has the patient developed?
(a) Avascular necrosis
(b) Coxa vara
(c) Secondary osteoarthritis
(d) Chondrolysis

70. Following a road traffic accident, a patient presents with bilateral femoral fractures and shock. The initial treatment would be to
(a) Start an IV line and start plasma expanders
(b) Do a complete physical examination to assess the extent of injuries
(c) Check for adequate airway and then treat shock
(d) Splint the fractures and start a blood transfusion immediately

71. 'Card test' tests the function of
(a) Median nerve
(b) Ulnar nerve
(c) Axillary nerve
(d) Radial nerve

72. Student's elbow is
(a) Trochlear bursitis
(b) Olecranon bursitis
(c) Lateral epicondylitis
(d) Medial epicondylitis

73. Calcification of menisci is seen in
(a) Hyperparathyroidism
(b) Chondrocalcinosis
(c) Renal osteodystrophy
(d) Acromegaly

ENT

74. **Waardenburg syndrome is characterized by all of the following features *EXCEPT***
 (a) Heterochromia of irides
 (b) Lateral displacement of inner canthi
 (c) Conductive deafness
 (d) White forelock

75. **Alderman's nerve is**
 (a) Tympanic branch of glossopharyngeal nerve
 (b) Auricular branch of vagus
 (c) Tonsillar branch of facial nerve
 (d) Chorda tympani nerve

76. **Malignant otitis externa is**
 (a) Malignant melanoma of external ear
 (b) Squamous cell carcinoma of external ear
 (c) Basal cell carcinoma of external ear
 (d) External ear canal infection spreading along bone and soft tissue of skull base

77. **Histopathological picture showing plasma cells, lymphocytes, eosinophils, large foam cells and Russell bodies is characteristic of**
 (a) Rhinoscleroma
 (b) Rhinosporidiosis
 (c) Lupus vulgaris
 (d) Wegener's granulomatosis

OPHTHALMOLOGY

78. **The tear film**
 (a) Is 100 u thick
 (b) Has three layers – mucous, aqueous and lipid
 (c) Has a normal break up time of 5–10 seconds
 (d) Does not contribute to refractive function of the eye

79. **Sjögren's syndrome results in**
 (a) Aqueous tear deficiency
 (b) Mucin deficiency
 (c) Meibomian dysfunction
 (d) Squamous metaplasia

80. **Quick dark adaptation occurs by wearing**
 (a) Red goggles
 (b) Green goggles
 (c) Blue goggles
 (d) Gray goggles

81. **A 25-year-old male complaints of progressive loss of vision of 10 years duration. On examination, the cornea shows bifurcating criss-cross lines associated with punctate opacities. Histology shows that the lesions are composed of amyloid. The most probable diagnosis is**
 (a) Schnyder dystrophy
 (b) Lattice dystrophy
 (c) Granular dystrophy
 (d) Reis-Buckler's dystrophy

82. **Oil droplet reflex on ophthalmoscopy is seen in**
 (a) Pellucid marginal degeneration
 (b) Keratoconus
 (c) Limbal girdle of Vogt
 (d) Terrien's marginal degeneration

83. **Which of the following is NOT an extraocular muscle?**
 (a) Inferior rectus
 (b) Levator palpebrae superioris
 (c) Orbicularis oculi
 (d) Inferior oblique

84. **Smokestack or inkblot appearance in fundus fluorescein angiography is seen in**
 (a) Central serous chorioretinopathy
 (b) Acute retinal necrosis
 (c) Sarcoidosis
 (d) Sickle cell retinopathy

85. **Rhegmatogenous retinal detachment occurs in**
 (a) Hypertension in pregnancy
 (b) Proliferative diabetic retinopathy
 (c) Eales' disease
 (d) High myopia

86. **Rosette cataract is seen in**
 (a) Ocular trauma
 (b) Retained iron foreign body
 (c) Uveitis
 (d) Long-term steroid usage

MICROBIOLOGY

87. **All the following infections due to nematodes result from ingestion of infective eggs *EXCEPT***
 (a) *Ascaris lumbricoides*
 (b) *Enterobius vermicularis*
 (c) *Strongyloides stercoralis*
 (d) *Trichuris trichiura*

88. **Microfilariae of the following parasites are found in blood *EXCEPT***
 (a) *Brugia malayi*
 (b) *Loa loa*
 (c) *Onchocerca volvulus*
 (d) *Wuchereria bancrofti*

89. Weil-Felix test is done to diagnose infections caused by
(a) *Mycoplasma*
(b) *Chlamydia*
(c) *Actinomyces*
(d) *Rickettsia*

90. The virus causing which of the following diseases produces both intranuclear and intracytoplasmic inclusion bodies?
(a) Chickenpox
(b) Rabies
(c) Smallpox
(d) Measles

91. Antibodies acting predominantly on the mucosal cells belong to
(a) IgG class
(b) IgM class
(c) IgE class
(d) IgA class

92. A 22-year-old software engineer was brought in an unconscious state to the casualty. Clinical examination revealed features suggestive of shock, DIC and multisystem failure. CSF and petechial rashes yielded gram-negative diplococcic, which subsequently grew on modified Thayer-Martin medium. This isolation is known to be associated with
(a) Waterhouse-Friderichsen syndrome
(b) Fitz-Hugh-Curtis syndrome
(c) Job's syndrome
(d) Toxic shock syndrome

93. All of the given drugs inhibit microbial cell wall synthesis *EXCEPT*
(a) Neomycin
(b) Vancomycin
(c) Meropenem
(d) Bacitracin

94. The specialized type of microscope, which enables quantitative measurements of the chemical constituents of cells is the
(a) Optical microscope
(b) Interference microscope
(c) Phase contrast microscope
(d) Polarization microscope

PATHOLOGY

95. Which type of immune response is responsible for caseation necrosis in TB?
(a) Cell-mediated immunity
(b) Delayed-type hypersensitivity
(c) Allergic reaction
(d) Immune complexes

96. The immune cells with CD16 and CD56 on their surface, which are important in immunological surveillance and natural defense against virus infected and malignant cells are
(a) Helper T cells
(b) Dendritic cells
(c) Natural killer cells
(d) Macrophages

97. The pH of the freshly collected blood in CPD solution bag is
(a) 7.1
(b) 7.3
(c) 7.4
(d) 7.6

98. Linear deposits of immunoglobulin on immunofluorescence microscopy is typical of
(a) Goodpasture's syndrome
(b) Wegener's granulomatosis
(c) Lupus nephritis
(d) IgA nephropathy

99. The following marker is used to assess the monoclonality in T cells
(a) Kappa and Lambda chain
(b) TCR gene rearrangement
(c) CD
(d) CD34

100. Neurotensinoma causes
(a) Cyanosis
(b) Hypertension
(c) Hyperkalemia
(d) Weight gain

101. The most common type of acute myeloid leukemia is
(a) Hypergranular promyelocytic leukemia
(b) Monocytic leukemia
(c) Myeloblastic leukemia
(d) Erythroleukemia

102. Which of the following disease is transmitted as an X-linked inheritance?
(a) Phenylketonuria
(b) Alport's syndrome
(c) Myotonic dystrophy
(d) Spinal muscular atrophy

103. The most common site of hypertensive intracranial hemorrhage is
(a) Putamen
(b) Midbrain
(c) Medulla
(d) Cerebrum

104. Which one of the following is NOT a feature of autosomal recessive disorder?
(a) Wide variation in phenotype within a family
(b) Males and females are equally affected
(c) Parents of an affected child are heterozygous carriers
(d) Display horizontal pattern in pedigrees

105. Macrophages containing PAS positive granules and rod-shaped bacilli in small intestinal mucosa are found in
(a) Agammaglobulinemia
(b) Tropical sprue
(c) Whipple's disease
(d) Celiac sprue

106. The RBC morphology in a peripheral blood smear in thalassemia trait resembles that of
(a) Vitamin B_{12} deficiency anemia
(b) Folate deficiency anemia
(c) Hereditary spherocytosis
(d) Iron deficiency anemia

107. E-cadherin is more often mutated in
(a) Diffuse type of gastric cancer
(b) Intestinal type of gastric cancer
(c) Malignant ulcer of stomach
(d) Erosive gastritis

108. The sites of endometriosis in order of frequency are
(a) Umbilicus, vulva, rectovaginal septum
(b) Pelvic peritoneum, ovaries, laparotomy scar
(c) Vagina, appendix, uterine ligaments
(d) Ovaries, uterine ligaments, rectovaginal septum

109. Atypical lymphoid cells in infectious mononucleosis are
(a) Monocytes
(b) CD lymphocytes
(c) Killer T cells
(d) Lymphoblasts

DERMATOLOGY, ANESTHESIOLOGY, PSYCHIATRY, RADIODIAGNOSIS

110. Satellite lesions are seen in
(a) Indeterminate leprosy
(b) Borderline leprosy
(c) Borderline tuberculoid leprosy
(d) Lepromatous leprosy

111. Vitiligo is seen in
(a) Blepharitis
(b) Vogt-Koyanagi-Harada syndrome
(c) Syphilitic uveitis
(d) Posner-Schlossman syndrome

112. Which one of these should NOT to be used in severe widespread psoriasis?
(a) Methotrexate
(b) Oral retinoids
(c) Cyclosporin
(d) Oral glucocorticoids

113. The most common plant causing airborne contact dermatitis is
(a) *Semecarpus anacardium*
(b) *Parthenium hysterophorus*
(c) *Croton*
(d) *Primula obconica*

114. The color code for nitrous oxide is
(a) White
(b) Green
(c) Blue
(d) Black

115. The best way of preventing hypotension during spinal anesthesia is
(a) Preloading with crystalloids
(b) Dopamine infusion
(c) Mephentermine
(d) Trendelenburg's position

116. Which of the following side effects is UNLIKELY with glycopyrrolate?
(a) Tachycardia
(b) Inhibition of salivation
(c) Suppression of gastric secretion
(d) Central anticholinergic syndrome

117. Thickened gastric folds on barium meal are seen in
(a) Leiomyosarcoma
(b) Scleroderma
(c) Amyloidosis
(d) Linitis plastica

118. In magnetic resonance imaging, paramagnetic substances cause
(a) Shortening of both T1 and T2 relaxation times
(b) Shortening of T2 relaxation time only
(c) Shortening of T1 relaxation time only
(d) No effect on T1 or T2 relaxation times

119. **Which of the following is NOT a radiological feature of progressive primary pulmonary TB?**
(a) Cavitating disease
(b) Pulmonary nodules
(c) Lobar collapse
(d) Bronchopneumonia

120. **Briquet's syndrome is characterized by**
(a) Multiple delusions
(b) Multiple mood symptoms
(c) Multiple somatic symptoms
(d) Multiple cognitive deficits

121. **After a single depressive episode**
(a) Full recovery is achieved in 5% of patients
(b) Most patients develop a manic episode
(c) There is about 50% chance of recurrence of depression
(d) Antidepressant can be stopped immediately

122. **Oedipus complex according to Sigmund Freud refers to**
(a) Striving for superiority
(b) Dream work
(c) Theory of instincts
(d) Child's love for the parent of opposite sex

123. **Agoraphobia is a disorder characterized by all of the following *EXCEPT***
(a) Visual hallucinations
(b) Avoidance of situations in which it is difficult to obtain help
(c) Presence of panic symptoms
(d) Avoidance of being outside alone

124. **The following is a life-threatening side effect associated with the use of clozapine**
(a) Pancreatitis
(b) Hypoglycemia
(c) Agranulocytosis
(d) Acute renal failure

125. **Which is true of panic disorder?**
(a) It is characterized by recurrent and unpredictable panic attacks
(b) The panic attacks always occur in specific situations
(c) Autonomic symptoms are rare in panic disorder
(d) The panic attacks evolve very slowly

FORENSIC

126. **The minimum blood alcohol level at or above which one can get punished for drunken driving under Indian Motor Vehicles Act is**
(a) 35 mg%
(b) 30 mg%
(c) 40 mg%
(d) 45 mg%

127. **The confirmatory test for blood is**
(a) Benzidine test
(b) Luminol test
(c) Leucomalachite green test
(d) Teichmann test

128. **In case of death due to starvation, at autopsy, the condition of the gallbladder will be**
(a) Distended with inspissated bile
(b) Empty
(c) Filled with mucus
(d) Filled with purulent fluid

129. **The term 'Grave wax' refers to**
(a) Embalming fluid
(b) Fluids of decomposition
(c) Saponification
(d) Soil contamination of a buried body

130. **Sarcoidosis is mimicked by chronic _______ poisoning**
(a) Mercury
(b) Beryllium
(c) Aluminum
(d) Lead

131. **'Declaration of Oslo' deals with**
(a) Abortion
(b) Torture
(c) Human experimentation
(d) Consumerism

132. **Which of the following is called 'Liquid Gold'?**
(a) Marijuana
(b) Amphetamine
(c) Lead
(d) Lysergic acid diethylamide

PREVENTIVE AND SOCIAL MEDICINE

133. Socialized medicine is
(a) Provision of health services to all as a constitutional right
(b) Study of health and disease in the population of a defined community
(c) Systematic investigation of community's health status and problems
(d) Organization of range of promotive, preventive and curative health services

134. The meal provided in mid-day meal program should supply at least
(a) 1/2 of proteins and 1/2 of the calories required per day
(b) 1/2 of proteins and 1/3 of the calories required per day
(c) 1/3 of proteins and 1/3 of the calories required per day
(d) 1/3 of proteins and 1/2 of the calories required per day

135. The disease for which vaccination certificate is required for international travel is
(a) Cholera
(b) Hepatitis
(c) Yellow fever
(d) Tetanus

136. All of the following statements are TRUE about the term 'disease control' *EXCEPT*
(a) Agent is permitted to persist at low levels
(b) Reducing the incidence of disease
(c) Interruption of the transmission of disease
(d) Focus is on primary and/or secondary prevention

137. Burning foot syndrome was described by
(a) Gopalan
(b) Ramalingaswamy
(c) Pauling
(d) Limann

138. Method of identifying missing case of disease in a population is
(a) Epidemiological surveillance
(b) Contact tracing
(c) Sentinel surveillance
(d) Contact survey

139. The 'physical quality of life index' takes into account all of the following factors *EXCEPT*
(a) Infant mortality
(b) Life expectancy at age one
(c) Literacy
(d) Income

140. According to Indian Biomedical Waste Rules, 1998, human anatomical waste (tissues, organs, body parts) are to be segregated in
(a) Yellow bags
(b) Black bags
(c) Red bags
(d) White bags

141. Maternal death is defined as death of a woman while pregnant or within
(a) 14 days of the termination of pregnancy
(b) 30 days of the termination of pregnancy
(c) 42 days of the termination of pregnancy
(d) 90 days of the termination of pregnancy

142. The index of operational efficiency of malaria control/eradication program is
(a) Annual falciparum incidence (AFI)
(b) Slide positivity rate (SPR)
(c) Annual parasite incidence (API)
(d) Annual blood examination rate (ABER)

143. Recommended level of fluorides in drinking water in our country is accepted as
(a) 0.5 mg/L
(b) 1.5 mg/L
(c) 2.5 mg/L
(d) 3.5 mg/L

144. The minimum recommended concentration of free chlorine (mg/L) in drinking water at the end of 1 hour is
(a) 0.1
(b) 0.5
(c) 1.0
(d) 1.5

ANATOMY, PHYSIOLOGY AND BIOCHEMISTRY

145. Right gastroepiploic artery is a branch of
(a) Right gastric artery
(b) Splenic artery
(c) Gastroduodenal artery
(d) Hepatic artery

146. The glabella may show the remains of the
(a) Anterior fontanel
(b) Posterior fontanel
(c) Metopic suture
(d) Lambdoid suture

147. **All are branches of thyrocervical trunk *EXCEPT***
(a) Inferior thyroid artery
(b) Suprascapular artery
(c) Superficial cervical artery
(d) Superior thyroid artery

148. **The cochlear nuclei belong to which type of nuclei**
(a) General visceral afferent
(b) General somatic afferent
(c) Special somatic afferent
(d) Special visceral afferent

149. **Primary sinusoidal dilatation of liver is also known as**
(a) Hepar lobatum
(b) Peliosis hepatis
(c) von Meyenburg complex
(d) Caroli's disease

150. **The common peroneal nerve can be rolled against the following part of the fibula**
(a) Styloid process
(b) Head
(c) Neck
(d) Shaft

151. **Following tarsal bone is devoid of muscular attachment**
(a) Talus
(b) Navicular
(c) Cuboid
(d) Medial cuneiform

152. **Ubiquitin is involved in**
(a) Intracellular proteolysis
(b) Electron transport chain
(c) Transport of ATP
(d) Protein folding

153. **Ghrelin is responsible for**
(a) Stimulation of appetite
(b) Suppression of appetite
(c) Stimulation of sleep
(d) Suppression of sleep

154. **The normal plasma osmolality (mOsmol/kg) is**
(a) 240–255
(b) 260–275
(c) 285–295
(d) 300–312

155. **The stomach motility is inhibited by**
(a) Histamine
(b) Angiotensin
(c) Acetylcholine
(d) Dopamine

156. **The magnitude of an electrical difference that exists across the membrane can be determined by**
(a) Gibbs-Donnan equation
(b) Henderson-Hasselbalch equation
(c) Nernst equation
(d) Fick's law

157. **All of the following are renal vasoconstrictors *EXCEPT***
(a) Angiotensin II
(b) Carbon monoxide
(c) Norepinephrine
(d) Endothelin

158. **Local anesthetics depress transmission first in**
(a) Group A α-fibers
(b) Group A β-fibers
(c) Group B fibers
(d) Group C fibers

159. **Ethanol increases urine output by**
(a) Inhibiting Na^+ reabsorption
(b) Suppressing ADH secretion
(c) Increasing glomerular filtration rate
(d) Suppressing H^+ secretion

160. **Vitamin K is necessary for the formation of the following factors by the liver *EXCEPT***
(a) Factor II
(b) Factor VII
(c) Factor IX
(d) Factor V

161. **In sickle cell anemia**
(a) Glutamate replaces valine
(b) Valine replaces glutamate
(c) Valine replaces aspartate
(d) Aspartate replaces valine

162. **The deficiency of ADAMTS13 enzyme is seen in**
(a) Idiopathic thrombocytopenic purpura
(b) Thrombotic thrombocytopenic purpura
(c) Hemolytic-uremic syndrome
(d) von Willebrand's disease

163. The rate-limiting step in the biosynthesis of catecholamines is catalyzed by
(a) Tyrosine hydroxylase
(b) Dopa decarboxylase
(c) Dopamine f3 hydroxylase
(d) Catechol-O-methyltransferase

164. Benedict's test will be positive in the urine after administration of
(a) Folic acid
(b) Ascorbic acid
(c) Pantothenic acid
(d) Retinoic acid

PHARMACOLOGY

165. Identify the cytoprotective agent that is used for reduction of renal toxicity associated with repeated administration of cisplatin
(a) Amifostine
(b) Estramustine
(c) Carboplatin
(d) Mesna

166. A 160 mg dose of a drug was administered IV and 80 mg was eliminated during the first 120 minutes. If the drug follows first-order elimination kinetics, how much of the drug will remain 6 hours after its administration?
(a) None
(b) 20 mg
(c) 10 mg
(d) 40 mg

167. PGF2α acts predominantly on the
(a) Myometrium
(b) Cervix
(c) Ovary
(d) Pituitary

168. Which among the following anti-HIV drugs is also used to treat viral hepatitis B?
(a) Enfuvirtide
(b) Lamivudine
(c) Efavirenz
(d) Ritonavir

169. Which of the following antitubercular drug requires dose modification in renal failure?
(a) INH
(b) Thiacetazone
(c) Rifampicin
(d) Ethambutol

170. Which among the following benzodiazepines has no active metabolite?
(a) Diazepam
(b) Lorazepam
(c) Flurazepam
(d) Prazepam

171. Which among the following drugs blocks platelet glycoprotein IIb/IIIa receptors?
(a) Abciximab
(b) Etanercept
(c) Adalimumab
(d) Infliximab

172. Bhopal gas tragedy is an example of
(a) Point source epidemic
(b) Continuous epidemic
(c) Propagated epidemic
(d) Slow epidemic

173. Which among the following drugs would be least appropriate for a hypertensive emergency?
(a) Enalapril
(b) Sodium nitroprusside
(c) Nitroglycerin
(d) Labetalol

174. The most common type of primary glomerular disease causing nephrotic syndrome in adults is
(a) IgA nephropathy
(b) Rapidly progressive glomerulonephritis
(c) Membranous glomerulonephritis
(d) Membranoproliferative glomerulonephritis

175. Carditis in rheumatic heart disease may show all of the following features *EXCEPT*
(a) MacCallum plaques
(b) Valve leaf thickening
(c) Bulky friable vegetations
(d) Fused chordae tendineae

176. Which of the following helps to visualize the corneal endothelium
(a) Focal illumination
(b) Retroillumination
(c) Specular reflection
(d) Sclerotic scatter

177. The first step in planning cycle for health is
(a) Fixing priorities
(b) Establishment of objectives and goals

(c) Analysis of the health situation
(d) Assessment of resources

178. First human liver transplantation was performed by
(a) Thomas Starzl
(b) Alexis Carrel
(c) Christiaan Barnard
(d) Halstead

179. Thiamin status of an individual can be detected by which of the following tests/enzymes in erythrocytes?
(a) Transaldolase
(b) Glucose-6-phosphatase
(c) Transketolase
(d) Enolase

180. What is the positive predictive value of the test in the following data?

Screening test results	Diagnosis		Total
	Diseased	Not diseased	
Positive	a	b	a + b
Negative	c	d	c + d
Total	a + c	b + d	a + b + c + d

(a) [a/(a + b)] × 100
(b) [a/(a + c)] × 100
(c) [a/(a + d)] × 100
(d) [b/(a + b)] × 100

COMED-K 2010

ANSWERS AND EXPLANATIONS

MEDICINE

1. **Answer is a (Microvascular complications of type 1 DM).**
Ref: Harrison's, 17th edition Pg 2285-86, Table 338-7.
Firstly, be aware of the ***micro- and macro-vascular complications given in flowchart below:***

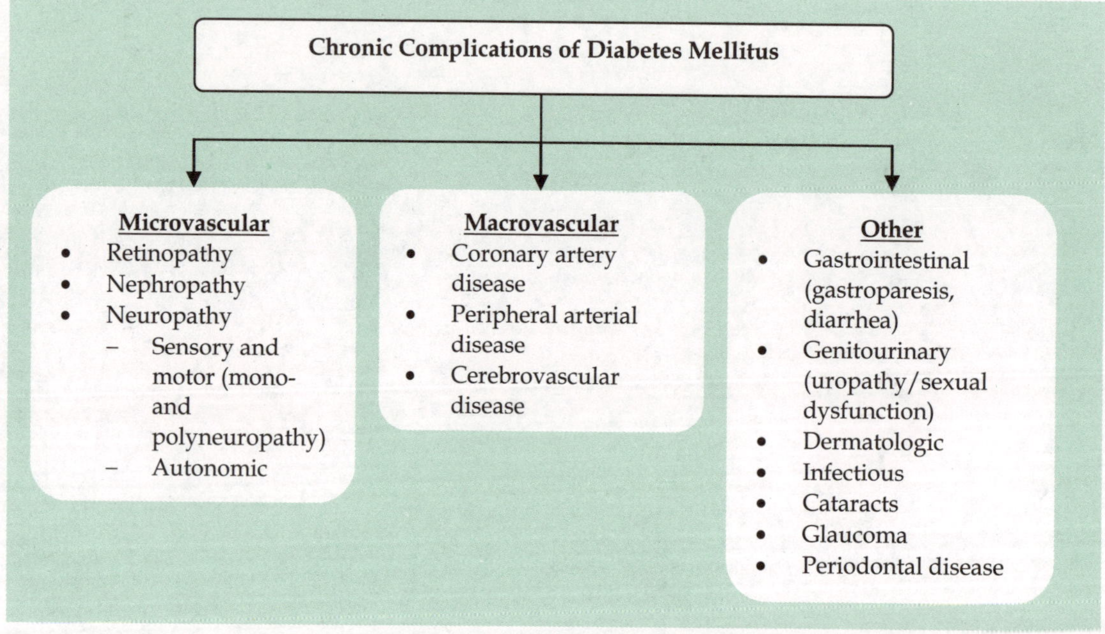

Direct quote:

*"The **Diabetes Control and Complications Trial (DCCT)** provided definitive proof that **reduction in chronic hyperglycemia** can prevent many of the early complications of **type 1 DM**. This large multicenter clinical trial randomized over 1,400 individuals with type 1 DM to either intensive or conventional diabetes management and prospectively evaluated the development of **retinopathy, nephropathy and neuropathy**" (all of which are **microvascular complications** as seen from flowchart above).*

- The DCCT demonstrated that improvement of glycemic control reduced
  - Non-proliferative and proliferative retinopathy
  - Microalbuminuria and clinical nephropathy
  - Neuropathy.

Another direct quote:
*"There was a **non-significant trend in reduction of macrovascular events** during the trial (most individuals were young and had a low risk of cardiovascular disease)".*

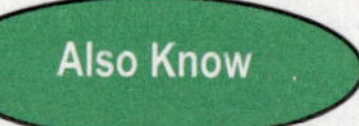

United Kingdom Prospective Diabetes Study (UKPDS)
- UKPDS studied *type 2 DM* patients for ***over 10 years.***

- UKPDS demonstrated that ***each percentage point reduction in A1C*** was associated with a ***35% reduction in microvascular complications***.
- ***Strict blood pressure control*** significantly reduced both macro- and micro-vascular complications.

2. **Answer is d (Malignancy).**
Ref: Harrison's, 17th edition Pg 286.

Direct quote:
"A detailed history may provide important clues regarding the etiology of the hypercalcemia. ***Chronic hypercalcemia*** *is* ***most commonly caused by primary hyperparathyroidism****, as opposed to the* ***second most common etiology of hypercalcemia, an underlying malignancy****".*

3. **Answer is c (HRCT lung).**
Ref: Harrison's, 17th edition Pg 1630.

- CT, especially with ***high-resolution images (HRCT)*** 1.0–1.5 mm thick, provides an excellent view of dilated airways. Consequently, it is NOW the ***standard technique for detecting or confirming the diagnosis of bronchiectasis***.

4. **Answer is b (Erythroplakia).**
Ref: Harrison's, 17th edition Pg 217, Table 32.1-32.4.

Erythroplakia (with or without white patches)	➢ Affects floor of mouth commonly in men; tongue and buccal mucosa in women ➢ Velvety, reddish plaque; occasionally mixed with white patches or smooth red areas ➢ ***High risk of squamous cell cancer*** ➢ Early biopsy essential
Fordyce 'spots'	➢ Affects buccal and labial mucosa ➢ Numerous small yellowish spots just beneath mucosal surface; no symptoms ➢ Due to hyperplasia of sebaceous glands ➢ Benign; remains without apparent change
Median rhomboid glossitis	➢ Congenital abnormality of tongue with ovoid, denuded area in median posterior portion of the tongue ➢ May be a/w candidiasis and may respond to antifungals
Erythema multiforme minor and major (Stevens-Johnson syndrome)	➢ Affects primarily the oral mucosa and the skin of hands and feet ➢ Intraoral ruptured bullae surrounded by an inflammatory area ➢ Lips may show hemorrhagic crusts ➢ The 'iris' or 'target' lesion on the skin is pathognomonic ➢ Patient may have severe signs of toxicity ➢ Onset very rapid; usually idiopathic, but may be associated with trigger such as drug reaction ➢ Condition may last 3–6 weeks; mortality with EM major 5–15% if untreated

5. **Answer is c (Ticks).**
Ref: Harrison's, 17th edition Pg 1236, Table 189-4.

- Kyasanur forest disease is a viral hemorrhagic fever found in Mysore, India and Western Siberia.

More About

Kyasanur forest disease

- Named after Kyasanur forest area in Shimoga district, Karnataka, where cases were first reported
- ***Tick-borne hemorrhagic fever***, seen in monkeys and humans and is genetically related to Russian spring summer encephalitis (RSSE)

- Reservoir hosts: Forest birds and small mammals
- Amplifier hosts: Monkeys
- ***Vector tick: H. spinigera***
- Major outbreak: In 1982 in Belthangady taluk, South Kanara; 1,142 human cases were reported with 104 deaths
- Russian counterpart of KFD is Omsk hemorrhagic fever

6. **Answer is b (Beta blockers).**
Ref: Harrison's, 17th edition Pg 1485.

Hypertrophic Cardiomyopathy (HOCM)

Drugs to be AVOIDED in HOCM	Drugs which CAN be used in HOCM
➢ Digitalis ➢ Diuretics ➢ Dihydropyridine calcium blockers ➢ Nitrates ➢ Vasodilators ➢ β-adrenergic agonists ➢ Alcohol ingestion	➢ Beta blockers ameliorate angina pectoris and syncope in one third to one half of patients ➢ Amiodarone (supraventricular and ventricular arrhythmias) ➢ Non-dihydropyridine calcium channel blockers (verapamil and diltiazem) and disopyramide may reduce the severity of outflow tract pressure gradients

Simple Summary

- ***HOCM*** is characterized by ***LV hypertrophy, typically of a non-dilated chamber, without obvious cause,*** such as hypertension or aortic stenosis.
- Two features of HOCM have attracted the greatest attention:
  - ❖ *Asymmetric LV hypertrophy,* often with *preferential hypertrophy of the interventricular septum*
  - ❖ A *dynamic LV outflow tract pressure gradient* related to narrowing of the subaortic area.
- The ubiquitous pathophysiologic abnormality is ***diastolic dysfunction***, which can be detected by Doppler tissue imaging.
- About *50% of all patients with HOCM* have a positive family history compatible with *autosomal dominant* transmission.
- Clinically:
  - ❖ ***Double or triple*** apical precordial impulse
  - ❖ **S4** (fourth heart sound)
  - ❖ *Rapidly rising* arterial pulse
  - ❖ ***Systolic murmur,*** which is typically harsh, diamond shaped and usually begins well after S1; murmur is best heard at the lower left sternal border as well as at the apex, where it is often more holosystolic and blowing in quality, no doubt, due to the mitral regurgitation that usually accompanies obstructive HOCM.
- Investigations:
  - ❖ ECG – LV hypertrophy and widespread deep, *broad Q waves*
  - ❖ *Chest X-ray* may be normal, although a mild-to-moderate increase in the cardiac silhouette is common
  - ❖ ***Echocardiogram,*** *gold standard for diagnosis,* which demonstrates LV hypertrophy, often with the septum > 1.3 times the thickness of the posterior LV free wall. The septum may demonstrate an unusual 'ground-glass' appearance, probably related to its myocardial fibrosis.
- Treatment – see above.

7. **Answer is a (Parathyroid).**
Ref: Harrison's, 17th edition Pg 2358.

Direct quote:

"*Primary hyperparathyroidism* is the most common manifestation of MEN 1, with an estimated penetrance of 95–100%."
"*Enteropancreatic tumors* are the second most common manifestation of MEN 1, with an estimated penetrance of 50%."

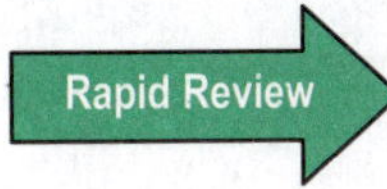

Multiple Endocrine Neoplasia (MEN) Syndromes

MEN 1 (Werner's syndrome), AD	• Parathyroid adenoma • Pancreatic islet cell tumor • Pituitary hyperplasia/adenoma
MEN 2A (Sipple's syndrome), AD	• Medullary carcinoma thyroid, parathyroid adenoma • Pheochromocytoma • MEN 2A with cutaneous amyloidosis • MEN 2A with Hirschsprung's disease • Familial MTC • Monitor calcitonin and calcium levels
MEN 2B or MEN 3, AD	• Medullary carcinoma thyroid • Pheochromocytoma • Mucosal and gastrointestinal neuromas • Marfan habitus, neuropathy
Mixed syndromes	• von Hippel-Lindau syndrome: Renal cell carcinoma, retinal angiomas, hemangioblastoma of CNS, Islet cell tumor, pheochromocytoma
Carney complex	• Myxomas of heart, skin and breast, spotty cutaneous pigmentation, testicular, adrenal and GH secreting pituitary tumors, peripheral nerve schwannomas

8. **Answer is a (Lying down posture).**
Ref: Harrison's, 17th edition Pg 1391; Dent Essentials, High yield NBDE Part 1 review, Kaplan Medical, 2007 edition Pg 173.

- Normally, the QRS axis ranges from –30° to +100°.
- ***Left axis deviation*** = An axis more negative than –30°.
- ***Right axis deviation*** = An axis more positive than +100°.

Left axis deviation	Right axis deviation
➢ Normal variant ➢ Left ventricular hypertrophy (more common) ➢ Block in the anterior fascicle of the left bundle system (left anterior fascicular block or hemiblock) ➢ Inferior myocardial infarction ➢ Expiration ➢ Lying down ➢ Obesity	➢ Normal variant (particularly in children and young adults) ➢ Spurious finding due to reversal of the left and right arm electrodes ➢ Right ventricular overload (acute or chronic) ➢ Infarction of the lateral wall of the left ventricle ➢ Dextrocardia ➢ Left pneumothorax ➢ Left posterior fascicular block ➢ Inspiration ➢ Tall lanky people ➢ Standing up

9. **Answer is d (γ-globulin).**
Ref: Textbook of Microbiology, CP Baveja, 3rd edition Pg 147.

- ***Primary immunodeficiencies*** result from abnormalities in the development of immune mechanisms. It consists of various ***γ-globulin deficiencies***.
- ***Secondary immunodeficiencies*** are due to consequence of some other disease, malnutrition, drugs and other processes that affect the functioning of the normal mature immune system.

10. **Answer is a (Peptic ulcer).**
Ref: KD Tripathi, 6th edition Pg 618; Textbook of Pharmacology, Seth, 2009 edition Pg V-67, 68.

- ***Niacin*** (***Nicotinic acid***) is a B group vitamin whose lipid lowering property is unrelated to its vitamin activity, its amide derivative nicotinamide (vitamin B_3) is ineffective.

- **Lipid changes during niacin therapy**
  - ***Plasma LDL-C*** decreases by 15–25%
  - ***Plasma triglycerides*** decreases by 20–50%
  - HDL increases by 15–35%
  - ***Fall in lipoprotein levels*** by 25% (this effect is not seen with any other hypolipidemic drug and is unique feature of niacin).

- **Adverse effects**
  - Prostaglandin mediated harmless flushing, dizziness, palpitation every time the drug is ingested or dose is increased – can be minimized by taking aspirin tablet 30 minutes before ingestion
  - Peptic ulcer can be activated
  - Pruritus, dry skin, acanthosis nigricans
  - Increased uric acid level
  - Decreased glucose tolerance.

- **Contraindications**
  - Absolute contraindications: Chronic liver disease and acute gout
  - Relative contraindications: Diabetes, hyperuricemia and peptic ulcer disease.

11. Answer is b (Respiratory acidosis).
Ref: Harrison's, 17th edition Pg 288, Fig 48-1.

- ***For detailed explanation,*** see ***Figure 48-1 in Harrison's, 17th/Pg 288,*** read ***Acid-base nomogram*** and the associated text adjacent to it (quite a detailed explanation, which would run into few paragraphs/pages and difficult to elaborate here).

12. Answer is a (Ascitic fluid neutrophil count is > 250/mm³).
Ref: Harrison's, 17th edition Pg 1979.

- **Spontaneous Bacterial Peritonitis** (SBP) is a *common and severe complication of ascites* characterized by ***spontaneous infection of the ascitic fluid*** without an intra-abdominal source.
- ***Bacterial translocation*** is the presumed mechanism for development of SBP.
- The ***most common organisms are Escherichia coli*** and other gut bacteria.
- ***If more than two organisms are identified,*** secondary bacterial peritonitis due to a perforated viscus should be considered.
- The ***diagnosis of SBP*** is made when the ascitic fluid sample has an ***absolute neutrophil count > 250/mm³***.
- Patients with ascites may present with *fever, altered mental status, elevated white blood cell count, and abdominal pain or discomfort, or they may present* ***without*** *any of these features.*
- Therefore, it is necessary to have a high degree of clinical suspicion and *peritoneal taps are important for making the diagnosis.*
- Treatment is with a ***second-generation cephalosporin***, with ***cefotaxime*** being the most commonly used antibiotic.
- ***Prophylaxis against SBP*** is recommended when a patient presents with ***upper GI bleeding*** since in patients with ***variceal hemorrhage***, the frequency of SBP is significantly increased.

13. Answer is a (Achalasia cardia).
Ref: Dunn's Surgical Diagnosis and Management: A Guide to General Surgical Care, David C Dunn, Pg 273.

- In ***achalasia cardia***, the patient is typically aged ***30–40 years*** and the condition is slightly ***more common in females.***
- H/o gradually progressive dysphagia over several years with spasms of epigastric pain radiating to the throat.
- Regurgitation of stagnant, undigested food occurs with foul belching.
- Aspiration occurs at night when patient lies down and it results in a fit of coughing – this is called ***nocturnal asthma.***
- Recurrent chest infections due to aspiration pneumonia are common.
- There may be ***loss of weight.***

Author's comment: *"The D/D is between gastroesophageal reflux (GERD) and achalasia cardia".*

14. **Answer is b (Leptospirosis).**
Ref: Davidson's, 20th edition Pg 288, Table 13.7; http://www.nlm.nih.gov/medlineplus/ency/article/001376.htm.

- ***Leptospirosis*** is caused by exposure to several types of the *Leptospira* bacteria, which can be found in ***fresh water*** that has been contaminated by animal urine. It occurs in warmer climates.
- Risk factors include:
  - ***Occupational exposure***—farmers, ranchers, slaughterhouse workers, trappers, veterinarians, loggers, sewer workers, rice field workers and military personnel
  - ***Recreational activities***—fresh water swimming, canoeing, kayaking and trail biking in warm areas
  - ***Household exposure***—pet dogs, domesticated livestock, rainwater catchment systems and infected rodents.
- Hawaii has the highest number of cases in the United States.
- In India, most outbreaks of leptospirosis are reported in coastal regions: Gujarat (Valsad district), Mumbai, Kerala, Chennai and the Andaman Islands.

15. **Answer is a (Muscular dystrophy).**
Ref: Interpreting Signs and Symptoms, Nursing Series, Lippincott Williams and Wilkins, 2007 edition Pg 278-79.

Waddling gait (duck-like walk) is an important sign of:

- Muscular dystrophy
  - Duchenne's
  - Becker's
- Spinal muscular atrophy
  - Werdnig-Hoffmann disease
  - Kugelberg-Welander syndrome
- Bilateral congenital hip displacement (rarely)

- ***Waddling gait*** may be present when the child begins to walk or may present later in life.
- The gait results from ***deterioration of the pelvic girdle muscles, primarily the gluteus medius, hip flexors and hip extensors***.
- Weakness in these muscles hinders stabilization of the weight bearing hip during walking, causing the opposite hip to drop and the trunk to lean towards that side in an attempt to maintain balance.

<u>**Also Note**</u>:

Ref: Davidson's, 20th edition Pg 1181.
- ***Rolling or Waddling gait***: Seen with *proximal muscle weakness.*
- ***'Like a drunken sailor' gait***: Broad-based gait seen in ***cerebellar ataxia*** (vermis lesions).

16. **Answer is c (Aortic stenosis, gastrointestinal bleeding and angiodysplasia of colon).**
Ref: http://en.wikipedia.org/wiki/Heyde's_syndrome

- ***Heyde's syndrome*** is a syndrome of ***aortic valve stenosis*** associated with ***gastrointestinal bleeding*** from ***colonic angiodysplasia***.
- It is named after ***Edward C Heyde***, who first described the association in 1958.
- It is due to the induction of ***von Willebrand disease type IIA*** by the valvular stenosis.

17. **Answer is a (Deltoid).**
Ref: Harrison's, 17th edition Pg 2866.

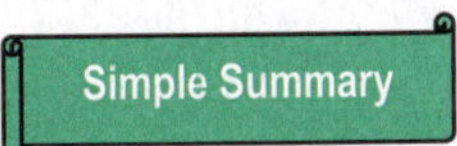

Facioscapulohumeral muscular dystrophy

- Autosomal dominant; deletion, distal 4q; onset before age 20.
- Other associations: *Deafness, Coats' (eye) disease.*

Types of weakness

- ***Facial weakness*** (difficulty with eye closure, whistling and impaired smile) may be *initial manifestation*.
- ***Weakness of the shoulder girdles***, rather than the facial muscles, usually brings the patient to medical attention.
- ***Scapular winging*** becomes apparent with attempts at abduction and forward movement of the arms.
- *Biceps and triceps muscles may be severely affected*, with ***relative sparing of the deltoid muscles***. ***Atrophy of the humeral muscles*** is characteristic.
- Weakness for wrist extension and foot drop may occur.

- Serum CK normal, EMG myopathic pattern.

18. Answer is d (Concurrent ethanol ingestion worsens the clinical features).
Ref: KD Tripathi, 6th edition Pg 387; Davidson's, 20th edition Pg 219.

- ***Methyl alcohol*** is added to rectified spirit in order to render it unfit for drinking.
- Unscrupulous mixing of methylated spirit with alcoholic beverages results in inadvertent methanol poisoning.
- Methanol is metabolized to ***formaldehyde and formic acid*** (by ***alcohol dehydrogenase***) causing profound ***metabolic acidosis*** and ***ocular toxicity*** (retinal damage due to formic acid).
- Death is due to *respiratory failure*.
- Diagnosed by presence of ***high anion gap, osmolal gap (> 10 mOsmol/L)***.
- Treatment: Antidotes [***oral ethanol***, IV ethanol – inhibit alcohol dehydrogenase; ***4-methylpyrazole (fomepizole)*** also inhibits alcohol dehydrogenase; hemodialysis].

Author's comment: *"Thus from the above explanation you see that oral ethanol is actually used as an antidote for methanol poisoning and hence option (d) is the answer"*.

19. Answer is a (Periampullary carcinoma).
Ref: See answer below.

Ref: Portable Signs and Symptoms, Lippincott Williams and Wilkins, 2007 edition Pg 327.

Direct quote:

"Carcinoma of the ampulla of Vater initially produces fluctuating jaundice, mild abdominal pain, a recurrent fever and chills. Occult bleeding may be the first sign".

Ref: Field Guide to Bedside Diagnosis, David S Smith, 2nd edition Pg 126.

Direct quote:

"Fluctuating jaundice occurs with toxins, ampullary carcinoma or gallstones".

20. Answer is d (Dermatitis herpetiformis).
Ref: Harrison's, 17th edition Pg 339, 1881-82.

Celiac Sprue and Dermatitis Herpetiformis (DH)

- DH consists of ***extremely itchy small papules and vesicles*** on elbows, knees, buttocks and posterior nuchal area (extensor surfaces).
- ***Almost all DH patients have:***
  - ➢ An associated, usually ***subclinical, celiac sprue (gluten-sensitive enteropathy)***.
  - ➢ Histologic changes in the small intestine consistent with celiac sprue.
- But, relatively few patients with celiac sprue have DH.
- ***Direct immunofluorescence*** is the ***gold standard of diagnosis: Granular IgA deposits*** at dermoepidermal junction.
- Mainstay of treatment is *Dapsone*.
- Strictly ***exclude gluten from diet*** (i.e. exclude wheat, rye, barley and oats).

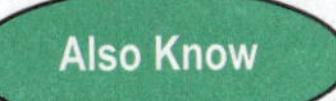

- Celiac sprue is also a/w ***type 1 DM*** and ***IgA deficiency*** (for more associations see *Box. No 22.45 in Davidson's 20th/pg 894*).
- Severe watery diarrhea without evidence of malabsorption in type 1 DM is ***'diabetic diarrhea'***.
- ***Collagen sprue***: A layer of collagen-like material is present beneath the basement membrane; patients do not respond to a gluten-free diet.
- ***Complications*** of celiac disease: ***T-cell lymphoma, small bowel Ca, squamous Ca esophagus***.

21. Answer is a (Thyroperoxidase antibody).
Ref: Harrison's, 17th edition Pg 2232; Davidson's, 20th edition Pg 757; Bailey, 25th edition Pg 776.

- ***Autoimmune hypothyroidism*** may be associated with a goiter (***Hashimoto's or goitrous thyroiditis***) or, at the later stages of the disease, minimal residual thyroid tissue (***atrophic thyroiditis***).
- In Hashimoto's thyroiditis, there is a marked lymphocytic infiltration of the thyroid with germinal center formation, atrophy of the thyroid follicles accompanied by oxyphil metaplasia, absence of colloid and mild-to-moderate fibrosis.
- In atrophic thyroiditis, the fibrosis is much more extensive, lymphocyte infiltration is less pronounced and thyroid follicles are almost completely absent. Atrophic thyroiditis likely represents the end stage of Hashimoto's thyroiditis rather than a distinct disorder.
- ***Thyroid peroxidase (TPO) antibodies*** are present in the serum of ***> 90% patients with Hashimoto's disease*** (direct quote in all three—*Harrison's, 17th/2232; Davidson's, 20th/757; Bailey, 25th/776*).

22. Answer is d (Acyclovir).
Ref: KD Tripathi, 6th edition Pg 776.

Postexposure Prophylaxis (PEP) of HIV [as per National Aids Control Organization (NACO)]

Basic (2 drug) regimen	**For low risk**
Zidovudine 300 mg + Lamivudine 150 mg	Twice daily for 4 weeks
Expanded (3 drug) regimen	
Zidovudine 300 mg + Lamivudine 150 mg + Indinavir (or another protease inhibitor)	Twice daily for 4 weeks Thrice daily for 4 weeks

<u>Low risk =</u>
- When the source is HIV positive, but asymptomatic with low HIV-RNA titer and high CD4 cell count.
- Exposure is through mucous membrane or superficial scratch, or through thin and solid needle.

<u>High risk =</u>
- When the source is asymptomatic AIDS patient with high HIV-RNA titer and low CD4 cell count.
- Exposure is through major splash or large area of contact of longer duration with mucous membrane, or abraded skin or through large bore hollow needle, deep puncture, visible patient's blood on needle.

<u>Note</u>:
- In advanced countries, where a large number of source HIV patients have received one or more anti-HIV regimens and may be harboring drug-resistant virus, alternative prophylactic regimens using ***stavudine, didanosine, abacavir, efavirenz*** or other drugs with which the source has not been treated have been used.
- ***Nevirapine*** is NOT recommended for PEP due to its hepatotoxic potential.
- ***Acyclovir*** is active ONLY against the Herpes group of viruses, so NO use in HIV PEP.

23. Answer is c (≥ 15%).
Ref: Davidson's, 20th edition Pg 656, 673, Fig 19.20, Box 19.22.

- When airflow obstruction is seen, spirometry should be repeated following ***inhaled short-acting β2-adrenoceptor agonists (salbutamol)***; *reversibility to normal is suggestive of asthma.*
- When a ***≥15% (and 200 mL) improvement in FEV1 is noted***, it confirms a diagnosis of asthma.

24. **Answer is a (6 mL/kg).**
Ref: Davidson's, 20th edition Pg 195, Box 8.20, 8.21.

Direct quote:

Optimal ventilation in ARDS
"Ventilation using positive end-expiratory pressure but limiting tidal volume to 5–7 mL/kg and accepting high $PaCO_2$ levels improves outcomes in ARDS".

Principles of Mechanical Ventilation in ARDS

- Optimum ventilator settings are
  - Pressure controlled
  - Long inspiratory to expiratory time
  - Positive end-expiratory pressure (PEEP)
- Allow $PaCO_2$ to rise (permissive hypercapnia) and tolerate lower oxygen saturations than normal (e.g. 88–90%)
- Avoid
  - Large tidal volumes (***ideally 6 mL/kg***)
  - Airway pressure of more than 35 cm H_2O
  - FiO_2 of more than 0.8 if possible
- Remember – high intrathoracic pressure compromise circulatory function, so oxygen delivery *may actually fall* inspite of improved oxygenation
- Management must be a balance between improving gas exchange. Minimizing the risk of subsequent pulmonary fibrosis due to lung injury and avoiding adverse circulatory effects.

25. **Answer is a (Scleroderma).**
Ref: http://www.scleroderma.org/medical/facial_articles/wood_2002_2_1.shtm#encoup

- ***Linear scleroderma 'en-coup-de saber'*** is the localized scleroderma that produces facial changes.
- 'En-coup-de sabre' is a ***French term*** which means ***'cut of the sword'.*** It is so named because its deep lesion or scarring ***resembles a saber wound.***
- Scleroderma *en-coup-de sabre* is confined to one side of the face and cranium (head) and may occur with or without facial hemiatrophy.
- Progressive hemifacial atrophy (PHA), or ***Parry-Romberg syndrome***, has considerable clinical overlap with *en-coup-de sabre.*
- Three phases of scleroderma *en-coup-de sabre* are:
  - The initial inflammatory phase
  - Induration
  - Subsequent atrophy of the skin and underlying tissues, including fat and fascia (fiber-like connective tissue).
- The ***MC early sign*** of scleroderma *en-coup-de sabre* is a painless furrow or indentation near the midline of the face, usually on the forehead or at the frontal hairline, which marks the boundary between normal and atrophic tissue.
- The line of thickened skin on the affected side of the face may spread to involve the cheek area, jaw, chin, neck and upper extremity.
- There may be ***CNS involvement*** (e.g. seizures, epilepsy, focal deficits, headaches), as well as various ***ocular changes*** on the affected side of the face (diminished vision, central corneal thickness, dilated pupil, Horner's syndrome, mydriasis, heterochromia iridis and uveitis).

26. **Answer is b (Propylthiouracil).**
Ref: Harrison's, 17th edition Pg 47.

- The ***treatment of choice for hyperthyroidism during pregnancy is propylthiouracil.*** Because it crosses the placenta, the minimum effective dose should be used to maintain free T4 in the upper normal range.

<u>Contraindicated in pregnancy</u>

- ➢ *Methimazole (and carbimazole)* crosses the placenta to a greater degree than propylthiouracil and has been a/w fetal aplasia cutis.
- ➢ ***Radioiodine*** because of effects on the fetal thyroid.

27. **Answer is c (Spinal cord disease)—answer verified with revised answer key.**
Ref: Harrison's, 17th edition Pg 297.

- ***Priapism** = **P**ersistent* and ***P**ainful erection*.

Conditions causing priapism

- □ *Sickle cell anemia* (MC cause in children): Priapism is due to infarction of the penile venous outflow tracts; permanent impotence is a frequent consequence
- □ *Leukemia (second MC cause in children)*
- □ Hypercoagulable states
- □ Spinal cord *injury*
- □ Injection of vasodilator agents into the penis.

28. **Answer is b (Double-contrast barium enema).**
Ref: Intestinal Polyps and Polyposis: From Genetics to Treatment and Follow-up, by GG Delani, Tomas S, et al. 2009. Pg 94.

- Radiology plays a critical role in the diagnosis and management of colorectal cancer.
- The ***double-contrast barium enema (DCBE)*** may be used for screening, especially for patients who are at higher than normal risk.
- It is also a method for diagnosing symptomatic colorectal cancer and for detecting complications such as obstruction and perforation.

29. **Answer is a (Perimembranous).**
Ref: OP Ghai, 7th edition Pg 40; Harrison's, 17th edition Pg 1450.

• *Ventricular septal defect (VSD)*	= ***MC congenital heart disease***; accounts for 1/3 of all congenital heart defects.
• *90% of VSDs*	= ***located in the membranous part*** of the ventricular septum with extension into the adjoining muscular part.
• *Gerbode defect*	= is rare—there is a communication between the left ventricle and right atrium.

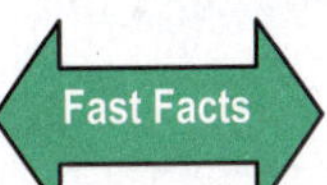

- ❖ 70–80% of VSDs have *spontaneous closure*
- ❖ In infants, failure to thrive, congestive cardiac failure are the MC features
- ❖ VSD is the MC congenital heart disease *complicated by IE*
- ❖ Physical findings
- ❖ Widely split, variable S2
- ❖ Pansystolic murmur at left sternal border
- ❖ Small VSD, loud murmur (Maladie de Roger)
- ❖ CXR: Biventricular hypertrophy, pulmonary plethora.

30. **Answer is d (Lymph).**
Ref: Digestive Involvement in Systemic Autoimmune Diseases, Josep F, Manueal RC, 2008 edition Pg 193.

Direct quote:

"Although HBsAg does not reveal the whole infective HBV particle, it can be detected in all kinds of human secretions including ***blood, serum, saliva, tears, sweat, urine, stool, semen, vaginal secretions and maternal milk****".*

31. **Answer is c (Infectious mononucleosis).**
Ref: Davidson's, 20th edition Pg 307; Harrison's, 17th edition Pg 1108.

- ***Epstein-Barr virus*** (EBV) is the cause of heterophile-positive ***infectious mononucleosis (IM)***.
- **Clinical features of IM**:
  - Fever, fatigue, malaise, myalgia
  - Pharyngitis (often the most prominent sign)
  - Splenomegaly
  - Lymphadenopathy (tender)
  - Jaundice.
- **Diagnosis of IM**:
  - 20% or more ***peripheral lymphocytes*** must have an ***atypical morphology***.
  - Serum ***must*** contain the ***characteristic heterophile antibody***. This antibody present during the acute illness and convalescence, agglutinates erythrocytes of other species (sheep and horse). It has a specific absorption pattern detected by the ***classical Paul-Bunnell titration*** or by a more convenient slide test such as the ***'Monospot' test***.
- **Treatment**: Consists of supportive measures, with rest and analgesia. REMEMBER, treatment with ampicillin results in a macular rash.

32. **Answer is a (Right lateral wall of ascending aorta).**
Ref: Robbins Pathology, 7th edition Pg 532-3; Davidson's, 20th edition Pg 607; Harrison's, 17th edition Pg 1563, Table 242-1.

- ***Acute aortic dissection*** is a catastrophic illness characterized by dissection of blood between and along the laminar planes of the media, with the formation of blood-filled channel within the aortic wall which often ruptures outward causing hemorrhage.
- ***In contrast to atherosclerotic and syphilitic aneurysm,*** aortic dissection may or may not be associated with marked dilatation of the aorta, hence the older term 'dissecting aneurysm' is discouraged.
- Aortic dissection is caused by a ***circumferential*** or less frequently, transverse tear of the intima.
- Sites:
  - Most common: Along the ***right lateral wall of the ascending aorta*** where the hydraulic shear stress is high
  - Another common site is the descending thoracic aorta just below the ligamentum arteriosum.

Also Know

DeBakey's classification	Stanford classification
➢ Type I: Dissection involves ascending to descending aorta. ➢ Type II: Limited to ascending and transverse aorta without descending aorta. ➢ Type III: Dissection involves descending aorta only.	➢ Type A involves ascending aorta (DeBakey I and II) and type B does not (DeBakey III).

Etiology of acute aortic dissection	*Pathology*
☐ Hypertension (80% of cases) ☐ Atherosclerosis ☐ Vasculitis (Takayasu's, Giant cell arteritis) ☐ Pregnancy ☐ Trauma (including cardiac catheterization)	Cystic medial degeneration: Most frequent histological lesion; the term *'cystic medial necrosis'* is inaccurate, because neither necrosis or cysts are present

SURGERY

33. Answer is c (Renal cell carcinoma).
Ref: Harrison's, 17th edition Pg 1798.

AD Polycystic Kidney

- ***APKD-1 gene*** on chromosome **16p** (*Mnemonic:"Polycystic kidney" word* = ***16*** *letters* = ***16p***).
- Does ***not manifest before 30 years.***
- Manifests disease as ***renomegaly, flank pain, hematuria, infection, hypertension, uremia.***
- Associated abnormalities:
  - ***Hepatic cysts*** (*MC extrarenal anomaly*); (also cysts are seen in spleen, pancreas, ovaries)
  - *Intracranial* ***berry aneurysms***
  - ***Colonic diverticula***
  - ***Mitral valve prolapse***
  - *Abdominal wall* and *inguinal hernias.*
- IVU—'***spider-leg***' deformity.

AR Polycystic Kidney

- *ARPKD gene—chromosome 6.*
- Diagnosed in *first year of life* presenting as *bilateral abdominal masses.*
- Death in neonatal period is MC due to *pulmonary hypoplasia.*
- A/w *congenital hepatic fibrosis.*

34. Answer is b (T4 N3c M0).
Ref: Harrison's, 17th edition Pg 566, Table 86-1.

- The given example falls into ***T4 N3c M0*** as per the staging of breast cancers—see below.

STAGING OF BREAST CANCER

Primary Tumor (T)
T0 No evidence of primary tumor
TIS Carcinoma *in situ*
T1 Tumor ≤ 2 cm
T1a Tumor > 0.1 cm but ≤ 0.5 cm
T1b Tumor > 0.5 but ≤ 1 cm
T1c Tumor > 1 cm but ≤ 2 cm
T2 Tumor > 2 cm but ≤ 5 cm
T3 Tumor > 5 cm
T4 Extension to chest wall, inflammation, satellite lesions, ulcerations.

Regional Lymph Nodes (N)
PN0(i-): No regional lymph node metastasis histologically, negative IHC
PN0(i+): No regional lymph node metastasis histologically, positive IHC, no IHC cluster greater than 0.2 mm
PN0(mol-): No regional lymph node metastasis histologically, negative molecular findings (RT-PCR)
PN0(mol+): No regional lymph node metastasis histologically, positive molecular findings (RT-PCR)
PN1: Metastasis in 1–3 axillary lymph nodes or in internal mammary nodes with microscopic disease detected by sentinel lymph node dissection, but not clinically apparent
PN1mi: Micrometastasis (> 0.2 mm, none > 2.0 mm)
PN1a: Metastasis in 1–3 axillary lymph nodes
PN1b: Metastasis in internal mammary nodes with microscopic disease detected by sentinel lymph node dissection, but not *clinically apparent*
PN1c: Metastasis in 1–3 axillary lymph nodes and in internal mammary lymph nodes with microscopic disease detected by sentinel lymph node dissection, but not clinically apparent (if associated with greater than three positive axillary lymph nodes, the internal mammary nodes are classified as PN3b to reflect increased tumor burden)
PN2: Metastasis in 4–9 axillary lymph nodes or in clinically apparent internal mammary lymph nodes in the *absence* of axillary lymph node metastasis
PN3a: Metastasis in ten or more axillary lymph nodes, or in infraclavicular lymph nodes, or in clinically apparent ipsilateral internal mammary lymph nodes in the *presence* of one or more positive axillary lymph nodes

PN3b: Metastasis in more than 3 axillary lymph nodes with clinically negative microscopic metastasis in internal mammary lymph nodes
PN3c: Metastasis in ipsilateral supraclavicular lymph nodes.

Distant Metastasis (M)
M0: No distant metastasis
M1: Distant metastasis (includes spread to ipsilateral supraclavicular nodes).

35. **Answer is a (Serum osmolality is more than 320 mOsmol/kg).**
Ref: Neurological and Neurosurgical Intensive Care, Alan HR, 2004 edition Pg 42.

- ***Mannitol*** is used routinely in cases of ***raised intracranial pressure***.
- However, it is frequently suggested that the ***use of mannitol be curtailed if serum osmolality exceeds 320 mOsmol/L → Direct myocardial depression*** and ***renal failure*** are feared.
- Despite frequent repetition of this tenet by authoritative sources, its validity has never been established.

More About

Therapeutic uses of mannitol	Contraindications to mannitol
• ***Promotion of diuresis*** in the prevention or treatment of the oliguric phase of acute renal failure before irreversible renal failure is established • ***Reduction of intracranial pressure*** and brain mass • ***Reduction of high intraocular pressure*** when the pressure cannot be lowered by other means • ***Promotion of urinary excretion*** of toxic materials	• Acute LVF, congestive heart failure • Anuria, acute tubular necrosis • Cerebral hemorrhage

36. **Answer is c (6).**
Ref: Stoelting and Miller's, Basics of Anesthesia, 5th edition 2007. Pg 175, Table 13-26 (adapted from the journal Anesthesiology 1999; 90:896-905).

Summary of fasting recommendations to reduce the risk of pulmonary aspiration (These recommendations apply to healthy patients undergoing elective operations)

Ingested Material	Minimum Fasting Period (applies to all ages)
Clear liquids (water, pulp free juices, carbonated beverages, clear tea, black coffee)	2 hours
Breast milk	4 hours
Infant formula	6 hours
Non-human milk	6 hours
Light meal (typically—toast and clear liquids; meals that include fried or fatty foods or meat may prolong the gastric emptying time)	6 hours

37. **Answer is b (Teratoma).**
Ref: Robbins Pathology, 7th edition Pg 1100.

- ***Struma ovarii*** is composed entirely of ***mature thyroid tissue***—a monodermal ***teratoma*** present in the ***ovary***.
- These thyroid neoplasms may overfunction causing ***hyperthyroidism***.

38. **Answer is c (Diagnosis of toxic megacolon).**
Ref: Atlas of Colonoscopy: Techniques, Diagnosis, Interventional Procedures. Helmut M, Jürgen B, Pg 94; Practical Pediatric GI Endoscopy, George G, Marvin Em, 2007 edition Pg 133 and 134, Table 7.1 and 7.2.

- As seen from table below colonoscopy is contraindicated in toxic megacolon.

Indications for colonoscopy in IBD (Ulcerative colitis and Crohn's disease)	Contraindications to colonoscopy
• Diagnosis • Differential diagnosis	• Peritonitis • Conditions with high risk of perforation

• Evaluation of extent and severity • Treatment monitoring • Unclear response to therapy • Evaluation of prognosis • Surveillance for colorectal cancer	– Fulminant colitis – Toxic megacolon – Recent surgical anastomoses • Inability to visualize mucosa – Poor bowel preparation – Massive GI bleeding • Associated medical problems – Sepsis – Absolute neutropenia – Respiratory and CVS distress

39. **Answer is a (Fundus of stomach).**
Ref: Harrison's Gastroenterology and Hepatology, Anthony FS and Longo, 2010 edition Pg 148.

- Patients suffering from shock, sepsis, massive ***bURns (CURling's ulcers)***, severe trauma, ***head injury (Cushing's ulcers)*** can develop acute erosive gastric mucosal changes or frank ulceration with bleeding.
- Classified as stress-induced gastritis or gastric ulcers, injury is most commonly observed in the acid-producing (fundus and body) portions of the stomach.
- Histologically stress injury does not contain inflammation or *H. pylori* – hence 'gastritis' here is a misnomer.

40. **Answer is a (Stomach).**
Ref: Tropical Hepatogastroenterology, BN Tandon, 2008 edition Elsevier Publications. Pg 21 and Table 1.13.

Direct quote:

"Several organs have been used as conduits to replace the esophagus after esophagectomy (stomach, colon, jejunum, myocutaneous grafts).
The ***stomach is the overwhelming favorite.***
The gastroepiploic arcade provides a good collateral blood supply and the robust submucosal plexus takes care of the blood supply at the fundus."

Comparison of replacements for esophagus (conduits) after esophagectomy

	Stomach	Colon (left)	Jejunum
Vascularity	Very good	Good	Uncertain
Length	Adequate	Adequate	Short
Ease	Easy	Tedious	Cumbersome
Anastomotic problems	+	++	+++
Reflux	++	–	+
Nutritional problems	+	–	–
Respiratory problems	+	–	–
Preoperative preparation	–	+	–

Author's comment: *"The above reference book author, BN Tandon is considered as the Father of Tropical Hepatogastroenterology"*.

41. **Answer is d (Drooping lily sign).**
Ref: www.ajronline.org/cgi/reprint/145/3/639.pdf (article titled "The Radiology of Hydatid Disease").

Signs of Pulmonary Hydatidosis on Chest X-ray

'Meniscus/crescent sign'	As the cyst enlarges, it erodes bronchioles. Air is introduced between the penicyst and laminated membrane and appears as a thin, lucent crescent in the upper part of the cyst: the crescent or meniscus sign or perivesicular pneumocyst. It is a sign of impending rupture and is an indication for urgent thoracotomy.
'Water lily', 'iceberg' or 'camalote' sign	When completely collapsed, the crumpled endocyst floats freely in the most dependent part of the pericyst cavity.

'Rising sun' sign	Daughter cysts may, rarely, be present and the appearance of a round daughter cyst in the lowest part of the cavity resembles the rising sun.
Cumbo's sign	When the parasite itself ruptures and air enters it, the endocyst is outlined by a double arch of air.
'Onion peel' sign	CT may show an onion-peel appearance.
'Serpent' sign	
'Whirl' sign	

Author's comment: *"No single textbook gives all these signs in one location; however the above journal article is a comprehensive giving the above signs, hence the above reference".*

42. **Answer is b (Chlamydia infection).**
Ref: Harrison's, 17th edition Pg 824.

Direct quote:

*"In sexually active men, under the age 35, **acute epididymitis is caused most frequently by C. trachomatis** and less commonly **by N. gonorrhoeae**".*

Also Know

- ☐ ***Acute epididymitis***, almost always ***unilateral***, produces ***pain, swelling and tenderness of the epididymis***, with or without symptoms or signs of urethritis.
- ☐ D/D = Testicular torsion, tumor and trauma.
- ☐ ***Ceftriaxone*** (250 mg as a single dose IM) followed by ***doxycycline*** (100 mg PO twice daily for 10 days) is effective for both *N. gonorrhoeae* or *C. trachomatis*.

Note

- ☐ ***Testicular torsion***, a surgical emergency, usually occurs in the second or third decade of life and produces a sudden onset of pain, elevation of the testicle within the scrotal sac, rotation of the epididymis from a posterior to an anterior position and absence of blood flow on Doppler examination or 99mTc scan.
- ☐ ***Prehn's sign: Elevation of the scrotum*** usually ***relieves pain in epididymo-orchitis***, but increases the pain in torsion of the testis (spermatic cord).

43. **Answer is a (Tumor size).**
Ref: Mayo Clinic Internal Medicine Textbook, by Thomas MH, 2007 edition Pg 662.

Direct quote:

"The ***number of axillary lymph nodes involved is the most important*** predictor of outcome. After nodal status, tumor size is the most important prognostic factor".

Author's comment: *"This is an often repeated question in the Karnataka PGET also. The above given reference is taken since the direct quote is given. However, **Harrison's, 17th/566 and Bailey and Love, 25th/841, also mention axillary nodal status and tumor size** as the most important prognostic factor".*

- ***Other prognostic variables*** are histological, grade, hormone receptor status, measures of tumor proliferation such as S-phase fraction, growth factor analysis and oncogene or oncogene product measurements.

44. **Answer is d (Pancreatic injury).**
Ref: Bailey and Love's, 25th edition Pg 348, 1137.

- The ***pancreas*** is not frequently damaged in blunt abdominal trauma due to its location in the ***retroperitoneum***.
- A ***forceful blow to the epigastrium*** may crush the body of the pancreas against the vertebral column.
- Blunt pancreatic trauma presents with ***abdominal pain radiating to the back***.
- CT scan will delineate the damage to the pancreas and the ***retroperitoneal hematoma*** may be seen.

45. **Answer is d (Abnormal gamma-glutamyl transferase).**
Ref: SRB's Manual of Surgery, Sriram Bhat, 2nd edition 2007, Jaypee, Pg 407.

Indications for choledochotomy

- Ultrasound shows stone in CBD
- Palpable stone in CBD
- CBD diameter > 10 mm
- Recent h/o jaundice with raised serum alkaline phosphatase level
- On table cholangiogram shows stone (using C-arm)

46. **Answer is b (Median sternotomy).**
Ref: Complications in Cardiothoracic Surgery: Avoidance and Treatment, Alex GL and Walter HM, 2nd edition Pg 38.

Direct quotes:

- Median sternotomy provides anterior mediastinal, bilateral pleural and lower cervical access. It is ideal in both elective and emergency situations including thoracic trauma.
- Superb exposure of the heart and the great vessels has made the incision the gold standard for cardiac surgery, particularly when cardiopulmonary bypass is indicated.
- Median sternotomy can be performed rapidly.
- It is safe and heals rapidly.
- Since it is less painful than thoracotomy, it compromises pulmonary function less, especially in the early postoperative period making it the ideal incision for patients with diminished pulmonary capacity.

Author's comment: *"An often repeated question in the Karnataka PGET also, The above direct quotes should be more than enough to tell you why median sternotomy is the best answers".*

OBG

47. **Answer is d (Angiotensin-converting enzyme inhibitors).**
Ref: KD Tripathi, 6th edition Pg 553; Dutta's obstetrics, 6th edition Pg 507, Table 33.6.

Antihypertensive drugs to be avoided during pregnancy	Antihypertensive drugs found safer during pregnancy
• ***Diuretics***: Tend to reduce blood volume, accentuate uteroplacental perfusion deficit (of toxemia), increase risk of fetal wastage, placental infarcts, miscarriage, stillbirth • ***ACE inhibitors, AT1 antagonists***: Risk of fetal damage, growth retardation • ***Non-selective beta blockers***: Propranolol implicated in causing LBW, decreased placental size, neonatal bradycardia and hypoglycemia • ***Sodium nitroprusside***	• Hydralazine • ***Methyldopa*** (central sympatholytic) • Dihydropyridine ***CCBs***: Discontinue before labor since they weaken uterine contractions • Cardioselective ***beta blockers*** and those with ISA: for example, atenolol, metoprolol, pindolol and acebutolol may be used if no other choice • Prazosin and clonidine—provided that postural hypotension can be avoided

- *Dutta's Obstetrics, 6th edition/Pg 506* mentions
  - ***Methyldopa is drug of first choice***; safe for both mother and fetus.
  - ***Labetalol can also be used; efficacy and safety equal to methyldopa.***
  - ***Sodium nitroprusside*** as drug of last resort for acute hypertension. Should be used in critical care for very short time. Fetal toxicity due to metabolites—cyanide and thiocyanate.

48. **Answer is c (Estrogen deficiency).**
Ref: Shaw's Gynecology, 14th edition Pg 106, 119, 130.

- ***Vulvovaginitis in children*** may be
  - Nonspecific due to ***foreign body*** inserted into vagina
  - ***Threadworm*** infection
  - *Gonococcus, E. coli, T. vaginalis, Candida, Chlamydia.*
- *Estrogen deficiency* causes *senile vaginitis* most commonly in postmenopausal women.

49. Answer is c (4–9%).
Ref: William's Obstetrics, 22nd edition Pg 611, Table 26.4.

Estimated risks for uterine rupture in women with previous cesarean delivery

Prior uterine incision	Estimated rupture
Low transverse	0.2–1.5%
Low vertical	1–7%
T-shaped	4–9%
Classical	4–9%

50. Answer is d (Infection of urethra).
Ref: Urological Oncology by Vinod HN, 2007 edition Pg 120.

Direct quote (from emedicine.com):

"***Urethritis***, has ***long been recognized as a cause of hematospermia***, especially in younger men".

- ***Hematospermia*** is defined as ***blood in the semen.***

Causes of hematospermia

Congenital	Infections
– Seminal vesicle (SV)/ejaculatory duct cysts	– Urethritis, prostatitis, epididymitis – Genitourinary TB – CMV, HIV – Schistosomiasis, hydatid – UTI – Condyloma of urethra and meatus
Obstruction	**Tumors**
– Prostatic and SV ejaculatory duct calculi – Postinflammatory SV cysts – SV diverticula – Urethral stricture – Utricle cyst – BPH	– Prostate, bladder, SV, urethra, testis, epididymis, melanoma
Vascular	**Trauma/Iatrogenic**
– Prostatic varices – Prostatic telangiectasia – Hemangioma – Posterior urethral veins – Excessive sexual intercourse – Masturbation	– Perineum – Testicle – Self-instrumentation – Post-hemorrhoid injection – TRUS biopsy – Venovenous fistula
Systemic	
– HTN, hemophilia, purpura, bleeding disorders, chronic liver disease, renovascular disease – Leukemia, lymphoma – Cirrhosis of liver, amyloidosis	

51. **Answer is d (It is treated with doxycycline).**
Ref: Shaw's Gynecology 14th edition Pg 132.

Types of Vaginitis

***Trichomonas* Vaginitis**	• ***Trichomonas vaginalis*** is actively motile and anaerobic. • Sexually transmissible; its ingress into the vagina is favored when the ***pH is raised (5–6)*** during menstrual period. • It is characterized by ***copious, green, frothy discharge***, which may be associated with ***foul odor* and *vulvar pruritus***. • On examination, punctuation on the cervix and vagina, classically called ***'strawberry cervix/vagina'*** is seen. • ***Diagnosis*** may be made by ***saline wet mount of the vaginal discharge***, which reveals highly motile trichomonads. • Treatment is with ***metronidazole***.
Candidal Vulvovaginitis	• *Caused by* ***Candida albicans***, which ***flourishes in an acid medium*** with an abundant supply of carbohydrate. It is therefore common in pregnancy, diabetes, use of OCPs, systemic steroids, antibiotics. • Clinically ***thick, white, curdy discharge with extreme vulvar itching***; white patches of cheesy material adherent to the vagina, which when removed leave multiple petechial-like hemorrhagic areas. • Diagnosis is by microscopic examination of the vaginal discharge in 10% KOH solution, which reveals candidal hyphae and buds. Cultures with Nickerson's medium may be used. • Treatment is by antifungal agents: Topical (azole creams) and/or systemic (fluconazole).
Bacterial Vaginosis	• This is caused by an overgrowth of a variety of bacterial species such as ***Gardnerella vaginalis* (MC)**, *Bacteroides, Peptostreptococcus* and *Mycoplasma hominis*. • *Gardnerella vaginalis* vaginitis is characterized by vaginal discharge with a ***'fishy/musty'* odor with *little vulvar irritation***. • ***Amsel criteria:*** Any three of the following four clinical abnormalities: 1. Objective signs of increased white homogeneous vaginal discharge. 2. A vaginal discharge pH of > 4.5. 3. Liberation of a distinct *fishy odor* (attributable to volatile amines such as trimethylamine) immediately after vaginal secretions are mixed with a 10% solution of KOH. 4. Microscopic demonstration of ***'clue cells'*** (vaginal epithelial cells coated with coccobacillary organisms, which have a granular appearance and indistinct borders) on a wet mount prepared by mixing vaginal secretions with normal saline in a ratio of ~1:1. • Treatment is by ***metronidazole***.
Herpes	• Usually occurs as ***vesicles*** on the genital region, about 1 week after infection. • There is tenderness, swollen glands and fever. The vesicles are ***extremely painful*** and heal in about 3 weeks. However, herpes is usually an external infection and does not fall under the category of vaginitis.
Atrophic Vaginitis (or 'Senile Vaginitis')	• Usually causes ***scant vaginal discharge with no odor, dry vagina and painful intercourse***. • These symptoms are usually due to ***decreased estrogen*** usually occurring during and after menopause.

52. **Answer is c (Norgestrel 0.30 mg and Ethinyl estradiol 30 μg).**
Ref: Dutta's Obstetrics, 6th edition Pg 565.

☐ *Mala-N* and *Mala-D* are oral contraceptive pills (*OCPs*).

• *Mala-N* contains norgestrel 0.3 mg and ethinyl estradiol 30 µg (0.03 mg) • Mala-*N* supplied *free* through all PHCs (*Mnemonic N = No* cost)	• *Mala-D* contains levonorgestrel 0.5 mg and ethinyl estradiol 30 µg (₹3/packet)

Note:

- *30 micrograms* = 30 × 10^{-6} g = 0.03 mg.

53. Answer is c (Controlled cord traction).
Ref: Dutta's Obstetrics, 6th edition Pg 141-143.

- ***Third stage of labor*** = Separation, descent and expulsion of the placenta with its membranes.
- Direct quote: "Desire to fiddle with the uterus or ***massage*** the uterus is to be ***strongly condemned***".
- ***Manual removal of placenta*** is attempted ONLY WHEN repeated ***controlled cord traction fails*** to deliver the placenta.

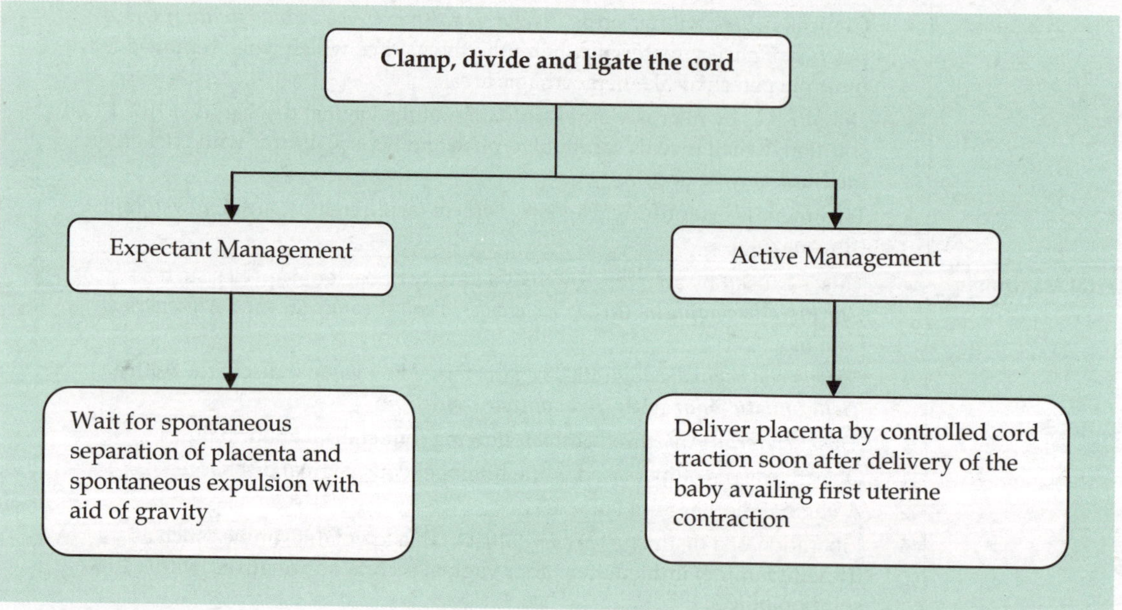

54. Answer is b (2 days).
Ref: Dutta's Obstetrics, 6th edition Pg 58.

Direct quote:

"In the early pregnancy, the doubling time of hCG concentrations in plasma is ***1.4–2 days****".*

More About

Human Chorionic Gonadotropin (hCG)

- Synthesized by the ***syncytiotrophoblast*** of the placenta.
- t½ = 1.5 days; by RIA it can be detected in the maternal serum or urine as early as ***8–9 days following ovulation***— used to detect pregnancy.
- Maximum blood and urine levels seen between 60 and 70 days of pregnancy; disappears from the circulation within 2 weeks following delivery.

- hCG ***maintains the corpus luteum*** (and thus progesterone) for the first trimester by acting like LH (otherwise no luteal cell stimulation and abortion results). In the second and third trimester, the placenta synthesizes its own estriol and progesterone and the corpus luteum degenerates.

55. Answer is a (Sacral agenesis).
Ref: Dutta's Obstetrics, 6th edition Pg 287.

- Chance of ***major congenital malformation*** is more if ***HbA1C values in the first trimester is*** ≥ 9.5%.

Major birth defects in infants of diabetic mothers

CNS and skeletal	Cardiac	Renal	Gastrointestinal	Others
Sacral agenesis Anencephaly Microcephaly Neural tube defects	VSD, ASD Coarctation of aorta TGV Cardiomegaly	Renal agenesis Hydronephrosis Ureteral duplication	Duodenal atresia Anorectal atresia	Single umbilical artery

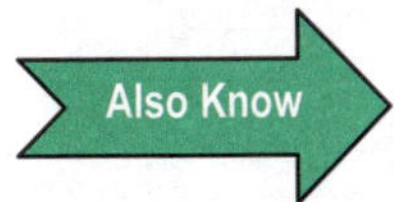

Clinical features of infant of diabetic mother

General	Cardiovascular
– Macrosomia – Normal head size – Increased subcutaneous fat – Birth trauma – Hairy pinna	– Cardiomegaly – Transient hypertrophic cardiomyopathy – Persistent fetal circulation
Others	**Metabolic**
– Renal vein thrombosis – Respiratory distress syndrome – Polycythemia – Increased risk of DM – Small (lazy) left colon syndrome – Increased incidence of Down syndrome	– Hypoglycemia Hypocalcemia – Hypomagnesemia – Hyperbilirubinemia

56. Answer is b (Carcinoma endometrium).
Ref: Harrison's, 17th edition Pg 527, 569.

- ***Tamoxifen is a partial estrogen receptor antagonist***; it has a *ten fold greater antitumor activity in breast cancer patients whose tumors express estrogen receptors* than in those who have low or no levels of expression.
- Side effects include:
  - A somewhat increased risk of estrogen related cardiovascular complications, such as ***thromboembolic phenomena***
  - A small increased incidence of ***endometrial carcinoma***, which appears after ***chronic use (usually > 5 years)***
  - Increased risk of ***cataract formation***
  - ***Tamoxifen retinopathy.***

PEDIATRICS

57. Answer is A [right bundle branch block].
Ref: OP Ghai, 7th edition Pg 398, 399 and Fig 14.8; Harrison's, 17th edition Pg 1459.

- <u>NOTE</u>: *"Widening of the S1 is most often due to complete right bundle branch block and the resulting delay in onset of the right ventricular pressure pulse" – Harrison's, 17th edition Pg 1385.*

Repeat Topic

Normal second heart sound (S2)

- Has two components A2 (aortic closure) and P2 (pulmonary closure).
- During expiration A2 and P2 are superimposed – so single sound is heard.
- During Inspiration A2 precedes P2 – so splitting occurs.
- A2 is louder than P2 except in infants below 3–6 months.

Abnormalities in splitting of S2

- Normal S2 is single in expiration (i.e. A2-P2 interval < 0.03s) and A2-P2 interval > 0.03s in inspiration.
- ***Wide splitting means*** A2-P2 interval > 0.03s during expiration.
- ***Wide variable splitting***: During inspiration, the A2-P2 interval increases further.
- ***Wide and fixed splitting***: The A2-P2 interval is the same in inspiration and expiration.

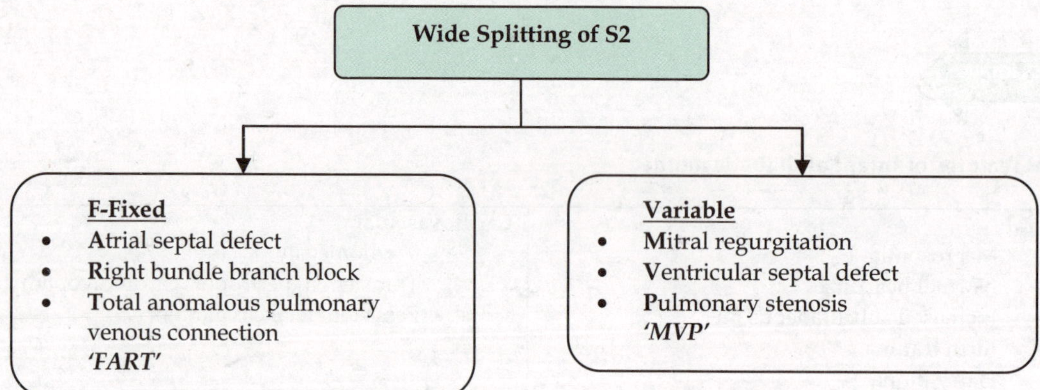

Note: ***Reversed/paradoxical splitting*** due to delayed left heart emptying (e.g. LBBB).

58. Answer is b (May show overinflation of the involved lung).
Ref: Encyclopedia of Diagnostic Imaging, Albert LB, 2008 edition Pg 728; Board Buster Clinical Cases: Steps 2 and 3, by George Jesse Taylor, LWW, 2004 edition Pg 42.

- ***Partial obstruction*** resulting in a ***'ball-valve' effect*** may cause ***overinflation of the distal lung segment***.
- Complete obstruction causes atelectasis.
- Most aspirated foreign bodies are radiolucent – in one study, 80% of the chest radiographs were normal.

59. Answer is a (Enterovirus).
Ref: Harrison's, 17th edition Pg 1205, Table 183.1; Park, 20th edition Pg 195, Table 2.

Infections causing diarrhea

Viruses	Bacteria	Others
Rotaviruses	*C. jejuni*	*E. histolytica*
Astroviruses	*E. coli*	*G. lamblia*
Adenoviruses	*Shigella*	Trichuriasis
Caliciviruses	*Salmonella*	*Cryptosporidium*
Coronaviruses	*V. cholerae*	Intestinal worms
Norwalk viruses	*V. parahaemolyticus*	
Enteroviruses	*B. cereus*	

Direct quotes (from Harrison's, 17th/1208)

"Several other viruses (e.g. *enteroviruses, reoviruses, pestiviruses and parvovirus B*) have been identified in the feces of patients with diarrhea, but their ***etiologic role in gastroenteritis has not been proven***".

"*Enteroviruses* are so named, because of their ability to multiply in the gastrointestinal tract. Despite their name, these viruses are ***NOT a prominent cause of gastroenteritis***".

60. Answer is d (Rotor syndrome).
Ref: Robbins Pathology, 7th edition Pg 887, Table 18.3; Nelson's Essentials of Pediatrics, 6th edition Pg 317; Oski's Pediatrics, 4th edition Pg 238.

Predominantly unconjugated hyperbilirubinemia
□ Excess bilirubin production
➢ Hemolytic anemia
➢ Resorption of blood from internal hemorrhage (GI tract bleeding, hematomas)
➢ Ineffective erythropoesis syndrome (pernicious anemia, thalassemia)
□ Reduced hepatic uptake
➢ Drug interference with membrane carrier systems
➢ Gilbert syndrome
□ Impaired bilirubin conjugation
➢ Physiologic jaundice of the newborn (decreased UGT1A1 activity, decreased excretion)
➢ Breast milk jaundice (prolonged neonatal jaundice)
➢ Congenital hypothyroidism/cretinism (prolonged neonatal jaundice)
➢ Crigler-Najjar syndrome types I and II
➢ Diffuse hepatocellular disease (viral or drug-induced hepatitis, cirrhosis)
Predominantly Conjugated hyperbilirubinemia
□ Dubin-Johnson syndrome
□ Rotor syndrome
□ Impaired bile flow

➲ ***Cretinism, breast milk jaundice***: ***Prolonged*** unconjugated hyperbilirubinemia.

61. Answer is a (High sodium and chloride levels in the sweat).
Ref: Harrison's, 17th edition Pg 1632-34.

- The case history given is that of ***cystic fibrosis*** **(CF)**.
- CF is an ***autosomal recessive*** disease resulting from mutations in the gene that encodes the ***CF transmembrane conductance regulator (CFTR) protein*** located on ***chromosome*** 7.
- This disease is characterized by:

Respiratory system	▪ Chronic bacterial infection of the airways that ultimately leads to bronchiectasis and bronchiolectasis ▪ > 95% of CF patients die of complications resulting from lung infection
Exocrine pancreatic insufficiency	▪ Protein and fat malabsorption, with frequent, bulky, foul-smelling stools
Intestinal dysfunction	▪ Abdominal distention, failure to pass stool and emesis. The abdominal flat plate can be diagnostic with small-intestinal air-fluid levels, a granuiar appearance representing meconium and a small colon—meconium ileus
Abnormal sweat gland function	▪ CF patients are not able to absorb NaCl from sweat as it moves through the sweat duct due to the inability to absorb Cl^- across the ductal epithelial cells; sweat Cl^- concentration > 70 mEq/L
Urogenital dysfunction	▪ Late onset of puberty is common in both males and females; some 20% of CF women are infertile; more than 95% of male patients with CF are azoospermic

62. Answer is c (Meconium peritonitis).
Ref: Chapman's Radiological D/D, 5th edition Pg 364-65.

Meconium peritonitis

- Antenatal bowel perforation results in ***aseptic peritonitis, which rapidly calcifies.***

- *Calcification occurs in the peritoneum itself* most commonly, but also in the bowel wall and scrotum.
- It may be a feature of *Hirschsprung's disease, small left colon syndrome* and a presenting feature of *cystic fibrosis.*

About the other choices

❖ *Meconium plug syndrome*—plugged meconium present in distal colon.
❖ *Hirschsprung's disease*—multiple dilated loops of small bowel seen.
❖ *Meconium aspiration*—affects the lungs and not the abdomen.

63. Answer is d (ABO incompatibility).
Ref: Dutta's Obstetrics, 6th edition Pg 497, 333.

- ***Non-immune hydrops fetalis (NIHF)*** is defined as the accumulation of extracellular fluid in tissues and serous cavities ***in conditions OTHER THAN Rh incompatibility***.
- With complete prevention of Rh problem, ***more than 75% of fetal hydrops is due to NIFH***.
- It is a/w
  - ➢ Increased skin thickness (> 5 mm)
  - ➢ Placental enlargement
  - ➢ Pericardial effusion
  - ➢ Pleural effusion
  - ➢ Ascites.

Causes of Hydrops Fetalis

- ■ **Immune hydrops fetalis** = Rh incompatibility, ABO incompatibility
- ■ **Non-immune hydrops fetalis**
  - – ***Chromosomal:*** Down's, Turner's, triploidy, aneuploidy
  - – ***Cardiac failure***: Arrhythmias (SVT, heart block), congenital heart disease, AV malformation
  - – ***Congenital infection***: TORCHeS, parvovirus B19
  - – ***Hematological:*** β-thalassemia, G6PD deficiency
  - – ***Congenital malformations***: Diaphragmatic hernia, renal abnormality (congenital nephrotic syndrome), lung malformation (adenomatous or lymphangiectasia)
  - – ***Placental and umbilical cord diseases***: Twin-to-twin transfusion, chorioangioma, umbilical vein thrombosis
  - – ***Malignancy***: Neuroblastoma
  - – ***Others***: Uncontrolled maternal diabetes, severe anemia, thyrotoxicosis, achondroplasia, hypoalbuminemia, hepatitis, meconium peritonitis
  - – ***Idiopathic*** (20%)

64. Answer is a (Constitutional).
Ref: OP Ghai, 7th edition Pg 17, 18.

❖ ***Short stature*** is defined as height below 3rd centile or more than 2 SD below the median height for that age and sex according to the population standard.
❖ ***50% cases = physiological (most common); constitutional or familial.***
❖ 50% cases = pathological.

Causes of pathological short stature

- Undernutrition (common)
- Chronic systemic illness (renal, CVS, GIT, severe chronic infections)
- Growth hormone deficiency
- Hypothyroidism
- Precocious/delayed puberty
- Skeletal dysplasia (achondroplasia, rickets)
- Genetic (Turner's, Down's).

65. Answer is a (Phenylketonuria).
Ref: OP Ghai, 7th edition Pg 628; Harrison's, 17th edition Pg 2470.

- The hyperphenylalaninemia result from ***impaired conversion of phenylalanine to tyrosine***.
- The most common and clinically important is ***phenylketonuria*** (frequency 1:10,000), which is an ***autosomal recessive*** disorder.
- Clinical features:
  - Child is usually ***normal at birth*** and in first month of life, but later:
    - Fail to attain early developmental milestones
    - Develop ***microcephaly***
    - Demonstrate progressive impairment of cerebral function
    - ***Hyperactivity, hyperkinesis, muscular hypertonia, seizures and severe mental retardation*** are major clinical problems later in life.
  - ***'Mousy/musty' odor*** of skin, hair and urine (due to phenylacetate accumulation)
  - Tendency to ***rashes and eczema***
  - ***Blond hair, blue eyes and fair skin*** (due to high phenylalanine levels which result in competitive inhibition of tyrosinase which converts tyrosine to melanin).
- ***Guthrie test*** or ferric chloride detects abnormal urinary metabolites of phenylalanine
- To prevent mental retardation, diagnosis and initiation of dietary treatment of classic phenylketonuria must occur *before the child is 3 weeks of age*.

66. **Answer is d (Exchange transfusion to remove ammonia).**
Ref: OP Ghai, 7th edition Pg 634; Harrison's, 17th edition Pg 2474.

- In ***hyperammonemic states*** (organic acidemias, urea cycle defects), therapy is aimed at stopping catabolism and ammonia production by providing adequate calories (***as intravenous glucose and lipids*** in the comatose patient) and, if needed, insulin.
- Excess nitrogen is removed by ***intravenous phenylacetate and benzoate*** (0.25 g/kg for the priming dose and subsequently as an infusion over 24 h) that conjugate with glutamine and glycine, respectively to form phenylacetylglutamine and hippuric acid, water-soluble molecules efficiently excreted in urine.
- ***Arginine*** (200 mg/kg/d) becomes an essential amino acid (except in arginase deficiency) and should be provided intravenously to resume protein synthesis.
- Appropriate dietary restriction of proteins (in acute stage 0.25 g/kg/d as ***mixture of essential amino acids*** and later 1–1.5 g/kg/d).
- ***Hemodialysis, peritoneal dialysis or hemofiltration*** should be instituted if serum ammonia *exceeds 500 mmol/L*.
- Sustained ammonia *levels > 800 mmol/L are a/w irreversible neurological damage*.

67. **Answer is b (Meticulous handwashing before and after contact with patients).**
Ref: Pediatric Critical Care Medicine: Basic Science and Clinical Evidence, Derek S Wheeler, Hector Wong, 2007 edition Pg 1482.

Direct quote:
"Numerous reviews have consistently demonstrated that appropriate **handwashing** *remains the* ***single most effective measure to decrease Staphylococcus aureus*** **infection**".

Another direct quote:
"***Handwashing is the most effective means of preventing spread*** *of Staphylococcus aureus" (Pediatric Board Certification Review, Katie S Fine, 2008 edition LWW, Pg 145).*

ORTHOPEDICS

68. **Answer is a (Chordoma).**
Ref: Maheshwari, 3rd edition Pg 216 and Fig 30.1e.

- ***Chordoma*** is a locally malignant, sometimes actually malignant tumor supposedly originating from the remnants of the notochord.
- The ***sacrum*** and cervical spine are commonest sites.
- It presents with ***persistent pain and swelling***, sometimes with a neurological deficit.

- ***Bone destruction*** is the only ***hallmark feature*** of this tumor.
- Treatment, if possible, is by complete excision; if not possible, by radiotherapy.

69. Answer is a (Avascular necrosis).
Ref: John Ebenezer's Orthopedics, 4th edition Pg 41, 417.

- ***Avascular necrosis of the femoral head (13%)*** and chondrolysis are usual complications of slipped capital femoral epiphysis.
- In avascular necrosis, patient complains of ***pain, develops limp with loss of movements***.
- ***X-rays of bone*** show ***dense changes in the bone, collapse and osteoarthritis*** features.

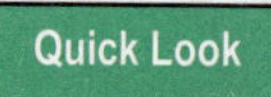

Slipped Capital Femoral Epiphysis

- MC affects ***boys aged 10–16 years***; 30% are bilateral; 50% of patients are obese (may be endocrine abnormality).
- Pain in the groin, limitation of internal rotation and abduction. Trendelenburg's sign may be positive.
- ***Trethowan's sign***: A line drawn along the superior surface of the neck, passes superior to the head unlike in a normal head where it passes bisecting the head.
- ***Capener's sign***: Normally, the posterior acetabular margin cuts across the medial corner of the metaphysis. But in slipped epiphysis the entire metaphysis remains lateral to the posterior acetabular margin.

70. Answer is c (Check for adequate airway and then treat shock).
Ref: Essential Orthopedics, Maheshwari, 3rd edition Pg 122.

- In ***closed fracture shaft of the femur***, an average of ***1,200–1,500 mL*** of blood is lost and may result in hypovolemic shock.
- Hence, all patients with this fracture should be on IV line with blood arranged in case need arises.
- A close watch should be kept on pulse and blood pressure during the early post injury period.

Also Know

❖ In ***pelvic fractures also excess blood loss can occur*** without obviously being visible externally and hence the first step would be to ***prevent shock by starting IV fluids***, ensuring patent airway and stabilizing the patient. Fracture repair will be the next step. Similar question is asked in various examinations.

71. Answer is b (Ulnar nerve).
Ref: Maheshwari, 3rd edition Pg 55.

• **Ulnar N**	– Injury results in ***partial claw hand*** – In ***Ulnar N injury*** there is ***paralysis of all the interossei and the medial two lumbricals*** Palsy tested by: – ***Froment's sign/Book test***: When the adductor pollicis (Ulnar N) paralyzed patient tries to hold the book by using the flexor pollicis longus (Median N) in place of adductor – ***Egawa test*** (weak dorsal interossei): Unable to abduct middle finger/fingers against resistance – ***Card test*** (weak palmar interossei): Unable to hold card between fingers *PAD = Palmars ADduct; DAB = Dorsals ABduct*

Also Know

• **Median N**	Palsy tested by: – ***Pointing index*** (Oschner's clasping test): Flexor digitorum superficialis and flexor digitorum profundus of the index finger are paralyzed

	– *Pen test:* Tests the abductor pollicis brevis – *Ape thumb* (simian deformity)
• **Radial N**	– Commonly injured in *fracture of the humeral shaft* – Injury is usually a *neuropraxia only* – Paralysis of the wrist, finger and thumb extensors (wrist drop), brachioradialis and the supinator. There is a sensory change in a small area on the radial side of the back of the hand. – For *wrist drop cock-up splint* may be needed – In neglected cases or where repair of divided nerve is impractical *modified Jones tendon transfer* is popular

72. **Answer is b (Olecranon bursitis).**
Ref: Essential Orthopedics, Maheshwari, 3rd edition Pg 256; Essential Orthopedics, RM Shenoy, 262.

- ***Olecranon bursitis*** is also called ***Student's (Miner's/draughtsman's) elbow***.

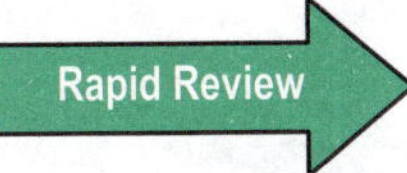

Other Named Bursitis

• Prepatellar bursitis	Housemaid's knee
• Infrapatellar bursitis	Clergyman's knee or Vicar's knee
• Ischial bursitis	Weaver's bottom
• On lateral malleolus	Tailor's ankle
• On great toe	Bunion
• Popliteal cyst	Morrant Baker's cyst
• Lateral end of clavicle	Porter's shoulder

Note:
- ***Jumper's knee***: Patellar tendonitis involving the lower pole of the patella due to overuse of patellofemoral extensor mechanism.

73. **Answer is b (Chondrocalcinosis).**
Ref: Chapman's radiological D/D, 5th edition Pg 410.

- ***Calcium pyrophosphate dihydrate deposition disease (CPPD)*** consists of 3 manifestations, which occurs singly or in combination:
  1. Crystal-induced acute synovitis (***acute gout***).
  2. ***Cartilage calcification*** (***chondrocalcinosis***).
  3. Structural joint abnormalities (***pyrophosphate arthropathy***).

- ☐ ***Chondrocalcinosis*** involves:
  – ***Fibrocartilage***: Especially menisci of the knee, triangular cartilage of the wrist, symphysis pubis and annulus fibrosus of the IV disk.
  – ***Hyaline cartilage***: Especially the wrist, knee, elbow and hip.

ENT

74. **Answer is c (Conductive deafness).**
Ref: Harrison's, 17th edition Pg 325, 200.

Waardenburg syndrome

- ☐ ***Piebaldism*** (***White forelock***; areas of ***hypomelanosis*** contain normally pigmented and hyperpigmented macules of various sizes)
- ☐ Congenital ***sensorineural deafness***
- ☐ ***Dystopia canthorum*** (lateral displacement of the inner canthi, but normal interpupillary distance)

- ***Heterochromatic irises***
- ***Broad nasal root***
- Mutations in three genes including two (*PAX-3* and *MITF*) that encode DNA-binding proteins

Fast Facts

Syndromic forms of hearing loss (sensorineural)

- Usher syndrome (retinitis pigmentosa and hearing loss)
- Pendred syndrome (thyroid organification defect and hearing loss)
- Alport's syndrome (renal disease and hearing loss)
- Jervell and Lange-Nielsen syndrome (prolonged QT interval and hearing loss), neurofibromatosis type 2 (bilateral acoustic schwannoma)
- MELAS (mitochondrial encephalopathy, lactic acidosis and stroke-like episodes)
- MERRF (myoclonic epilepsy and ragged red fibers)
- Progressive external ophthalmoplegia.

75. Answer is b (Auricular branch of vagus).
Ref: Logan Turner's ENT, 10th edition Pg 218-220.

- The **auricular branch of the vagus nerve** is often termed the **Alderman's nerve** or **Arnold's nerve.**

76. Answer is d (External ear canal infection spreading along bone and soft tissue of skull base).
Ref: Harrison's, 17th edition Pg 208.

Invasive otitis externa (malignant or necrotizing otitis externa)

- A potentially life-threatening disease.
- Occurs MC in elderly ***diabetics and immunocompromised*** patients.
- MC caused by ***P. aeruginosa.***
- The disease begins in the external canal, progresses slowly over weeks to months and often is difficult to distinguish from a severe case of chronic otitis externa, because of the presence of ***purulent otorrhea and an erythematous swollen ear and external canal.***
- Severe, ***deep-seated otalgia*** is often noted (and can help differentiate invasive from chronic otitis externa).
- Characteristic finding: ***Granulation tissue in the posteroinferior wall of the external canal, near the junction of bone and cartilage.***
- If left unchecked, the infection can ***migrate to the base of the skull*** (resulting in skull-base osteomyelitis) and on to the ***meninges and brain,*** with a high associated mortality rate.
- **Treatment**:
  - ***External ear canal should be cleaned*** and a biopsy specimen of the granulation tissue within the canal (or of deeper tissues) should be obtained for culture.
  - IV antibiotic therapy for *P. aeruginosa*: The regimen typically includes an ***antipseudomonal penicillin or cephalosporin*** (e.g. piperacillin or ceftazidime) with an ***aminoglycoside***.
  - ***Antibiotic drops*** containing an agent active against *Pseudomonas* (e.g. ciprofloxacin) are usually prescribed and are ***combined with glucocorticoids*** to reduce inflammation.

77. Answer is a (Rhinoscleroma).
Ref: Maqbool's ENT Textbook, 11th edition Pg 198.

- ***Rhinoscleroma*** is a chronic progressive granulomatous disease of the respiratory tract caused by ***Klebsiella rhinoscleromatis*** (***Frisch bacillus***).
- Worldwide distribution: In India, common in ***UP, MP, Mumbai, Delhi and Punjab*** and elsewhere in Central and Eastern Europe and South America.

- Histology of lesion shows a picture of granuloma characterized by ***plasma cells, lymphocytes*** and ***eosinophils*** among which are scattered ***large foam cells*** (***Mikulicz cells***) with vacuolated cytoplasm and mononuclear cells with nucleus (***Russell bodies***) having an eosinophilic cytoplasm and enveloping large quantities of Frisch organisms.
- ***Stages***: *Prodromal stage* (catarrhal) → *Atrophic stage* (resembling atrophic rhinitis) → *Nodular stage* (bluish red nodules) → *Stenotic stage* (nostrils get stenosed).
- ***Treatment*** is by *antibiotics* (streptomycin/tetracycline/rifampicin) *for 2–3 months* depending upon the response. Steroids may be necessary. In late stages, surgery is necessary to clear the airway.

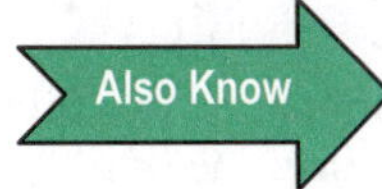

- ☐ ***PAS positive inclusions*** containing immunoglobulin are frequently seen in the cytoplasm (***Russell bodies***) or nucleus (***Dutcher bodies***) of plasmacytoid cells in ***multiple myeloma***.

OPHTHALMOLOGY

78. **Answer is b (Has three layers—mucous, aqueous and lipid).**
Ref: Kanski's Clinical Ophthalmology, 6th edition Pg 210.

Precorneal Tear Film

Layer	**Secreted by**	**Mnemonic**
• Outer **L**ipid layer	**Me**ibomian glands	*'Love Me'*
• Middle **A**queous layer	Lacrimal and accessory lacrimal glands	*'Always'*
• Inner **M**ucin layer	Conjunctival **G**oblet cells	*'My Girl'!*

<u>**About the other choices:**</u>

- ❖ ***Normal tear film break up time*** is ***more than 10 seconds***.
- ❖ Tear film is a ***part of the refractive surface of the eye***—acts like a tear lens.
- ❖ ***Normal tear film thickness*** is about ***500–1,000 microns***.

79. **Answer is a (Aqueous tear deficiency).**
Ref: Kanski's Clinical Ophthalmology, 6th edition Pg 207, Table 7.1.

Types of Dry Eyes

☐ **Aqueous deficiency**	• Due to lacrimal gland disease by – ***Sjögren's syndrome*** (Keratoconjunctivitis sicca: Triad of ***dry eyes, dry mouth and rheumatoid arthritis***) – Lacrimal gland inflammation – Drugs – Collagen vascular disease – Sarcoidosis – Ocular cicatricial pemphigoid – Radiation – Chemical burns – Graft vs host disease
☐ **Mucin deficiency**	• Due to goblet cells disease by – Conjunctival scarring (alkali burns, trachoma, pemphigoid) – Hypovitaminosis A – Drug induced

☐ **Lipid deficiency**	• Due to meibomian gland disease from – Blepharitis – Meibomitis – Anhidrotic ectodermal dysplasia (congenital absence of meibomian glands)

80. Answer is a (Red goggles).
Ref: Anatomy and Physiology of the Eye, Khurana, 2nd edition Pg 214 and Fig. 6.80.

- It has been common practice in occupations in which work has to be performed under dim illumination (ex: ***pilots during night flying***) to keep the eyes exposed to red light by ***use of red goggles*** in an effort to ***preserve the dark adaptation of the retina***.
- The possible explanation of the effect of red goggles is that *their use prevents the short waves of the spectrum (blue end of the spectrum)* from reaching the rods and thus *preventing their bleaching* (since only the rods are affected by the blue end of the spectrum).
- Therefore, in order that the sensitivity of the rods mechanism be maintained, the blue end of the spectrum must be eliminated.

81. Answer is b (Lattice dystrophy).
Ref: Kanski, 6th edition Pg 293-300.

Corneal dystrophies – Stromal dystrophies

Lattice dystrophy	Granular dystrophy	Macular dystrophy
AD	AD	AR
Criss-crossing lattice lines like network	Bread crumb-like sharply demarcated deposits spring limbus	Poorly delineated dense spots involving limbus
Amyloid deposits	Hyaline deposits	Glycosaminoglycans deposits

82. Answer is b (Keratoconus).
Ref: Parson's, 20th edition Pg 203.

KERATOCONUS

Early signs	Late signs
– Keratoscopy/Placido's disk: Irregular rings – Retinoscopy: ***Scissor reflex*** – Direct ophthalmoscopy: ***Oil drop sign*** – *Vogt's striae* (Vertical lines) – Prominent corneal nerves	– ***Fleischer's ring***: Iron deposition in epithelium at base of cone – ***Munson's sign***: Bulging of lower lid when patient looks down – ***Charleaux sign***: Arrowhead reflex on torchlight examination – Corneal scarring
Etiology	**Treatment**
– Chromosomal disorders (Down's syndrome) – Connective tissue disorders (Marfan's syndrome) – Cutaneous disorders (atopic dermatitis, allergic eye disease – due to constant eye rubbing) – Contact lens wear – Congenital eye anomalies (aniridia, Leber's amaurosis) *'5 Cs'*	– Hard (RGP) contact lenses – Optical penetrating keratoplasty (has excellent success) – Newer treatments: ➲ Rose K contact lens ➲ INTACS (**INT**r**AC**orneal ring **S**egments) ➲ DALK (**D**eep **A**nterior **L**amellar **K**eratoplasty) ➲ C3R (**C**orneal **C**ollagen **C**ross linking with **R**iboflavin eye drops)

__Note__: Some similar terms
- ☐ ***Oil drop cataract***: Seen in ***galactosemia***
- ☐ ***Kayser-Fleischer*** ring: Seen in ***Wilson's disease*** due to *copper deposition in Descemet's membrane.*

83. **Answer is c (Orbicularis oculi).**
Ref: Short answer questions for the MRCOphth, by Nathaniel KC, Petros C. 2005 edition Pg 136.

Direct quote:

"Some consider levator palpebrae superioris to be an extraocular muscle, but its function, elevation of upper lid is quite different to that of recti or oblique muscles."

Author's comments: *This answer has been confirmed with another reference also (Neuroscience in medicine, P Michael Conn, 3rd edition 2008. Pg 556. Surprisingly not found in all standard ophthalmology textbooks!).*

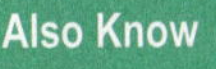

Six extraocular muscles are (4 recti and 2 obliques):
- Superior rectus
- Inferior rectus
- Medial rectus
- Lateral rectus
- Superior oblique
- Inferior oblique.

Nerve supply of extraocular muscles
- ☐ **LR6(SO4)3**: Means Lateral rectus (abducens, CN VI); Superior oblique (trochlear CN IV); all others including levator palpebrae (oculomotor, CN III).

Actions of extraocular muscles:

Muscle	Primary action	Subsidiary action
• Medial rectus	Adduction	
• Lateral rectus	Abduction	
• Superior rectus	Elevation	Intorsion and adduction
• Inferior rectus	Depression	Extorsion and adduction
• Superior oblique	Intorsion	Depression and abduction
• Inferior oblique	Extorsion	Elevation and abduction

Easy method of remembering EOM actions

The actions of extraocular muscles are frequently asked in PG entrance examinations. It is a straight forward question and should be answered correctly.

Basic concepts
- Primary action is the action when the eye is in the primary position.
- Subsidiary actions are the additional effects on the position of the eye.

Read and remember the below statements.

Horizontal recti have only one action (i.e. primary action only)
- Medial rectus: Adduction
- Lateral rectus: Abduction.

AND
- *All other muscles have one primary and two subsidiary actions.*

AND
- *Primary action of oblique muscles is torsion (intorsion or extorsion).*

AND
- *Primary action of superior rectus is elevation and inferior rectus is depression.*

After going through the above statements,

- JUST Remember the mnemonic **'SINRAD'**, which means: All **S**uperiors are **IN**tortors; All **R**ecti (obviously I am talking about only the 2 *vertical* recti) are **AD**ductors.
- The mnemonic also implies (inferiors are extortors and obliques are abductors), but you don't need to remember this.
- Superior oblique—'copying (in examination) muscle'; inferior oblique—'stargazer's muscle'.
- With the above knowledge read the above table once; now take a paper and write down the actions once without looking. IT WORKS. And you will not forget even if you want to!

84. Answer is a (Central serous chorioretinopathy).
Ref: Parson's, 20th edition Pg 238-39.

Central Serous Retinopathy

☐ **Etiology**	– Localized serous detachment of retina at macula due to RPE pump failure – Affects ***young males*** with *type A personality, hypertensives*, aggravated by *systemic steroid usage*; may be a/w *optic disc pit*
☐ **Clinically**	– Moderately blurred vision correctable with weak 'plus' lens, central positive scotoma ('something blocking vision'), micropsia, ***ring reflex at macula***
☐ **Treatment**	– Diagnosed by ***fluorescein angiogram***—shows ***MC smokestack pattern or inkblot pattern*** – Usually ***resolves spontaneously***

85. Answer is d (High myopia).
Ref: Parson's, 20th edition Pg 311-317.

Retinal Detachment (RD)

☐ **Rhegmatogenous RD**	– ***MC type of RD***; due to ***tear/break*** in retina – MC in ***high myopes*** due to frequent ***lattice degeneration*** – ***Photopsia/flashes*** (more temporally) and floaters present – Loss of vision like a 'curtain coming across field of vision' – ***Schaeffer's sign*** 'Tobacco dust' in vitreous (anterior vitreous pigments)
☐ **Tractional RD**	– 2nd MC type – Due to ***proliferative vitreoretinopathy***—mechanical pull on the retina – MC in ***diabetics***
☐ **Exudative RD**	– No tear/break – Causes are ***choroidal tumors, toxemia of pregnancy, malignant hypertension, Harada's disease*** – No photopsia/floaters – ***Shifting of subretinal fluid*** is the hallmark

86. Answer is a (Ocular trauma).
Ref: Parson's, 20th edition Pg 367.

- ***Blunt trauma*** (concussion) to the eye typically results in a ***rosette*** (flower or star shaped) ***cataract***.

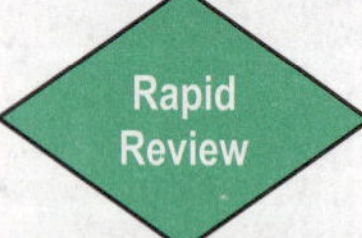

Type of cataract	Comment
• **Blue dot cataract**	MC congenital cataract; no significant visual symptoms
• **Radiation cataract**	Posterior subcapsular cataract
• **Steroid-induced cataract**	Posterior subcapsular cataract
• **Sunflower cataract**	Chalcosis (excess copper accumulation in lens)
• **Traumatic cataract**	Rosette cataract, Vossius ring (pigments on anterior lens capsule due to constricted pupil striking lens during blunt trauma)

• **After cataract**	Posterior capsule opacification, Elschnig's pearls, Soemmering's ring
• **Anterior lenticonus**	**AL**port's syndrome
• **Complicated cataract**	Due to any disease process in eye (e.g. uveitis), polychromatic lustre, bread crumb appearance
• **Christmas tree cataract**	Myotonic dystrophy
• **Glass blowers cataract**	Heat cataract, infrared rays
• **Posterior subcapsular cataract**	Even in the early stages, vision is usually impaired owing to the position of the opacity near the nodal point of the eye; more blurring in bright sunlight and headlights of oncoming cars
• **Nuclear cataract**	'Second sight' due to induced myopia – person who was using glasses to read earlier will be able to read better without glasses
• **Oil drop cataract**	Galactosemia
• **Posterior polar**	Early visual impairment since located at nodal point of the eye; high risk of posterior capsule rupture during surgery
• **Zonular (lamellar) cataract**	Hypocalcemia, Riders are seen
• **Snowflake cataract**	Diabetes mellitus
• **Diabetic cataract**	In diabetes mellitus, the glucose in lens is converted to sorbitol by aldose reductase → diabetic cataract. Aldose reductase inhibitors are being studied to prevent diabetic cataract.

MICROBIOLOGY

87. Answer is c (*Strongyloides stercoralis*).
Ref: Harrison's, 17th edition Pg 1321-22 and Table 210-1.

Direct quote:
"Humans acquire ***strongyloidiasis*** when ***filariform larvae*** in fecally contaminated soil ***penetrate the skin or mucous membranes***".

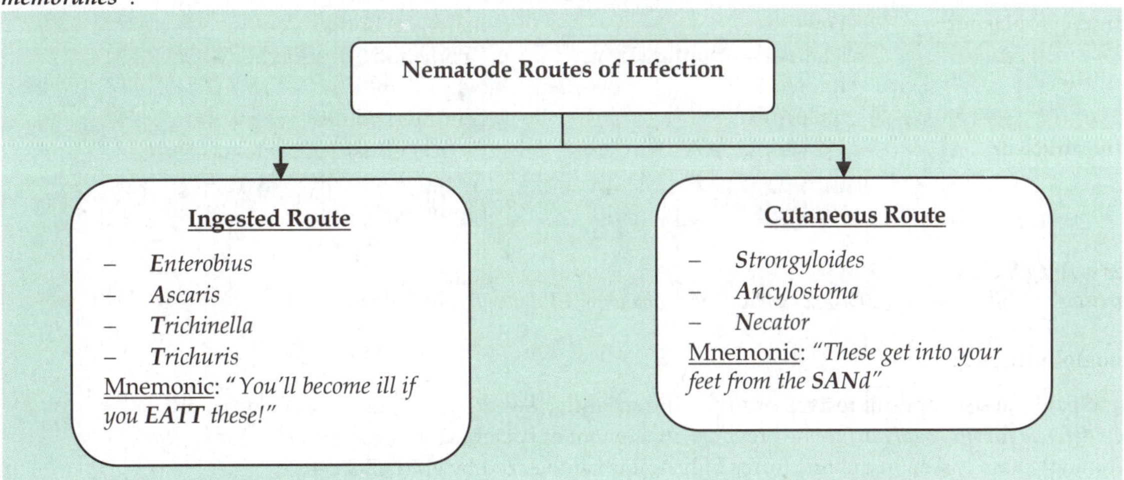

88. Answer is c (*Onchocerca volvulus*).
Ref: Harrison's, 17th edition Pg 211-1.

- ***Onchocerciasis*** (***river blindness***) is transmitted by S***imulium flies (black fly)***.
- Microfilaria are present in the skin and eye, but not in peripheral blood. Definitive diagnosis depends on the detection of an adult worm in an excised nodule or, more commonly of microfilariae in a skin snip.
- Clinical features:
  - ☐ Skin: Pruritus, rash, dermatitis (sowdah).
  - ☐ Ocular: Keratitis, scleritis, secondary glaucoma, uveitis, retinitis.
  - ☐ Lymph nodes: Inguinal and femoral lymphadenopathy (hanging groin).
- Treatment: Ivermectin.

89. **Answer is d (Rickettsia).**
Ref: Textbook of Microbiology, CP Baveja, 3rd edition Pg 391.

- ***Weil-Felix reaction*** is a ***heterophile agglutination test, which*** detects anti-rickettsial antibodies that cross react with certain non-motile *Proteus* strains OX 19, OX 2 and OX K. The basis of the test is the sharing of an alkali stable carbohydrate antigen of some rickettsia with non-motile strains of *Proteus, P. vulgaris* OX 19 and OX 2, and *P. mirabilis* OX K. The *Proteus* organisms are used as antigens.
- The test is of ***no value*** in the diagnosis of ***rickettsialpox***.

Weil-Felix reaction in diagnosis of rickettsial diseases

Disease	Agglutination with *Proteus* strain		
	OX 19	OX 2	OX K
Epidemic typhus	++++	±	–
Brill-Zinsser disease	±	–	–
Endemic typhus	+++	±	–
Spotted fever group	++	++	–
Scrub typhus	–	–	+++
Rickettsialpox	–	–	–

90. **Answer is d (Measles).**
Ref: Textbook of Microbiology, CP Baveja, 3rd edition Pg 468.

- For isolation of ***measles virus***, throat washings, nasopharyngeal swab, blood and conjunctival swab may be used. These specimens are cultured on primary human embryo kidney, monkey kidney or human amnion cells.
- Cytopathic changes may take 7–10 days to develop.
- The appearance of mutlinucleated giant cells (cytopathic effect) containing ***both intranuclear and intracytoplasmic inclusion bodies*** suggests ***presence of measles virus***.

Viral Inclusion Bodies

Intracytoplasmic	**Fowlpox**	: Bollinger, Borrell's body
	Molluscum contagiosum	: Henderson-Peterson body
	Rabies	: Negri bodies
	Smallpox	: Guarnieri bodies
Intranuclear	**Cowdry type A**	: Herpes virus, Yellow fever
	Cowdry type B	: Adenovirus, polio virus
	Varicella	: Lipschutz body

91. **Answer is d (IgA class).**
Ref: Harrison's, 17th edition Pg 2036; Textbook of Microbiology, CP Baveja, 3rd edition Pg 102.

Immunoglobulin A

- Principal Ig in secretions of respiratory and GI tract and in sweat, saliva, tears and colostrums
- ***Key defense for mucosal surfaces*** – prevents attachment of bacteria and viruses to mucosa
- J (joining) chain is seen in dimeric forms of IgA, it is synthesized by epithelial cells
- When aggregated binds polymorphs and activates complement through alternate pathway.

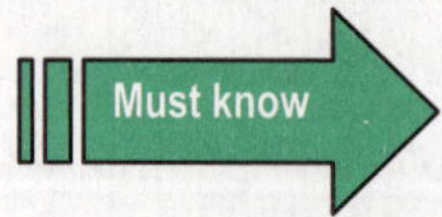

Biological properties of Immunoglobulins

- **IgG** : Placental transfer, secondary Ab for most antipathogen responses
- **IgA** : Secretory immunoglobulin
- **IgM** : Primary Ab responses, complement activation
- **IgD** : Marker for mature B cells
- **IgE** : Allergy, antiparasite responses, reaginic hypersensitivity

92. **Answer is a (Waterhouse-Friderichsen syndrome).**
Ref: Harrison's, 17th edition Pg 912.

- ***Neisseria meningitidis*** is the etiologic agent of two life-threatening diseases: Meningococcal meningitis and fulminant meningococcemia.
- Meningococci are ***gram-negative aerobic diplococci***.
- Definitive diagnosis is established by recovering *N. meningitidis*, its antigens, or its DNA from normally sterile body fluids (e.g. blood, ***CSF*** or synovial fluid) or from ***skin lesions***—cultured on ***Thayer-Martin medium of Mueller-Hinton medium***.
- The ***Waterhouse-Friderichsen syndrome*** is a dramatic example of ***DIC-induced microthrombosis, hemorrhage and tissue injury***.
- Although overt adrenal failure is infrequently documented in patients with fulminant meningococcemia, patients may have partial adrenal insufficiency and be unable to mount the normal hypercortisolemic response to severe stress or cosyntropin stimulation.
- Almost all patients who die from fulminant meningococcemia have adrenal hemorrhages at autopsy.

About the other choices:

- **Staphylococcal toxic shock syndrome toxin 1 (TSST 1):** A ***superantigen*** binds to a constant region of the T cell receptor, non-specifically activating T lymphocytes resulting in unregulated inflammation; acquired from ***contaminated tampons*** in menstruating women or from infected wounds; leads to systemic hypotension, tachycardia.
- **Job's syndrome**: Multiple abscesses of the skin and viscera due to increase susceptibility of unknown cause to staphylococcal infection.
- **Fitz-Hugh-Curtis syndrome:** Gonococcal perihepatitis in women with a history of gonococcal salpingitis.

93. **Answer is a (Neomycin).**
Ref: KD Tripathi, 6th edition Pg 668.

Classification of antimicrobials by mechanism of action

Inhibit cell wall synthesis	**Cause leakage from cell membranes**	**Inhibit protein synthesis**	**Cause misreading of m-RNA code and affect permeability**
– Penicillins – Cephalosporins – Cycloserine – Vancomycin – Bacitracin	– Polypeptides—polymyxins, colistin, bacitracin – Polyenes—Amphotericin B, Nystatin, hamycin	– Tetracyclines – Chloramphenicol – Erythromycin – Clindamycin – Linezolid	– Aminoglycosides—streptomycin, gentamicin, ***neomycin***, etc.
Inhibit DNA gyrase	**Interfere with DNA function**	**Interfere with DNA synthesis**	**Interfere with intermediary metabolism**
– Fluoroquinolones—ciprofloxacin and others	– Rifampin, metronidazole	– Acyclovir – Zidovudine	– Sulfonamides – Sulfones – Trimethoprim – Pyrimethamine – Ethambutol

94. **Answer is b (Interference microscope).**
Ref: Textbook of Microbiology, CP Baveja, 3rd edition Pg 10, 11.

- ***Interference microscope*** is useful for revealing cell organelles and for quantitative measurements of the chemical constituents of the cell such as lipids, proteins and nucleic acids.
- ***Optical microscope (light microscope)*** contains a light source and a compound lens system. It has magnification and resolving power. Resolving power is defined as the ability of the lens system to distinguish two objects as separate rather than one.

- ***Phase contrast microscope*** improves the contrast and makes evident the internal structure of cells, which differ in thickness or refractive index.
- ***Polarization microscope***: Image formation in polarizing microscope is based on the ability of polarized light to visualize birefringence. Used to study mitotic spindle fibers in dividing cells; actin and myosin filaments; plasma membrane and mitochondria.
- ***Dark field (dark ground) microscope***: Reflected light is used instead of transmitted light; useful for seeing spirochetes.
- ***Fluorescent microscope***: Specimens are exposed to light of shorter wavelength (UV light), which results in emission of a longer wavelength visible light. Bacteria stained with fluorescent dye (auramine, rhodamine) become visible as brightly glowing objects in a dark background.
- ***Electron microscope***: A beam of electrons is used instead of the beam of light used in optical microscope.

PATHOLOGY

95. Answer is a (Cell-mediated immunity).
Ref: Robbins pathology, 7th edition Pg 215.

Hypersensitivity Reactions

Type	Name	Examples
1. Type 1	Anaphylactic reaction Mediated by IgE	• Anaphylaxis • Atopic bronchial asthma • Angioedema • Allergic rhinitis, urticaria, hay fever
2. Type 2	Cytotoxic-cytolytic reaction Antibody mediated Mediated by IgG and IgM	• Transfusion reaction • Hemolytic anemia • Erythroblastosis fetalis • Certain drug reactions • Goodpasture's syndrome • Myasthenia gravis • ITP • Rheumatic fever
3. Type 3	Immune complex reaction Antigen-antibody complex activates complement	• Acute serum sickness (large amounts of foreign serum) • Chronic serum sickness – SLE • Arthus reaction • Certain forms of acute glomerulonephritis • Hypersensitivity pneumonitis
4. Type 4	Delayed hypersensitivity ***Cell-mediated reaction*** T cell mediated	• Mantoux test • Tuberculoid leprosy • Contact dermatitis • Transplant rejection (graft-versus-host disease) • Multiple sclerosis, Guillain-Barré syndrome, Hashimoto's thyroiditis
'ACID' = Types 1, 2, 3, 4 hypersensitivity reactions		

96. Answer is c (Natural killer cells).
Ref: Robbins pathology, 7th edition Pg 200.

- ***Natural killer (NK) cells*** recognize antigens on target, e.g. on tumor cells and lyse targets.
- It is important in ***resistance to virus infection and malignancy***.
- Identified by two cell surface molecules, ***CD16 and CD56*** are widely used to identify NK cells.
- CD 16 is the Fc receptor for IgG and it endows NK cells with another function, the ability to lyse IgG-coated target cells (antibody-dependent cytotoxicity).

97. Answer is c (7.4).
Ref: http://www.tpub.com/content/armymedical/MD0845/MD08450042.htm

- Concentrations of 2,3-DPG are affected by pH.
- The ***initial pH of blood collected in CPD*** and measured at the temperature of storage is approximately **7.4–7.5**.
- As stored red blood cells metabolize glucose to lactate, hydrogen ions accumulate, plasma pH falls and 2,3-DPG declines.

98. Answer is a (Goodpasture's syndrome).
Ref: Harrison's, 17th edition Pg 1788.

- Patients who develop autoantibodies directed against glomerular basement antigens frequently develop a glomerulonephritis termed ***antiglomerular basement membrane (anti-GBM) disease***.
- ***Goodpasture's syndrome*** = lung hemorrhage + glomerulonephritis (a pulmonary-renal syndrome).
- In Goodpasture's syndrome, the presence of anti-GBM antibodies and complement is recognized on biopsy by ***linear immunofluorescent staining for IgG*** (rarely IgA).

99. Answer is b (TCR gene rearrangement).
Ref: http://www.clinlabnavigator.com/Tests/TCellReceptorGeneRearrange.html

- T lymphocytes recognize and respond to foreign antigens by means of specific ***T cell receptors (TcR)***.
- The human genome does not contain enough unique DNA sequences to code for the vast repertoire of receptors needed to recognize all the foreign antigens a person is exposed to during their lifetime.
- To overcome this limitation, TcR genes undergo a complex series of DNA rearrangements to produce more than 1 billion unique receptors.
- Two types of TcR have been identified. The ***alpha-beta receptor is expressed on 95% of mature T cells***, whereas the remaining 5% of T cells express a gamma-delta receptor.
- In leukemia or lymphoma, detection of a TcR gene rearrangement indicates that a monoclonal population of T cells is present.
- The percentage of difficult to classify T cell lineage disorders is higher than B cell disorders. Often, T cell disorders cannot be definitely diagnosed by morphology and flow cytometry. ***T-lineage disorders lack a phenotypic marker of clonality such as the kappa and lambda light chain restriction in B lineage*** disorders. ***Sometimes*** T cell clonality can be inferred when the lymphocytes express a predominance of CD4 or CD8 antigens.
- ***Molecular analysis of the beta TcR gene rearrangements provides the most definitive assessment of T cell clonality***.
- TcR gene rearrangements are useful in the diagnosis of T cell malignancies such as T cell ALL and lymphoblastic lymphoma, mycosis fungoides, Sézary syndrome, T cell PLL/CLL and adult T cell leukemia. A pathologist interprets the results.

100. Answer is none.
Ref: See below with answer.

http://www.endotext.org/guthormones/guthormone10/guthormoneframe10.htm

- ***Neurotensinomas*** probably are best characterized as yet another tumor that is capable of causing the ***WDHHA*** (watery diarrhea, hypokalemia, hypochlorhydria and acidosis) syndrome. ***Edema, hypotension and flushing*** should increase the suspicion of a neurotensinoma.

http://emedicine.medscape.com/article/276943-overview

- ***Neurotensinomas*** can cause ***hypotension, hypokalemia, weight loss, flushing and diabetes***. These tumors are usually malignant.

101. Answer is c (Myeloblastic leukemia).
Ref: Harrison's, 17th edition Pg 678, Table 104-1.

French-American-British (FAB) Classification	Incidence
M0: Minimally differentiated leukemia	5%
M1: Myeloblastic leukemia without maturation	20%

COMED-K 2010 ANSWERS

M2: Myeloblastic leukemia with maturation	*30%*
M3: Hypergranular promyelocytic leukemia	10%
M4: Myelomonocytic leukemia M4Eo: Variant: Increase in abnormal marrow eosinophils	20%
M5: Monocytic leukemia	10%
M6: Erythroleukemia (Di Guglielmo's disease)	4%
M7: Megakaryoblastic leukemia	1%

102. Answer is b (Alport's syndrome).
Ref: Harrison's 17th edition Pg 1794.

Direct quote:
*"Approximately 85% of patients with Alport's syndrome have an **X-linked inheritance** of mutations in the ∝ 5(IV) collagen chain on chromosome Xq22–24".*

Features of Alport's syndrome:
- Hematuria
- Thinning and splitting of the Glomerular Basement Membranes
- Mild proteinuria (< 1–2 g/24 h)
- Chronic glomerulosclerosis, leading to renal failure
- Sensorineural deafness
- Anterior lenticonus
- Mental retardation or leiomyomatosis (rarely).

Must know

Inherited Disorders (*Ref: Robbins, 7th edition Pg 151, Table 5-1, 5-2, 5-3*)

System	Autosomal dominant	Autosomal recessive	X-linked recessive
Skeletal	Marfan's syndrome Ehlers-Danlos syndrome (some variants) Osteogenesis imperfecta Achondroplasia	Ehlers-Danlos syndrome (some variants) Alkaptonuria	Duchenne muscular dystrophy
Nervous	Huntington's disease Neurofibromatosis Myotonic dystrophy Tuberous sclerosis	Friedreich ataxia Neurogenic muscular atrophies Spinal muscular atrophy	Fragile-X syndrome
Metabolic	Familial hypercholesterolemia Acute intermittent porphyria	Cystic fibrosis Phenylketonuria Galactosemia Homocystinuria Lysosomal storage diseases α-1 antitrypsin deficiency Wilson disease Hemochromatosis Glycogen storage disease	Hunters syndrome Diabetes insipidus Lesch-Nyhan syndrome
Hematopoietic	Hereditary spherocytosis von Willebrand disease	Sickle cell anemia Thalassemias	Hemophilia A and B Chronic granulomatous disease

			Glucose-6-phosphate deficiency
Gastrointestinal	Familial polyposis coli		
Urinary	Polycystic kidney disease		
Endocrine		Congenital adrenal hyperplasia	
Immune			Agammaglobulinemia Wiskott-Aldrich syndrome

"As a general rule most structural abnormalities are autosomal dominant, whereas most enzymatic/biochemical abnormalities are autosomal recessive".

103. Answer is a (Putamen).
Ref: Harrison's, 17th edition Pg 2532, 2534.

- ***Intraparenchymal hemorrhage*** is the ***most common type of intracranial hemorrhage***. It accounts for ~10% of all strokes and is associated with a 50% case fatality rate.

Simple Summary

Location	Clinical features
☐ **Putaminal hemorrhage**	– ***MC site for hypertensive hemorrhage* (50–60% cases)** *(Harrison's, 17th/2532)* – Contralateral hemiparesis is sentinel sign since adjacent internal capsule is damaged
☐ **Thalamic hemorrhage**	– Contralateral hemiparesis – Prominent sensory deficit involving all modalities – Ocular disturbances
☐ **Pontine hemorrhage**	– Deep coma with quadriplegia usually occurs over a few minutes – Prominent decerebrate rigidity – 'Pin-point' (1 mm) pupils – Hyperpnea, severe hypertension and hyperhidrosis are common – Death often occurs within a few hours, but small hemorrhages are compatible with survival – Hemorrhages are compatible with survival
☐ **Cerebellar hemorrhage**	– Rarely – Develop over several hours – Occipital headache – Repeated vomiting – Ataxia, paralysis of conjugate lateral gaze toward the side of hemorrhage

- ***Treatment***:
  - ➢ Evacuation of supratentorial hematomas does not appear to improve outcome when compared with medical management.
  - ➢ For ***cerebellar hemorrhages, a neurosurgeon should be consulted immediately*** to assist with the evaluation; most ***cerebellar hematomas > 3 cm in diameter will require surgical evacuation.***

104. Answer is a (Wide variation in phenotype within a family).
Ref: Medical genetics for the Modern Clinician, Judith A Westman, 2006 edition Pg 80.

Autosomal Recessive

❖ ***Both parents*** of affected child are ***usually heterozygous symptomatic*** (one copy of mutated gene and one copy of normal/functional gene) ***carriers***

- ***Males and females*** are ***equally affected***
- Visually the autosomal recessive pedigree shows a ***horizontal pattern***
- Consanguineous partners have an increased risk of sharing the same genetic mutation and an increased risk of having affected children
- Unaffected parents who have one affected child have a 25% risk of having an affected child with each subsequent pregnancy
- The unaffected sibling of an affected individual has a 2 in 3 risk of being a carrier assuming that both parents are unaffected
- The gene product is commonly an enzyme.

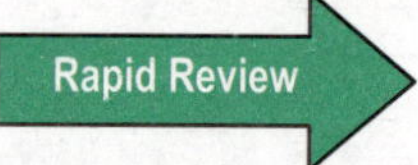

Autosomal Dominant

- Males and females are equally affected
- Affected males and females are equally capable of transmitting the trait
- An affected person usually have atleast one affected parent
- An affected person has a 50% chance of transmitting the trait to any offspring
- The gene product is commonly a non-enzymatic protein.

X-linked Recessive

- Males are MC affected
- All daughters of affected males are carriers
- Females are affected if they have a structural X cytogenetic abnormality or 45X or have an affected father and carrier mother
- No male-to-male transmission occurs
- Carrier females have a 50% risk of transmitting the trait to their sons and a 50% risk of transmitting carrier status to their daughters.

X-linked Dominant

- Both males and females may be affected, but females are more evident
- Females are less severely affected, because of random X inactivation and mosaicism
- The pedigree may vary similar to an autosomal dominant pedigree, but without any male-to-male transmission.

105. Answer is c (Whipple's disease).

Ref: Harrison's, 17th edition Pg 1880, Table 288-7.

- The typical pathologic finding in ***Whipple's disease*** is that the lamina propria contains ***PAS macrophages*** containing the characteristic small ***bacilli*** *(Tropheryma whipplei).*

<u>**More about Whipple's disease**</u>

- Whipple's disease is a chronic multisystem disease associated with *diarrhea, steatorrhea, weight loss, arthralgia* (migratory large-joint arthropathy) and *central nervous system (CNS) and cardiac* problems; it is caused by the bacteria ***Tropheryma whipplei***.
- Whipple's disease ***can be confused with*** the PAS-positive macrophages containing *M. avium* complex, which may be a cause of diarrhea in AIDS.
- The presence of *T. whipplei* bacillus *outside of macrophages is a more important indicator of active disease* than is their presence within the macrophages.
- *T. whipplei* has now been ***successfully grown in culture***.
- Treatment: Prolonged use of antibiotics. The current drug of choice is ***double-strength trimethoprim/sulfamethoxazole*** for approximately 1 year (chloramphenicol is second choice).
- PAS-positive macrophages can persist following successful treatment and the presence of bacilli outside of macrophages is indicative of persistent infection or an early sign of recurrence.

106. Answer is d (Iron deficiency anemia).
Ref: Harrison's, 17th edition 640, 99-5.

- Profound ***microcytosis with hypochromia*** and minimal anemia ***resembling iron deficiency*** is seen in thalassemia trait.

107. Answer is a (Diffuse type of gastric cancer).
Ref: Encyclopedia of medical genomics and proteomics, Vol 1, by Jurgen F and M Podda, Pg 600, Taylor and Francis publishers.

Direct quote:
"Frequent somatic mutations in ***E-cadherin (CDH1)*** have been particularly implicated in the carcinogenesis of gastric carcinomas (in 40–83% of ***sporadic diffuse type gastric cancer.*** BUT NOT in sporadic intestinal type gastric cancer)".

Also Know

- ***Hereditary diffuse gastric cancer syndrome*** (HDGC) is an ***autosomal dominant*** inherited cancer susceptibility syndrome with high penetrance for gastric cancer caused by ***germline truncating mutation in the E-cadherin (CDH1) tumor-suppressor gene.***
- The syndrome is characterized by ***early, diffuse, multifocal, submucosal involvement***, rendering *endoscopy and random biopsy inaccurate.*
- *Once a carrier is identified*, ***prophylactic total gastrectomy is the only effective treatment.***

108. Answer is d (Ovaries, uterine ligaments, rectovaginal septum).
Ref: Mosby's guide to women's health: A handbook for health professionals, by Tolu Oyelowo, 2007 edition Pg 94, fig 15-1; Cracking the boards, USMLE stpe2, Th Princeton review, 2nd edition Pg 149.

Common sites of endometriosis in decreasing order of frequency:
(1) Ovary (2) Cul-de-sac (3) Uterosacral ligaments (4) Broad ligaments (5) Fallopian tubes (6) Uterovesical fold (7) Round ligaments (8) Vermiform appendix (9) Vagina (10) Rectovaginal septum (11) Rectosigmoid colon (12) Cecum (13) Ileum (14) Inguinal canals (15) Abdominal scars (16) Ureters (17) Urinary bladders (18) Umbilicus (19) Vulva (20) Peripheral sites.

Also Know

- ***Spleen*** is ***NOT*** involved; it is relatively immune to endometriosis.

109. Answer is b (CD lymphocytes).
Ref: Harrison's, 17th edition Pg 1106-07.

Laboratory findings in infectious mononucleosis

- ***Lymphocytosis*** (with > 10% ***atypical lymphocytes***)
  - These are ***enlarged lymphocytes*** that have abundant cytoplasm, vacuoles, indentations of the cell membrane.
  - ***CD8+ cells*** *predominate among the atypical lymphocytes.*
- *Low-grade neutropenia* and *thrombocytopenia* are common during the first month of illness.
- *Elevated WBC count* (10,000–20,000/μL) during the 2nd or 3rd week of illness.
- *Liver function* is abnormal in > 90% of cases.
- *Serum aminotransferases and alkaline phosphatase* are usually mildly *elevated.*
- *Serum bilirubin is elevated* in ~40% of cases.

DERMATOLOGY, ANESTHESIOLOGY, PSYCHIATRY, RADIODIAGNOSIS

110. Answer is c (Borderline tuberculoid leprosy).
Ref: OP Ghai, 7th edition Pg 661, Table 24.8 and Fig 24.23.

Types of Leprosy

□ **Lepromatous leprosy**	– ↓↓ ***cell-mediated immunity*** (CMI) and ***bacillary load is*** ↑↑ (lepromin test negative) – Collections of bacilli are also found in the liver, spleen and bone marrow, but no visceral organ system dysfunction has been a/w this presence – Histology shows clear subepidermal free zone, foamy macrophages laden with acid-fast bacilli (***Virchow or lepra cells***) and many intracellular bacilli, frequently in spheroidal masses (***globi***). Epithelioid cells and giant cells are NOT found – Symmetric, poorly marginated, multiple infiltrated nodules and plaques or diffuse infiltration; xanthoma-like – Dermatofibroma papules; leonine facies and eyebrow alopecia. Hypesthesia a late sign; nerve palsies variable; acral, distal, symmetric anesthesia common – *M. leprae* PGL-1 antibodies present in 95%
□ **Tuberculoid leprosy**	– ↑↑ ***cell-mediated immunity*** and ***bacillary load*** **is** ***low*** (lepromin test positive) – Histology shows ***non-caseating granuloma*** with epithelioid and giant cells
□ **Indeterminate leprosy**	– Sensory loss is usually absent, peripheral nerves are normal; lesions may heal spontaneously in a year or two
□ **Borderline tuberculoid leprosy (BT)**	– ***Satellite lesions*** are seen – Nerve abscesses MC in BT leprosy
□ **Borderline leprosy**	– All kinds of ***bizarre lesions*** in single patient distributed asymmetrically; saucer-shaped lesions are seen – Epithelioid cells seen

111. Answer is b (Vogt-Koyanagi-Harada syndrome).
Ref: Harrison's, 17th edition Pg 325.

- Systemic diseases that should be considered in a patient with skin findings suggestive of ***vitiligo***
  - □ ***Vogt-Koyanagi-Harada syndrome*** (aseptic meningitis, non-traumatic uveitis, tinnitus, hearing loss and/or dysacusis)
  - □ **Scleroderma**
  - □ **Onchocerciasis**
  - □ ***Melanoma-associated leukoderma.***

Note:

❖ ***Posner-Schlossman syndrome*** = glaucomatocyclitis crisis = hypertensive uveitis = uveitis + glaucoma, recurrent, in young patients.

112. Answer is d (Oral glucocorticoids).
Ref: Harrison's, 17th edition Pg 316.

Direct quote:

*"**Oral glucocorticoids** should NOT be used for the treatment of psoriasis due to the potential for developing life-threatening pustular psoriasis when therapy is discontinued".*

Various systemic agents can be used for severe, widespread psoriatic disease:
- Methotrexate (oral antimetabolite)
- Acitretin (oral retinoid)
- Cyclosporine (oral calcineurin inhibitor).

113. Answer is b *(Parthenium hysterophorus).*
Ref: Manual of Dermatologic Therapeutics, Kenneth AA, Jeffrey TS, 7th edition 2007. Pg 59; Atlas of Clinical Dermatology, Anthony Du Vivier, Phillip McKee, 3rd edition 2002. Pg 66.

Direct quote:
*"**In India,** Parthenium hysterophorus **is the most common cause of ABCD**".*

- ***Airborne Contact Dermatitis (ABCD)*** is caused when an allergen that is aerosolized comes into contact with sensitized individuals. Frequent involvement will be in a characteristic distribution on the face, V of neck, hands and forearms and hand dermatitis.
- In ***USA, composite plant pollen*** is a frequent cause of ABCD.
- *Parthenium hysterophorus* was ***imported into India from Texas.***

114. Answer is c (Blue).
Ref: Understanding Anesthesia, By Peter J Simpson, Mansukh T Popat, 4th edition Pg 68. Elsevier publications.

Color of Medical Gas Cylinders

❖ **Oxygen**	Black body with white shoulder
❖ **Nitrous oxide**	Blue
❖ **Entonox**	Blue body with white/blue quartered shoulders
❖ **Cyclopropane**	Orange
❖ **Ethylene**	Red
❖ **Halothane bottle**	Amber
❖ **Helium**	Brown
❖ **Air (medical)**	Gray with white and black valve
❖ **Carbon dioxide**	Gray with gray valve

115. Answer is a (Preloading with crystalloids).
Ref: Lee's Synopsis of Anesthesia, 13th edition Pg 510.

Direct quote:
*"Prophylactic **volume loading with colloid solutions (500–1,000 mL) prior to spinal injection has consistently maintained blood pressure** and volume expansion in both surgical and obstetric patients owing to a sustained increase in intravascular volume, maternal cardiac output and uteroplacental blood flow".*

116. Answer is d (Central anticholinergic syndrome).
Ref: KD Tripathi, 6th edition; Lee's Anesthesia, Pg 17.

- ***Glycopyrrolate*** is a longer acting ***quaternary atropine substitute.***
- It is a ***potent antisecretory and antibradycardic drug;*** acts rapidly and is *less likely to produce central effects.*
- Quaternary compounds ***do not penetrate the brain*** and eye; central and ocular effects are not seen after parenteral/oral administration.
- ***Glycopyrrolate*** does NOT cross the blood brain or placental barrier; so ***DOES NOT CAUSE central anticholinergic*** effects.
- Hence, glycopyrrolate is used as ***preanesthetic medication.***

117. Answer is c (Amyloidosis).
Ref: MCQs in Clinical Radiology, Prabhakar Rajaiah, Jaypee Brothers Medical Publishers (P) Ltd, Pg 48.

Stomach fold thickening on barium meal is caused by
- Amyloidosis
- Eosinophilic enteritis
- Lymphoma
- Metastasis
- Zollinger-Ellison syndrome

Note:
- Tongue thickening ***(macroglossia)*** is seen in ***AL amyloidosis.***
- *GAVE*: Gastric Antral Vascular Ectasia is seen in ***scleroderma*** (***watermelon stomach***).

118. Answer is a (Shortening of both T1 and T2 relaxation times).
Ref: Step By Step MRI, Jagan Mohan Reddy, V Prasad, Pg 78-79, Taylor and Francis publishers.

Pathological change and effects of relaxation time

T1 shortened	T2 shortened	T1 prolonged	T2 prolonged
– Lipid – Paramagnetic substance (copper, iron, manganese) – Mucus – Cholesterol – Postradiation changes (after 2 weeks) – Hemorrhage (methemoglobin) – Increases protein content – Melanin	– Air – Calcium – Cortical bone – Paramagnetic substance – Fat	– Air – Calcium – Cortical bone – Edema – Demyelination – Neoplasia	–

119. Answer is b (Pulmonary nodules).
Ref: Pediatric Radiography, Maryann H, Stephen B, 2003 edition Pg 37.

- ***Progressive pulmonary TB*** most commonly occurs during ***infancy*** as a result of the primary infection not being contained and subsequently progresses to:
  - ***Bronchopneumonia***
  - ***Lobar pneumonia*** (usually middle or lower lobe)
  - ***Cavitation.***
- In contrast, pulmonary TB in older infants and children is usually asymptomatic illness with minimal abnormalities demonstrated on chest radiograph, while adolescent infection will follow more closely the typical adult appearances with upper lobe opacification and possible cavitation.

120. Answer is c (Multiple somatic symptoms).
Ref: Kaplan and Sadock's Study Guide and Self-examination Review in Psychiatry, 8th edition Pg 185.

Direct quote:

"In the early 1960s, two studies confirmed the original findings of a definable clinical syndrome demonstrating diagnostic stability of the multisymptomatic concept of hysteria. In 1970, the eponym ***Briquet's syndrome*** *was proposed to denote multisymptomatic hysteria. Ironically after the decision was made to incorporate Briquet's syndrome as part of the new diagnostic nomenclature, an unrelated decision was made to drop all eponyms. Hence, a new name* ***somatization disorder*** *had to be created".*

Somatoform disorders	Somatization disorder (Briquet's syndrome)
• These are characterized by physical symptoms without a sufficient organic cause. A person with somatoform disorder is not malingering and not delusional, but truly believes that he/she has a physical problem.	➢ *Multiple somatic symptoms* with *no physical disorder* ➢ Symptoms should be present for *at least 2 years* for diagnosis ➢ Involves multiple systems

• It consists of: 1. ***Somatization Disorder (Briquet's synd)*** 2. Hypochondriasis 3. Body dysmorphic disorder 4. Pain disorder 5. Somatoform autonomic dysfunction.	➢ Presence of *conversion* symptoms is *common* ➢ Onset before 30 years, usually chronic and lifelong disorder ➢ Symptoms are increased by stressful life events.

121. **Answer is c (There is about 50% chance of recurrence of depression).**
Ref: Psychiatry Essentials for Primary Care, by Robert KS, James LS, American College of Physicians, 21 edition 2008. Pg 46.

Direct quote:

"The recurrence rate after 1 (depressive) episode is 50–85%".

- For the first, uncomplicated depressive episode, the patient should receive full therapeutic dose of the chosen antidepressant for a ***period of 6–12 months, after achieving full remission.***

122. **Answer is d (Child's love for the parent of opposite sex).**
Ref: Niraj Ahuja's Psychiatry, 6th edition Pg 224.

- According to ***Sigmund Freud***, psychosexual phases of development consist of 4 stages—***oral phase, anal phase, phallic (oedipal) phase*** and ***genital phase.***
- ***Oedipus complex*** consists of *aggressive impulses towards the father*; named after the Greek tragedy Oedipus Rex, in which Oedipus unknowingly kills his father and *marries his mother* unaware of their true identities).
- Oedipus complex usually resolves by identification with the father, attempting to adopt his characteristics.
- In females, they develops *penis envy* (discontent with female genitalia following a fantasy that they result from loss of penis). This is theorized by Freud to lead to wish to 'receive' the penis and to bear a child. Resolution occurs by identification with the mother. This phase has been called ***Electra complex***.

123. **Answer is a (Visual hallucinations).**
Ref: Niraj Ahuja's Psychiatry, 6th edition Pg 98-100.

Agoraphobia
- ***MC type of phobia*** seen in ***clinical practice***; MC in ***females.***
- It is characterized by
  - ➢ ***Anxiety about being in places or situations from which escape might be difficult*** or in ***which help may not be available*** in the event of having a ***panic attack***
  - ➢ ***Anxiety*** of ***being outside the home alone***
  - ➢ ***Anxiety*** or ***of being in public places.***
- Depression, depersonalization and obsessional thoughts are more common in agoraphobia than in other phobias.

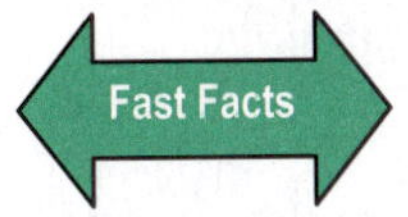

Social Phobia
Case example: A 30-year-old, real-estate agent is uncomfortable, because he must take a client to a dinner in a restaurant. Although he knows the client well, he is so afraid that he will make a mess while eating and embarrass himself that he says he is not hungry and sips water from a glass instead.
- ***Social phobia*** is a persistent ***fear of social performances*** in which the individual is exposed to unfamiliar people or to possible scrutiny by others and fears that he/she will act in a way, which will be humiliating or embarrassing.
- Examples are ***fear of blushing (erythrophobia), fear of vomiting or passing urine in public place.***

Simple (specific) phobias
- Fear induced by the presence or anticipation of a *specific* object or situation—see box below.

PHOBIAS	
❖ *Acrophobia*	= Fear of heights
❖ *Zoophobia*	= Fear of animals
❖ *Arachnophobia*	= Fear of spiders
❖ *Xenophobia*	= Fear of strangers
❖ *Algophobia*	= Fear of pain
❖ *Claustrophobia*	= Fear of closed places
❖ *Sitophobia*	= Fear of eating

124. Answer is c (Agranulocytosis).
Ref: Davidson's, 20th edition Pg 243; Harrison's, 17th edition Pg 2722.

- The model first-generation antipsychotic agent is ***clozapine***, a dibenzodiazepine that has a greater potency in blocking the ***5HT2*** than the D2 receptor and a much higher affinity for the ***D4*** than the D2 receptor.

Advantages of clozapine	Side effects of clozapine
➤ Approximately 30% of patients who do not benefit from conventional antipsychotic agents will have a ***better response to clozapine*** ➤ Clozapine has superiority to other antipsychotic agents ***in preventing suicide*** ➤ It is ***most appropriate for treatment-resistant schizophrenia*** ➤ As clozapine may take some time to improve symptoms in domains such as social functioning, clinicians should consider a minimum trial period of 6 months ➤ Unlike other antipsychotics, clozapine does NOT cause a rise in prolactin level.	➤ Neutropenia and ***agranulocytosis (monitor blood counts)*** ➤ Weight gain and diabetes ➤ Epileptic seizures and ➤ Cardiac problems such as cardiomyopathy.

125. Answer is a (It is characterized by recurrent and unpredictable panic attacks).
Ref: Niraj Ahuja's Psychiatry, 6th edition Pg 97.

Panic disorder

- *Etiology*:
  - Mean age of onset is *25 years*
  - MC in *women*
  - Often accompanied by agoraphobia
  - *Genetic factors* are involved (first degree relatives have a 4–7 times greater chance of having panic disorder)
  - May occur soon after divorce/marital separation
  - ***Usually there is no apparent precipitating factor.***
- Panic disorder is a/w *separation anxiety disorder* of childhood; a/w *mitral valve prolapse; a/w depression* in approximately *50%* of patients.
- *Characteristics:*
  - Panic attacks, defined as ***episodic periods*** of anxiety symptoms that have a ***sudden onset*** and increase in intensity over a period of approximately 10 minutes—palpitations, sweating, tremors, dyspnea, chest pain, nausea, fear of losing control (***autonomic symptoms***).
- Panic attacks occur approximately *twice weekly* and last approximately *30 minutes*. Between attacks, the patient fears having another attack (anticipatory anxiety). For diagnosis, at least 1 month of worry about attacks should be present.
- Treatment:
  - ***For immediate relief*** or anticipatory anxiety, benzodiazepines, particularly *alprazolam* with gradual withdrawal over 8–12 months.
  - ***For maintenance***, SSRIs, tricyclics, MAOIs. Psychological treatment: Systemic desensitization and cognitive therapy are useful.

FORENSIC

126. Answer is b (30 mg%).
Ref: Narayan Reddy's FMT, 23rd edition Pg 288.

- ***In India***, the law has made it an offense for a person to drive a motor vehicle above a specified blood alcohol level—***30 mg% (S.185 Motor Vehicle Act, 1985)***.

127. Answer is d (Teichmann test).
Ref: Fundamentals of Forensic Science, by Max, MH, Pg 238, 2nd edition 2010; Principles of Medical Physiology, Sabysachi Sircar, 2008 edition Pg 139.

- Two microchemical tests for hemoglobin are ***sensitive and confirmatory for blood***
  - ***Teichmann*** test
  - ***Takayama*** test (hemochromogen test).
- Presumptive tests for blood
  - Benzidine test
  - LMG test
  - Luminol test.

128. Answer is a (Distended with inspissated bile).
Ref: Narayan Reddy's FMT, 23rd edition Pg 156.

Postmortem appearances in starvation

- *Rigor mortis* sets in and disappears *early*.
- Trophic skin changes are common.
- *Hair and nails* are dry, brittle and lusterless.
- Extreme emaciation and general reduction in size and weight of all organs *EXCEPT brain*.
- *Fat* of female breast and orbits spared till late.
- *Muscles* are atrophied and darker due to increased lipochrome.
- *Heart* is small from brown atrophy and chambers are empty.
- *Lungs* are pale and collapsed and exude very little blood when cut.
- *Liver* is atrophied and may show necrosis due to protein deficiency.
- ***Gallbladder is distended with bile.***
- *Spleen* is shrunken.
- *Kidneys* show atrophy of the nephron.
- *Stomach* and intestines show atrophy of all coats and mucosa is stained with bile.
- *Bowel* contains offensive fluid and gas.
- *Urinary bladder* is empty.

129. Answer is c (Saponification).
Ref: http://en.wikipedia.org/wiki/Saponification; Essential Forensic Biology, Alan Gunn, 2009 edition Pg 25.

- **Saponification** can also refer to the other soft tissue in a ***conversion of the fat of a corpse into adipocere***, often called ***"grave wax."***
- This process is more common where the amount of fatty tissue is high, the agents of decomposition are absent or only minutely present and the ***burial ground is particularly alkaline***.

130. Answer is b (Beryllium).
Ref: Harrison's, 17th edition Pg 1615.

- ***Beryllium*** is a light-weight metal with tensile strength, has good electrical conductivity and is valuable in the control of nuclear reactions through its ability to quench neutrons.
- Although beryllium may produce an acute pneumonitis, it is far more commonly associated with a ***chronic granulomatous inflammatory disease that is similar to sarcoidosis***.

- Unless one inquires specifically about occupational exposures to beryllium in the manufacture of ***alloys, ceramics or high-technology electronics*** in a patient with sarcoidosis, one may miss entirely the etiologic relationship to the occupational exposure.
- ***What distinguishes chronic beryllium disease (CBD) from sarcoidosis*** is evidence of a specific cell-mediated immune response (i.e. ***delayed hypersensitivity) to beryllium***.
- The test that usually provides this evidence is the ***beryllium lymphocyte proliferation test (BeLPT)***.
- Chronic beryllium disease is one of the best studied examples of gene-environment interaction. Susceptibility to CBD is highly associated with ***HLA-DP*** alleles possessing a glutamic acid in position 69 of the β-chain.

131. Answer is a (Abortion).
Ref: http://125.16.62.44/intranet/eip/legislation/uploads/WMA%20Declaration%20of%20Oslo.pdf

Declaration of Oslo (Statement on Therapeutic Abortion)
- Adopted by the 24th World Medical Assembly, Oslo, Norway, 1970
- 'Therapeutic abortion' (may be performed in circumstances) 'where the vital interests of the mother conflict with those of the unborn child'.

Also Know

- The **Declaration of Helsinki** was developed by the World Medical Association (WMA), as a set of ethical principles for the medical community regarding human experimentation and is widely regarded as the ***cornerstone document of human research ethics.***

132. Answer is b (Amphetamine).
Ref: Modern Medical Toxicology, 3rd edition 2005, Pg 103.

- The term ***"liquid gold"*** is ***slang for urine of amphetamine addicts,*** which is collected and sold on the streets of USA.
- Since a significant proportion of ingested amphetamine is excreted unchanged in the urine, consuming the latter is an economical way of amphetamine intake!!!

Rapid Review

VOCABULARY OF DRUG ABUSERS

• Amphetamines	Speed; whiz; billy; pink champagne
• Amyl nitrate	Goldrush; poppers; snappers
• Barbiturates	Barbs; idiot pills
• Cocaine	Coke; Charlie; uncle; Rock, crack; nuggets; wash; gravel; snow
• Dihydrocodeine	Dfs
• Drug-induced sleep	Gauching; nodding; going on the nod
• Drug intoxication	Stoned; wiped out; bladdered
• Heroin (+/- cocaine)	Smack; the nasty; gear; brown; Harry; scag
• Ecstasy (MDMA)	XTC; echo; disco biscuit; love drug; methylenedioxy-methamphetamine
• Febrile reaction	Bad hit
• *Injecting*	
➤ Subcutaneous	Skin popping
➤ IM	Muscle popping
➤ Subclavian	Pocket shot
➤ Failed	Miss
• LSD	Acid trips; cardboard; tabs
• Marijuana	Weed; pot; draw; ganja; grass; resin; Mary; Hash
• Methadone	Mud
• Phencyclidine (PCP)	Angel dust; KJ; ozone; missile, peace pill, hog
• Physeptone ampules	Amps
• Smoking cocaine	Bonging

• Smoking heroin	Chasing the dragon
• Temazepam	Temazies; eggs; jellies
• White heroin	China white
• Opiate withdrawal	Turkeying; clucking
• Zopiclone	Zim-Zims

PREVENTIVE AND SOCIAL MEDICINE

133. Answer is d (Organization of range of promotive, preventive and curative health services).
Ref: Park, 20th edition Pg 44.

- The term ***social medicine*** was first introduced by Jules Guerin, a French physician in 1848.
- By derivation, social medicine is "***the study of man as a social being in his total environment***".
- Social medicine by derivation is concerned with the health of groups of people and individuals within these groups with a ***view to create, promote, preserve and maintain optimum health***.

134. Answer is b (1/2 of proteins and 1/3 of the calories required per day).
Ref: Park, 20th edition Pg 500.

- In view of the limited finances in India, it is recommended that the ***mid-day school meal*** should provide at least ***1/3 of the daily calorie requirement*** and about ***1/2 of the daily protein requirement*** of the child.

135. Answer is c (Yellow fever).
Ref: Park, 20th edition Pg 248.

- Measures designed to restrict the spread of yellow fever are specified in the ***"International Health Regulations" of WHO***.
- All travelers (including infants) exposed to the risk of ***yellow fever*** or passing through endemic zones of yellow fever must possess a ***valid international certificate of vaccination*** against yellow fever before they are allowed to enter yellow fever 'receptive' areas.
- If no such certificate is available, the traveler is placed on *quarantine* in a *mosquito proof ward for 6 days* from the date of leaving an infected area.
- If the traveler arrives before the certificate becomes 'valid' he is isolated till the certificate becomes valid.

136. Answer is c (Interruption of the transmission of disease).
Ref: Park, 20th edition Pg 37.

- The term 'disease control' describes (ongoing) operations aimed at *decreasing*
  - ➢ *Incidence of the disease*
  - ➢ Duration of the disease and consequently the risk of transmission
  - ➢ Effects of infection, including both physical and psychosocial complications
  - ➢ Financial burden to the community.
- Control activities may focus on *primary prevention or secondary prevention*; the concept of tertiary prevention is comparatively less relevant to control the efforts.
- In disease control, the *disease agent is permitted to persist in the community at a level where it ceases to be a public health problem* according to the tolerance of the local population.
- *A state of equilibrium becomes established* between the disease agent, host and environment components of the disease process.
- An excellent embodiment of this concept is *malaria control*, which is distinct from malaria eradication.

137. Answer is a (Gopalan).
Ref: http://en.wikipedia.org/wiki/Burning_feet_syndrome

- ***Burning feet syndrome***, also known as ***Grierson-Gopalan syndrome***, is a medical condition that causes severe burning and aching of the feet, hyperesthesia and vasomotor changes of the feet that leads to excessive sweating.
- It can even affect the eyes, causing scotoma and amblyopia.

- It occurs more frequently in women, commonly between 20 and 40 years of age.
- Generally due to *deficiency in B complex vitamins;* also seen in *uremia* and as *autosomal dominant* condition.

138. Answer is c (Sentinel surveillance).
Ref: Park, 20th edition Pg 38.

- No routine notification system can identify all cases of infection or disease. A method for ***identifying the missing cases*** and thereby ***supplementing the notified cases*** is required. This is known as ***'sentinel surveillance'***.
- The sentinel data is extrapolated to the entire population to estimate the disease ***prevalence in the total population.***
- The advantages of such system are the *reporting biases are minimized* and the feedback of information to the providers is issued.

139. Answer is d (Income).

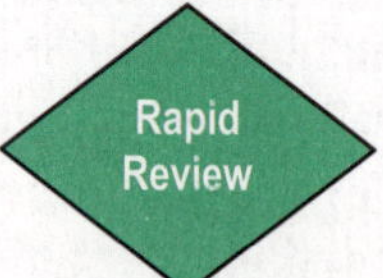

Summary of "Indicators"

■ **Physical quality of life index (PQLI)**	• Infant mortality rate • Life expectancy at age 1 • Literacy ***'ILL'*** • PQLI in India is 65
■ **Human development Index (HDI)**	• Longevity (life expectancy at birth) • Income (real GDP per capita or purchasing power) • Knowledge/Education (adult literacy rate and mean years of schooling) ***'LIKE'*** • High HDI ≥ 0.800; Medium HDI 0.500–0.799; Low HDI < 0.500 • HDI for India is 0.545 (***medium HDI*** category); ***rank 132***
■ **Sullivan's index**	• Expectation of life ***'free of disability'*** • Computed by subtracting from the life expectancy the probable duration of bed disability and inability to perform major activities • One of the most advanced indicators currently available
■ **Disability adjusted life year (DALY)**	• It expresses years of life lost to premature death and years lived with disability adjusted for the severity of the disability. One DALY is one lost year of healthy life • ***Measure used to express global burden of disease***
■ **Health adjusted life expectancy (HALE)**	• It is based on life expectancy at birth, but includes an adjustment for time spent in poor health. It means equivalent number of years in full health that a newborn can expect to live based on current rates of ill health and mortality

140. Answer is a (Yellow bags).
Ref: Park, 20th edition Pg 697,698.

Biomedical Waste disposal

Color Coding	Waste Material
Yellow plastic bag	Human anatomical waste, biopsied tissue, enucleated eyes, pus, etc.
Red plastic bag	Soiled dressings, bandages, infected cotton, gauze
Blue plastic bag	Plastic syringes without needles, plastic tubes, catheters, urine/blood bags, gloves
Black plastic bag	Discarded medicines and cytotoxic drugs
Puncture proof container	Needles, blades, sharps, broken glass

141. Answer is c (42 days of the termination of pregnancy).
Ref: Dutta's Obstetrics, 6th edition Pg 602.

Definition of maternal deaths:

- Death of a woman ***while pregnant or within 42 days of termination of pregnancy*** irrespective of the duration and the site of pregnancy from any cause related to or aggravated by the pregnancy or its management, but not from accidental or incidental causes.

142. Answer is d [Annual blood examination rate (ABER)].
Ref: Park, 20th edition Pg 227, 228.

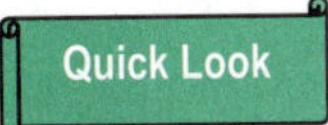

Measurement of malaria

Pre-eradication era: Here the magnitude of the malaria problem in a community used to be determined mostly from the reports of ***clinically diagnosed malaria cases***. The classical malariometric measures are given below. These ***classical measures*** may provide the needed information, i.e. ***the trend of the disease***.

Spleen rate	• Percentage of children between 2 and 10 years showing enlargement of spleen. • Adults are excluded since splenomegaly in adults may be due to various other causes. • The spleen rate is widely used for ***measuring the endemicity of malaria*** in a community.
Average enlarged spleen	• Denotes average size of the enlarged spleen; a further refinement of the spleen rate.
Parasite rate	• Percentage of children between 2–10 years showing malaria parasites in their blood films.
Parasite density index	• Average degree of parasitemia in a well-defined group of population. • Only the positive slides are included in the denominator.
Infant parasite rate (IPR)	• Percentage of infants below the age of 1 year showing malaria parasites in their blood films. • ***Most sensitive index of recent malaria transmission*** in a locality. • If the ***IPR is zero for 3 consecutive years in a locality, it is regarded as absence of malaria transmission***, even though the Anopheline vectors may remain.
Proportional case rate	• Since the morbidity rate is difficult to determine except in conditions where the diagnosis and reporting of each case is carried to perfection, proportional case rate is used. • Defined as the number of cases diagnosed as clinical malaria for every 100 patients attending the hospitals and dispensaries. • This is a crude index since the cases are not related to the time/space distribution.

Eradication era: Here, the ***microscopic diagnosis of malaria*** cases became the main method of diagnosis. These parameters are unlikely to reveal the true epidemiological picture unless the case detection machinery is fully supervised and very efficient. The parameters are:

Annual parasite incidence (API)	• It is a ***sophisticated measure of malaria incidence in a community***. It is based on intensive active and passive surveillance and cases are confirmed by blood examination. • *API* = confirmed cases during 1 year/population under surveillance × 1,000.
Annual blood examination rate (ABER)	• *ABER* = No. of slides examined/population × 100. • The WHO expert committee on malaria in 1964 recommended that the monthly number of slides examined should be at least 1% of the

	population. In the modified plan of operation (MPO) the minimum prescribed is ***10% of the population in a year.*** • ABER is an ***index of operational efficiency.***
□ **Annual falciparum incidence**	• Data are collected separately for total malaria cases and falciparum cases.
□ **Slide positivity rate and slide falciparum rate**	• Provide information on the ***trend of malaria transmission.***

143. Answer is a (0.5 mg/L).
Ref: Park, 20th edition Pg 540.

- The ***recommended level of fluorides in drinking water*** in the country is accepted as ***0.5–0.8 mg/L.***

Quick Look

- In ***most parts of India,*** the fluoride content of drinking water is about ***0.5 mg/L.***
- In ***endemic areas*** it may be as high as ***3–12 mg/L.***
- ***Foods*** rich in fluorides are ***sea fish, cheese and tea.***
- 96% of fluorine in body is found in the ***bones and teeth.***
- ***Dental fluorosis***—at levels above 1.5 mg/L, mottling of dental enamel, chalk white teeth best seen on permanent upper incisors.
- ***Skeletal fluorosis***—at levels of 3-6 mg/L.
- Crippling fluorosis—> 10 mg/L
- ***Genu valgum***—a special type of fluorosis in AP and Tamil Nadu; seen in people shoes ***staple diet is sorghum (jowar).***
- ***Nalgonda technique*** is used for ***defluoridation of water.***

144. Answer is b (0.5).
Ref: Park, 20th edition Pg 625.

- The ***minimum recommended concentration of free chlorine is 0.5 mg/L for 1 hour.*** The free residual chlorine provides a margin of safety against subsequent microbial contamination such as may occur during storage and distribution. The sum of the chlorine demand of the specific water plus the free residual chlorine of 0.5 mg/L constitutes the correct dose of chlorine to be applied.

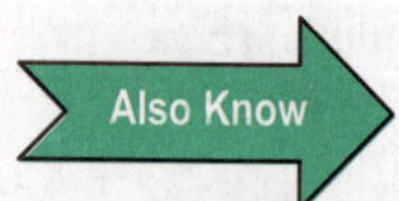

Other points about chlorination of water

- The ***chlorine demand*** of the water is the difference between the amount of chlorine added to the water and the amount of residual chlorine remaining at the end of a specific period of contact (usually 60 minutes), at a given temperature and pH of water. In other words, it is the amount of chlorine that is needed to destroy bacteria and to oxidize all the organic matter and ammonia substances present in the water.
- The point at which the chlorine demand of the water is met is called ***'break point'.*** If further chlorine is added beyond the breakpoint, free chlorine (HOCl and OCl) begins to appear in the water.
- ***Orthotolidine test*** (OT) enables both free and combined chlorine in the water to be determined with speed and accuracy.
- ***OT arsenite*** test is a modification of the OT test to determine the free and combined chlorine residual separately.

ANATOMY, PHYSIOLOGY AND BIOCHEMISTRY

145. Answer is c (Gastroduodenal artery).
Ref: BD Chaurasia, Vol 2, Pg 228.

Branches of Celiac A. are

◻ **Common Hepatic A.**	Gives rise to – Right gastric A. – Cystic A. – Right and left hepatic branches – Gastroduodenal A. gives right gastroepiploic A.; Superior pancreaticoduodenal A.; Supraduodenal artery.
◻ **Left Gastric A.**	Smallest branch of celiac A. It runs along the lesser curvature of the stomach It gives few esophageal branches also
◻ **Splenic A.**	Largest branch of celiac A. is an end artery. Its branches are: – Pancreatic branches – Short gastric branches – Left gastroepiploic

146. Answer is c (Metopic suture).
Ref: Gray's Anatomy, 2005 edition Pg 455.

- The ***glabella may show the remains of the interfrontal (metopic) suture***, which is present in 9% of adult skulls, where it ascends to the coronal suture, indicating that the frontal bone is the result of fusion of two halves.

147. Answer is d (Superior thyroid artery).
Ref: BD Chaurasia, Vol 3, Pg 143.

Branches of the subclavian artery are:
1. Vertebral artery.
2. Internal thoracic artery.
3. ***Thyrocervical trunk,*** which divides into three branches:
   - Inferior thyroid
   - Suprascapular
   - Superficial cervical artery.
4. Costocervical trunk, which divides into two branches:
   - Superior intercostal
   - Deep cervical artery.
5. Dorsal scapular artery.

Note:
◻ ***Superior thyroid artery*** is the first branch of the ***external carotid artery***.

148. Answer is c (Special somatic afferent).
Ref: BD Chaurasia, Vol 2, Pg 260.

Somatic efferent nuclei	Special visceral efferent (branchial efferent) nuclei	General visceral efferent nuclei
– Oculomotor nucleus – Trochlear nucleus – Abducent nucleus – Hypoglossal nucleus	– Motor nucleus of trigeminal nerve – Nucleus of facial nerve – Nucleus ambiguous	– Edinger-Westphal nucleus – Superior salivatory nucleus – Inferior salivatory nucleus – Lacrimatory nucleus – Dorsal nucleus of vagus
Visceral afferent nuclei	**General somatic afferent nuclei**	**Special somatic afferent nuclei**
– Nucleus of the solitary tract	– Main sensory nucleus of the trigeminal nerve – Spinal nucleus of the trigeminal nerve – Mesencephalic nucleus of the trigeminal nerve	– Cochlear nuclei – Vestibular nuclei

149. Answer is b (Peliosis hepatis).
Ref: Textbook of Hepatology, Vol 1, Juan Rodes, Pg 1412, 3rd edition 2007.

- ***Peliosis hepatis, sinusoidal dilatation, perisinusoidal fibrosis and nodular regenerative hyperplasia*** may coexist.
- The ***peliotic cavities consist of dilated sinusoids*** and the space of Disse.

About the other choices

- **von Meyenburg Complex:** ***Bile duct hamartomas*** that are relatively common benign lesions. They are of no clinical importance, except that they mimics metastasis or microabscess.
- **Caroli disease** is a rare, autosomal recessive developmental disorder characterized by non-obstructive ***saccular or multifocal dilatation of intrahepatic bile ducts,*** multiple intrahepatic calculi and is associated with infantile and adult polycystic kidney disease and cystic renal dysplasia.
- **Hepar lobatum**: Syphilitic cirrhosis; scarred ***gummatous liver in tertiary syphilis***.

150. Answer is c (Neck).
Ref: BD Chaurasia, Vol 2, pg 26.

- The ***common peroneal nerve*** can be rolled against the ***neck of the fibula***.
- Injury to this nerve can give rise to ***foot drop***.

151. Answer is a (Talus).
Ref: BD Chaurasia, Vol 2, pg 28.

- The ***talus is devoid of muscular attachments,*** but numerous ligaments are attached to it because it takes part in three joints.

152. Answer is a (Intracellular proteolysis).
Ref: Vasudevan's Biochemistry, 5th edition Pg 176.

- Intracellular protein breakdown also occurs independent of lysosomes. This involves ***ubiquitin***.
- It is so called because it is seen in all cells abundantly.
- Ubiquitin attached proteins are immediately broken down.
- Ubiquitin tagged proteins are degraded in ***proteasomes*** inside the cells.
- Ciechanover, Hershko and Rose were awarded Nobel Prize in 2004 for their discovery of ubiquitin-mediated protein degradation.

153. Answer is a (Stimulation of appetite).
Ref: Vasudevan's Biochemistry, 5th edition Pg 338; Ganong's Physiology, 23rd edition Pg 384, 448.

Polypeptides Involved in Regulating the Appetite for Food

Increased food intake	Decreased food intake
➢ AGRP	➢ α-MSH
➢ β-endorphin	➢ Bombesin
➢ ***Ghrelin***	➢ CART
➢ Galanin	➢ CCK
➢ GHRH	➢ CRH
➢ MCH	➢ CGRP
➢ Neuropeptide Y	➢ Glucagon
➢ Orexin A	➢ GLP-1,2
➢ Orexin B	➢ GRP
	➢ Leptin
	➢ Neurotensin
	➢ Oxytocin
	➢ Peptide YY
	➢ Somatostatin

154. Answer is c (285–295).
Ref: Vasudevan's Biochemistry, 5th edition Pg 374.

Direct quote:

*"The **osmolality of plasma varies from 285 to 295 mOsmol/kg**. It is maintained by the kidney, which excretes water or solute as the case may be".*

155. Answer is d (Dopamine).
Ref: Bailey and Love's, 25th edition Pg 1048, Table 60.1.

Substances stimulating and inhibiting stomach motility

Stimulate motility	Inhibit motility
➢ Acetylcholine	➢ VIP
➢ 5-HT	➢ Enkephalin
➢ Histamine	➢ Nitric oxide
➢ Substance P	➢ Noradrenaline
➢ Substance K	➢ Dopamine
➢ Motilin	➢ Somatostatin
➢ Gastrin	Mnemonic: *"VENNDS"*
➢ Angiotensin	

156. Answer is c (Nernst equation).
Ref: Ganong's Physiology, 23rd edition Pg 7.

- Because at equilibrium, the distribution of permanent ions across the membrane is asymmetric, an ***electrical difference exists across the membrane whose magnitude can be determined*** by the ***Nernst equation***.

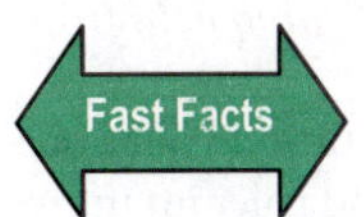

- ***Donnan and Gibbs*** showed that, in the presence of a non-diffusible ion, the ***diffusible ions distribute themselves*** so that at equilibrium their concentrations are equal. This is the ***Gibbs-Donnan equation***.
- ***Fick's law of diffusion***: The ***magnitude of the diffusing tendency*** from one region to another is directly proportional to the cross-sectional area across which, diffusion is taking place and the concentration gradient or chemical gradient, which is the difference in concentration of the diffusing substance divided by the thickness of the boundary.
- ***Henderson-Hasselbalch equation***: Deals with the ***buffering capacity*** of acids and bases.

157. Answer is b (Carbon monoxide).
Ref: Ganong's Physiology, 23rd edition Pg 644, 564.

- There is growing evidence that ***carbon monoxide as well as nitric oxide produces local dilation*** in blood vessels.
- ***Endothelin 1*** is one of the ***most potent vasoconstrictor agents*** yet isolated—it is found in ***brain and kidneys***.

Regulation of Renal blood flow

Renal vasoconstrictors	Renal vasodilators
Norepinephrine	Dopamine
Angiotensin II	Acetylcholine
Endothelin 1	Carbon monoxide

158. Answer is d (Group C fibers).
Ref: Ganong's Physiology, 23rd edition Pg 90, Table 4-3.

Susceptibility of Mammalian A, B and C Nerve Fibers

Susceptibility to	Most susceptible
Pressure	A
Hypoxia	B
Cocaine (Local Anesthetics)	C

Mnemonic: *"ABC = PHC"*

159. Answer is b (Suppressing ADH secretion).
Ref: Ganong's Physiology, 23rd edition Pg 659, Table 38-10.

- ***Ethanol and water*** act as diuretics by ***inhibiting vasopressin (ADH) secretion.***
- For mechanism of action of other diuretics see the above table in Gaing's 23rd/659.

160. Answer is d (Factor V).
Ref: Vasudevan's Biochemistry, 5th edition Pg 292.

Vitamin K dependant clotting factors are

- Factor 2 = Prothrombin
- Factor 7 = SPCA
- Factor 9 = Christmas factor
- Factor 10 = Stuart-Power factor

161. Answer is b (Valine replaces glutamate).
Ref: Harrison's, 17th edition Pg 637.

- The ***sickle cell syndromes*** are caused by a mutation in the β-globin gene that changes the ***sixth amino acid from glutamic acid to valine.***
- ***HbS*** ($\alpha 2\beta 2^{6Glu\rightarrow Val}$) polymerizes reversibly when deoxygenated to form a gelatinous network of fibrous polymers that *stiffen the RBC membrane, increase viscosity and cause dehydration* due to potassium leakage and calcium influx.

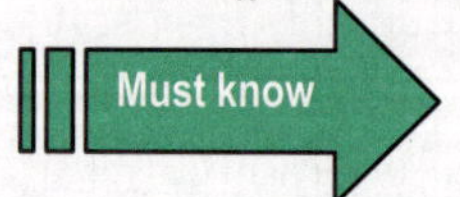

Hemoglobin Variants

Hemoglobin	Point mutation position at	Amino acid substitution
• **HbS**	β6	Glu → Val
• **HbC**	β6	Glu → Lys
• **HbE**	β26	Glu → Lys

162. Answer is b (Thrombotic thrombocytopenic purpura).
Ref: Harrison's, 17th edition Pg 722, Figure 109-4.

Pathogenesis of thrombotic thrombocytopenic purpura (TTP)

- Normally the ultra-high molecular weight multimers of von Willebrand factor (vWF) produced by the endothelial cells are processed into smaller multimers by a plasma metalloproteinase called ***ADAMTS13.***
- In ***Thrombotic Thrombocytopenic Purpura*** (***TTP***) the ***activity of the protease is inhibited*** and the ultra-high molecular weight multimers of vWF initiate platelet aggregation and thrombosis.

163. Answer is a (Tyrosine hydroxylase).
Ref: KD Tripathi, 6th edition Pg 117.

- Catecholamines are synthesized from the amino acid phenylalanine. Tyrosine hydroxylase is the rate limiting enzyme. See box below.

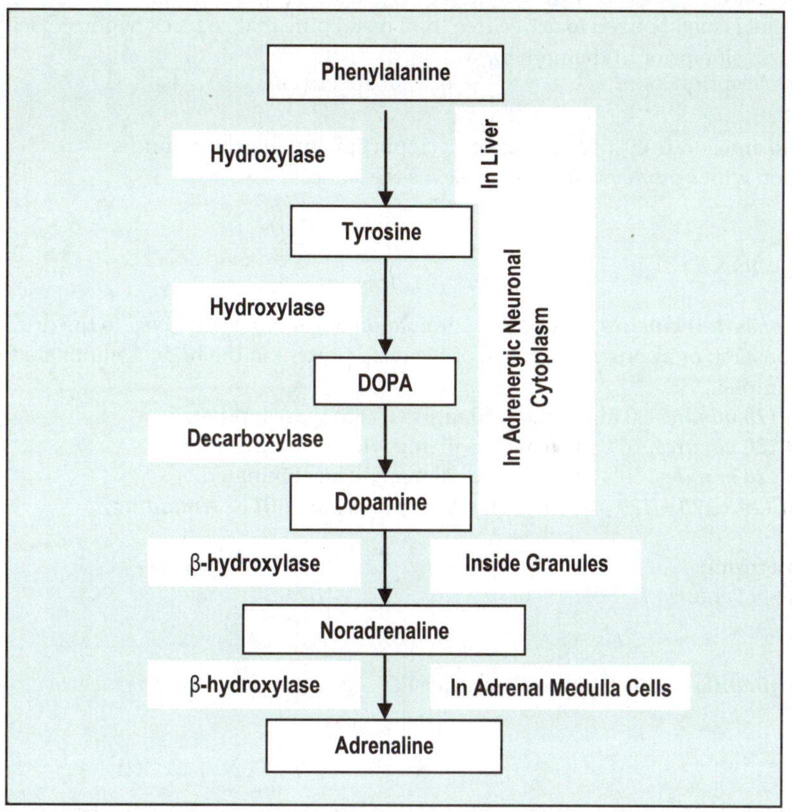

164. Answer is b (Ascorbic acid).
Ref: Vasudevan's Biochemistry, 5th edition Pg 310.

- ***Ascorbic acid*** is readily absorbed from the GIT.
- The vitamin is *excreted in the urine*.
- Since ***vitamin C is a strong reducing agent***, the ***Benedict's test will be positive*** in the urine sample after vitamin C administration.

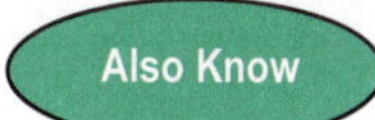

- ***Benedict's test*** is a ***semiquantitative*** test for the ***detection of reducing sugars*** in the urine.
- Any reducing sugar (any substance with free aldehyde or keto group) will give a positive test; hence this test is ***not specific for glucose***.
- Benedict's reagent contains ***sodium carbonate, copper sulfate and sodium citrate***.
- On adding Benedict's reagent to urine
  - ***Blue*** = ***absence*** of reducing sugars
  - Green = 0.5%
  - Yellow = 1.0%
  - Orange = 1.5%
  - Red = 2% or more (1% = 1 g/100 mL).

PHARMACOLOGY

165. Answer is a (Amifostine).
Ref: CMDT 2008, Pg 1312.

- ***Amifostine*** is used for ***prophylaxis of cisplatin-induced nephrotoxicity***.

- It is a prodrug that is metabolized to active free thiol metabolite that reduces nephrotoxicity.
- It is used as IV infusion prior to chemotherapy.

Note:

➲ *Mesna* is used to ameliorate cystitis caused by cyclophosphamide or ifosfamide.
➲ Bladder irrigation with ***acetylcysteine*** also achieves the same.

166. Answer is b (20 mg).
Ref: KD Tripathi, 6th edition Pg 31.

- ***First order (exponential) kinetics***: The rate of elimination is *directly proportional* to the drug concentration, clearance (CL) remains constant; or a constant ***fraction*** of the drug present in the body is eliminated in unit time.
- In the given example:
  - ➲ In the ***first 120 minutes*** 80 mg (out of 160 mg; i.e. 50%) was eliminated.
  - ➲ In the ***next 120 minutes***, 50% of 80 mg, i.e. 40 mg will be eliminated.
  - ➲ In the ***next 120 minutes***, 50% of 40 mg, i.e. 20 mg will be eliminated.
- So ***at the end of 120 + 120 + 120 = 360 minutes (6 hours) 20 mg will be remaining.***

167. Answer is a (Myometrium).
Ref: Dutta's Obstetrics, 6th edition Pg 504.

Direct quote:

*"**PGF2α acts predominantly on the myometrium**, while PGE2 acts mainly on the cervix due to its collagenolytic property".*

More About

- ☐ Prostaglandins (PGs) of the E and F series in the uterus is a prerequisite for labor both in term and preterm.
- ☐ PGs are ***paracrine/autocrine hormones*** as they act locally, at the site of their production:
  - ❖ ***Decidua*** is the main source of ***PGF2α***
  - ❖ ***Fetal membranes*** (***amnion***) produce ***PGE2***
  - ❖ ***Myometrium*** mainly produce ***PGI2***.
- ☐ ***PGE2*** is at least ***5 times more potent than PGF2α.***
- ☐ Local application of ***PGE2 gel*** is the ***'gold standard'*** for ***cervical ripening***.
- ☐ Uses of PGs in obstetrics:
  - ➢ Induction of labor (MTP and missed abortion)
  - ➢ Termination of molar pregnancy
  - ➢ Induction of labor
  - ➢ Cervical ripening prior to induction or abortion of labor
  - ➢ Acceleration of labor
  - ➢ Management of atonic PPH (refractory cases)
  - ➢ Medical management of tubal ectopic pregnancy.

168. Answer is b (Lamivudine).
Ref: Harrison's, 17th edition Pg 1758.

- ***Lamivudine***: The first of the nucleoside analogues to be approved, the dideoxynucleoside ***lamivudine, inhibits reverse transcriptase activity of both HIV and HBV*** and is a potent and effective agent for patients with chronic hepatitis B.
- ***HBV DNA titer*** is *markedly reduced* and *biochemical as well as histological indices of liver function improves.*
- Point mutation in HIV reverse transcriptase and HBV DNA polymerase gives rise to rapid lamivudine resistance.

169. Answer is d (Ethambutol).
Ref: KD Tripathi, 6th edition Pg 742.

- ***Ethambutol*** is excreted in urine by glomerular filtration and tubular secretion; plasma t1/2 is approximately 4 hours.
- ***Caution is required*** in its use with ***renal disease***.

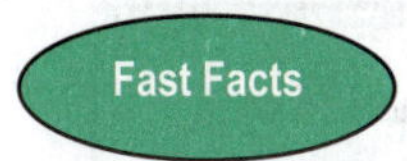

Antimicrobials needing dose reduction/avoidance in renal failure

Reduce dose even in mild failure	Reduce dose only in moderate-to-severe failure	Drugs to be AVOIDED
– Aminoglycosides	– Metronidazole	– Cephalothin
– Amphotericin B	– Carbenicillin	– Talamoicllin
– Cephalosporins	– Cotrimoxazole	– Nalidixic acid
– Ethambutol	– Fluoroquinolones	– Tetracyclines (except doxycycline)
– Vancomycin	– Aztreonam	
– Flucytosine	– Clarithromycin	– Nitrofurantoin
	– Meropenem	
	– Imipenem	

170. Answer is b (Lorazepam).
Ref: KD Tripathi, 6th edition Pg 450, 396.

- ***Lorazepam*** is unique in that it DOES NOT produce any active metabolite.
- It is used for short lasting anxiety states, panic, OCD and tension syndromes.

171. Answer is a (Abciximab).
Ref: KD Tripathi, 6th edition Pg 610-11.

Abciximab
- ***Antithrombotic*** (monoclonal antibody), ***platelet aggregation inhibitor*** (by binding to ***glycoprotein IIb/IIIa receptor***).
- ***Used as*** adjunct in ***percutaneous coronary interventions*** (e.g. PTCA) for *prevention of acute cardiac ischemic complications.*
- Side effects are bleeding (most common), thrombocytopenia, hypotension, bradycardia, pleurisy/pleural effusion, leukocytosis, peripheral edema, pneumonia and hypersensitivity reactions (due to human antichimeric antibody).
- For monitoring of treatment, PT (or APTT) may be used.

Etanercept
- ***Etanercept*** is a dimeric fusion protein of the tumor necrosis factor receptor (TNFR) linked to the Fc portion of human IgG1.
- Etanercept binds specifically to ***tumor necrosis factor (TNF) and blocks its interaction*** with cell surface TNF receptors.
- Used subcutaneously in adult: ***Rheumatoid arthritis***, ***ankylosing spondylitis*** and ***psoriatic arthritis*** patients.

Adalimumab
- Recombinant ***anti-TNF antibody*** used in rheumatoid arthritis.

Infliximab
- A ***chimeric monoclonal antibody,*** which binds and neutralizes TNFα, used in rheumatoid arthritis.

172. Answer is a (Point source epidemic).
Ref: Park, 20th edition Pg 61.

- The 'unusual' occurrence in a community or region of a disease/specific health-related behavior (smoking) or other health related events (traffic accidents) in excess of expected occurrence are called ***epidemic***.
- An arbitrary limit of ***two standard errors from the endemic frequency*** is used to define the epidemic threshold for common diseases.

■ **Point source epidemic**	• **Common source/Single exposure epidemics.** • The resultant cases all develop within one incubation period of the disease (e.g. in an epidemic of food poisoning). • The epidemic tends to be explosive with clustering of cases within a narrow interval of time; the epidemic curve rises and falls rapidly with no secondary waves (e.g. ***Bhopal gas tragedy*** *in India, Minamata disease in Japan*).
■ **Continuous epidemic**	• **Multiple/Repeated exposure epidemic.** • Example *Gonorrhea*, a well of contaminated water, *Legionnaire's* disease.
■ **Propagated epidemic**	• Usually of infectious origin (polio, hepatitis A); person-to-person transmission occurs; also through arthropods/animal reservoir. • High secondary attack rate occurs. • Cases occur later than known length of incubation period. • Slow transmission occurs in areas with good herd immunity.

173. Answer is a (Enalapril).
Ref: KD Tripathi, 6th edition Pg 553.

- Systolic BP > 180 mm Hg or diastolic BP > 120 mm Hg with evidence of active end organ damage is termed ***'hypertensive emergency'***, while the same elevation of BP without signs of end organ damage is termed ***'hypertensive urgency'***.

Drugs used in HTN emergencies and urgencies are:
1. ***Sodium nitroprusside***: Drug of choice for most emergencies; needs infusion pump; most effective drug.
2. ***Glyceryl trinitrate***
3. ***Diazoxide***
4. ***Hydralazine***: Avoid in patients with MI or aortic dissection.
5. ***Esmolol***
6. ***Phentolamine***: α1 + α2 blocker; drug of choice in hyperadrenergic states such as hypertensive episodes in pheochromocytoma, cheese reaction, clonidine withdrawal.
7. ***Labetalol***
8. ***Furosemide***

Drugs, which were used earlier ***BUT NOT NOW***
- ☐ **Nifedipine**: Inability to control rate and degree of fall in BP.
- ☐ **Captopril** and **clonidine**: Unsatisfactory.

174. Answer is c (Membranous glomerulonephritis).
Ref: Robbin's Pathology, 7th edition Pg 979.

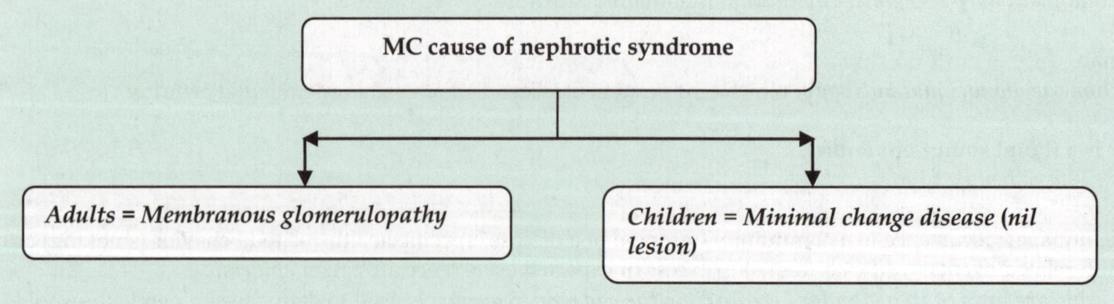

175. Answer is c (Bulky friable vegetations).
Ref: Robbin's Pathology, 7th edition Pg 593-94, Fig 12-24.

Pathologic features of rheumatic heart disease

- ❖ Inflammatory focus: *Aschoff* bodies
- ❖ *MacCallum plaques*: Subendocardial lesions usually in left atrium
- ❖ *Small vegetations* (verrucae): Only 1–2 mm size
- ❖ Leaflet *thickening*, commissural *fusion* and shortening and *thickening of chordae tendineae.*

176. Answer is c (Specular reflection).
Ref: Parson's, 20th edition Pg 113.

- ***Specular reflection*** is a type of view using slit lamp, which helps in seeing ***corneal endothelium***.
- ***Specular microscope*** is used to visualize and count ***corneal endothelial cells***.

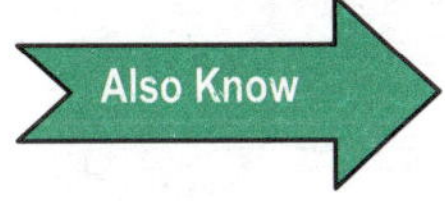

- ☐ ***Focal illumination***: For direct observation of the illuminated point.
- ☐ ***Retroillumination***: Light reflects off the retina and highlights media opacities such as cataracts, corneal blood vessels, corneal scars.
- ☐ ***Scleral scatter***: For viewing opacities in the cornea.

177. Answer is c (Analysis of the health situation).
Ref: Park, 20th edition Pg 772.

The steps in planning cycle are:

i. Analysis of the health situation.
ii. Establishment of objectives and goals.
iii. Assessment of resources.
iv. Fixing priorities.
v. Write-up of formulated plan.
vi. Programming and implementation.
vii. Monitoring.
viii. Evaluation.

178. Answer is a (Thomas Starzl).
Ref: Harrison's, 17th edition Pg 1984; Organ Transplantation, David Petechuk, 2006 edition Pg 180; Transplantation Surgery, Nadey SH, 2001 edition (Table given is derived from all the mentioned references).

- Pioneered in the 1960s by Starzl at the University of Colorado and later at the University of Pittsburgh and by Calne in Cambridge, England; liver transplantation is now performed routinely worldwide.

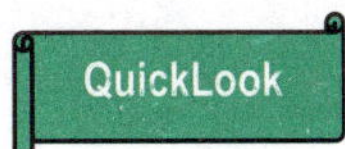

"FIRSTS" in organ transplantation

Organ transplant	By (name)	Date
Corneal	Edward Zim	1906
Kidney	RH Lawler	1950
Liver	Thomas Starzl	1961
Lung transplant	James Hardy	1963
Pancreas	Richard Lillehei	1966
Heart	Christiaan Barnard	1967
Heart, lung	Denton Cooley	1968

179. Answer is c (Transketolase).
Ref: Vasudevan's Biochemistry, 5th edition Pg 119, 295.

- In ***thiamine deficiency, transketolase*** activity is reduced.
- Transketolase is an enzyme, which uses thiamine as a cofactor.

180. Answer is a {[a/(a+b)] × 100}.
Ref: Park, 20th edition.

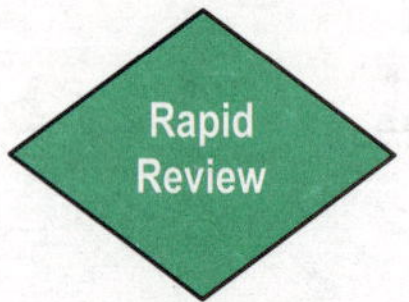

ANALYSIS OF DIAGNOSTIC TESTS

Test result	Disease	
	Disease ⊕	Disease –
⊕	a (true positive)	b (false positive)
–	c (false negative)	d (true negative)

• **Sensitivity**	– The test's ability to all people with disease who truly have the disease (true positives) = ***a / a + c × 100*** = 1 – false negative rate – Most acceptable screening tests are > 80% sensitive – A false negative is a negative test in a patient with the disease
• **Specificity**	– The test's ability to correctly identify all people without disease, i.e. those who do not have the disease (true negatives) = ***d / b+d × 100*** = 1 – false positive rate – Used as confirmatory test after a positive screening test – Most acceptable confirmatory tests are > 85% specific – Example HIV testing; screen with ELISA (sensitive, high false positive rate, low threshold); confirm with Western blot (specific, high false negative rate, high threshold)
• **Predictive value**	– Reflects the diagnostic power of the test
• **Positive predictive value**	– Proportion of positive test results that are true positive, i.e. the probability that a person with a positive test actually has the disease = ***a / a + b × 100***
• **Negative predictive value**	– Proportion of negative test results that are true negative, i.e. the probability that a person with a negative test actually is disease free = ***d / c + d × 100***

COMED-K 2009

COMED-K 2009 QUESTIONS

MEDICINE

1. **Dissecting hematoma is a clinical complication occurring in**
   (a) Turner's syndrome
   (b) Klinefelter's syndrome
   (c) Down syndrome
   (d) Marfan syndrome

2. **Beryllium exposure is associated with**
   (a) Pulmonary fibrosis
   (b) Granulomatous lung disease
   (c) Lung cancer
   (d) Chronic bronchitis

3. **Adenosine deaminase in CSF is significantly higher in**
   (a) Tuberculous meningitis
   (b) Bacterial meningitis
   (c) Viral meningitis
   (d) Syphilitic meningitis

4. **All of the following are signs of cerebellar disease *EXCEPT***
   (a) Resting tremors
   (b) Past pointing
   (c) Nystagmus
   (d) Ataxic gait

5. **Excessive production of aldosterone results in**
   (a) Metabolic acidosis
   (b) Severe hypotension
   (c) Potassium retention
   (d) Depressed plasma renin

6. **A 62-year-old patient has been diagnosed with a restrictive pulmonary disease. Which of his following lung measurements is likely to be normal?**
   (a) FEV_1
   (b) FVC
   (c) FEV_1/FVC
   (d) FRC

7. **An example of chronic myeloproliferative disorder is**
   (a) Neutrophilic leukemoid reaction
   (b) Essential thrombocythemia
   (c) Plasmacytosis
   (d) Hairy cell leukemia

8. **All of the following drugs can be used for the prophylaxis of migraine *EXCEPT***
   (a) Propranolol
   (b) Sumatriptan
   (c) Amitriptyline
   (d) Flunarizine

9. **The drug of choice for the treatment of *Pneumocystis jiroveci (Pneumocystis carini)* pneumonia is**
   (a) Lamivudine
   (b) Co-trimoxazole
   (c) Doxycycline
   (d) Itraconazole

10. **Giant 'v' wave on examination of the jugular venous pulse is suggestive of**
    (a) Atrial flutter with changing block
    (b) Tricuspid incompetence
    (c) Ventricular septal defect
    (d) Pulmonary stenosis

11. **Kimmelstiel-Wilson disease is a feature of**
    (a) Amyloidosis
    (b) Diabetic glomerulosclerosis
    (c) Systemic lupus erythematosus
    (d) Fibrillary glomerulonephritis

12. **An arterial blood gas report of pH: 7.00; PaO_2: 60 mm Hg; $PaCO_2$: 80 mm Hg; HCO_3: 28**
    (a) Respiratory acidosis with normoxemia
    (b) Metabolic acidosis with normoxemia
    (c) Metabolic acidosis with hypoxemia
    (d) Respiratory acidosis with hypoxemia

13. **Paradoxical undressing occurs with**
    (a) Heat stroke
    (b) Hypothermia
    (c) Hyperthermia
    (d) Hyperpyrexia

14. **The most common cause of bronchopulmonary aspergillosis is**
    (a) *Aspergillus fumigatus*
    (b) *Aspergillus clavatus*
    (c) *Aspergillus flavus*
    (d) *Aspergillus niger*

15. **Bibasilar velcro crackles occur in**
    (a) Acute pulmonary edema
    (b) Acute bronchopneumonia
    (c) Pulmonary fibrosis
    (d) Pulmonary embolism

16. **A mill wheel type of murmur during laparoscopy suggests**
(a) Tension pneumothorax
(b) Intra-abdominal bleeding
(c) Gas embolism
(d) Pre-existing valvular disease

17. **An increase in serum bilirubin level on prolonged fasting is seen in**
(a) Dubin-Johnson syndrome
(b) Gilbert's syndrome
(c) Pancreatic tumors
(d) Crigler-Najjar syndrome

18. **Sexual ambiguity may be seen in which of the following conditions?**
(a) Androgen insensitivity
(b) Pure gonadal dysgenesis
(c) Swyer syndrome
(d) Mixed gonadal dysgenesis

19. **The following are single gene disorders *EXCEPT***
(a) Hemochromatosis
(b) Cystic fibrosis
(c) William's syndrome
(d) Huntington's disease

20. **Multifactorial inheritance is known in**
(a) Neurofibroma
(b) Hemophilia
(c) Cardiac septal defects
(d) Hypophosphatemic rickets

21. **Isolated deletion of which chromosome causes myelodysplastic syndrome?**
(a) 2q
(b) 5q
(c) 8q
(d) 11q

22. **Of the following vasculitides, coronary artery aneurysms are most often seen in**
(a) Kawasaki disease
(b) Giant-cell arteritis
(c) Wegener's granulomatosis
(d) Leukocytoclastic vasculitis

23. **All are true regarding progressive supranuclear palsy *EXCEPT***
(a) Tremors
(b) Unsteadiness
(c) Dysarthria
(d) Gaze palsy

SURGERY

24. **Cobra head appearance is described for**
(a) BPH
(b) Bladder tumor
(c) Vesical calculus
(d) Ureterocele

25. **Heller's operation is done for**
(a) Achalasia cardia
(b) Pyloric stenosis
(c) Hirschsprung's disease
(d) Crohn's disease

26. **The commonest systemic abnormality associated with renal cell carcinoma is**
(a) Hypertension
(b) Polycythemia
(c) Elevated ESR
(d) Pyrexia

27. **In the management of symptomatic benign prostatic hyperplasia with finasteride the period of trial required for determining a satisfactory response is**
(a) 1 month
(b) 2 months
(c) 4 months
(d) 6 months

28. **Saccular diverticulum of extrahepatic bile duct in choledochal cyst is classified as**
(a) Type I
(b) Type II
(c) Type III
(d) Type IV

29. **In exocrine pancreatic cancer, the commonest tumor marker to be elevated is**
(a) CA 125
(b) CEA
(c) CA 15-3
(d) CA 19-9

30. **The site of mucosal tear in Mallory-Weiss syndrome is**
(a) Stomach
(b) Small intestine
(c) Colon
(d) Esophagus

31. **The triad of diabetes, gallstones and steatorrhea is associated with which one of the following tumors?**
(a) Gastrinomas
(b) Somatostatinomas
(c) VIPomas
(d) Glucagonomas

32. **Which of the following is NOT associated with elevation of prostatic specific antigen?**
(a) Acute prostatitis
(b) BPH
(c) Prostatic intraepithelial neoplasm
(d) Prostatic needle biopsy

33. **The most common complication of transurethral resection of the prostate is**
(a) Erectile dysfunction
(b) Retrograde ejaculation
(c) Urinary incontinence
(d) Urethral stricture disease

34. **Complications of total parenteral nutrition include all *EXCEPT***
(a) Hyperglycemia
(b) Hypoglycemia
(c) Hypochloremic alkalosis
(d) Electrolyte abnormalities

35. **A tumor arising in a burns scar is likely to be**
(a) Basal cell carcinoma
(b) Squamous cell carcinoma
(c) Malignant melanoma
(d) Fibrosarcoma

36. **Pneumatosis intestinalis is diagnostic of**
(a) Ileal perforation
(b) Necrotizing enterocolitis
(c) Meconium ileus
(d) Colonic aganglionosis

37. **Toxic megacolon is seen in**
(a) Carcinoma colon
(b) Gastrocolic fistula
(c) Ulcerative colitis
(d) Amebic colitis

OBSTETRICS AND GYNECOLOGY

38. **Fern pattern in cervical mucus is due to high**
(a) Potassium chloride
(b) Sodium chloride
(c) Calcium chloride
(d) Protein content

39. **Characteristics of the fertile phase of the menstrual cycle include all of the following *EXCEPT***
(a) Peak levels of estrogen
(b) Clear, abundant cervical mucus
(c) Ovulation
(d) Production of progesterone

40. **Intrauterine exposure of diethylstilbestrol is associated with**
(a) Squamous cell carcinoma of cervix
(b) Adenocarcinoma of endometrium
(c) Clear cell adenocarcinoma of vagina
(d) Sarcoma of uterus

41. **Medical termination of pregnancy can be done by a registered medical practitioner if the gestation period is less than**
(a) 8 weeks
(b) 12 weeks
(c) 20 weeks
(d) 24 weeks

42. **Which of the following methods of contraception suppresses ovulation as its primary mechanism of action?**
(a) Medicated intrauterine device (IUD)
(b) Levonorgestrel
(c) Mifepristone
(d) Gonadotropin releasing hormone (GnRH) agonists

43. **Infants born to mothers who are heavy drinkers are at increased risk of which of the following problems?**
(a) Mental retardation
(b) Chronic liver disease
(c) Excessive birthweight
(d) Chorioretinitis

44. **The minimum number of antenatal visits advised to pregnant women is**
(a) Three
(b) Six
(c) Seven
(d) Nine

45. **Perinatal mortality is expressed in terms of**
(a) Deaths/1,000 total births
(b) Deaths/1,000 live births
(c) Deaths/10,000 total births
(d) Deaths/10,000 live births

46. **Which clotting factors decrease during pregnancy?**
(a) 1 and 3
(b) 11 and 13
(c) 10 and 12
(d) 7 and 8

47. **Hydrops fetalis may be caused by all the following, *EXCEPT***
(a) Congenital heart block
(b) Cystic hygroma
(c) Congenital varicella syndrome
(d) Congenital nephrosis

48. **Lactation suppression in hypertensive postpartum patient is achieved by**

(a) Bromocriptine
(b) Estrogen alone
(c) Estrogen and testosterone
(d) Breast binder and analgesics

49. The primary site of hematopoiesis in the fetus before midpregnancy is
(a) Bone
(b) Liver
(c) Spleen
(d) Lung

PEDIATRICS

50. In children the most commonly recognized form of familial hyperlipidemia is
(a) Hypertriglyceridemia
(b) Hypercholesterolemia
(c) Hyperchylomicronemia
(d) Combined hyperlipidemia

51. Thrombocytopenia, macerated skin lesions, rash and periostitis in a newborn are seen in
(a) Erythroblastosis fetalis
(b) Cytomegalovirus infection
(c) Syphilis
(d) HIV infection

52. Amount of ORS to be given in the first 4 hours to a child with some dehydration is
(a) 50 mL/kg body wt
(b) 75 mL/kg body wt
(c) 100 mL/kg body wt
(d) 200 mL/kg body wt

53. In a child with acute liver failure, the most important abnormal serum biochemical test that indicates poor prognosis is
(a) Increasing transaminases
(b) Increasing bilirubin
(c) Increasing prothrombin time
(d) Reversal of serum albumin-globulin ratio

54. Deficiency of which element can lead to syndrome of growth failure, anemia and hypogonadism?
(a) Calcium
(b) Copper
(c) Zinc
(d) Magnesium

55. Which of the following is NOT a feature of hypothyroidism?
(a) Mental retardation
(b) Large head
(c) Calf muscle hypertrophy
(d) Microcephaly

56. Early strict toilet training can result in
(a) Nocturnal enuresis
(b) Encopresis
(c) Night terror
(d) Temper tantrums

57. A 2 year child is classified as having pneumonia, if the respiratory rate is more than
(a) 30/min
(b) 40/min
(c) 50/min
(d) 60/min

58. The likely diagnosis in a child with limb pain and pancytopenia is
(a) Aplastic anemia
(b) Acute lymphocytic leukemia
(c) Rheumatic fever
(d) Rheumatoid arthritis

ORTHOPEDICS

59. The ossification center of pisiform bone appears at the age of
(a) 10–11 years
(b) 12–13 years
(c) 14–15 years
(d) 15–16 years

60. Onion peel radiologic appearance is seen typically in
(a) Ewing's sarcoma
(b) Osteosarcoma
(c) Fibrosarcoma
(d) Aneurysmal bone cyst

61. Which of the following is not a sign of active rickets?
(a) Prominent fontanelle
(b) Hot cross bun sign
(c) Saddle nose
(d) Caries teeth

62. Which of the following is NOT a risk factor for avascular necrosis of head of femur?
(a) Alcohol
(b) Smoking
(c) Obesity
(d) Chondromyxoid fibroma

63. 'Telescopic fingers' occur in
(a) Rheumatic arthritis
(b) Rheumatoid arthritis
(c) Psoriatic arthritis
(d) Reiter's arthritis

64. **Aviator fracture is**
   (a) Fracture of neck of talus
   (b) Fracture of scaphoid
   (c) Fracture of calcaneus
   (d) Fracture of 5th metatarsal

65. **The deforming force in a Bennett's fracture is due to the action of**
   (a) Abductor pollicis longus
   (b) Flexor pollicis brevis
   (c) Opponens pollicis
   (d) Extensor pollicis brevis

66. **A cut injury of the ulnar nerve results in**
   (a) Total claw hand
   (b) Paralysis of all lumbricals
   (c) Paralysis of all interossei
   (d) Paralysis of all slips of the flexor digitorum profundus

OPHTHALMOLOGY

67. **Rubella cataract is seen as**
   (a) Posterior polar cataract
   (b) Nuclear cataract
   (c) Blue dot cataract in young
   (d) Cuneiform cataract

68. **Which vitamin deficiency produces progressive external ophthalmoplegia?**
   (a) Vitamin A
   (b) Vitamin C
   (c) Vitamin D
   (d) Vitamin E

69. **Immunoglobulin which is present in the human aqueous is**
   (a) IgA
   (b) IgD
   (c) IgG
   (d) IgM

70. **Corneal sensation is diminished in**
   (a) Band keratopathy
   (b) Exposure keratitis
   (c) Phlyctenular keratitis
   (d) Dendritic keratitis

71. **Open angle glaucoma causes**
   (a) Sudden loss of vision
   (b) Difficulty in dark adaptation
   (c) Amaurosis fugax
   (d) Uniocular diplopia

72. **Siderosis bulbi is often associated with**
   (a) Glaucoma
   (b) Keratitis
   (c) Papillitis
   (d) Band keratopathy

73. **Roth spots are seen in**
   (a) Hypertension
   (b) Septicemia
   (c) Diabetes
   (d) Central retinal occlusion

74. **Topical sodium cromoglycate is useful in treatment of**
   (a) Phlyctenular conjunctivitis
   (b) Vernal catarrh
   (c) Subconjunctival hemorrhage
   (d) Trachoma

75. **Grid laser photocoagulation is indicated in**
   (a) Ischemic maculopathy
   (b) Clinically significant macular edema
   (c) Macular hole
   (d) Proliferative diabetic retinopathy

EAR, NOSE AND THROAT

76. **Pulsatile tinnitus is present in**
   (a) Meniere's disease
   (b) Presbycusis
   (c) Otosclerosis
   (d) Glomus jugulare tumor

77. **Otomycosis is caused by**
   (a) *Aspergillus niger*
   (b) *Histoplasma capsulatum*
   (c) *Rhinosporidium seeberi*
   (d) *Cryptococcus neoformans*

78. **Spiral ganglion and organ of corti is fully developed in a fetus by**
   (a) 20 weeks
   (b) 25 weeks
   (c) 30 weeks
   (d) 35 weeks

PATHOLOGY

79. **Birbeck granules in the cytoplasm is characteristic of**
   (a) Neutrophil
   (b) Natural killer cells
   (c) Eosinophil
   (d) Langerhans cells

80. The stain used for the demonstration of reticulocyte is
(a) Wright stain
(b) Brilliant cresyl blue
(c) Alcian blue
(d) Giemsa stain

81. The commonest site for extragonadal germ cell tumor is
(a) Retroperitoneum
(b) Sacrococcygeal region
(c) Pineal gland
(d) Mediastinum

82. The gene that predisposes to retinoblastoma is located at
(a) Chromosome 13q14
(b) Chromosome 15q11
(c) Chromosome lip 13
(d) Chromosome 22q11

83. Mediastinal lymph node calcification is seen in which one of the following?
(a) Metastatic neoplasm
(b) Lymphoma
(c) Sarcoidosis
(d) Bronchiectasis

84. Most specific histological lesion in diabetic nephropathy is
(a) Glomerular crescents
(b) Immune complex deposition
(c) Occlusion of glomeruli with fibrin caps
(d) Nodular glomerulosclerosis

85. 'Onion skin' fibrosis of bile duct is seen in
(a) Primary biliary cirrhosis
(b) Primary sclerosing cholangitis
(c) Extrahepatic biliary fibrosis
(d) Congenital hepatic fibrosis

86. The LE cell in Romanowsky-stained preparation is a/an
(a) Monocyte
(b) Neutrophil
(c) Eosinophil
(d) Lymphocyte

87. von Willebrand factor is produced by
(a) Liver
(b) Platelets
(c) Endothelial cells
(d) Spleen

88. Which of these types of asbestos is LEAST associated with mesothelioma?
(a) Chrysotile
(b) Crocidolite
(c) Amosite
(d) Tremolite

89. A low mean corpuscular volume with a normal red cell distribution width suggests
(a) Iron deficiency anemia
(b) β-thalassemia trait
(c) Anemia of chronic disease
(d) Sideroblastic anemia

90. Ruffled membrane is seen in
(a) White fibrous cartilage
(b) Osteoblast
(c) Osteoclast
(d) Elastic cartilage

91. Xanthogranulomatous pyelonephritis is often associated with infection by
(a) *Proteus*
(b) *E. coli*
(c) *H. influenzae*
(d) *Klebsiella*

92. In lobar pneumonia, the presence of fibrinosuppurative exudate with disintegration of red cells is seen in the stage of
(a) Congestion
(b) Red hepatization
(c) Gray hepatization
(d) Resolution

93. Mikulicz cells and Russell bodies is diagnostic of
(a) Hodgkin's disease
(b) Rhinosporidiosis
(c) Chordoma
(d) Rhinoscleroma

94. Endodermal sinus tumor is characterized by
(a) Schiller-Duval body
(b) Psammoma body
(c) Call-Exner bodies
(d) Homer-Wright rosettes

MICROBIOLOGY

95. Romana's sign occurs in
(a) Babesiosis
(b) Leishmaniasis
(c) Trypanosomiasis
(d) Schistosomiasis

96. Which one of the following viruses produces both intranuclear and intracytoplasmic inclusion bodies?

(a) Chicken pox
(b) Rabies
(c) Small pox
(d) Measles

97. Transplantation between genetically different members of the same species is termed as
(a) Autograft
(b) Isograft
(c) Allograft
(d) Xenograft

98. Toxic shock syndrome is caused by
(a) *Staphylococcus aureus*
(b) Group B *Streptococcus*
(c) *Pseudomonas aeruginosa*
(d) *Clostridium difficile*

99. The following immunoglobulin DOES NOT fix to complement
(a) IgE
(b) IgM
(c) IgA
(d) IgG

100. All the following can be used to grow human viruses *EXCEPT*
(a) Continuous cell lines
(b) Suckling mice
(c) Embryonated egg
(d) Enriched media

101. Which one of the following test is used for the diagnosis of *Giardia lamblia* infection?
(a) Enterotest
(b) Casoni's test
(c) Parasite F test
(d) Napier's test

102. Which one of the following enteric organisms is anaerogenic and non-motile?
(a) *Shigella sonnei*
(b) *Salmonella typhi*
(c) *Proteus mirabilis*
(d) *Klebsiella pneumoniae*

PHARMACOLOGY

103. Which among the following is the drug of choice for Clostridium difficile-induced colitis?
(a) Gentamicin
(b) Ciprofloxacin
(c) Metronidazole
(d) Linezolid

104. Imatinib mesylate is most useful in the treatment of
(a) Chronic lymphoid leukemia
(b) Chronic myeloid leukemia
(c) Acute myeloid leukemia
(d) Acute lymphoid leukemia

105. The chief compound in cannabis is
(a) 9-Δ-tetrahydrocannabinol
(b) 6-Δ-tetrahydrocannabinol
(c) 5-Δ-tetrahydrocannabinol
(d) 4-Δ-tetrahydrocannabinol

106. Topical azelaic acid is used in
(a) Hyperpigmentary disorders
(b) Dermatophyte infections
(c) Vitiligo
(d) Mixed infections

107. Which among the following anti-HIV drugs is also used to treat viral hepatitis B?
(a) Enfuvirtide
(b) Lamivudine
(c) Efavirenz
(d) Ritonavir

108. Purple toe syndrome is associated with which of the following drugs?
(a) Warfarin
(b) Phenytoin
(c) Theophylline
(d) Thalidomide

109. Combination of ampicillin and gentamicin is an example of
(a) Indifference
(b) Synergy
(c) Antagonism
(d) Bacterial symbiosis

110. The drug of choice for the treatment of gonorrhea in a pregnant patient allergic to β-lactam antibiotics is
(a) Piperacillin
(b) Ceftriaxone
(c) Spectinomycin
(d) Ciprofloxacin

111. Which of the following drugs is a long-acting somatostatin analog?
(a) Leuprolide
(b) Somatropin
(c) Goserelin
(d) Octreotide

112. Proton pump inhibitors suppress gastric acid secretion by inhibition of

(a) HVCl⁻-ATPase pump
(b) H^+/K^+-ATPase pump
(c) Na/Cl^--ATPase pump
(d) Na/K^+-ATPase pump

113. Which of the following premedications is associated with extrapyramidal side effects?
(a) Metoclopramide
(b) Cimetidine
(c) Scopolamine
(d) Glycopyrrolate

PREVENTIVE AND SOCIAL MEDICINE

114. 17D vaccine is used for the prevention and control of
(a) Yellow fever
(b) Japanese encephalitis
(c) Hemorrhagic fever
(d) Dengue

115. The most heat sensitive vaccine is
(a) Measles
(b) Hepatitis B
(c) DPT
(d) OPV

116. In severe heat strain the heat stress index (HIS) is
(a) 10–30
(b) 40–60
(c) 70–90
(d) 100

117. Calculate the prevalence if incidence is 2 cases per 1,000 population per year and mean duration is 4 years
(a) 8 cases per 1,000 population
(b) 2 cases per 1,000 population
(c) 0.5 cases per 1,000 population
(d) 32 cases per 1,000 population

118. Among the principles of primary health care, the one which is NOT included is
(a) Intersectoral coordination
(b) Appropriate technology
(c) Equitable distribution
(d) Information, education and communication

119. Point source epidemic tends to
(a) Continue over one incubation period
(b) Produce multiple peaks in the epidemic curve
(c) Be explosive
(d) Tail off gradually

120. Communicability is best measured by
(a) Serial interval
(b) Case fatality rate
(c) Secondary attack rate
(d) Generation time

121. The vector which transmits trench fever
(a) Tick
(b) Mite
(c) Flea
(d) Louse

122. The pulse polio immunization (PPI) was first launched in India in the year
(a) 1995
(b) 1996
(c) 1999
(d) 2000

123. As compared to cow's milk, human milk has a higher content of
(a) Fat
(b) Sugar
(c) Protein
(d) Calcium

124. The minimum recommended concentration of free chlorine in drinking water at the end of 1 hour (mg/L) is
(a) 0.1
(b) 0.5
(c) 1.0
(d) 1.5

FORENSIC MEDICINE

125. Dark brown postmortem lividity is seen in
(a) Aniline poisoning
(b) Carbon-monoxide poisoning
(c) Phosphorus poisoning
(d) Cyanide poisoning

126. In India the age of consent for marriage of a female is
(a) 15 years
(b) 16 years
(c) 18 years
(d) 20 years

127. Diaphanous test is the test to detect
(a) Pregnancy
(b) Stoppage of respiration
(c) Stoppage of circulation
(d) Presence of blood

DERMATOLOGY

128. Gottron's papules are
(a) Erythematous papules on cheeks
(b) Erythema seen over elbows and knees
(c) Periorbital lesions
(d) Violaceous papules over knuckles

129. Intraepidermal bullae are seen in
(a) Pemphigoid
(b) Pemphigus
(c) Dermatitis herpetiformis
(d) Light reaction

130. Subcutaneous granuloma is a feature of
(a) Chancroid
(b) Secondary syphilis
(c) Lymphogranuloma venereum
(d) Donovanosis

131. Seborrheic dermatitis is frequently seen in
(a) Lipid storage disorders
(b) Psoriasis vulgaris
(c) Hypertension
(d) Parkinson's disease

132. Urticarial lesions are best described as
(a) Non-pruritic
(b) Bullous
(c) Evanescent
(d) Macular

133. The most important pathogen involved in non-gonococcal urethritis is
(a) *Chlamydia trachomatis*
(b) *Trichomonas vaginalis*
(c) *Ureoplasma ureolyticum*
(d) Herpes simplex

RADIOLOGY

134. 'Rim' and 'ball' nephrograms in intravenous urography are seen in
(a) Normal kidneys
(b) Acute obstructive nephropathy
(c) Chronic obstructive nephropathy
(d) Chronic renal failure

135. Which of the following is a cause of a unilateral hyperlucent lung on chest radiography?
(a) Poland syndrome
(b) Asthma
(c) Acute bronchiolitis
(d) Pleural effusion

136. 'Stipple sign' seen in transitional cell carcinoma of the renal collecting system is *best* demonstrated by
(a) Intravenous urography
(b) Retrograde pyeloureterography
(c) Radionuclide scan
(d) Ultrasound scan

137. Calcific hepatic metastases are seen in
(a) Adenocarcinoma of the colon
(b) Carcinoid tumors
(c) Renal cell carcinoma
(d) Lymphoma

138. 'Shrinking lung' is a feature of
(a) Rheumatoid arthritis
(b) Systemic lupus erythematosus
(c) Systemic sclerosis
(d) Polymyositis

139. Square root sign is characteristic of
(a) Dilated cardiomyopathy
(b) Restrictive cardiomyopathy
(c) Constrictive pericarditis
(d) Cardiac tamponade

ANESTHESIA

140. Which among the following is NOT used for surface anesthesia?
(a) Lignocaine
(b) Procaine
(c) Tetracaine
(d) Benzocaine

141. Which anesthetic gas is contraindicated in the presence of pneumothorax?
(a) Halothane
(b) Isoflurane
(c) Nitrous oxide
(d) Chloroform

142. The incidence of unpleasant dreams associated with emergence from ketamine anesthesia can be reduced by administration of
(a) Atropine
(b) Scopolamine
(c) Physostigmine
(d) Diazepam

143. Earliest sign of systemic absorption of local anesthetic is
(a) Convulsions
(b) Circulatory collapse
(c) Circumoral numbness
(d) Respiratory arrest

144. Treatment of choice in obstructive sleep apnea is
(a) Nebulization
(b) Home oxygen treatment
(c) Respiratory stimulants
(d) Domiciliary CPAP

145. Pulse less electrical activity of heart can be seen in poisoning with drug
(a) Flumazenil
(b) Naloxone
(c) Propoxyphene
(d) Glucagon

PSYCHIATRY

146. All of the following can be considered as treatment for anxiety disorder *EXCEPT*
(a) Buspirone
(b) Benzodiazepines
(c) Serotonin reuptake inhibitors
(d) Dopaminergic blockers

147. The lower level of normal IQ while defining mental retardation is
(a) 60
(b) 70
(c) 80
(d) 90

148. Bruxism is
(a) Walking during sleep
(b) Nocturnal enuresis
(c) Grinding of teeth during sleep
(d) Sleep apnea

149. All of the following are considered to be negative symptoms of schizophrenia *EXCEPT*
(a) Apathy
(b) Ambivalence
(c) Auditory hallucinations
(d) Affective flattening

150. Voyeurism is a sexual perversion characterized by
(a) Sexual pleasure derived from observing people in sexual acts
(b) Sexual focus on children
(c) Sexual focus on pain
(d) Sexual focus from non-living objects

151. Tactile hallucination is seen in poisoning with
(a) Carbolic acid
(b) Cannabis
(c) Cocaine
(d) Chloral hydrate

ANATOMY, PHYSIOLOGY AND BIOCHEMISTRY

152. The dartos muscle is innervated by
(a) Ilioinguinal nerve
(b) Iliohypogastric nerve
(c) Sympathetic nerves
(d) Pudendal nerve

153. Which of the following muscles is enclosed within the clavipectoral fascia?
(a) Pectoralis major
(b) Serratus anterior
(c) Coracobrachialis
(d) Subclavius

154. Macula densa is present in
(a) Collecting tubule
(b) Proximal convoluted tubule
(c) Distal convoluted tubule
(d) Loop of Henle

155. The sensory supply of the tube and ovary is from
(a) D6–D8
(b) D8–D10
(c) D10–D12
(d) L2–L4

156. As viewed from the right atrium, the floor of the fossa ovalis is formed by
(a) Septum primum
(b) Septum secundum
(c) Endocardial cushions
(d) Tricuspid valve orifice

157. The rhombencephalon includes all *EXCEPT*
(a) Midbrain
(b) Pons
(c) Medulla oblongata
(d) Cerebellum

158. The thoracic duct crosses the posterior mediastinum at the level of which vertebral body?
(a) T5
(b) T6
(c) T7
(d) T8

159. The principal steroid secreted by testes is
(a) Testosterone
(b) Dihydrotestosterone
(c) Androstenedione
(d) Dehydroepiandrosterone

160. **Resting membrane potential of a neuron is**
(a) -9 mV
(b) -50 mV
(c) -70 mV
(d) -100 mV

161. **Oxyhemoglobin dissociation curve is shifted to left in**
(a) Metabolic acidosis
(b) Hypercapnia
(c) Hypothermia
(d) Increased 2–3 DPG levels

162. **The basis of Korotkoff sound is related to**
(a) Aortic valve closure
(b) Production of heart sound
(c) Arterial turbulence
(d) Arterial valve expansion

163. **The only neuron in retina showing action potentials are**
(a) Rods and cones
(b) Bipolar cells
(c) Amacrine cells
(d) Ganglion cells

164. **Which one of the following hormone decreases Na^+-K^+-ATPase activity**
(a) Thyroid hormone
(b) Aldosterone
(c) Dopamine
(d) Insulin

165. **The cell which forms blood-testis barrier is**
(a) Spermatogonia
(b) Primary spermatocyte
(c) Leydig cell
(d) Sertoli cell

166. **Surfactant is produced by**
(a) Pulmonary alveolar macrophages
(b) Plasma cells
(c) Type I pneumocytes
(d) Type II pneumocytes

167. **The saliva in healthy people contains**
(a) No bacteria
(b) Up to 10^8/mL anaerobic bacteria
(c) Up to 10^8/mL aerobic bacteria
(d) Up to 10^3/mL bacteria

168. **All the following hormones have receptors on the plasma membrane of target tissues *EXCEPT***
(a) Thyrotropin
(b) Glucagon
(c) Estradiol
(d) Epinephrine

169. **Sarcomere is the area between**
(a) Two consecutive I bands
(b) Two adjacent Z lines
(c) A band and I band
(d) Two H zones

170. **The following is an example of a primarily inhibitory amino acid**
(a) Glutamate
(b) Aspartate
(c) Glycine
(d) Somatostatin

171. **Northern blotting is used for analysis of**
(a) DNA
(b) RNA
(c) Proteins
(d) Polysaccharides

172. **The parameter used as an index of lipid peroxidation is the level of**
(a) Ascorbic acid
(b) Hydrogen peroxide
(c) Malondialdehyde
(d) Volatile fatty acids

173. **The completeness of a 24-hour urine collection is best assessed by the simultaneous measurement of urinary**
(a) Volume
(b) Urea
(c) Creatinine
(d) pH

174. **During standard plasma electrophoresis, a protein that moves ahead of albumin is**
(a) Fibrinogen
(b) α-fetoprotein
(c) Hemopexin
(d) Retinol-binding protein

175. **Plasma ceruloplasmin is a**
(a) α-1 globulin
(b) α-2 globulin
(c) β-1 globulin
(d) β-2 globulin

176. **Heme to bilirubin conversion is carried out by**
(a) Heme oxygenase
(b) Heme reductase

(c) Heme isomerase
(d) Heme hydrolase

177. **Glycated hemoglobin reflects blood glucose of preceding**
(a) 0–1 week
(b) 2–3 weeks
(c) 4–5 weeks
(d) 6–8 weeks

178. **Which of the following act through tyrosine kinase receptor?**
(a) Insulin
(b) Glucagon
(c) Growth hormone
(d) Follicle stimulating hormone

179. **The amino acid that produces kinks in the b pleated structure of proteins is**
(a) Glycine
(b) Serine
(c) Proline
(d) Alanine

180. **The enzyme level used for evaluation of myopathies is**
(a) Gamma-glutamyl transferase (GGT)
(b) Creatine kinase (CK)
(c) Lactic dehydrogenase (LDH)
(d) Alanine amino transferase (ALT)

COMED-K 2009

ANSWERS AND EXPLANATIONS

MEDICINE

1. **Answer is d (Marfan syndrome).**
   Ref: Harrison's, 17th edition Pg 1565.

- The four major acute aortic syndromes include aortic rupture, aortic dissection, intramural hematoma and penetrating atherosclerotic ulcer.
- The presentations of aortic dissection and its variants are the consequences of intimal tear, ***dissecting hematoma***, occlusion of involved arteries and compression of adjacent tissues.

Risk factors that predispose to aortic dissection

❖ Systemic hypertension, a coexisting condition in 70% of patients ❖ Cystic medial necrosis ❖ ***Marfan syndrome*** (major cause of morbidity and mortality) ❖ Ehlers-Danlos syndrome ❖ Inflammatory aortitis (i.e. Takayasu's arteritis, giant cell arteritis)	❖ Congenital aortic valve anomalies (e.g. bicuspid valve) ❖ Coarctation of the aorta ❖ A history of aortic trauma ❖ Otherwise normal women during the third trimester of pregnancy

2. **Answer is b (Granulomatous lung disease).**
   Ref: Harrison's, 17th edition Pg 1615.

Repeat Qn

- See ***answer no. 130 in COMED-K 2010 answers*** for detailed explanation.

3. **Answer is a (Tuberculous meningitis).**
   Ref: Current Diagnosis and Treatment in Neurology, 2006 edition Pg 422.

- In ***TB meningitis, adenosine deaminase levels are elevated***, but are not entirely specific for tuberculosis.

CSF Findings in Meningitis

	Bacterial (pyogenic) meningitis	**Tuberculous meningitis**	**Viral meningitis**
Opening pressure (mm H_2O)	200–500	180–300	< 250
Appearance	Often turbid	Opalescent (fibrin web)	Usually clear
Cells	PMNs	Lymphocytes	Lymphocytes
Glucose	Low	Very low	Normal
Protein	High	Normal to high	Normal

4. **Answer is a (Resting tremors).**
Ref: Davidson's, 17th edition Pg 1179, 1196.

- Rest tremor is pathognomonic of Parkinson's disease – pill rolling tremor.

Features of Cerebellar Lesions

a. Lack of coordination on same side of the body
b. ***'Intention tremor':*** Initial part of the treatment is normal, but as the target is approached, the accuracy of the movement deteriorates, producing an 'intention' tremor
c. ***'Past pointing':*** The distances of targets are misjudged (dysmetria) resulting in past pointing
d. ***Dysdiadochokinesis:*** The ability to produce rapid, accurate, regularly alternating movements is impaired
e. ***Ataxia:*** The central vermis of the cerebellum is concerned with gait and posture. Disorders of this part therefore produce ataxic gait
f. ***Nystagmus:*** Cerebellar and brainstem lesions can commonly cause nystagmus

5. **Answer is d (Depressed plasma renin).**
Ref: Harrison's, 17th edition Pg 2260.

- The criteria for the diagnosis of ***primary aldosteronism*** are:

(1) ***Diastolic hypertension*** without edema.
(2) ***Hyposecretion of renin*** (as judged by low plasma renin activity levels) that fails to increase appropriately during volume depletion (upright posture, sodium depletion).
(3) ***Hypersecretion of aldosterone*** that does not suppress appropriately in response to volume expansion.

- Clinically:
  - Hypersecretion of aldosterone increases the renal distal tubular exchange of intratubular sodium for secreted potassium and hydrogen ions, with progressive depletion of body potassium and development of hypokalemia.
  - Most patients have diastolic hypertension, which may be very severe and headaches. The hypertension is probably due to the increased sodium reabsorption and extracellular volume expansion.
  - *Potassium depletion* is responsible for the muscle weakness and fatigue and is due to the effect of potassium depletion on the muscle cell membrane.
  - Metabolic alkalosis and elevation of serum bicarbonate are caused by hydrogen ion loss into the urine and migration into potassium-depleted cells.

6. **Answer is c (FEVl/FVC).**
Ref: Harrison's, 17th edition Pg 1588.

Changes in Pulmonary Function Tests in Obstructive and Restrictive Disease States Compared to Normal Lung

Measurements	Obstructive	Restrictive
TLC	↑	↓
FVC	↑	↓
RV	↑	↓
FRC	↓↓	↓
FEV_1	↓	↓
FEV_1/FVC	↓	Normal or ↑

FEV_1, one-second forced expiratory volume; FRC, functional reserve capacity; FVC, functional vital capacity; RV, residual volume; TLC, total lung capacity; ↑, increase; ↓, decrease; ↓↓, large decrease.

7. **Answer is b (Essential thrombocythemia).**
Ref: Davidson's, 20th edition Pg 1055.

- *Myeloproliferative disorders* are a group of chronic conditions characterized by clonal proliferation of:
  - Marrow erythroid precursors (*polycythemia rubra vera*)
  - Megakaryocytes (*primary thrombocythemia and myelofibrosis*)
  - Myeloid cells (*chronic myeloid leukemia*).

8. **Answer is b (Sumatriptan).**
   Ref: Harrison's, 17th edition Pg 102, Table 15-7.

- Stimulation of 5-HT1B/1D receptors can stop an acute migraine attack.
- Ergotamine and dihydroergotamine are non-selective receptor agonists, while the '***triptans' are selective* 5-HT1B/1D *receptor agonists*.**
- A variety of triptans (e.g. naratriptan, rizatriptan, eletriptan, sumatriptan, zolmitriptan, almotriptan, frovatriptan) are now available for the treatment of acute migraine.
- **Preventive treatments in migraine**
  - Pizotifen
  - Beta blockers – propranolol
  - Tricyclics – amitriptyline, dothiepin, nortriptyline
  - Anticonvulsants – topiramate, valproate, gabapentin
  - Serotonergic drugs – methysergide, flunarizine.

9. **Answer is b (Co-trimoxazole).**
   Ref: Harrison's, 17th edition Pg 1170, Table 182-8.

- First choice drug for ***Pneumocystis jiroveci* pneumonia** is *trimethoprim sulfamethoxazole* (*co-trimoxazole*)
- Alternatives are dapsone, pyrimethamine, aerosolized pentamidine.

10. **Answer is b (Tricuspid incompetence).**
    Ref: Davidson's, 17th edition Pg 521, Box 5, Pg 628.

Jugular Venous Pulse (JVP)

The ***right internal jugular vein is the best vein*** for ***accurate estimation*** of the central venous pressure. The waves in the normal JVP are:

• *a wave*	Atrial contraction
• *c wave*	Bulging of tricuspid valve into right atrium during right ventricular isovolumetric systole
• *v wave*	Increasing volume of blood in the right atrium during ventricular systole as the tricuspid valve is closed
• *x descent*	Atrial relaxation and downward displacement of tricuspid valve during ventricular systole
• *y descent*	Opening of tricuspid valve and rapid inflow of blood into right ventricle

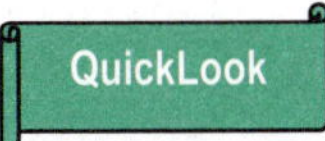

Abnormalities of JVP

❖ **Raised JVP with normal waveform**	Fluid overload, right heart failure
❖ **Raised JVP with absent pulsation**	SVC obstruction (edema of head and neck, collateral veins and absent venous pulsation)
❖ **Large a wave**	Tricuspid stenosis, pulmonary stenosis/hypertension, some cases of left ventricular hypertrophy (Bernheim effect)

❖ Cannon a wave	Complete heart block, junctional rhythm, atrioventricular dissociation with ventricular tachycardia.
❖ Absent a wave	Atrial fibrillation
❖ Systolic giant (*cv*) waves	*Tricuspid regurgitation, look for earlobe movement*
❖ Slowly descent	Tricuspid stenosis
❖ Deep x and y descents	Constrictive pericarditis and pericardial tamponade

11. Answer is b (Diabetic glomerulosclerosis).
Ref: Harrison's, 17th edition Pg 1792.

Repeat Topic

- Within 1–2 years after the onset of clinical ***diabetes***, morphologic changes appear in the kidney.
- This expansion in mesangial matrix can be associated with the development of *mesangial sclerosis*. Some patients also develop eosinophilic, PAS+ nodules called ***nodular glomerulosclerosis*** or ***Kimmelstiel-Wilson nodules***.
- Also ***see answer no. 35 in the same COMED-K 2009 answers*** above.

12. Answer is d (Respiratory acidosis with hypoxemia).
Ref: Davidson's, 20th edition Pg 657, Fig 19.10.

13. Answer is b (Hypothermia).
Ref: Harrison's, 17th edition Pg 135.

- Patients with ***hypothermia*** may be confused or combative; these symptoms abate more rapidly with rewarming than with the use of restraints.
- **A classic example of maladaptive behavior in patients with hypothermia is** *'paradoxical undressing'*, **which involves the inappropriate removal of clothing in response to a cold stress.**

14. Answer is a (*Aspergillus fumigatus*).
Ref: Harrison's, 17th edition Pg 1607.

- ***Bronchopulmonary aspergillosis*** **(BPA)** is uncommon and results from an allergic pulmonary reaction to *inhaled spores of* ***Aspergillus fumigatus*** and, occasionally, other *Aspergillus* species.
- A ***skin prick test to A. fumigatus is always positive***, whereas serum *Aspergillus* precipitins are low or undetectable.
- Characteristically, there are ***fleeting eosinophilic infiltrates in the lungs***, particularly in the ***upper lobes***. As airways become blocked with mucoid plugs rich in eosinophils, patients may cough up brown plugs and have hemoptysis.
- BPA may result in ***bronchiectasis***, particularly affecting central airways, if not suppressed by corticosteroids. Asthma is controlled in the usual way by inhaled corticosteroids, but it is necessary to give a course of oral corticosteroids if there is any sign of worsening or pulmonary shadowing is found.
- Treatment with the oral antifungal itraconazole is beneficial in preventing exacerbations.

15. Answer is c (Pulmonary fibrosis).
Ref: Current Diagnosis and Treatment in Pulmonary Medicine, Pg 110.

- In ***idiopathic pulmonary fibrosis***, physical examination may reveal digital clubbing and the presence of ***bibasilar fine inspiratory crackles*** (so called 'dry' or ***'velcro'*** crackles).

16. Answer is c (Gas embolism).
Ref: Lee's anesthesia, 13th edition Pg 339; Urology secrets, Martin Resnick, Andrew Novick, 3rd edition Pg 123.

- The appearance of a ***'mill wheel murmur'*** is a ***classic sign of gas embolism***.
- Although typical, the mill wheel murmur is not the earliest sign of venous gas embolism.
- An ***exponential rapid decrease in end tidal*** CO_2 within the space of a dozen breaths is the ***earliest sign of gas embolus***, which results from a sudden interruption of pulmonary blood flow by the embolus.

- Auscultation of mill wheel murmur, severe hypotension and a sudden decline in oxygen saturation appear somewhat later and are more ominous findings.
- Although a rare occurrence, *gas embolism remains one of the most dreaded complications associated with* ***laparoscopy***.
- Hence ***for all laparoscopies, capnometric monitoring*** is routinely used.

17. Answer is b (Gilbert's syndrome).
Ref: Pediatric gastrointestinal disease, Vol 1, Alan Walker, Pg 1349.

- A characteristic, but poorly understood finding in ***Gilbert's syndrome is the exaggerated rise in serum bilirubin associated with fasting***.
- Normal individuals can double their serum bilirubin levels, while fasting, **BUT** ***in Gilbert's syndrome a more pronounced increase occurs***.

18. Answer is d (Mixed gonadal dysgenesis).
Ref: Harrison's, 17th edition Pg 2342.

- ***Mixed gonadal dysgenesis*** typically results ***from 45,X/46,XY mosaicism***.
- The phenotype of patients with this condition varies considerably.
- Although some patients have a predominantly female phenotype with somatic features of TS, streak gonads and Müllerian structures, most 45,X/46,XY individuals have a male phenotype and testes and the diagnosis is made incidentally after amniocentesis or during investigation of infertility.
- In practice, ***most children referred for assessment have ambiguous genitalia and variable somatic features***.

19. Answer is c (William's syndrome).
Ref : Cleveland Clinics Internal medicine, Pg 119.

- ***Single gene disorder*** is due to single mutated gene. This may be autosomal dominant (e.g. Huntington's disease), autosomal recessive (e.g. cystic fibrosis, hemochromatosis), X-linked dominant, X-linked recessive, Y linked and mitochondrial inheritance.
- ***Polygenic/complex/multifactorial inheritance*** is seen in heart disease and diabetes.
- ***William's syndrome*** is ***not inherited***; it is caused by ***deletion of a part of chromosome 7***, which can happen randomly.

20. Answer is c (Cardiac septal defects).
Ref: Manual of Clinical Problems in Cardiology with Annotated Key References, 6th edition Pg 330; Harrison's, 17th edition Pg 1458.

- ***Congenital Heart Disease*** is generally the result of aberrant embryonic development of a normal structure or failure of such a structure to progress beyond an early stage of embryonic or fetal development.
- ***Most patients with congenital heart disease have a multifactorial inheritance pattern*** in which a discrete cardiac abnormality (i.e. VSD, ASD or PDA) occurs without abnormalities in other organs.
- Recognized ***chromosomal aberrations and mutations of single genes account for < 10%*** of all cardiac malformations.

21. Answer is b (5q).
Ref: Robbins Pathology, 7th edition Pg 695.

- Chromosomal abnormalities in myelodysplastic syndrome include ***monosomy 5 and monosomy 7, deletions of 5q and 7q, trisomy 8 and deletions of 20q***.

22. Answer is a (Kawasaki disease).
Ref: Harrison's, 17th edition Pg 2130.

- ***Kawasaki disease*** (mucocutaneous lymph node syndrome).
- Features are:
  - Acute, febrile, multisystem disease of children (80% of cases < 5 years of age, with the peak incidence at ≤ 2 years).
  - Non-suppurative cervical adenitis.
  - Changes in the skin and mucous membranes such as edema; congested conjunctiva; erythema of the oral cavity, lips and palms; and desquamation of the skin of the fingertips.

- Although the disease is generally benign and self-limited, it is associated with ***coronary artery aneurysms in ~25% of cases***, with an overall case-fatality rate of 0.5–2.8%.
- These complications usually occur ***between the 3rd and 4th week of illness*** during the convalescent stage. Vasculitis of the coronary arteries is seen in almost all the fatal cases that have been autopsied.

23. Answer is a (Tremors).
Ref: Harrison's, 17th edition Pg 2559.

- ***Progressive supranuclear palsy*** (PSP) is characterized by:
  - Akinetic rigid parkinsonism
  - Dizziness, unsteadiness, slowness and falls
  - Pseudobulbar dysarthria (incoherent verbal speech).
- ***Tremor is distinctly uncommon.***
- ***Supranuclear eye movement abnormalities*** affecting downgaze occur first, followed by variable limitations of upward and horizontal eye movement.
- Because the vestibular ocular reflex ('doll's eyes' maneuver) and the Bell's reflex (elevation and abduction of eyes on attempted lid closure) are intact, these abnormalities are termed supranuclear.

SURGERY

24. Answer is d (Ureterocele).
Ref: Bailey and Love, 25th edition Pg 1290.

- ***Ureterocele*** is a cystic enlargement of the intramural ureter, which is thought to result from congenital atresia of the ureteric orifice. Although present from childhood, the condition is not recognized until adult life.
- The ***'adder head'/'cobra head'*** on ***excretory urography*** is typical.
- Treatment should be avoided unless there are symptoms resulting from infection.

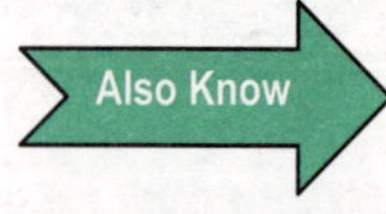

- ☐ ***Flower-vase*** appearance on IVU: ***Horseshoe*** kidney
- ☐ ***Spider-leg*** appearance on IVU: ***Polycystic*** kidney.

25. Answer is a (Achalasia cardia).
Ref: Bailey and Love, 25th edition Pg 1037.

- ***Heller's cardiomyotomy*** is done for the treatment of ***achalasia cardia***.

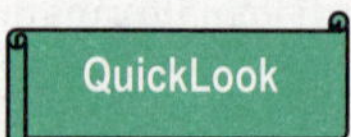

Few named surgeries

Surgery/Surgeon name	Performed for
Ramstedt's pyloromyotomy	Infantile pyloric stenosis
Thiersch's, Delorome's, Altemier's	Full thickness prolapse of the rectum
Lord's and Jaboulay's	Hydrocele
Whipple's	Pancreaticoduodenectomy for Ca head of pancreas
Billroth I and II	Gastrectomy for peptic ulcers
Kasai procedure	Extrahepatic biliary atresia, type II and III
Notaras	Lateral anal sphincterotomy for anal fissure

26. Answer is c (Elevated ESR).
Ref: Harrison's, 17th edition Pg 572, Table 90-4.

Incidence of signs and symptoms in patients with renal cell cancer

- Increased ESR = 55%
- Pyrexia and hypertension = 20%
- Erythrocytosis/polycythemia = 3%.

Note:

- The *classic triad* of hematuria, flank pain and flank mass is present ONLY IN *10–20% of patients*.

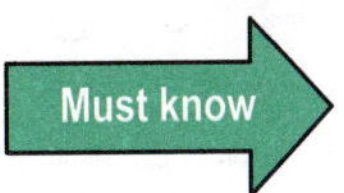

Renal Cell Carcinoma (RCC) – (syn: *Hypernephroma, Grawitz Tumor*)

• *Risk factors* ➢ Cigarette smoking ➢ Acquired cystic disease of the kidney a/w end stage renal disease ➢ Tuberous sclerosis ➢ Polycystic kidney disease ➢ von-Hippel-Lindau disease	• *M:F = 2:1* • *Originates from proximal tubule cells* • *MC adenocarcinoma* • *MC* occurs at the *upper pole of kidney*

- 5 variants are clear cell tumors (75%); chromophilic tumors; chromophobic tumors; oncocytic tumors and collecting duct or Bellini duct tumors.

Clinical features	Paraneoplastic syndromes
• *Hematuria* • Flank *pain* • Flank *mass* • *Fever* • Weight loss • *Anemia* • *Varicocele-left* sided *(as left renal vein is more often compressed)*	• Erythrocytosis • Hypercalcemia • *Stauffer's syndrome*: Non-metastatic reversible hepatic dysfunction • Acquired dysfibrinogenemia • Nephrotic syndrome

- Spread: It is *prone to grow into the renal vein*; may also be seen in the *lungs* as *cannonball metastases*.
- *CT scanning* is the *most valuable* imaging test for renal cell carcinoma. It confirms the character of the mass and further stages the lesion with respect to regional lymph nodes, renal vein or hepatic involvement. It also gives valuable information on the contralateral kidney (function, bilaterality of neoplasm).
- *MRI and duplex Doppler ultrasonography* are excellent methods of assessing for the presence and *extent of tumor thrombus within the renal vein* or vena cava in selected patients.

- **Robson system** is used for staging renal cell carcinoma:
  - *Stage I*: Tumors are confined to the kidney
  - *Stage II*: Tumors extend through the renal capsule, but are confined by Gerota's fascia
  - *Stage III:* Tumors involve the renal vein or vena cava (stage IIIA) or the hilar lymph nodes (stage IIIB)
  - *Stage IV*: Tumors that are locally invasive to adjacent organs (excluding the adrenal gland) or distant metastases

- The standard management for *stage I and stage II tumors* and selected cases of stage III disease is *radical nephrectomy*.
- RCC responds *poorly to chemotherapy and radiotherapy; Vinblastine* is the single most effective agent, with short-term partial response rates of 15%. Alpha *interferon* and *interleukin-2* have shown promising results.
- RCC is one of the several tumors in which *spontaneous regressions have been reported anecdotally*.

Note:

- ***Bellini duct carcinomas*** are *very rare;* believed to arise from collecting ducts in renal medulla; affect *younger patients* and have a *very aggressive* clinical course.

27. Answer is d (6 months).
Ref: Harrison's, 17th edition Pg 600; Bailey and Love, 25th edition Pg 1350.

- Medical therapies for BPH include

1. ***Finasteride and other 5 alpha-reductase inhibitors***
   - Act by ***blocking the conversion of testosterone to dihydrotestosterone***
   - Impacts upon the epithelial component of the prostate, resulting in ***reduction in size of the gland*** and improvement in symptoms
   - ***6 months of therapy*** is required ***for maximum effects on prostate size*** (20% reduction) and symptomatic improvement.
   - ***Increases urine flow rates***
   - ***Lower baseline PSA levels by 50%*** (an important consideration when using PSA to guide biopsy recommendations).

2. **α-Adrenergic blockers such as terazosin, tamsulosin**
   - Act by relaxing the smooth muscle of the bladder neck and increasing peak urinary flow rates
   - No data show that these agents influence the progression of the disease
   - ***Tamsulosin*** causes ***intraoperative floppy iris syndrome,*** which causes difficulty during cataract surgery.

28. Answer is b (Type II).
Ref: Pediatric body CT, Marilyn G Siegel. Pg 209; Palanivelu's textbook of surgical laparoscopy.

- ***Choledochal cyst*** **is *a congenital dilatation of the extrahepatic or intrahepatic biliary tree.***

❖ Type I (80–90%)	Cystic dilatation (type IA), focal segmental dilatation (type IB) and fusiform dilatation (type IC)
❖ Type II	***Saccular diverticulum*** of the ***extrahepatic*** bile duct
❖ Type III	Choledochocele (cystic dilatation of the intraduodenal portion of the common bile duct)
❖ Type IV	Dilatation of intrahepatic and extrahepatic bile ducts (IVA) and multiple cystic dilatations (IVB)
❖ Type V	Caroli's disease (cystic dilatation) of the intrahepatic bile ducts

29. Answer is d (CA 19-9).
Ref: Harrison's, 17th edition Pg 587.

- The ***most widely used serum marker in pancreatic cancer is cancer-associated antigen 19-9 (CA 19-9).***

More About CA 19-9

- CA 19-9 has a reported ***sensitivity and specificity of about 80–90%*** and is suggestive, rather than confirmatory, of the diagnosis of pancreatic cancer.
- CA 19-9 can be elevated in patients ***with jaundice without pancreatic cancer.***
- ***Very high levels of CA 19-9*** are sometimes found in patients with ***inoperable disease.***
- In advanced disease, patients treated with chemotherapy who had high pretreatment levels of CA 19-9 have also been found to have a worse survival, whereas those patients whose levels of marker fell with treatment had a better outcome.
- In cancers with elevated ***CA 19-9, serial evaluation of this marker is useful for monitoring responses to treatment.***
- *In patients with completely resected tumors,* ***follow-up with CA 19-9 is useful for detecting recurrence.***

30. Answer is a (Stomach).
Ref: Bailey and Love, 25th edition Pg 1016.

Mallory-Weiss syndrome:

- ***Mucosal tear*** usually caused by vomiting, retching or vigorous coughing.
- The tear usually is ***a vertical split in the gastric mucosa***, immediately below the squamocolumnar junction ***at the cardia in 90% of cases*** (on ***lesser curvature***).
- ***In only 10% is the tear in the esophagus.***
- Patients present with upper gastrointestinal bleeding, which may be severe.
- In most patients, ***bleeding ceases spontaneously***; continued bleeding may respond to vasopressin therapy or angiographic embolization. Surgery is rarely needed.

31. **Answer is b (Somatostatinomas).**
    Ref: Harrison's, 7th edition Pg 2355.

- The ***somatostatinoma syndrome*** is due to a neuroectodermal tumor that secretes excessive amounts of somatostatin and is characterized by:
  - ***Diabetes mellitus***
  - ***Gallstones*** (cholelithiasis)
  - ***Diarrhea***
  - ***Steatorrhea***
- ***The above symptoms*** are ***improved by octreotide treatment.***

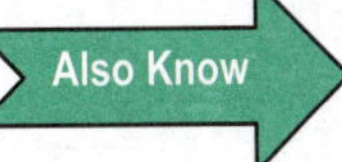

- ***Pancreatic Somatostatinomas*** are ***frequently (70–92%) metastatic at presentation.***
- ***Small-intestinal somatostatinomas:*** The presence of psammoma bodies in a duodenal tumor should particularly raise suspicion; 30–70% have metastases.
- ***Surgery is the treatment of choice*** for those without widespread hepatic metastases.

32. **Answer is c (Prostatic intraepithelial neoplasm).**
    Ref: Harrison's, 17th edition Pg 594; Diagnostic ultrasound, Vol 1, John PM, 2nd edition Pg 901, Table 3.

- ***Prostate-specific antigen (PSA)*** and acid phosphatase are *produced in the epithelial cells.*
- PSA is a kallikrein-like serine protease that causes liquefaction of seminal coagulum.
- It is *produced by both non-malignant and malignant epithelial cells.*
- PSA is prostate-specific, **NOT** prostate cancer–specific.

Serum PSA increases may occur from:
– Prostatitis
– BPH
– Prostatic infarct
– Prostate cancer
– Performance of a prostate biopsy (can increase PSA levels up to ten fold for 8–10 weeks); cystoscopy, TURP
– Sexual activity

- The ***serum PSA level is NOT affected by*** digital rectal examination and ***is NOT elevated in prostatic intraepithelial neoplasia.***

33. **Answer is b (Retrograde ejaculation).**
    Ref: Bailey and Love, 25th edition Pg 1352.

- ***Impotence*** in men with good sexual function before TURP is uncommon (after TURP).
- ***Retrograde ejaculation occurs commonly after TURP (> 50%)*** because of disruption to the bladder mechanism.

34. Answer is c (Hypochloremic alkalosis).
Ref: Bailey and Love, 25th edition Pg 232-33, summary Box 17.4.

Complications of parenteral nutrition

- *Related to nutrient deficiency*
  - ***Hypoglycemia***, *hypocalcemia, hypophosphatemia, hypomagnesemia* (refeeding syndrome)
  - Chronic deficiency syndromes (essential fatty acids, zinc, mineral and trace elements).
- *Related to overfeeding*
  - Excess glucose: ***Hyperglycemia***, hyperosmolar dehydration, hepatic steatosis, hypercapnia, increased sympathetic activity, fluid retention, electrolyte abnormalities
  - Excess fat: Hypercholesterolemia and formation of lipoprotein X, hypertriglyceridemia, hypersensitivity reactions
  - Excess amino acids: ***Hyperchloremic metabolic acidosis***, hypercalcemia, aminoacidemia, uremia.
- *Related to sepsis*
  - Catheter related sepsis
  - Possible increased predisposition to systemic sepsis.
- *Related to line*
  - On insertion: Pneumothorax, damage to adjacent artery, air embolism, thoracic duct damage, cardiac perforation or tamponade, pleural effusion, hydromediastinum
  - Long-term use: Occlusion, venous thrombosis.

Note:

❖ *Hypochloremic hypokalemic metabolic alkalosis* is typically seen in vomiting following *pyloric stenosis*.

35. Answer is b (Squamous cell carcinoma).
Ref: Surgery: Pre-Test Self Assessment and Review, Lillian S Kao, Pg 91.

- ***Marjolins ulcer*** refers to a ***squamous cell carcinoma*** that develops in a chronic wound such as a:
  - ➢ ***Previous burn scar***
  - ➢ ***Venous ulcer***
  - ➢ ***Sinus tract secondary to osteomyelitis.***
- Although others like basal cell carcinoma, melanoma and other malignancies can occur, ***squamous cell carcinoma is most common.***

36. Answer is b (Necrotizing enterocolitis).
Ref: Bailey and Love, 25th edition Pg 88.

- ***Necrotizing enterocolitis*** is an *acquired inflammatory condition of neonatal gut*, mostly *premature infants*; it is NOT congenital.

Simple Summary

Pathogenesis	Signs	Treatment
– Immaturity – Formula feeds – Bacterial infection – Impaired gut blood flow	– Abdominal distension – Bloody stools – Bilious aspirates with signs of systemic sepsis – Patchy or extensive ***pneumatosis intestinalis*** *progresses to necrosis and perforation of gut* – Variable length of small and large bowel may be involved, colon may also be involved	– Milder cases responds to antibiotics, gut rest and parenteral nutrition – Severe cases need urgent intestinal resection of infarcted bowel

37. Answer is c (Ulcerative colitis).
Ref: Robbins pathology, 7th edition Pg 849-50.

Crohn's Disease and Ulcerative Colitis Compared

	Crohn's disease (CD)	Ulcerative colitis (UC)
• Site of involvement	***Entire GI tract*** may be involved (mouth to anus) with ***'skip' areas*** ***Distal ileum*** MC involved All layers of bowel wall involved (***transmural***); ***Granulomas; creeping fat***	***Continuous*** disease beginning at rectum and extending possibly as far as distal ileum ***Only mucosa and submucosa affected*** (mucosal) ***Crypt abscesses***
• Symptoms	***Watery*** diarrhea Abdominal pain, weight loss	***Bloody*** diarrhea Abdominal pain, urgency, tenesmus, weight loss, nausea, vomiting
• Clinically	Palpable right lower quadrant Abdominal mass Perianal fissures and fistula ***Oral ulcers*** Fever	Fever, abdominal tenderness, Orthostatic hypotension, tachycardia, ***gross rectal bleeding***
• Laboratories	***ASCA frequently positive,*** pANCA rarely positive Hemoccult positive stool Biopsy diagnostic	ASCA rarely positive, ***pANCA frequently positive*** Biopsy diagnostic
• Radiology	Skip lesions, Colonic ulcers ***Cobblestoning*** mucosa Strictures ***'String sign of Kantor'*** on Ba swallow	Continuous involvement Fine mucosal ulcers (double contour) Pseudopolyps, friable mucosa ***'Lead pipe' colon*** without haustra and colon shortening
• Complications	Abscess formation ***Fistula*** and fissure common Malabsorption (since ileal disease)	Increased risk of ***colon cancer*** Hemorrhage Bowel obstruction Toxic megacolon
• Treatment	Mesalamine, broad spectrum antibiotics, corticosteroids, immunosuppressives, surgical resection of severely affected areas, flares and remissions, recurrence after colectomy	Mesalamine, supplemental iron, corticosteroids, immunosuppressives, total colectomy is curative

To remember features of Crohn's disease you could imagine:

- *"**2 obsessed** (abscesses) **fish** (fissures and fistulas) **skipping** (skip lesions) on a **cobblestoned** (cobblestones) path **fully penetrated** (transmural) **fat** (creeping fat) **grandma's** (granuloma) house wall. She caught them with a **string** (strictures, String sign) and ate them and got **ulcers at both ends** (mouth and perianal) and screamed **'AMMA'!** (Abdominal Mass and MAlabsorption)".*

OBSTETRICS AND GYNECOLOGY

38. Answer is b (Sodium chloride).
Ref: Shaw's gynecology, 14th edition Pg 194.

Fern test

- A specimen of ***cervical mucus*** obtained by platinum loop or pipette is spread on a clean glass slide and allowed to dry.
- When viewed under the low power of microscope, it shows ***during the estrogenic phase***, a characteristic pattern of ***fern formation***.
- This fern disappears after ovulation and if previously present, its disappearance is presumptive evidence of corpus luteum activity.
- The ferning is ***due to the presence of sodium chloride secreted in the mucus under estrogenic effect***.

39. Answer is d (Production of progesterone).
Ref: Shaw's gynecology, 14th edition Pg 29-30.

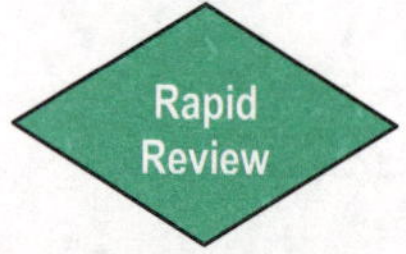

MENSTRUAL PHYSIOLOGY

ProliFerative (Follicular) phase (Days 1–14; Follicular phase can vary in length)

Begins on 1st day of menstrual cycle
↓
FSH stimulates growth of Graafian (ovarian) follicle
↓
Granulosa cells of the ovarian follicle secrete estradiol
↓
Estradiol induces endometrial proliferation and further increases FSH and LH secretion due to positive feedback effect of the pituitary

Ovulation (Day 15)

Ovulation occurs 14 days before menses, regardless of cycle length (i.e. ovulation day = menstruation day–14)
↓
Estrogen surge occurs day before ovulation, which stimulates LH and inhibits FSH
↓
A sudden rise in LH (i.e. LH surge) induces ovulation
↓
Cervical mucus increases in quantity and becomes less viscous and highly elastic (*spinnbarkeit*) and more penetrable by sperm; 'ferning' occurs due to estrogen action

- Mittelschmerz – blood from ruptured follicle causes peritoneal irritation that can mimic appendicitis.
- OCPs prevent estrogen surge, LH surge → ovulation does not occur.

Secretory (luteal) phase (Days 15–28, Luteal phase is usually a constant 14 days)

The residual follicle (i.e. corpus luteum) begins to develop and synthesizes estrogen and progesterone
↓
Progesterone stimulates endometrial glandular secretion and vascular development in anticipation of fertilized egg
↓
Basal body temperature increases due to effect of progesterone
↓
If the ovum is not fertilized, the corpus luteum regresses, progesterone and estradiol levels decrease and endometrium is sloughed off (i.e. menses)

40. Answer is c (Clear cell adenocarcinoma of vagina).
Ref: Shaw's gynecology, 14th edition Pg 45.

- ***Adenocarcinoma (clear cell carcinoma)*** was seen in the vagina in children whose mothers took ***diethylstilbestrol*** for threatened abortion.
- It is ***not seen nowadays*** as this is replaced by safer progesterone treatment.

41. Answer is b (12 weeks).
Ref: Park, 20th edition Pg 435.

- ***MTP*** can be performed by one registered medical practitioner if duration of pregnancy is less than ***12 weeks*** and if between 12 and ***20 weeks***, opinion of two registered medical practitioners is necessary.

42. Answer is d [Gonadotropin releasing hormone (GnRH) agonists].
Ref: Shaw's gynecology, 14th edition Pg 214.

- Daily administration of ***gonadotropin releasing hormone agonists (buserelin) prevents ovulation***
- The drug is on trial for its contraceptive effect.

43. Answer is a (Mental retardation).
Ref: Harrison's, 17th edition Pg 2726.

- ***Heavy drinking during pregnancy*** results in the rapid placental transfer of both ethanol and acetaldehyde, which may have serious consequences for fetal development.
- It is advisable for pregnant women to abstain from alcohol completely.

Fetal alcohol syndrome

- Facial changes with epicanthal eye folds
- Poorly formed ear concha
- Small teeth with faulty enamel
- Cardiac atrial or ventricular septal defects
- Aberrant palmar crease and limitation in joint movement
- Microcephaly with mental retardation.

44. Answer is a (Three).
Ref: Park, 20th edition Pg 450.

- ***Ideally*** the mother should attend the antenatal clinic once a month during the first 7 months, twice a month during the next month; and thereafter once a week, if everything is normal.
- A high proportion of mothers in India are from the lower socioeconomic group and many of them are working women. Attendance at the antenatal clinic may mean loss of daily wages. Consequently it is difficult for them to visit the antenatal clinic so often.
- In these cases, ***a minimum of 3 visits covering the entire period of pregnancy should be the target as shown below***:
  - ☐ 1st visit at 20 weeks or as soon as the pregnancy is known
  - ☐ 2nd visit at 32 weeks
  - ☐ 3rd visit at 36 weeks.

45. Answer is b (Deaths/1,000 live births).
Ref: Park, 20th edition Pg 484.

- The WHO expert committee on the Prevention of perinatal Mortality and Morbidity (1970) recommended a more precise formulation for ***perinatal mortality*** – "late fetal (28 weeks gestation and more) and early neonatal (1st week) ***deaths*** weighing over 1,000 g at birth expressed as ***ratio per 1,000 live births*** weighing over 1,000 g at birth".
- Perinatal mortality rate in India for the year 2006 is about 37 per 1,000 total births.

46. Answer is b (11 and 13).
Ref: Dutta's obstetrics, Pg 57.

- In ***pregnancy fibrinogen level is raised***
- There is an ***increase in activities of clotting factors 10, 9, 8, 7 and 2***
- Levels of ***factor 11 and 13 are slightly decreased.***

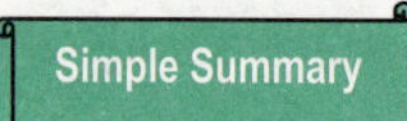

Simple Summary

Physiological Response of Mother to Pregnancy

❖ **Cardiovascular changes**	↑ cardiac output, heart rate and stroke volume ↑ blood flow to many tissues and organs Compression of vena cava in supine position decreased venous return, cardiac output and BP (supine hypotensive syndrome)
❖ **Hematological**	↑ blood volume, red cell mass and plasma volume ↑ blood fibrinogen, ESR (about 4 times) ↑ plasma (Hb), (iron) ↓ plasma (transferrin) and total iron-binding capacity ↓ fibrinolytic activity ↓ whole body hematocrit Levels of all coagulation factors except XI and XIII are increased Clotting time and bleeding time unaffected Neutrophil leukocytosis occurs
❖ **Respiratory changes**	↑ tidal volume by 40% ↑ oxygen consumption by 20–30% ↑ basal metabolic rate by 25–30% ↓ residual volume ↓ lung volumes
❖ **Renal**	↑ renal blood flow by 25% ↑ GFR by 50% ↑ clearance of urea, uric acid and creatinine (glucose and amino acids may be lost in the urine)
❖ **Plasma proteins**	↓ plasma protein concentration ↑ β-globulin ↓ albumin (g/100 mL) ↓ albumin: Globulin ratio (normal 1.7:1 is diminished to 1:1)
❖ **Endocrine**	↑ placental hormone production ↑ plasma thyroxine and TBG
❖ **Nutrition**	↑ total serum lipids, triglycerides, cholesterol, phospholipids ↑ 15% calorie requirement ↑ 50% protein requirement ↑ requirement for folate, calcium, phosphorus, Mg^{2+}, iron, vitamins A and C, zinc and iodine

Note:

❖ In pregnancy absolute plasma protein content is increased, but plasma protein concentration decreases due to dilutional effect.

47. Answer is c (Congenital varicella syndrome).
Ref: Dutta's obstetrics, 6th edition Pg 497, 333; Robbins pathology, 7th edition Pg 484-87.

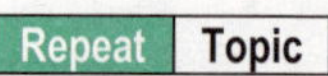

Repeat Topic

- See *answer no. 63 in COMED-K 2010 answers* for detailed explanation.

48. Answer is d (Breast binder and analgesics).
Ref: The 5-minute Obstetrics and Gynecology Consult, Puala J Adams, Pg 348, 2008 edition Dutta's obstetrics, 6th edition Pg 150.

- ***Lactation suppression becomes necessary***
  - If the baby is born dead
  - If the baby dies in the neonatal period
  - If the mother does not like to feed the baby
  - If breastfeeding is contraindicated.
- Management:
  - Mechanical: ***Firm brassiere of binder; Cold compress and analgesics*** for effective to stop lactation when it has already begun; ***breast compression bandage*** and analgesics are necessary. The normal decline in prolactin postpartum in non-lactators occurs in 10–14 days.
  - ***Bromocriptine***: Dopamine agonist and ***inhibits prolactin secretion***; associated with early return of ovulation and hence contraception necessary; ***although bromocriptine has a hypotensive effect, severe hypertension with subsequent stroke has been reported in the postpartum period, hence not FDA approved.***
  - ***Hormone treatment is ineffective***: Ethinyl estradiol or combination of testosterone and ethinyl estradiol; risk of thromboembolic manifestation and late postpartum blood loss present.
  - ***Decreasing fluids is ineffective.***

49. Answer is b (Liver).
Ref: Rudloph's pediatrics, 21st edition Pg 1519.

Hematopoiesis in Fetus

The anatomic sites of hematopoiesis undergo developmental changes during embryonic and fetal life

↓

RBC formation can be observed within the developing blood vessels of the ***yolk sac at 2 weeks*** of gestation

↓

By 8 weeks of gestation the site of RBC formation begins to ***shift to the sinusoids of the liver***, where granulocyte precursors and megakaryocytes are also seen; ***Hematopoiesis in the liver is maximal at 5 months*** and declines thereafter

↓

Hematopoiesis in the ***bone marrow*** is evident by the 5th month of gestation and this becomes the ***predominant site of hematopoiesis during the rest of gestation and later***

PEDIATRICS

50. Answer is d (Combined hyperlipidemia).
Ref: Nutrition in Pediatrics, Basic Science, Clinical Applications, Christopher Duggan, Pg 677.

- ***Familial combined hyperlipidemia*** is the ***most common type of inherited hyperlipidemia***
- It is ***autosomal dominant*** and is found in ***1 in 100*** individuals.

51. Answer is c (Syphilis).
Ref: Harrison's, 17th edition Pg 1042.

- Early manifestations, which appear within the first 2 years of life (often at 2–10 weeks of age), are infectious and resemble the manifestations of severe secondary syphilis in the adult.

Early manifestations of congenital syphilis		
– **Rhinitis or 'snuffles'** (*earliest sign* **appearing 2–6 weeks after birth)** – **Skin changes**	– Bone changes: osteochondritis, osteitis and *periostitis* – Hepatosplenomegaly	– CNS invasion by *T. pallidum* is detectable in 22% of infected neonates – Neonatal death is usually

– **Bullae (syphilitic pemphigus), vesicles,** *superficial desquamation,* **petechiae and (later)** *papulosquamous lesions,* **mucous patches and** *condylomata lata*	– Lymphadenopathy – Anemia – Jaundice – ***Thrombocytopenia*** – Leukocytosis	due to pulmonary hemorrhage, secondary bacterial infection or severe hepatitis

❖ **Late manifestations**, which appear after 2 years and are non-infectious and is largely subclinical—characterized by
- *Interstitial keratitis*
- Bilateral knee effusions (***Clutton's joints***)
- Periostitis
- Eighth nerve deafness
- Recurrent arthropathy
- Destruction of hard palate and bony nasal septum.

❖ **Residual stigmata**: *Classic stigmata include*
- *Hutchinson's teeth* (centrally notched, widely spaced, peg-shaped upper central incisors)
- *'Mulberry' molars* (sixth-year molars with multiple, poorly developed cusps)
- *Saddle nose* and
- *Saber shins (Saber tibia).*

52. Answer is b (75 mL/ kg body wt).
Ref: Park, 20th edition Pg 197.

- When obvious signs of dehydration exist the water deficit is somewhere between 50 and 100 mL/kg body wt.
- If the child's weight is known, the amount of ORS solution required for rehydrating during the first 4 hours may be calculated by setting the deficit at ***approximately 75 mL/kg.***

53. Answer is c (Increasing prothrombin time).
Ref: Diseases of the Liver, Sheila Sherlock, Pg 357.

Poor prognostic factors for children with fulminant hepatic failure requiring listing for liver transplantation are:
- Non-A-G hepatitis (seronegative hepatitis)
- Rapid onset of coma with progression to grade II or IV hepatic coma
- Diminishing liver size
- ***Persistent coagulopathy*** (***prothrombin time*** > 50s/control; INR > 4) MOST IMPORTANT
- ***Falling transaminases***
- ***Increasing bilirubin*** (> 300 mmol/L).

Note:
❖ The height of serum bilirubin and transaminases are POOR indicators of prognosis.

54. Answer is c (Zinc).
Ref: OP Ghai, 7th edition Pg 92.

- ***Zinc deficiency***: The typical syndrome of zinc deficiency in humans consists of ***growth retardation, hypogonadism*** and ***anemia***. Other major symptoms include diarrhea, hair loss, anorexia, dermatitis, impaired immune function, impaired taste perception and skeletal abnormalities.
- ***Acrodermatitis enteropathica*** is an autosomal recessive syndrome caused by impaired intestinal absorption of zinc.
- ***Copper deficiency***: Anemia, growth retardation, defective keratinization and pigmentation of hair, hypothermia, degenerative changes in aortic elastin, osteopenia, mental deterioration.
- ***Calcium deficiency*** may cause *tetany* characterized by muscle cramps, numbness and tingling in limbs. Rickets and osteoporosis may occur with chronic deficiency.
- ***Magnesium deficiency*** results in tetany, irritability and hypo- or hyper-reflexia.

55. Answer is d (Microcephaly).
Ref: OP Ghai, 7th edition Pg 481, 483.

Clinical features of hypothyroidism

Congenital	Acquired
➢ Open posterior fontanelle (large head)	➢ Growth retardation
➢ Umbilical hernia	➢ Delayed skeletal maturation
➢ Edematous characteristic facies	➢ Delayed dental development
➢ Constipation	➢ Delayed puberty
➢ Pallor	➢ Myopathy
➢ Hypothermia	➢ Enlarged sella
➢ Large tongue	➢ Pseudotumor cerebri
➢ Rough dry skin	
➢ Hypotonia	
➢ Large abdomen	

56. Answer is a (Nocturnal enuresis).
Ref: Continence and Incontinence, Paul S smith, Linda J Smith, 1987 edition Pg 140.

- ***Early, strict or inconsistent training*** have been proposed as factors in ***nocturnal enuresis***.

57. Answer is b (40/min).
Ref: Park, 20th edition Pg 155, Table 4.

Classification of pneumonia in child aged 2 months to 5 years

Severe pneumonia	Pneumonia	No pneumonia: cough or cold
Chest in drawing (if also recurrent wheezing go directly to treat wheezing)	No chest in drawing and *fast breathing* (50/min or more if child 2 months up to 12 months; 40/min or more if child 12 months up to 5 years)	*No chest in drawing and no fast breathing* (less than 50/min if child 2 months up to 12 months; less than 40/min if child 12 months up to 5 years)

58. Answer is b (Acute lymphocytic leukemia).
Ref: OP Ghai, 7th edition Pg 581.

- ***Infants and young children with acute lymphoblastic leukemia (ALL) may present with a limp or refusal to walk.***
- The clinical features of ALL are those of bone marrow infiltration with leukemic cells (bone marrow failure) and the extent of extramedullary disease spread.
- Common features include manifestations of ***anemia, neutropenia and thrombocytopenia***.
- Children with aplastic anemia may also have pancytopenia, however limb pain may ***not*** be a presenting feature.
- Rheumatic fever and rheumatoid arthritis do not present with pancytopenia.

ORTHOPEDICS

59. Answer is b (12–13 years).
Ref: The juvenile skeleton, Louise Scheuer, Pg 481.

- ***Pisiform ossification*** center is first seen by 8–10 years
- Pisiform ossification ***complete by 12 years***.

60. Answer is a (Ewing's sarcoma).
Ref: Essentials of Orthopedics, RM Shenoy, Pg 190.

- ***Ewings sarcoma:*** Affects boys < 15 years; affects diaphysis of long bones, flat bones; pain and swelling of few weeks to months present.

- X-ray—***onion skin appearance***; extremely aggressive with early metastases, but ***responds to chemotherapy—curable tumor*** especially in children < 11 years; anaplastic small blue malignant tumor; chromosome ***11:22 translocation.***

61. Answer is d (Caries teeth).
Ref: OP Ghai, 7th edition Pg 81.

Signs of rickets

- Relative or absolute deficiency of vitamin D; presents by 3–6 months, almost always < 2 years; increased uncalcified osteoid in the immature skeleton.
- Changes at the growth plate
  a. Widened growth plate.
  b. *Fraying, splaying* and *cupping of metaphysis* (distal ends of radius and ulna) = *earliest change.*
  c. *Epiphyseal separation* is MC in *renal rickets.*
  d. *Rachitic rosary* = cupping of anterior ends of ribs and, on palpation, abnormally large costochondral junctions.
  e. Looser's zones *uncommon* in children.
  f. On treatment, *Müller's lines* in the widened space at the site of zone of preparatory calcification are the first sign of healing.
- Changes due to bone softening (deformities)
  a. Bowing of long bones.
  b. Triradiate pelvis.
  c. *Harrison's sulcus* = indrawing of the lower part of the chest wall because of soft ribs.
  d. Scoliosis, biconcave vertebral bodies, basilar invagination.
  e. *Craniotabes* = flattening of the occiput and accumulating osteoid in the frontal and parietal regions.
  f. ***Hot cross bun sign:*** *Frontoparietal bossing and prominent fontanelle.*
  g. ***Saddle nose, Olympic front*** may also be seen.
- General changes
  a. ↓ bone density = uncommon.
  b. Retarded bone maturation and growth.
  c. Delayed teeth eruption.

62. Answer is d (Chondromyxoid fibroma).
Ref: http://emedicine.medscape.com/article/386808-overview; Ref: Orthopedic rehabilitation science: principles for clinical management of bone, Katie Lindson, Pg 136, Table 10-2.

Diseases or conditions associated with or leading to avascular necrosis

• Trauma—fracture of the femoral neck – Slipped capital femoral epiphysis (obesity is risk factor) – Proximal femoral epiphysiolysis – Dislocation of the femoral head – Epiphyseal compression – Vascular trauma – Burns – Radiation exposure • Hemoglobinopathies – Sickle cell disease – Hemoglobin S or hemoglobin C hemoglobinopathy – Polycythemia • Local infiltrative disease – Gaucher's disease – Infection – Neoplasms	• Alcoholism, cigarette smoking • Pregnancy • Hypercholesterolemia • Pancreatitis • Chronic renal failure • Collagen vascular diseases (SLE) • Gout and hyperuricemia • Hemodialysis • Hypercoagulable states, DIC, thrombophlebitis • Hyperparathyroidism • Organ transplantation • Caisson disease—Dysbaric osteonecrosis • Fabry's disease • Giant cell arteritis • Idiopathic

• Hypercortisolism – Corticosteroid medications – Cushing disease • Congenital and developmental – Congenital dislocation of the hip – Ehlers-Danlos syndrome – Hereditary dysostosis – Legg-Calvé-Perthes' disease	

63. **Answer is c (Psoriatic arthritis).**
Ref: Current Diagnosis and Treatment in Rheumatology, Pg 413; Davidson's, 20th edition Pg 1109-10.

Psoriatic arthritis

- NO juxta-articular osteoporosis, i.e. preserved bone density (unlike RA)
- Periosteal new bone particularly in the hands and feet
- Asymmetrical destruction of distal interphalangeal *(DIP)* joint with ankylosis
- Resorption of terminal tufts with ***'pencil in cup'*** deformity; ***Ivory phalanx***
- ***'Opera glass hand'*** (***main en lorgnette—telescoping*** *of one bone into its neighbor*)
- Destruction of first toe interphalangeal joint with periosteal reaction and bony proliferation at distal phalangeal base (pathognomonic)
- Asymmetrical syndesmophytes (lower cervical to upper lumbar spine)
- Squaring of vertebrae in lumbar spine; paravertebral soft tissue calcifications
- Bilateral asymmetric sacroiliitis; a/w HLA B-27 antigen, negative rheumatoid factor.

64. **Answer is a (Fracture of neck of talus).**
Ref: Essentials of Orthopedics, RM shenoy, Pg 60.

- Anderson in 1911, gave the name ***'Aviator's fracture'*** *to the* ***fracture of neck of talus*** since he found these injuries in aviators when they crashed with their machine
- The ***foot resting on the rudder took the impact*** of extreme dorsiflexion, plantar flexion or inversion thereby causing injuries of the talus.

65. **Answer is A (Abductor pollicis longus).**
Ref: Essentials of Orthopedics, RM Shenoy, Pg 18.

- ***Bennett's fracture*** is an oblique fracture occurring at the base of the first metacarpal bone (thumb metacarpal) with subluxation of the carpometacarpal joint
- Mechanism of injury is an axial loading of a partially flexed thumb metacarpal (e.g. delivery of a punch with a clenched fist)
- Displacements:
  - The ulnar fragment remains in place and the radial fragment is displaced as follows:
    - The volar ulnar triangular fragments is held in place by the volar oblique ligament
    - The radial distal fragment is displaced radially, dorsally and proximally ***by the pull of the abductor pollicis longus tendon***.

66. **Answer is c (Paralysis of all interossei).**
Ref: Essentials of orthopedics, RM Shenoy, Pg 142.

- ***Only Ulnar nerve Injury*** results in ***partial claw hand; if both ulnar and median nerves are involved*** (low ulnar and low median; high ulnar and low median) the deformity of ***total or combined claw hand*** otherwise called the 'simian hand' develops.
- In ***Ulnar N injury*** there is ***paralysis of all the interossei and the medial two lumbricals.***

- Palsy tested by:
  - ***Froment's sign/book test***: When the adductor pollicis (Ulnar. N) is paralyzed patient tries to hold the book by using the flexor pollicis longus (Median.N) in place of adductor.
  - ***Egawa test*** (weak dorsal interossei)—unable to abduct middle finger/fingers against resistance.
  - ***Card test*** (weak palmar interossei)—unable to hold card between fingers.

"PAD = Palmars ADduct; DAB = Dorsals ABduct"

OPHTHALMOLOGY

67. Answer is b (Nuclear cataract).

Ref: Parsons' Diseases of the Eye, 20th edition Pg 256.

- A progressive type of congenital cataract ***originally nuclear***, is associated with the occurrence of ***rubella (German measles)*** in the mother if the infection is contracted in the ***second and sometimes in the 3rd month of pregnancy***.
- The virus reaches the fetus before it has developed a immunological defense mechanism so that extensive parasitism occurs.
- The virus interferes with the translation of DNA into RNA.
- Pathologically, the ***lens nucleus is found to be necrotic*** and the whole lens becomes opaque. ***Retinitis of the salt and pepper type*** may be seen at posterior pole.
- Unless all lens matter is removed, aspiration of the cataract may be followed by a chronic inflammatory endophthalmitis associated with presence of residual lens matter.

Other anomalies in congenital rubella

- Patent Ductus Arteriosus
- Multiple peripheral pulmonary artery stenoses
- Microphthalmos
- Micrencephaly
- Mental retardation
- Deafness
- Dental anomalies

68. Answer is d (Vitamin E).

Ref: Manual of Neurologic Therapeutics, Martin Samuels, 7th edition Pg 491; Harrison's, 17th edition Pg 448.

Vitamin E Deficiency

- Dietary deficiency of ***vitamin E*** does not exist. Vitamin E deficiency is seen in:
  - Severe and prolonged malabsorptive diseases, such as celiac disease or after small-intestinal resection
  - Children with cystic fibrosis or prolonged cholestasis may develop vitamin E deficiency characterized by areflexia and hemolytic anemia
  - Children with abetalipoproteinemia cannot absorb or transport vitamin E and become deficient quite rapidly
  - A familial form of isolated vitamin E deficiency also exists; it is due to a defect in the tocopherol transport protein.
- Clinically:
  - ***Vitamin E deficiency*** causes ***axonal degeneration of the large myelinated axons*** and results in posterior column and spinocerebellar symptoms
  - ***Peripheral neuropathy*** is initially characterized by areflexia, with progression to an ataxic gait and by decreased vibration and position sensations
  - ***Progressive external ophthalmoplegia***, skeletal myopathy and pigmented retinopathy are also be features of vitamin E deficiency.

69. Answer is c (IgG).

Ref: Textbook of Ophthalmology, Sunita Agarwal, Vol 1, 1st 2002 edition Pg 63.

- ***Normally IgG is present in aqueous humor at a concentration of about 3 mg/100 mL.***
- ***IgA, IgM and IgD*** are ***NOT present*** commonly in detectable amounts.
- However in inflammatory conditions of the anterior segment of the eye IgG increases and IgM and IgA also become detectable.
- ***Regarding complement activity***, normal human aqueous contains only ***functional C2, C6 and C7 fractions***.

70. Answer is d (Dendritic keratitis).

Ref: Parsons' Disease of the Eye, 20th edition Pg 116, 194.

- ***Corneal sensation is diminished*** after any gross disorder, but the change is of diagnostic significance in certain cases, ***particularly herpes keratitis*** where minimal corneal changes are accompanied by a gross diminution of sensation.
- In all cases of ***dendritic ulcer***, the cornea is relatively insensitive.

71. Answer is b (Difficulty in dark adaptation).

Ref: Parsons' Disease of the Eye, 20th edition Pg 275.

- ***Primary open angle glaucoma*** is usually asymptomatic and patients may have non-specific complaints such as ***headache*** and ***frequent changes in presbyopic correction***.
- Some may notice a ***scotoma*** especially present in the inferior field and some may experience ***difficulty in dark adaptation***.
- Other necessary features to make a diagnoses are:
  - ***IOP*** > 21 mm Hg
  - Optic nerve head changes
  - Visual field defects
  - Defects in the retinal nerve fiber layer.

72. Answer is a (Glaucoma).

Ref: Parsons' Disease of the Eye, 20th edition Pg 373.

- ***Iron foreign body*** in the eye causes ***siderosis bulbi***.
- Earliest manifestation is *iron deposition in the anterior capsule of the lens*—eventually leads to *cataract*. Iris becomes reddish brown in color and mydriasis occurs. Retinal degeneration resembling retinitis pigmentosa occurs.
- ***Secondary glaucoma of the chronic type is a common late complication*** and unless the foreign body is removed, optic atrophy develops and most of these eyes go blind.

73. Answer is b (Septicemia).

Ref: Manual of Ocular Diagnosis and Therapy, Deborah PL, Pg 437, Table 15.4.

Roth spots consist of ***retinal hemorrhage with white centers***; they are seen in

- Infective endocarditis
- Anemia
- Leukemia
- HIV retinopathy
- Septicemia bacterial metastatic endophthalmitis.

74. Answer is b (Vernal catarrh).

Ref: Parsons' Disease of the Eye, 20th edition Pg 172-73.

Vernal conjunctivitis (Spring catarrh)

Clinical features	Treatment
– Affects children/young adults – Type I hypersensitivity reaction due to external allergens – Intense itching, mucoid 'stringy/ropy' discharge (Maxwell Lyon sign) – Cobblestone papillae on undersurface of upper eyelid – Horner Trantas spots at limbus; corneal 'shield ulcer' may be seen; pseudogerontoxon	– Mast cell stabilizers (sodium *cromoglycate*, olopatadine) – Limited topical corticosteroids; – Topical cyclosporine – Cool compress

75. **Answer is b (Clinically significant macular edema).**
Ref: Parsons' Disease of the Eye, 20th edition Pg 297, Table 20.1; Modern Ophthalmology, LC Dutta, 3rd edition, Vol 3, Pg 1613, 1617.

- ***Clinically Significant Macular Edema (CSME)*** can be treated by either ***focal or grid laser*** photocoagulation *(Dutta 1613, 1617).*
- ***Macular hole:*** Some cases resolve spontaneously with no treatment. In many cases, vitreous surgery is required to ease the vitreous traction and an internal tamponade with gas to close the hole and restore useful vision.
- Isolated ischemic maculopathy is NOT treated with laser *(Diabetic retinopathy, Gabriele E Lang, Vol 39, Pg 61 in Developments in Ophthalmology Series).*

Type of retinopathy	Therapy	Indications
Background	Control of diabetes, regular review	All
Maculopathy - CSME	Focal photocoagulation	Discrete areas of leakage on fluorescein angiography
Diffuse leak around the macula - Circinate	Grid laser Focal photocoagulation	
Preproliferative retinopathy	Frequent review	
Proliferative retinopathy	Panretinal photocoagulation	NVE/NVD
Advanced diabetic eye disease	Vitreoretinal surgery with photocoagulation	Persistent vitreous hemorrhage, tractional retinal detachment

EAR, NOSE AND THROAT

76. **Answer is d (Glomus jugulare tumor).**
Ref: Maqbool's ENT textbook, 11th edition Pg 262.

Glomus Jugulare Tumor

- Also called ***Chemodectoma, Non-chromaffin Paraganglioma***. F:M = 5:1; ***Pulsatile, roaring tinnitus***.
- Profuse spontaneous hemorrhage often occurs; in early stage TM appears reddish with a ***rising sun*** appearance.
- ***Browne's sign:*** Increasing the pressure in the external auditory canal by the Siegle's speculum makes the tumor mass more prominent and red, with increased pulsations.

77. **Answer is a (*Aspergillus niger*).**
Ref: Maqbool. ENT textbook, 11th edition Pg 53.

- ***Otomycosis*** is ***fungal otitis externa*** due to ***Aspergillus niger***, *Aspergillus fumigatus*, etc. More common in *hot and humid climates, swimming in infected water predisposes.*
- Clinical features: ***Itching and irritation***, dull pain, *scanty discharge*. Otoscopy reveals canal to be blocked by *debris resembling wet newspaper or blotting paper or grayish black cotton wool*-like masses.

- Treatment: Removal of fungus mass in external canal by *microsuction*. Local *nystatin or clotrimazole drops* may be used and treatment has to be *continued for at least 3 weeks after apparent cure* in order to eradicate fungal spores.

78. **Answer is b (25 weeks).**
Ref: Ballenger's Otorhinolaryngology: Head and Neck Surgery, 17th edition Pg 24.

- By the ***25th week of gestation the organ of Corti and spiral ganglion is fully differentiated***.

PATHOLOGY

79. **Answer is d (Langerhans cells).**
Ref: Robbins pathology, 7th edition Pg 701.

- ***Langerhans cell histiocytosis*** earlier referred to as ***Histiocytosis X*** consists of:

1. ***Unifocal LCH—Eosinophilic granuloma***.
2. ***Multifocal LCH—Hand-Schuller-Christian disease***, consisting of triad of calvarial bone defects, diabetes insipidus and exophthalmos.
3. ***Acute disseminated LCH—Letterer-Siwe syndrome***, seen in infants.

- The tumor cells in each are ***derived from dendritic cells*** and express HLA-DR, S-100 and CD1a. They have abundant, often vacuolated cytoplasm and vesicular nuclei containing linear grooves or folds.
- The presence of ***Birbeck granules in the cytoplasm is characteristic***.
- Under electron microscope, Birbeck granules have a pentalamelar, rodlike, tubular appearance and sometimes a dilated terminal end (***tennis racket-like appearance***).
- As Birbeck granules are not seen in all tumor cells by EM, the detection of ***S-100 and CD1a*** expression by immunohistochemical techniques aids in the diagnosis.

80. **Answer is b (Brilliant cresyl blue).**
Ref: Atlas of Clinical hematology, By Helmut Loeffler et al. Pg 8.

- ***Heilmeyer's reticulocyte stain*** consists of ***brilliant cresyl blue solution*** in physiologic saline.

81. **Answer is d (Mediastinum).**
Ref: Encyclopedia of diagnostic imaging, Albert LB, Pg 1110, 2008 edition.

- The ***mediastinum is the most common site of extragonadal germ cell tumors***—most common within the ***anterior mediastinum***.
- They can also arise in the retroperitoneum and sacrococcygeal region.

82. **Answer is a (Chromosome 13ql4).**
Ref: Harrison's, 17th edition Pg 413, Table 63-4, 401.

- Cytogenetic abnormality of ***Retinoblastoma*** is located at: ***13q14.11*** (deletion).
- In many cancer syndromes, there is an inherited *predisposition* to tumor formation. In these instances, a germline mutation is inherited in an autosomal dominant fashion inactivating one allele of an autosomal tumor-suppressor gene.
- If the second allele is inactivated by a somatic mutation or by epigenetic silencing in a given cell, this will lead to neoplastic growth (***Knudson two-hit model***). Thus, the defective allele in the germline is transmitted in a dominant mode, though tumorigenesis results from a biallelic loss of the tumor-suppressor gene in an affected tissue.
- The ***classic example to illustrate this phenomenon is retinoblastoma***, also this two-hit model applies to other inherited cancer syndromes such as MEN-1 and NF type 2.

More about Retinoblastoma (RB)

- ***MC primary intraocular tumor*** of ***childhood.***
- 40% RB is hereditary, 30% RB is bilateral.
- Pathologically: Exophytic, endophytic or diffuse infiltrating types. Flexne**R**-Wintersteine**R** true **R**osette and Fleurettes seen in retinoblastoma. Homer Wright pseudorosette is found in neuroblastoma or medulloblastoma and rarely in RB. *Increased aqueous LDH* with aqueous to serum LDH ratio > 1.0 indicates retinoblastoma. Total tumor necrosis → *spontaneous regression*, rare.
- Clinically: ***Leukocoria*** (white pupillary reflex/cat's eye reflex) is the MC presenting sign, *second MC is strabismus*, others include glaucoma retinal detachment, pseudouveitis with hypopyon (masquerade syndrome), proptosis.
- Treatment: Enucleation for large tumors; for medium to small tumors chemotherapy with plaque radiotherapy (brachytherapy).
- ***Reese Ellworth*** classification of RB relates to visual prognosis.
- MC second tumor in RB patients is ***osteogenic sarcoma.***
- ***Trilateral RB = RB + Osteogenic sarcoma + pinealoblastoma.***

83. Answer is c (Sarcoidosis).
Ref: Robbins' Pathology, 7th edition Pg 738.

- In ***sarcoidosis, lymph nodes are involved in almost all cases***, specifically in the hilar and mediastinal nodes, but any other node in the body may be involved.
- Nodes are characteristically enlarged, discrete and sometimes ***calcified.***

84. Answer is d (Nodular glomerulosclerosis).
Ref: Robbins pathology, 7th edition Pg 992.

- ***Nodular glomerulosclerosis*** also called ***Kimmelstiel-Wilson disease*** or ***intercapillary glomerulosclerosis is highly, but not completely specific for diabetes.***
- ***Approximately 15–30% patients*** with ***long-term diabetes develop nodular glomerulosclerosis*** and in most instances is associated with renal failure.

85. Answer is b (Primary sclerosing cholangitis).
Ref: The autoimmune diseases, By Noel R Rose, Pg 769, Fig 55.4.

- ***Onion skin fibrosis*** is the ***characteristic lesion seen in primary sclerosing cholangitis,*** but is rarely seen in percutaneous liver biopsies.

86. Answer is b (Neutrophil).
Ref: Robbins pathology, 7th edition Pg 230.

- The ***LE cell is any phagocytic leukocyte (neutrophil or macrophage)*** that has engulfed the denatured nucleus of an injured cell.
- The demonstration of LE cell in vitro was ***used in the past as a test for SLE.***
- With new techniques for detection of antinuclear antibodies however, <u>this test is now largely of historical interest</u>.
- Sometimes LE cells are found in pericardial or pleural effusions in patients.

87. Answer is c (Endothelial cells).
Ref: Robbins pathology, 7th edition Pg 126, 513.

- ***von Willebrand factor (vWF)*** is a ***product of normal endothelium***; it is not specifically synthesized after endothelial injury.
- vWF is an essential cofactor for platelet binding to collagen and other surfaces.
- Endothelial cells uniquely contain ***Weibel Palade bodies*** that are membrane bound storage organelles containing vWF.

88. Answer is a (Chrysotile).
Ref: Robbins pathology, 7th edition Pg 735.

- There are 2 ***distinct generic forms of asbestos***
  - ***Serpentine*** (curly and flexible fibers): Chrysotile accounts for 90% of asbestos used in industry
  - ***Amphibole*** (straight, stiff and brittle fibers): Crocidolite, amosite, tremolite, anthophyllite and actinolite.
- ***Amphiboles, even though less prevalent are more pathogenic than chrysotiles***, particularly with respect to induction of malignant pleural tumors (***mesotheliomas***).
- Amphibole exposure correlates with mesothelioma.

89. Answer is b (β-thalassemia trait).
Ref: Wintrobe's Clinical hematology, Vol 1, 12th edition Pg 4.

- ***Red cell distribution width (RDW)*** is a red cell measurement that quantitates cellular volume heterogeneity reflecting the range of red cell sizes within a sample.
- RDW has been proposed to be useful in early classification of anemia as it becomes abnormal earlier in nutritional deficiency anemias than other red cell parameters, especially in case of iron deficiency anemia.
  - ➲ Uncomplicated iron deficiency anemia = HIGH RDW, normal or low MCV
  - ➲ Uncomplicated heterozygous beta-thalassemia (thalassemia trait, thalassemia minor) = NORMAL RDW, low MCV

90. Answer is c (Osteoclast).
Ref: Robbins pathology, 7th edition Pg 1275; Rubin's pathology, Raphael Rubin, 2008 edition Pg 1088.

- ***Osteoclasts*** are multinucleated cells that contain lysosomes and many hydrolytic enzymes. They are found in small depressions termed ***Howship's lacunae*** on bone surfaces. Osteoclast is the cell responsible for bone resorption.
- By electron microscopy, they form a ***ruffled polarized plasmalemmal membrane*** when the cell is in contact with and is actively degrading bone.

91. Answer is a (*Proteus*).
Ref: Robbins pathology, 7th edition Pg 1001.

- ***Xanthogranulomatous pyelonephritis*** is an unusual and relatively rare form of chronic pyelonephritis characterized by the accumulation of foamy macrophages intermingled with plasma cells, lymphocytes, polymorphonuclear leukocytes and occasional giant cells.
- ***Often associated with Proteus infections*** and obstruction, the lesions sometimes produce large, yellowish-orange nodules that may be confused with renal cell carcinoma.

92. Answer is c (Gray hepatization).
Ref: Robbins pathology, 7th edition Pg 750.

Stages of lobar pneumonia

- ***Stage of congestion:*** Heavy, boggy, red lung; vascular engorgement, intra-alveolar fluid with few neutrophils and numerous bacteria.
- ***Stage of red hepatization:*** Massive confluent exudation with red cells (congestion), neutrophils and fibrin filling the alveolar spaces. On gross examination the lobe now appears distinctly red, firm and airless, with a liver-like consistency, hence the term hepatization.
- ***Stage of gray hepatization:*** Progressive disintegration of red cells and the persistence of fibrinosuppurative exudate giving the gross appearance of a grayish brown dry surface.
- ***Stage of resolution:*** Consolidated exudates undergoes enzymatic digestion to produce a granular, semi-fluid debris that is reabsorbed, ingested by macrophages coughed up or organized by fibroblasts growing into it.

93. Answer is d (Rhinoscleroma).
Ref: Ballenger's Otorhinolaryngology, Head and Neck Surgery, 17th edition Pg 891.

Repeat Qn

- See *answer no. 77 in COMED-K 2010 answers* for detailed explanation.

94. Answer is a (Schiller-Duval body).
Ref: Robbins pathology, 7th edition Pg 1101.

- ***Endodermal sinus tumor*** is the second most common malignant tumor of germ cell origin.
- It is thought to be derived from differentiation of malignant germ cells towards extraembryonic yolk sac structure.
- Similar to the yolk sac the tumor is rich in α-fetoprotein and α-1 antitrypsin.
- Its characteristic histological architecture is a glomerulus-like structure composed of a central blood vessel enveloped by germ cells within a space lined by germ cells – ***Schiller-Duval body***.

About the other choices

- ***Psammoma body*** – Papillary thyroid carcinoma, Serous cystadenoma of ovary, Meningioma.
- ***Call exner bodies*** – ***Granulosa cell tumor*** of ovary.
- ***Homer Wright rosettes*** – pseudorosette seen in ***neuroblastoma.***

MICROBIOLOGY

95. Answer is c (Trypanosomiasis).
Ref: Harrison's, 17th edition Pg 1301.

- ***Chagas' disease*** is caused by ***Trypanosoma cruzi***.
- *T. cruzi* is transmitted among its mammalian hosts by hematophagous triatomine insects, often called **Reduviid bugs**.
- The first signs of acute Chagas' disease develop at least 1 week after invasion by the parasites. When the organisms enter through a break in the skin, an indurated area of erythema and swelling (the chagoma), accompanied by local lymphadenopathy, may appear.
- ***Romaña's sign*** – the classic finding in acute Chagas' disease, which consists of unilateral painless edema of the palpebrae and periocular tissues – can result when the conjunctiva is the portal of entry.
- Therapy for Chagas' disease is unsatisfactory. For many years, only two drugs – ***nifurtimox and benznidazole*** – have been available for this purpose. Unfortunately, both drugs lack efficacy and often cause severe side effects.

96. Answer is d (Measles).
Ref: Textbook of Microbiology, CP Baveja, 3rd edition Pg 468.

Repeat Qn

- See *answer no. 90 in COMED-K 2010 answers* for detailed explanation.

97. Answer is c (Allograft).
Ref: Textbook of Microbiology, CP Baveja, 3rd edition Pg 163.

Types of grafts

Autograft	From self
Syngeneic graft/isograft	From identical twin or clone (i.e. genetically identical with recipient)
Allograft /homograft	From non-identical member of same species
Xenograft	From different species

98. Answer is a (*Staphylococcus aureus*).
Ref: Harrison's, 17th edition Pg 875.

Common Illnesses Caused By *Staphylococcus Aureus*

Toxin-mediated Illnesses	Musculoskeletal Infections	Respiratory Tract Infections
– Toxic shock syndrome – Food poisoning – Staphylococcal scalded-skin syndrome	– Septic arthritis – Osteomyelitis – Pyomyositis – Psoas abscess	– Ventilator-associated or nosocomial pneumonia – Septic pulmonary emboli – Postviral pneumonia (e.g. influenza) – Empyema
Skin and Soft Tissue Infections – Folliculitis – Furuncle, carbuncle – Cellulitis – Impetigo – Mastitis – Surgical wound infections – Hidradenitis suppurativa	**Bacteremia and its Complications** – Sepsis, septic shock – Metastatic foci of infection (kidney, joints, bone, lung) – Infective endocarditis	**Infective Endocarditis** – Injection drug use–associated – Native-valve – Prosthetic-valve – Nosocomial
Device-related Infections (e.g. intravascular catheters, prosthetic joints) – Invasive infections Associated with community-acquired MRSA – Necrotizing fasciitis		

99. Answer is a (IgE).
Ref: Textbook of Microbiology, 3rd edition CP Baveja, Pg 101, Table 13.1.

- *IgE and IgD do not* fix complement.

Properties of Immunoglobulins

1. IgG	– ***Most abundant Ig*** (80%), distributed in blood and interstitial fluids – Main Ig in ***secondary immune response*** – Only Ig that ***crosses placenta***, so the ***major protective Ig in neonate*** – Opsonizes bacteria, neutralizes bacterial toxins and viruses, coats cells prior to killing by killer cells – ***Activates complement*** via ***classical pathway***
2. IgA	– Principal Ig in ***secretions of respiratory and GI tract*** and in sweat, saliva, tears and colostrums – ***Key defense for mucosal surfaces***—prevents attachment of bacteria and viruses to mucosa – J (joining) chain is seen in dimeric forms of IgA, it is synthesized by epithelial cells – When aggregated binds polymorphs and ***activates complement via alternate pathway***
3. IgM	– Macroglobulin made up of 5 monomeric Ig subunits linked by a J chain—Massive, Maximum molecular weight – Mainly intravascular – Major Ig of ***primary immune response*** (priMary = IgM)

	– Does not cross placenta, fetal production of high levels of IgM may be of diagnostic significance (e.g. rubella) – ***Activates complement*** via ***classical pathway*** – Blood group antibodies are IgM
4. IgD	– Unclear function – Found on ***surface of many B cells*** and in serum
5. IgE	– Mediates ***immediate (type I) hypersensitivity reactions*** by inducing the release of mediators from mast cells and basophils when exposed to allergens; mediates immunity to worms by activating eosinophils. – Least abundant Ig

100. Answer is d (Enriched media).
Ref: Textbook of Microbiology, CP Baveja, 3rd edition Pg 411-12.

- The methods employed for the cultivation of viruses are:
  - ***Animal inoculation*** (infant/suckling mice)
  - ***Embryonated egg inoculation*** (routes used are chorioallantoic membrane, allantoic cavity, amniotic sac and yolk sac)
  - ***Tissue culture*** (organ culture, explant culture, cell cultures such as primary cell cultures, diploid cell strains and continuous cell lines).

101. Answer is a (Enterotest).
Ref: Nursing Laboratory and Diagnostic Tests Demystified, James Keogh, chapter 23, Pg 505.

- The ***enterotest*** **(Giardiasis String Test)** determines if the patient has ***giardiasis*** by sampling fluid in the ***duodenum***.
- The patient ***swallows a gelatin capsule attached to a string***. The string is taped on the outside of the patients cheek while the capsule dissolves in the stomach and duodenum. The string is then removed and examined under the microscope for the presence of *Giardia intestinalis*.

102. Answer is a *(Shigella Sonnei)*.
Ref: Textbook of Microbiology, CP Bavja, 3rd edition Pg 257.

- ***Shigella are***
  - ***Non-motile*** (unique among enterobacteriaceae in lacking a flagella)
  - ***Anaerogenic*** (do not produce gas from sugars)
  - ***Non-lactose fermenters***.

PHARMACOLOGY

103. Answer is c (Metronidazole).
Ref: KD Tripathi, 6th edition Pg 799, 673.

- ***Clostridium difficile (Pseudomembranous) enterocolitis*** (superinfection) is a unique colon infection that is acquired almost exclusively ***in association with antimicrobial use*** (*clindamycin, tetracyclines, aminoglycosides, co-trimoxazole*) and the consequent disruption of the normal colonic flora; more common after colorectal surgery.
- The organism produces an ***enterotoxin,*** which damages gut mucosa forming plaques.
- ***Oral Metronidazole is more effective, more convenient, less toxic and therefore preferred over vancomycin.***

104. Answer is b (Chronic myeloid leukemia).
Ref: KD Tripathi, 6th edition Pg 828.

- ***Imatinib mesylate*** is a novel antineoplastic drug that ***inhibits the protein kinases*** in ***chronic myeloid leukemia (CML)*** cells and the ones that are activated by platelet derived growth factor (PDGF) receptor, stem cell receptor and c-kit receptor found in ***gastrointestinal stromal tumors (GIST)***.
- ***Striking success*** has been obtained in ***chronic phase of CML***, as well as in accelerated phase and in ***metastatic kit positive GIST***.
- **Adverse effects**: Fluid retention, edema, abdominal pain, myalgia, liver damage.

105. Answer is a (9-Δ-tetrahydrocannabinol).
Ref: KD Tripathi, 6th edition Pg 438.

- ***Cannabis*** is derived from the hemp plant, ***Cannabis sativa***; the ***pistillate*** form of the ***female plant*** is most important in cannabis production.
- ***9-Δ-tetrahydrocannabinol*** is the active principle of ***Cannabis indica*** (marijuana).
- Cannabis is the *drug of abuse having* ***lowest toxicity***.
- *Effects of use*: Low dose *impairs memory and complex motor activity*, alters sensory and time perception, causes *conjunctival reddening* and may *increase sexual desire*; at high doses causes psychotic symptoms and paranoia; chronic use causes decreased sexual functioning, lung problems due to smoking, decreased motivation (i.e. the ***'amotivational syndrome'***); *flashback phenomenon*; ***reverse tolerance***.

Various forms of cannabis use

- ***Bhang***—the dried leaves—is generally taken by the oral route, acts slowly.
- ***Ganja***—the dried female inflorescence—is more potent and is smoked: effects are produced almost instantaneously.
- ***Charas***—dried resinous extract from the flowering tops and leaves—most potent, smoked with tobacco, also called 'hashish'.

106. Answer is a (Hyperpigmentary disorders).
Ref: KD Tripathi, 6th edition Pg 852.

- ***Azelaic acid*** is a drug for ***acne*** that is also effective in ***hyperpigmentary disorders including melasma***
- It appears to act by ***inhibiting the enzyme tyrosinase***
- However it is a weak demelanising agent with reversible demelanising action
- It is used as a 10 or 20% cream. The only side effect is mild and transient local irritation.

107. Answer is b (Lamivudine).
Ref: KD Tripathi, 6th edition Pg 457; Harrison's, 17th edition Pg 1958.

Repeat Qn

- See ***answer no. 168 in COMED-K 2010 answers*** for detailed explanation.

108. Answer is a (Warfarin).
Ref: Medical toxicology, 3rd edition Pg 616.

- The ***purple toe syndrome*** has been attributed to ***cholesterol crystal emboli*** released as a result of ***Warfarin-induced bleeding*** into atherosclerotic plaques.
- It usually occurs 3–10 weeks after initiation of therapy.
- ***Purple discoloration of the plantar surface of the toes and feet*** occurs with pain and tenderness, it may be bilateral.

109. Answer is b (Synergy).
Ref: KD Tripathi, 6th edition Pg 677.

- ***Two bactericidal drugs*** are frequently ***additive and sometimes synergistic*** if the organism is sensitive to both, e.g.:
  - Penicillin/***Ampicillin*** + streptomycin/***gentamicin*** for enterococcal SABE.
  - Penicillins by acting on the cell wall may ***enhance the penetration of the aminoglycoside*** into the bacterium.

COMED-K 2009 ANSWERS

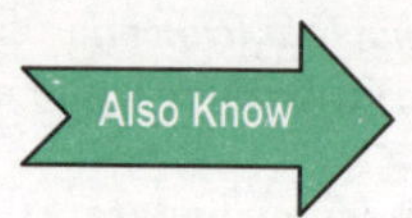

Synergism: When the action of one drug is facilitated by another, they are said to be synergistic. Synergism can be:

1) **Additive**: The effect of two drugs is in the same direction and simply adds up, i.e.

Effect of drugs A + B = Effect of drug A + effect of drug B

Additive drug combinations
Aspirin + Paracetamol (as analgesic/antipyretic)
Nitrous oxide + halothane (as general anesthetic)
Amlodipine + atenolol (as antihypertensive)
Glibenclamide + metformin (as hypoglycemic)
Ephedrine + theophylline (as bronchodilator)

Side effects of the components of an additive pair may be different—do not add up. Thus, the combination is better tolerated than the higher dose of one component.

2) **Supra-additive (potentiation)**: The effect of combination is greater than the individual effects of the components

Effect of drugs A + B > effect of drug A + effect of drug B

This is always the case when one component is inactive as such.

Supra-additive drug combinations	
Drug pair	**Basis of potentiation**
Acetylcholine + Physostigmine	Inhibition of breakdown
Levodopa + Carbidopa/Benserazide	Inhibition of peripheral metabolism
Adrenaline + Cocaine/Desipramine	Inhibition of neuronal uptake
Sulfamethoxazole + Trimethoprim	Sequential blockade
Antihypertensives (Enalapril + Hydrochlorothiazide)	Tackling two contributory factors
Tyramine + MAO inhibitors	Increasing releasable CA store

110. Answer is c (Spectinomycin).
Ref: Harrison's, 17th edition Pg 919.

- ***Spectinomycin*** has been an alternative regimen for the treatment of uncomplicated ***gonococcal infections*** in *penicillin-allergic* ***pregnant patients***.

111. Answer is d (Octreotide).
Ref: Harrison's, 17th edition Pg 2211.

- Octreotide acetate is an eight amino acid synthetic somatostatin analogue.
- In contrast to native somatostatin, the analogue is relatively resistant to plasma degradation. It has a 2 hour serum half-life and possesses ***forty-fold greater potency than native somatostatin to suppress Growth Hormone (GH)***.
- Octreotide is administered by ***subcutaneous*** route.
- The ***long-acting somatostatin depot*** formulations, ***octreotide and lanreotide*** are the ***preferred medical treatment*** *for patients with* ***acromegaly***.
- Somatostatin analogues exert their therapeutic effects through ***SSTR-2 and -5 receptors***, both of which are invariably expressed by GH-secreting tumors.

112. Answer is b (H^+/K^+-ATPase pump).
Ref: KD Tripathi, 6th edition Pg 631.

- ***Proton pump inhibitors*** include omeprazole, esomeprazole, lansoprazole, pantoprazole and rabeprazole.

- Proton pump inhibitors react covalently with SH groups of the ***H^+-K^+-ATPase enzyme and inactivate it irreversibly***.
- After diffusing into the parietal cell from the blood, it gets concentrated in the acidic pH of the canaliculi because the charged forms generated are unable to diffuse back. Moreover it gets tightly bound to the enzyme.
- These features and the specific localization of the H^+-K^+-ATPase enzyme to the apical membrane of the parietal cells confer high degree of selectivity of action to omeprazole.
- Acid secretion resume only when new H^+-K^+-ATPase is synthesized.

113. Answer is a (Metoclopramide).

Ref: KD Tripathi, 6th edition Pg 644, 379.

- ***Metoclopramide*** is a ***prokinetic agent*** used as an ***antiemetic***.
- It acts through both dopaminergic and serotonergic receptors. Its mechanism of actions are:
  - ***D2 antagonism***: Central antidopaminergic (D2) action of metoclopramide on the CTZ is clearly responsible for its antiemetic property. Other manifestations of D2 blockade are antagonism of apomorphine-induced vomiting, ***CPZ-like extrapyramidal effects*** and hyperprolactinemia.
  - ***5-HT4 antagonism***: It acts in the GIT to enhance ACh release from myenetric motor neurons. This results from 5-HT4 receptor activation on primary afferent neurons of the ENS via interneurons. The gastric hurrying and LES tonic effects are mainly due to this action, which is synergized by bethanechol and attenuated by atropine.
  - ***5-HT3 antagonism***: Central 5-HT3 action appears to be significant only when larger doses are used to control chemotherapy-induced vomiting.
- **Adverse effects** of metoclopramide:
  - Sedation, dizziness, loose stools, *muscle dystonias (especially in children)*
  - Long-term use can cause *parkinsonism, galactorrhea* and *gynecomastia.*

PREVENTIVE AND SOCIAL MEDICINE

114. Answer is a (Yellow fever)

Ref: Park, 20th edition Pg 247.

Yellow Fever Vaccine

- Approved vaccine is the live attenuated vaccine ***–17D vaccine***.
- Sensitivity of the lyophilized 17D vaccine to heat is major drawback to the use of this vaccine in mass campaigns in tropical countries.
- It should be stored between +5 and -30°C, preferably ***below 0°C*** until reconstituted with sterile, ***cold physiological saline diluent*** provided. Reconstituted vaccine not used within half an hour should be discarded.
- Vaccine is ***given SC at the insertion of deltoid*** in a single dose of 0.5 mL irrespective of age.
- ***Immunity appears to begin on the 7th day*** and *lasts for more than 35 years* and possibly for life.
- Revaccination after 10 years is ***recommended for international travel***.
- *Cholera and yellow fever vaccines* together or within 3 weeks interfere with each other, so whenever possible they should be given *3 weeks or more apart*.

115. Answer is d (OPV).

Ref: Park, 20th edition Pg 101.

- Among the vaccines, ***polio is the MOST sensitive to heat*** requiring ***storage at –20 degrees centigrade***.
- Vaccines, which **must be *stored in the freezer*** compartment are polio and measles.
- Vaccines, which **must be *stored in the cold part* BUT NEVER *be allowed to freeze*** are typhoid, DPT, tetanus toxoid, DT, BCG and diluents.

More About Vaccines

☐ Live Attenuated Vaccines (LAV)	OPV, MMR (Measles, Rubella) Hepatitis A, Rotavirus, Yellow fever, Live JE
☐ Vaccines CI in immunodeficiency	All Live Attenuated Vaccines
☐ Freeze Dried (Purely Lyophilized vaccines)	BCG, MMR, Measles, Rubella, Hepatitis A, Varicella, Rotavirus, Rabies, Inactivated JE, MPSV, Yellow fever
☐ Vaccines with Saline as Diluent	BCG, Yellow fever; All other freeze dries vaccines use sterile water as diluent
☐ Vaccines to be protected from light	BCG, DPT, MMR, HPV, Varicella, Rotavirus, Measles
☐ Vaccines to be given subcutaneously (SC) only	MMR, Varicella, JE, Yellow fever

116. Answer is b (40–60).
Ref: Park, 20th edition Pg 654.

- ***Heat stress index (HSI)*** represents the ***percentage of heat storage capacity of an average man.***

HSI value	Interpretation
0	No thermal stress
10–30	Moderate to mild heat strain
40–60	Severe heat strain
70–90	Very severe heat strain
100	Upper limit of heat tolerance

117. Answer is a (8 cases per 1,000 population).
Ref: Park, 20th edition Pg 57.

- Incidence is the number of new cases occurring in a defined population during a specified period of time. It is expressed as per 1,000 per year. Incidence is a rate.
- Incidence is not affected by the duration of disease, the use of incidence is generally restricted to acute conditions.
- Examples of special incidence rates are attack rate, secondary attack rate, hospital admission rate, etc.

☐ Prevalence refers specifically to all current cases (old and new) existing at a given point in time or over a period of time in a given population. Prevalence is a ratio.
☐ Longer the duration of the disease, the greater its prevalence (e.g. TB).
☐ If a disease has high mortality and high case fatality (rapid death) or easily curability (rapid recovery) → it implies that the disease is acute and of a very short duration → prevalence will be low.

➲ Relationship between prevalence and incidence can be expressed as
Prevalence = Incidence duration; P = I × D.

Hence in the given question, Prevalence = *2 cases per 1,000 population per year* × *4 years* = ***8 cases per 1,000 population per year.***

118. Answer is d (Information, education and communication).
Ref: Park, 20th edition Pg 792.

- The *principles of primary health care* are:
  (1) Equitable distribution.
  (2) Community participation.
  (3) Intersectoral coordination.
  (4) Appropriate technology.

119. Answer is c (Be explosive).
Ref: Park, 20th edition Pg 61.

Repeat Topic

Common source epidemics	Propagated epidemics
– Single exposure or 'point-source' epidemics – Continuous or multiple exposure epidemics	– Person to person – Arthropod vector – Animal reservoir

Common source single exposure epidemics (point source) epidemics

- The exposure to the disease agent is brief and essentially ***simultaneous***; the resultant cases all develop within one incubation period of the disease (e.g. an epidemic of food poisoning).
- The epidemic curve rises and falls rapidly with ***no secondary waves.***
- The curve has usually ***one peak***.
- The epidemic ***tends to be explosive***, there is ***clustering of cases*** within a narrow interval of time.
- Examples are ***Bhopal gas tragedy*** and ***Minamata disease in Japan***.

Common source continuous or repeated exposure epidemics

- Examples are a ***prostitute with gonorrhea, a well of contaminated water***, etc.

120. Answer is c (Secondary attack rate).
Ref: Park, 20th edition Pg 95.

- ***Secondary attack rate*** was ***initially developed to measure the spread of infection*** within a family, household or any closed aggregate of persons who have had contact with a case or disease.
- It is also useful to determine whether a disease of unknown etiology (e.g. Hodgkin's disease) is communicable or not; and in evaluating the effectiveness of control measures such as isolation and immunization.

121. Answer is d (Louse).
Ref: Harrison's, 17th edition Pg 989.

Arthropod-borne Diseases

Arthropod	Diseases transmitted
Mosquito	See separate table below
Housefly	Typhoid and paratyphoid fever, diarrhea, dysentery, cholera, gastroenteritis, amoebiasis, helminthic infestations, poliomyelitis, conjunctivitis, trachoma, anthrax, yaws, etc.
Sandfly	Kala-azar, oriental sore, sandfly fever, oroya fever
Louse	Epidemic typhus, relapsing fever, trench fever
Rat flea	Bubonic plague, endemic typhus, chiggerosis, *Hymenolepis diminuta*
Hard tick	Tick typhus, viral encephalitis, viral fevers, viral hemorrhagic fever (e.g. Kyasanur forest disease), tularemia, tick paralysis, human babesiosis
Soft tick	Q fever, relapsing fever
Blackfly	Onchocerciasis
Reduviid bug	Chagas' disease
Tsetse fly	Sleeping sickness

Trombiculid mite	Scrub typhus, Rickettsial-pox
Itch-mite	Scabies
Cyclops	Guinea-worm disease, fish tapeworm *(D. latum)*
Cockroaches	Enteric pathogens

122. Answer is a (1995).

Ref: Park, 20th edition Pg 378.

- ***Pulse polio immunization (PPI) program*** was launched in India in the year **1995**.
- PPIs are when oral polio vaccine is given to all children in the country on a single day, regardless to previous immunization. PPI is carried out on 'National immunization days' (NIDs) every year in ***December and January***.
- The 1st PPI started on ***9th December 1995*** targeting all children < 3 years, but later on age group was increased to ***all children < 5 years***.
- The dose of OPV during PPIs are extra doses, which supplement and do not replace the doses received during routine immunization services.
- A country will be declared polio free only *when no new cases will be reported for 3 consecutive years*.
- ***Vaccine vial monitor*** use in PPI started after ***1998*** for efficacy.
- In view of rapid progress in polio eradication India 5 national rounds (targeting 165 million children) and one such national round for high incidence states conducted in 2004.

123. Answer is b (sugar).

Ref: Park, 20th edition Pg 463, 545.

	Cow's milk	Human Milk
Lactose (g)	4.4	7.4
Proteins (g)	3.2	1.1
Fat (g)	4.1	3.4
Calcium (mg)	120	28
Iron (mg)	0.2	1.0
Water (g)	87	88
Energy (kCal)	67	65
Carbohydrate (g)	4.4	7.4

Author's comments: *"Breast milk and Breastfeeding are important from both PSM and pediatrics – be through with this".*

124. Answer is b (0.5).

Ref: Park, 20th edition Pg 625.

Repeat Qn

- See ***answer no. 144 in COMED-K 2010 answers*** for detailed explanation.

FORENSIC MEDICINE

125. Answer is c (Phosphorus poisoning).

Ref: Narayan Reddy's FMT, 23rd edition Pg 81.

Postmortem Lividity (Postmortem Hypostasis, Livor Mortis)

- Bluish purple/purplish red discoloration, which appears under the skin of the dependant parts of the body ***due to capillovenous distension***.
- ***Pressure points are spared***.
- It appears 1–3 hours after death, is usually well developed within 4 hours and reaches a maximum between 6 and 12 hours.
- When coagulation in capillaries takes place, the stains become permanent and this is known as ***fixation of postmortem staining***. This usually occurs in about 6 hours.

Poisoning	Color of hypostasis
Carbon monoxide	: Cherry red
Hydrocyanic acid	: Bright red
Phosphorus	: Dark brown
Aniline, nitrates, potassium chloride/bicarbonate, nitrobenzene	: Red brown

126. Answer is c (18 years).
Ref: Narayan Reddy's FMT, 23rd edition Pg 48.

- In India, a ***female under 18 years*** and ***a male under 21 years*** cannot contract marriage.

127. Answer is c (Stoppage of circulation).
Ref: AIDS to forensic medicine and toxicology, 9th edition Pg 2007.

- ***Cessation of circulation*** is a sign of death. It may be determined by:
  - ***Magnus test***: Placing a ligature around the base of the finger.
  - ***Icard test***: Injecting a solution of fluorescein.
  - ***Diaphanous test***: Looking through the web of the fingers through a bright light.

DERMATOLOGY

128. Answer is d (Violaceous papules over knuckles).
Ref: Harrison's, 17th edition Pg 2696.

Dermatomyositis (DM)

➢ Presentation	– ***Heliotrope rash***: MC manifestation of DM. It is a *purple red* discoloration of upper eyelids. – ***Gottrons papules***: Violaceous flat-topped papules over bony prominences, particularly the *metacarpophalangeal* joints, the proximal *interphalangeal* joints and/or the distal interphalangeal joints. – ***Dowling's lines***: Linear erythematosquamous lesions on the dorsal surface of the fingers over the metacarpals. – ***Poikiloderma*** may occur on exposed skin such as the extensor surfaces of the arm, the 'V' of the neck or the upper back *(Shawl sign)*. – *Facial* (malar) erythema, *periungual telangiectases,* scalp involvement (violaceous, psoriasiform dermatitis and non-scarring alopecia), hyperkeratosis of the palms ***('mechanic's hands')*** may occur in DM. – With the exception of the heliotrope rash, the eruption of dermatomyositis is *photodistributed and is photoexacerbated,* but photosensitivity is not common.

➢ Treatment	– Therapy of the muscle component involves the use of corticosteroids with or without an immunosuppressive agent. – The skin disease is treated with sun avoidance, sunscreens, topical corticosteroids, antimalarial agents and/or methotrexate.

129. Answer is b (Pemphigus).

Ref: Robbins pathology, 7th edition Pg 1260.

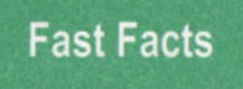

Immunologically Mediated Blistering Skin Diseases

Many of these disorders are due to autoimmune mechanisms. Clinically they are characterized by morbidity (pain, pruritus, disfigurement) and mortality (largely due to loss of epidermal barrier function and/or secondary infection). Blister formation is due to loss of cohesion between epidermal cells (acantholysis). The mainstay of treatment is systemic glucocorticoids ± immunosuppressives.

Disease	Clinical features	Histology
Pemphigus vulgaris (PV)	***Flaccid*** blisters, which rupture easily leaving denuded skin; ***Nikolsky's sign+***; ***Mouth*** (~90% have oromucosal involvement at sometime), scalp, face, neck, axilla, trunk affected; lesions usually heal without scarring.	Blisters formed in suprabasal layer of epidermis (***intraepidermal***).
Pemphigus foliaceus (PF)	Crusts and shallow erosions on scalp, central-face, neck, upper chest and back. Mucus membrane lesions are ***rare***. Associated with thymoma/myasthenia. Drug-induced pemphigus resembles PF (penicillamine MC, captopril, rifampin, piroxicam, penicillin, phenobarbital).	Blister formed in superficial layers of epidermis (subcorneal).
Bullous pemphigoid (BP)	Large ***tense blisters*** on flexor surfaces, oromucosal lesions. Direct immuno-fluorescence microscopy of the normal-appearing perilesional skin shows linear deposits of IgG and/or C3 in the epidermal BMZ	Blister formed in subepidermal region, eosinophil-rich.
Dermatitis herpetiformis	Extremely itchy small papules and vesicles on elbows, knees, buttocks and posterior nuchal area (extensor surfaces). Almost all patients have an associated, usually subclinical, gluten sensitive enteropathy. More than 90% express the HLA B8/DRW3 and HLA DQW2. Mainstay of treatment is dapsone. Strictly exclude gluten from the diet. Granular IgA deposits in dermal papillae of perilesional skin observed by direct immunofluorescence is the gold standard of diagnosis.	Subepidermal blister with neutrophils in the dermal papillae.
Linear IgA disease	Extremely itchy small papules and vesicles on extensor surfaces, occasionally larger arciform blisters. Linear band of IgA at BMZ.	Subepidermal blister with neutrophils in the dermal papillae.
Cicatricial pemphigoid	Erosive and/or blistering lesions of mucous membranes and possibly the skin; scarring at some sites.	Subepithelial blister and may or may not be a/w a mononuclear cell-rich infiltrate.

130. Answer is d (Donovanosis).
Ref: Dermatology, by Otto Braun Falco, 2nd edition 2000. Pg 293, Table 5.11.

- In ***donovanosis (granuloma inguinale) subcutaneous granulomas*** may form, which may be mistaken for enlarged lymph nodes—hence the name 'pseudobubo'.

131. Answer is d (Parkinson's disease).
Ref: Harrison's, 17th edition Pg 315.

- Although it is ***frequently*** seen in patients with ***Parkinson's disease***, in those who have had ***cerebrovascular accident*** and in those with ***HIV infection***, the overwhelming majority of individuals with ***seborrheic dermatitis*** have no underlying disorder.

132. Answer is c (Evanescent).
Ref: Harrison's, 17th edition Pg 312, Fig 52-11; 330.

- Urticaria (hives) are ***transient lesions*** that are composed of a central wheal surrounded by an erythematous halo.
- Individual lesions are round, oval or figurate and are ***often pruritic***. Acute and chronic urticaria has a wide variety of allergic etiologies and reflect edema in the dermis. Urticarial lesions can also be seen in patients with mastocytosis (***urticaria pigmentosa, Darier's sign***), hyperthyroidism and systemic-onset juvenile idiopathic arthritis (Still's disease).
- Discrete and confluent, edematous, erythematous ***papules and plaques*** are characteristic of this whealing eruption.

133. Answer is a (*Chlamydia trachomatis*).
Ref: Harrison's, 17th edition Pg 823.

- ***Non-gonococcal urethritis*** refers to urethritis where gonococci cannot be demonstrated by microscopy or culture.
- ***Most common cause*** in 30–50% is ***Chlamydia trachomatis***.

RADIOLOGY

134. Answer is c (Chronic obstructive nephropathy).
Ref: Uroradiology, Pg 74.

- ***Rim nephrogram*** = Rim of cortex receiving collateral blood flow from capsular, peripelvic and periureteric vessels; most specific indicator of renovascular compromise; 2–4 mm peripheral band of cortical opacification.
- Causes:
  - Acute total main renal artery occlusion: Seen in 50% cases with renal infarction
  - Renal vein thrombosis
  - Acute tubular necrosis
  - ***Severe chronic urinary obstruction***
- D/D—severe hydronephrosis.

135. Answer is a (Poland syndrome).
Ref: Chapman's Aids to radiological D/D, 5th edition Stephen Davies, 2009. Pg 168.

D/D of Unilateral Hypertransradiant hemithorax

- ***Rotation***—poor technique, scoliosis—the hypertransradiant hemithorax is on the side to which the patient is turned.
- ***Chest wall***
  - Mastectomy (absent breast)
  - Poliomyelitis (atrophy of pectoral muscles)
  - ***Poland's syndrome*** (unilateral congenital absence of pectoral muscles +/- rib defects, syndactyly).
- ***Pleura***
  - Pneumothorax.
- ***Lungs***
  - Compensatory emphysema
  - Airway obstruction
  - Unilateral bullae
  - Swyer James (McLeod's) syndrome: Late sequelae of childhood bronchiolitis
  - Congenital lobar emphysema.

136. Answer is a (Intravenous urography).
Ref: Imaging of Kidney Cancer, By Ali Guermazi, Pg 128.

- On ***intravenous urography (IVU) renal transitional cell Ca*** manifests as a filling defect within the contrast enhanced renal collecting system. Filling defects may be single or multiple, smooth, irregular or stippled.
- The ***'stipple sign'*** refers to tracking of contrast material into the interstices of a papillary lesion. This sign however may also be seen with blood clots and fungal balls and should be interpreted with caution.

137. Answer is a (Adenocarcinoma of the colon).
Ref: Chapman's Aids to radiological D/D, Stephen Davies, 2009. Pg 168.

- ***Calcification*** is uncommon in hepatic metastases, but ***colloid carcinoma of the rectum, colon or stomach*** may ***calcify most frequently***.
- It may be amorphous, stippled, granular, flaky and solitary/multiple.

138. Answer is b (Systemic lupus erythematosus).
Ref: Harrison's, 17th edition Pg 2078.

- Life-threatening ***pulmonary manifestations of SLE*** include
  - Interstitial inflammation leading to fibrosis
  - ***Shrinking lung syndrome***
  - Intra-alveolar hemorrhage.
- All of these probably require early aggressive immunosuppressive therapy as well as supportive care.
- The ***most common pulmonary manifestation of SLE is pleuritis with or without pleural effusion***. This manifestation, when mild, may respond to treatment with non-steroidal anti-inflammatory drugs (NSAIDs); when more severe, patients require a brief course of glucocorticoid therapy. Pulmonary infiltrates also occur as a manifestation of active SLE and are difficult to distinguish from infection on imaging studies.

139. Answer is c (Constrictive pericarditis).
Ref: Harrison's, 17th edition Pg 1493.

- In ***constrictive pericarditis***, the ventricular pressure pulses in both ventricles exhibit characteristic ***'square root' sign*** during diastole.

ANESTHESIA

140. Answer is b (Procaine).
Ref: KD Tripathi, 6th edition Pg 351, 357.

- Procaine is ***NOT*** a surface anesthetic.
- Procaine is a low potency, short duration acting injectable anesthetic; practically not used now since lignocaine is available.
- Procaine was the first synthetic local anesthetic.

Classification of surface anesthetics

Soluble	Insoluble
❖ Cocaine	❖ Benzocaine
❖ Lidocaine	❖ Butyl aminobenzoate (Butamben)
❖ Tetracaine	❖ Oxethazaine
❖ Benoxinate	

141. Answer is c (Nitrous oxide).
Ref: KD Tripathi, 6th edition Pg 371.

- ***Nitrous oxide*** *can expand pneumothorax* and other abnormal air pockets in the body—hence ***contraindicated in pneumothorax***.

142. Answer is d (Diazepam).
Ref: Goodman and Gilman's, Manual of Pharmacology and Therapeutics, Pg 231, 2007 edition.

Ketamine

• Pharmacology	– A phencyclidine derivative – Produces an anesthetic state frequently called *'dissociative anesthesia'* which implies that the patient is detached from their surroundings – ***Vivid hallucinations are common during recovery (emergence delirium)*** and can be minimized by concurrent use of benzodiazepines
• Systemic Effects	– ↑↑ *BP, IOP, ICT*; may be dangerous for hypertensives and in ischemic heart disease; since heart rate, BP, cardiac output are well-maintained even in *shocked patients*, it is *useful in emergency surgery*; laryngeal reflexes are better maintained and *bronchodilation* occurs; it ↓ salivation
• Advantages	– Ketamine can also be administered by *IM* injection even when venous access is difficult – Common procedures undertaken with ketamine anesthesia include minor to intermediate orthopedic surgery (especially distal arm or lower leg surgery including manipulation of fractures), gynecological surgery (e.g. dilatation and curettage and other minor surgical procedures), drainage of abscesses, debridement of burns, change of dressings

143. Answer is c (Circumoral numbness).
Ref: Cousins and Bridenbaugh's Neural Blockade in Clinical Anesthesia and Pain Medicine, Michael J Cousins, 4th edition Pg 114.

- **Feature of systemic absorption of local anesthetics**
  - ***Perioral numbness or paresthesia***, lightheadedness, muscular twitching, tinnitus, visual disturbances—***classical initial features***.
  - Later—convulsions, coma, respiratory arrest and finally cardiovascular arrest may follow.

144. Answer is d (Domiciliary CPAP).
Ref: Harrison's, 17th edition Pg 667.

- *Continuous positive airway pressure* **(CPAP)** and *mandibular repositioning splint* **(MRS)** are the *two most widely used* and *best evidence-based therapies for* ***obstructive sleep apnea***.
- Direct comparisons in randomized control trials indicate better outcomes with CPAP in terms of apneas and hypopneas, nocturnal oxygenation, symptoms, quality of life, mood and vigilance.
- Adherence to CPAP is generally better than to an MRS and there is evidence that CPAP improves driving, whereas there are no such data on MRSs. Thus, ***CPAP is the current treatment of choice***.
- However, MRSs are evidence-based second-line therapy in those who fail CPAP. In younger, thinner patients, maxillomandibular advancement should be considered.

145. Answer is c (Propoxyphene).
Ref: Pediatrics, by Lucy M Osborn, Pg 247.

- ***Pulseless electrical activity***, also called ***electromechanical dissociation*** is the condition in which peripheral pulses are not palpable, but heart shows some electrical activity on ECG other than ventricular tachycardia and ventricular fibrillation.
- Causes are:

'4 T's'	*'4 H's'*
❖ Tension pneumothorax ❖ Cardiac tamponade ❖ Pulmonary thromboembolism ❖ Toxins (beta blockers, calcium channel blockers, digitalis)	❖ Hypoxia ❖ Hypovolemia ❖ Hypothermia ❖ Hypokalemia

PSYCHIATRY

146. Answer is d (Dopaminergic blockers).
Ref: Harrison's, 17th edition Pg 2712.

- Treatment of anxiety disorders includes:
  - ***Benzodiazepines***
  - ***Antidepressants***
  - ***Buspirone*** (5-HT1A partial agonist; very long-acting; low abuse (dependence/withdrawal) potential; no sedation, anticonvulsant or muscle relaxant properties. Used for generalized anxiety disorder, chronic anxiety).

147. Answer is b (70).
Ref: Niraj Ahuja's psychiatry, 6th edition Pg 169.

- ***Intelligence quotient (IQ)*** = Mental age (MA) divided by chronological age (CA) multiplied by 100, i.e.

IQ = MA/CA × 100; according to Stanford-Binet

- Stanford-Binet and Wechsler are the most famous test of IQ.

Classification of Mental Retardation (MR)

Grade	IQ
Mild	50–70
Moderate	35–49
Severe	20–34
Profound	< 20

148. Answer is c (Grinding of teeth during sleep).
Ref: Harrison's, 17th edition Pg 178.

- ***Bruxism*** is an involuntary, ***forceful grinding of teeth during sleep*** that affects 10–20% of the population. The patient is usually unaware of the problem.

149. Answer is c (Auditory hallucinations).
Ref: Niraj ahuja's psychiatry, 6th edition Pg 60, 63.

- **Positive symptoms of schizophrenia**
  - These are characterized by *excessive function*
  - Positive symptoms include ***delusions, hallucinations, strange behavior and talkativeness***
  - These *symptoms respond well to treatment with antipsychotic agents.*
- **Negative symptoms of schizophrenia**
  - These are characterized by decreased function
  - Negative symptoms ***respond better*** **to** ***atypical antipsychotics*** such as ***clozapine***, olanzapine, quetiapine and risperidone.
  - Negative symptoms include
    - ❖ Affective flattening
    - ❖ Attention impairment
    - ❖ Avolition apathy (lack of initiative)
    - ❖ Anhedonia (inability to experience pleasure)
    - ❖ Asociality (social withdrawal)
    - ❖ Alogia (lack of speech output).

150. Answer is a (Sexual pleasure derived from observing people in sexual acts).
Ref: Narayan Reddy's FMT, 23rd edition Pg 197.

- ***Voyeurism or scoptophilia*** is the counterpart of exhibitionism.
- The voyeur, so called 'peeping tom' must see people undress in order to be sexually satisfied.
- In this there is a morbid desire to look at the sexual organs or other usually clothed body parts of one of the opposite sex or to ***watch sexual intercourse as a source of sexual gratification***.

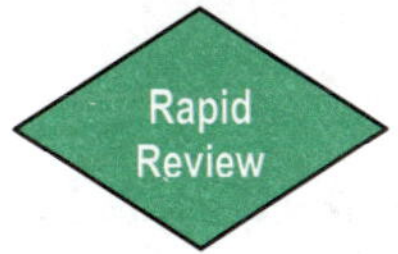

Summary of Sexual Paraphilias

Paraphilias (sexual deviations or sexual perversions) refer to preferential use of unusual objects of sexual desire or engagement in unusual sexual activity over a period of at least 6 months, causing impairment in occupational or social functioning.

■ **Fetishism**	Sexual preference for ***inanimate objects*** (e.g. women's shoes, stockings, bras, rubber sheets).
■ **Transvestism**	Men gaining sexual gratification from ***wearing women's clothing***, particularly undergarments.
■ **Exhibitionism**	Almost exclusively seen in males; Persistent method of sexual arousal by ***revealing one's genitals*** to unsuspecting women so that they will be shocked. This is followed by masturbation to achieve orgasm.
■ **Frotteurism**	Obtaining sexual gratification by rubbing the penis against a woman who is nonconsenting and unaware (e.g. ***in crowded buses***).
■ **Sadism or masochism**	Obtaining sexual pleasure from giving (sadism) or receiving (masochism) ***physical pain or humiliation.***
■ **Voyeurism**	Obtaining sexual pleasure from ***secretly watching people*** (often with binoculars) undressing or engaging in sexual activity.
■ **Pedophilia**	Obtaining sexual gratification through fantasies or behaviors with ***children of the opposite or same sex***; the pedophile must be at least 16 years of age and 5-year older than the victim.
■ **Zoophilia (Bestiality)**	Persistent and significant involvement in sexual activity with ***animals.***
■ **Telephone scatologia**	Gaining sexual pleasure from making telephone calls to unsuspecting women and engaging them in conversations of a sexual nature.
■ **Miscellaneous**	Sexual arousal with ***urine (urophilia); corpses (necrophilia); feces (coprophilia); enemas (klismaphilia)***, etc.

151. Answer is c (Cocaine).
Ref: Davidson's, 20th edition Pg 213.

- ***Cocaine*** (hydrochloride) is usually purchased as a white crystalline powder or colorless crystals. ***'Crack'*** is cocaine that has been separated from its hydrochloride base, free melted and smoked in a pipe or mixed with tobacco in a cigarette to give a rapid onset of effect similar to IV use.
- Any amount over 1g is potentially fatal.
- ***Mild-to-moderate intoxication***: Euphoria, agitation, cerebellar signs, dilated pupils, aggression, vomiting, pallor. Headache, cold sweats, pyrexia, twitching, tachycardia, hallucinations and hypertension.

- *Severe intoxication*: Convulsions coma, muscular paralysis, stroke, hypertension.
- A ***toxic psychosis*** occurs with high levels of consumption and ***tactile hallucinations (formication)*** may be prominent.

ANATOMY, PHYSIOLOGY AND BIOCHEMISTRY

152. Answer is c (Sympathetic nerves).
Ref: BD Chaurasia, Vol 2, Pg 184.

- The ***dartos muscle is involuntary*** and is ***supplied by sympathetic fibers*** passing through the ***genital branch of the genitofemoral nerve.***
- ***Dartos muscle helps in regulation of temperature within the scrotum.***

153. Answer is d (Subclavius).
Ref: BD Chaurasia, Vol 1, Pg 29.

- The ***clavipectoral fascia*** is a fibrous sheet situated deep to the clavicular portion of the pectoralis major muscle.
- It ***extends from*** the clavicle above to the axillary fascia below:
  - ☐ Its ***upper part splits*** to enclose the ***subclavius*** muscle
  - ☐ Its ***lower part splits*** to enclose the ***pectoralis minor*** muscle.
- The upper part of this fascia is thick and is called the costocoracoid ligament.

154. Answer is d (Loop of Henle).
Ref: Harrison's, 17th edition Pg 1742.

- Tubuloglomerular feedback changes the rate of filtration and tubular flow by reflex vasoconstriction or dilatation of the afferent arteriole.
- Tubuloglomerular feedback is mediated by specialized cells in the ***thick ascending limb of the loop of Henle*** called the ***macula densa*** that act as sensors of solute concentration and flow of tubular fluid.

155. Answer is c (D10–D12).
Ref: BD Chaurasia, Vol 2. Pg 260.

156. Answer is a (Septum primum).
Ref: Essential anatomy, Keith moore. Pg 126.

- Found in the right atrium of the heart, the ***fossa ovalis is an embryonic remnant of the foramen ovale,*** which normally closes shortly after birth.
- The muscular part of the atrial septum is derived from the septum secundum fused with the septum primum.
- The ostium secundum is covered by the septum secundum.
- The limbus fossae ovalis is the free border of the septum secundum.
- The ***floor of the fossa ovalis is formed of septum primum:*** It is thin and membranous and forms the flap valve mechanism.

157. Answer is a (Midbrain).
Ref: BD Chaurasia, Vol 1, Pg 311.

Parts of Developing Brain

- The cavity of the developing brain shows three dilatations, craniocaudally these are given in the table below.

Developing brain		**Adult derivatives**
Prosencephalon (Forebrain)	→ Telencephalon (Endbrain)	→ Cerebral hemispheres and lateral ventricle
	→ Diencephalon	→ Thalamus, hypothalamus, optic stalk, posterior pituitary and 3rd ventricle

Mesencephalon	→ Midbrain	→ Aqueduct
Rhombencephalon (Hindbrain)	→ Metencephalon	→ Pons and cerebellum and 4th ventricle
	→ Myelencephalon	→ Medulla oblongata

158. Answer is a (T5).
Ref: BD Chaurasia, Vol 1, Pg 199.

Highlights of Thoracic Duct

- ***Largest lymphatic vessel*** in the body
- Extends from the upper part of the abdomen to the lower part of the neck, crossing the posterior and superior parts of the mediastinum
- About ***18 inches long***
- Has a beaded appearance due to the many valves in its lumen.

Course of Thoracic Duct

- It begins as a continuation of the upper end of the cisterna chyli (near the lower border of T12) and enters the thorax through the aortic opening in the diaphragm
- It then ascends through the posterior mediastinum ***crossing from the right side to the left at the level of the T5***. It then runs through the superior mediastinum along the left edge of the esophagus and reaches the neck
- In the neck it arches laterally (at the level of the transverse process of C7)
- Finally it descends in front of the first part of the left subclavian vein and ends by opening into the angle of junction between the left subclavian and left internal jugular veins.

159. Answer is a (Testosterone).
Ref: Ganong, 23rd edition Pg 406.

- ***Testosterone the principal hormone of the testis*** is a C19 steroid with an –OH group in the 17 position.
- It is ***synthesized from cholesterol in the Leydig cells*** and is also formed from *androstenedione secreted by the adrenal cortex.*
- 98% of testosterone in plasma is bound to proteins. 65% is bound to a β-globulin called gonadal steroid-binding globulin (GBG) and 33% to albumin.

160. Answer is c (–70 mV).
Ref: Ganong, 23rd edition Pg 84.

- In ***neurons***, the ***resting membrane potential is usually about –70 mV,*** which is close to the equilibrium potential for K^+.

161. Answer is c (Hypothermia).
Ref: Davidson's, 20th edition Pg 184; Ganong, 23rd edition Pg 611.

Shift of curve to right (Hb easily **R**eleases O_2) *'**R**ight shift **R**eleases'*	**Shift of curve to left** (Hb does not release O_2 easily → tissue hypoxia)
↑ P**C** O_2 **A**nemia; high **A**ltitudes; **A**cidosis (↓ pH) ↑ 2,3-**D**PG **E**xercise ↑ **T**emperature (acidosis) **Right** shift <u>Mnemonic</u> = *'CADET face **Right**'*	↓ PC O_2 ↓ 2,3-DPG ↓ Temperature ↑ pH (alkalosis) Fetal Hb (HbF) Methemoglobin and carboxyhemoglobin Rare hemoglobinopathies (Chesapeake and Heathrow)

162. Answer is c (Arterial turbulence).
Ref: Principles of Medical Physiology, Sabysachi Sircar, Pg 256.

- In the auscultatory method of measuring blood pressure a stethoscope is placed over the brachial artery in the cubital fossa
- Sounds called ***Korotkoff sounds*** appear at the systolic pressure and disappear at the diastolic pressure
- These sounds have ***been attributed to turbulence caused by partial occlusion of the artery.***

163. Answer is d (Ganglion cells).
Ref: Ganong, 23rd edition Pg 190.

- The eye is unique in that the receptor potential of the photoreceptors (rods and cones) and the electrical responses of most of the other neural elements in the retina are local, graded potentials and it is ***only in the ganglion cells that all-or-none action potentials*** transmitted over appreciable distances ***are recorded***.
- These ***action potentials in the ganglion cells*** are transmitted to the brain.

164. Answer is c (Dopamine).
Ref: Diseases of kidney and urinary tract, Robert WS, 8th edition 2007. Pg 251.

- ***Dopamine inhibits Na^+K^+ATPase activity.***

165. Answer is d (Sertoli cell).
Ref: Harrison's, 17th edition Pg 2312.

- The seminiferous tubules are convoluted, closed loops with both ends emptying into the rete testis, a network of progressively larger efferent ducts that ultimately form the epididymis. The seminiferous tubules total about 600 m in length and comprise about two thirds of testis volume. The walls of the tubules are formed by polarized Sertoli cells that are apposed to peritubular myoid cells.
- ***Tight junctions between Sertoli cells*** create a ***blood-testis barrier.***

166. Answer is d (Type II Pneumocytes).
Ref: Ganong, 23rd edition Pg 597.

SurfacTanT

- Dipalmitoyl lecithin
- Produced by Type **II** pneumocytes
- ↓ alveolar surface tension
- ↑ compliance
- ↓ work of inspiration

167. Answer is b (Up to 10^8/mL anaerobic bacteria).
Ref: Biotherapeutic agents and infectious diseases, Gary Elmer, Pg 86.

- Saliva contains a mixture of microorganisms from the buccal epithelium, the dorsum of the tongue, the tooth surfaces, the gingival crevices and the tonsillar crypts.
- The ***number of microorganisms in saliva is 10^8–10^9 CFU/mL*** and the ***relative proportion of anaerobic to aerobic numbers is 10:1***.
- The ***predominant bacteria are*** *Veillonella,* lactobacilli, *Actinomyces, Bacteroides, Prevotella,* porphyromonas and fusobacteria.

168. Answer is c (Estradiol).
Ref: Textbook of Biochemistry, Vasudevan, 5th edition Pg 380, Table 36.1.

Hormones that bind to intracellular receptors

- Glucocorticoids
- Mineralocorticoids
- Estrogens
- Progesterone
- Androgens
- Calcitriol
- Thyroxine

169. Answer is b (Two adjacent Z lines).
Ref: Ganong, 23rd edition Pg 95.

Physiologic Anatomy of Muscle Fiber

- Each muscle fiber is a single cell that is long, multinucleated, cylindric and surrounded by a cell membrane, the **sarcolemma**. The muscle fiber is in turn made up of myofibrils, in turn made up of individual filaments, made up of contractile proteins.
- Muscle contractile proteins are **actin**, **myosin**, **troponin** (I, T, C) and **tropomyosin**.
- **Troponin**: Present in skeletal and cardiac muscles, but not smooth muscle. Has 3 subunits:
  1. Troponin **T**: binds to **T**ropomyosin.
  2. Troponin **I**: **I**nhibits myosin-actin interaction.
  3. Troponin **C**: binds **C**alcium and brings about **C**ontraction by removing effect of tropomyosin.
- Differences in the refractive indexes of the various parts of the skeletal muscle are responsible for the cross striations seen.
- The lIghter **I** band is divided by the dark Z line and the dArker **A** band is divided by the lighter H line. *"**HAZI** = H line is in A band and Z line is in I band".*
- ***The area between two adjacent Z lines is a sarcomere.***
- **Actinin** binds actin to the Z lines.
- **Titin** connects Z lines to the M-lines and provides scaffolding to the sarcomere.
- **Desmin** binds the Z lines to the plasma membrane.
- **Sarcotubular system**: T tubules and sarcoplasmic reticulum.
- **Motor unit**: Each single motor neuron and the muscle fiber innervates is called motor unit.

170. Answer is c (Glycine).
Ref: Ganong, 23rd edition Pg 140, 142; Harrison's, 17th edition Pg 2479.

- ***Glycine*** is the major ***inhibitory neurotransmitter*** in ***spinal cord***
- ***GABA*** is the major ***inhibitory mediator in the brain***, including being responsible for presynaptic inhibition
- ***Glutamate*** is the main ***excitatory transmitter in the brain and spinal cord***.

171. Answer is b (RNA).
Ref: Textbook of Biochemistry, Vasudevan, 5th edition Pg 454.

• *Northern blotting*	To demonstrate specific *RNA*
• *Southern blotting*	To detect a specific segment of *DNA* in the whole genome
• *Western blotting*	*Proteins* (not nucleic acids) are identified

Mnemonic: 'North Rotis, South Dosas'.

172. Answer is c (Malondialdehyde).
Ref: Textbook of Biochemistry, Vasudevan, 5th edition Pg 165, 355; Molecular and cellular mechanisms of toxicity, F Matteis, Pg 51.

Lipid peroxidation

- In vitro, ***lipid peroxidation would lead to rancidity*** of fats and oils.
- In vivo, the membrane lipids are more liable to attack by free radicals and produce damage to the integrity of the membrane.
- In naturally occurring lipids, antioxidants (including vitamin E) prevent the lipid peroxidation.
- Degradation products of lipid peroxidation is ***malondialdehyde, which is used as an index of lipid peroxidation.***

173. Answer is c (Creatinine).

Ref: Pediatric nephrology and urology: the requisites in pediatrics, Bernard SK, Pg 313.

- Whenever a child is able to cooperate, a timed ***24-hour urine collection*** will provide more complete information, including assessment of daily urine volume.
- ***Completeness of the collection is assessed by the creatinine excretion rate*** in mg/kg/24 h.

174. Answer is d (Retinol-binding protein).

Ref: Textbook of Biochemistry, Vasudevan, 5th edition Pg 241, Table 21.1.

- ***Electrophoresis*** is a commonly used separation technique.
- The term electrophoresis refers to movement of charged molecules under influence of an applied current.
- It is used to ***separate variety of compounds*** like proteins, lipoproteins, hemoglobins, etc.
- ***Prealbumin moves faster than albumin*** on electrophoresis and hence it is named so. It is more appropriately named ***transthyretin*** or thyroxine-binding prealbumin.
- ***Retinol-binding Protein (RBP)*** carries vitamin A. It is a low molecular weight protein and so is liable to be lost in the urine. To prevent this loss, RBP is attached with prealbumin, hence it also moves faster than albumin.

175. Answer is b (α-2 globulin).

Ref: Textbook of Biochemistry, Vasudevan, 5th edition Pg 242.

- ***Ceruloplasmin*** is ***blue*** in color (latin, ceruleus = blue).
- It is an ***α-2 globulin*** with molecular weight of 160,000 Daltons.

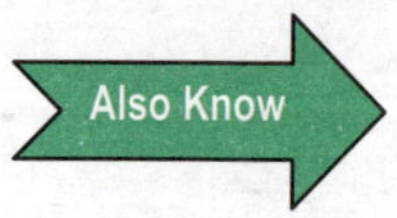

- It is synthesized in the ***liver***. It contains ***6–8 copper atoms*** per molecule.
- Ceruloplasmin is also called ***ferroxidase***, an enzyme which ***helps in incorporation of iron into transferrin***.
- 90% of copper content of plasma is bound with ceruloplasmin and 10% with albumin.
- Copper is bound with albumin loosely and so easily exchanged with tissues. Hence, ***transport protein for copper is albumin***.
- ***Ceruloplasmin*** is an important ***antioxidant*** in plasma.
- ***Lowered levels of ceruloplasmin*** is seen in ***Wilson's disease, malnutrition, nephrosis and cirrhosis***.
- Ceruloplasmin is an ***acute phase protein***. So, its level in blood is increased in all inflammatory conditions, collagen disorders and in malignancies.

176. Answer is a (Heme oxygenase).

Ref: Textbook of Biochemistry, Vasudevan, 5th edition Pg 265.

- The end products of ***heme catabolism*** are the ***bile pigments bilirubin and biliverdin***.
- Heme is degraded primarily by a microsomal enzyme system; heme oxygenase.

177. Answer is d (6–8 weeks).

Ref: Harrison's 17th edition Pg 2296.

- Measurement of ***glycated hemoglobin*** is the standard method for assessing long-term glycemic control

- When plasma glucose is consistently elevated, there is an increase in non-enzymatic glycation of hemoglobin; this alteration ***reflects the glycemic history over the previous 2–3 months***, since erythrocytes have an average life span of 120 days.

178. Answer is a (Insulin).
Ref: Harrison's, 17th edition Pg 2278.

- Once insulin is secreted into the portal venous system, ~50% is degraded by the liver
- ***Unextracted insulin*** enters the systemic circulation where it binds to receptors in target sites
- ***Insulin binding to its receptor stimulates intrinsic tyrosine kinase activity***, leading to receptor autophosphorylation and the recruitment of intracellular signaling molecules.

179. Answer is c (Proline).
Ref: Biology, By Raven, 2005, 7th edition Tata Mc Graw Hill. Pg 41.

- Special function amino acids have unique individual properties:
  - Methionine is often the first amino acid in a chain of amino acids
  - ***Proline causes kinks in chains***
  - Cysteine links chains together.

180. Answer is b [Creatine kinase (CK)].
Ref: Textbook of Biochemistry, Vasudevan, 5th edition Pg 54.

- ***Creatine kinase (CK)*** was called creatine phosphokinase in old literature
- ***Estimation of total CK is employed in muscular dystrophies*** and ***MB isoenzyme in acute myocardial infarction***.

Elevated Creatine Kinase

- Muscular dystrophies
- Crush injury
- Fractures
- Acute cerebrovascular accidents

About the other choices

- ***LDH level*** is 100 times more in RBCs and hence even minor hemolysis will increase LDH levels. In *myocardial infarction*, H4 isoenzyme is raised.
- ***Gamma-glutamyl transferase*** will increase in *alcoholic liver disease.*
- ***Alanine aminotransferase*** or SGPT is raised in *acute hepatitis.*

NOTES

COMED-K 2008

COMED-K 2008 QUESTIONS

MEDICINE

1. **Which of the following tests is most sensitive for detecting early diabetic nephropathy?**
   (a) Serum creatinine
   (b) Creatinine clearance
   (c) Microalbuminuria
   (d) Ultrasonography

2. **Unilateral steppage gait occurs in all *EXCEPT***
   (a) L5 radiculopathy
   (b) Sciatic neuropathy
   (c) Peroneal neuropathy
   (d) Distal polyneuropathy

3. **The drug of choice in paroxysmal supraventricular tachycardia is**
   (a) Digoxin
   (b) Adenosine
   (c) Nifedipine
   (d) Esmolol

4. **Which of the following tools can be used for self-monitoring of asthma?**
   (a) Spirometer
   (b) Peak flow meter
   (c) Plethysmograph
   (d) Ventilator

5. **In an asthmatic patient which of the following pulmonary functions would show the greater improvement on inhaling a bronchodilator?**
   (a) Tidal volume
   (b) FEV1
   (c) FEF 25–75%
   (d) FVC

6. **Increased frequency of HLA-B27 is seen in all the following diseases *EXCEPT***
   (a) Ankylosing spondylitis
   (b) Reiters syndrome
   (c) Acute anterior uveitis
   (d) Myasthenia gravis

7. **Wilson's disease is characterized by**
   (a) Low serum ceruloplasmin and low urinary copper
   (b) Low serum ceruloplasmin and high urinary copper
   (c) High serum ceruloplasmin and low urinary copper
   (d) High serum ceruloplasmin and high urinary copper

8. **The ECG change seen in hyperkalemia is**
   (a) Narrowing of the QRS complex
   (b) Increased amplitude of P waves
   (c) Narrowing and peaking of T waves
   (d) Prominent U waves

9. **Digoxin can accumulate to toxic levels in patients with**
   (a) Renal insufficiency
   (b) Chronic hepatitis
   (c) Advanced cirrhosis
   (d) Chronic pancreatitis

10. **Antigliadin antibodies are detectable in**
    (a) Tropical sprue
    (b) Whipple's disease
    (c) Celiac disease
    (d) Intestinal lymphoma

11. **Thrombocytopenia due to increased platelet destruction is seen in**
    (a) Aplastic anemia
    (b) Cancer chemotherapy
    (c) Acute leukemia
    (d) Systemic lupus erythematosus

12. **Refeeding edema is due to increased release of**
    (a) Growth hormone
    (b) Glucocorticoids
    (c) Insulin
    (d) Thyroxine

13. **Fetal erythropoiesis first occurs at what week of gestation?**
    (a) 6 weeks
    (b) 10 weeks
    (c) 12 weeks
    (d) 14 weeks

14. **The drug used in the treatment of idiopathic hypercalciuria is**
    (a) Allopurinol
    (b) Furosemide
    (c) Acetazolamide
    (d) Thiazide

15. **The systolic ejection murmur in hypertrophic obstructive cardiomyopathy is diminished when a patient**
    (a) Performs the Valsalva maneuver
    (b) Lies down

(c) Inhales amyl nitrite
(d) Stands up

16. **Multiple sites of narrowing of peripheral pulmonary artery occurs with**
(a) Roseola
(b) Rubeola
(c) Rubella
(d) Rocio virus disease

17. **Which of the following drugs is most likely to cause myocardial depression?**
(a) Morphine
(b) Thiopental
(c) Etomidate
(d) Ketamine

18. **The tumor causing polycythemia due to erythropoietin production is**
(a) Cerebellar hemangioma
(b) Medulloblastoma
(c) Ependymoma
(d) Oligodendroglioma

19. **Hemiparesis is NOT a feature of**
(a) Carotid artery occlusion
(b) MCA occlusion
(c) ACA occlusion
(d) Vertebral artery occlusion

20. **Which one of the following causes of hypoxemia is NOT corrected by giving supplemental oxygen?**
(a) Ventilation-perfusion mismatch
(b) Alveolar hypoventilation
(c) Impairment of diffusion
(d) Right-to-left shunt

21. **The single most useful clinical sign of severity of pneumonia in a person without underlying lung disease is**
(a) Temperature more than 38.5°C
(b) Heart rate more than 100/min
(c) Systolic BP less than 90 mm Hg
(d) Respiratory rate less than 30/min

22. **Microalbuminuria is defined as protein levels of**
(a) 100–150 mg/L
(b) 151–200 mg/L
(c) 201–300 mg/L
(d) 301–600 mg/L

23. **All are true of cerebral salt wasting *EXCEPT***
(a) Increased urine output
(b) Low intravascular volume
(c) Low uric acid in serum
(d) Decreased vasopressin levels

SURGERY

24. **The most common tumor of the minor salivary gland is**
(a) Mucoepidermoid carcinoma
(b) Acinic cell carcinoma
(c) Adenoid cystic carcinoma
(d) Pleomorphic adenocarcinoma

25. **Which one of the following is used as an irrigation solution during transurethral resection of the prostate?**
(a) 1.5% glycine
(b) Physiological saline
(c) Ringer's lactate
(d) 5% dextrose

26. **Prepyloric or channel ulcer in the stomach is termed as**
(a) Type 1
(b) Type 2
(c) Type 3
(d) Type 4

27. **The tumor marker for endodermal sinus tumor is**
(a) HCG
(b) Human placental lactogen
(c) CA 125
(d) Alpha-fetoprotein

28. **The most common benign tumor of the lung is**
(a) Hamartoma
(b) Alveolar adenoma
(c) Teratoma
(d) Fibroma

29. **Gray Turner's sign (flank discoloration) is seen in**
(a) Acute pyelonephritis
(b) Acute cholecystitis
(c) Acute pancreatitis
(d) Acute peritonitis

30. **The most common organism isolated in emphysematous pyelonephritis is**
(a) *E. coli*
(b) *Proteus*
(c) *Pseudomonas*
(d) *Klebsiella*

31. **Delphic nodes are**
(a) Pretracheal
(b) Paratracheal
(c) Supraclavicular
(d) Posterior triangle

32. **Pendred's syndrome is due to a defect in**
(a) Chromosome 7p
(b) Chromosome 7q
(c) Chromosome 8p
(d) Chromosome 8q

33. **The Reynold's pentad of fever, jaundice, right upper quadrant pain, septic shock and mental status change is typical of**
(a) Cholangitis
(b) Hepatitis
(c) Cholecystitis
(d) Pancreatitis

34. **The drug that has the fastest onset of action in benign prostatic hyperplasia is**
(a) Finasteride
(b) Tamsulosin
(c) Dutasteride
(d) Flutamide

35. **In a 6-year-old child with burns involving the whole of head and trunk, the estimated body surface area of burns is**
(a) 44%
(b) 52%
(c) 55%
(d) 58%

OBSTETRICS AND GYNECOLOGY

36. **The screening test for gestational diabetes mellitus that has the highest sensitivity is**
(a) Glycosylated Hb
(b) Blood fructosamine
(c) 50 g glucose challenge test
(d) Random blood sugar

37. **Dose of anti-D gamma globulin following first trimester abortion is**
(a) 50 μg
(b) 100 μg
(c) 200 μg
(d) 300 μg

38. **The best predictor of ovulation is**
(a) Estrogen peak
(b) Follicle-stimulating hormone (FSH) surge
(c) Onset of the LH surge
(d) Preovulatory rise in progesterone

39. **Partogram is used to**
(a) Assess the fetal well-being in labor
(b) Assess the condition of the baby at birth
(c) Record the events of pregnancy
(d) Assess the progress of labor

40. **All the following are used in first trimester MTP *EXCEPT***
(a) Dilation and evacuation
(b) Ru486
(c) Suction and evacuation
(d) Ethacridine extra amniotic

41. **Commonest tumor of the cervix is**
(a) Squamous cell Ca
(b) Adenocarcinoma
(c) Sarcoma
(d) Adenoacanthoma

42. **Oral contraceptive pill of choice in a lactating woman is**
(a) Monophasic pill
(b) Biphasic pill
(c) Triphasic pill
(d) Mini pill

PEDIATRICS

43. **Commonest cause of heart failure in infancy is**
(a) Myocarditis
(b) Rheumatic fever
(c) Cardiomyopathy
(d) Congenital heart disease

44. **Subacute sclerosing panencephalitis (SSPE) is associated with**
(a) Mumps
(b) Chickenpox
(c) Herpes
(d) Measles

45. **The earliest clinical sign of vitamin A deficiency is**
(a) Conjunctival xerosis
(b) Corneal xerosis
(c) Bitot's spots
(d) Keratomalacia

46. **Acute and recurrent pancreatitis is reported to occur in**
(a) Homocystinuria
(b) Maple syrup urine disorder
(c) Methylmalonic acidemia
(d) Tyrosinemia

47. **Which of the following drugs can help the patent ductus arteriosus prior to surgery for pulmonary stenosis in a neonate?**
(a) Alprostadil
(b) Indomethacin
(c) Carboprost
(d) Misoprostol

48. **The recommended drug for the prophylaxis of influenza A and B is**
(a) Acyclovir
(b) Ganciclovir
(c) Amantadine
(d) Foscarnet

49. **Congenital long QT syndrome is associated with neonatal**
(a) Sinus bradycardia
(b) Sinus tachycardia
(c) Supraventricular tachycardia
(d) Ventricular tachycardia

50. **An increase in protein without pleocytosis in cerebrospinal fluid is seen in**
(a) Froin's syndrome
(b) Guillain-Barré syndrome
(c) Pyogenic meningitis
(d) Tuberculous meningitis

ORTHOPEDICS

51. **Which of the following conditions is predominant in females?**
(a) Talipes equinovarus
(b) Cleft palate
(c) Congenital hip dislocation
(d) Pyloric stenosis

52. **The following are associated with fibular hemimelia *EXCEPT***
(a) Short tibia
(b) Anterior bowing of the leg
(c) Equinovalgus deformity of the foot and ankle
(d) Presence of polydactyly

53. **Which of the following tendons is lengthened in posteromedial soft tissue release for idiopathic congenital talipes equinovarus?**
(a) Tibialis anterior
(b) Tibialis posterior
(c) Extensor digitorum longus
(d) Flexor hallucis longus

54. **Most common medial meniscal tear is**
(a) Longitudinal tear
(b) Oblique tear
(c) Radial tear
(d) Horizontal tear

55. **Spina ventosa is caused by**
(a) Tuberculosis
(b) Leprosy
(c) Brucellosis
(d) Sickle cell disease

56. **Mucin clot test is done to detect**
(a) Mucin in stool
(b) Protein in CSF
(c) Hyaluronate in synovial fluid
(d) Protein in pleural fluid

57. **Association of sexual precocity, multiple cystic bone lesions and endocrinopathies are seen in**
(a) McCune-Albright syndrome
(b) Granulosa cell tumor
(c) Androblastoma
(d) Hepatoblastoma

ENT AND OPHTHALMOLOGY

58. **Recruitment phenomenon is seen in**
(a) Otosclerosis
(b) Meniere's disease
(c) Acoustic nerve schwannoma
(d) Otitis media with effusion

59. **Trotter's triad is seen in carcinoma of**
(a) Maxilla
(b) Larynx
(c) Nasopharynx
(d) Ethmoidal sinus

60. **A 28-year-old male complains of glare in both eyes. The cornea shows whorl like opacities of the epithelium. He also gave a history of long-term treatment with amiodarone. The most likely diagnosis is**
(a) Terrien's marginal degeneration
(b) Cornea verticillata
(c) Band-shaped keratopathy
(d) Arcus juvenilis

61. **All are causes of papilledema *EXCEPT***
(a) Cerebral tumors
(b) Friedreich's ataxia
(c) Cavernous sinus thrombosis
(d) Cerebral abscess

62. **Under the National Program for Control of Blindness, the goal is to reduce the prevalence of blindness to a level of**
(a) 0.1%
(b) 0.3%
(c) 0.5%
(d) 1%

63. **Spontaneous absorption of lenticular material is seen in**
(a) Myotonic dystrophy
(b) Hallermann-Streiff syndrome
(c) Aniridia
(d) Persistent hyperplastic primary vitreous

64. **The following are grades of binocular single vision, *EXCEPT***
(a) Simultaneous macular perception
(b) Fusion
(c) Stereopsis
(d) Suppression

65. **Swinging flash light test is used to examine**
(a) Cornea
(b) Pupil
(c) Lens
(d) Conjunctiva

66. **The first line of treatment of open-angle glaucoma is**
(a) Timolol
(b) Pilocarpine
(c) Epinephrine
(d) Carbonic anhydrase inhibitor

67. **The following bacteria can invade intact corneal epithelium *EXCEPT***
(a) *Neisseria gonorrhoeae*
(b) *Haemophilus influenzae*
(c) *Staphylococcus aureus*
(d) *Listeria* species

68. **Argon laser trabeculoplasty is done in**
(a) Open-angle glaucoma
(b) Secondary glaucoma
(c) Angle-recession glaucoma
(d) Angle-closure glaucoma

69. **Objective assessment of the refractive state**
(a) Retinoscopy
(b) Gonioscopy
(c) Ophthalmoscopy
(d) Keratoscopy

70. **Amaurosis fugax refers to occlusion of**
(a) Middle cerebral artery
(b) Retinal artery
(c) Renal vessels
(d) Mesenteric vessels

DERMATOLOGY, ANESTHESIOLOGY, RADIOLOGY AND PSYCHIATRY

71. **Perioral pallor and Dennie's line are seen in**
(a) Atopic dermatitis
(b) Chronic actinic dermatitis
(c) Blood dyscrasias
(d) Perioral contact dermatitis

72. **The causative agent of favus is**
(a) *Microsporum audouinii*
(b) *Microsporum canis*
(c) *Trichophyton mentagrophyte*
(d) *Trichophyton schoenleinii*

73. **Mycetoma is caused by the following agents *EXCEPT***
(a) *Allescheria boydii*
(b) *Madurella mycetoma*
(c) *Trichosporon beigelii*
(d) *Nocardia asteroides*

74. **Moth-eaten alopecia is seen in**
(a) Black dot tinea
(b) Telogen effluvium
(c) Alopecia areata
(d) Secondary syphilis

75. **Pitting of nails can be seen in**
(a) Tinea unguium
(b) Alopecia areata
(c) Androgenetic alopecia
(d) Peripheral vascular disease

76. **Antipsychotic induced 'akathisia' is characterized by**
(a) Rigidity
(b) Tremor
(c) Spasm of muscle/muscle group
(d) Restlessness

77. **Gustatory hallucinations are most commonly associated with**
(a) Temporal lobe epilepsy
(b) Grand mal epilepsy
(c) Anxiety disorders
(d) Tobacco dependence

78. **Early and reliable indication of air embolism during anesthesia can be obtained by continuous monitoring of**
(a) ECG
(b) Blood pressure
(c) End tidal CO_2
(d) Oxygen saturation

79. **The following is a life-threatening side effect associated with the use of clozapine**
(a) Pancreatitis
(b) Hypoglycemia
(c) Agranulocytosis
(d) Acute renal failure

80. **Agoraphobia is a disorder characterized by all *EXCEPT***
(a) Visual hallucinations
(b) Avoidance of situations in which it occurs
(c) Presence of panic symptoms
(d) A voidance of being outside alone

81. **Long-term use of lithium is associated with the following endocrine abnormality**

(a) Hypothyroidism
(b) Diabetes mellitus
(c) Hyperthyroidism
(d) Cushing's syndrome

82. Kienböck disease is due to avascular necrosis of the
(a) Talus
(b) Lunate
(c) Pisiform
(d) Medial tibial condyle

83. 'Bird of prey' sign is seen in the radiographic barium examination of
(a) Gastric volvulus
(b) Intussusception
(c) Sigmoid volvulus
(d) Cecal volvulus

84. Central stellate scar on CT scans are seen in
(a) Renal hemangiomas
(b) Renal oncocytomas
(c) Wilms' tumor
(d) Papillomas

85. Linear striations are typically seen in
(a) Vertebral myeloma
(b) Vertebral lymphangiomas
(c) Vertebral metastases
(d) Vertebral hemangiomas

86. Bone infarcts are seen in
(a) Iron deficiency anemia
(b) Thalassemia
(c) Sickle cell anemia
(d) Hereditary spherocytosis

87. Which of the following inhalation anesthetics should be avoided in middle ear surgery, when tympanic grafts are used?
(a) Halothane
(b) Nitrous oxide
(c) Ether
(d) Isoflurane

88. Which of the following local anesthetics is also an antiarrhythmic?
(a) Procaine
(b) Lignocaine
(c) Bupivacaine
(d) Cocaine

89. Which among the following general anesthetic causes cardiovascular stimulation?
(a) Thiopental
(b) Ketamine
(c) Midazolam
(d) Etomidate

90. Heimlich valve is used for drainage of
(a) Pneumothorax
(b) Hemothorax
(c) Empyema
(d) Malignant pleural effusion

91. A ventilator pressure relief valve stuck in closed position can result in
(a) Barotrauma
(b) Hypoventilation
(c) Hypoxia
(d) Hyperventilation

92. Nipple shadows on chest radiographs characteristically have a sharp
(a) Lateral margin
(b) Medial margin
(c) Inferior margin
(d) Superior margin

93. All the following are the radiological features of osteomalacia *EXCEPT*
(a) Triradiate pelvis
(b) Milkman's fractures
(c) Osteopenia
(d) Lytic lesions

94. At the end of 1 year of age, the number of carpal bones seen in the skiagram of the hand is
(a) Nil
(b) 1
(c) 2
(d) 3

FORENSIC MEDICINE

95. The species origin of blood can be detected by
(a) Benzidine test
(b) Takayama test
(c) Spectroscopy
(d) Precipitin test

96. The poison that can be detected after death in hair is
(a) Lead
(b) Copper
(c) Mercury
(d) Arsenic

97. Copper sulfate poisoning manifests with
(a) Acute hemolysis
(b) High anion gap acidosis
(c) Peripheral neuropathy
(d) Rhabdomyolysis

98. Sex can be established by examining hair root cells for the presence of

(a) Davidson body
(b) Barr body
(c) Golgi body
(d) Medullary index

99. Fetishism is a sexual perversion characterized
(a) Sexual focus on children
(b) Sexual focus on genital rubbing
(c) Sexual pleasure from pain
(d) Sexual pleasure derived from non-living things

100. Postmortem rigidity first starts in
(a) Eyelids
(b) Neck
(c) Upper limbs
(d) Lower limbs

101. In normal conditions of temperature and atmosphere, the rate of cooling of dead body is
(a) 1.0°F/hour
(b) 1.5°F/hour
(c) 2.0°F/hour
(d) 2.5°F/hour

102. Among the secondary changes in tooth the most useful one for age determination is
(a) Attrition
(b) Secondary dentin deposition
(c) Root resorption
(d) Root transparency

PATHOLOGY

103. The commonest gastric polyp is
(a) Hyperplastic polyp
(b) Inflammatory polyp
(c) Adenomatous polyp
(d) Part of familial polyposis

104. Periodic acid Schiff stain shows block positivity in
(a) Myeloblasts
(b) Lymphoblasts
(c) Monoblasts
(d) Megakaryoblasts

105. Berger nephropathy disease is due to mesangial deposition of
(a) Fibrin and C3
(b) IgD and C3
(c) IgE and C3
(d) IgA and C3

106. Bilateral renal cell carcinoma is seen in
(a) Eagle-Barrett syndrome
(b) Beckwith-Wiedemann syndrome
(c) von Hippel-Lindau disease
(d) Bilateral angiomyolipoma

107. Onion skin thickening of arteriolar wall is seen in
(a) Atherosclerosis
(b) Medial calcific sclerosis
(c) Hyaline arteriosclerosis
(d) Hyperplastic arteriosclerosis

108. The interstitial lung disease (ILD) showing granulomas on lung biopsy is
(a) Usual interstitial pneumonitis
(b) Sarcoidosis
(c) Diffuse alveolar damage
(d) Desquamative interstitial pneumonia

109. Pawn ball megakaryocytes are characteristic of
(a) Myelodysplastic syndrome
(b) Idiopathic thrombocytopenic purpura
(c) Thrombotic thrombocytopenic purpura
(d) Chloramphenicol toxicity

110. The most common site of ectopic pheochromocytoma is
(a) Organ of Zuckerkandl
(b) Bladder
(c) Filum terminale
(d) Celiac plexus

111. The commonest clinical pattern of basal cell carcinoma is
(a) Nodular
(b) Morpheaform
(c) Superficial
(d) Keratotic

112. In myocardial infarction, microscopic picture of coagulation necrosis with neutrophilic infiltration is seen in
(a) 4–12 hours
(b) 12–24 hours
(c) 1–3 days
(d) 3–7 days

113. Replication of EBV occurs in cells expressing
(a) CD4
(b) CD8
(c) CD21
(d) CD15

MICROBIOLOGY

114. Buruli ulcer is caused by
(a) *Mycobacterium ulcerans*
(b) *Mycobacterium marinum*
(c) *Mycobacterium kansasii*
(d) *Mycobacterium fortuitum*

115. Fecal leukocytes are absent in all the following *EXCEPT*
(a) Giardiasis
(b) Cryptosporidiosis
(c) Campylobacter infection
(d) Clostridium perfringens infection

116. The antibody produced during primary immune response is
(a) IgM
(b) IgG
(c) IgA
(d) IgE

117. Pneumonia alba is due to
(a) *Klebsiella*
(b) Streptococci
(c) *Treponema pallidum*
(d) Staphylococci

118. Which virus given below is not a teratogenic virus?
(a) Rubella
(b) Cytomegalovirus
(c) Herpes simplex
(d) Measles

119. An emerging viral pathogen causing pyelonephritis in kidney allografts is
(a) Molluscum contagiosum
(b) Herpes simplex virus
(c) Polyomavirus
(d) Influenza virus

120. Which one given below is a DNA virus?
(a) Poliovirus
(b) Adenovirus
(c) Parvovirus
(d) Hepatitis A virus

121. Which of immunoglobulins is associated with allergic disorders?
(a) IgG
(b) IgM
(c) IgA
(d) IgE

122. Which immunoglobulin crosses placenta?
(a) IgM
(b) IgA
(c) IgG
(d) IgD

123. Duffy blood group antigen negativity confers protection against infection by
(a) *Plasmodium falciparum*
(b) *Plasmodium ovale*
(c) *Plasmodium vivax*
(d) *Plasmodium malariae*

124. Vascular involvement and thrombosis is seen in
(a) Coccidioidomycosis
(b) Aspergillosis
(c) Mucormycosis
(d) Histoplasmosis

125. Undulant fever is caused by
(a) *Salmonella typhi*
(b) *Staphylococcus aureus*
(c) *Brucella melitensis*
(d) *Coxiella burnetii*

PHARMACOLOGY

126. Which among the following is *not* an adverse effect of furosemide?
(a) Hypokalemia
(b) Ototoxicity
(c) Hypercalcemia
(d) Hyperuricemia

127. Which one of the following is direct thrombin inhibitor?
(a) Enoxaparin
(b) Dalteparin
(c) Fondaparinux
(d) Argatroban

128. Metrifonate is effective against
(a) Amebiasis
(b) Leishmaniosis
(c) Schistosomiasis
(d) Giardiasis

129. Which among the following drug is safest in a patient allergic to penicillin?
(a) Cephalexin
(b) Imipenem
(c) Cefepime
(d) Aztreonam

130. Which of the following anti-tumor agents works by impairing de novo purine synthesis?
(a) Hydroxyurea
(b) 5-fluorouracil
(c) Methotrexate
(d) Allopurinol

131. Selenium sulfide is indicated for treating
(a) Tinea versicolor
(b) Tinea corporis
(c) Mixed mycotic infections
(d) Candidiasis only

132. **All of the following are tumor necrosis factor blocking agents *EXCEPT***
(a) Adalizumab
(b) Etanercept
(c) Infliximab
(d) Abciximab

133. **Which of the following does *not* increase neuromuscular blockade?**
(a) Clindamycin
(b) Lincomycin
(c) Streptomycin
(d) Erythromycin

134. **In case of drug that follows first order elimination**
(a) The rate of elimination is constant
(b) The elimination half-life varies with dose
(c) The clearance varies with dose
(d) The rate of elimination varies directly with dose

135. **Which among the following is a cell cycle specific antineoplastic drug?**
(a) Cyclophosphamide
(b) Doxorubicin
(c) Methotrexate
(d) Cisplatin

PREVENTIVE AND SOCIAL MEDICINE

136. **Among the pulses, the highest quantity of protein is present in**
(a) Green gram
(b) Red gram
(c) Soybean
(d) Black gram

137. **The maximum hours of work per week prescribed under the Factories Act is**
(a) 42
(b) 48
(c) 54
(d) 60

138. **Mineral oils are used in mosquito control measure as a**
(a) Personal protection method
(b) Larvicide
(c) Adulticide
(d) Space spray

139. **'Maldon teeth' is due to**
(a) Lead
(b) Fluoride
(c) Calcium
(d) Phosphorus

140. **The most common form of diabetic neuropathy is**
(a) Acute mononeuropathy
(b) Autonomic neuropathy
(c) Polyradiculopathy
(d) Distal symmetric polyneuropathy

141. **Bhopal gas tragedy is an example of**
(a) Point source epidemic
(b) Continuous epidemic
(c) Propagated epidemic
(d) Slow epidemic

142. **Sling psychrometer is used for measuring**
(a) Air velocity
(b) Rain fall
(c) Median radiant temperature
(d) Relative humidity

143. **Emporiatrics deals with the health**
(a) Farmers
(b) Travelers
(c) Industrial workers
(d) Mine workers

144. **The anopheles species most commonly found in coastal regions is**
(a) *Anopheles philippinensis*
(b) *Anopheles stephensi*
(c) *Anopheles fluviatilis*
(d) *Anopheles minimus*

145. **The recommended content of iodine in salt at the consumer level is**
(a) 10 ppm
(b) 15 ppm
(c) 20 ppm
(d) 30 ppm

146. **Yellow fever is absent in India because**
(a) Climatic conditions are not favorable
(b) Virus is not present
(c) Vector mosquito is absent
(d) Population is immune

147. **The objective of National Population Policy 2000 is to bring Total Fertility Rate to replacement levels by the year**
(a) 2005
(b) 2010
(c) 2015
(d) 2020

148. **Cu T 380A IUCD should be replaced once in**
(a) 4 years
(b) 6 years
(c) 8 years
(d) 10 years

149. Case-control study is a type of
(a) Descriptive epidemiological study
(b) Analytic study
(c) Longitudinal study
(d) Experimental epidemiological study

150. A full course of immunization against tetanus with 3 doses of tetanus toxoid, confers immunity for how many years?
(a) 5
(b) 10
(c) 15
(d) 20

151. Time required for development of parasite from the gametocyte to sporozoite stage in mosquito is called
(a) Extrinsic incubation period
(b) Intrinsic incubation period
(c) Generation time
(d) Median incubation period

152. The limit of loudness expressed as decibels that people can tolerate without substantial damage to their hearing is
(a) 55
(b) 65
(c) 75
(d) 85

153. The dangerous particle size causing pneumoconiosis varies from
(a) 100–150 μm
(b) 50–100 μm
(c) 10–50 μm
(d) 1–5 μm

ANATOMY, PHYSIOLOGY AND BIOCHEMISTRY

154. The principal polypeptide that increase food intake are the following *EXCEPT*
(a) Neuropeptide-Y
(b) Leptin
(c) Orexin-A
(d) B-endorphin

155. Ghrelin is responsible for
(a) Stimulation of appetite
(b) Suppression of appetite
(c) Stimulation of sleep
(d) Suppression of sleep

156. Normal portal vein pressure is
(a) < 3 mm Hg
(b) 3–5 mm Hg
(c) 5–10 mm Hg
(d) 10–12 mm Hg

157. The cofactor required for the activity of sulfite oxidase is
(a) Copper
(b) Selenium
(c) Molybdenum
(d) Zinc

158. CAMP action mediates all *EXCEPT*
(a) Glucagon
(b) Follicle-stimulating hormone
(c) Luteinizing hormone
(d) Estrogen

159. Gartner's duct is remnant of
(a) Mullerian duct
(b) Wolffian duct
(c) Cloacal duct
(d) Epoophoron

160. Which of the following types of nerve fibers carry pain?
(a) Aa
(b) Ab
(c) Ag
(d) Ad

161. The last tributary of the azygos vein is
(a) Right superior intercostal vein
(b) Hemiazygos vein
(c) Right bronchial vein
(d) Accessory azygos vein

162. Alpha fetoprotein is genetically and structurally related to
(a) Albumin
(b) Transferrin
(c) Fibrinogen
(d) Growth hormone

163. Which of the following *does not* cause an increase in serum amylase?
(a) Pancreatitis
(b) Carcinoma lung
(c) Renal failure
(d) Cardiac failure

164. Proximal convoluted tubule have which
(a) Aquaporin 1
(b) Aquaporin 2
(c) Aquaporin 5
(d) Aquaporin 9

165. The supraoptic nucleus of the hypothalamus is believed to control the secretion of which of the following hormones?
(a) Antidiuretic hormone
(b) Oxytocin
(c) Growth hormone
(d) Adrenocorticotropic

166. The estimation of 3-methylhistidine in urine is used to study
(a) Status of folate in the body
(b) Renal disease
(c) Skeletal muscle mass
(d) Protein absorption in the gut

167. Facial angle is a rough index of the degree of development of the
(a) Jaws
(b) Nose
(c) Brain
(d) Eyes

168. The preganglionic parasympathetic fibers to the parotid gland travel in
(a) Lesser petrosal nerve
(b) Greater petrosal nerve
(c) Deep petrosal nerve
(d) Internal carotid nerve

169. von Brunn's nest is seen in
(a) Normal urothelium
(b) Transitional cell carcinoma
(c) Squamous cell carcinoma
(d) Adenocarcinoma

170. Which of the following amino acids is purely ketogenic?
(a) Phenylalanine
(b) Leucine
(c) Proline
(d) Tyrosine

171. Which of the following laryngeal muscles is supplied by the external laryngeal nerve?
(a) Posterior cricoarytenoid
(b) Lateral cricoarytenoid
(c) Cricothyroid
(d) Thyroarytenoid

172. Which muscle is an abductor of the vocal cords
(a) Transverse arytenoid
(b) Oblique arytenoid
(c) Lateral thyroarytenoid
(d) Posterior cricoarytenoid

173. Biosynthesis of the enzyme pyruvate carboxylase is repressed by
(a) Insulin
(b) Glucagon
(c) Cortisol
(d) Epinephrine

174. The raphe nuclei located in lower pons and medulla secrete the following neurotransmitter
(a) Norepinephrine
(b) Dopamine
(c) Serotonin
(d) Acetylcholine

175. Superior colliculus is concerned with
(a) Olfaction
(b) Hearing
(c) Vision
(d) Pain sensation

176. Sclera is thinnest at
(a) Limbus
(b) Insertion of recti
(c) Posterior pole
(d) Equator

177. A major lipid of mitochondrial membrane is
(a) Lecithin
(b) Inositol
(c) Plasmalogen
(d) Cardiolipin

178. The single most important sign in suspecting early Volkmann's ischemic contracture is
(a) Pallor of fingers
(b) Pain
(c) Obliteration of pulse
(d) Paralysis of involved muscles

179. In the mucosal cells, triglycerides are formed primarily in the
(a) Rough endoplasmic reticulum
(b) Smooth endoplasmic reticulum
(c) Golgi apparatus
(d) Ribosomes

180. The epithelial lining of the urethra below the opening of the ejaculatory ducts is
(a) Stratified cuboidal epithelium
(b) Stratified columnar epithelium
(c) Transitional epithelium
(d) Stratified squamous epithelium

COMED-K 2008

ANSWERS AND EXPLANATIONS

MEDICINE

1. **Answer is c (Microalbuminuria).**

Ref: Harrison's, 17th edition Pg 1792, 2288, Fig 338-10; Davidson's, 20th edition Pg 841, Box 21.50, 21.51, 21.52, 21.53, Fig 21.17.

Direct quote:

"Glomerular hyperperfusion and renal hypertrophy occur ***in the first years after the onset of DM*** and are associated with ***an increase of the glomerular filtration rate (GFR)***. During the first 5 years of DM, thickening of the glomerular basement membrane, glomerular hypertrophy and mesangial volume expansion occur as the GFR returns to normal. ***After 5–10 years*** of type 1 DM, ***~40% of individuals begin to excrete small amounts of albumin in the urine.***"

Author's comments: *"Thus the earliest abnormality is hyperfiltration (increased GFR) and the earliest manifestation of the disease is microalbuminuria—that should make it clear."*

More About

- ***Microalbuminuria*** = Albuminuria in the range of ***30–300 mg/24 h*** in a 24-h collection or 30–300 μg/mg creatinine in a spot collection (preferred method).
- ***Type 1 and Type 2 DM:*** *Microalbuminuria appears 5–10 years after onset.*
- ***Microalbuminuria indicates incipient diabetic nephropathy*** and calls for aggressive management at which stage the disease may be ***potentially reversible*** (i.e. microalbuminuria can regress).
  - ***Type 2 DM***: Patients may present with *advanced diabetic nephropathy*.
  - ***Type 2 DM + Microalbuminuria = ↑ risk of cardiovascular events*** and death.
  - ***Type 2 DM***: 60% patients with DN have diabetic retinopathy.
  - ***Type 1 DM***: > 90% patients with DN have diabetic retinopathy. Thus do not forget to screen for retinopathy in type 1 DM.

Current recommendations for microalbuminuria testing:

- Type 1 DM: Annually from 5 years after diagnosis.
- Type 2 DM: Annually from the time of diagnosis.

Risk factors for developing diabetic nephropathy

- Hyperglycemia, dyslipidemia, HTN, smoking
- Long duration of diabetes
- Presence of other microvascular complications (retinopathy)
- Ethnicity (e.g. Pima Indians, Asian races)
- Family h/o diabetic nephropathy

Schematic of progression of renal abnormalities in DM

Thickening of glomerular basement membrane (at the time of microalbuminuria)

↓

Accumulation of matrix material in mesangium

↓

Nodular glomerulosclerosis (***Kimmelstiel-Wilson nodule***, characteristic of DN)

↓

End-stage renal disease (ESRD, time from microalbuminuria to EESRD is 10–20 years)

Prevention of diabetic nephropathy

- Strict blood glucose control
- Control of BP
- ***ACE inhibitors*** in type 1 DM
- ***ACE inhibitors*** or ***Angiotensin receptor blockers*** (ARBs) in type 2 DM.

2. **Answer is d (Distal polyneuropathy).**
Ref: Atlas of adult physical diagnosis, Dale Berg, Pg 190.

- ***Steppage gait*** is observed in patients who have ***foot drop*** due to peripheral neurologic disorders. It is:
  - *Usually unilateral*
  - Due to *injury to common peroneal nerve* at the level of fibular head in lateral portion of the knee.

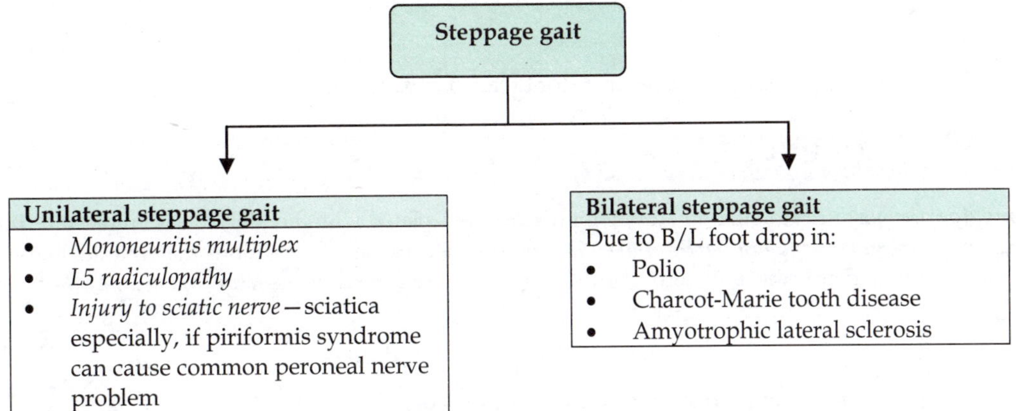

3. **Answer is b (Adenosine).**
Ref: KD Tripathi, 6th edition Pg 518.

Direct quote:
*"An attack of PSVT can be terminated by IV injection of verapamil diltiazem, esmolol or digoxin; BUT **most cardiologists NOW prefer adenosine.**"*

- ***Paroxysmal supraventricular (atrial) tachycardia*** is a regular, fast (160–220 beats per minute) heart rate that begins and ends suddenly, and originates in heart tissue other than that in the ventricles.
- When PSVT is not terminated by vagal maneuvers, short-term management involves ***intravenous adenosine***; advantages are:
  - Adenosine is a short-acting drug that blocks AV node conduction and it terminates 90% of tachycardias
  - Its rapid onset of action (usually within 10–25 seconds via a peripheral vein) and action lasts < 1 minute (short half-life of 10 seconds)
  - Efficacy equivalent to or better than verapamil
  - Safe in wide QRS tachycardia (verapamil is unsafe)
  - No hemodynamic deterioration (can be given to patients with hypotension, CHF or those receiving beta blockers).

4. **Answer is b (Peak flow meter).**
Ref: Davidson's, 20th edition Pg 673; Harrison's, 17th edition Pg 1602.

- A ***peak flow meter*** is a ***small, inexpensive, hand-held device used to manage asthma*** by monitoring airflow through the bronchi and thus the degree of obstruction in the airways.
- Ideally patients should be instructed to *record peak flow readings after rising in the morning and before retiring in the evening.*
- A ***diurnal variation in PEF*** (the lowest values being recorded in the morning) of ***more than 20% is considered diagnostic*** and the magnitude of variability provides some indication of disease severity.

Note:

A layman's guide to peak flow meter: "A peak flow meter for a patient with asthma is like a thermometer for a patient with a fever. Peak flow meters help to determine how open your airways are, rather than guessing just how you 'feel'. In some cases when you are not feeling well, you may feel 'hot' or 'feverish' but when you take your temperature with a thermometer, it is normal. With asthma, sometimes you may feel your breathing is 'tight' or your chest may feel 'heavy', but you are having normal lung function. The peak flow meter can help you determine whether your sense of chest tightness is really an airway change or not, just like the thermometer helps you to determine, if your hot feeling is really a fever."

5. **Answer is b (FEV1).**
Ref: Davidson's, 20th edition Pg 656, 673, Fig 19.20, Box 19.22.

Repeat Topic

- See ***answer no. 23 in COMED-K 2010 answers*** for detailed explanation.

6. **Answer is d (Myasthenia gravis).**
Ref: Harrison's, 17th edition Pg 2109.

- ***Spondyloarthropathies*** are inflammatory joint diseases associated with the MHC class I molecule ***HLA-B27***.
- The term ***seronegative spondyloarthropathy*** is used because this set of conditions may mimic rheumatoid diseases such as rheumatoid arthritis, BUT serological (blood) tests are ***typically negative for rheumatoid factor***.

HLA-B27 associated conditions

- Ankylosing spondylitis (Marie-Strumpell disease).
- Reactive arthritis (Reiter's syndrome)
- Enteropathic arthritis associated with inflammatory bowel disease
- Psoriatic arthritis
- Isolated acute anterior uveitis.

Also Know

Other autoimmune disease HLA associations

- Grave's disease : DR3
- *Myasthenia gravis* : DR3
- Rheumatoid arthritis : DR4
- Type 1 diabetes : DR3/DR4.

7. **Answer is b (Low serum ceruloplasmin and high urinary copper).**
Ref: Harrison's, 17th edition Pg 1981.

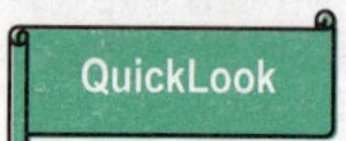

Wilson's Disease (Hepatolenticular Degeneration)

Etiology	Diagnosis
• ***AR***, inherited disorder of copper homeostasis; a/w ***mutation in ATP7B gene*** → results in ***excess accumulation of copper*** in ***liver*** and ***brain***	• ↓ ***ceruloplasmin level*** • ↑ ***urinary excretion of copper*** • ↑ ***hepatic copper level*** • Liver biopsy may show acute or chronic hepatitis or cirrhosis

	• MRI of the brain may show evidence of increased basal ganglia, brainstem and cerebellar copper even early in the course of the disease
Clinically	**Treatment**
• ***Liver-related features*: *Chronic hepatitis, hepatic steatosis and cirrhosis*** in ***adolescents and young adults*** • ***CNS features***: Indicates that liver disease is present and include ***speech disorders*** and various ***movement disorders*** • Eye: ***Kayser-Fleischer rings*** in the periphery of cornea—***copper deposition in Descemet's membrane***; best seen by ***slit lamp examination***	• Early in the treatment phase, ***restriction of dietary copper*** (shellfish, organ foods, nuts, mushrooms and chocolate) may be of value copper chelating medications such as ***D-penicillamine*** and ***trientine*** Oral ***zinc acetate*** competes with copper absorption in the gut and induces ***metallothionein*** in the intestine, which then sequesters copper and promotes fecal copper excretion

- Also see ***answer no. 24 in COMED-K 2009 answers*** for further details on serum ceruloplasmin.

8. **Answer is c (Narrowing and peaking of T waves).**
Ref: Harrison's, 17th edition Pg 284, 1395.

- ***ECG is essential*** and ***may be instrumental in diagnosing hyperkalemia*** in the appropriate clinical setting.
- ECG changes have a sequential progression of effects, which roughly correlate with the potassium level, but potentially life-threatening arrhythmias can occur without warning at almost any level of hyperkalemia.
  - Early changes of hyperkalemia include:
    - ***Peaked/Tall tented/ T waves***
    - Shortened QT interval
    - ST-segment depression.
  - These changes are followed by bundle-branch blocks causing a:
    - ***Widening of the QRS complex***
    - Increases in the PR interval
    - ***Decreased amplitude of the P wave.***
  - These changes reverse with appropriate treatment.
  - Without treatment:
    - The P wave eventually disappears
    - QRS morphology widens to resemble a ***'sine wave'***
    - Ventricular fibrillation or asystole follows.

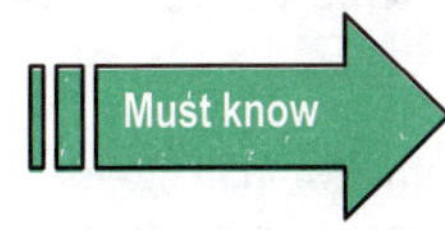

ECG Changes in Various Conditions—a Summary

Hypokalemia	Prominent *U-waves*, small T-waves, ventricular bigeminy.
*Hyper***calcemia**	*Shortens* Q-T interval.
*Hypo***calcemia**	*Lengthens* Q-T interval.
Subarachnoid hemorrhage	Marked QT prolongation with deep, wide T-wave inversions (*'CVA T-wave'*).
Hypothermia	Convex elevation of J point (*J waves or Osborn waves*).
Pericardial effusion	Total *electrical alternans* (often with tamponade).
TCA overdose	Sinus tachycardia with QRS and QT prolongation.
'Torsades de pointes' (QTC prolongation)	Seen with *hypokalemia, hypomagnesemia, various antiarrhythmic drugs (especially quinidine), phenothiazines and tricyclic antidepressants, liquid protein diets, intracranial events, third-degree AV block, drug interactions (erythromycin and terfenadine).*
Digoxin effect	*Shortened QT interval* with a characteristic 'scooping' of the ST-T wave complex, ST depression and inverted T-wave in V5-V6.

➲ **Pulmonary embolism**	Sinus tachycardia with an otherwise normal ECG is *commonest*. There may be deep S-waves in I, pathological Q-waves in III, inverted T-waves in III (*'SIQIIITIII'*), strain pattern V1-V3, right axis deviation, RBBB, atrial fibrillation.
➲ **Wolff-Parkinson-White (WPW) syndrome**	A wide QRS complex associated with a relatively short PR interval and slurring of the initial part of the QRS (***delta wave***), the latter effect due to aberrant activation of ventricular myocardium (by ***bundle of Kent***, accessory pathway from atria to ventricles bypassing VA node). Digoxin and verapamil are *contraindicated in WPW* syndrome since these drugs increase conduction in the accessory pathway.
➲ **Syndrome a/w prolonged QT interval**	*Romano-ward syndrome* (AD) and *Jervell Lange-Nielsen syndrome* (AR, associated with congenital deafness).
➲ **Lev's disease and Lenegre's disease**	Degenerative diseases commonly responsible for damage to the specialized conducting system and produce AV block usually associated with bundle branch block.
➲ **Left axis deviation (LAD)**	An axis more negative than 30° is referred to as LAD; may occur as a normal variant, but is more commonly a/w left ventricular hypertrophy, a block in the anterior fascicle of the left bundle system (left anterior fascicular block or hemiblock) or inferior MI.
➲ **Right axis deviation (RAD)**	An axis more positive than 100° is referred to as RAD. RAD also may occur as a normal variant (particularly in children and young adults), as a spurious finding due to reversal of the left and right arm electrodes, or in conditions such as right ventricular overload (acute or chronic), infarction of the lateral wall of the left ventricle, dextrocardia, left pneumothorax, or left posterior fascicular block.
➲ **Right bundle branch block (RBBB)**	More common than LBBB; RBBB occurs with heart disease, both congenital (e.g. atrial septal defect) and acquired (e.g. valvular, ischemic).
➲ **Left bundle branch block (LBBB)**	LBBB is often a marker of one of four underlying conditions: Ischemic heart disease, long-standing hypertension, severe aortic valve disease and cardiomyopathy.

9. Answer is a (Renal insufficiency).
Ref: KD Tripathi, 6th edition Pg 498.

- In patients with ***decreased kidney function (renal insufficiency)*** the half-life of ***digoxin*** is considerably longer—***dose has to be reduced.***

  OR
- Change to a different glycoside (such as digitoxin, which although having a much longer elimination half-life of around 7 days, is mainly eliminated from the body via the liver and thus not affected by changes in renal function).

☐ Also ***see answer no. 169 in COMED-K 2010 answers*** for antimicrobials needing dose reduction/avoidance in renal failure.

10. Answer is c (Celiac disease).
Ref: Harrison's, 17th edition Pg 1880.

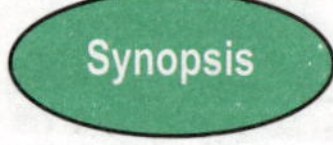

Celiac Disease

- ***Etiology***: It is caused by a immunologic reaction to gluten protein found in wheat, rye and barley. A/w HLA-DQ2 or DQ8; A/w dermatitis herpetiformis.
- Antibodies present are
  - ☐ ***Antigliadin IgA***

- ☐ ***Anti-tissue transglutaminase (tTG)*** and ***IgA anti-endomysium antibodies*** (AEA)—both have 90–95% sensitivity and 90–95% specificity.
- ***Clinically***: Small intestinal malabsorption disease; diarrhea, steatorrhea, weight loss, abdominal distention, weakness, muscle wasting or growth retardation (in children < 2 years).

> - ***Diagnosis***: ***Confirmed*** by ***small intestinal (duodenal/jejunal) biopsy***. Changes are restricted to the mucosa and include:
>   1. Absence or reduced height of villi, resulting in a flat/blunted appearance.
>   2. Increased loss of villous cells in a/w with increased crypt cell proliferation, resulting in crypt hyperplasia and loss of villous structure, with consequent villous, but not mucosal, atrophy.
>   3. Cuboidal appearance and nuclei that are no longer oriented basally in surface epithelial cells and increased intraepithelial lymphocytes.
>   4. Increased lymphocytes and plasma cells in the lamina propria.
> - The presence of a characteristic histologic appearance that reverts toward normal following the initiation of a gluten-free diet establishes the diagnosis of celiac sprue.

- ***Treatment***: Removal of gluten from diet.
- An increased incidence of both gastrointestinal and non-gastrointestinal neoplasms as well as intestinal lymphoma exists in patients with celiac sprue.

11. Answer is d (Systemic lupus erythematosus).
Ref: Davidson's, 20th edition Pg 1017, 1056.

Thrombocytopenia due to decreased production

- Vitamin B_{12} or folic acid deficiency
- *Leukemia* or myelodysplastic syndrome
- Decreased production of thrombopoietin by the liver in liver failure.
- Sepsis, systemic viral or bacterial infection
- Dengue fever can cause thrombocytopenia by direct infection of bone marrow megakaryocytes as well as immunological shortened platelet survival
- Hereditary syndromes:
  - Congenital amegakaryocytic thrombocytopenia (CAMT)
  - Thrombocytopenia absent radius syndrome
  - Fanconi anemia
  - Bernard-Soulier syndrome, associated with large platelets
  - May-Hegglin anomaly, the combination of thrombocytopenia, pale-blue leukocyte inclusions and giant platelets
  - Gray platelet syndrome
  - Alport's syndrome.

Thrombocytopenia due to increased platelet destruction

- Idiopathic thrombocytopenic purpura (ITP)
- Thrombotic thrombocytopenic purpura (TTP) and hemolytic-uremic syndrome (HUS)
- Disseminated intravascular coagulation (DIC)
- Paroxysmal nocturnal hemoglobinuria (PNH)
- Antiphospholipid syndrome
- *Systemic lupus erythematosus* (SLE)
- Post-transfusion purpura
- Neonatal alloimmune thrombocytopenia (NAITP)
- Splenic sequestration of platelets due to hypersplenism
- Dengue fever has been shown to cause shortened platelet survival and immunological platelet destruction
- HIV.

Thrombocytopenia due to direct myelosuppression
- Valproic acid
- Methotrexate
- Carboplatin
- Interferon
- Other *chemotherapy* drugs.

12. **Answer is c (Insulin).**
Ref: Harrison's, 17th edition Pg 460, 476.

- ***Refeeding edema** or **Refeeding syndrome*** is a syndrome consisting of metabolic disturbances that occur as a result of reinstitution of nutrition to patients who are starved or severely malnourished.
- ***Renourishment*** is the process of *avoiding refeeding syndrome*. The syndrome was first described in Japanese war prisoners after the Second World War.
- Refeeding syndrome usually occurs within 4 days of starting to feed. Patients can develop fluid and electrolyte disorders, especially ***hypophosphatemia***, along with neurologic, pulmonary, cardiac, neuromuscular and hematologic complications.
- Most effects result from a sudden shift from fat to carbohydrate metabolism and a ***sudden increase in insulin levels after refeeding***, which leads to increased cellular uptake of phosphate. This syndrome can occur at the beginning of treatment for anorexia nervosa when patients are reintroduced to a healthy diet. The shifting of electrolytes and fluid balance increases cardiac workload and heart rate. This can lead to acute heart failure.
- Patients at risk of refeeding syndrome include: Chronic alcoholics, drug abusers, the chronically malnourished (particularly the elderly), patients with anorexia nervosa, patients with prolonged nil by mouth or fasting times coupled with depletion or physiological stress.

13. **Answer is b (10 weeks).**
Ref: Dutta's Obstetrics, 6th edition Pg 42.

- Hematopoiesis is demonstrated in the embryonic phase first in the ***yolk sac by the 14th day***.
- By ***10th week liver*** becomes the major site.
- Gradually the RBC production sites extend to the spleen and bone marrow and at term, bone marrow becomes the major site of RBC production.

14. **Answer is d (Thiazide).**
Ref: Harrison's, 17th edition Pg 1816, 1818.

- ***Hydrochlorothiazide*** and other *thiazide – type* diuretics are the agents most frequently used to treat ***hypercalciuria***.
- May be used in children with hypercalciuria > 4 mg/kg/day that do not respond to dietary modifications.
- It may also be used in children who are at high risk for urinary stones (e.g. previous urinary stone, strong family history of stones) or decreased bone density on a low calcium diet.

15. **Answer is b (Lies down).**
Ref: Harrison's, 17th edition Pg 1484.

Murmur of Hypertrophic Obstructive Cardiomyopathy (HOCM)

- ***Systolic ejection murmur of HOCM*** typically is a systolic ***ejection crescendo-decrescendo murmur***, which is best heard between the apex and left sternal border and radiates to the suprasternal notch but not to the carotid arteries or neck.

Murmur diminishes with	Murmur increases with
▪ ↑ in preload (e.g. mueller maneuver, squatting) ▪ ↑ in afterload (e.g. handgrip, passive leg raising, pregnancy)	▪ ↓ in preload (e.g. valsalva maneuver, nitrate administration, diuretic administration, sudden standing) or with ▪ ↓ in afterload (e.g. vasodilator administration)

16. **Answer is c (Rubella).**
Ref: Harrison's, 17th edition Pg 1463.

Direct quote:

"***Multiple sites of narrowing of the peripheral pulmonary arteries*** are a feature of ***rubella embryopathy*** and may occur with both the familial and sporadic forms of supravalvular aortic stenosis."

- ***Patent ductus arteriosus*** is the ***most frequent lesion in maternal rubella syndrome*** along with ***peripheral pulmonary artery stenosis.***

17. **Answer is b (Thiopental).**
Ref: Lee's synopsis of Anesthesia, 13th edition Pg 154.

- ***Thiopentone*** directly ***depresses the contractile force of the heart***; it increases heart rate, coronary blood flow and the oxygen demand of the heart.
- Patients with *cardiac disease (particularly those with stenotic heart valve lesions) are at risk from the cardiovascular depressant effects of thiopentone.*

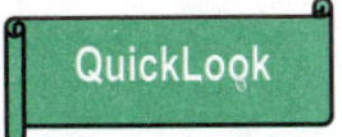

Systemic effects of sodium thiopentone

CNS	**CVS**
– Sedation – Anesthesia – Respiratory depression – Anticonvulsant action – Retrograde amnesia – Depression of vasomotor center	– ↓ myocardial contractility – ↓ cardiac output – Hypotension – Tachycardia
Respiratory system	**Other actions**
– Respiratory depression – ↓ sensitivity to raised CO_2 Laryngeal reflexes remain intact	– ↓ intracranial tension (ICT) and – ↓ intraocular pressure (↓ IOP) – *Uterine tone* is *UNAFFECTED*

18. **Answer is a (Cerebellar hemangioma).**
Ref: Harrison's, 17th edition Pg 2607.

- ***Erythropoietin*** produced by ***hemangioblastomas*** may result in ***polycythemia.***
- ***Cerebellar hemangioblastomas*** are a part of the ***von Hippel-Lindau syndrome.***

19. **Answer is d (Vertebral artery occlusion).**
Ref: Harrison's, 17th edition Pg 2526.

Direct quote:

"***Hemiparesis is NOT a feature of vertebral artery occlusion,*** *however, quadriparesis may result from occlusion of the anterior spinal artery.*"

Note:

➢ Nearly 85% of ischemic stroke patients have hemiparesis, but not in vertebral artery occlusion as seen above.

20. **Answer is d (Right-to-left shunt).**
Ref: Harrison's, 16th edition Pg 291, 1503-04.

Right-to-left shunt

- From a physiological point of view, this cause of hypoxi resembles intrapulmonary right to left shunting, but is caused by congenital heart disease such as TOF, TGA and Eisenmenger's syndrome.
- The PaO_2 (O_2 in arterial blood) in these cases cannot be restored with inspiration of 100% O_2.

Low PO_2 not correctable with O_2	Low PO_2 correctable with O_2
Shunts	V/Q mismatch
Alveolar collapse (atelectasis)	Airway disease (asthma, COPD)
Intra-alveolar filling (pneumonia/pulmonary edema)	Interstitial lung disease
Intracardiac shunt	Alveolar disease
Vascular shunt in lungs	Pulmonary vascular disease

21. Answer is None of the above.
Ref: Harrison's, 16th edition Pg 1532.

- Single ***most useful sign of the severity of pneumonia is a respiratory rate of > 30/min*** in a patient without underlying lung disease.
- Of the several measures of pneumonia severity, the simplest is the British Thoracic Society rule, which relies on 3 clinical findings and one laboratory finding as given below:
  - ***Respiratory rate*** > 30/min
  - ***BP***: Diastolic < 60 mm Hg or Systolic < 90 mm Hg
  - ***Confusion***
  - ***Urea*** > 7 mmol/L.

Author's Comments: *"The option 'd' should have been respiratory rate > 30 /min – looks like a printing mistake in the original question paper."*

22. Answer is c (201–300 mg/L).
Ref: Harrison's, 17th edition Pg 1792, 2288, fog 338-10; Davidson's, 20th edition Pg 841, Box 21.50, 21.51, 21.52, 21.53, Fig 21.17.

Repeat **Topic**

- See ***answer no. 1 above in the same COMED-K 2008 answers***.

23. Answer is d (Decreased vasopressin levels).
Ref: Cecil's Internal medicine, 23rd edition Pg 932.

- As noted, head injury and intracranial hemorrhage can induce a state of negative sodium balance through urinary losses, with clinical parameters consistent with hypovolemia—***'cerebral salt wasting'***.
- The hypovolemia ***induces release of AVP*** coupled with ingestion or administration of hypotonic fluids tends to produce hyponatremia, which is quite severe.
- In these patients, ***urine sodium concentrations can be impressively high***, thereby increasing tendency to hyponatremia
- Because of the setting of intracranial pathology and because the degree of hypovolemia may escape clinical detection, this condition is difficult to distinguish from hyponatremia caused by SIADH.

SURGERY

24. Answer is c (Adenoid cystic carcinoma).
Ref: Bailey and Love, 25th edition Pg 757; Robbins pathology, 7th edition Pg 791.

Salivary gland tumors—frequency and distribution

Type	Location	Frequency	Malignant
Major	Parotid	Common	15–30%
	Submandibular	Uncommon	50%
	Sublingual	Very rare	85%
Minor	Upper aerodigestive tract	Rare	90%

- While *adenoid cystic carcinoma* accounts for only 25% of carcinomas arising in the salivary glands, this type of tumor comprises the majority (50–70%) of all neoplasms arising in the minor salivary glands.

Fast Facts

- ***MC site*** of ***salivary gland tumor*** = ***parotid*** (65–80%).
- MC parotid gland tumor = ***pleomorphic adenoma.***
- MC salivary gland tumor overall also = ***pleomorphic adenoma.***
- The likelihood of salivary gland tumor being ***malignant*** is more or less ***inversely proportional to the size of the gland*** – i.e. ***malignant tumors are most common in*** minor salivary glands > ***sublingual gland*** > submandibular gland > parotid glands.
- ***Warthin's tumor (adenolymphoma)***—benign—almost ***fully limited to parotid*** gland only; MC in ***smokers***.
- ***Mucoepidermoid*** carcinoma—***MC malignant tumor of salivary glands.***
- ***Adenoid cystic carcinomas*** has tendency to invade ***perineural spaces***; MC found in the minor salivary glands (***palate***).
- **Clinical features of malignant salivary tumors**:
  - Facial nerve weakness
  - Rapid enlargement of swelling
  - Induration and/or ulceration of overlying skin
  - Cervical node enlargement.
- Three ***cranial nerves are at risk during removal of the submandibular*** gland:
  - Marginal mandibular branch of facial nerve
  - Lingual nerve
  - Hypoglossal nerve.

25. Answer is a (1.5% glycine).
Ref: Bailey and Love, 25th edition Pg 1350-51.

- ***TURP*** is a cystoscopic procedure used to alleviate the symptoms of bladder outflow obstruction, usually caused by benign prostatic hypertrophy (BPH).
- The operation is performed under direct vision using a diathermy current passed through a loop of wire at the tip of a resectoscope, which is inserted into the bladder through the patient's urethra. This enables the hypertrophied prostate to be resected in pieces and washed out using an irrigation solution.
- The ***most commonly used irrigation fluid is 1.5% isotonic glycine solution***, which has the advantages of ***being optically clear and non-electrolytic*** (and therefore does not conduct electric current).
- The ***risks of hyponatremia are also reduced.***

26. Answer is c (Type 3).
Ref: General surgery board review, Michael SG, Larry AS, 3rd edition Pg 17.

Types of Gastric Ulceration

- Type 1 : A single gastric ulcer
- Type 2 : Simultaneous gastric and duodenal ulcers
- Type 3 : Pyloric ***channel*** ulcer
- Type 4 : A gastric ulcer near the GE junction

- The ***type 1 or 4 gastric ulcers*** are a/w l*ow* ***or normal gastric acid secretion***, whereas type 3 and type 4 ulcers are a/w increased gastric acid secretion.

27. Answer is d (Alpha-fetoprotein).
Ref: Robbins pathology, 7th edition Pg 1101; Shaw's gynecology, 14th edition Pg 380.

- ***Endodermal sinus tumor (EST)***, also known as ***yolk sac tumor (YST)***, is a member of the germ cell tumor group of cancers. Endodermal sinus tumor like the yolk sac is rich in ***alpha-fetoprotein (AFP)*** and alpha-1-antitrypsin and can be monitored by AFP.
- Serum levels of AFP can be followed from the preoperative period through the course of chemotherapy.
- When elevated, AFP has excellent predictability that persistent disease is present.

28. Answer is a (Hamartoma).
Ref: Harrison's, 17th edition Pg 561.

- ***Hamartoma*** is the ***MC benign tumor of the lung*** (90%).
- On CXR, pulmonary hamartomas characteristically appear as well-defined ***solitary pulmonary nodules***, which may show varying patterns of calcification:
  - Irregular popcorn
  - Stippled
  - Curvilinear pattern
  - Or even a combination of all three.
- ***Popcorn calcification*** is virtually ***diagnostic of hamartoma***.

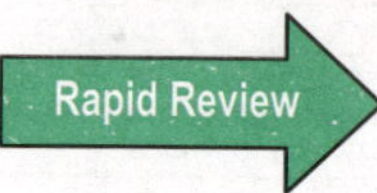

Lung Cancer

- Presents with cough, hemoptysis, bronchial obstruction, wheezing, pneumonic 'coin' lesions on X-ray film
- Risk factors: Tobacco/smoking, asbestos.

Type	Characteristics
Squamous cell Ca	• Central location • MC lung cancer in Cigarette smokers • Hilar-mass arising from bronchus; Cavitation; direct extension to hilar lymph nodes • PN: Parathyroid like activity (PTHrP) – hyperCalcemia; dermatomyositis • Histology: Keratin Pearls and Intercellular Bridges • MC Lung Ca detected by positive sputum Cytology • MC Lung Ca leading to PanCoast tumor • Cavitating, Central, Cigarette, hyperCalcemia • *Best prognosis* • Treatment: Surgery

Adeno Ca	• *Peripheral* • MC lung cancer in *non-smokers and females* • Develops in site of prior pulmonary inflammation or injury • Wide metastases, *a/w asbestosis*; pleural effusions show ↑ hyaluronidase levels • 2 types are bronchial and bronchioloalveolar • Histology: Clara cells, type 2 pneumocytes • PN: *DIC, thrombophlebitis, microangiopathic hemolytic anemia* • *Good prognosis*
Small cell (oat cell) Ca	• Central • *Rapidly growing*, early distant metastases • PN: *SIADH, Ectopic GH and ACTH secretion, peripheral neuropathy, Eaton-Lambert syndrome* • MC lung Ca causing *SVC syndrome* • Neoplasm of neuroendocrine Kulchitsky cells—small blue round cell tumor • Responsive to *chemotherapy* (cisplatin and etoposide)
Large cell Ca	• *Peripheral* • Highly undifferentiated *anaplastic* tumor • *Poor prognosis* • Less tendency to metastasize • PN: *Gynecomastia* • Less responsive to chemotherapy • Treat surgically

PN = Paraneoplastic syndrome; SVC = Superior vena cava; SIADH = Syndrome of inappropriate secretion of ADH; DIC = Disseminated intravascular coagulation.

1. **Pancoast tumor:** Carcinoma that occurs in the apex of the lung and may affect cervical sympathetic plexus causing ***Horner's syndrome.***
2. **SVC syndrome**: Characterized by swelling of face and arm, most often on the right side and elevated JVP. Treated with radiation therapy.
3. **Trousseau's syndrome**: A ***hypercoagulable state*** seen MC with adenocarcinoma.
4. **Eaton-Lambert syndrome**: autoantibodies against calcium channels, clinically similar to myasthenia, except that ***muscle fatigue improves with repeated stimulation***.

29. Answer is c (Acute pancreatitis).
Ref: Bailey and Love, 25th edition Pg 967t, 1140.

- The ***Gray-Turner sign*** is a ***reddish-brown discoloration along the flanks*** resulting from ***retroperitoneal blood*** dissecting along tissue planes. More commonly, patients may have a ruddy erythema in the flanks secondary to extravasated pancreatic exudate. This sign takes ***24–48 hours to appear*** and predicts a severe attack of ***acute pancreatitis***.
- Other causes include:
  - Blunt abdominal trauma
  - Ruptured abdominal aortic aneurysm
  - Ruptured/Hemorrhagic ectopic pregnancy
  - Spontaneous bleeding secondary to coagulopathy (congenital or acquired).

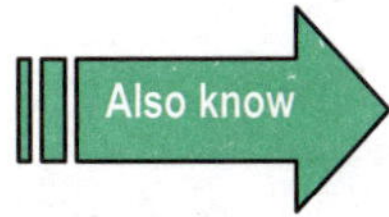

Other Important Signs in Patients with Abdominal Pain

Cullen's sign	Bluish periumbilical discoloration; seen in ***retroperitoneal hemorrhage*** (hemorrhagic pancreatitis, abdominal aortic aneurysm rupture)

Murphy's sign:	In ***acute cholecystitis,*** deep inspiration or cough during subcostal palpation of the RUQ usually produces increased pain and inspiratory arrest
Markle's sign:	A maneuver ***to detect peritoneal irritation*** is tested by the heel jar test. The patient stands on his/her toes, then allows his/her heels to hit the floor thus jarring the body and causing abdominal pain in ***peritonitis*** (also positive in appendicitis)
Kehr's sign:	Severe left shoulder pain; seen in ***Splenic rupture, Ectopic pregnancy rupture***
Courvoisier's sign:	Palpable gallbladder and jaundice; seen in ***Ca head of pancreas***
Virchow's sign:	Palpable ***left supraclavicular fossa lymph node;*** seen in ***stomach carcinoma*** (or abdominal malignancy)

30. Answer is a (*E. coli*).
Ref: Harrison's, 17th edition Pg 1826.

Emphysematous Pyelonephritis
- MC in ***diabetic*** patients, often in concert with ***urinary obstruction and chronic infection.***
- Characterized by a rapidly progressive clinical course, with high fever, leukocytosis, renal parenchymal necrosis and accumulation of fermentative gases in the kidney and perinephric tissues. Most patients also have polyuria and glycosuria.
- ***E. coli causes most cases.***
- Gas in tissues is often seen on plain films and is best confirmed and localized by CT.
- Surgical resection of the involved tissue in addition to systemic antimicrobial therapy is usually needed to prevent a fatal outcome in emphysematous pyelonephritis.

Emphysematous cystitis
- MC in ***diabetic*** patients, usually in association with ***E. coli*** or other facultative gram-negative rods and often ***in relation to bladder outlet obstruction.***
- Patients are less severely ill and have less rapidly progressive disease than those with emphysematous pyelonephritis. The patient typically reports abdominal pain, dysuria, frequency and (in some cases) pneumaturia.
- CT shows gas within ***both*** the bladder lumen and the bladder wall.
- Generally, conservative therapy with systemic antimicrobial agents and relief of outlet obstruction are effective, but some patients do not respond to these measures and require cystectomy.

31. Answer is a (Pretracheal).
Ref: Bailey and Love, 25th edition Pg 771.

- A ***midline prelaryngeal/pretracheal lymph node,*** adjacent to the thyroid gland, enlargement of which indicates thyroid disease.
- This node gets its name from Greek mythology. The ***Oracle of Delphi,*** called Pythria, was a Priestess who would answer questions posed to her, never concealing nor revealing the truth.
- Thus, an enlarged Delphian node may or may not indicate the presence of thyroid cancer.

32. Answer is b (Chromosome 7q).
Ref: Harrison's, 17th edition Pg 2225.

- Mutation of the ***PENDRIN gene*** causes ***Pendred's syndrome,*** an **autosomal recessive** disorder characterized by:
  - *Defective organification of iodine*
  - ***Goiter***
  - ***Sensorineural deafness*** (typically associated with a malformation of the inner ear bony labyrinth, referred to as ***Mondini cochlea***)
- Linkage of Pendred's syndrome to ***chromosome 7q22-31.1*** was first established in 1996.

33. Answer is a (Cholangitis).
Ref: First Aid for the USMLE, Step 2 CK, 7th edition Pg 176.

- ***Reynolds pentad*** is seen in ***ascending/acute suppurative cholangitis.***

Reynolds' pentad

Charcot's triad (jaundice, fever, right upper quadrant pain)
+
Hypotension (shock)
+
An ***altered mental state***

- ***Charcot's*** triad is also seen in cholangitis.

34. Answer is b (Tamsulosin).
Ref: KD Tripathi, 6th edition Pg 136.

- Two classes of drugs are available to treat benign prostatic hypertrophy (BPH):
  - ***α-1-adrenergic blockers*** (terazosin, doxazosin, tamsulosin): Decrease tone of prostate, bladder neck muscles
  - ***5-α-reductase inhibitor*** (finasteride)—arrest growth/reduce size of prostate.
- The ***α-1-blockers afford faster and greater symptomatic relief (<u>within 2 weeks</u>)*** than *finasteride,* which takes nearly *6 months* for clinical improvement.
- Flutamide is an oral antiandrogen drug primarily used to treat prostate cancer and not BPH.

35. Answer is a (44%).
Ref: Bailey and Love, old 21st edition Pg 145.

- According to Lund and Browder chart:
  - ☐ Head: Front and back = 13%
  - ☐ Neck: Front and back = 2%
  - ☐ Trunk: Front and Back = 26%.
- Adding the above values (13 + 2 + 26 = 41%)
- 41 is closest to 44. Hence A is the answer.

OBSTETRICS AND GYNECOLOGY

36. Answer is c (50 g glucose challenge test).
Ref: Harrison's, 17th edition Pg 46; Dutta's obstetrics, 6th edition Pg 285.

- A typical two-step strategy for establishing the diagnosis of gestational diabetes involves administration of a ***50 g oral glucose challenge*** with a single serum glucose measurement at 60 minutes.
- If the plasma glucose is < 7.8 mmol/L (< 140 mg/dL), the test is considered normal.
- Serum glucose > 7.8 mmol/L (>140 mg/dL) warrants administration of a 100 g oral glucose challenge with serum glucose measurements obtained in the fasting state and at 1, 2 and 3 hours.
- Other tests (e.g. *maternal HbA1C, random postprandial or fasting blood sugar level or fructosamine level*) are <u>NOT</u> *recommended because of <u>low sensitivity</u>.*

37. Answer is a (50 μg).
Ref: Dutta's obstetrics, 6th edition Pg 334.

- To prevent active immunization of the Rh-negative yet immunized mother, Rh-anti-D immunoglobulin (IgG) is administered IM to the mother following childbirth and abortion.
- **Dose of anti D-IgG:**
  - ☐ Following childbirth/delivery: full dose of 300 μg.
  - ☐ Following induced abortion, spontaneous abortion, ectopic pregnancy or chorionic villous biopsy in ***first trimester*: *50 μg within 72 hours*.**
  - ☐ Women with pregnancy beyond 12 weeks: full dose of 300 μg.

38. Answer is c (Onset of the LH surge).
Ref: Shaw's gynecology, 14th edition Pg 195.

- ***LH surge*** from the ***anterior pituitary*** gland ***occurs 24 hours before ovulation.***
- Not only does the ***LH surge help in predicting ovulation*** but the approximate time of ovulation can be gauged and coitus around this time ***can improve the chances of conception.***
- Gauging the time of ovulation has therapeutic implications in the in vitro fertilization and artificial insemination.
- RIA of the morning sample of urine and blood give the LH results in 3 hours

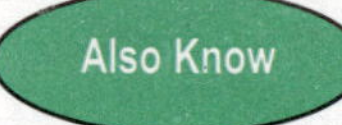

Other Tests for Ovulation

1. **Basal body temperature test (BBT)**
   - ❖ BBT falls by about 0.5°F at the time of ovulation.
   - ❖ Subsequently ***during the progestational half of the cycle, the temperature is slightly raised*** above the preovulatory level and the rise is of the order of 0.5–1°F.
   - ❖ If the patient conceives, the temperature remains elevated at this level and does not fall as it would during a menstrual cycle.
   - ❖ This phenomenon is due to the thermogenic action of progesterone and hence presumptive evidence of a functioning corpus luteum and hence ovulation.

2. **Fern test**
   - ❖ During estrogenic phase the cervical mucus shows ***ferning due to effect of NaCl secreted under estrogen*** influence.
   - ❖ This ferning disappears after ovulation and if previously present is presumptive evidence of a corpus luteum activity.

3. **Ultrasound**
   - ❖ Ultrasound has now become the ***standard procedure for monitoring maturation of the Graafian follicle*** and in ***detecting imminent ovulation in the in vitro fertilization*** and timing intercourse.

39. Answer is d (Assess the progress of labor).
Ref: Dutta, 6th edition Pg 403, 528.

- ***Normal partogram*** plots the ***cervical dilatation in the Y axis*** against the ***time duration on the X axis,*** i.e. dilatation of the cervix in centimeters against time in hours.
- ***Friedman*** classically proposed that ***this is sigmoid shaped in normal labor.***
- ***Action line*** is drawn ***4 hours to the right of the alert line.***
- The main purpose of the partogram is to avoid prolonged labor and intervene within time.
- It is the ***best method to assess progression of labor.***

40. Answer is d (Ethacridine extra amniotic).
Ref: Dutta, 6th edition Pg 174 and Pg 565.

Methods of termination of pregnancy

First trimester (up to 12 weeks)	Second trimester (13–20 weeks)
Surgical ❖ Manual vacuum aspiration (MVA) ❖ Suction evacuation ❖ Surgical evacuation and/or curettage ❖ Dilation and evacuation: Rapid/Slow method **Medical** ❖ Mifepristone (RU486) ❖ Mifepristone and misoprostol (PGE1) ❖ Methotrexate and misoprostol ❖ Tamoxifen and misoprostol	❖ Dilation and evacuation (13–14 weeks) ❖ Intrauterine instillation of hyperosmotic solutions – Intra-amniotic hypertonic urea (40%), saline (20%) – Extra-amniotic *ethacridine lactate*, prostaglandins (PGE2, PGF2α) ❖ Prostaglandins PGE1 (misoprostol), 15 methyl PGF2α (carboprost), PGE2 (dinoprostone) and their analogues (used intravaginally, IM or intra-amniotically) ❖ Oxytocin infusion high dose used along with either of the above two methods ❖ Hysterotomy (abdominal) — less commonly done

41. Answer is a (Squamous cell Ca).
Ref: Harrison's, 17th edition Pg 608.

- Approximately ***70% of invasive cervix cancers*** are ***squamous cell tumors***, 20–25% are adenocarcinomas and 2–5% are adenosquamous with epithelial and glandular structures.

42. Answer is d (Mini pill).
Ref: Shaw's gynecology, 14th edition Pg 210.

Mini pill (progestin only pill)
Advantages
➲ ***Can be used in lactating women. No adverse effect on lactation — often called 'lactation pill'.*** ➲ Can be prescribed in patients having hypertension, diabetes mellitus, fibroids, epilepsy, smoking and in patients with h/o thromboembolism. ➲ Side effects of estrogen in the combined pill are totally eliminated; easy to take as there is no on and off regime. ➲ Can be prescribed to women over 35 years and smokers; those with focal migraine. ➲ As regards to return of fertility, it is faster than in combined pill users, because ovulation is not suppressed in all cases.
Contraindications
☐ Previous ectopic pregnancy, breast and genital cancers, ovarian cysts, abnormal vaginal bleeding, active liver and arterial disease, porphyria, liver tumor, valproate, spironolactone and meprobamate.

PEDIATRICS

43. Answer is d (Congenital heart disease).
Ref: In a Page: Pediatric signs and symptoms, Jonathan ET, et al. Pg 85, 2004 edition; Braunwald's cardiology, Pg 212.

- The most likely causes of CHF depend on the age of the child:
  - ☐ ***CHF in the fetus*** or hydrops, can be detected by performing fetal echocardiography. In this case, CHF may represent underlying anemia (e.g. Rh sensitization, fetal-maternal transfusion), arrhythmias (usually supraventricular tachycardia) or myocardial dysfunction (myocarditis or cardiomyopathy).

- *Neonates and infants younger than 2 months* are the ***most likely group to present with CHF related to congenital structural heart disease***. The systemic or pulmonary circulation is often dependent on the patency of the ductus arteriosus, especially, if the patient presents in the first few days of life. In these patients, prompt cardiac evaluation is mandatory. Nonetheless, respiratory illnesses, anemia and known or suspected infection must be considered and appropriately managed.
- ***In older children***, CHF may be caused by left-sided obstructive disease (aortic stenosis or coarctation); rheumatic fever, myocardial dysfunction (myocarditis or cardiomyopathy); hypertension; renal failure; or more rarely, arrhythmias or myocardial ischemia.

44. Answer is d (Measles).
Ref: Harrison's, 17th edition *Pg 1215, Table 185-1.*

Subacute sclerosing panencephalitis (SSPE)

- *Rare complication of measles* (1 in 100,000)
- Seen usually when measles occurs in infancy; seen 5–10 years later
- A chronic, progressive encephalitis that affects primarily children and young adults
- Caused by a persistent infection of ***immune resistant measles virus***.

Other Complications of Measles

- Otitis media
- Pneumonia
- Croup
- Gastroenteritis
- Acute encephalitis
- Cervical adenitis

45. Answer is a (Conjunctival xerosis).
Ref: Park, 20th edition Pg 532.

- ***Conjunctival xerosis*** is the ***first clinical sign of vitamin A deficiency***.

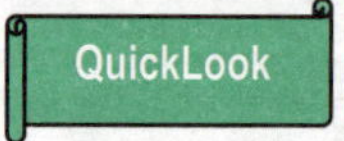

WHO Classification of Vitamin A Deficiency.

XN	*Night Blindness is the earliest symptom* of vitamin A deficiency, which is often reported by the mother as reduced visual acuity of the child in the evening and the night-time.
X1A	***Conjunctival xerosis*** or drying of the conjunctiva.
X1B	***Bitot's spots*** on the conjunctiva.
X2	***Corneal xerosis*** or dryness of the cornea with a granular looking surface.
X3A	***Keratomalacia*** involving ***< 1/3 of the cornea***. Cornea becomes dry, thin and soft and then ulcerates.
X3B	Keratomalacia involving ***> 1/3 of cornea.***
XF	*Fundoscopic changes* visible on ophthalmoscopy (Uyemura fundus).
XS	***Corneal Scarring*** compromising severely on visual acuity.

46. Answer is c (Methylmalonic acidemia).
Ref: http://www.ncbi.nlm.nih.gov/bookshelf/br.fcgi?book=gene&part=mma

Kahler et al. Pancreatitis in patients with organic acidemias. J Pediatr. 1994; 124: 239–43 (Pubmed).

- The incidence of ***pancreatitis*** in isolated ***methylmalonic acidemia*** is unknown, but it is a well-recognized complication (Kahler et al, 1994). It can occur acutely or chronically.
- Because pancreatitis can manifest non-specifically, with vomiting and abdominal pain, it may be under-recognized.

47. Answer is a (Alprostadil).
Ref: KD Tripathi, 6th edition Pg 182.

- ***Alprostadil*** is a prostaglandin (*PGE1*) that is used for the ***temporary maintenance of PDA*** in patients with ductal dependent congenital heart disease till surgery is done; ***apnea*** occurs in few cases.

Note:

- ***Alprostadil*** injected directly into the corpus cavernosum using affine needle produces ***penile erection*** lasting 1–2 hour to perform intercourse; most commonly used drug in patients not responding to PDE-5 inhibitors.

48. Answer is c (Amantadine).
Ref: Harrison's, 17th edition Pg 1131, Table 180-2.

- Antiviral medications for ***influenza treatment and prophylaxis***:
- The *neuraminidase inhibitors* (***oseltamivir*** and ***zanamivir***) inhibit the action of influenza neuraminidase, thereby blocking the release of infectious virion particles from the infected cell surface.
- The *adamantanes* (***amantadine*** and ***rimantadine***) bind to the M2 protein ion channels on the viral envelope, which interferes with release of viral nucleic acid into the host cell.

49. Answer is a (Sinus bradycardia).
Ref: Neonatal Cardiology By Michael Artman, David F Tetal, 2002 edition Pg 179.

ECG abnormalities present in long QT syndrome

- Prolongation of QTc interval
- Sinus bradycardia
- T-wave abnormalities (T-wave alternans)
- Episodic torsades de pointes

50. Answer is b (Guillain-Barré syndrome).
Ref: Harrison's, 17th edition Pg 2669.

- In ***Guillain-Barré syndrome*** , typically, the CSF findings on lumbar puncture is suggestive of demyelination (i.e. increased protein > 45 mg/dL within 3 weeks of onset) without evidence of active infection *(lack of CSF pleocytosis)*, as originally noted by Guillain and Barré—***albuminocytological dissociation.***

D/D of Albuminocytological Dissociation

- Heavy metal intoxication (lead encephalopathy)
- Porphyria
- Botulism
- Spinal cord compression (Froin syndrome)
- Post-diphtheritic paralysis

ORTHOPEDICS

51. Answer is c (Congenital hip dislocation).
Ref: John Ebnezer's orthopedics, 4th edition Pg 494.

4 Fs of Congenital hip dislocation (CDH)

- Female preponderance
- First borns affected
- Familial (20%)
- Faulty intrauterine position (breech in 30–50%)

Also Know

- CDH is now called Developmental Dysplasia of Hip
- Incidence of CDH is 1 per 1,000 live births
- Left hip affected more commonly (67%)
- 1/3 cases are bilateral.

52. **Answer is d (Presence of polydactyly).**
Ref: Limb Lengthening and Reconstructive Surgery By S ***Ilizarov****, SR Rozburch, 2007 edition CRC Press, Pg 454.*

- ***Fibular hemimelia*** is the ***most common long-bone congenital absence or hypoplasia.***

Associated anomalies of fibular hemimelia

☐ Coxa vara ☐ Proximal femoral focal deficiency – Associated femoral shortening adds to limb length discrepancy – At skeletal maturity, this averages about 5 inches (12 cm) ☐ Ankle instability ☐ Lateral column deficiency of the foot	☐ *Equinovarus/valgus foot* (+/- absent lateral rays) ☐ Tarsal coalition ☐ *Short tibia with anterior tibial bowing* ☐ Abnormality of the distal tibial physis ☐ Deficiency in muscles on the peroneal side of the leg

53. **Answer is b (Tibialis posterior) and d (Flexor hallucis longus).**
Ref: John Ebnezer's orthopedics, 4th edition Pg 509; Maheshwari, 3rd edition Pg 197.

Structures released in posteromedial soft tissue release (Turco procedure) For CTEV

- **On the medial side**
  - Lengthening of the tibialis posterior, flexor hallucis longus and flexor digitorum longus muscle
  - Release of talonavicular ligament, spring ligament and superficial part of deltoid ligament
  - Release of interosseous talocalcaneal ligament, capsules of naviculocuneiform and first tarsal cuneiform joints.
- **On plantar side**
  - Plantar fascia
  - Release of abductor hallucis and flexor digitorum brevis.
- **On posterior side**
  - Z-plasty of tendon Achilles to lengthen it
  - Posterior capsulotomy of the ankle and subtalar joints
  - Release of posterior talofibular and calcaneofibular ligaments.

54. **Answer is a (Longitudinal tear).**
Ref: The Meniscus By Hilippe Beaufils, 2010 edition Pg 47; Apley's system of orthopedics and fractures, 8th edition Pg 48; Orthopedic pathology, Vincent JV et al, 2nd edition Pg 715.

- ***Most meniscus tears are usually longitudinal***, usually affecting the posterior segment of the meniscus.
- Because of structural differences, ***bucket-handle type of longitudinal tears are more common in the medial meniscus***.

Smillie's classification of medial meniscus injury

- ***Vertical or Longitudinal tears:***
  - Includes complete tear (bucket handle tear), peripheral attachment tear and segmental tears.
  - More commonly due to traumatic injuries in younger persons.
- ***Horizontal tears:***
  - More commonly degenerative tears in persons > 40 years of age.
  - Could be posterior, middle or anterior.
- Cystic degeneration.
- Congenital abnormalities.

More About

- The ***medial meniscus is more prone to injury*** than the lateral meniscus as it is connected to the medial collateral ligament and the joint capsule and so is less mobile.
- Mechanism of injury: ***A rotational force when a flexed knee extends***; e.g. any forces impacting from the outer surface of the knee, such as ***rugby tackle.***
- Medial meniscal injuries are often also a/w injuries to the anterior cruciate ligament.
- ***Lateral meniscus is less commonly injured*** since— it is smaller in diameter, thicker in periphery, wide, more mobile, attached to both cruciate ligaments and stabilized posteriorly to the femoral condyle by popliteus.

Tests for medial meniscus injury

- McMurray's test
- Apley's compression test
- Apley's distraction test
- Steinmann's sign
- Helfet sign
- Duck Waddle test

55. Answer is a (Tuberculosis).

Ref: John Ebnezer's Orthopedics, 4th edition Pg 572-73

- Boyer is credited with the first anatomical description of ***spina ventosa (spina = short bone; ventosa = inflated with air)*** in the short long bones in 1803, while Nélaton proved the ***tuberculous etiology*** of the condition in 1837.

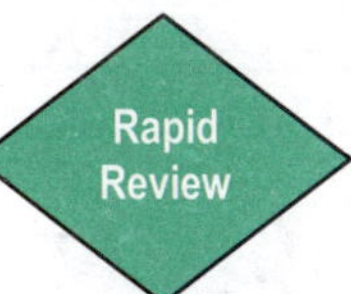

Summary of Musculoskeletal TB

Tissue	Disease	Remarks
Bone		
1. Long bone	**TB osteomyelitis**	***Tibia*** commonly affected; lots of lytic lesions, minimal new bone formation unlike pyogenic osteomyelitis; thin watery discharge; multiple sinuses.
2. Short bone (phalanges)	**TB dactylitis**	Also called ***spina ventosa.***
3. Spine	**TB spondylitis**	Also called ***Pott's disease; MC site of skeletal TB***; bacilli reach spine through paravertebral (*Batson's*) plexus; ***Paradiscal type*** is MC; MC symptom is ***back pain***; on X-ray reduction of disk space is earliest sign; Anterior type of vertebral TB may show erosion of anterior part of the body, much the same as that in aneurysm of aorta—***aneurysmal sign***; TB spine with neurological involvement is ***Pott's paraplegia***—MC in ***thoracic spine.***

Joints		
1. Arthritis	**TB arthritis**	***Hip joint*** commonly affected; MC in children/adolescents; pain referred to knee severe at night (***night cries***); ***true shortening*** of lower limb present, ***Thomas test*** used to detect fixed flexion deformity of hip. Shoulder joint TB may not produce any pus/cold abscess – ***'Caries sicca'***.
2. Synovium	**Synovial TB**	***Knee joint*** commonly affected; begins in synovium; long standing TB knee causes ***triple subluxation*** (flexion of knee, posterior subluxation and external rotation of tibia); ***X-ray*** essentially ***normal.***
Others		
1. Tendon (synovium)	**TB tenosynovitis**	***Compound palmar ganglion*** (of flexor tendons at wrist).
2. Bursae	**TB bursitis**	Trochanteric bursitis.

56. Answer is c (Hyaluronate in synovial fluid).
Ref: Medical Laboratory Technology, Ramnik Sood, 5th edition Pg 281.

- The ***viscosity of synovial fluid*** is because of its high concentration of ***hyaluronic acid***.
- The viscosity of the fluid can be assessed by allowing a drop of synovial fluid to fall slowly from the tip of a needle, or by placing a drop between the thumb and forefinger (of a gloved hand), and slowly separating them.
- The quantity and quality of mucin (and therefore hyaluronic acid) can be assessed using ***a mucin clot test***.
- The mucin clot test (***Ropes test***) is a semi-quantitative measure of polymerization that is evaluated after acetic acid precipitation of protein.
- In general, when a joint is inflamed, hyaluronic acid is depleted and the viscosity of the fluid is reduced. A drop of fluid from an osteoarthritic joint may form a string only 1–2 cm long.
- Inflammation in the joint space damages the hyaluronic polymers, shortening them. Thus, the 'mucin clot' is:
  - GOOD in osteoarthritis, trauma and hemophilic arthritis
  - FAIR in subacute and chronic inflammatory diseases such as lupus or rheumatoid arthritis
  - POOR TO VERY POOR in septic and acute crystalline arthritis.

57. Answer is a (McCune-Albright syndrome).
Ref: Harrison's, 17th edition Pg 2413.

McCune-Albright syndrome

- *Polyostotic fibrous dysplasia*
- *Café au lait* skin pigmentation
- *Precocious puberty* (gonadotropin independent)

ENT AND OPHTHALMOLOGY

58. Answer is b (Meniere's disease).
Ref: Maqbool's ENT textbook, 11th edition Pg 106.

- ***Cochlear recruitment*** in ***Meniere's disease*** confirms a cochlear localization of ***receptive hearing loss***.
- Vestibular recruitment is analogous to cochlear recruitment and may be seen in 6.7–100% patients with Meniere's disease.
- Recruitment patients often find normal loudness of sounds extremely painful and too loud for their tolerance. Often with an older person, having difficulty in hearing they would say "Speak up a bit... I can't hear you" and then after you speak up they say, "Don't shout! I'm not deaf"!

- A person with recruitment may not be able to hear high frequency sounds, below 50 dB (decibels), but may find any sounds above 80 dB uncomfortable and liable to produce *distortion*.

More About Meniere's disease

☐ **Pathogenesis**	– Faulty absorption of endolymph by endolymphatic sac.
☐ **Clinically**	– Usually unilateral; F:M = 3:1; affects 35–60 years age group. – Attacks of ***episodic vertigo, fluctuating sensorineural hearing loss, tinnitus and aural fullness***. – ***Diplacusis*** (same sound perceived as different pitch in two ears). – ***Hennebert's sign***: Vertigo and nystagmus experienced by patient during pressure induced excursion of the stapedial foot plate. – ***Tulio's phenomenon***: Subjective imbalance and nystagmus observed in response to loud noise exposure due to distended saccule lying against the stapedial foot plate.
☐ **Investigations**	– On pure tone audiometry, low frequency sensorineural hearing loss present (rising type curve). – On electrocochleography, summating potential: Action potential, i.e. SP:AP ↑ (> 50%). – SISI score > 70% (N < 15%). – Tone decay test—normally there is decay of < 20 dB. – ***Recruitment is positive.***
☐ **Treatment**	– ***Low salt*** diet, ***diuretics***, short course of ***glucocorticoids*** and intratympanic gentamicin, vasodilators of inner ear-like ***betahistine***.
☐ **Variants**	– ***Lermoyez syndrome*** = variant of Meniere's disease, SNHL improves suddenly during attacks of vertigo. – ***Cochlear hydrops*** = only cochlear symptoms are present, no vertigo.

59. Answer is c (Nasopharynx).
Ref: Maqbool's ENT textbook, 11th edition Pg 416.

- Named after, Wilfred Trotter of London, Trotter's triad is a triad of:
  - Decreased hearing (conductive deafness)
  - Mandibular neuralgic pain
  - Impaired soft palate mobility-asymmetry of soft palate.
- Seen due to local spread of nasopharyngeal carcinoma.

60. Answer is b (Cornea verticillata).
Ref: Parson's, 20th edition Pg 206.

- **Vortex Keratopathy or Cornea Verticillata** consists of symmetric, bilateral, *whorl-like pattern* of powdery, white or yellow corneal *epithelial* deposits.
- It appears in a vortex fashion in the ***inferocentral cornea*** and swirls outwards ***sparing the limbus***.
- The corneal changes are ***not of much visual significance*** and may be incidentally noticed on examination.

Causes of Cornea Verticillata

- Fabry's disease
- *Amiodarone*
- Chloroquine
- Amodiaquine
- Meperidine
- Indomethacin
- Chlorpromazine
- Tamoxifen

61. Answer is b (Friedreich's ataxia).
Ref: Parson's, 20th edition Pg 329-335.

- ***Papilledema*** is an ***optic disk swelling that is secondary to elevated intracranial pressure***.
- The term 'papilledema' should NOT be used to describe optic disk swelling with underlying infectious, infiltrative or inflammatory etiologies.

Causes of papilledema	Ocular causes of disk edema
❖ Any tumors or space-occupying lesions of the CNS ❖ Idiopathic intracranial hypertension ❖ Decreased CSF resorption (e.g. venous sinus thrombosis, inflammatory processes, meningitis, subarachnoid hemorrhage) ❖ Increased CSF production (tumors) ❖ Obstruction of the ventricular system ❖ Cerebral edema/encephalitis ❖ Craniosynostosis	❖ Papillitis ❖ Optic neuritis ❖ Anterior ischemic optic neuropathy ❖ Diabetic papillopathy ❖ Optic disk drusen (disk edema like)

62. Answer is b (0.3%).
Ref: Park, 20th edition Pg 375, 555.

- The ***National Program for Control of Blindness (NPCB)*** was launched in ***1976*** as a 100% centrally sponsored and incorporates the earlier Trachoma Control Program that was started in 1963.
- It aims to reduce the ***prevalence of blindness*** (1.49% in 1986–1989) to ***less than 0.3%.***

63. Answer is b (Hallermann-Streiff syndrome).
Ref: Shields' Textbook of glaucoma, 3rd edition Pg 266.

Hallermann-Streiff syndrome – features

- *Ocular*: Microphthalmos (bilateral); proptosis; nystagmus; strabismus; ***cataracts which may resorb spontaneously and lead to glaucoma***; bilateral optic atrophy; coloboma of optic disk, choroid and iris; keratoglobus; microcornea; antimongoloid slant; iris atrophy; uveitis; blue sclera; persistent pupillary membrane; secondary glaucoma.
- *Systemic*: Malformations of skull (brachycephaly), facial skeleton and jaws; erupted teeth at birth; diminished hair growth; hyperextensibility of joints; short stature; skin atrophy; mental deficiency; predisposition to upper airway compromise; obstructive sleep apnea.

64. Answer is d (Suppression).
Ref: Kanski's Clinical Ophthalmology, 6th edition Pg 487.

There are ***three grades of binocular vision as given by Worth's classification***:

- ***Grade I: Simultaneous macular perception*** is the most elementary type of binocularity. It occurs when the visual cortex perceives separate stimuli to the two eyes at the same time and concerns itself essentially with the absence of suppression. SMP is not the same as superimposition, whereby the two different pictures are seen simultaneously in the same direction. SMP in the true sense just represents simple sensory fusion.
- *Grade II:* It represents ***true fusion*** with some amplitude. Not only are the two images fused, but some effort is made to maintain this fusion in spite of difficulties. Thus the second grade implies a motor response added to simple sensory fusion.
- *Grade III:* In the highest type of binocularity, not only are the images of the two eyes fused, but they are blended to produce a ***stereoscopic effect (stereopsis)***. This involves a perceptual synthesis at a higher level.
- These three grades are not necessarily mutually exclusive, since fusion in the periphery, even showing motor responses, may exist coincidentally with the total absence of simultaneous foveal perception.

Note:

☐ *Suppression:* It is a neurophysiological active inhibitory mechanism in which when corresponding retinal areas are stimulated by dissimilar stimuli or when non-corresponding retinal areas are stimulated by similar stimuli, one or the other is temporarily inhibited or suppressed to prevent confusion or diplopia respectively. Suppression is foveal in order to tackle confusion and extrafoveal in order to avoid diplopia.

65. Answer is b (Pupil).
Ref: Parson's diseases of the eye, 20th edition Pg 119-20.

- The ***Relative Afferent Pupillary Defect (RAPD) or Marcus-Gunn Pupil*** is an extremely significant and highly objective clinical finding in the examination of the visual system.
- The ***'swinging flashlight test'*** is probably the ***best test for identifying an RAPD***.
- In this test, a strong, steady light is used. The light is shined into one eye and then quickly switched to the other. This is repeated back and forth, until one of four conclusions is reached (listed below). Since light in one pupil causes both pupils to constrict, quickly switching from one eye to the other will give a 'relative' indication of the functioning of each eye and optic nerve. If both eyes are equally dysfunctional, no 'relative' defect would be found. The results of the test include:
  - *No RAPD*: Both pupils constrict equally without evidence of pupillary redilation with the 'swinging flashlight test', except possibly for 'hippus'. Hippus refers to non-rhythmic fluctuations in pupillary size when there is a steady illumination.
  - *Mild RAPD*: One pupil shows a weak initial constriction, followed by dilation to a greater size.
  - *Moderate RAPD*: One pupil shows sustained constriction, followed by dilation to a greater size.
  - *Severe RAPD*: One pupil shows an immediate dilation to a greater size.

66. Answer is a (Timolol).
Ref: Parson's diseases of the eye, 20th edition Pg 286.

- ***Latanoprost*** is the most frequently prescribed drug for glaucoma (especially in developed countries) and is emerging as the ***favored first-line antiglaucoma drug***.
- ***Beta-blockers are still the most popular antiglaucoma agents (especially in India)***, as the first therapy of choice in open-angle glaucoma.
- ***Miotics (pilocarpine)*** are ***rapidly falling out of favor*** because of their local effects and the need to instill them up *to four times daily*.
- ***Epinephrine*** is NO LONGER AVAILABLE as an antiglaucoma drug.
- ***Topical carbonic anhydrase inhibitors, dorzolamide and brinzolamide*** are usually ***used as adjuncts***, and they need thrice daily instillations and are ***only occasionally satisfactory as monotherapy***.

67. Answer is c (*Staphylococcus aureus*).
Ref: Parson's, 20th edition Pg 187; Kanski, 6th edition Pg 254.

- ***Bacteria*** that ***invade intact corneal epithelium*** are
  - *Neisseria*
  - *Corynebacterium*
  - *Listeria and*
  - *H. influenzae*

68. Answer is a (Open-angle glaucoma).
Ref: Kanski, Clinical Ophthalmology, 5th edition Pg 287.

- ***Trabeculoplasty*** is a treatment used for ***primary open-angle glaucoma***. It involves laser application to the trabecular meshwork to enhance outflow of aqueous humor.
- It is not useful in angle-closure/narrow-angle glaucoma, since the trabecular meshwork is not visible in these cases.
- The types of trabeculoplasty are given below.

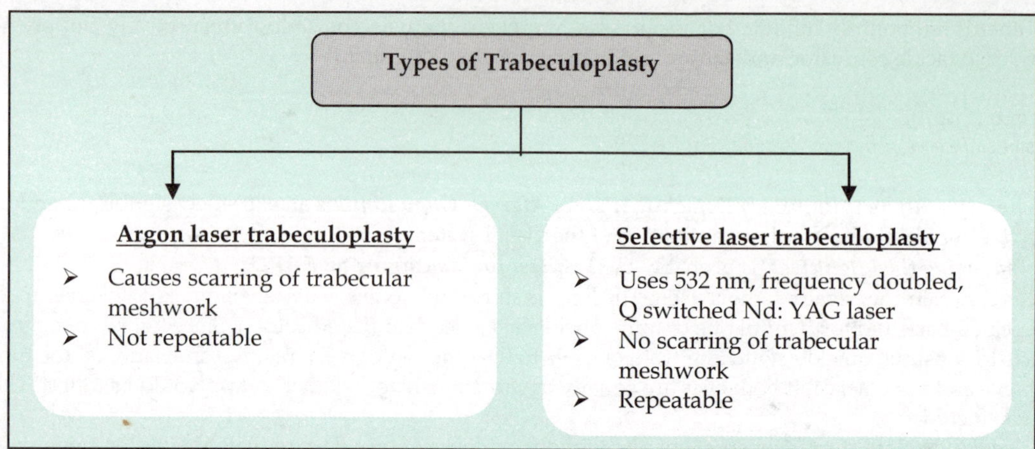

69. **Answer is a (Retinoscopy).**
Ref: Parson's diseases of the eye, 20th edition Pg 61.

- ***Retinoscopy*** is a technique to obtain an objective measurement of the refractive condition of a patient's eyes.
- ***Ophthalmoscopy*** is to see the fundus of the eye.
- ***Gonioscopy*** is to see the angle of the eye.
- ***Keratoscopy*** is to see the refractive power (curvature) of the cornea.

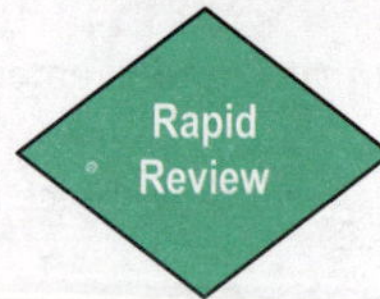

PROCEDURES AND INSTRUMENTATION

1. Retinoscopy	To determine refractive error of eye
2. Gonioscopy	To view angle of anterior chamber
3. Pachymetry	Measures thickness of cornea
4. Keratometry	To measure the curvature of the cornea
5. Campimetry/Perimetry	Measures field of vision
6. Specular microscope	For corneal endothelial cell count and endothelial study
7. Confocal microscope	To study corneal layers, useful in acanthameba keratitis
8. Optical coherence tomography (OCT)	To study retinal nerve fiber layers, useful in glaucoma and macular pathology
9. Heidelberg Retina Tomogram (HRT)	
10. GDX	To study retinal nerve fiber layers—used in glaucoma only
11. Corneal topography	To study corneal surface; done to diagnose keratoconus, done prior to LASIK
12. Tonography	Measures facility of aqueous outflow
13. Ultrasound biomicroscope (UBM)	To view angle structures and to classify the type of glaucoma; useful in opaque corneas to view anterior segment structures and up to 5 mm depth
14. B scan ultrasound	For posterior segment evaluation (vitreous and retina)
15. A scan ultrasound	For axial length calculation, which is used in IOL power calculation before cataract surgery
16. Fundus fluorescein angiography	To visualize retinal vessels and retinal pathology

70. Answer is b (Retinal artery).
Ref: Harrison's 17th edition Pg 186.

- **Amaurosis Fugax** refers to a transient ischemic attack of the retina that results in *transient monocular blindness*, a term used interchangeably with amaurosis fugax.
- Patients describe a rapid fading of vision like a curtain descending, sometimes affecting only a portion of the visual field.
- Amaurosis fugax usually occurs from ***an embolus that becomes stuck within a retinal arteriole***.
- If the embolus breaks up or passes, flow is restored and vision returns quickly to normal without permanent damage.
- With prolonged interruption of blood flow, the inner retina suffers infarction. Ophthalmoscopy reveals zones of whitened, edematous retina following the distribution of branch retinal arterioles.
- ***Complete occlusion of the central retinal artery*** produces arrest of blood flow and a ***milky retina*** with a ***cherry-red fovea***.
- Emboli are composed of either cholesterol (Hollenhorst plaque), calcium or platelet-fibrin debris. The most common source is an atherosclerotic plaque in the carotid artery or aorta.

DERMATOLOGY, ANESTHESIOLOGY, RADIOLOGY AND PSYCHIATRY

71. Answer is a (Atopic dermatitis).
Ref: Harrison's, 17th edition Pg 313.

- In patients with localized disease, ***atopic dermatitis*** may be suspected because of a typical personal history, family history or the presence of cutaneous stigmata of AD such as:
  - ***Perioral pallor***
  - An extra fold of skin beneath the lower eyelid (***Dennie's line***)
  - ***Increased palmar skin markings***
  - Increased incidence of ***skin infections***, particularly with *Staphylococcus aureus*
  - ***Prominent pruritus*** and is exacerbated by dry skin
  - *Lichenification* (secondary to rubbing and scratching).

72. Answer is d (*Trichophyton schoenleinii*).
Ref: http://emedicine.medscape.com/article/1090828-overview

- ***Favus*** is a superficial dermatophyte infection usually caused by ***T. schoenleinii***.
- The ***scutulum***, a yellow cup-shaped crust that surrounds a hair and pierces its center, is characteristic.
- Treatment is with oral griseofulvin and shampoos (ketoconazole, selenium sulfide).

73. Answer is c (*Trichosporon beigelii*).
Ref: Harrison's 17th edition Pg 1265.

- ***Mycetoma*** is a chronic suppurative infection that begins in the subcutaneous tissue and *spreads to fascia and bone*.

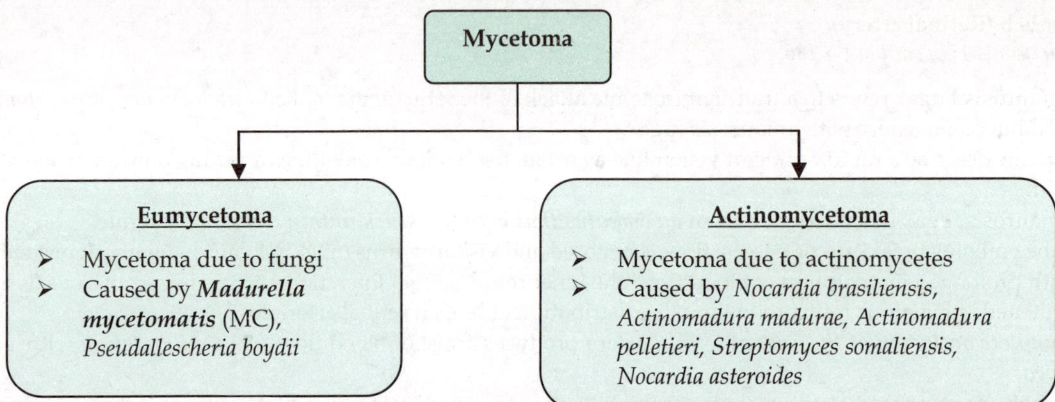

- Both diseases are characterized by ***abscesses containing grains*** composed of ***large aggregates of filaments*** (fungal or actinomycete).
- Traumatic inoculation is responsible for initial infection.

Note:

- ***Trichosporon beigelii*** is a minor component of normal skin flora and is widely distributed in nature. *T. beigelii* is regularly associated with the soft nodules of ***white piedra*** and has been involved in a variety of opportunistic infections in the immunosuppressed patient.
- ***Disseminated infections*** are most frequently a/w immunosuppression.
- Infections in ***non-immunosuppressed patients*** include:
  - Postsurgical ***endophthalmitis***
  - ***Endocarditis*** usually following insertion of prosthetic cardiac valves
  - ***Peritonitis*** in patients on continuous ambulatory peritoneal dialysis (CAPD) and IV abuse.

74. Answer is d (Secondary syphilis).
Ref: Harrison's, 17th edition Pg 323.

- Scattered, poorly circumscribed patches of ***alopecia with a 'moth-eaten' appearance*** are a manifestation of the ***secondary stage of syphilis***.

Also Know

- ***Telogen effluvium***—generalized hair loss caused by pregnancy, certain drugs, high fever or stress.
- ***Androgenic alopecia***—also known as male-pattern baldness.
- ***Trichotillomania***—manually pulling the hair out caused by a psychological disorder.
- Non-scarring type of alopeciain SLE may be localized to the frontal scalp, eventually resulting in multiple short hairs ***('lupus hairs')***.

75. Answer is b (Alopecia areata).
Ref: Harrison's, 17th edition Pg 323, Table 54-5.

- ***Pitting of nails*** may occur as a result of imperfect nail plate formation in the matrix area.

Pitting of nails may be a/w:

- Psoriasis
- Lichen planus
- Alopecia areata
- Eczema
- Idiopathic

76. Answer is d (Restlessness).
Ref: KD Tripathi, 6th edition Pg 431.

- ***Akathisia*** is a frequent and common adverse effect of treatment with ***antipsychotic (neuroleptic) drugs***.
- This syndrome consists of subjective feeling of ***inner restlessness and the urge to move about*** as well as objective components (rocking while standing or sitting, lifting feet as if marching on the spot and crossing and uncrossing the legs while sitting), ***but without anxiety***.

77. Answer is a (Temporal lobe epilepsy).
Ref: The Handbook of Juvenile Forensic Psychology By Neil Ribner, 2002 edition Pg 157.

- ***Gustatory hallucination*** is the ***sensation of taste*** in the absence of a gustatory stimulus; may be seen in
  - Temporal lobe epilepsy
  - Migraine
  - Schizophrenia
  - Cocaine intoxication.

78. Answer is c (End tidal CO_2).
Ref: Lee's anesthesia, 13th edition Pg 339.

Repeat Topic

- Venous ***air embolism*** may occur during any operative procedure in which the operative site is above the level of the heart and non-collapsible veins are exposed to atmospheric pressure or when air or any other gas is introduced under pressure into a body cavity (laparoscopy).
- ***Determination of end tidal CO_2 ($ETCO_2$)*** concentration to confirm adequate ventilation is useful during all anesthetic procedures, but particularly so for general anesthesia.
- ***A rapid fall of $ETCO_2$ is a sensitive indicator of air embolism***, a major complication of sitting craniotomies.
- Also ***see answer no. 94 in COMED-K 2009 answers***.

79. Answer is c (*Agranulocytosis*).
Ref: Davidson's, 20th edition Pg 243; Ref: Harrison's, 17th edition Pg 2722.

Repeat Question

- **See *answer no. 124 in COMED-K2010 answers*** for detailed explanation.

80. Answer is a (Visual hallucinations).
Ref: Niraj Ahuja's Psychiatry, 6th edition Pg 98-100.

Repeat Question

- See ***answer no. 123 in COMED-K 2010 answers*** for detailed explanation.

81. Answer is a (Hypothyroidism).
Ref. Harrison's, 17th edition Pg 2236; KD Tripathi, 6th edition Pg 35, 435.

Side effects of lithium

- ***Acute toxicity***: *Lithium causes* ***tremors***; *treatment of choice* is *hemodialysis*. Osmotic diuretics and sodium bicarbonate infusion promote Li excretion.
- Renal ***diabetes insipidus*** (thirst and polyuria).
- ***Hypothyroidism*** may occur.
- ***Leukocytosis.***
- ***Contraindicated in pregnancy*** (***Ebstein anomaly*** in neonate).

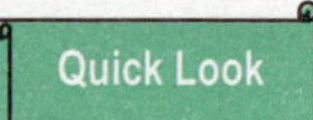

- **Therapeutic blood level** of lithium = 0.8–1.2 mEq/L.
- Since the margin of safety with lithium is narrow, monitoring of serum lithium concentration is essential for optimal therapy.

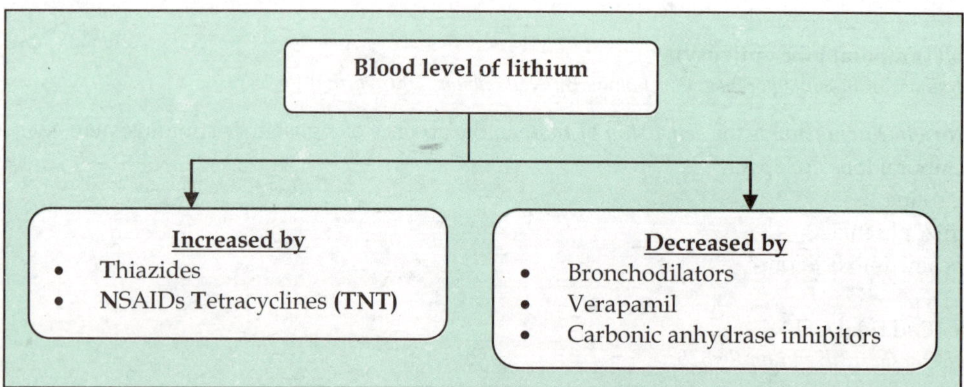

82. **Answer is b (Lunate).**
Ref: Essential orthopedics, Maheshwari, 3rd edition Pg 269.

- Specifically, ***Kienbock's disease*** is another name for ***avascular necrosis*** with fragmentation and collapse of the ***lunate***.

Types of Osteochondritis and Nomenclature

Crushing (due to avascular necrosis)	
• HiP joint	Perthe's
• Meta**tarsal**	**Frie**berg ***(Fried Meat)***
• Navicu**LAR**	**Koh**LER
• **Lunate**	Kienbock ***(Keen lunatic)***
• Thoracic Spine	*Scheur***mann**'s ***(Sure man,*** *nice* ***T Shirt)***
• **Cap**itulum	**Pan**ner's ***(PanCap)***
Traction epiphysitis (chronic strain injuries)	
• Tibial Tuberosity	Osgood-SchlaTTer
• **Calcaneum**	**Sever *(Severely Calc****ulative* ***Calcaneum!)***
• **Lower pole of patella**	Sinding-Larsen's
Splitting (osteochondritis dissecans)	
• Femoral condyles	--
• Elbow (capitulum)	--
• Ankle (talus)	--

Author's comments: *"You must remember the names of these osteochondritis – use the mnemonics given or make your own, useful in every Karnataka PGET and any entrance examination."*

83. **Answer is c (Sigmoid volvulus).**
Ref: Grainger and Allison Radiology, 4th edition Pg 988; ASI textbook of surgery, Pg 512.

Radiological features of sigmoid volvulus

- **Bird's beak or bird-of-prey sign**: Single contrast barium enema examination is adequate because the barium readily enters the empty rectum and usually encounters a complete stenosis, which is likened to a beak.

- A markedly distended sigmoid loop, which assumes a ***bent inner tube or inverted U***-shaped appearance, with the limbs of the sigmoid loop directed towards the pelvis.
- **Coffee bean sign**: The involved bowel walls are edematous and the contiguous walls form a dense white line on radiographs. This line is surrounded by the curved and dilated gas filled lumen resulting in a coffee bean-shaped structure.
- **Liver overlap sign**: The colonic haustra are lost and progressive distension elevates the sigmoid loop under one of the diaphragms.
- **Northern exposure sign**: A dilated sigmoid colon that ascends to the transverse colon is said to be reliable sign of sigmoid volvulus on a supine abdominal radiograph.

84. Answer is b (Renal oncocytomas).

Ref: Genitourinary radiology, The requisites, Ronald JZ, 2nd edition 2004 Pg 101.

- ***Renal oncocytomas*** are usually ***isoechoic to the kidney*** with well-demarcated margins.
- Masses that exceed 6 cm in diameter may have areas of ***central necrosis***.
- A central scar typical of oncocytoma may be visible with US.
- With CT or MRI these lesions appear well circumscribed and have homogenous enhancement patterns with ***pseudocapsule***.
- As these lesions enlarge, a ***central stellate scar*** may be detectable ***with CT or MRI***.
- Although this scar is typical of oncocytoma, it is not diagnostic and ***RCC may have an identical appearance***.

85. Answer is d (Vertebral hemangiomas).

Ref: Essential orthopedics, Maheshwari, 3rd edition Pg 215.

X-ray findings in *vertebral hemangiomas* include:

- Vertebral body: Vertical striations ('ivory')
- Skull: 'Sunburst' or 'sunrise'
- Long bone: 'Soap bubble' or honeycomb, which may surround a joint

86. Answer is c (Sickle cell anemia).

Ref: Harrison's, 17th edition Pg 638, Table 99.2.

X-ray findings in sickle cell anemia

1. Deossification due to marrow hyperplasia	❖ ***'H-shaped vertebrae'*** or 'fish vertebrae' ❖ Decreased bone density in skull with widened diploic space ❖ Rib notching
2. Thrombosis and ***bone infarction***	❖ Avascular Necrosis, esp. femoral head ❖ Periosteal reaction ***('bone within bone')***
3. Secondary osteomyelitis	❖ *Staphylococcus aureus* > ***Salmonella*** ❖ Dactylitis = ***'hand foot syndrome'***
4. Growth effects	❖ Bone shortening secondary to diminished blood supply

87. Answer is b (Nitrous oxide).

Ref: Clinical Anesthesiology by Morgan, 4th edition Pg 779; Pediatric anesthesia, Edward Doyle, 2007 edition Pg 252.

- ***Tympanoplasty and other middle ear surgeries*** are usually performed under general endotracheal anesthesia.
- *During tympanoplasty the middle ear is open* to the atmosphere and there is no pressure build up. Once the surgeon has placed a *tympanic membrane graft the middle ear becomes a closed space*.

- If nitrous oxide is allowed to diffuse into this space, middle ear pressure will rise and the ***graft may be displaced***. Hence ***nitrous oxide should be avoided***.
- Similarly *nitrous oxide* should be *avoided during laparoscopy*.

88. Answer is b (Lignocaine).
Ref: KD Tripathi, 6th edition Pg 513.

- ***Lignocaine*** is the most widely used ***local anesthetic***.
- In addition it is used as a ***popular antiarrhythmic in ICUs***.

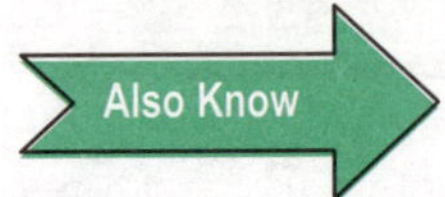

- ❖ The most prominent cardiac (antiarrhythmic) action of lignocaine is ***suppression of automaticity in ectopic foci***.
- ❖ Lignocaine is a ***blocker of inactivated Na⁺ channels***, but does not delay channel recovery (channel recovery time < 1 s) – ***subclass IB***.
- ❖ It does not depress AV conduction or prolong (or even shorten) APD, ERP and Q-T.
- ❖ It is used ***only in ventricular tachyarrhythmias***.
- ❖ ***Good drug in emergency setting*** (e.g. Flowing acute MI, digitalis toxicity, during cardiac surgery, etc.)
- ❖ It is *ineffective in atrial arrhythmias*.

89. Answer is b (Ketamine).
Ref: KD Tripathi, 6th edition Pg 376.

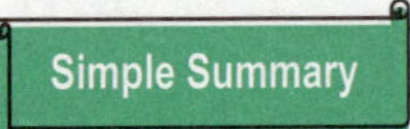

Ketamine

Pharmacology
– A phencyclidine derivative; produces an anesthetic state frequently called ***'dissociative anesthesia'***, which implies that the patient is detached from their surroundings – ***Vivid hallucinations*** are common during recovery ***(emergence delirium)*** and can be minimized by concurrent use of benzodiazepines (e.g. midazolam).
Systemic Effects
– ↑↑ *BP, IOP, ICT* – May be dangerous for hypertensive and in ischemic heart disease – ***Heart rate, BP, cardiac output are elevated (due to sympathetic stimulation)*** and well-maintained even in *shocked patients*, it is *useful in emergency surgery* – Laryngeal reflexes are better maintained and *bronchodilatation* occurs; it ↑ salivation.
Advantages
– Ketamine can also be administered by *IM* injection even when venous access is difficult. – Common procedures undertaken with ketamine anesthesia include minor to intermediate orthopedic surgery (especially distal arm or lower leg surgery including manipulation of fractures), gynecological surgery (e.g. dilatation, curettage and other minor surgical procedures), drainage of abscesses, debridement of burns, change of dressings.

90. Answer is a (Pneumothorax).
Ref: Morgan's clinical anesthesia, 2003 edition Pg 987.

- A ***flutter valve*** also known as the ***Heimlich valve*** after its inventor, Henry Heimlich is a one way valve used in respiratory medicine to prevent air from traveling back along a chest tube.
- It is most commonly used to help ***remove air from a pneumothorax***.

91. Answer is a (Barotrauma).

Ref: Review of clinical anesthesia By Neil Roy Connelly , 5th edition Pg 131.

Direct quote:

"A ventilator pressure relief valve stuck in closed position can cause ***barotrauma***".

- Whenever a ventilator is used, the circle system pressure relief valve should be closed or functionally removed from the circuit.
- Ventilators commonly used in anesthesia, contain their own pressure-relief valves that remain closed during inspiration so that positive pressure can be generated. When the bellows are filled during expiration, circuit pressure rises and ventilator pressure relief valve opens. ***Sticking of this valve*** results in abnormally elevated airway pressure and hence has chances of ***barotrauma to the lungs***.

92. Answer is a (Lateral margin).

Ref: http://www.ajronline.org/cgi/reprint/145/3/521.pdf (Miller WT, et al. The troublesome nipple shadow. AJR 1985 (September); http://www.radrounds.com/photo/nipple-shadows-on-chest-xray

Classic Nipple Shadows

- Bilateral symmetric
- Fuzzy margins with radiolucent halo or ***sharp lateral,*** but poorly defined medial margins
- Characteristic location (fifth or sixth anterior ribs or near bottom of breast shadow)

93. Answer is d (Lytic lesions).

Ref: Davidson's, 20th edition Pg 1076, Box 25.5; Pg 1127; Essential Orthopedics, Maheshwari, 3rd edition Pg 263.

Radiology of Osteomalacia

- X-rays appear to be of ***'poor quality'***! i.e. not sharply defined—***osteopenia*** on X-ray or decreased bone mineral density.
- Diffuse ***rarefaction*** of bones.
- ***Looser's zones*** (pseudofractures): Radiolucent zones occurring at fracture sites; MC pubic rami, axillary border of scapula, ribs and medial cortex of neck of femur.
- ***Triradiate pelvis*** in females.
- ***Protrusio acetabuli.***
- ***Milkman's fractures.***

QuickLook

- ***Osteomalacia*** = literally means 'softening of bones'; is the adult counterpart of rickets.
- The hypocalcemia and hypophosphatemia that accompany ***vitamin D deficiency*** result in impaired mineralization of bone matrix proteins → osteomalacia.

Laboratory diagnosis of vitamin D deficient osteomalacia

- Low or low-normal serum Ca^{2+} and P^{+}
- ***Raised serum alkaline phosphatase***
- Low 25(OH)D
- Raised Parathormone (PTH)

Note:

- ***Osteomalacia*** is a/w ***proximal myopathy***.
- ***Lytic lesions*** are usually a feature of ***metastases***.

94. Answer is c (2).

Ref: http://education.yahoo.com/reference/gray/subjects/subject/56; http://education.yahoo.com/reference/gray/illustrations/figure?id=234

- The **carpal bones** are each ossified from a single center and ossification proceeds in the following order:

Ossification Year	Carpal Bones
During the 1st year	Capitate and hamate, the capitate earlier
During the 3rd year	Triangular
During the 5th year	Lunate and greater multangular, the lunate earlier
During the 6th year	Navicular
During the 8th year	Lesser multangular
About the 12th year	Pisiform

FORENSIC MEDICINE

95. Answer is d (Precipitin test).

Ref: Narayan Reddy's FMT, 23rd edition Pg 216.

- ***Precipitin test*** is used to test *whether blood-stains are related to human or not.*
- Serum for this test is obtained from rabbits, which have produced antibodies to destroy a small quantity of human blood injected into them.
- A drop of this anti-human serum is added to suspect blood, which will precipitate its protein if it is of human origin.
- The precipitin test is sensitive and will work on small traces of blood.
- The test is also known as the ***Uhlenhuth test*** after the German scientist who developed it.
- For other tests of blood, ***see answer no. 127 in Karnataka 2010 answers***.

96. Answer is d (Arsenic).

Ref: Narayan Reddy's FMT, 23rd edition Pg 269.

- Arsenic is the ***most popular homicidal poison*** because:
  - ☐ It is cheap, easily available
  - ☐ Colorless, odorless, tasteless—can be easily administered with food or drink
  - ☐ Small quantity is required to cause death
  - ☐ Onset of symptoms is gradual and ***simulates cholera***.
- However disadvantages are:
  - ☐ It delays putrefaction
  - ☐ Can be detected in completely decomposed bodies
  - ☐ Can be found in bones, hair and nails for a long time
  - ☐ Can be detected in charred bones or ashes.

Arsenic poisoning

❖ **Chemical nature**	– Metallic arsenic is ***not*** poisonous, as it is not absorbed from the alimentary canal. – Arsenic or white arsenic is arsenious oxide or arsenic trioxide (Sankhya or Somalkhar) – Copper arsenite is ***Scheele's green***; Copper acetoarsenite is ***Paris green*** – Arsenic combines with ***sulfhydryl enzymes*** and interferes with cell metabolism – Most popular homicidal poison
❖ **Acute poisoning**	– Resembles cholera, gastroenteritic type; ***garlic*** odor – When acute arsenic poisoning is suspected, X-ray of the abdomen may reveal ingested arsenic, which is ***radio-opaque*** – Arsenic is rapidly cleared from blood and distributed to various organs and tissues. Blood sample is useful only in acute poisoning

❖ **Chronic poisoning**	– Skin and nail changes, such as hyperkeratosis, ***'rain drop'*** hyperpigmentation , exfoliative dermatitis and ***Mee's*** lines (transverse white striae of the fingernails) – Sensory and motor ***polyneuritis*** manifesting as numbness and tingling in a 'stocking-glove' distribution – ***Subendocardial hemorrhages*** of the left ventricle – ***Stomach*** mainly affected and shows red-velvety appearance – Chronic consumption of water containing arsenic at high concentrations leads to vasospasm and peripheral vascular insufficiency culminating in ***'blackfoot disease'***, a gangrenous condition affecting the extremities – Risk of skin cancer and possibly of ***cancers*** of the lung, liver (angiosarcoma), bladder, kidney and colon
❖ **Tests**	– **MAR**sh test and Reinsch tests are positive – Arsenic can be detected in completely decomposed bodies, since it is present in hair, nails and bones
❖ **Treatment**	– Freshly prepared hydrated ferric oxide (Fe_2O_3) is ***arsenic antidote***; Dialyzed iron maybe used as substitute – **Alkalis should not be given as they increase the solubility of arsenic**

97. Answer is a (Acute hemolysis).
Ref: Narayan Reddy's FMT, 23rd edition Pg 270-71.

- Ingestion of ***copper sulfate (blue vitriol)*** is an uncommon mode of poisoning in the Indian subcontinent. Cases are ***mainly suicidal*** in nature.
- The clinical course of the copper sulfate intoxicated patient is often complex involving ***intravascular hemolysis, jaundice and renal failure***.
- ***Intravascular hemolysis*** appears ***12–24 h following ingestion of copper sulfate.***
- Hemolytic anemia, is caused either by direct red cell membrane damage or indirectly as a result of the inactivation of enzymes (including glutathione reductase), which protect against oxidative stress.
- Copper ions can oxidize heme iron to form methemoglobin. This blood loses its oxygen carrying capacity. Clinically cyanosis and chocolate brown blood may be seen.

98. Answer is b (Barr body).
Ref: Narayan Reddy's FMT, 23rd edition Pg 33.

- In those species (including humans) in which sex is determined by the presence of the Y or X chromosome, a ***Barr body is the inactive X chromosome in a female cell*** or the inactive Z in a male (Lyon, 2003), rendered inactive in a process called Lyonization.
- The Lyon hypothesis states that in cells with multiple X chromosomes, all but one is inactivated during mammalian embryogenesis (Lyon, 1961). This happens early in embryonic development at random in mammals.
- A dark pack of sex chromatin, called ***Barr body, is seen in the interphase nucleus of all female mammals.***
- Normally – males never have a Barr body and women always have one.

<u>Note</u>:

❖ In females, neutrophil leukocytes contain a small nuclear appendage of drumstick form ***(Davidson body)*** in up to 6% of cells.

99. Answer is d (Sexual pleasure derived from non-living things).
Ref: Narayana Reddy's FMT, 23rd edition Pg 196.

Repeat Topic

- ***Fetishism*** is the ***use of an inanimate object or a specific part of the body*** for ***physical or mental sexual stimulation.***
- Also see ***answer no. 150 in COMDED-K 2009 answers*** for summary of sexual paraphilias.

100. Answer is a (Eyelids).
Ref: Narayan Reddy's FMT, 23rd edition Pg 82.

Postmortem Rigidity or Rigor Mortis (RM)

- Occurs due to ***ATP depletion***.
- **Appears first in involuntary muscles of heart**; then it begins in the ***eyelids*** >> neck >> lower jaw >> muscle of face >> muscle of chest and UL >> abdomen >> LL muscle.
- Time of onset of RM—***in India it begins in 1–2 hours after death*** and takes further 1–2 hours to develop.
- Duration of RM—in India it lasts usually 24–48 hours in winter and 18 to 36 hours in summer. It last for 2–3 days in temperate regions.
- Early RM occurs in death due to strychnine poisoning, cholera, cancers, TB, typhoid, fatigue/exhaustion before death (due to rapid ATP depletion).
- ***Delayed RM*** occurs in death due to
  - Arsenic poisoning
  - Apoplexy
  - Pneumonia
  - Asphyxia.
- RM *does not occur in a fetus of less than 7 months*.

101. Answer is b (1.5°F/hour).
Ref: Forensics demystified, by David Fishcer, Barry AJ Fischer, 2006 edition Pg 69.

- ***Algor mortis (cooling of dead body)*** is the rate at which a body loses heat and in a normal room temperature environment it is ***1.5°F/hour***.

102. Answer is d (Root transparency).
Ref: Narayan Reddy's, FMT, 23rd edition Pg 43.

Gustafson's method: Age estimation of adult over 21 years depends upon the physiologic changes in each of the dental tissues:

- Attrition
- Paradentosis
- Secondary dentin
- Cementum apposition
- Root resorption
- ***Transparency of the root***: ***Most reliable*** of all criteria.

PATHOLOGY

103. Answer is a (Hyperplastic polyp).
Ref: Robbins Basic pathology, 7th edition Pg 821.

- ***Hyperplastic polyp*** ('regeneration polyp', 'inflammatory polyp') is *the* ***most common type*** of gastric polyp (75–90%)
- ***Histology***: Proliferated gastric mucosa with acute and chronic inflammatory infiltrates in lamina propria
- ***Location***: Randomly distributed in stomach and may be associated with chronic atrophic gastritis and pernicious anemia
- On examination, findings include: Sharply delineated polyp with smooth circular border; 'Mexican hat sign': stalk seen in face overlying the head of the polyp; sessile/pedunculate; usually multiple usually < 1 cm; no contour defect in stomach.

104. Answer is b (Lymphoblasts).
Ref: Rubin's pathology, Pg 745.

- In Acute Lymphoblastic Leukemia (ALL), blasts with ***L1 or L2 morphology showing block PAS positivity*** are classified as ***lymphoblasts***.

105. Answer is d (IgA and C3).
Ref: Harrison's, 17th edition Pg 1788.

- ***Berger*** first described the glomerulonephritis termed ***IgA nephropathy***.
- It is classically characterized by ***episodic hematuria*** associated with the deposition of ***IgA in the mesangium***.
- *IgM, IgG, C3* or immunoglobulin light chains may be ***codistributed with IgA***.

106. Answer is c (von Hippel-Lindau disease).
Ref: Harrison's, 17th edition Pg 592, 1800.

- ***Renal cell carcinoma*** with clear cell histologic features, which may be bilateral, ***develops in nearly 40% of patients with von Hippel-Lindau (VHL) disease*** and is a ***major cause of death among these patients***.
- ***Deletions of 3p*** occur commonly in renal cell carcinoma associated with VHL disease.
- The high risk of renal cell carcinoma mandates periodic surveillance (usually yearly in adults) by either CT or MRI.
- Other associations of VHL disease:
  - Pheochromocytoma
  - Pancreatic cysts and islet cell tumors
  - Retinal angiomas
  - Central nervous system hemangioblastomas
  - Endolymphatic sac tumors
  - Epididymal cystadenomas.

More About

- ***Beckwith-Wiedemann syndrome***: Macrosomia, macroglossia, omphalocele.
- ***Eagle-Barrett syndrome (Prune-Belly syndrome)***:
  - A partial or complete lack of abdominal muscles. There may be wrinkly folds of skin covering the abdomen.
  - Undescended testicles in males.
  - Urinary tract abnormality such as unusually large ureters, distended bladder, accumulation and backflow of urine from the bladder to the ureters and the kidneys.
  - Frequent urinary tract infections due to the inability to properly expel urine.

107. Answer is d (Hyperplastic arteriosclerosis).
Ref: Robbin's pathology, 7th edition Pg 529-30.

Vascular Pathology in Hypertension

Hyaline arteriolosclerosis	Hyperplastic arteriolosclerosis
➤ Associated with *mild diabetes and mild hypertension*. ➤ Endothelial injury → migration of circulating monocytes and other inflammatory cells, which engulf lipoproteins and oxidized LDL → production of inflammatory mediators → continued inflammation and build of cholesterol → formation of ***plaques***.	➤ A concentric lamellar ***onion-skin reduplication*** of intimal smooth muscle cells. ➤ Characteristic of *malignant hypertension*. ➤ Frequently associated with *fibrin deposition* and wall necrosis (necrotizing arteriolitis).

108. Answer is b (Sarcoidosis).
Ref: Harrison's, 17th edition Pg 1644.

- **Granulomatous Lung Disease:** This process is characterized by an accumulation of T lymphocytes, macrophages and epithelioid cells organized into discrete structures (granulomas) in the lung parenchyma. The granulomatous lesions can progress to fibrosis. Many patients with granulomatous lung disease remain free of severe impairment of lung function or, when symptomatic, they improve after treatment. The main differential diagnosis is between ***sarcoidosis*** and ***hypersensitivity pneumonitis***.

- Histologically, involvement of both lung and lymph nodes occurs in nearly all instances of ***sarcoidosis***. Multiple sarcoid nodules are scattered in the interstitium, particularly in relation to lymphatics, i.e. in the bronchovascular bundle and in the lobular septa. There is increased cellularity of the alveolar walls, owing to infiltrate of mononuclear cells.
- The central part of the ***granuloma*** is fibrotic and surrounded by ***palisaded histiocytes***. In about 60% cases, ***Schaumann bodies*** (laminated calcified proteinaceous concretions) and ***asteroid bodies*** (stellate inclusions within giant cells) are found. Giant cells at the periphery resemble those of the tuberculosis.
- The cuff of lymphocytes that surrounds the histiocytes is inconspicuous, compared with tuberculosis, hence the term ***'naked tubercle'***.
- Granulomas also occur in the airways and occasionally may be so prominent as to lead to airway obstruction (endobronchial sarcoid). Pulmonary lesions have strong tendency to heal, so that only hyalinized scars may be seen microscopically.

109. Answer is a (Myelodysplastic syndrome).

Ref: Robbins pathology, 7th edition Pg 695, 696 figure; Pathology pretest, Earl Brown, 270.

- ***Dysmegakaryocytopoiesis*** with discrete megakaryocyte nuclei lacking lobation (***'pawn ball' nuclei***) are seen in ***myelodysplastic syndrome***.

110. Answer is a (Organ of Zuckerkandl).

Ref: Robbin's pathology, 7th edition Pg.1218.

- The ***Organ of Zuckerkandl*** (close to origin of the inferior mesenteric artery) is of pathological significance in the adult as the ***most common extra-adrenal site of pheochromocytoma.***

Also Know

- ***Over 90% of pheochromocytomas*** are located ***within the adrenal glands*** and 98% are within the abdomen.
- Extra-adrenal pheochromocytomas develop in the paraganglion chromaffin tissue of the sympathetic nervous system. They may occur anywhere from the base of the brain to the urinary bladder.
- Common locations for *extra-adrenal pheochromocytomas include the organ of Zuckerkandl*, bladder wall, heart, mediastinum and carotid and glomus jugulare bodies.

111. Answer is a (Nodular).

Ref: Bailey and Love, 25th edition Pg 609.

Types of basal cell carcinoma (BCC)

Localized BCC	Generalized BCC
• Nodular • Nodulocystic • Cystic • Pigmented • Nevoid	• Superficial • Multifocal • Superficial spreading • Infiltrative • Morphoeic • Ice pick • Cicatrizing

- ***Nodular and nodulocystic*** variants account for ***90% of BCCs***.

112. Answer is b (12–24 hours).

Ref: Robbins, pathology, 7th edition Pg 577-581.

- For the first ~30 minutes no change at all can be seen by gross examination or by light microscopy in histopathology.
- *On electron microscopy:*
  - Reversible phase (first 30 minutes): Relaxed myofibrils, glycogen depletion and mitochondrial swelling.
  - Irreversible phase (after first 30 minutes): Sarcolemal disruption, mitochondrial amorphous densities.

Time from onset	Gross examination	Microscopically	Comments
2–3 hours		Wavy myocardial fibers Staining defect with tetrazolium or basic fuchsin dye	
4–12 hours		Coagulation necrosis with loss of cross striations, contraction bands, edema, hemorrhage, early neutrophilic infiltrate	
18–24 hours	Pallor of myocardium	Continuing coagulation necrosis, pyknosis of nuclei, marginal contraction bands	Risk for arrhythmia
24–72 hours	Pallor with some hyperemia	Total loss of nuclei and striations dense neutrophilic infiltrate	
3–7 days	Hyperemic border with central yellowing	Macrophage and mononuclear infiltration begin, fibrovascular response begins	Risk for ventricular wall rupture
10–21 days	Maximally yellow and soft with vascular margins	Fibrovascular response Prominent granulation tissue	
6 weeks	White fibrosis	Fibrosis	Risk for ventricular aneurysm

113. Answer is c (CD21).
Ref: Harrison's 20th edition Pg 1079, 1106.

- ***Epstein-Barr virus (EBV)*** glycoprotein gp350 binds to the B lymphocyte complement receptor CD21 and then engages major histocompatibility complex (MHC) class II molecules as a coreceptor.
- The ***EBV receptor (CD21)*** on the surface of B cells is also the receptor for the C3d component of complement. EBV infection of epithelial cells results in viral replication and production of virions. When B cells are infected by EBV in vitro, they become transformed and can proliferate indefinitely.

MICROBIOLOGY

114. Answer is a (*Mycobacterium ulcerans*).
Ref: Harrison's, 17th edition Pg 1031.

- ***Buruli ulcer*** is a disease caused by infection with ***Mycobacterium ulcerans****; in* tropical and subtropical climates
- Infection leads to extensive destruction of skin and soft tissue with the formation of ***large ulcers usually on the legs or arms***.

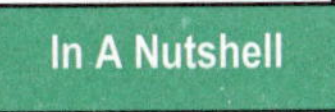

ATYPICAL MYCOBACTERIA (Runyon classification)

Classification	Infection and comments
1. Photochromogens	*M. kansasii, M. simiae, M. asiaticum*
2. Scotochromogens	*M. scrofulaceum* [Pigmented colonies, even in the dark; Scrofula (cervical adenitis) in children]
3. Non-photochromogens	*M. intracellulare* (a/w AIDS), *M. avium, M. xenopi (epididymitis)*

4. Rapid growers (*Grow within 7 days)*	*M. chelonae* (Porcine heart valves), *M. fortuitum, M. szulgai* (subcutaneous bursitis)
5. Skin pathogens	*M. ulcerans (Buruli ulcer); M. marinum (swimming pool granuloma)*

115. Answer is c (Campylobacter infection).

Ref: Harrison's, 17th edition Pg 814, Table 122-1.

Gastrointestinal Pathogens and Features of Acute Diarrhea

Mechanism	Location and Illness	Stool Findings	Examples of Pathogens Involved
Non-inflammatory (enterotoxin)	Proximal small Bowel; Watery diarrhea	NO fecal leukocytes; mild or no increase in fecal lactoferrin	*V. cholerae*, ETEC (LT and/or ST), EAEC, *C. perfringens, Bacillus cereus, S. aureus, Aeromonas hydrophila, Plesiomonas shigelloides*, rotavirus, norovirus, enteric adenoviruses, *Giardia lamblia, Cryptosporidium, Cyclospora,* microsporidia
Inflammatory (invasion or cytotoxin)	Colon or distal small bowel; ***Dysentery or inflammatory diarrhea***	***Fecal polymorphonuclear leukocytes;*** substantial increase in fecal lactoferrin	*Shigella, Salmonella,* ***C. jejuni,*** EHEC, EIEC, *Y. enterocolitica, V. parahaemolyticus, Cl. difficile, E. histolytica*
Penetrating	Distal small Bowel; Enteric fever	Fecal mononuclear leukocytes	*Salmonella typhi*

ETEC = enterotoxigenic *E. coli;* EAEC = enteroaggregative *E. coli; EHEC* = enterohemorrhagic *E. coli; EIEC* = enteroinvasive *E. coli.*

116. Answer is a (IgM).

Ref: Textbook of Microbiology, 3rd edition CP Baveja, Pg 101, Table 13.1.

Repeat Topic

- ***The primary immune response***: The immune response occurring on the first exposure to an antigen. After a lag or latent period of from 3 to 14 days depending on the antigen, specific antibodies appear in the blood. There is a ***peak of IgM production lasting several days*** followed immediately by a peak of IgG production.
- See ***answer no. 50 in Karnataka 2009 answers*** for detailed summary table on immunoglobulins.

117. Answer is c (*Treponema pallidum*).

Ref: Pediatric infectious disease secrets, Joel Dk, Pg 199, 2003 edition.

- ***Pneumonia alba***: A fatal desquamative ***pneumonia of the newborn due to congenital syphilis,*** with fatty degeneration of the lungs.

118. Answer is d (Measles).

Ref: Park, 20th edition Pg 92.

- A ***teratogen*** is an agent, such as a virus, a drug, or radiation that causes malformation of an embryo or fetus.
- ***Teratogenic viral infections*** are: ***TORCH*** infections
  - TOxoplasmosis
  - Rubella virus
  - Cytomegalovirus
  - Herpes virus.

119. Answer is c (Polyomavirus).

Ref: Harrison's, 17th edition Pg 1781, Table 276.5.

- The ***polyoma group (BK, JC, SV40)*** is another class of DNA viruses that ***can become dormant in kidneys and can be activated by immunosuppression***.
- When reactivation occurs with BK there is a 50% chance of progressive fibrosis and *loss of the graft within 1 year by the activated virus*.
- The ***use of tacrolimus has been a/w the highest risk***.

Opportunistic Infections in the Renal Transplant Recipient		
Peritransplant (< 1 month)	**Early (1–6 months)**	**Late (> 6 months)**
❖ Wound infections	❖ *Pneumocystis carinii*	❖ *Aspergillus*
❖ Herpes virus	❖ Cytomegalovirus	❖ *Nocardia*
❖ Oral candidiasis	❖ *Legionella*	❖ BK virus (polyoma)
❖ Urinary tract infection	❖ *Listeria*	❖ Herpes zoster
	❖ Hepatitis B, C	❖ Hepatitis B, C

120. Answer is b (Adenovirus) and c (Parvovirus).
Ref: Textbook of Microbiology, CP Baveja, 3rd edition Pg 418.

CLASSIFICATION OF DNA VIRUSES

Capsid symmetry	Virion: Enveloped or Naked	Physical type of Nucleic acid	Virus family
Icosahedral	Naked	SS	Parvoviridae
		DS circular	Papovaviridae
		DS	Adenoviridae
	Enveloped	DS	Herpesviridae
Complex	Complex coats	DS	Poxviridae
		DS circular	HepaDNAviridae

CLASSIFICATION OF RNA VIRUSES

Capsid symmetry	Virion: Enveloped or Naked	Physical type of Nucleic acid	Virus family
Icosahedral	Naked	SS	PicoRNAviridae
		DS segmented	Reoviridae
	Enveloped	SS	Togaviridae
Unknown or complex	Enveloped	SS	Flaviviridae
		SS segmented	Arenaviridae
		SS	Coronaviridae
		SS	Retroviridae
Helical	Enveloped	SS segmented	Bunyaviridae
		SS segmented	Orthomyxoviridae
			Paramyxoviridae
			Rhabdoviridae

Inferences from the above tables are

■ **DNA virus**	– Herpes, Hepadna, Adeno, Parvo, Papilloma, Polyoma, Pox viruses. "***HHAPPPPy** viruses*" – All are double stranded (dsDNA) *except* Parvovirus single stranded (ss DNA) – Naked DNA viruses are Parvo, Adeno, Papilloma, Polyoma viruses **(*"PAPP"*)** – All replicate in the nucleus *except* Pox (carries own DNA-dependent RNA polymerase) – All are linear except Hepadna (partial circular), Papilloma, Polyoma (circular) – All are icosahedral *except* Poxvirus (complex)

■ RNA virus	– All are single stranded (ssRNA) *except* Reovirus (double stranded, dsRNA) – Naked RNA viruses are **Picorna**, **Calici** and **Reoviruses** ***('PCR')*** – All replicate in cytoplasm *except* influenza and reoviruses – Segmented RNA viruses are **Bunya**, **Orthomyxo**, **Arena**, **Retroviruses** ***('BOAR')***

121. Answer is d (IgE).
Ref: Textbook of Microbiology, 3rd edition CP Baveja, Pg 101, Table 13.1.

Repeat Topic

- ***Immunoglobulin E (IgE)*** plays an important role in ***allergy*** and is especially associated with ***type 1 hypersensitivity***.
- See ***answer no. 50 in COMED-K 2009 answers*** for detailed summary table on immunoglobulins.

122. Answer is c (IgG).
Ref: Textbook of Microbiology, 3rd edition CP Baveja, Pg 101, Table 13.1.

Repeat Topic

- *IgG* is the only isotype that ***can pass through the human placenta***, thereby providing ***natural passive immunity to the fetus*** in utero and the newborn.
- See ***answer no. 50 in Karnataka 2009 answers*** for detailed summary table on immunoglobulins.

123. Answer is c (*Plasmodium vivax*).
Ref: Park, 20th edition Pg 225.

Direct quote:
"Persons whose RBCs are 'Duffy negative' are resistant to P. vivax infection."

Also Know

❖ Newborns have considerable resistance to *P. falciparum* infection due to high levels of HbF.
❖ Patients with sickle cell trait, thalassemia and G-6-PD deficiency are relatively immune to malaria.

124. Answer is c (Mucormycosis).
Ref: Harrison's, 17th edition Pg 1261.

- ***Mucormycosis*** (***zygomycosis***) is a serious, relatively uncommon invasive fungal infection.
- MC in ***uncontrolled diabetics, immunocompromised patients*** and ***iron overload syndromes*** (particularly those associated with hemodialysis).
- In diabetic patients with elevated blood sugar levels and acidemia, the spores germinate, hyphae develop and the fungi begin an inexorable march throughout the lung tissue, ***invading blood vessels*** and surrounding tissues.
- ***As blood vessels become involved, thrombosis occurs***, tissue necrosis results and the fungi continue to grow in this devitalized tissue.
- Involvement includes:
  - ➢ Rhinocerebral mucormycosis—***cavernous sinus thrombosis*** is a grave complication.
  - ➢ Pulmonary mucormycosis
  - ➢ GI mucormycosis
  - ➢ Cutaneous mucormycosis

125. Answer is c (*Brucella melitensis*).
Ref: Harrison's, 17th edition Pg 1124.

- ***Brucellosis*** is called ***undulant fever*** from the remittent character of its fever or from its resemblance to malaria and typhoid (e.g. typhomalarial fever, intermittent typhoid).
- ***Brucella melitensis*** is the main species of bacteria that cause brucellosis.

- Humans are commonly infected with the *Brucella* organism through ingestion of ***contaminated milk*** or dairy products.

Synonyms of brucellosis
- Malta fever
- Mediterranean fever
- Gibraltar fever
- Cyprus fever

Note: *"Maltese cross" appearance* is seen in *babesiosis*, no connection with brucellosis.

PHARMACOLOGY

126. Answer is c (Hypercalcemia).

Ref: KD Tripathi, 6th edition Pg 566-67.

Adverse reactions of furosemide

Gastrointestinal System	CNS	Hematologic
– ***Pancreatitis*** – Intrahepatic cholestatic jaundice – Anorexia, nausea, vomiting, headache	– ***Ototoxicity*** – Paresthesias – Vertigo, dizziness, – Blurred vision, xanthopsia	– Aplastic anemia (rare) – Thrombocytopenia – Agranulocytosis (rare) – Hemolytic anemia – Leukopenia, anemia
Others	**CVS**	**Dermatologic**
– *Hyperglycemia* – *Hyperuricemia* – *Hypokalemia* – Hypomagnesemia – *Hypocalcemia* – Metabolic alkalosis – Muscle spasm/weakness – Urinary bladder spasm – Thrombophlebitis	– Orthostatic hypotension may occur and be aggravated by alcohol, barbiturates or narcotics	– Exfoliative dermatitis – Erythema multiforme purpura – Photosensitivity – Pruritus, urticaria, rash – Systemic vasculitis – Interstitial nephritis – Necrotizing angiitis – Fever

127. Answer is d (Argatroban).

Ref: Harrison's, 17th edition Pg 721, 743.

- Argatroban is a ***direct thrombin inhibitor*** that *reversibly binds to the thrombin* active site. It does not require the cofactor antithrombin III for antithrombotic activity. It exerts its anticoagulant effects *by **inhibiting thrombin-catalyzed or thrombin-induced reactions**,* including fibrin formation and activation of coagulation factors V, VIII and XIII.
- It *also inhibits the effect of thrombin on protein C activation and platelet aggregation.*
- Uses:
  - As an anticoagulant for ***prophylaxis or treatment of thrombosis*** in patients with ***heparin induced thrombocytopenia*** (HIT)
  - In patients with or at risk for HIT undergoing percutaneous coronary intervention.

Note:

- ***Fondaparinux, enoxaparin and dalteparin*** are ***low-molecular-weight heparins***.

Simple Summary

All About Anticoagulant Drugs

Drug	Mechanism	Role/Comments	Adverse Effects
Heparin	Activates *antithrombin III, which* ↓ the activity of thrombin and Xa and prevents clot formation. Monitor PTT.	Immediate anticoagulation for MI, DVT, PE, stroke and postoperative prophylaxis for DVT and PE; dialysis, ↓ post-MI thrombus risk, safer in pregnancy (does not cross placenta).	*Thrombocytopenia* (HIT), hemorrhage, osteoporosis; hypersensitivity, narrow therapeutic window, short half-life; for heparin reversal use *protamine sulfate.*
Low-molecular-weight heparin – Eno*X*aparin – Dalteparin	Binds to *factor **Xa*** to prevent clot formation. Can give SC and without laboratory monitoring. 2–4 times longer half-life.	Postoperative prophylaxis for DVT and PE, *safest option during pregnancy.*	Hemorrhage, fever and rare thrombocytopenia; not easily reversible.
Direct thrombin inhibitors – Lepirudin – Argatroban – Bivalirudin	*Highly selective inhibitors of thrombin* to suppress activity of factors V, IX and XIII and platelet aggregation.	Alternative to heparin for anticoagulation in patients *with* h/o *HIT.*	Hemorrhage and hypotension.
Direct factor Xa inhibitors – Fondaparinux	Highly selective inhibition of factor Xa *without activity against thrombin.*	DVT prophylaxis, anticoagulation following acute DVT or PE.	Hemorrhage, fever, *anemia, edema*, rash, constipation.
Warfarin (Coumadin)	Impairs synthesis and carboxylation of vitamin K dependent of factors II, VII, IX and X and protein C and protein C and protein S. Affects Extrinsic pathway and ↑ PT. Follow PT/INR values.	*Long-term anticoagulation* post-thrombotic event or in cases of ↑ thrombus risk (postsurgery, Afib, artificial valves); long half-life; metabolized by cytochrome P-450 pathway.	Hemorrhage, numerous *drug interactions* and *teratogenicity (Conradi syndrome).*
Aspirin – ASA, Acetyl – Salicylic Acid	Acetylates and irreversibly inhibits cyclooxygenase (both COX-a and COX-2) to prevent conversion of arachidonic acid to thromboxane A_2→ *Inhibits platelet aggregation.*	↓ thrombus risk in CAD and post-MI, ↓ post-operative thrombus risk. Antipyretic, analgesic, anti-inflammatory, anti-platelet.	↑ risk of hemorrhagic stroke and *GI ulceration and bleeding*, tinnitus, *Reye's syndrome.*
Thienopyridines – Clopidogrel – Ticlopidine	*Block ADP receptors* to suppress fibrinogen binding and platelet adhesion to injury sites.	↓ risk of repeat MI or stroke in patients with prior MI, stroke, or PVD; ↓ thrombus risk in coronary stenting.	↑ risk of hemorrhage and *GI bleeding, neutropenia (ticlopidine).*
GP IIb/IIIa inhibitors – Abciximab	Inhibit platelet aggregation by binding to platelet *GP IIb/IIIa* receptors.	↓ risk of thrombus in unstable angina or following PTCA.	↑ risk of hemorrhage, nausea, back pain and hypotension.
Adenosine reuptake inhibitors – Dipyridamole	*Inhibit activity of adenosine deaminase and phosphodiesterase* to inhibit platelet aggregation.	Used in combination with ASA in patients with recent stroke or with warfarin following artificial heart valve replacement.	Dizziness, headache and nausea.

128. Answer is c (Schistosomiasis).
Ref: Harrison's, 17th edition Pg 123 (electronic).

- ***Metrifonate*** is effective in the treatment of urinary ***schistosomiasis***.
- ***In 2000 the WHO stopped recommending metrifonate*** for treating urinary schistosomiasis because the drug did not appear to be as effective as the ***treatment of choice, praziquantel***.
- *Praziquantel requires only one dose* and is operationally more convenient, while metrifonate requires three doses at 14-day intervals. This could be a strong reason for stopping metrifonate use, especially in rural community-based treatment programs, where it is difficult to give multiple doses.

Caution:
- ***Metrifonate*** is an ***organophosphorus (OP)*** compound and a prodrug that is converted non-enzymatically to dichlorvos (2,2-dichlorovinyl dimethyl phosphate, DDVP), a highly active chemical that irreversibly inhibits the acetylcholinesterase enzyme.
- Schistosomal cholinesterase is more susceptible to dichlorvos than is the corresponding human enzyme.
- 2.5 months are required for erythrocyte cholinesterase levels to return to normal.
- Hence *metrifonate treated persons should not be exposed to neuromuscular blocking agents or organophosphate insecticides* for at least 48 h after treatment.

129. Answer is d (Aztreonam).
Ref: KD Tripathi, 6th edition, Basic pharmacology, Janet Stringer.

- There is ***limited cross-reactivity between aztreonam*** and other beta-lactam antibiotics, and it is generally considered ***safe to administer aztreonam to patients with hypersensitivity to penicillins***.

130. Answer is c (Methotrexate).
Ref: Harrison's, 17th edition Pg 526.

- ***Methotrexate*** competitively and reversibly ***inhibits dihydrofolate reductase (DHFR)***, an enzyme that participates in the tetrahydrofolate synthesis → dTMP and therefore ↓ ***DNA and protein synthesis***.
- Folic acid is needed for the *de novo* synthesis of the nucleoside thymidine, required for DNA synthesis. Also, folate is needed for purine base synthesis, ***so all purine synthesis will be inhibited***.
- ***Folinic acid (leucovorin, citrovorum factor)*** rescue for doses over 100 mg/m^2.

Side Effects (SE) of Methotrexate
– Bone marrow suppression
– Oral and gastrointestinal ulceration (mucositis)
– ***Acute renal failure***
– Idiosyncratic ***pneumonitis***
– ***Hepatotoxicity*** *(macrovesicular fatty change)*
– Rash
– ↑ *toxicity when effusions* (pleural effusion, ascites) *are present*
– SE with ***intrathecal*** use of MTX are ***arachnoiditis*** (within hours); *neurotoxicity* (a few weeks later) and *necrotizing demyelinating leukoencephalopathy* (a few years later)

131. Answer is a (Tinea versicolor).
Ref: Harrison's, 17th edition Pg 326, Table 54-10.

- ***Topical selenium sulfide*** lotion 2.5% is used to treat ***tinea (pityriasis) versicolor***.
- Other agents include topical and systemic imidazoles (ketoconazole, itraconazole, fluconazole).

More About Tinea Versicolor

- *Caused by **Malassezia furfur***
- ***Oval, scaly, macules*** and patches on the ***chest, shoulders and back***. On dark skin, they appear ***hypopigmented***, while on light skin they are slightly hyperpigmented (*versi* means several); **"Coup d' ongle" sign of Besnier** is seen; *catheter-acquired sepsis* due to *M. furfur* develops in patients (esp. neonates) receiving intravenous lipid.
- KOH preparation from scaling lesions will show short ***cigar-butt hyphae*** and round spores, the so-called ***"spaghetti and meatballs" or "bacon and eggs" appearance***.
- Under *Wood's light* the lesions <u>DO NOT</u> fluoresce or appear *yellow-green/coppery-orange.*

132. Answer is d (Abciximab).
Ref: Harrison's, 17th edition Pg 2044, Table 308-16.

- ***Etanercept, infliximab and adalimumab*** are ***TNF blocking drugs (immunomodulators)*** used in treatment various chronic autoimmune diseases [rheumatoid arthritis (RA), etc.].
- ***Abciximab*** is a monoclonal antibody with that non-competitively ***inhibits platelet aggregation by blocking glycoprotein (GP) IIb/IIIa receptor***.
- ***Anakinra*** is a recombinant ***interleukin-1 inhibitor*** used for RA.

133. Answer is d (Erythromycin).
Ref: KD Tripathi, 6th edition Pg 721-22.

- All ***aminoglycosides*** including ***streptomycin*** can ***induce or potentiate neuromuscular block*** (NMB).
- Mechanism involves interference with calcium and inhibition of release of acetylcholine at the presynaptic membrane.
- The reaction has been associated with severely ill patients, associated with rapid administration, concurrent use of NMB agents (d-TC, succinylcholine, decamethonium), hypocalcemia and aminoglycoside accumulation or overdosage.
- ***Clindamycin*** may prolong the effects of neuromuscular-blocking drugs.
- ***Lincomycin*** has been shown to have neuromuscular blocking properties that may enhance the action of other neuromuscular blocking agents.

134. Answer is d (The rate of elimination varies directly with dose).
Ref: KD Tripathi, 6th edition Pg 31.

First order (exponential) kinetics	Zero-order (linear) kinetics
• The rate of elimination is directly proportional to the drug concentration	• The rate of elimination remains constant irrespective of drug concentration
• Clearance remains constant	• Clearance decreases with increase in concentration
• A constant fraction of the drug present in the body is eliminated in unit time	• A constant amount of the drug is eliminated in unit time
	Examples: – Phenytoin – Ethyl alcohol – Warfarin – Tolbutamide – Theophylline

135. Answer is c (Methotrexate).
Ref: KD Tripathi, 6th edition Pg 830.

- *Cell cycle specific* anticancer drugs ***kill only actively dividing cells.***
- Their toxicity is generally expressed in S phase.

Cell cycle	Drugs
G1	Vinblastin
S	Methotrexate, cytarabine, 6-TG, 6-MP, hydroxyurea, mitomycin C, doxorubicin, daunorubicin
G2	Daunorubicin, bleomycin, etoposide, topotecan
M	Vincristine, Vinblastine, Paclitaxel, Docetaxel

PREVENTIVE AND SOCIAL MEDICINE

136. Answer is c (Soybean).
Ref: Park, 20th edition Pg 544.

- ***Soybeans*** are the ***richest among pulses.***
- It contains about ***40% of protein,*** 20% of fat and 4% of minerals.
- The *limiting amino acid* is ***methionine.***

137. Answer is b (48).
Ref: Park, 20th edition Pg 720.

- The ***Factories Act*** (1948) has prescribed a ***maximum of 48 working hours per week, not exceeding 9 hours per day*** with rest for at least half hour after 5 hours of continuous work.
- The total number of hours of work in a week *including overtime shall not exceed 60.*

More About

- ☐ ***Factory*** is an establishment employing *10 or more workers where power is used* and *20 or more workers where power is not used.*
- ☐ Employment of children ***below the age of 14 years is prohibited.***

138. Answer is b (Larvicide).
Ref: Park, 20th edition Pg 676.

Classification of mosquito control measures

Anti-larval measures	– Environmental control – Chemical control: Mineral oils, Paris green, Synthetic insecticides – Biological control
Anti-adult measures	– Residual sprays – Space sprays – Genetic control
Protection against mosquito bites	– Mosquito net – Screening – Repellents

- ❖ ***Mineral oil*** or alcohol-based surface products and other surface films are put on water to kill mosquito larvae and pupae.
- ❖ These ***larvicides*** spread out and form a thin layer over the surface of the water where mosquito larvae or pupae are present.
- ❖ Mineral oils suffocate the mosquito larva or pupa by preventing them from breathing.

139. Answer is b (Fluoride).

Ref: http://www.jstor.org/pss/3860089;http://www.ncbi.nlm.nih.gov/pmc/articles/PMC2530276/pdf/postmedj00584-0039.pdf

- The relation between fluoride in drinking water and a reduced incidence of dental decay is probably one of the best established links between geochemistry and disease.
- In ***Britain***, unusual ***mottling of teeth was described in patients of Maldon*** where the prevalence of caries teeth was less compared with other districts.
- This was explained due to water from Maldon containing more fluoride compared to elsewhere.

140. Answer is d (Distal symmetric polyneuropathy).

Ref: Harrison's, 17th edition Pg 2289.

- The ***most common form of diabetic neuropathy is distal symmetric polyneuropathy.***
- It most frequently presents with distal sensory loss, but up to 50% of patients do not have symptoms of neuropathy.
- Hyperesthesia, paresthesia and dysesthesia also may occur.

<u>About the other choices</u>

- ☐ ***Diabetic polyradiculopathy*** is a syndrome characterized by severe disabling pain in the distribution of one or more nerve roots. It may be accompanied by motor weakness.
- ☐ ***Mononeuropathy*** (dysfunction of isolated cranial or peripheral nerves) is *less common than polyneuropathy* in DM and presents with pain and motor weakness in the distribution of a single nerve. A vascular etiology has been suggested, but the pathogenesis is unknown.
- ☐ ***Autonomic neuropathy***: Individuals with long-standing type 1 or 2 DM may develop signs of autonomic dysfunction involving the cholinergic, noradrenergic and peptidergic (peptides such as pancreatic polypeptide, substance P, etc.) systems. DM-related autonomic neuropathy can involve multiple systems, including the cardiovascular, gastrointestinal, genitourinary, sudomotor and metabolic systems.

141. Answer is a (Point source epidemic).

Ref: Park, 20th edition Pg 61.

Repeat Question

- See ***answer no. 172 in COMED-K 2010 answers*** for detailed explanation.

142. Answer is d (Relative humidity).

Ref: Park, 20th edition Pg 655.

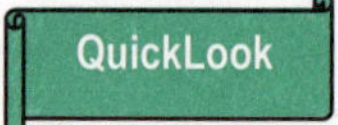

Instrument	Used for measuring
• Sling psychrometer	Relative humidity of air
• *A*nemometer	*A*ir velocity
• *K*ata thermometer	*K*(c)ooling power of the air
• Globe thermometer	Mean radiant temperature of surroundings

143. Answer is b (Travelers).

Ref: Park, 20th edition Pg 816-17.

- ***Travel medicine*** or ***emporiatrics*** is the branch of medicine that deals with the prevention and management of health problems of ***international travelers.***

144. Answer is b (*Anopheles stephensi*).
Ref: Park, 20th edition Pg 674.

Areas of distribution of female *Anopheles* mosquito

Plains	*A. culicifacies, A. philippinensis*
Coastal regions	*A. stephensi, A. sundaicus*
Foot-hill regions	*A. fluviatilis, A. minimus*
Urban areas	*A. stephensi*
Rural areas	*A. culicifacies*

145. Answer is b (15 ppm).
Ref: Park, 20th edition Pg 557.

- In India, the ***level of iodization***, is fixed under the Prevention of Food Adulteration Act (PFA) and is ***not less than 30 ppm at the production point*** and ***not less than 15 ppm at the consumer level***.

More Info

- ***Himalaya goiter belt***—World's largest goiter belt extending from Kashmir to Naga hills, about 2,400 km.
- Currently no less than ***170 million people are estimated to be affected by goiter*** in India.
- In one particular ***district (Gonda) of Uttar Pradesh*** known to be highly endemic, the ***prevalence of neonatal hypothyroidism*** has been measured at extremely high ***rate of 15%***.
- ***"Two-in-one" salt*** = common salt fortified with ***iron and iodine***.
- Four essential components of the national goiter control program = iodized salt or oil, monitoring and surveillance, manpower training and mass communication.
- ***WHO's regional strategy*** for control of IDD has as its principal objective the ***reduction of prevalence of goiter in areas of endemicity to 10% or below by the year 2000***.

146. Answer is b (Virus is not present).
Ref: Park, 20th edition Pg 247-48.

- ***India is a yellow fever 'receptive' area***, i.e. an area in which yellow fever does not exist, but where conditions would permit its development if introduced.
- The *population of India is unvaccinated and susceptible* to yellow fever.
- The vector *Aedes aegypti is found in abundance*.
- The *climatic conditions are favorable* in most parts of India for its transmission.
- The *common monkey in India (Macaus spp) is susceptible* to yellow fever.
- The ***missing link in the chain of transmission is the virus of yellow fever***, which does ***NOT*** seem to occur in India.
- Hence International Health Regulations require a ***valid certificate of vaccination against yellow fever*** for all travelers exposed to yellow fever before they enter a receptive zone like India.
- The validity of the certificate begins 10 days after date of vaccination and extends up to 10 years.

147. Answer is b (2010).
Ref: Park, 20th edition Pg 423.

National Population Policy (NPP) 2000—Objectives
■ **Immediate objective**: To address the unmet needs for contraception, health care infrastructure and health personnel and to provide integrated service delivery for basic reproductive and child health care.
■ **Medium-term objective**: To ***bring the TFR to replacement levels by 2010***, through vigorous implementation of intersectoral operational strategies.

■ **Long-term objective** is ***to achieve a stable population by 2045***, at a level consistent with the requirements of sustainable economic growth, social development and environmental protection.

148. Answer is d (10 years).
Ref: Dutta's Obstetrics, 6th edition Pg 534-35.

Summary of lifespan of IUCDs

Generation	Example	Lifespan
I	Lippe's loop	5 years
II	Cu-T-200	3 years
	Multiload -25U	3 years
	Nova-T	5 years
	Multiload 375	5 years
	Cu-T 380A	10 years
III	Progestasert	1 year
	Mirena (LNG-20, levonorgestrel)	7–10 years

149. Answer is b (Analytic study).
Ref: Park, 20th edition Pg 67.

Analytical epidemiology consists of two distinct types of observational studies
- ☐ ***Case-control study*** – retrospective study
- ☐ ***Cohort study*** – prospective longitudinal study

About the other choices

- ➲ ***Experimental epidemiology*** in modern medicine means ***randomized controlled trials.***
- ➲ ***Descriptive epidemiology*** deals with following basic questions: 'Where is the disease occurring? When is it occurring? Who is getting the disease?'.

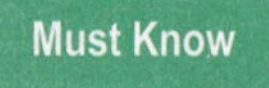

Comparison of the two types of analytical studies

	Case-control study	Cohort study
1.	Proceed from "effect to cause"	Proceeds from "cause to effect"
2.	Suitable for rare diseases	Suitable for common diseases
3.	Short study time	Prolonged study time
4.	Smaller number of subjects	Large number of subjects
5.	Yields only odds ratio	Yields incidence rates, relative risk as well as attributable risk
6.	More chance for bias	Less selection bias occurs
7.	Relatively inexpensive	Expensive
8.	No volunteer subjects needed	Regular follow-up of participants needed

150. Answer is b (10).
Ref: Textbook of Microbiology, CP Baveja, 3rd edition Pg 232.

- A full course of ***three doses of tetanus toxoid*** confers immunity for a period of ***at least 10 years***.
- A 'booster' dose of toxoid is recommended after 10 years.

151. Answer is a (Extrinsic incubation period).

Ref: Park, 20th edition Pg 224.

- The period of time required for the development of the parasite ***from the gametocyte to sporozoite stage*** in the body of mosquito is about 10–20 days depending on favorable conditions of atmospheric temperature and humidity.
- This period is called ***"extrinsic incubation period"***.

152. Answer is d (85).

Ref: Park, 20th edition Pg 648.

- A daily exposure of *85 dB* is the ***maximum limit*** that people can tolerate without substantial damage to their hearing.

153. Answer is d (1–5 μm).

Ref: Park, 20th edition Pg 711.

- Dust within the ***size range of 0.5–3 microns***, is a health hazard producing, after a variable period of exposure, a lung disease known as ***pneumoconiosis***.

ANATOMY, PHYSIOLOGY AND BIOCHEMISTRY

154. Answer is b (Leptin).

Ref: Vasudevan's biochemistry, 5th edition Pg 338; Ganong's physiology, 23rd edition Pg 384, 448.

Repeat Topic

- See ***answer no. 153 in Karnataka 2010 answers*** for detailed explanation.

155. Answer is a (Stimulation of appetite).

Ref: Vasudevan's biochemistry, 5th edition Pg 338; Ganong's physiology, 23rd edition Pg 384, 448.

Repeat Topic

- See ***answer no. 153 in Karnataka 2010 answers*** for detailed explanation.

156. Answer is C (5–10 mm Hg).

Ref: Davidson's, 20th edition Pg 957.

- Normal pressure in the ***portal vein is 5–10 mm Hg***.
- *Patients developing clinical features of complications of portal hypertension* usually have ***portal venous pressures above 12 mm Hg***.

157. Answer is c (Molybdenum).

Ref: Nutritional Biochemistry, Tom Brody 1999, 2nd edition Pg 819.

Molybdenum cofactor is associated with the enzymes
- ***Sulfite oxidase***
- ***Xanthine dehydrogenase/oxidase***
- ***Aldehyde oxidase***

158. Answer is d (Estrogen).

Ref: Vasudevan's biochemistry, 5th edition Pg 380, Table 36.1.

- Binding of hormone to receptor initiates a series of events, which leads to generation of so-called ***second messengers*** within the cell (the hormone is the first messenger).
- The second messengers then trigger a series of molecular interactions that alter the physiologic state of the cell. Another term used to describe this entire process is ***signal transduction***.
- Currently, four second messenger systems are recognized in cells, as summarized in the table below. Note that not only do multiple hormones utilize the same second messenger system, but a single hormone can utilize more than one system.

Second messenger	Examples of hormones, which utilize this system
Cyclic AMP	**ACTH**, FSH, LH, MSH, PTH, ADH, HCG, TSH, CRH, Glucagon, Calcitonin, Catecholamines
Cyclic GMP	**ANF** (Atrial natriuretic factor), Nitric oxide
Calcium and/or phosphatidylinositol	**TRH**, GnRH, Catecholamines, Acetylcholine, CCK, Gastrin, Vasopressin, Oxytocin
Tyrosine kinase	Insulin, somatomedin, several growth factors
Intracellular receptors	Glucocorticoids, mineralocorticoids, estrogens, progesterone, androgens, calcitriol, thyroxine

159. Answer is b (Wolffian duct).

Ref: Urologic pathology, Robert OP, Isabel AS, Charles JD, 2009 edition Pg 1.

- In females, the mesonephric (Wolffian) duct regresses after its role in the urinary tract.
- BUT, it can be found as vestigial remnants in the:
  - ☐ *Gartner's* duct
  - ☐ Rudimentary tubules in ovarian hilum
  - ☐ Walls of fallopian tubes and uterus as paroophoron
  - ☐ Hydatids of *Morgagni.*

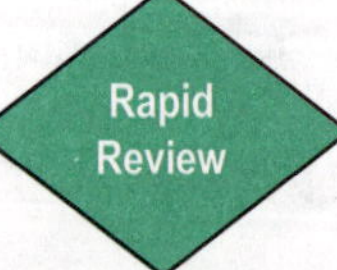

Genital Homologues in Male and Female

Male	Undifferentiated	Female
Glans penis	← Genital tubercle →	Glans clitoris
Corpus spongiosum Bulbourethral glands of Cowper Prostate gland	← Urogenital sinus →	Vestibular bulbs Greater vestibular glands of Bartholin Urethral and paraurethral glands of Skene
Ventral shaft of penis (penile urethra)	← Urogenital folds →	Labia minora
Scrotum	← Labioscrotal swelling →	Labia majora
Gubernaculum testis	← Gubernaculum →	Ovarian and round ligaments
(SEED) Seminal vesicles Epididymis Ejaculatory duct Ductus deferens	← Mesonephric (Wolffian) duct →	Duct of epoophoron

Appendix of testis Prostatic utricle	← Paramesonephric (Mullerian) duct→	Fallopian tube Uterus and Upper part of vagina.

REMNANTS OF

Ductus arteriosus Q	Ligamentum arteriosum
Ductus venosusQ	Ligamentum venosum
Left umbilical veinQ	Ligamentum teres of Liver
Right umbilical vein	Disappears
Vitello intestinal ductQ	Meckel's diverticulum
UrachusQ	Median umbilical ligament
Obliterated umbilical artery	Medial Umbilical fold
Inferior epigastric artery	Lateral umbilical fold (epigastric fold)
Proximal part of umbilical A	Superior vesical AQ
Distal part of umbilical A	Lateral umbilical ligamentQ
Left common cardinal vein	Oblique vein of left atriumQ

160. Answer is d (Ad).

Ref: Ganong's Physiology, 23rd edition Pg 89.

Nerve fiber type and their functions

Fiber type	Function
A-alpha	Proprioception, somatic motor
A-beta	Touch, pressure, motor
A-gamma	Motor to muscle spindles
A-delta	Pain, cold touch
B	Preganglionic autonomic
C-dorsal root	Pain, temperature, some mechanoreception
C sympathetic	Post-ganglionic sympathetic

Mnemonic: D= Delta; D= "Dard (pain in Hindi)"

Note:

➲ ***Fiber diameter and conduction velocity*** are ***maximum*** in ***A-alpha***.

161. Answer is c (Right bronchial vein).

Ref: Essential anatomy, Keith Moore, 2005 edition Pg 123.

- The ***azygos system of veins*** is considered to be the azygos vein, along with its left-sided counterparts, the hemiazygos vein and the accessory hemiazygos vein. Together, they form an anastomosis between the superior vena cava to the inferior vena cava.
- It can be noted that the azygos system of veins exists because the superior vena cava and the inferior vena cava are not continuous. While the aorta travels downward (continuously) through the mediastinum, supplying blood to the intercostal spaces, the vena cava does not exist at the level of the heart. Thus, the azygos venous system makes up for this deficiency of the vena cava.
- ***Tributaries:*** The azygos vein receives the right subcostal and intercostal veins, the upper three or four of these latter opening by a common stem, the highest superior intercostal vein. It receives the hemiazygos veins, several esophageal, mediastinal and pericardial veins, and ***near its termination, the right bronchial vein***.

162. Answer is a (Albumin).

Ref: Vasudevan's Biochemistry, 5th edition Pg 472.

- ***Alpha-fetoprotein (AFP)*** is ***fetal albumin*** and ***has similarities to adult albumin***.
- AFP is a tumor marker and is increased in:
  - ❖ Hepatocellular Ca
  - ❖ Germ cell tumor
  - ❖ Teratocarcinoma of ovary
  - ❖ Pregnancy with fetal malformations of neural tube.

163. Answer is d (Cardiac failure).
Ref: Harrison's, 17th edition Pg 2004, Table 306.2.

Causes of Hyperamylasemia and Hyperamylasuria

Pancreatic Disease	
I. Pancreatitis including complications of pancreatitis II. Pancreatic trauma III. Pancreatic carcinoma	
Non-pancreatic Disorders	
I. Renal insufficiency II. Salivary gland lesions A. Mumps, calculus B. Irradiation sialadenitis C. Maxillofacial surgery III. "Tumor" hyperamylasemia A. Carcinoma of the lung, esophagus B. Breast carcinoma, ovarian carcinoma	IV. Macroamylasemia V. Burns VI. Diabetic ketoacidosis VII. Pregnancy VIII. Renal transplantation IX. Cerebral trauma X. Drugs: Morphine
Other Abdominal Disorders	
I. Biliary tract disease: cholecystitis, choledocholithiasis II. Intra-abdominal disease A. Perforated or penetrating peptic ulcer B. Intestinal obstruction or infarction	C. Ruptured ectopic pregnancy D. Peritonitis E. Aortic aneurysm F. Chronic liver disease G. Postoperative hyperamylasemia

164. Answer is a (Aquaporin 1).
Ref: Ganong's Physiology, 23rd edition Pg 652.

- Rapid diffusion of water across cell membranes depends on the presence of water channels, integral membrane proteins called aquaporins.
- To date, ***13 aquaporins*** have been cloned, only 4 aquaporins (aquaporins 1, 2, 3, 4) play a key role in the kidney.
- ***Aquaporin 1*** is localized to both the basolateral and apical membrane of the ***proximal tubules***.
- The vasopressin-responsive water channels in the ***collecting ducts is Aquaporin 2***.

165. Answer is a (Antidiuretic hormone).
Ref: KD Tripathi, 6th edition Pg 574.

- ***Vasopressin (antidiuretic hormone, ADH)*** is synthesized in the ***hypothalamic (supraoptic and paraventricular)*** nerve cell bodies as large precursor peptide along with its binding protein (neurophysin) and is transported down the axons to nerve endings in the pars nervosa (***posterior pituitary***).

166. Answer is c (Skeletal muscle mass).
Ref: Sport Nutrition: An introduction to energy and performance, Askar J, Michael G, 2010 edition Pg 177.

- ***3-methylhistidine*** is a derivative of the amino acid, histidine, found mainly in the ***contractile proteins of muscle (myosin and actin)***.
- When proteins are degraded, 3-methyhistidine cannot be recycled within the muscle and is excreted in the urine.
- The amount of 3-methylhistidine in urine is therefore ***a measure of contractile protein breakdown***.
- ***Meat and fish*** contain a relatively large amount of 3-MH and could cause erroneous results.

- Although the technique has several limitations, it is regarded as a ***relatively easy and non-invasive way to get an idea of muscle protein breakdown***.

167. Answer is c (Brain).

Ref: http://en.wikipedia.org/wiki/Petrus_Camper

- ***Petrus Camper*** is also known for his theory of the ***"facial angle"*** in connection with ***intelligence***.
- According to this technique, the facial angle is the angle formed by the intersection of the orbitomeatal (Frankfurt) plane with the nasion-pogonion line (inner lower angle), which establishes the anteroposterior relation of the mandible to the upper face at the orbitomeatal plane.
- Measuring this angle was thought to determine the ***intelligence*** of animals and human beings.

168. Answer is a (Lesser petrosal nerve).

Ref: Bailey and Love, 25th edition Pg 752-60.

- Secretion of saliva by the parotid gland is controlled by ***preganglionic parasympathetic fibers originating in the inferior salivatory nucleus of brain*** → the ***glossopharyngeal nerve (CN IX)*** → travel along the ***tympanic nerve (of Jacobson)*** → pass through the tympanic plexus (located in the middle ear) → and then travel in the ***lesser petrosal nerve*** until they reach the → ***otic ganglion***.
- After synapsing in the otic ganglion, the ***postganglionic fibers*** travel as part of the ***auriculotemporal nerve*** [a branch of the mandibular nerve (V_3)] to reach the parotid gland.
- Sympathetic nerves originating from Superior Cervical Ganglion reach the gland with blood vessels.
- Parasympathetic stimulation produces water rich serous saliva.
- Sympathetic stimulation leads to the production of low volume enzyme rich saliva.
- There is no inhibitory nerve supply to the gland.

169. Answer is a (Normal urothelium).

Ref: Essentials of anatomic pathology, Laing Chang, David GB, 2nd edition 2006. Pg 1186.

von Brunn's nests

- Occur in ~85% of autopsy patients.
- Represent a ***normal variant of bladder mucosa***.
- Solid nests of ***urothelium*** project into lamina propria.
- May contain luminal eosinophilic secretions

170. Answer is b (Leucine).

Ref: Textbook of Biochemistry, Vasudevan, 5th edition Pg 214, 220.

- A *ketogenic amino acid* is an amino acid that can be converted into ketone bodies through ketogenesis.
- A *glucogenic amino acid* is an amino acid that can be converted into glucose through gluconeogenesis.

• Essential amino acids (Aa's) • **(PVT, TIM, HALL)**	PVT—Phenylalanine (Phe); Valine (Val); Threonine (Thr) TIM—Tryptophan (Try); Isoleucine (Ile); Methionine (Met) HALL—Histidine (His); Arginine (Arg), Leucine (Leu); Lysine (Lys)
• Ketogenic Aa's • Glucogenic Aa's • Glucogenic/Ketogenic	Leu, Lys Met, Val, Arg, His Ile, Phe, Tyr, Thr
• Acidic Aa's • Basic Aa's	Asp, Glu (Monoamino-dicarboxylic acids) Arg (**most basic**), Lys, His
• Sulfur containing Aa's	**Me**thionine, **C**ysteine, **Cy**stine (Sulfur is **MeCCy**)
• Aromatic Aa's	**His**tidine, **Phe**nylalanine, **T**yrosine, **T**ryptophan (**His PheTT** have aroma)

• Aa's with **ALI**phatic side chains	Alanine, Leucine, Isoleucine, Glycine, Valine **(ALI-GV)**
• Aa's with hydroxyl (OH) groups	Serine, Threonine, Tyrosine **(OH! - STT)**
• Imino acids	Proline

171. Answer is c (Cricothyroid).
Ref: BD Chaurasia, Vol 3, Pg 152.

Muscles of larynx are

– Cricothyroid	***Only*** intrinsic muscle lying on the external aspect of larynx; tensor of larynx; supplied by ***external laryngeal nerve***—all are unique features, ***remember***!
– Posterior Cricoarytenoid	Only **AB**ductor of vocal cords (opens the glottis). ***Mnemonic:*** *"Police Captured all* ***AB****ductors"*
– Lateral cricoarytenoid, Transverse arytenoids	Adductor of vocal cords (close the glottis)
– Thyroarytenoid	Upper part = thyroepiglotticus, lower part = vocalis

❖ **Motor N supply:** All the intrinsic muscles of the larynx are supplied by the *recurrent laryngeal nerve*, except the ***Cricothyroid by the External laryngeal nerve***.

❖ **Sensory N supply:** Internal laryngeal nerve supplies mucous membrane above level of vocal folds. RLN supplies it **below** the level of vocal folds.

Note:

☐ The ***superior laryngeal nerve divides into external laryngeal nerve,*** which supplies the cricothyroid and the ***internal laryngeal nerve,*** which supplies mucous membrane above level of vocal folds.

172. Answer is d (Posterior cricoarytenoid).
Ref: BD Chaurasia, Vol 3, Pg 152.

- See ***previous answer above*** for detailed explanation.

173. Answer is a (Insulin).
Ref: Textbook of Biochemistry, Vasudevan, 5th edition Pg 96, Fig 9.33.

- Similar to other gluconeogenic enzymes, ***pyruvate carboxylase*** is:
  - ☐ ***Positively regulated by glucagon and glucocorticoids***
  - ☐ ***Negatively regulated by insulin.***

174. Answer is c (Serotonin).
Ref: Harrison's, 17th edition Pg 2479, Table 360.2.

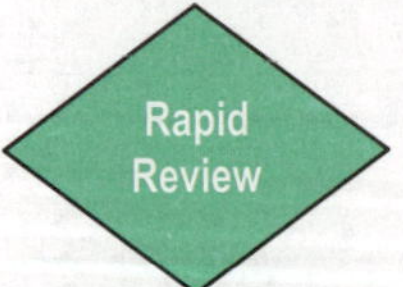

Principal Classic Neurotransmitters

Neurotransmitter	Physiologic Anatomy	Clinical Aspects
• **Serotonin**	Pontine raphe nuclei → widespread projections	Mood disorders (SSRIs improve depression) Migraine pain pathway

	Medulla/Pons → dorsal horn of spinal cord	Pain pathway
• **Acetylcholine**	Motor neurons in spinal cord → neuromuscular junction Basal forebrain → widespread cortex Interneurons in striatum Autonomic nervous system (preganglionic and postganglionic sympathetic)	Acetylcholinesterases (nerve gases) Myasthenia gravis antibodies to ACh receptor) Congenital myasthenic syndrome (mutations in Ach receptor subunits) Lambert-Eaton syndrome (antibodies to Ca channels impair ACh release) Botulism (toxin disrupts ACh release by exocytosis) Alzheimer's disease (selective cell death) AD frontal lobe epilepsy (mutations in CNS ACh receptor) Parkinson's disease (tremor)
• **Dopamine**	Substantia nigra → striatum (nigrostriatal pathway) Substantia nigra → limbic system and widespread cortex Arcuate nucleus of hypothalamus → anterior pituitary (via portal veins)	Parkinson's disease (selective cell death) MPTP parkinsonism (toxin transported into neurons) Addiction, behavioral disorders Inhibits prolactin secretion
• **Norepinephrine (NE)**	Locus coeruleus (pons) → limbic system, hypothalamus, cortex Medulla → locus coeruleus, spinal cord Postganglionic neurons of sympathetic nervous system	Mood disorders (MAO inhibitors and tricyclics increase NE and improve depression) Anxiety Orthostatic tachycardia syndrome (mutations in NE transporter)
• **γ-amino butyric acid (GABA)**	Major inhibitory neurotransmitter in brain; Widespread cortical interneurons and long projection pathways	Stiff person syndrome (antibodies to glutamic acid decarboxylase, the biosynthetic enzyme for GABA) Epilepsy (gabapentin and valproic acid increase GABA)
• **Glycine**	Major inhibitory neurotransmitter in spinal cord	Spasticity Hyperekplexia (myoclonic startle syndrome) due to mutations in glycine receptor
• **Glutamate**	Major excitatory neurotransmitter; located throughout CNS, including cortical pyramidal cells	Seizures due to ingestion of domoic acid (a glutamate analogue) Rasmussen's encephalitis (antibody against glutamate receptor 3) Excitotoxic cell death

175. Answer is c (Vision).

Ref: Ganong's physiology, 23rd edition Pg 199.

- The ***superior colliculi,*** which regulate saccades are innervated by ***M fibers from the retina***.
- They also receive extensive innervation from the cerebral cortex.
- Each superior colliculus has a ***map of visual space*** plus a map of the body surface and a map or sound in space.

COMED-K 2008 ANSWERS

- The *superior colliculi are constantly active positioning the eyes,* and they have one of the highest rates of blood flow and metabolism of any region of the brain.

Note:

- ☐ *Inferior colliculi* are the centers for *auditory reflexes*.

176. Answer is b (Insertion of recti).
Ref: Ophthalmology, Duker-Yanoff, 3rd edition Pg 1301.

- *Sclera* is *thinnest just before the insertion of the recti* muscles.

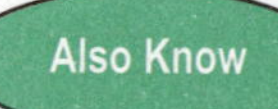

Insertions of Rectus Muscles from the Limbus

Superior rectus	7.7 mm
Lateral rectus	6.9 mm
Inferior rectus	6.6 mm
Medial rectus	5.5 mm
"SLIM"	

177. Answer is d (Cardiolipin).
Ref: Textbook of Biochemistry, Vasudevan, 5th edition Pg 78.

- ***Cardiolipin (bisphosphatidyl glycerol)*** is typically present in metabolically active cells of the ***heart and skeletal muscle,*** in the ***membranes of their mitochondria,*** mostly in the ***inner membrane*** and consists roughly 20% of its lipids.
- Patients with anti-cardiolipin antibodies (Antiphospholipid syndrome) can have recurrent thrombotic events even early in their mid-late teen years.
- Cardiolipin from a cow heart is used as an antigen in the Wassermann test for syphilis.
- ***Barth syndrome*** is a rare genetic disorder that was recognized in the 1970s to cause infantile death. It has a mutation in the gene coding for tafazzin, an enzyme involved in the biosynthesis of cardiolipin.

178. Answer is b (Pain).
Ref: Maheshwari, 3rd edition Pg 84-85.

- Early diagnosis of ***Volkmann's ischemia*** is of extreme importance. The following are some of the early signs:
  - ➲ Complaint of ***severe pain in forearm***
  - ➲ ***Stretch pain***: Pain on flexor aspect of forearm when the fingers are extended passively.

179. Answer is b (Smooth endoplasmic reticulum).
Ref: Ganong's Physiology, old 19th edition Pg 453; The Pleura in health and disease, Jacques C, 1985 edition Pg 288.

- Electron microscopic studies of chylomicron formation (Sabesin and Frase, 1977) reveal that ***triglyceride globules are first visible in the smooth endoplasmic reticulum of the intestinal mucosal cell.***

Author's Comments: *"The above question references are from old editions, since there they are found as direct quotes."*

Rough ER	Smooth ER
– Granules of ribosomes are attached to the cytoplasm side of the membrane	– Granules of ribosome are absent
– Concerned with protein synthesis	– Synthesis of lipids, especially phospholipids and cholesterol – Site of cholesterol synthesis – Site of detoxification process

180. Answer is b (Stratified columnar epithelium).

Ref: Imaging Pelvic floor disorders, by Jaap Stoker et al, 2nd revised edition Pg 15.

Urethral part	Lining epithelium
❖ Preprostatic and proximal prostatic urethra	Urothelium (transitional epithelium) of bladder
❖ Below the ejaculatory ducts ❖ Membranous urethra ❖ Proximal penile urethra	Stratified columnar epithelium (Pseudo)
❖ Distal penile urethra	Stratified squamous epithelium

NOTES

COMED-K 2007

COMED-K 2007 QUESTIONS

MEDICINE

1. **In alcoholic hepatitis, the specific enzyme raised is**
   (a) Alanine aminotransferase (ALT)
   (b) Aspartate aminotransferase
   (c) Alkaline phosphatase (ALP)
   (d) Gamma-glutamyl transpeptidase (GGT)

2. **All of the following drugs may be used in hypertensive crisis *EXCEPT***
   (a) Nifedipine
   (b) Labetalol
   (c) Furosemide
   (d) Pindolol

3. **All are features of Plummer-Vinson syndrome *EXCEPT***
   (a) Esophageal web
   (b) Iron deficiency
   (c) Achalasia cardia
   (d) Dysphagia

4. **The definitive diagnosis of *Pneumocystis carinii* pneumonia is**
   (a) Serological tests
   (b) Chest X-ray
   (c) Finding cysts in tissue specimen
   (d) CT scan of thorax

5. **Antiglomerular basement membrane antibodies are seen in**
   (a) Goodpasture syndrome
   (b) Henoch-Schönlein purpura
   (c) Heymann nephritis
   (d) Systemic lupus erythematosus

6. **Antimicrobials that produce hemolysis in G6PD deficiency**
   (a) Ciprofloxacin
   (b) Nitrofurantoin
   (c) Norfloxacin
   (d) Mandelamine

7. **Magnesium level in blood increases in**
   (a) Uncontrolled diabetes mellitus
   (b) Liver cirrhosis
   (c) Kidney failure
   (d) Chronic alcoholism

8. **Hemobilia is characterized by all *EXCEPT***
   (a) Jaundice
   (b) Biliary colic
   (c) Melena
   (d) Fever

9. **The test of choice to detect perivalvular abscess of the aortic valve is**
   (a) MRI of heart
   (b) Transesophageal echo with Doppler
   (c) Ventriculography
   (d) CT chest

10. **HLA-B27 histocompatibility antigen is correlated with**
   (a) Sjögren's disease
   (b) Ankylosing spondylitis
   (c) Felty's syndrome
   (d) Scleroderma

11. **The earliest symptom in primary biliary cirrhosis is**
   (a) Jaundice
   (b) Pruritus
   (c) Melanosis
   (d) Vomiting

12. **The drug used in the treatment of complications of multiple sclerosis is**
   (a) Rifampicin
   (b) Isoniazid
   (c) Ethambutol
   (d) Streptomycin

13. **Amphotericin may be administered mixed in any of the following *EXCEPT***
   (a) Glucose infusion
   (b) Mannitol infusion
   (c) Saline infusion
   (d) Lipid complex (ABLC)

14. **The following are autosomal dominant disorders *EXCEPT***
   (a) Myotonic dystrophy
   (b) von Willebrand disease
   (c) Hemochromatosis
   (d) Marfan syndrome

15. **Most common manifestation of cardiac lupus is**
   (a) Myocarditis
   (b) Libman-Sacks endocarditis

(c) Pericarditis
(d) Aortic regurgitation

16. The earliest case of severe acute respiratory syndrome (SARS) was reported in
(a) China
(b) Singapore
(c) Vietnam
(d) Toronto

17. Cortical lesions are usually accompanied by word blindness due to involvement of
(a) Angular gyrus
(b) Lateral geniculate body
(c) Occipital cortex
(d) Edinger-Westphal nucleus

18. Which cholesterol is designated 'good cholesterol'?
(a) VLDL
(b) LDL
(c) HDL
(d) IDL

19. MRI is the investigation of choice in all of the following *EXCEPT*
(a) Syringomyelia
(b) Brainstem tumors
(c) Skull bone tumors
(d) Multiple sclerosis

20. Crohn's disease can be seen in
(a) Jejunum only
(b) Colon only
(c) Terminal ileum and right side of colon
(d) Mouth to anus

21. Bronchiectasis is associated with which syndrome?
(a) α-1 antitrypsin deficiency
(b) Kartagener syndrome
(c) Stevens-Johnson syndrome
(d) Stickler syndrome

22. The triad of diabetes, gallstones and steatorrhea is associated with which one of the following tumors?
(a) Glucagonomas
(b) Somatostatinoma
(c) VIPomas
(d) Gastrinoma

23. Which needle is used for pleural biopsy?
(a) Vim-Silverman needle
(b) Abram's needle
(c) Abraham's
(d) Osgood's

24. Conn's syndrome is characterized by
(a) Hyperinsulinism
(b) Hyperthyroidism
(c) Hypoadrenalism
(d) Hyperaldosteronism

25. The ECG of a patient with an artificial pacemaker in the right ventricle shows
(a) Right bundle branch block with narrow QRS complex
(b) Right bundle branch block with narrow QRS complex
(c) Left bundle branch block with broad QRS complex
(d) Left bundle branch block with narrow QRS complex

SURGERY

26. Which of the following nerves lie closest to the Wharton's duct surgery?
(a) Hypoglossal
(b) Lingual
(c) Chorda tympani
(d) Facial

27. Common congenital anomaly of midgut is
(a) Hirschsprung's disease
(b) Omphalocele
(c) Duodenal atresia
(d) Meckel's diverticulum

28. The Meckel's diverticulum is situated within about __________ cm from the ileocecal valve
(a) 25
(b) 60
(c) 75
(d) 100

29. Which of the following is the most common non-alcoholic cause of acute pancreatitis?
(a) Thiazides
(b) Hypercalcemia
(c) Hyperlipidemia
(d) Gallstones

30. The commonest cause of acute pancreatitis is
(a) Biliary calculi
(b) Alcohol abuse
(c) Infective
(d) Idiopathic

31. The most accurate method of diagnosis of gastro-esophageal reflux disease is
(a) Barium swallow
(b) Endoscopy

(c) 24-hour pH recording
(d) Esophageal manometry

32. The most common complication of transurethral resection of the prostate is
(a) Erectile dysfunction
(b) Retrograde ejaculation
(c) Urinary incontinence
(d) Urethral stricture disease

33. The commonest anterior mediastinal tumor is
(a) Aneurysm of ascending aorta
(b) Neurogenic tumor
(c) Thymoma
(d) Bronchogenic cyst

34. The predominant constituent of the pale yellow gallstones in the gallbladder is
(a) Mucin glycoprotein
(b) Calcium carbonate
(c) Cholesterol
(d) Calcium phosphate

35. The commonest site of lymphoma in the gastrointestinal system is
(a) Small bowel
(b) Stomach
(c) Large intestine
(d) Esophagus

36. Which vessel is most commonly associated with posterior duodenal ulcer?
(a) Right gastroepiploic artery
(b) Common hepatic artery
(c) Gastroduodenal artery
(d) Superior mesenteric artery

37. Sump syndrome occurs most commonly after
(a) Cholecystojejunostomy
(b) Choledochoduodenostomy
(c) Mirizzi's syndrome
(d) Choledochojejunostomy

38. The competence of the deep venous system is diagnosed clinically by performing, which of the following tests?
(a) Pratt's test
(b) Schwartz's test
(c) Perthes' test
(d) Brodie-Trendelenburg test

39. Which of the following organs is the most common site of origin of the tumor associated with the Zollinger-Ellison syndrome?
(a) Duodenum
(b) Lymph nodes
(c) Spleen
(d) Gallstones

40. Which of the following anemias is a risk factor for the development of gastric cancer?
(a) Pernicious anemia
(b) Megaloblastic anemia
(c) Aplastic anemia
(d) Hemolytic anemia

41. All are features of irritable bowel syndrome *EXCEPT*
(a) Vomiting
(b) Pain abdomen
(c) Diarrhea
(d) Constipation

42. The minimum amount of normal perfused liver parenchyma necessary to be left intact when a hepatic resection is planned is
(a) 10%
(b) 20%
(c) 50%
(d) 75%

43. In a highly selective vagotomy, the vagal supply is severed to
(a) Proximal two thirds of stomach
(b) Antrum
(c) Pylorus
(d) Whole of stomach

44. A patient with Ca cheek has tumor of 2.5 cm located close to and involving the lower alveolus. A single mobile homolateral node measuring 6 cm is palpable. Based on these clinical findings TNM stage of tumor is
(a) T1N1M0
(b) T2N2M0
(c) T3N1M0
(d) T4N2M0

45. Thyroid carcinoma with pulsating vascular skeletal metastasis is
(a) Follicular
(b) Anaplastic
(c) Medullary
(d) Papillary

46. The normal narrowing in the middle of the esophagus is due to
(a) Azygos vein
(b) Hemiazygos vein
(c) Right mainstem bronchus
(d) Left mainstem bronchus

47. Lucid interval is classically seen in
(a) Intracerebral hematoma
(b) Acute subdural hematoma
(c) Chronic subdural hematoma
(d) Extradural hematoma

48. The most important use of transrectal ultrasonography is for
(a) Screening for prostate cancer
(b) Distinguishing prostate cancer from benign prostatic hyperplasia
(c) Systemic prostate biopsy in suspected prostate cancer
(d) Guiding transurethral resection of prostate cancer

49. Which of the following diagnostic techniques is most specific for pulmonary thromboembolism?
(a) Pulmonary angiography
(b) Ventilation lung scanning
(c) Perfusion lung scanning
(d) Arterial blood gas analysis

50. Thyroid storm after operation is due to
(a) Inadequate control of hyperthyroidism
(b) Massive bleeding
(c) Recurrent laryngeal nerve injury
(d) Postoperative infection

OBG

51. The commonest type of genital tuberculosis in OBG is
(a) Endosalpingitis
(b) Exosalpingitis
(c) Endometritis
(d) Interstitial salpingitis

52. Stein-Leventhal syndrome is
(a) Pelvic endometriosis
(b) Polycystic ovarian disease
(c) Functioning granulosa cell ovarian tumor
(d) Endometrial hyperplasia

53. Senile vaginitis is due to
(a) Gonococcal infection
(b) Cancer cervix
(c) Diabetes
(d) Estrogen deficiency

54. Chronic treatment with Tamoxifen can cause carcinoma of
(a) Ovary
(b) Endometrium
(c) Cervix
(d) Vulva

55. Puerperal pyrexia is defined as
(a) Temperature of 99°F within 24 hours of delivery
(b) Temperature of 99°F 24 hours after delivery
(c) Temperature of 100.4°F 24 hours after delivery
(d) Temperature of 102°F after 45 days of delivery

56. Maternal mortality ratio is the number of maternal deaths that result from the reproductive process
(a) Per 100,000 live births
(b) Per 100,000 total births
(c) Per 10,000 live births
(d) Per 10,000 total births

57. Age of gestation when ovaries and testis are first distinguishable
(a) 4 weeks
(b) 8 weeks
(c) 12 weeks
(d) 16 weeks

PEDIATRICS

58. A 2-year-old child with a head circumference of 55 cm is likely to have had intrauterine infection due to
(a) Rubella
(b) Toxoplasmosis
(c) Herpes
(d) Hepatitis B

59. Antistreptolysin O (ASO) test is used for the diagnosis of
(a) Rheumatoid arthritis
(b) Typhoid fever
(c) Rheumatic fever
(d) Rickettsial fever

60. All the following factors affect the APGAR score *EXCEPT*
(a) Prematurity
(b) Maternal sedation
(c) Neurological condition of the baby
(d) Mode of delivery

61. Koplik spots is a feature of
(a) Rubella
(b) Measles
(c) Mumps
(d) Tetanus

62. Chvostek's sign is a contraction of facial muscles and upper lip when the examiner taps the facial nerve in front of the ear. A positive sign suggests, which of the following conditions?

(a) Hypercalcemia
(b) Hypocalcemia
(c) Hyperkalemia
(d) Acidosis

63. **90% of brain growth is achieved by the**
(a) 2nd year
(b) 3rd year
(c) 5th year
(d) 15th year

64. **Which is the commonest site for extrapulmonary TB?**
(a) Pleura
(b) Lymph node
(c) Intestine
(d) Meninges

65. **Child changes a rattle from one hand to another at the age of**
(a) 3 months
(b) 6 months
(c) 9 months
(d) 1 year

66. **One of the following statement is false regarding complications of protein energy malnutrition**
(a) Hyperglycemia
(b) Hypothermia
(c) Septic shock
(d) Electrolyte imbalance

67. **In adrenogenital syndrome, the diagnostic criteria are following *EXCEPT***
(a) Karyotyping 46XX
(b) Serum 17-hydroxy progesterone is normal
(c) Urinary pregnanetriol is increased
(d) Normal internal genital organs

68. **Pneumatoceles often develop in children after pneumonia due to the following organism**
(a) *Klebsiella*
(b) *Streptococcus*
(c) *Staphylococcus aureus*
(d) *Haemophilus influenzae*

69. **Non-immune hydrops fetalis is caused by all *EXCEPT***
(a) Parvo B19 virus
(b) Chromosomal abnormalities
(c) α-thalassemia
(d) ABO incompatibility

70. **Respiratory distress syndrome is due to defect in the biosynthesis of**
(a) Dipalmitoyl lecithin
(b) Dipalmitoyl cephalin
(c) Dipalmitoyl serine
(d) Dipalmitoyl inositol

71. **Failure to initiate and maintain spontaneous respiration following birth is clinically k/a**
(a) Birth asphyxia
(b) Respiratory distress syndrome (RDS)
(c) Respiratory failure
(d) Pulmonary edema

ORTHOPEDICS

72. **The most common vertebral lesion seen in spinal tuberculosis is**
(a) Central cystic type
(b) Anterior type
(c) Paradiscal
(d) Posterior spinal disease

73. **Which of the following joint findings is most suggestive of an inflammatory, rather than an osteoarthritic, cause of joint pain?**
(a) Painful range of motion
(b) Crepitus
(c) Bony articular enlargement
(d) Swelling and warmth

74. **In Erb-Duchene paralysis, the injury is limited to**
(a) 2nd and 3rd cervical nerves
(b) 3rd and 4th cervical nerves
(c) 4th and 5th cervical nerves
(d) 5th and 6th cervical nerves

75. **Gunstock deformity occurs in**
(a) Supracondylar fracture of femur
(b) Intercondylar fracture of femur
(c) Supracondylar fracture of humerus
(d) Distal radial fractures

76. **Myositis ossificans is**
(a) Worm calcification
(b) Callus formation
(c) Regenerate
(d) Post-traumatic ossification

77. **In Bennett's fracture, the following bone is injured**
(a) 1st metacarpal
(b) 2nd metacarpal
(c) 3rd metacarpal
(d) 4th metacarpal

78. Onion skin pattern of cortical bone formed by tumor is characteristic of
(a) Giant cell tumor
(b) Osteosarcoma
(c) Chondrosarcoma
(d) Ewing's sarcoma

79. Surgical neck of humerus is related to
(a) Ulnar nerve
(b) Radial nerve
(c) Median nerve
(d) Axillary nerve

80. Which of Dens fractures is most common?
(a) Type I
(b) Type II
(c) Type III
(d) Type IV

81. Ewing's sarcoma is common in
(a) 1st decade
(b) 2nd decade
(c) 6th decade
(d) 9th decade

82. Erb's point is formed by
(a) C4 and C5
(b) C5 and C6
(c) C6 and C7
(d) C8 and T1

OPHTHALMOLOGY AND ENT

83. A primary deviation less than the secondary deviation is seen in
(a) Concomitant squint
(b) Paralytic squint
(c) Spastic squint
(d) Acute squint

84. Commonest site of otosclerosis is
(a) Round window
(b) Oval window
(c) Utricle
(d) Ossicles

85. The parasympathetic secretomotor nerve supply to the nose is via
(a) Anterior ethmoid nerve
(b) Greater palatine nerve
(c) Vidian nerve
(d) Inferior orbital nerve

86. The type of laser employed for treating posterior capsule thickening is
(a) Krypton
(b) Excimer laser
(c) Argon laser
(d) YAG laser

87. Photopsia occurs in
(a) Iritis
(b) Cyclitis
(c) Choroiditis
(d) Retinitis

88. Vossius ring is seen in
(a) Cornea
(b) Lens
(c) Vitreous
(d) Retina

89. Fleischer ring is seen in
(a) Tay-Sachs disease
(b) Keratoconus
(c) Siderosis bulbi
(d) Contusion injury

90. The aqueous flare is best seen by
(a) Streak retinoscope
(b) Operating microscope
(c) Biomicroscope
(d) Ophthalmoscope

91. 'Malignant otitis externa' is caused by
(a) Rhabdomyosarcoma
(b) Squamous cell carcinoma
(c) Stewarts granuloma
(d) *Pseudomonas aeruginosa*

92. In Marfan's syndrome lens dislocation is commonly
(a) Upwards
(b) Downwards
(c) Superotemporally
(d) Nasally

93. Sympathetic ophthalmia is characterized by
(a) Lisch nodules
(b) Busacca nodules
(c) Koeppe nodules
(d) Dalen-Fuchs nodules

FORENSIC MEDICINE

94. There is no criminal responsibility below the age of
(a) 5 years
(b) 7 years

(c) 10 years
(d) 12 years

95. **Fracture dislocation of 2nd and 3rd cervical vertebrae is common in**
(a) Partial hanging
(b) Lynching
(c) Judicial hanging
(d) Throttling

96. **If death of a patient occurs during surgery due to the negligence of the surgeon, then he can be charged under**
(a) 299 IPC
(b) 300 IPC
(c) 304 (A) IPC
(d) 304 (B) IPC

97. **Which of the following poisons has only local actions?**
(a) Sulfuric acid
(b) Carbolic acid
(c) Oxalic acid
(d) Phosphorus

98. **Formication is associated with _____ abuse**
(a) Alcohol
(b) Cocaine
(c) Benzodiazepines
(d) Analgesics

99. **With reference to an incised wound all the following are true *EXCEPT***
(a) It has clean cut margins
(b) Bleeding is generally less than in laceration
(c) Tailing is often present
(d) Length of injury does not correspond with the length of the blade

100. **Mineralization of teeth begins at**
(a) Crown and progresses towards root
(b) Root and progresses towards crown
(c) Simultaneously at root and crown
(d) Begins in the center

PATHOLOGY

101. **Popcorn type of Reed-Sternberg cell is seen in the following type of Hodgkin's lymphoma**
(a) Lymphocyte rich
(b) Mixed cellularity
(c) Lymphocyte predominant
(d) Lymphocyte depletion

102. **The form of vascular disease responsible for malignant hypertension is**
(a) Hyaline arteriolosclerosis
(b) Arteriosclerosis obliterans
(c) Hyperplastic arteriolosclerosis
(d) Medial calcific sclerosis

103. **Antihistone antibodies are characteristic of**
(a) Drug-induced lupus
(b) Cardiac lupus
(c) Lupus nephritis
(d) MCTD

104. **Neutrophilic leukocytosis is seen in all *EXCEPT***
(a) Sepsis
(b) Myocardial infarction
(c) Pyogenic osteomyelitis
(d) Hay fever

105. **In sickle cell anemia, the mutational event responsible for the mutation of beta chain is**
(a) Crossing over
(b) Point mutation
(c) Insertion
(d) Deletion

MICROBIOLOGY

106. **Toxic shock syndrome is due to**
(a) Septic abortion
(b) Forgotten tampons
(c) IUCD
(d) Pelvic examination

107. **The causative agent of *Tinea cruris* is**
(a) *Trichophyton concentricum*
(b) *Cladosporium werneckii*
(c) *Malassezia furfur*
(d) *Epidermophyton floccosum*

108. ***Chlamydia trachomatis* infection causes the following *EXCEPT***
(a) Pneumonitis
(b) Rhinitis
(c) Conjunctivitis
(d) Urethritis

109. **Hepatitis C virus resembles to which of the following virus groups?**
(a) Picrona
(b) Herpes
(c) Hepadna
(d) Flavi

110. Arthus phenomenon is an example of which hypersensitivity?
(a) Type I
(b) Type II
(c) Type III
(d) Type IV

111. Which of the following response is found in atopic individuals?
(a) IgM response
(b) IgE response
(c) IgA response
(d) Hypogammaglobulinemia

112. Tetanus toxoid given during antenatal period will protect
(a) Only the child
(b) Only the mother
(c) Both mother and child
(d) Partially

113. Which of the following is the most specific test to diagnose syphilis?
(a) VDRL
(b) Wassermann
(c) RPR
(d) FTA-ABS

114. Which of the following mycobacteria can cause disease in HIV positive patient with a CD4 count of 600/cu mm?
(a) *M. tuberculosis*
(b) *M. avium* intracellulare
(c) *M. chelonae*
(d) *M. fortuitum*

PHARMACOLOGY

115. Effective for common gram-negative anaerobes
(a) Aztreonam
(b) Doxycycline
(c) Vancomycin
(d) Tobramycin

116. Drug of choice for methicillin-resistant *Staphylococcus aureus* (MRSA) is
(a) Ceftriaxone
(b) Ceftazidime
(c) Ampicillin
(d) Vancomycin

117. Podophyllin is used in the treatment of
(a) Genital warts
(b) Common warts
(c) Molluscum contagiosum
(d) Herpes simplex

118. A patient who is using a direct-acting sympathomimetic agent as a decongestant is most likely to be taking
(a) Ephedrine
(b) Amphetamine
(c) Phenylephrine
(d) Metaraminol

119. Depolarizing neuromuscular blockade is associated with
(a) Fasciculations
(b) Fade on tetanic stimulation
(c) Enhancement by volatile anesthetic agents
(d) Antagonized by acetylcholine

120. Oxytocin-induced myometrial contractions are inhibited by all of the following *EXCEPT*
(a) Ergometrine
(b) Terbutaline
(c) Magnesium
(d) Halothane

121. Cilastatin is an inhibitor of
(a) β-lactamase
(b) Dehydropeptidase
(c) Transpeptidase
(d) Peptidyl transferase

122. cAMP action mediates all *EXCEPT*
(a) Glucagon
(b) FSH
(c) LH
(d) Estrogen

PREVENTIVE AND SOCIAL MEDICINE

123. Mid-day meal contains
(a) 1/2 of proteins and 1/2 of the calories required per day
(b) 1/2 of proteins and 1/3 of the calories required per day
(c) 1/3 of proteins and 1/3 of the calories required per day
(d) 1/3 of proteins and 1/2 of the calories required per day

124. Maternal mortality rate in India is close to
(a) 1 per 1,000 live births
(b) 3–4 per 1,000 live births
(c) 8 per 1,000 live births
(d) 10 per 1,000 live births

125. According to the concept of the iceberg phenomenon of diseases, all of the following statements about the submerged portion of the iceberg are true *EXCEPT*

(a) It includes subclinical cases
(b) It includes carriers
(c) It constitutes undiagnosed reservoir of infection
(d) Diagnosis can be made with available techniques

126. The incubation period of leprosy is
(a) 2–4 days
(b) 2–4 weeks
(c) 2–4 months
(d) 2–4 years

127. Most common drug resistance in tuberculosis, in India, is found for
(a) INH
(b) Rifampicin
(c) Streptomycin
(d) Ethambutol

128. Hind milk is richer in
(a) Carbohydrate
(b) Protein
(c) Fat
(d) Minerals

129. In triage, green color indicates
(a) Ambulatory patients
(b) Dead/Moribund patients
(c) High priority treatment or transfer
(d) Medium priority or transfer

130. What is the standard dose of PPD for Mantoux test?
(a) 5 TU
(b) 10 TU
(c) 15 TU
(d) 20 TU

131. The period of training for a village health guide is
(a) 1 month
(b) 3 months
(c) 6 months
(d) 12 months

132. To find out whether the water has been properly chlorinated, the test used is
(a) Horrock's test
(b) Orthotolidine test
(c) Presumptive coliform test
(d) Total bacterial count

133. The non-modifiable risk factor for hypertension is
(a) Obesity
(b) Age
(c) Salt intake
(d) Environmental stress

134. Validity of an indicator means
(a) It should actually measure what it is supposed to measure
(b) The answer should be same, if measured by different persons in similar circumstances
(c) Indicators should reflect changes in the situation concerned
(d) Indicators should have ability to obtain data needed

135. The Millennium Development Goals (MDG) is to be achieved by the year
(a) 2010
(b) 2015
(c) 2020
(d) 2030

136. The number of new cases occurring in a defined population during a specified period of time is called
(a) Period prevalence
(b) Point prevalence
(c) Prevalence
(d) Incidence

137. Disbursement of old age pension by the government is
(a) Social assistance
(b) Social welfare
(c) Social insurance
(d) Social defense

138. A patient with tubercular pleural effusion falls under category of WHO grading TB PSM
(a) I
(b) II
(c) III
(d) IV

139. The life expectancy in India as per 2001 census is PSM
(a) 55 years
(b) 63 years
(c) 70 years
(d) 75 years

DERMATOLOGY, ANESTHESIA, RADIOLOGY, PSYCHIATRY

140. Scrambled egg appearance is seen in RADIO
(a) Carcinoma stomach
(b) Carcinoma gallbladder
(c) Pancreatic carcinoma
(d) Renal carcinoma

141. The first modality of sensation to be lost in leprosy is
(a) Touch
(b) Pain

(c) Temperature
(d) Joint sense

142. Dennie-Morgan fold is seen in
(a) Dermatomyositis
(b) Systemic lupus erythematosus
(c) Psoriasis vulgaris
(d) Atopic dermatitis

143. Cobblestone appearance is seen in
(a) Ulcerative colitis
(b) Crohn's disease
(c) Appendicitis
(d) Carcinoma rectum

144. Classical 'raindrop' lesions are seen in
(a) Burkitt's lymphoma
(b) Hodgkin's lymphoma
(c) Multiple myeloma
(d) Hemophilia

145. Rigler's sign is seen in
(a) Ulcerative colitis
(b) Crohn's disease
(c) Megacolon
(d) Pneumoperitoneum

146. Herald patch is the first feature of
(a) Pityriasis rosea
(b) Pemphigus
(c) Psoriasis
(d) Leprosy

147. Adequate recovery of neuromuscular function after reversal is indicated by
(a) Minute volume
(b) Respiratory rate
(c) Tidal volume
(d) Head lift for 3 seconds

148. Depressive delusions that the world and everything related to it cease to exist is called
(a) Persecutory delusion
(b) Delusion of infidelity
(c) Nihilistic delusion
(d) Delusion of reference

149. Histrionic personality disorder is recognized by
(a) Withdrawn behavior
(b) Extrovert with excessive emotionality and attention seeking
(c) Extrovert with emotional warmthness
(d) Obsessive features

150. A person who is very rigid, inflexible and loves order and discipline, can be categorized as
(a) Hysterical
(b) Anankastic
(c) Affective
(d) Explosive

151. Early and reliable indication of air embolism during anesthesia can be obtained by continuous monitoring of
(a) ECG
(b) Blood pressure
(c) End tidal CO_2
(d) Oxygen saturation

152. A mentally ill person smells pleasant or unpleasant odor when none is present. This is an example of
(a) Illusion
(b) Delusion
(c) Obsession
(d) Hallucination

153. Munro microabscesses are characteristically seen in
(a) Lichen planus
(b) Lupus erythematosus
(c) Psoriasis
(d) Seborrheic dermatitis

154. Obsessive compulsive disorder is distinguished from psychosis by the absence of
(a) Ritualistic behavior
(b) Perceptual anomalies
(c) Anxiety
(d) Violent behavior

155. Hypotension during anesthesia may be due to
(a) CO_2 retention
(b) Isoflurane
(c) Pancuronium
(d) Vecuronium

156. The local anesthetic with the longest duration of action is
(a) Procaine
(b) Bupivacaine
(c) Lidocaine
(d) Mepivacaine

157. A 78-year-old patient is anesthetized for resection of a liver tumor. After induction and tracheal intubations, a 20 gauge arterial line is placed and connected to a transducer, which is located 20 cm below the level of heart. The system is zeroed at the stopcock located at the wrist, while the patient's arm is stretched out on

an arm board. How will the arterial line pressure compare with the true blood pressure?

(a) It will be 20 mm Hg higher
(b) It will be 15 mm Hg higher
(c) It will be the same
(d) It will be 15 mm Hg lower

158. Pseudohypertrophic pulmonary osteoarthropathy

(a) Periostitis of femur
(b) Persistent pathological changes
(c) Related to underlying carcinoma in the body
(d) None of the above

ANATOMY, PHYSIOLOGY, BIOCHEMISTRY

159. The fourth heart sound is caused by

(a) Closure of aortic and pulmonary valves
(b) Vibrations in the ventricular wall during systole
(c) Ventricular filling
(d) Closure of the mitral and tricuspid valves

160. All of the following are inhibitors of cytochrome oxidase *EXCEPT*

(a) Carbon monoxide
(b) Amytal
(c) Cyanide
(d) Azide

161. All the following are signs of cerebellar disease *EXCEPT*

(a) Resting tremors
(b) Past pointing
(c) Nystagmus
(d) Ataxic gait

162. Carbon dioxide transported in blood mostly as

(a) Carboxyhemoglobin
(b) In combination with plasma proteins
(c) Bicarbonate
(d) Carbonic acid dissolved in plasma

163. Power grip of the hand depends on

(a) Short flexor of fingers
(b) Lumbricals of hand
(c) Long flexors of fingers
(d) Palmaris brevis

164. The abductors of the vocal cords are

(a) Transverse arytenoid
(b) Oblique arytenoid
(c) Lateral thyroarytenoid
(d) Posterior cricoarytenoid

165. Which of the following nerves accompanies the profunda brachii artery?

(a) Ulnar
(b) Musculocutaneous
(c) Radial
(d) Median

166. The dicrotic notch on the aortic pressure curve is caused by

(a) Closure of pulmonary valve
(b) Rapid filling of left ventricle
(c) Closure of aortic valve
(d) Contraction of atria

167. The preganglionic parasympathetic fibers to the parotid gland travel in

(a) Lesser petrosal nerve
(b) Great petrosal nerve
(c) Deep petrosal nerve
(d) Internal carotid nerve

168. Stomach derives its blood supply from all these arteries directly or indirectly *EXCEPT*

(a) Splenic artery
(b) Hepatic artery
(c) Superior mesenteric artery
(d) Celiac axis

169. Bell's palsy is paralysis of

(a) UMN V nerve
(b) UMN VII nerve
(c) LMN V nerve
(d) LMN VII nerve

170. The center of ossification of which of the following is used as medicolegal evidence for fetal viability?

(a) Head of femur
(b) Distal end of femur
(c) Greater trochanter
(d) Lesser trochanter

171. von Willebrand factor is produced by

(a) Liver
(b) Platelets
(c) Endothelial cells
(d) Spleen

172. Which of the following types of nerve fibers carry pain?

(a) A alpha
(b) A beta
(c) A gamma
(d) A delta

173. The activities of all the following enzymes are increased in starvation *EXCEPT*

(a) Pyruvate kinase
(b) Pyruvate carboxylase

(c) Phosphoenolpyruvate carboxykinase
(d) Glucose-6-phosphatase

174. Cholecalciferol produces all of the following effects *EXCEPT*
(a) Synthesis of new calcium-binding proteins
(b) Induction of osteocalcin for bone mineralization
(c) Regulation of parathyroid secretion
(d) Increase calcium and phosphate excretion

175. Cutaneous vasoconstriction is mediated by
(a) Sympathetic adrenergic nerves
(b) Sympathetic cholinergic nerves
(c) Parasympathetic cholinergic
(d) Somatic nerves

176. Serum creatine kinase-3 (CK-3) is elevated in
(a) Muscular dystrophy
(b) Myocardial infarction
(c) Alcoholic cirrhosis
(d) Brain tumors

177. Copper is a constituent of the enzyme
(a) Lysyl oxidase
(b) Glucose oxidase
(c) Xanthine oxidase
(d) Transketolase

178. The principle that in a spinal cord dorsal roots are sensory and the ventral roots are motor is known as
(a) Laplace's law
(b) Bell-Magendie law
(c) Frank-Starling law
(d) Weber-Fechner law

179. Immunity acquired due to injection of immunologically competent lymphocytes is termed as
(a) Innate immunity
(b) Adoptive immunity
(c) Active immunity
(d) Local immunity

180. Following is a clinical feature of cerebellar disease
(a) Paralysis
(b) Sensory deficit
(c) Ataxia
(d) Resting tremors

COMED-K 2007

ANSWERS AND EXPLANATIONS

MEDICINE

1. **Answer is d [Gamma-glutamyl transpeptidase (GGT)].**
Ref: Harrison's, 19th edition Pg 2053, Table 363-2.

Laboratory diagnosis of alcoholic fatty liver and alcoholic hepatitis

Test	Comment
AST	Increased two-to seven-fold, < 400 U/L, ***greater than ALT***
ALT	Increased two-to seven-fold, < 400 U/L
AST/ALT (Dertis ratio)	Usually > 1
GGTP	***Not specific*** to alcohol, easily inducible, elevated in all forms of fatty liver
Bilirubin	May be markedly increased in alcoholic hepatitis despite modest elevation in alkaline phosphatase

- ***Gamma-glutamyl transferase*** is not a specific indicator of ***alcohol-induced liver damage*** *(Harrison's, 19th/1992); BUt increased serum GGT levels are seen in alcoholic hepatitis.*

2. **Answer is d (Pindolol).**
Ref: Harrison's, 17th edition Pg 1561, Table 241-9.

Antihypertensive agents that are useful in hypertensive crises/hypertensive emergencies

• Hypertensive encephalopathy	Nitroprusside, nicardipine, labetalol
• Malignant hypertension (when IV therapy is indicated)	Labetalol, nicardipine, nitroprusside enalaprilat
• Stroke	Nicardipine, labetalol, nitroprusside
• Myocardial infarction/Unstable angina	Nitroglycerin, nicardipine, labetalol esmolol
• Acute left ventricular failure	Nitroglycerin, enalaprilat, loop diuretics (furosemide)
• Aortic dissection	Nitroprusside, esmolol, labetalol
• Adrenergic crisis	Phentolamine, nitroprusside
• Preeclampsia/Eclampsia of pregnancy	Hydralazine, labetalol, nicardipine
• Postoperative hypertension	Nitroglycerin, nitroprusside, labetalol, nicardipine

3. **Answer is c (Achalasia cardia)**
Ref: Harrison's, 17th edition Pg 570.

Plummer-Vinson syndrome (Paterson-Kelly syndrome)

- Esophageal (hypopharyngeal, postcricoid) *webs*
- *Iron deficiency anemia*
- MC in *middle-aged women*
- *Premalignant* condition (leads to esophageal *squamous cell Ca*)

4. **Answer is c (Finding cysts in tissue specimen).**
Ref: Harrison's, 17th edition Pg 1172; Davidson's, 20th edition Pg 391.

- A ***definitive diagnosis of PCP requires demonstration of the organism*** in samples obtained from induced sputum (30–80% sensitivity), bronchoalveolar lavage (90%), transbronchial biopsy (95%) or open lung biopsy (100%).

About the other choices:

❖ ***Regarding Chest X-ray***: The most common finding on chest X-ray is either a *normal film,* if the disease is suspected early or a *faint bilateral interstitial infiltrate.* The classic finding of a dense perihilar infiltrate is unusual in patients with AIDS. In patients with PCP who have been receiving aerosolized pentamidine for prophylaxis, one may see an X-ray picture of upper lobe cavitary disease, reminiscent of TB. Other less common findings on chest X-ray include lobar infiltrates and pleural effusions.

❖ ***Regarding serology***: PCR of bronchoalveolar lavage fluid, induced sputum or saliva is sensitive and specific, but DOES NOT distinguishes active from treated infection or colonization.

❖ ***Regarding CT***: HRCT has a high sensitivity in HIV-infected patients with PCP. A negative (normal or unchanged) CT scan alone DOES NOT rule out PCP.

5. **Answer is a (Goodpasture syndrome).**
Ref: Harrison's, 17th edition Pg 1788.

- ***Goodpasture syndrome***: The cause is ***antiglomerular basement membrane antibodies*** directed against antigens in glomerular and pulmonary alveolar basement membranes.
- The target epitopes for this autoimmune disease lie in the quaternary structure of ***a3 NC1 domain of collagen IV***.
- The presence of anti-GBM antibodies and complement is recognized on biopsy by ***linear immunofluorescent staining for IgG*** (rarely IgA).
- Clinical manifestations include:
  - ➢ ***Nephritic*** syndrome
  - ➢ ***Pneumonitis*** with ***hemoptysis*** (hemorrhagic pneumonitis)
  - ➢ Peak incidence in men in their mid 20s
  - ➢ RPGN ***crescentic morphology***.

6. **Answer is b (Nitrofurantoin).**
Ref: Harrison's, 17th edition Pg 657, Table 101-5.

Drugs that Carry Risk of Clinical Hemolysis in Persons with G-6-PD Deficiency

	Definite Risk	**Possible Risk**
Antimalarials	Primaquine Dapsone/Chlorproguanil	Chloroquine
Sulfonamides / Sulfones	Sulfamethoxazole Dapsone	Sulfasalazine Sulfadimidine
Antibacterial / Antibiotics	Co-trimoxazole Naldixic acid Nitrofurantoin Niridazole	Ciprofloxacin Norfloxacin
Antipyretic / Analgesics	Acetanilide Phenazopyridine (pyridium)	Aspirin (high dose > 3 g/d)
Other	Naphthalene Methylene blue	Vitamin K analogues Ascorbic acid > 1 g Rasburicase

7. **Answer is c (Kidney failure).**
Ref: Davidson's, 20th edition Pg 441.

Direct quote:

"***Hypermagnesemia*** nearly ***always involves acute or chronic*** ***renal failure***".

Other causes of hypermagnesemia

- Adrenocortical insufficiency
- Increased intake of medications containing magnesium (antacids, laxatives, enemas).

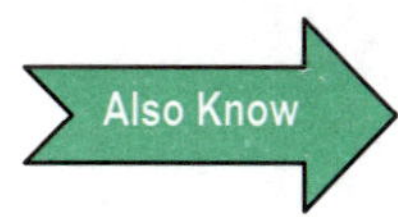

Causes of hypomagnesemia

Inadequate intake	Starvation, malnutrition (especially alcoholism), parenteral alimentation
Excessive losses	
Gastrointestinal	Prolonged vomiting, nasogastric aspiration, chronic diarrhea/laxative abuse, malabsorption, small bowel bypass surgery, fistulae
Urinary	Diuretic therapy (loop, thiazide), alcohol, tubulotoxic drugs (Genticyn, cisplatin), volume expansion (primary hyperaldosteronism), diabetic ketoacidosis, postobstructive diuresis, recovery from ATN, inherited tubular transport defect (Bartter's syndrome, Gitelman's syndrome)
Complex formation	Acute pancreatitis, foscarnet therapy, hungry bone syndrome

8. **Answer is d (Fever).**
Ref: http://www.ncbi.nlm.nih.gov/pubmed/7025304

- ***Hemobilia***: ***Hemorrhage in or through the biliary tract***, due to trauma, inflammation, cholelithiasis, vascular disease or neoplasms.
- Clinical features include:
  - ☐ ***Jaundice***
  - ☐ Right upper quadrant abdominal pain (***biliary colic***)
  - ☐ ***Hematemesis*** and ***melena.***

9. **Answer is b (Transesophageal echo with Doppler).**
Ref: Harrison's, 17th edition Pg 796.

Direct quote:

"***Transesophageal echocardiography with color Doppler*** *is the* ***test of choice*** *to detect* ***perivalvular abscesses*** *(sensitivity, ≥ 85%)*".

- ***Perivalvular infection*** is ***most common with aortic valve infection***.
- Occurs in 10–15% of native valve and 45–60% of *prosthetic valve infections* is suggested by:
  - ➲ Persistent unexplained fever during appropriate therapy
  - ➲ New ECG conduction disturbances
  - ➲ Pericarditis.
- Occasionally, perivalvular infections are cured medically.
- ***Surgery*** is warranted when fever persists, fistulae develop, prostheses are dehisced and unstable and invasive infection relapses after appropriate treatment.

10. **Answer is b (Ankylosing spondylitis).**
Ref: Harrison's, 17th edition Pg 2109.

Repeat Topic

- Refer ***answer no. 6*** in ***COMED-K 2008 answers.***

11. **Answer is b (Pruritus).**
Ref: Harrison's, 17th edition Pg 1974.

- ***Primary biliary cirrhosis (PBC)*** is a disease characterized by inflammatory destruction of the small bile ducts within the liver. PBC eventually leads to cirrhosis of the liver.
- ***Pruritus is seen in approximately 50% of patients at the time of diagnosis*** and can be debilitating.
- Pruritus that presents prior to the development of jaundice indicates severe disease and a poor prognosis.

12. **Answer is b (Isoniazid).**
Ref: http://www.mult-sclerosis.org/mstreatments.html; http://www.msinfowiki.ca/index.php?title=Isoniazid

- ***Intention Tremor*** is quite common in ***multiple sclerosis*** (MS) though it is associated with a number of other conditions including Parkinson's disease, trapped peripheral nerves and some drug treatments.
- Intention Tremor is related to Ataxia and in MS it is often caused by lesions in the cerebellum.
- Intention Tremor is commonly detected by neurologists using finger to nose tests. The neurologist holds up his or her finger and you move your finger from your nose to his or her finger and back to your nose.
- ***Isoniazid*** has been used to treat ***intention tremor in multiple sclerosis***.

13. **Answer is c (Saline infusion).**
Ref: KD Tripathi, 6th edition Pg 758-59.

Administration of Amphotericin B

- ***Orally for intestinal candidiasis***; also ***topically for vaginitis, otomycosis***, etc.
- For systemic mycoses: It is available as dry powder along with DOC for extemporaneous dispersion before use.
- It is first suspended in 10 mL water and then ***diluted to 500 mL with glucose solution*** (***saline tends to make the suspension coarse***).
- New amphotericin B formulations:
  - Amphotericin B ***lipid complex*** (ABLC)
  - Amphotericin B ***colloidal dispersion*** (ABCD)
  - ***Liposomal*** Amphotericin B (small unilamellar vesicles, SUV).
- ***Mannitol*** given concurrently with amphotericin B (slow IV infusion) may ***reduce nephrotoxicity***.

14. **Answer is c (Hemochromatosis).**
Ref: Robbins, 7th edition Pg 151, Table 5-1, 5-2, 5-3.

- ***Hereditary hemochromatosis*** is an ***autosomal recessive single gene disorder***, (HFE gene on ***chromosome 6p***).

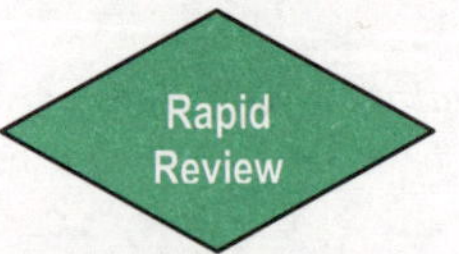

Inherited Disorders

System	Autosomal dominant	Autosomal recessive	X-linked recessive
Skeletal	Marfan's syndrome Ehler-Danlos syndrome (some variants) Osteogenesis imperfecta Achondroplasia	Ehler-Danlos syndrome (some variants) Alkaptonuria	Duchenne muscular dystrophy
Nervous	Huntington's disease Neurofibromatosis Myotonic dystrophy Tuberous sclerosis	Friedrich ataxia Neurogenic muscular atrophies Spinal muscular atrophy	Fragile-X syndrome
Metabolic	Familial hypercholesterolemia	Cystic fibrosis Phenylketonuria	Hunters syndrome Diabetes insipidus

	Acute intermittent porphyria	Galactosemia Homocystinuria Lysosomal storage diseases α-1 antitrypsin deficiency Wilson disease Hemochromatosis Glycogen storage disease	Lesch-Nyhan syndrome
Hematopoietic	Hereditary spherocytosis von Willebrand disease	Sickle cell anemia Thalassemias	Hemophilia A and B Chronic granulomatous disease Glucose-6-phosphate deficiency
Gastrointestinal	Familial polyposis coli		
Urinary	Polycystic kidney disease		
Endocrine		Congenital adrenal hyperplasia	
Immune			Agammaglobulinemia Wiskott-Aldrich syndrome

"As a general rule most structural abnormalities are autosomal dominant, whereas most enzymatic/biochemical abnormalities are autosomal recessive."

15. Answer is c (Pericarditis).
Ref: Harrison's, 17th edition Pg 1079.

- In SLE, ***pericarditis*** is the ***most frequent cardiac manifestation***; it usually ***responds to anti-inflammatory therapy*** and *infrequently* leads to tamponade.
- More serious cardiac manifestations are:
  - Myocarditis
  - ***Libman-Sacks fibrinous endocarditis***.

16. Answer is c (Vietnam).
Ref: http://www.who.int/csr/sars/sarsfaq/en/

Direct quote from above WHO website is given below:

Q : Where and when was the first case of SARS reported?
A : On 26 February, a man was admitted to hospital in ***Hanoi*** (capital of Vietnam) with high fever, dry cough, myalgia (muscle soreness) and mild sore throat. Over the next 4 days he developed increasing breathing difficulties, severe thrombocytopenia (low platelet count) and signs of adult respiratory distress syndrome requiring ventilator support.

17. Answer is c (Occipital cortex).
Ref: Harrison's, 17th edition Pg 165.

Pure alexia without agraphia (word blindness)

- This is the ***visual equivalent of pure word deafness***.
- The lesions (usually a combination of damage to the ***left occipital cortex*** and to a posterior sector of the corpus callosum—the splenium) interrupt the flow of visual input into the language network.
- There is usually a right hemianopia, but the core language network remains unaffected. The patient can understand and produce spoken language, name objects in the left visual hemifield, repeat and write.
- However, the patient acts as if illiterate when asked to read even the simplest sentence, because the visual information from the written words (presented to the intact left visual hemifield) cannot reach the language network. Objects in the left hemifield may be named accurately because they activate non-visual associations in the right hemisphere, which, in turn, can access the language network through transcallosal pathways anterior to the splenium.

- Patients with this syndrome may also lose the ability to name colors, although they can match colors. This is known as a *color anomia*.
- The ***most common etiology of pure alexia*** is a vascular lesion in the territory of the posterior cerebral artery or an infiltrating neoplasm in the ***left occipital cortex*** that involves the optic radiations as well as the crossing fibers of the splenium.

Pure Word Deafness

- The most common causes are either bilateral or left-sided middle cerebral artery strokes affecting the ***superior temporal gyrus***. The net effect of the underlying lesion is to interrupt the flow of information from the unimodal auditory association cortex to Wernicke's area. Patients have no difficulty understanding written language and can express themselves well in spoken or written language.
- They have no difficulty interpreting and reacting to environmental sounds, since primary auditory cortex and subcortical auditory relays are intact. Since auditory information cannot be conveyed to the language network, however, it cannot be decoded into lexical representations and the patient reacts to speech as if it were in an alien tongue that cannot be deciphered.
- Patients cannot repeat spoken language, but have no difficulty naming objects. In time, patients with pure word deafness teach themselves lip reading and may appear to have improved. There may be no additional neurologic findings, but agitated paranoid reactions are frequent in the acute stages. Cerebrovascular lesions are the most frequent cause.

18. **Answer is c (HDL).**
Ref: Textbook of Biochemistry, Vasudevan, 5th edition Pg 157.

HDL	LDL
– ***HDL*** is antiatherogenic and 'protective' in nature—hence HDL is called ***'good cholesterol'***. – HDL = High Density Lipoprotein = Highly Desirable Lipoprotein; ***H = Healthy***!	– ***LDL***, especially oxidized and glycated LDL creates a procoagulant surface on the endothelium, causing blood clot formation. – LDL is atherogenic and gets deposited in blood vessels—hence LDL is ***'bad cholesterol'***. – LDL = Low Density Lipoprotein = Lethally Dangerous Lipoprotein; ***L = Lousy***!

19. **Answer is c (Skull bone tumors).**
Ref: Harrison's, 17th edition Pg 2490.

- MRI is investigation of choice in soft tissue pathology, whereas for bone imaging CT is the investigation of choice.

Advantages of MRI	Advantages of CT scan
– No ionizing radiation. – They have much higher detail in the soft tissues. – Contrast of the images can be changed. Small changes in the radiowaves and the magnetic fields can completely change the contrast of the image. Different contrast settings will highlight different types of tissue. – Ability to change the imaging plane without moving the patient. Most MRI machines can produce images in any plane. – Contrast agents can also be used in MRI. – For purposes of tumor detection and identification, MRI is generally superior.	– CT is very good for imaging bone structures. – In CT scan, the time taken for total testing is shorter than taken by MRI. – CT scan is cheaper than MRI. – Some patients who have received certain types of surgical clips, metallic fragments, cardiac monitors or pacemakers cannot receive MRI. – MRI cannot be done in patients who are claustrophobic as the patient has to remain inside the machine for about 20–45 minute.

20. **Answer is d (Mouth to anus).**
Ref: Harrison's, 17th edition Pg 1888.

Repeat Topic

- In ***Crohn's disease*** any part of the gastrointestinal tract from ***mouth to anus*** may be involved in the chronic granulomatous process, but the ***terminal ileum is the region most frequently affected***.
- For more about the differences between Crohn's disease and ulcerative colitis please see ***answer no. 115 in COMED-K 2009 answers***.

21. Answer is b (Kartagener syndrome).

Ref: Harrison's, 17th edition Pg 1629.

Kartagener syndrome
❖ Situs inversus
❖ Bronchiectasis
❖ Sinusitis

- Primary ciliary dyskinesia is responsible for manifestations of Kartagener syndrome.
- Because normal sperm motility also depends on proper ciliary function, males are with Kartagener syndrome are generally ***infertile.***

22. Answer is b (Somatostatinoma).

Ref: Harrison's, 17th edition Pg 2355.

- ***Somatostatinomas*** are associated with excessive production of somatostatin by tumor cells of ***D-cell origin*** and they are frequently a/w a ***classic clinical pentad*** of:
  - Cholelithiasis (gallstones)
  - Diarrhea
  - Steatorrhea
  - Weight loss
  - Diabetes mellitus, hypochlorhydria and achlorhydria.

23. Answer is b (Abram's needle).

Ref: http://www.pulmononline.org/previousissues/pulmon-jan-apr-05/percutaneous.html

- The ***Abram's pleural biopsy punch/needle***, unlike some other pleural biopsy instruments is a cutting needle. The outer needle has a cutting groove into which tissue either prolapses or is aspirated. The cutting trocar is then advanced, cutting the biopsy. The needle is then removed, reopened and the specimen taken out.
- ***Osgood needle—*** used for bone marrow biopsy and transfusion.
- ***Vim-Silverman needle***—cannula or needle, for taking tissue specimens, particularly used for biopsies from liver or kidney.

24. Answer is d (Hyperaldosteronism).

Ref: Harrison's, 17th edition Pg 2262.

- In ***primary hyperaldosteronism,*** the cause for the excessive aldosterone production resides within the adrenal gland—*aldosterone-producing adrenal adenoma* ***(Conn's syndrome)***.
- In ***secondary hyperaldosteronism,*** the stimulus is extra-adrenal—an appropriately increased production of aldosterone in response to ***activation of the renin-angiotensin system***.

25. Answer is c (Left bundle branch block with broad QRS complex).

Ref: Pediatric Cardiology for practitioners, Myung K Park, 2008 edition Pg 449; Pocket Guide to ECG diagnosis, Edward K Chung, 2001, 2nd edition Pg 404.

- The position and number of spikes on the ECH rhythm strip are used to recognize different types of pacemakers.

- Thus, a pacemaker may be classified as ventricular pacemaker, atrial pacemaker or P-wave triggered ventricular pacemaker:
  - When the pacemaker stimulates the atrium, the resulting P-wave demonstrates an abnormal P axis.
  - When the pacemaker stimulates the *ventricle, wide QRS complexes* result:
    - The ventricle that is stimulated (or ***the ventricle on which the pacemaker electrode is placed) can be identified by the morphology of the QRS complexes***:
      - With the pacemaker on the *right ventricle* = a ***left bundle branch block*** (LBBB) pattern results.
      - With the pacemaker on the *left ventricle* = a ***right bundle branch block*** (RBBB) pattern results.

Author's comments: "Excellent explanation given in the above textbook – given as a direct quote here."

SURGERY

26. Answer is b (Lingual).
Ref: Bailey and Love's, 25th edition Pg 755.

- Care should be taken to avoid damage to the ***Lingual nerve*** when excising the Wharton's duct, since it lies in close proximity to the duct.

Also Know

- Three ***cranial nerves are at risk during removal of the submandibular*** gland:
  - Marginal mandibular branch of facial nerve
  - Lingual nerve
  - Hypoglossal nerve.

27. Answer is d (Meckel's diverticulum).
Ref: Bailey and Love's, 25th edition Pg 1158.

- ***Meckel's diverticulum*** is the ***MC congenital abnormality of the small intestine***; it is caused by an ***incomplete obliteration of the vitelline duct (i.e. omphalomesenteric duct)*** – i.e. it represents the patent intestinal end of the vitellointestinal duct.

Fast Facts

Rule of 2's - Meckel's diverticulum

- It is present in about *2%* of subjects
- Its length is about *2 inches*
- Usually *2 feet (60 cm)* proximal to the ileocecal valve and occurs on the antimesenteric border of the ileum
- *Present in 2%* of the population

- Meckel's diverticulum is typically lined by ileal mucosa, but *other tissue types are also found* with varying frequency, ***ectopic gastric mucosa*** in about 50%.
- A Meckel's diverticulum ***possesses all 3 coats of the intestinal wall*** and ***has its own blood supply***. It is therefore *vulnerable to infection* and *obstruction* in the same way as the appendix.

28. Answer is b (60).
Ref: Bailey and Love's, 25th edition Pg 1158.

Repeat Topic

- Refer ***previous answer*** for detailed explanation.

29. Answer is d (Gallstones).
Ref: Harrison's, 17th edition Pg 2006-07.

Direct Quote:

*"**Gallstones** continue to be the leading cause of acute pancreatitis in most series **(30–60%)**. **Alcohol is the second most common cause**, responsible for 15–30% of cases in the United States".*

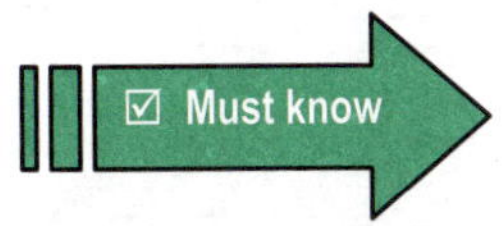

Etiology of acute pancreatitis (Mnemonic: "GET SMASHED")

➢ Gallstones ➢ Ethanol ➢ Trauma ➢ Steroids ➢ Mumps ➢ Autoimmune (PAN) ➢ Scorpion venom ➢ Hyperlipidemia (raised Ca^{2+}, hypothermia) ➢ ERCP (also emboli) ➢ Pregnancy	➢ Drugs – Asparaginase – Azathioprine – Didanisone – Diuretics – Exenatide – Mercaptopurine – OCPs – Pentamidine – Tetracycline – Valproic acid

30. Answer is a (Biliary calculi).
Ref: Harrison's, 17th edition Pg 2006-07.

Repeat Topic

- Refer ***previous answer above*** for detailed explanation.

31. Answer is c (24-hour pH recording).
Ref: GERD: reflux to esophageal adenocarcinoma, by Para Chandrasoma, Tom R DeMeester, Pg 302.

- The present gold standards for the diagnosis of gastroesophageal reflux are considered to be the ***24-hour pH test and newer multichannel impedance studies***.
- ***Ambulatory 24-hour pH monitoring*** registers the amount and frequency of acid in the esophagus and allows correlation with symptoms such as heartburn and pain. A probe is placed into the esophagus, which records the acid level in both the esophagus and stomach for a full 24 hours. This is the ***MOST ACCURATE METHOD OF OBJECTIVELY DETECTING REFLUX AND GERD***.

32. Answer is b (Retrograde ejaculation).
Ref: Mebust WK, et al. Transurethral Prostatectomy: Immediate and postoperative complications. J Urol 141: 243, 1989 – Journal reference; Bailey and Love, 25th edition Pg 1352.

Complications of TURP

- Retrograde ejaculation (50–100%)
- Failure to urinate (6.7%)
- Bleeding (3.3%)
- Infection (2.3%)
- Impotence (0–40%)

- Urethral stricture (2.5%)
- Incontinence
- TURP syndrome—mild 2%, severe 0.5%.

33. Answer is c (Thymoma).
Ref: Robbins Pathology, 7th edition Pg 707; Bailey and Love, 25th edition Pg 892.

- ***Thymoma*** is the commonest tumor of the anterior mediastinum and is locally invasive in 30–50% of cases.
- ***Thymoma*** is also the most common mediastinal tumor accounting for ***25% of the total.***

Note:

- ***Middle mediastinum***: Lymphoma
- ***Posterior mediastinum***: Neurogenic tumors.

34. Answer is c (Cholesterol).
Ref: Robbins Pathology, 7th edition Pg 930.

- ***Pure cholesterol stones are pale yellow*** and have a glistening crystalline center with a radiating appearance.
- Pigment stones are small, dark stones made of bilirubin.
- ***Black pigment stones***: Contain mucin glycoprotein; found in sterile gallbladder bile.
- ***Brown pigment stones***: Found in infected intrahepatic or extrahepatic ducts.

35. Answer is b (Stomach).
Ref: Harrison's, 17th edition Pg 573.

- The ***stomach is the most common extranodal site of lymphoma*** and is also the ***MC site of gastrointestinal lymphoma***.
- Gastrointestinal lymphomas typically present with non-specific signs and symptoms attributable to the site of involvement.
- Primary lymphoma of the stomach is relatively uncommon, accounting for < 15% of gastric malignancies and ~2% of all lymphomas.

36. Answer is c (Gastroduodenal artery).
Ref: Clinical Anatomy by regions, Richard Snell, 8th edition Pg 227.

- Majority of duodenal ulcers occur within 2 cm of pylorus in duodenal bulb:
  - ***Posterior ulcers—more likely to bleed*** because it ***erodes into gastroduodenal artery***
  - ***Anterior ulcers***—most likely to ***perforate*** (refer free air under diaphragm on upright abdominal radiograph).

37. Answer is b (Choledochoduodenostomy).
Ref: http://emedicine.medscape.com/article/187001-overview

- ***Sump syndrome***: A complication of ***side-to-side choledochoduodenostomy*** in which the lower end of the CBD at times acts as a diverticulum, resulting in stasis, trapping of food particles and infection.
- Often the *same symptoms that are present before the operation recur* or postoperative symptoms such as Colicky pain, bloating, nausea and vomiting occur.
- There is pain on palpation of the RUQ and sometimes jaundice.

38. Answer is c (Perthes' test).
Ref: en.wikipedia.org/wiki/Perthes'_test

- The following three tests may be helpful to distinguish primary and secondary varicosities:
  - ***Perthes' test***—to determine valvular competence in the ***deep femoral vein***
  - ***Brodie-Trendelenburg test***—to determine valvular incompetence in the saphenofemoral system
  - ***Percussion test***—to determine valvular competence in the great saphenous vein.

39. **Answer is a (Duodenum).**
Ref: Harrison's, 17th edition Pg 2109; Davidson's, 20th edition Pg 890.

Repeat Topic

- ***Zollinger-Ellison Syndrome*** consists of ***severe peptic ulcer*** diathesis secondary to ***gastric acid hypersecretion*** due to ***unregulated gastrin release*** from a ***non-β cell endocrine tumor (gastrinoma).***
- ***Age affected*** = 30–50 years.
- ***Etiology***: Gastrinomas are classified into ***sporadic tumors (MC)*** and those ***a/w multiple endocrine neoplasia (MEN) type I.***
- ***Location***: Over 80% of these tumors are found within the hypothetical ***gastrinoma triangle*** (confluence of the cystic and common bile ducts superiorly, junction of the second and third portions of the duodenum inferiorly, and junction of the neck and body of the pancreas medially).
- ***Duodenal tumors constitute the MC non-pancreatic lesion***; between 50% and 75% of gastrinomas are found here *(HPIM 17th, 2109).*
- Primary gastrinomas may arise in the pancreas (25%), ***duodenal wall (45%)*** or lymph nodes (5–15%) and in other locations or of unknown primary in 20% *(CMDT, chapter 15).*
- Around 90% of tumors occur in the pancreatic head or ***proximal duodenal wall, the latter site being more common*** *(Davidsons, 20th edition 890).*

Author's Comments: *"The above three direct quotes make it clear that the duodenum is the MC site of gastrinoma causing ZES".*

Clinically

- ***Peptic ulcers***, usually solitary and located in the duodenal bulb; isolated gastric ulcers do not occur.
- ***Gastric acid hypersecretion*** can cause direct intestinal mucosal injury and pancreatic enzyme inactivation, resulting in diarrhea, steatorrhea and weight loss; nasogastric aspiration of stomach acid stops the diarrhea.
- ***Suspect ZES*** when:
  - *Increased fasting gastrin levels* are a/w ulcers refractory to standard therapies
  - Giant ulcers (> 2 cm)
  - Ulcers located distal to the duodenal bulb (***postbulbar ulcer***), multiple duodenal ulcers
  - Frequent *ulcer recurrences*
  - Ulcers associated with *diarrhea*
  - Ulcers occurring *after ulcer surgery*
  - Patients with *ulcer complications*
  - Patients with *hypercalcemia* or family histories of ulcers (suggesting MEN 1); ulcers occurring in absence of *H. pylori* and NSAIDs usage.

Laboratory Findings

- ***Most sensitive and specific*** test: ***Increased fasting serum gastrin concentration*** (> 150 pg/mL).
- Gastric acid hypersecretion is present (pH < 3.0).
- ***IV secretin*** (2 units/kg) produces a rise in serum gastrin of over 200 pg/mL within 2–30 minutes in 85% of patients with gastrinoma.

Imaging

- ***Somatostatin Receptor Scintigraphy*** has a sensitivity (> 80%) for tumor detection that exceeds all other imaging studies combined. If SRS is positive for tumor localization, further imaging studies are NOT necessary.
- In patients with negative SRS, endoscopic ultrasonography (EUS) may be useful to detect small gastrinomas in the duodenal wall, pancreas or peripancreatic lymph nodes.

Treatment

- *Metastatic disease*: In patients with multiple hepatic metastases, initial therapy should be directed at controlling hypersecretion. Oral proton pump inhibitors.
- *Localized disease*: Cure can be achieved only if the gastrinoma can be resected before hepatic metastatic spread has occurred.

Note:
Gastrinoma triangle (Psaros triangle): 90% of gastrinomas are found here.

40. Answer is a (Pernicious anemia).

Ref: Harrison's, 17th edition Pg 572.

Risk factors for gastric carcinoma
• *H.pylori* infection
• Chronic Atrophic gastritis
• Blood group A
• Pernicious Anemia
• Adenomatous polyps
• Smoking and Alcohol
• Nitrosamines in smoked fish
• Menetrier's disease
• Postantrectomy:15–20 years after Billroth II anastomosis

41. Answer is a (Vomiting).

Ref: Harrison's, 17th edition Pg 1899.

- ***Pain or abdominal discomfort*** is a key symptom for the diagnosis of Irritable bowel syndrome (IBS). These symptoms should be improved with defecation and/or have their onset associated with a change in frequency or form of stool.
- ***Painless diarrhea or constipation*** does not fulfill the diagnostic criteria to be classified as IBS. Supportive symptoms that are not part of the diagnostic criteria include *defecation straining, urgency or a feeling of incomplete bowel movement, passing mucus and bloating/gas/flatulence.*
- ***Alteration in bowel habits is the most consistent clinical feature in IBS***. The most common pattern is constipation alternating with diarrhea, usually with one of these symptoms predominating.
- A small percentage of patients with IBS more commonly than others have gastroesophageal reflux, symptoms relating to the genitourinary system, psychological symptoms, fibromyalgia, headache and backache.

42. Answer is b (20%).

Ref: Hepatobiliary cancer, Leslie HB, 2001 edition, Pg 145.

- Hepatic resection is appropriate treatment for a variety of benign and primary or secondary malignant hepatic lesions. In appropriate patients with malignant disease, resection generally offers the best opportunity for long-term survival or cure. In patients with benign tumors, resection is safe and effective when carried out for symptoms directly related to the tumor.
- In a healthy, non-cirrhotic patient, up to 80% of the functional parenchyma can be removed with a reasonable expectation of subsequent regeneration.

43. Answer is a (Proximal two thirds of stomach).

Ref: Operative anatomy By Carol EH Scott-Conner, David L Dawson, 3rd edition Pg 380.

- Unlike other forms of vagotomy, this version only disables the nerve fibers, which control acid-secreting glands, while leaving other vagus nerve functions undisturbed.
- Highly selective vagotomy (HSV), also referrred to as parietal cell vagotomy or proximal gastric vagotomy, divides only the vagus nerves supplying the proximal two thirds of stomach.
- **There are four basic types of vagotomy procedures:**
  - ☐ Truncal or total abdominal vagotomy. The main vagal trunks are divided and surgery is accompanied by a drainage procedure, such as pyloroplasty
  - ☐ Selective (total gastric) vagotomy. The main vagal trunks are dissected to the point where the branch leading to the biliary tree divides and there is a cut at the section of vagus close to the hepatic branch. This procedure is rarely indicated or performed
  - ☐ Highly selective vagotomy (HSV): It selectively deprives the parietal cells of vagal nerves and reduces their sensitivity to stimulation and the release of acid. It does not require a drainage procedure. The branches of

Latarjet's nerve are divided from the esophagogastric junction to the crow's foot along the lesser curvature of the stomach

- Thoracoscopic vagotomy: Performed through the third, sixth and seventh left intercostal spaces, the posterior vagus trunk is isolated, clipped and a segment excised.

44. Answer is d (T4N2M0).
Ref: http://www.oncologychannel.com/oralcancer/staging.shtml

TNM Staging of Oral Cancer

Primary Tumor (T)

TX	Primary tumor cannot be assessed
T0	No evidence of primary tumor
sTis	Carcinoma *in situ*
T1	Tumor 2 cm or less in greatest dimension
T2 dimension	Tumor more than 2 cm, but not more than 4 cm in greatest
T3	Tumor more than 4 cm in greatest dimension
T4	*Tumor invades adjacent structures (e.g. through cortical bone, into maxillary sinus, skin, pterygoid muscle, deep muscle of tongue)*

Nodal Involvement (N)

NX	Regional lymph nodes cannot be assessed
N0	No regional lymph node metastasis
N1	Metastasis in a single ipsilateral lymph node, 3 cm or less in greatest dimension
N2	*Metastasis in a single ipsilateral lymph node, more than 3 cm, but not more than 6 cm in greatest dimension*; or in multiple ipsilateral lymph nodes, none more than 6 cm in greatest dimension; or in bilateral or contralateral lymph nodes, none more than 6 cm in greatest dimension
N2a	Metastasis in a single ipsilateral lymph node, more than 3 cm, but not more than 6 cm in greatest dimension
N2b	Metastasis in multiple ipsilateral lymph nodes, none more than 6 cm in greatest dimension
N2c	Metastasis in bilateral or contralateral lymph nodes, none more than 6 cm in greatest dimension
N3	Metastasis in a lymph node more than 6 cm in greatest dimension

Distant Metastasis (M)

MX	Distant metastasis cannot be assessed
M0	No distant metastasis
M1	Distant metastasis

Stage Grouping

Stage 0	Tis N0 M0
Stage I	T1 N0 M0
Stage II	T2 N0 M0
Stage III	T3 N0 M0; T1 or T2 or T3 N1 M0
Stage IV	Any T4 lesion or Any N2 or N3 lesions or Any M1 lesion

45. Answer is a (Follicular).
Ref: Textbook of surgery, S Das, 1st edition, Pg 213.

- Vascular invasion is characteristic for follicular carcinoma and therefore distant metastasis is more common. Distant metastasis may occur in a small primary.
- Lung, bone, brain, liver, bladder and skin are potential sites of distant spread.
- Lymph node involvement is far less common than in papillary carcinoma.

46. Answer is d (Left mainstem bronchus).
Ref: IB Singh's Histology, 229, Bailey and Love, 25th edition Pg 1009.

Constrictions of the esophagus

Distance from incisor teeth	Structure causing constriction	Problems associated
• 15 cm	→ Cricopharyngeal sphincter	Foreign body lodgment
• 25 cm	→ Aortic Arch → Left main Bronchus	Perforation during endoscopy
• 40 cm	→ Diaphragm entry	Malignancy

Mnemonic: *"Children And Adults Love Burgers at McDonald's"*; ***15, 25, 40 cm.***

High Yield Info

Surgical and Applied Anatomy of Esophagus

- 25 cm long; occupies the ***posterior mediastinum***
- Extends from the cricopharyngeal sphincter to the cardia of the stomach (45 cm from teeth to cardia of stomach); 1.25 cm of this tube lies below the diaphragm
- Is the narrowest region of the alimentary tract except for the vermiform appendix
- Lined by ***stratified squamous non-keratinizing epithelium,*** which is replaced by specialized columnar epithelium (lower 3 cm) at the level of the hiatus similar to gastric mucosa, but without oxyntic and peptic cells
- Serosa is absent in esophagus
- The parasympathetic nerve supply to esophagus is mediated by vagus through an extrinsic and intrinsic plexus. The intrinsic plexus has no Meissner's network, which is present elsewhere through the alimentary canal and only Auerbach's plexus is present.

Esophagus	Blood Supply	Muscle	Lymph
• Upper 1/3	Inferior Thyroid A.	Striated	Deep cervical
• Middle 1/3	Thoracic Aorta	Striated/Smooth	Mediastinal
• Lower 1/3	Left Gastric A.	Smooth	Gastric

Mnemonic: *"In Testing Times Always think Life's Good!"*

47. Answer is d (Extradural hematoma).
Ref: Harrison's, 17th edition Pg 2599.

- ***Epidural or extradural hematoma*** is a type of traumatic brain injury in which a buildup of blood occurs between the dura mater and the skull bone.
- A ***lucid interval*** is especially characteristic of an epidural hematoma.
- After the injury, the patient is momentarily dazed or knocked out and then becomes ***relatively lucid (regains consciousness)*** for a period of time, which can last minutes or hours. Thereafter, there is rapid decline as the blood collects within the skull, causing a rise in intracranial pressure, which damages brain tissue.

Must Know

Difference Between Epidural and Subdural Hemorrhage

Epidural (extradural) hematoma	Subdural hematoma
❖ Usually *arterial blood* accumulates between skull bone and dura	❖ *Venous blood* accumulates between dura and arachnoid
❖ Usually rupture of ***middle meningeal artery*** after trauma to *temporal* bone	❖ Rupture of torn superficial bridging veins between cerebral cortex and sinuses
❖ Brief unconsciousness followed by **LUC**id interval for several hours	❖ Occur in elderly and alcoholics after relatively minor trauma

❖ CT scan: convex mass *"EXtradural = convEX; Always give LUCy EXtra attention!"*	❖ Concave (crescent shaped) mass, which is less dense than epidural since blood is diluted with CSF

48. Answer is c (Systemic prostate biopsy in suspected prostate cancer).
Ref: Harrison's, 17th edition Pg 596.

- ***TransRectal Ultrasonography (TRUS)*** is the imaging technique most frequently used to assess the primary tumor, but ***its chief use is directing prostate biopsies***, NOT staging.
- No TRUS finding consistently indicates cancer with certainty.

49. Answer is a (Pulmonary angiography).
Ref: Harrison's, 17th edition Pg 1654.

- ***Computed tomography (CT) of the chest with intravenous contrast is the principal imaging test for the diagnosis of pulmonary embolism (PE).***
- Multidetector-row spiral CT acquires all chest images with ≤ 1 mm resolution during a short breath hold. This generation of CT scanners can image small peripheral emboli. ***Sixth-order branches can be visualized*** with ***resolution superior to conventional invasive contrast pulmonary angiography***.
- The CT scan also obtains excellent images of the RV and LV and can be used for risk stratification as well as a diagnostic tool.

> - Chest CT with contrast (see above) has ***virtually replaced invasive pulmonary angiography as a diagnostic test***
> - ***Lung scanning*** (ventilation perfusion scan) is now a ***second-line diagnostic test*** for PE

Author's Comments: *"Since the choice contains only pulmonary angiogram and no CT chest with contrast – go for **pulmonary angiogram, it is the gold standard**, go for that. Also if both CT chest and pulmonary angiogram are present in the choices go for angiogram as the answer".*

Also Know

Chest X-ray signs in pulmonary embolism

Embolism without infarction (90%)	Embolism with infarction (10%)
▪ ***Normal chest***; plate-like atelectasis; segmental/lobar consolidation; Pleural effusion ▪ ***Westermark sign*** (focal oligemia in the embolized zone) ▪ ***'Knuckle' sign*** (abrupt tapering off of an occluded vessel distally) ▪ Local widening of artery by impacted embolus	▪ ***Hampton hump*** (a peripheral, pleural based, wedged-shaped density above the diaphragm) ▪ Pleural effusion (50%) ▪ ***'Melting' sign*** (regression of consolidation from periphery to center; appears within days to weeks) ▪ ***Fleischner*** lines ▪ Plate-like atelectasis; cardiomegaly/CHF; elevated hemidiaphragm; no air bronchogram

❖ Best known sign of pulmonary embolism on ***echocardiography***: ***McConnell's sign*** – *hypokinesis of right ventricle-free wall* with normal motion of RV apex.

50. Answer is a (Inadequate control of hyperthyroidism).
Ref: KD Tripathi, 6th edition Pg 253; Bailey and Love, 25th edition Pg 791; Harrison's, 17th edition Pg 2237.

Thyrotoxic crisis (thyroid storm)

☐ Precipitating *factors*:
- Acute illness (e.g. stroke, infection, trauma, diabetic ketoacidosis), surgery (especially on the thyroid) or radioiodine treatment of a patient with partially treated or untreated hyperthyroidism.

- ***Post-thyroid surgery:*** Now uncommon secondary to preventative measures; manipulation of the thyroid gland during thyroidectomy historically caused a flood of hormone release, often resulting in highly toxic blood levels. Exacerbations of thyrotoxicosis are still seen in patients taken too soon to surgery, but are unusual in the antithyroid drug-controlled patient.
- The decreased incidence of thyroid storm can be largely attributed. To the improved methods of diagnosis and therapy available today. In most cases, thyrotoxicosis is recognized before extreme debilitation occurs and is treated by measures of predictable therapeutic value. Patients are routinely made euthyroid before surgery or treatment with 131-I. Under present-day therapy, using thiocarbamides, the glands have only minimal amounts of stored hormone, in contrast to the iodized gland facing the surgeons of 6 decades ago.
- Postoperative storm, formerly the most frequent kind of storm, has now been largely eliminated.

□ **Clinical features**:
- A rare, life-threatening ***acute exacerbation of hyperthyroidism***—accompanied by fever, delirium, seizures, coma, vomiting, diarrhea and jaundice.
- The mortality rate due to cardiac failure, arrhythmia or hyperthermia is as high as 30%, even with treatment.

□ **Management**:
- ***Measures that reduce thyroid hormone synthesis***:
  - ***Non-selective beta blockers (propranolol):*** Most valuable measure; give dramatic symptomatic relief (reduce tachycardia and other adrenergic manifestations); reduce peripheral conversion of T4 → T3
  - Large doses of ***propylthiouracil*** should be given orally or by nasogastric tube or per rectum; the drug's inhibitory action on T4 → T3 conversion makes it the antithyroid drug of choice
  - 1 hour after the first dose of propylthiouracil, ***stable iodide*** is given to block thyroid hormone synthesis via the Wolff-Chaikoff effect (the delay allows the antithyroid drug to prevent the excess iodine from being incorporated into new hormone). A saturated solution of ***potassium iodide, sodium iodide or ipodate or iopanoic acid***, may be given orally
  - ***Diltiazem (calcium channel blocker)*** may be added, if tachycardia not controlled by propranolol alone.
- ***Supportive treatment***:
  - IV fluids, cool patient with ice packs, administer oxygen, diuretics for cardiac failure, digoxin for uncontrolled atrial fibrillation, sedation and IV hydrocortisone.

Note:
- ***Before the availability of beta blockers***, drugs that deplete catecholamine stores such as ***reserpine and guanethidine*** were used with some success.

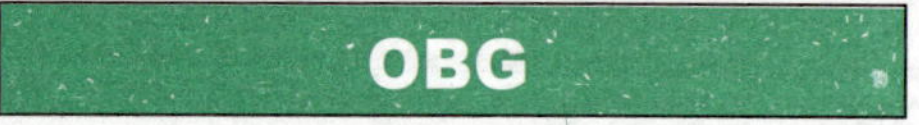

51. Answer is a (Endosalpingitis).
Ref: Shaw's gynecology, 14th edition Pg 137.

In ***tuberculosis, fallopian tube is the most commonly involved portion*** of the genital tract in over 90% of all genital tubercular lesions.

Types
- Tuberculaous endosalpingitis: Most common variety
- Tubercular exosalpingitis: Described as tobacco pouch appearance, frozen pelvis
- Interstitial salpingitis.

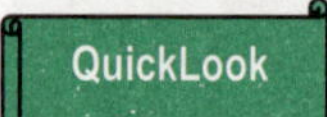

Hysterosalpingogram features of fallopian TB are:
- Rigid non-peristaltic pipe-like tube called lead pipe appearance
- Beading and variation in filling density
- Calcification of tube
- Cornual block
- A jagged fluffiness of tubal outline

- Vascular or lymphatic intravasation of the dye
- Tobacco pouch and dilated distal end of the tubes.

52. Answer is b (Polycystic ovarian disease).
Ref: Shaw's gynecology, 14th edition Pg 102, 189, 264.

POLYCYSTIC OVARIAN DISEASE (Stein-Leventhal syndrome)

- Clinically:
  - ↑ LH production leads to ***anovulation***, hyperandrogenism due to deranged steroid synthesis. ***Enlarged bilateral cystic ovaries*** manifest clinically with ***amenorrhea, infertility, obesity and hirsutism***
  - A/w ***insulin resistance***. ↑ ***risk of endometrial cancer***.
- Tests:
  - ↑ LH, ↓ FSH, LH:FSH ratio > 3; ↑ testosterone; ↑ DHEA and androstenedione
  - Positive progestin challenge (administration of progestin causes uterine bleeding within 5 days of administration).
- Treatment:
  - Weight loss, OCPs, gonadotropin analogs, clomiphene, metformin (for insulin resistance) or surgery (laparoscopic ovarian drilling, endoscopic ovarian cauterization, CO_2 laser vaporization of cysts).

53. Answer is d (Estrogen deficiency).
Ref: Shaw's gynecology, 14th edition Pg 119.

- ***Senile or atrophic vaginitis*** is an inflammation or irritation of the vagina caused by thinning and shrinking of the tissues of the vagina, and decreased lubrication of the vaginal walls
- This is due to a ***lack /deficiency of estrogen*** and is common in postmenopausal women
- It usually causes ***scant vaginal discharge with no odor, dry vagina and painful intercourse***.

54. Answer is b (Endometrium).
Ref: Harrison's, 17th edition Pg 607.

- **Side effects of tamoxifen include:**
  - ❖ Increased risk of endometrial cancer two fold in postmenopausal women who have not had a hysterectomy thrombosis
  - ❖ Abnormal growth of uterine tissue (endometriosis)
  - ❖ Stroke
  - ❖ Fertility issues
  - ❖ Hair and nail thinning

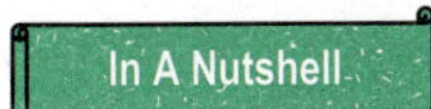

Other risk factors for carcinoma endometrium

Category	Risk factors
• Prolonged unopposed estrogen exposure	– Endometrial hyperplasia – Early menarche-late menopause – Nulliparity – Obesity (peripheral conversion to estrogen) – Estrogen replacement therapy – Tamoxifen (anti- and pro-estrogenic activity) – Chronic anovulation – Secondary infertility
• Family history	– Lynch type 2 syndrome, i.e. a higher incidence of endometrial, ovarian, breasts and colonic cancer
• Associated medical conditions	– Diabetes, hypertension

55. Answer is c (Temperature of 100.4°F 24 hours after delivery).
Ref: Dutta's obstetrics, 6th edition Pg 433.

- ***Puerperal pyrexia*** is defined as the presence of a ***fever that is greater than or equal to 38°C (100.4°F)*** in a woman ***within 14 days of giving birth***.

56. Answer is a (Per 100,000 live births).
Ref: Park, 20th edition Pg 481.

- Refer ***answer no. 124 below*** for detailed explanation.

57. Answer is b (8 weeks).
Ref: CPDT, 14th edition Pg 833.

- The gonads develop from a bipotential analogue in the genital ridge of celomic cavity.
- The primordial germ cells, which will become oocyte and spermatocyte arise in the yolk sac and migrate to the genital ridge by 4th week after conception, when the ***gonads are identifiable between 4 and 8 weeks of gestation***.
- Differentiation into an ovary or testis occurs by 7–9 weeks.

PEDIATRICS

58. Answer is b (Toxoplasmosis).
Ref: Washington Manual Pediatrics, 2012 edition, Pg 314.

- **The rule of 3s and 9s for head circumference:**
  - ***Birth***: 35 cm
  - ***3 months***: 40 cm
  - ***3 years***: 50 cm
  - ***9 years to adult***: 55 cm.

- So the child in the given question has macrocephaly; ***toxoplasmosis*** can lead to ***hydrocephalus and microcephaly***.

59. Answer is c (Rheumatic fever).
Ref: Op Ghai, 7th edition Pg 374-75.

- ***Antistreptolysin O antibodies*** will be raised ***after infection with streptococci***. Levels greater than 200 units/mL are considered significant.
- Measurement can be useful diagnostically, if recent infection with streptococci is known to be important in etiology.
- Streptococcal infections include:
  - ***Rheumatic fever***
  - Poststreptococcal glomerulonephritis
  - Scarlet fever
  - Erysipelas.

Also Know

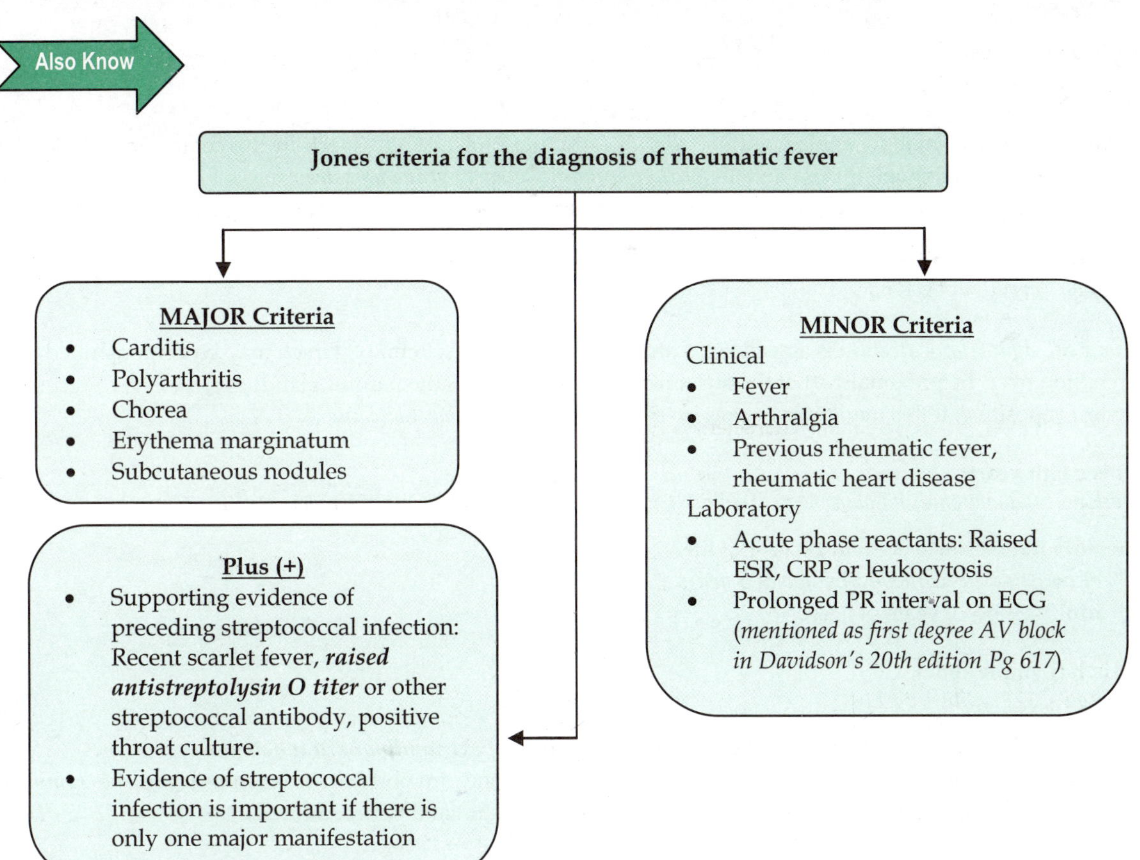

60. **Answer is d (Mode of delivery).**
Ref: OP Ghai, 7th edition Pg 107.

APGAR SCORE

	0	1	2
Appearance (color)	Blue or pale	Body pink, extremities blue	Pink
Pulse (heart rate)	0	< 100	> 100
Grimace to catheter in nose (reflex stimulation)	No response	Grimace	Cries, coughs or sneezes
Activity (muscle tone)	Flaccid	Some flexion	Actively moving extremities
Respiratory *effort (not rate)*	0	Slow irregular	Good crying

- *Normal APGAR score* = 8–10 at 1 minute after birth; < 7 indicates asphyxia.

Factors affecting Apgar score:

– Prematurity	– Spinal cord trauma
– Drugs—sedatives, narcotics, magnesium sulfate	– Lungs—diaphragmatic hernia
– A/c cerebral trauma	– Airway—choanal atresia
– Precipitate labor	– Congenital pneumonia (GBS)
– Congenital myopathy	– Maternal acidosis
– Congenital neuropathy	– High fetal catecholamine levels
– CNS anomaly	– Some full-term infants

61. Answer is b (Measles).
Ref: OP Ghai, 7th edition Pg 185.

- ***Koplik's spots*** are small, irregular, red spots with a minute bluish white speck in the center of each seen on the ***buccal mucosa*** and lingual mucosa and are ***pathognomonic of early stage measles***.
- They are named after Henry Koplik (1858–1927), an American pediatrician who first described them in 1896.

62. Answer is b (Hypocalcemia).
Ref: OP Ghai, 7th edition Pg 486.

- ***Chvostek' sign***: ***Hypocalcemia*** is associated with increased neural excitability, which may be demonstrated by gentle percussion over the proximal part of the facial nerve (as it exits from the parotid gland).
- The test is positive, if this maneuver evokes involuntary *facial muscular twitching*.

63. Answer is c (5th year).
Ref: Developmental anatomy and physiology of children, a practical approach, by Carol Chamley, Pg 116 .

- The ***brain*** doubles its weight in 1st year of life.
- ***90% of adult size*** is achieved by ***age of 5 years***.
- Full adult size by 10 years of age.

64. Answer is b (Lymph node).
Ref: Harrison's, 17th edition Pg 1101.

- ***Tuberculous Lymphadenitis*** is the ***most common presentation of extrapulmonary tuberculosis.***
- In ***order of frequency***, the extrapulmonary sites most commonly involved in tuberculosis are the ***lymph nodes***, pleura, genitourinary tract, bones and joints, meninges, peritoneum and pericardium.

65. Answer is b (6 months).
Ref: OP Ghai, 7th edition Pg 23-31.

- Child transfers objects from one hand to other at the age range of ***6 months***.

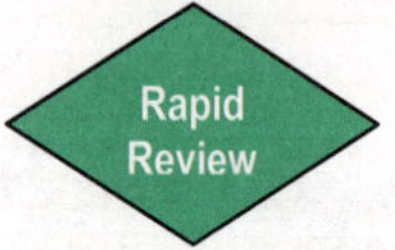

Developmental milestones

Age	Gross motor	Fine motor	Language	Social
1 month	**Momentarily lifts head when prone**	Has tight grasp, follows objects to midline	Responds to sound of bell	Regards face intently
2 months	Holds head in midline Lifts chest when prone	No longer clenches fist tightly, follows objects past midline	Smiles after being stoked or talked to	Recognizes parent, **social smile**
3 months	**Head holding achieved**	Follows moving objects in a circular fashion, converges and focuses	Coos (produces long vowel sounds in a musical fashion), laughs aloud	Reaches for familiar people or objects, anticipates feeding
4–5 months	**Rolls over**, sits with support	Grasps objects/rattle crudely	Orients to voice/bell (localizes laterally); 'ah-goo', razzes	Enjoys looking around environment
6 months	Takes foot to mouth, lifts head and upper chest with support	Transfers objects from one hand to another	Babbles	**Stranger anxiety**, smiles back at mirror image of self

9 months	**Sits unassisted** (8 months), crawls, cruises, pulls to stand	**Uses pincer grasp, probes with forefinger, holds feeding bottle**	Responds to name, says **mama/dada** (non-specific)	Responds to social play, plays pat-a-cake, starts to explore environment (9–10 months)
10 months	Pulls from supine to sitting; from sitting to standing, stands holding furniture		Understands to some extent, e.g. 'where is mama'	
12 months		Gives hand held objects to mother when asked, turns 2–3 pages at a time	Says 'mama, dada' (specific)	imitates actions
15 months	**Walks well** without support, walks backwards and sideways		Uses 3–5 words meaningfully	Temper tantrums, separation anxiety
18 months	Starts to run, climb stairs with help	Makes a tower of 3–4 cubes, scribbles spontaneously, may draw a vertical line	About 10 words spoken including name	Copies parents in tasks, toilet training started
2 years	Runs well, climbs stairs alone; walks on tiptoes (30 months)	Makes a tower of 6–7 cubes, turns one page of a book at a time, may draw horizontal line	Points to at least one named body part, simple **2** word sentences made ('2 words at 2 years')	Follows **2**-step commands
3 years	Pedals **tri**cycle, jumps with both feet off ground, **can alternate feet** when climbing stairs	Make a tower of 9–10 cubes, draws (copies) a **circle**	**Uses plurals,** 3 **word sentences** ('3 words at 3 years')	Dresses and undresses partially buttons/unbuttons
4 years	Hops, alternates feet going downstairs *('At 4 u hop off the floor')*	Draws (copies) a **Cross**	Knows colors	**Buttons clothing fully**, plays with other children
5 years	Jumps on one foot, heel to toe walk	Draws (copies) a **Square**		**Dresses without supervision**

66. Answer is a (Hyperglycemia).
Ref: OP Ghai, 7th edition Pg 67.

- Malnutrition is any physical condition resulting either from an inappropriate or inadequate diet, such as a diet that either provides too much or too little of necessary nutrients or from a physical inability to absorb or metabolize nutrients.
- Complications include:
  - Anemia
  - Vitamins deficiency
  - Infections
  - Spontaneous hypoglycemia
  - Disorder of water and electrolyte.

67. Answer is b (Serum 17-hydroxy progesterone is normal).
Ref: Harrison's, 17th edition Pg 2345; http://en.wikipedia.org/wiki/Congenital_adrenal_hyperplasia

- The term ***adrenogenital syndrome*** was applied to both sex-steroid producing tumors and severe forms of CAH for much of the 20th century, before some of the forms of CAH were understood.

- ***Congenital adrenal hyperplasia (CAH),*** which also dates to the first half of the century, has become the preferred term to reduce ambiguity and to emphasize the underlying pathophysiology of the disorders.
- CAH is a genetic disorder, which involves deficiency in one of enzymes required in steroid hormone synthesis.
- In enzyme defects associated with cortisol deficiency, hyperplasia of adrenal gland may occur due to excessive stimulation by ACTH.
- When enzyme deficiency leads to virilization of affected females (masculinization of external genitalia) disorder sometimes referred to as adrenogenital syndrome.
- Wolffian duct development consistently absent in virilized females, who, therefore, have normal internal sex organs.
- Why development is not stimulated by excess androgen is not understood, but high local concentrations created by testes may be required.
- The ***most common block is the 21-hydroxylase block,*** which accounts for more than 90% of all CAH cases. The steroid that accumulates is 17-hydroxyprogesterone. This is an easy diagnostic test to do in the newborn period. The blood spot, which is taken at 5 days, can be tested for 17-hydroxyprogesterone.

68. Answer is c (*Staphylococcus aureus*).
Ref: OP Ghai, 7th edition Pg 353; Harrison's, 17th edition Pg 876, 1622.

- ***Multiple pneumatoceles*** are characteristically found in X-ray films of the lung in pneumonia due to ***Staphylococcus and Klebsiella.***
- ***Pneumatoceles*** suggest infection due to ***Staphylococcus.***
- ***40–60%*** of children with ***staphylococcal pneumonia*** have ***pneumatoceles.***

69. Answer is d (ABO incompatibility).
Ref: Dutta's obstetrics, 6th edition Pg 497, 333.

Repeat Topic

- See ***answer no. 63 in COMED-K 2010*** answers for detailed explanation.

70. Answer is a (Dipalmitoyl lecithin).
Ref: Ganong, 23rd edition Pg 597; OP Ghai, 7th edition Pg 143.

Repeat Topic

- Respiratory distress syndrome is common in babies < 34 weeks of gestation and is due to surfactant deficiency.
- Also see ***answer no. 166 in Karnataka 2010 answers.***

71. Answer is a (Birth asphyxia).
Ref: Dutta's obstetrics, 6th edition Pg 469.

- In common clinical practice, ***asphyxia neonatorum*** means non-establishment of satisfactory pulmonary respiration at birth.

ORTHOPEDICS

72. Answer is c (Paradiscal).
Ref: Maheshwari, 3rd edition Pg 172.

- **Types of vertebral TB:**
  - ➲ ***Paradiscal – commonest*** type
  - ➲ Central
  - ➲ Anterior
  - ➲ Posterior.

More About TB Spine

- TB spine is also called ***Pott's disease***
- ***Spine is MC site of skeletal TB***
- Bacilli reach spine through paravertebral (*Batson's*) plexus
- ***Paradiscal type*** is MC
- MC symptom is ***back pain***; on X-ray reduction of disk space is earliest sign
- Anterior type of vertebral TB may show erosion of anterior part of the body, much the same as that in aneurysm of aorta—***aneurismal sign***
- TB spine with neurological involvement is ***Pott's paraplegia***—MC in ***thoracic spine.***

73. **Answer is d (Swelling and warmth).**
Ref: Harrison's, 17th edition Pg 2150-51, Fig 325-1.

Inflammatory disorders (infection with *Neisseria gonorrhoea* or *Mycobacterium tuberculosis*), crystal induced (gout, pseudogout), immune related [rheumatoid arthritis (RA), systemic lupus erythematosus (SLE)], reactive (rheumatic fever, Reiter's syndrome), may be identified by:

- ☐ Any of the four ***cardinal signs of inflammation*** (erythema, warmth, pain or swelling)
- ☐ Systemic symptoms (fatigue, fever, rash, weight loss)
- ☐ Laboratory evidence of inflammation [elevated erythrocyte sedimentation rate (ESR) or C-reactive protein (CRP), thrombocytosis, anemia of chronic disease or hypoalbuminemia]

Non-inflammatory disorders (osteoarthritis) are often characterized by:

- ☐ Pain ***without synovial swelling or warmth***
- ☐ ***Absence*** of inflammatory or systemic features
- ☐ Crepitus and painful range of motion due to joint degeneration
- ☐ Daytime gel phenomena rather than morning stiffness
- ☐ Bony enlargement of affected joints
- ☐ Normal (for age) or negative laboratory investigations

74. **Answer is d (5th and 6th cervical nerves).**
Ref: Dutta's obstetrics, 6th edition Pg 486.

Erb-Duchenne palsy	Klumpke's paralysis
– Follows trauma during delivery or blow to shoulder – ***Upper trunk*** of brachial plexus ***(C5, C6) injury*** – ***Waiter's/Porter's/Policeman's tip deformity***—arm adducted and internally rotated, elbow extended and forearm pronated – Sensory changes are absent if C5 only is involved, but if C6 also involved, an area of anesthesia is present over outer side of the arm – Mororeflex and biceps jerk are absent on the affected side; ipsilateral diaphragmatic involvement may be present – Preganglionic lesions have worse prognosis	– Hyperextension injury (falling person trying to catch an object) or trauma during birth – **Lower trunk** of brachial plexus lesion ***(C8, T1)*** – Intrinsic hand muscle weakness and claw hand may be seen – When T1 is involved there may be a ipsilateral Horner's syndrome (sympathetic involvement)

75. **Answer is c (Supracondylar fracture of humerus).**
Ref: Essential orthopedics, Maheshwari, 3rd edition Pg 84.

- ***Malunion*** is the ***commonest late complication*** of ***supracondylar fracture of the humerus*** and results in a ***cubitus varus (gunstock)*** deformity.

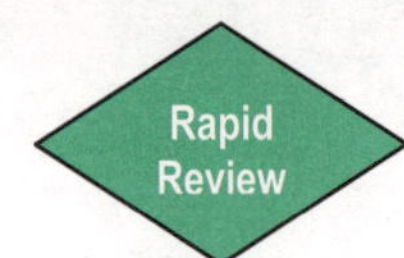

Characteristic Deformities by Injuries

Deformity	Injury
❖ Flattening of shoulder	Shoulder dislocation (anterior)
❖ Cubitus varus (*Gunstock deformity)*	Supracondylar # humerus
❖ Cubitus valgus	# Lateral condyle humerus
❖ Dinner fork (Velpeau's) deformity	Colles #
❖ Abduction, external rotation	Anterior hip dislocation
❖ **F**lexion, **AD**duction, **I**nternal **R**otation **(FADIR)**	Posterior hip dislocation (MC hip dislocation)
❖ Coxa vara	Trochanteric #
❖ Genu valgum	Condylar fractures of tibia (bumper fracture)
❖ External rotation of leg	# Neck of femur; trochanteric #
❖ Mallet finger	Avulsion of insertion of extensor tendon from distal phalanx
❖ Gamekeeper's thumb	Ulnar collateral ligament injury
❖ Winging of scapula	Injury to long thoracic nerve of bell (N. to serratus anterior)
❖ Tardy ulnar nerve palsy	# Lateral condyle of humerus

76. Answer is d (Post-traumatic ossification).
Ref: Essential Orthopedics, Maheshwari, 3rd edition Pg 42.

- ***Myositis ossificans*** is a benign, ***ossifying soft tissue lesion*** typically occurring within skeletal muscle. Patients are usually adolescents and young adults; myositis ossificans is rare in children under 10 years of age. The most frequent symptoms and signs are pain and tenderness with a soft tissue mass. Approximately, 80% of cases arise in the large muscles of the extremities.
- *Myositis ossificans traumatica* is produced as an insult (crushing injury) to muscle against bone. A hematoma (bloody mass) is formed against the periosteum, and subsequently calcification and ossification occurs.

77. Answer is a (1st metacarpal).
Ref: Maheshwari, Essential orthopedics, 3rd edition Pg 99.

- A ***Bennett's fracture*** is an ***intra-articular fracture*** of the proximal end ***(base) of the thumb (first) metacarpal***. The resulting bone fragment is held by the intermetacarpal ligament.
- The base of the metacarpal is *displaced laterally by the pull of the abductor pollicis longus.*

Note:
- ***Rolando's fracture***: ***Intra-articular fracture*** across the ***base of the first metacarpal***.

78. Answer is d (Ewing's sarcoma).
Ref: Essential Orthopedics, Maheshwari, 3rd edition Pg 221; John Crawford Adams, Outline of Orthopaedics, 12th edition Pg 91.

- ***Ewing's sarcoma*** is MC in ***second decade*** (affects boys < 15 years)
- ***Also called*** endothelial sarcoma of bone
- Affects ***diaphysis*** of long bones (humerus, tibia), flat bones (pelvis)
- Pain and swelling of few weeks to months present
- X-ray—***onion skin appearance***
- ***Extremely aggressive*** with early metastases, but ***responds to chemotherapy—curable tumor*** especially in children < 11 years
- Anaplastic ***small blue*** malignant tumor
- Chromosome ***11:22 translocation.***

79. **Answer is d (Axillary nerve).**
Ref: BD Chaurasia, Vol 1, Pg 39.

- The axillary nerve innervates teres minor and deltoid.
- It wraps around the surgical neck of the humerus and is endangered by fractures of the surgical neck. The axillary nerve may also be injured in anterior dislocations of the shoulder joint or compression of the axilla with a crutch.
- Injury to the axillary nerve results in:
  - Paralysis of the teres minor and deltoid muscles. Abduction of the shoulder is impaired.
  - Loss of sensation over a small part of the lateral upper arm.

80. **Answer is b (Type II).**
Ref: http://www.wheelessonline.com/ortho/dens_fracture

- ***Dens fractures*** are the result of severe forces including rotation across the cervical spine:

Anderson and D'Alonzo's classification of dens fractures

Type I	Thin radiolucent area ***above*** the base of the dens	Stable fracture
Type II	Radiolucent line ***at*** the base of the dens	Most common, most unstable and the most severe
Type III	Thin radiolucent line ***under*** the base of the dens which arcs upward	Stable fracture

81. **Answer is b (2nd decade).**
Ref: Essential Orthopedics, Maheshwari, 3rd edition Pg 221.

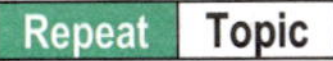

- Refer ***answer no. 78 above*** for detailed explanation.

82. **Answer is b (C5 and C6).**
Ref: Dutta's obstetrics, 6th edition Pg 486.

Repeat Topic

- ***Erb's point*** is the site in the lateral root of brachial plexus. It is ***formed by the union of C5 and C6 roots,*** which later converges together.
- Refer ***answer no. 74 above*** for detailed explanation.

Note:
- In ***cardiology, Erb's point*** refers to the ***third intercostal space*** on the left sternal border where S2 is best auscultated.

OPHTHALMOLOGY AND ENT

83. **Answer is b (Paralytic squint).**
Ref: Parson's, 20th edition Pg 391, Table 26.1.

- If secondary deviation is greater than primary deviation the squint is paralytic. This is because increased innervation is required by the paretic muscle to move the eye into a certain position and this same amount of innervation goes to the normal muscle in the other eye, causing the secondary deviation to be greater than primary deviation.

Differences between incomitant squint and comitant squint

Clinical features	Incomitant strabismus (paralytic or restrictive)	Comitant squint
Magnitude of squint	Varies with eye position	Same in all positions
Diplopia	Usually present	Usually absent
Ocular movements	Restricted	Full

False projection	Present	Absent
Abnormal head posture	Usually present	Absent
Secondary deviation	More than primary	Equal to primary

84. Answer is b (Oval window).
Ref: Maqbool, 11th edition Pg 88.

- ***Fissula ante fenestram*** is the ***most common site*** for ***otosclerosis***.
- It is a **2–3 *mm area in front of the oval window*** up to the processus cochleariformis where remnants of the embryonic cartilage may persist, which may later lead to new bone formation in susceptible cases.

More About Otosclerosis

❖ **Etiopathogenesis**	–	AD, *family h/o deafness* ++ in 70% cases; *common in Indians and whites;* M:F = 1:2 in *15–35 year age* group; *pregnancy* may *initiate or aggravate* otosclerosis
	–	This is a disease of the bony labyrinth in which *vascular spongy bone formation* near the oval window causes fixation or ankylosis of the footplate of the stapes
	–	*MC site is fissula ante fenestram* in front of the oval window
❖ **Clinically**	–	*MC cause of non-suppurative conductive deafness in the adult*
	–	Main symptom is *progressive deafness usually bilateral. Tinnitus* is present in *80%* cases
	–	*Paracusis Willsii* (Lombard effect) is present: It is the ability to hear better in noisy surroundings as people talk louder in a noisy place
	–	Otoscopy reveals normal intact and mobile tympanic membrane in most cases
	–	In some *(2%)* cases *flamingo pink tinge* may be seen due to vascular otospongiotic mass and is called positive *Schwartze's sign*
	–	Systemic associations: *van der Hoeve's syndrome:* Otosclerosis with blue sclera and pathologic bone fractures; *Paget's disease*
❖ **Investigations**	–	*Rinne's test is negative* and *Weber is lateralized to the more affected ear* (conductive deafness)
	–	*Gelle's test is negative*
	–	Cookie-bite curve shows that there is greatest degree of hearing loss in mid-frequency range
	–	*Cahart's notch in BC at 2000 Hz* is present in some cases
❖ **Treatment**	–	*Stapedectomy with artificial prosthesis is the surgery of choice*. Here, the stapes including its footplate is removed
	–	*Hearing aids* that amplify the sound waves and this overcomes the resistance to sound transmission
	–	*Cochlear otosclerosis* is treated by *fluoride therapy*

85. Answer is c (Vidian nerve).
Ref: Dhingra, 3rd edition Pg 169, 170.

- Nose is innervated by the:
  - ➢ Olfactory nerve
  - ➢ Sensory: Branches of the ophthalmic and maxillary divisions of the trigeminal nerve
  - ➢ Autonomic: Parasympathetic secretomotor fibers and sympathetic fibers.
- The autonomic nerve supply to the nose regulates vascular tone, turbinate congestion and nasal secretion.
- Parasympathetic fibers synapse in the sphenopalatine ganglion before innervating nasal mucosa. These fibers travel with the facial nerve, exiting at the geniculate ganglion as the greater superficial petrosal nerve.
- The ***vidian nerve (nerve of pterygoid canal)*** is formed by the union of the greater superficial petrosal and deep petrosal nerves, and carries the fibers to the sphenopalatine ganglion, where they synapse.

86. **Answer is d (YAG laser).**
Ref: Parson's diseases of the eye, 20th edition Pg 268; Pg 568, Appendix II.

- ***Posterior capsule opacification (PCO)*** = *'after cataract' or 'secondary cataract'* → occurs after *extracapsular cataract extraction* (ECCE).
- In ECCE, the posterior capsule and part of the anterior capsule are left behind in situ. The remnant part of anterior capsule continues to fulfill its function of forming new lens fibers—these fibers become opaque.

> ☐ ***Sommering's ring***: Sometimes, the lens fibers enclosed between the two layers of capsule form a dense ring behind the iris.
> ☐ ***Elschnig's pearls***: The subcapsular cells proliferate and instead of forming lens fibers, develop into large balloon-like cells, which fill up to the pupillary aperture.

- After cataract is treated by ***Nd:YAG laser capsulotomy,*** which clears the membrane centrally.
- Tough membranes may require removal with vitreous scissors or Ziegler knife.

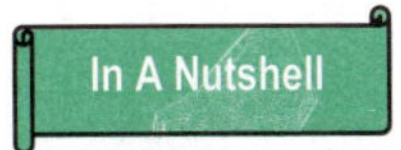

Lasers in Ophthalmology

	Laser	Clinical application	Wavelength
1.	Nd:YAG (neodymium-doped yttrium-aluminum-garnet)	Posterior capsulotomy, iridotomy, vitreolysis	1,064
2.	Frequency-doubled Nd:YAG	Cyclophotocoagulation, retinal photocoagulation	532
3.	Argon green	Trabeculoplasty, iridoplasty, pupillomydriasis, retinal photocoagulation (most widely used)	514
4.	Diode laser	Retinal photocoagulation	800
5.	Krypton red	Retinal photocoagulation	714
6.	Excimer (argon fluoride)	LASIK, LASEK, PRK (photorefractive keratectomy), phototherapeutic keratectomy (PTK)	193
7.	Femtosecond laser (neodymium-glass)	LASIK (bladeless LASIK), lamellar corneal surgery	1,053

87. **Answer is c (Choroiditis).**
Ref: Parson's, 20th edition Pg 321.

- ***Photopsia*** is a phenomenon in which the patient perceived *flashes of light* or has a sensation of flickering lights.
- This could be an indicator of ***developing retinal tear or retinal detachment***.
- Photopsiae are also seen in ***posterior uveitis/choroiditis due to retinal irritability***.

88. **Answer is b (Lens).**
Ref: Parson's disease of the eye, 20th edition Pg 367.

- ***Vossius ring:*** A circular ring of pigment on the anterior lens surface due to ***impression of the contracted pupil on the lens***, produced by force of the blow ***(trauma)*** driving the cornea and iris backwards.
- ***Traumatic cataract*** is usually ***unilateral, rosette shaped*** and can be ***lamellar***.

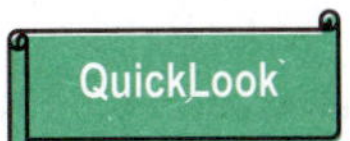

Other 'Rings' in Ophthalmology

	Ring	Seen in
1.	**Fleischer's ring**	Keratoconus—iron deposition in corneal epithelium
2.	**Kayser-Fleischer ring (K-F ring)**	Wilson's disease (copper in the Descemet's membrane best seen on slit lamp)

3.	**Weiss ring**	Posterior vitreous detachment
4.	**Wessley's ring**	Immune ring in cornea viral/disciform keratitis
5.	**Vossius ring**	A circular ring of pigment on the anterior lens surface due to ***impression of the contracted pupil on the lens,*** produced by force of the blow ***(trauma)*** driving the cornea and iris backwards
6.	**Retinal 'ring reflex'**	Central serous retinopathy
7.	**Limbal ring**	A metal ring sutures to the limbus and X-ray is taken to locate the position of intraocular metallic foreign body in relation to the ring
8.	**Capsule tension ring (CTR) or endocapsular ring**	To stabilize the capsular bag during IOL implantation into the capsular bag

89. Answer is b (Keratoconus).
Ref: Parson's, 20th edition Pg 204.

- ***Fleischer's ring***—partial or complete ***iron deposition ring in deep epithelium*** encircling the base of the cone, characteristic in eyes with ***keratoconus.***
- Appears as ***yellowish to dark brown-colored ring.***
- Best seen using ***cobalt blue light.***
- Also see ABOVE ANSWER for other rings in ophthalmology.

90. Answer is c (Biomicroscope).
Ref: Parson's 20th edition Pg 118, Fig 11.12.

- ***Aqueous flare:*** The release of protein following breakdown of the blood-aqueous barrier renders the aqueous no longer optically clear ***(Brownian movement or Tyndall phenomenon).*** The path of a light shone across the anterior chamber is defined in the aqueous. A sharp-focussed beam and careful observation are needed.
- It is best demonstrated on the ***slit lamp biomicroscope*** examination, by a narrow beam of light passed obliquely to the plane of the iris and observing in ***dark room*** after dark adaptation of examiner for 10–20 seconds.
- Flare is graded from 0 to +4.

<u>**About the other choices**</u>

- Ophthalmoscope is used to view the fundus (retina)—direct and indirect ophthalmoscopes.
- Streak retinoscope is used for retinoscopy—to objectively assess the refractive power of the eye.
- Operating microscope is obviously used for microsurgery of the eye.

91. Answer is d (*Pseudomonas aeruginosa*).
Ref: Harrison's, 17th edition Pg 208.

Repeat Topic

- Refer ***answer no. 76 in COMED-K 2010 answers*** for detailed explanation.

92. Answer is c (Superotemporally).
Ref: Parson's, 20th edition Pg 215, 322.

- The pathophysiologic mechanism of lens subluxation from congenital causes varies depending on the condition. The direction of displacement in each case is characteristic, although not completely diagnostic:
  - In ***Marfan's syndrome,*** the lenses tend to displace ***superotemporally*** due to abnormal collagen vascular tissue and faulty lens zonules. It is typically present at birth and is nonprogressive. Because the zonules are still attached to the lens, some accommodation remains.
  - ***Homocystinuria,*** a defect in amino acid metabolism, results in brittle zonules that rupture. This allows the lens to displace ***inferonasally*** or even into the anterior chamber. There is no accommodation and the condition may progress.
  - ***Simple ectopia lentis*** is an autosomal dominant condition where the lenses are dislocated ***superotemporally,*** but there are no other associated systemic abnormalities.

➲ ***Ectopia lentis et pupillae*** is likewise an isolated inherited condition, albeit autosomal-recessive, where the ***lenses displace temporally in opposite directions***.

93. **Answer is d (Dalen-Fuchs nodules).**
Ref: Parson's, 20th edition Pg 374-76.

Sympathetic Ophthalmia

Etiology:
- Bilateral ***granulomatous uveitis*** occurring between 2 weeks and several years after penetrating trauma to eye.
- Eye with penetrating injury/eye surgery is called 'exciting eye'. Fellow eye is called 'sympathizing eye'.

Clinically:
- ***Earliest symptom*** is decreased accommodation (ciliary body involvement).
- ***Earliest sign*** in the sympathizing eye is retrolental cells/anterior vitreous cells.
- ***Dalen fuchs*** nodules are seen.
- If the injured eye is unsalvageable, enucleation should be done within 2 weeks.

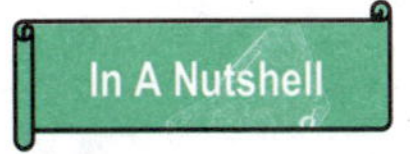

Iris Nodules

❖ KoePPe's nodules (at PuPillary border)	Granulomatous iridocyclitis
❖ BuSacca's nodules (on iris Surface)	Granulomatous iridocyclitis
❖ Lisch nodules	Neurofibromatosis
❖ Brushfield's spots	Down syndrome
❖ Iris pearls	Leprosy

FORENSIC MEDICINE

94. **Answer is b (7 years).**
Ref: Narayan Reddy's FMT, 23rd edition Pg 47.

- It may be noted that ***children below the age of 7 years*** are deemed to be ***incapable of criminal offence*** as per *section 82. IPC* (Indian Penal Code).

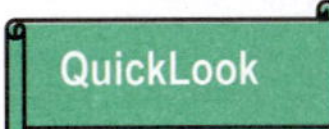

Other IPC Sections

IPC 44	Injury
IPC 84	Insanity
IPC 92	Implied consent
IPC 191	Perjury
IPC 197	Issuing or signing a false certificate (imprisonment for 7 years)
IPC 299	Culpable homicide
IPC 300	Murder
IPC 304-A	Criminal negligence
IPC 304-B	Dowry death
IPC 320	Grievous hurt
IPC 375	Rape
IPC 88-93	Legal protection to medical doctors

95. **Answer is c (Judicial hanging).**
Ref: Narayan Reddy's FMT, 23rd edition Pg 162.

- In *judicial hanging,* the posterior arch of the axis is snapped clean off and remains fixed to the third vertebra, while the atlas, the odontoid process and the anterior arch of the axis remain fixed to skull.
- *Fracture dislocation between C2 and C3* occurs in *modern judicial hanging* and in some instances of traffic accidents.
- Most likely, the forces involved in judicial hanging are much greater than those sustained by many motor vehicle accident victims and the spinal disruption between C2 and C3 caused by judicial hanging is considerably greater.

96. Answer is c [304 (A) IPC].
Ref: Narayan Reddy's FMT, 23rd edition Pg 162.

- **Section 304 (A) IPC: Causing death by negligence** – "whoever causes the death of any person by doing any rash or negligent act not amounting to culpable homicide, shall be punished with imprisonment of either description for a term, which may extend to 2 years or with fine, or with both".
- Examples are:
  – Amputation of wrong limb or wrong finger
  – Leaving instruments tubes or sponges in the abdomen
  – Performing criminal abortion.
- Also refer ***answer no. 94 above*** for detailed list of IPC sections.

97. Answer is a (Sulfuric acid).
Ref: Goldfrank's toxicology, Pg 349.

- Poisons may exert a ***two-fold action***. This may be either local or remote, or both local and remote.
- The ***local action of a poison*** is usually one of corrosion, inflammation or a direct effect upon the sensory or motor nerves.
- The ***remote actions of poisons*** are usually of a specific character, though some writers group the remote effects of poisons under two heads and speak of the common and the specific remote effects of a poison. The local action of a poison of the corrosive class is usually so well marked and obvious that the fact of the administration of a poison of this class is generally unmistakable.
- The ***symptoms produced by the mineral acids and the alkalies are almost altogether referable to local action***; but some corrosive poisons, such as carbolic acid, produce, besides a local action, remote and specific constitutional effects.

98. Answer is b (Cocaine).
Ref: Niraj Ahuja's Psychiatry, 6th edition Pg 50-51.

- ***Cocaine*** is called psychoactive because its actions modify the body's normal synaptic transmission. Its euphoric high is the result of its action on the dopamine system (although its reinforcing qualities, while not yet completely understood, have recently been linked to serotonin as well).
- The long-term effect is what is called ***'cocaine paranoia'***. It is characterized by dysphoria, hallucinations, paranoid psychosis, extreme delusions and irrational behavior.
- Also, many suffer from ***formication*** or the hallucination that ants, insects or snakes are crawling on or under the skin. Some people have actually bled to death trying to pick imaginary bugs out from under their skin, due to cocaine withdrawal.

99. Answer is b (Bleeding is generally less than in laceration).
Ref: Narayan Reddy's FMT, 23rd edition Pg 100.

Characters of incised wounds

- ***Margins*** are ***well defined, clean cut*** and everted.
- ***Length is greater*** than its width and depth, and has no relation to the cutting edge of the weapon for it may be drawn to any distance.

- Width is greater than the edge of the weapon causing it, due to retraction of divided tissues.
- Shape is usually ***spindle shaped*** due to greater retraction of the edges in the center.
- ***Hemorrhage is usually more*** as the vessels are cleanly cut; spurting of blood occurs if an artery is cut.
- Incised wounds are deeper at their beginning, since more pressure is exerted on the knife at this point—***head of the wound***; towards the end of the wound it becomes increasingly shallow—***tail of the wound***.

100. Answer is a (Crown and progresses towards root).
Ref: Textbook of Dental and Oral histology and embryology with MCQs by Chandra, 2004 edition, Pg 62.

- The ***process of mineralization starts from the cusps and incisal edges of the crown*** and progresses cervically.

PATHOLOGY

101. Answer is c (Lymphocyte predominant).
Ref: Robbin's pathology, 7th edition Pg 585.

Hodgkin's Lymphoma Types

Type	Prognosis	Comments
Nodular sclerosing (70%)	Excellent	***MC type; lacunar cells, collagen banding;*** women > men; young adults
Mixed cellularity	Intermediate	Numerous ***Reed Sternberg*** cells
Lymphocyte predominant	Excellent	***Popcorn cells (L and H cells),*** < 35-year-old males, cervical or axillary ***lymphadenopathy***
Lymphocyte depleted (rare)	Poor	***Older males*** with disseminated disease; RS cells high relative to lymphocytes

102. Answer is c (Hyperplastic arteriolosclerosis).
Ref: Robbin's pathology, 7th edition Pg 529-30.

Repeat Topic

- Refer ***answer no. 107 in COMED-K 2008 answers*** for detailed explanation.

103. Answer is a (Drug-induced lupus).
Ref: Harrison's, 17th edition Pg 2076, Table 313-1.

- ***Antihistone antibodies*** are more frequent in ***drug-induced lupus*** than in SLE.
- Drugs causing drug-induced SLE:
  - Antiarrhythmics ***procainamide*** (MC), disopyramide and propafenone
  - Antihypertensive: ***Hydralazine***, ACE inhibitors and beta blockers
  - Antithyroid propylthiouracil
  - Antipsychotics chlorpromazine and lithium
  - Anticonvulsants carbamazepine and phenytoin
  - Antibiotics isoniazid, minocycline and macrodantin; the antirheumatic sulfasalazine
  - Diuretic hydrochlorothiazide
  - Antihyperlipidemics lovastatin and simvastatin; and interferons and TNF inhibitors.
- Linkage with ***HLA-DR4*** is present.

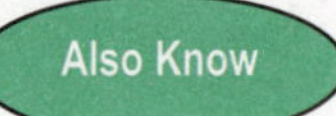

Autoantibodies in Connective Tissue Diseases

Disease	Immunologic marker	Comments
• **SLE**	*ANA (95% sensitivity)*	***Best screening test*** A negative test virtually excludes SLE A positive test, while non-specific increases post-test probability of SLE titer does not correlate with disease activity Also positive in drug-induced lupus, RA, scleroderma, Sjögren's syndrome
	Anti-dsDNA antibodies (60% sensitivity)	High titer correlate with nephritis and clinical activity Decreasing titer correlates with worsening renal disease
	Anti-Smith (Anti-Sm) antibodies	SLE specific/pathognomonic
• **Drug-induced lupus**	***Antihistone*** antibodies	Highly specific for ***drug-induced lupus***
• **Scleroderma**	Anti-Scl-70 antibody	
• **CREST syndrome**	Anticentromere antibodies	**C**alcinosis, **R**aynaud's syndrome, **E**sophageal dysmotility, **S**clerodactyly, **T**elangiectasia **(limited scleroderma)**
• **Mixed connective tissue disease (MCTD)**	Antiribonucleoprotein (anti-RNP)	
• **Sjögren's syndrome**	Anti-Ro (SS-A) Anti-La (SS-B)	If anti-Ro positive in SLE, risk of neonatal lupus and congenital heart block
• **Rheumatoid arthritis**	RF (70% sensitivity)	HLA-DR4 common, titer does not correlate with disease activity
• **Polymyositis or dermatomyositis**	ANA anti-Jo-1 antibodies	

104. Answer is d (Hay fever).

Ref: Harrison's, 17th edition Pg 379.

- Neutrophilic leukocytosis (***neutrophilia***) results from increased neutrophil production, increased marrow release or defective margination.
- The ***most important acute cause of neutrophilia is infection***.

Causes of neutrophilia

1. Increased production	• Idiopathic • Drug induced – glucocorticoids, G-CSF • Infection – bacterial, fungal, sometimes viral • Inflammation – thermal injury, tissue necrosis, myocardial and pulmonary infarction, hypersensitivity states, collagen vascular diseases • Myeloproliferative diseases – myelocytic leukemia, myeloid metaplasia, polycythemia vera
2. Increased marrow release	• Glucocorticoids • Acute infection (endotoxin) • Inflammation – thermal injury
3. Decreased or defective margination	• Drugs – epinephrine, glucocorticoids, non-steroidal anti-inflammatory agents • Stress, excitement, vigorous exercise • Leukocyte adhesion deficiency type 1 (integrin β □chain, CD18); leukocyte adhesion deficiency type 2 (select in ligand, CD15s, sialyl-Lewisx)

4. Miscellaneous	• Metabolic disorders—ketoacidosis, acute renal failure, eclampsia, acute poisoning • Drugs—lithium • Other—metastatic carcinoma, acute hemorrhage or hemolysis

Note:
- ***Eosinophils*** are the predominant ***inflammatory cells in allergic reactions and parasitic infestations***—eosinophilia occurs in allergies such as asthma, hay fever, hives, parasitic infections, polyarteritis nodosa and Hodgkin's lymphoma.

105. Answer is b (Point mutation).
Ref: Harrison's, 17th edition Pg 635-641.

- ***Point mutations = change of single nucleotide in the DNA.***
- Single nucleotide changes (point mutations) in the sequence of a gene can result in changes in the amino acid sequence of a protein produced from the mutated gene. One of the ***most well-studied examples*** of the effects of a mutation on the sequence of a protein involves hemoglobin.
- A ***point mutation creates*** an altered form of hemoglobin that produces the genetic disorder called ***sickle-cell disease.***
- Sickle-cell disease results from a point mutation in the second nucleotide of the codon GAA, which results in a change in the amino acid at position 6 in the beta chain of hemoglobin (valine at position 6 instead of the glutamic acid that is normally present).

MICROBIOLOGY

106. Answer is b (Forgotten tampons).
Ref: Harrison's, 17th edition Pg 877.

Staphylococcal Toxic Shock Syndrome
- TSS was first recognized as a disease in children in 1978
- The disease gained attention in the early 1980s, when a nationwide (USA) outbreak occurred among young, otherwise healthy, menstruating women
- Epidemiologic investigation demonstrated that these cases were ***associated with menstruation and the use of a highly absorbent tampon*** that had recently been introduced to the market
- Subsequent studies established the role of TSST-1 in these illnesses
- Manifested by fever, hypotension, tachycardia, erythroderma and skin desquamation.

107. Answer is d (*Epidermophyton floccosum*).
Ref: Textbook of Microbiology, CP Baveja, 3rd edition Pg 536.

- ***Tinea cruris***, a pruritic superficial fungal infection of the groin and adjacent skin (jockey's itch), is the second most common clinical presentation for dermatophytosis.
- The most common etiologic agents for tinea cruris include *Trichophyton rubrum* and ***Epidermophyton floccosum***; less commonly *Trichophyton mentagrophytes* and *Trichophyton verrucosum* are involved.
- Tinea cruris is a contagious infection transmitted by fomites, such as contaminated towels or hotel bedroom sheets or by autoinoculation from a reservoir on the hands or feet (tinea manuum, tinea pedis, tinea unguium).
- The etiologic agents produce keratinases, which allow invasion of the cornified cell layer of the epidermis. The host immune response may prevent deeper invasion.
- Risk factors for initial infection or reinfection include wearing tight fitting or wet clothing or undergarments.

108. Answer is b (Rhinitis).
Ref: Harrison's, 17th edition Pg 1074-1076.

Species of genus *Chlamydia* and disease caused

Species	Disease caused
■ *C. trachomatis*	
A, B, Ba and C	– *Trachoma*
D to K	– ***Non-gonococcal urethritis*** – ***Epididymitis*** – ***Reiter's*** syndrome – ***Cervicitis*** – Urethral syndrome in women – Pelvic inflammatory disease (***PID***) – ***Inclusion conjunctivitis*** in the newborn ('paratrachoma')
L1, L2 and L3	– ***Lymphogranuloma venereum*** and ***hemorrhagic proctocolitis***
■ *C. psittaci*	– ***Psittacosis***
■ *C. pneumoniae* (the old TWAR)	– ***Pneumonia*** – ***Atherosclerotic cardiovascular disease*** and – Asthma

109. Answer is d (Flavi).

Ref: Harrison's, 17th edition Pg 1080.

- The ***Hepatitis C virus*** is a small (50 nm in size), enveloped, *single stranded, positive sense RNA* virus in the family ***Flaviviridae***.

Virus	Family
Hepatitis A	: PicoRNAvirus
Hepatitis B	: HepaDNAviridae
Hepatitis C and G	: Flaviviridae
Hepatitis E	: Caliciviridae

- All hepatitis viruses are RNA ***except hepatitis B***.
- Remember like, HIV, hepatitis B is also a biohazard; '**BaD** virus (**B=DNA**)'.

110. Answer is c (Type III).

Ref: Textbook of Microbiology, CP Baveja, 3rd edition Pg 152-158.

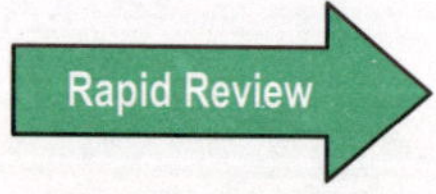

Hypersensitivity Reactions

Type	Name	Examples
1. **Type 1**	Anaphylactic reaction Mediated by IgE	• Anaphylaxis • Atopic bronchial asthma • Angioedema • Allergic rhinitis, urticaria, hay fever
2. **Type 2**	Cytotoxic-cytolytic reaction Antibody mediated Mediated by IgG and IgM	• Transfusion reaction • Hemolytic anemia • Erythroblastosis fetalis • Ceratin drug reactions • Goodpasture syndrome • Myasthenia gravis • ITP • Rheumatic fever
3. **Type 3**	Immune complex reaction Antigen-antibody complex activates complement	• Acute serum sickness (large amounts of foreign serum) • Chronic serum sickness—SLE • ***Arthus reaction***

		• Certain forms of acute glomerulonephritis • Hypersensitivity pneumonitis
4. Type 4	Delayed hypersensitivity Cell-mediated reaction T cell mediated	• Mantoux test • Tuberculoid leprosy • Contact dermatitis • Transplant rejection (graft versus host disease) • Multiple sclerosis, Gullain-Barré syndrome, Hashimoto's thyroiditis
'ACID' = Types 1, 2, 3, 4 hypersensitivity reactions		

111. Answer is b (IgE response).

Ref: Textbook of Microbiology, 3rd edition CP Baveja, Pg 101, Table 13.1.

Repeat Topic

- ***Immunoglobulin E (IgE)*** plays an important role in ***allergy*** and is especially associated with ***type I hypersensitivity***.
- Refer ***answer no. 50 in COMED-K 2009 answers*** for detailed summary table on immunoglobulins.

112. Answer is c (Both mother and child).

Ref: Harrison's, 17th edition Pg 900.

- Tetanus spores infect women and children through unsafe or unclean deliveries, accounting for an estimated 5% of maternal deaths and 14% of neonatal deaths.
- Tetanus toxoid vaccines ***can prevent infections*** and save the lives of ***mothers and infants alike***.
- Pregnant women should receive at least two doses of tetanus toxoid.

113. Answer is d (FTA-ABS).

Ref: Textbook of Microbiology, CP Baveja, 3rd edition Pg 361-363.

- The ***fluorescent treponemal antibody-absorption (FTA-ABS) test is used to confirm the diagnosis***. The FTA-ABS technique is ***more sensitive and specific*** than either the VDRL or the RPR test, but it is too expensive to be used for routine screening. FTA-ABS better suited as a confirmatory assay for syphilis infection after another method tests positive for the syphilis bacteria.
- The principal screening tests for syphilis are the Venereal Disease Research Laboratory ***(VDRL) test*** and the rapid plasma reagin ***(RPR) test***.
- These screening tests detect a rise in antibody titers following infection. The sensitivity of both tests is influenced by characteristic fluctuations in antibodies during the three stages of the disease. Antibody titers often are not significantly elevated in the early primary stages of syphilis and they may return to normal in latent and tertiary syphilis.
- The ***Wassermann test*** is a complement-fixation (complement system) antibody test for syphilis, named after the bacteriologist August von Wassermann. The reaction is not actually specific to syphilis and will produce a positive reaction to other diseases, including malaria, tuberculosis and numerous other diseases. It is possible for an infected individual to produce no reaction and for a successfully treated individual to continue to produce a reaction (called Wassermann fast or fixed).

114. Answer is a *(M. tuberculosis)*.

Ref: Davidson's, 20th edition Pg 384, Box 14.7.

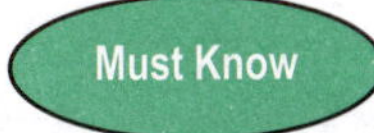

Correlation between CD4 count and HIV associated diseases

> 500 cells/mm^3	• Acute primary infection • Recurrent vaginal candidiasis • Persistent generalized lymphadenopathy
< 500 cells/mm^3	• Pulmonary TB

	• Pneumococcal pneumonia • Herpes zoster • Oropharyngeal candidiasis • Oral hairy leukoplakia • Extraintestinal salmonellosis • Kaposi's sarcoma • HIV-associated ITP • Cervical intraepithelial neoplasia II-III • Lymphoid interstitial pneumonitis
< 200 cells/mm^3	• *Pneumocystis jirovecii (carinii)* pneumonia • Mucocutaneous herpes simplex
< 100 cells/mm^3	• Cryptosporidium • Microsporidium • Esophageal candidiasis • Military/Extrapulmonary TB • HIV-associated wasting • Peripheral neuropathy
< 50 cells/mm^3	• CMV retinitis/GI disease • Disseminated MAC infection

PHARMACOLOGY

115. Answer is a (Aztreonam).

Ref: KD Tripathi, 6th edition Pg 708' Harrison's, 17th edition Pg 861, Table 127-6.

Drug	Spectrum
Aztreonam	Hospital-acquired infections caused by ***facultative gram-negative bacilli*** and ***Pseudomonas*** in penicillin-allergic patients
Tobramycin	Combined with a penicillin for staphylococcal, enterococcal or viridans streptococcal endocarditis; combined with a β-lactam antibiotic for gram-negative bacteremia; pyelonephritis
Vancomycin	Bacteremia, endocarditis and other serious infections due to MRSA; pneumococcal meningitis; antibiotic-associated pseudomembranous colitis
Doxycycline	Acute bacterial exacerbations of chronic bronchitis, granuloma inguinale, brucellosis (with streptomycin), tularemia, glanders, melioidosis, spirochetal infections caused by *Borrelia* (Lyme disease and relapsing fever), plague, ehrlichiosis, chlamydial infections, rickettsial infections, mild CAP, skin and soft tissue infections caused by gram-positive cocci

116. Answer is d (Vancomycin).

Ref: Harrison's, 17th edition Pg 879.

Direct quote

"***Vancomycin remains the drug of choice for the treatment of MRSA*** infections. Because it is less bactericidal than the β-lactams, it should be used only after careful consideration in patients with a history of β-lactam allergies".

117. Answer is a (Genital warts).

Ref: Harrison's, 17th edition Pg 1119.

- ***Condyloma acuminata,*** (venereal warts) are caused by human papilloma virus (HPV).
- Topically applied ***podophyllum preparations as well as podofilox*** may also be used for venereal warts.

118. Answer is c (Phenylephrine).

Ref: KD Tripathi, 6th edition Pg 121.

- ***Sympathomimetics*** are drugs with action similar to that of adrenaline or sympathetic stimulation.
  - ***Direct Sympathomimetics***: Acts directly as agonists on alpha and/or beta receptors
  - ***Indirect Sympathomimetics***: Act on adrenergic neuron to release noradrenaline, which then acts on the adrenoceptors.

Classification of sympathomimetics

Direct acting	Indirect acting	Mixed
➢ Adrenaline	➢ Tyramine	➢ Ephedrine
➢ Noradrenaline	➢ Amphetamine	➢ Dopamine
➢ Isoprenaline		➢ Mephentermine
➢ Phenylephrine		
➢ Methoxamine		
➢ Xylometazoline		
➢ Salbutamol		
➢ Many others		

119. Answer is a (Fasciculations).
Ref: KD Tripathi, 6th edition Pg 342.

- The neuromuscular blockade by the ***classic pathway (depolarizing)***, begins when a drug binds to a subunit of the nicotinic receptors like the molecule of acetylcholine does.
- In the beginning, an initial opening of the ion channel produces a contraction (***fasciculation***).
- After this, the depolarization of muscular membrane is sustained (persistent depolarization), since the drug is not broken by acetylcholinesterase, leading to neuromuscular block.

120. Answer is a (Ergometrine).
Ref: KD Tripathi, 6th edition Pg 323-24.

- Tocolytics ***are drugs, which are used to decrease uterine motility. They have been used to delay or postpone labor, arrest threatened abortion and in dysmenorrhea.***

TOCOLYTICS

These are drugs that ***decrease uterine motility***. They have been used to delay or ***postpone labor, arrest threatened abortion and in dysmenorrhea***.

1. ***Calcium channel blockers***: Especially nifedipine.
2. ***Adrenergic agonists*** (beta 2 agnoists like ritodrine)—increased maternal mortality, DO NOT use in mother with DM, heart disease, on beta blockers or steroids.
3. ***Atosiban*** (*oxytocin antagonist*).

– ***NO LONGER reommended:*** *Prostaglandin synthesis inhibitors (indomethacin);* ***Ethyl alcohol****; Magnesium sulfate; progesterone, general anesthetics, nitrates.*

<u>**Note**</u>:
- ***Ergometrine*** is an amine ergot alkaloid that ***stimulates contractions of uterine*** and vascular smooth muscle.

121. Answer is b (Dehydropeptidase).
Ref: KD Tripathi, 6th edition Pg 708-09.

- The main drug in the ***carbapenem*** class is a drug called ***Imipenem***—this drug has excellent, quite broad antimicrobial activity against both gram positive and gram-negative organisms, anaerobes and pseudomonas infections.
- Imipenem is given with a molecule called ***cilastatin***, which is an inhibitor of the renal enzyme dehydropeptidase—this renal enzyme would otherwise break down the drug too quickly and would make the drug ineffective in the

treatment of UTIs – thus by giving imipenem with the cilastatin, the half life of the drug is prolonged and it can be used to treat UTIs.

122. Answer is d (Estrogen).
Ref: Textbook of biochemistry, Vasudevan, 5th edition Pg 380, Table 36.1.

Second messenger	Hormones
cAMP	ACTH, FSH, LH, MSH, PTH, ADH, TSH, CRH, glucagon, catecholamines, calcitonin
cGMP	ANF (atrial natriuretic factor)
Calcium or phosphatidylinositol (PIP2)	TRH, GnRH, acetylcholine, CCK, gastrin, vasopressin, oxytocin
Tyrosine kinase	Insulin
Intracellular receptors	Glucocorticoids, mineralocorticoids, estrogens, progesterone, androgens, calcitriol, thyroxine

PREVENTIVE AND SOCIAL MEDICINE

123. Answer is b (1/2 of proteins and 1/3 of the calories required per day).
Ref: Park, 20th edition Pg 500.

Repeat Topic

- Refer *answer no. 134 in COMED-K 2010 answers* for detailed explanation.

124. Answer is b (3–4 per 1,000 live births).
Ref: Park, 20th edition Pg 481.

- "*As of 1989*, the estimated maternal mortality rate (MMR) is about *3–4 per 100 live births*".
- For the *year 2003, the MMR was 301 per 100,000*.
- The maternal mortality rate measures the risk of women dying from puerperal causes and is *defined as* (total number of female deaths due to complications of pregnancy/childbirth or within 42 days of delivery from 'puerperal causes' in an area during a given year)/total number of live births in the same area and year) × 1,000.
- Ideally, the denominator should include all deliveries and abortions.
- The *MMR should be expressed as a rate per 1,000 live births*.
- In developed countries, the MMR has decreased substantially; because of this decline they use the multiplying factor *100,000 instead of 1,000* to avoid fractions in calculating MMR.

125. Answer is d (Diagnosis can be made with available techniques).
Ref: Park, 20th edition Pg 37, 123.

- The *'iceberg of disease'* is a metaphor emphasizing that for virtually every health problem the number of cases of disease ascertained (those visible) is outweighed by those not discovered (those invisible).
- Diseases may be mild or even 'silent' – one of the many explanations for undiagnosed disease in the community. This phenomenon is described by the metaphor of the iceberg of disease.
- For most health problems there are large number of undiscovered or misdiagnosed cases of disease.
- Serious and killing disorders such as diabetes, atrial fibrillation and hypertension are other good examples of this iceberg phenomenon.
- Cases that have been correctly diagnosed can be likened to the tip of the iceberg, visible and easily measured.
- In most diseases, as with the iceberg, the larger presence lurks unseen, unmeasured and easily forgotten.

126. Answer is d (2–4 years).
Ref: Park, 20th edition Pg 275.

- Leprosy has a long incubation period, an average of 3-5 years or more for lepromatous cases.
- Tuberculoid form is thought to have a shorter incubation period.

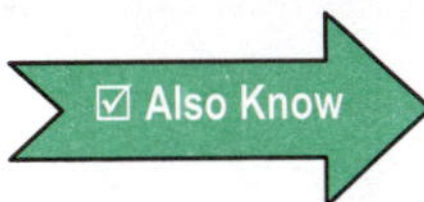

Incubation Periods (IP)

Short IP (< 7 days)	Medium IP (7–21 days)	Long IP (> 21 days)
• Influenza: 8–72 h • Cholera: 1–2 d • Anthrax: 1–3 d • Bacillary dysentery: 1–7 d • Diphtheria: 2–6 d • Pneumonic plague: 1–3 d • Bubonic plague: 2–7 d • Yellow fever: 3–6 d • Meningococcal meningitis: 3–4 d • Kyasanur forest disease: 3–8 d	• Trachoma: 5–12 d • Whooping cough (pertussis): 7–14 d • Polio: 7–14 days (3–35 d) • Measles: 10 d • Typhoid: 10–14 d (3 d–3 weeks) • Chickenpox: 14–16 d • Rubella: 2–3 weeks (18 d) • Mumps: 2–3 weeks (18 d)	• Hepatitis A: 15–45 d • Hepatitis B: 45–180 d • Ascariasis: about 2 months • Malaria: 3 weeks • Filariasis: 8–16 months • TB: Months to years • Leprosy: Months to years

127. Answer is a (INH).
Ref: Park, 20th edition Pg 173.

- The global project in Tuberculosis Drug Resistance Surveillance by the WHO/International Union against TB and Lung diseases during the period 1999–2002 included three centers from India—North Arcot (Tamil Nadu), Raichur (Karnataka) and Wardha (Maharashtra) over a period of 3–10 months for new cases only. Resistance was found as below.

Anti-TB drug	Incidence of resistance
INH (isoniazid)	15.2–23.4%
Rifampicin	0.5–2.8%
Ethambutol	1–4.6%
Streptomycin	7.2–12.4%

Also Know

- ☐ **Primary (pretreatment) resistance:** Resistance shown by the bacteria in a patient, who has not received the drug in question before.
- ☐ **Secondary (acquired) resistance:** Here, the bacteria were sensitive to the drug at the beginning of treatment, but became resistant during the course of treatment with it.

MDR-TB (Multidrug Resistant TB)	XDR-TB (Extensively Drug Resistant TB)
• Strain of TB that is ***at least resistant to INH or rifampicin*** • Now DOTS PLUS is used for MDR-TB	MDR-TB + Resistant to fluoroquinolone + Resistant to one or more of these second line injectable drugs (amikacin, capreomycin, kanamycin)

128. Answer is c (Fat).
Ref: Avery's diseases of the newborn, 8th edition, Pg 1060, 2005.

- ***Hindmilk*** has the ***highest concentration of fat*** and is released after several minutes of nursing. It is similar in consistency to cream and will have a ***soporific (sleepy) effect on the baby***.
- Hindmilk is important for the baby to feel satisfied and to gain adequate weight, especially in premature babies.

129. Answer is a (Ambulatory patients).
Ref: Park, 20th edition Pg 701.

- ***Triage*** consists of ***rapidly classifying the injured on the basis of the severity of their injuries*** and the likelihood of their survival with ***prompt medical intervention***.

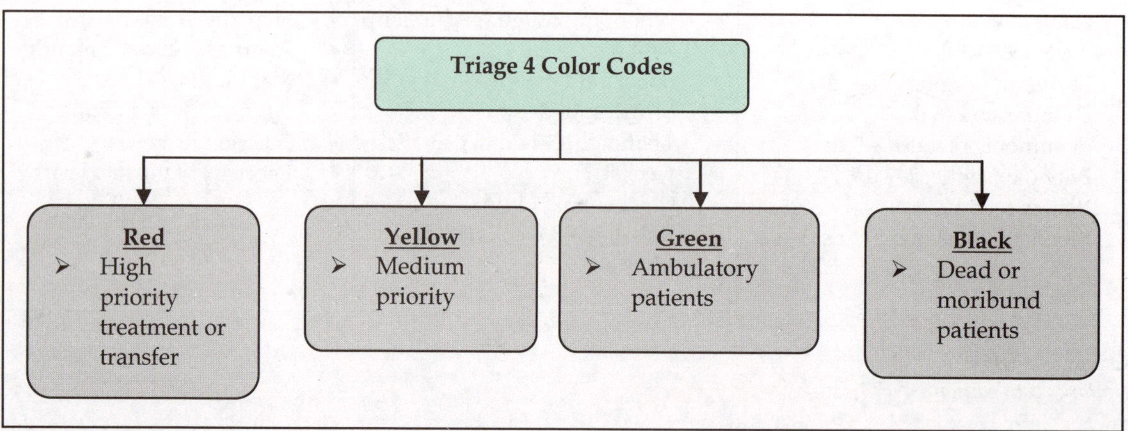

130. Answer is a (5 TU).
Ref: Harrison's, 17th edition Pg 1019.

- ***Mantoux test***: A standard dose of **5 *Tuberculin units*** (0.1 mL) is injected intradermally and read 72 hours later. A person who has been exposed to the bacteria is expected to mount an immune response in the skin containing the bacterial proteins.
- ***WHO*** advocates a preparation known as ***'PPD-RT 23 with Tween 80'***.
- The reaction is read by measuring the diameter of induration across the forearm (horizontal transverse diameter of induration) in millimeters.
- No induration should be recorded as '0 mm'. Erythema (redness) should not be measured:
  - ➢ Reaction > 10 mm are considered 'positive'
  - ➢ Reaction < 6 mm are considered 'negative'
  - ➢ Reaction between 6 and 9 mm are considered 'doubtful' (may be due to MTB or atypical mycobacteria).

Note:
- ■ For routine testing ***in India 1 TU is used***—if this is present among the choices it will be the best answer—Park, 20th.
- ■ In some countries 5 TU is used—Harrison's mentions 5 TU.

131. Answer is b (3 months).
Ref: Park, 20th edition Pg 802.

- The village health guide is a person with an aptitude for social service and is not full time government functionary.
- The guidelines for their selection are:
  - ❖ They should be permanent residents of the community preferably women
  - ❖ Able to read and write with minimum education of up to 6th standard
  - ❖ Acceptable to all sections of the community
  - ❖ Should be able to spare at least 2–3 hours every day for community work.
- Their training is arranged in the nearest primary health center, subcenter or any other suitable place for the ***duration of 200 hours, spread over the period of 3 months***.

132. Answer is b (Orthotolidine test).
Ref: Park, 20th edition Pg 626.

- ***Orthotolidine test (OT)*** enables both ***free and residual chlorine in the water to be determined with both speed and accuracy***.
- ***Orthotolidine arsenite test*** is a modification of the OT test to determine the free and residual chlorine separately.

Note:
- ❖ Horrock's apparatus is used to estimate the chlorine demand of well water.
- ❖ Presumptive coliform count is used to determine the drinking quality of water.

133. Answer is b (Age).
Ref: Park, 20th edition Pg 326.

Non-modifiable risk factors for HTN	Modifiable risk factors for HTN
☐ *Age*: High BP risk increases with age	☐ Obesity
☐ *Race/ethnicity*: High BP common among blacks; complications, such as stroke and heart attack, also are MC in blacks	☐ Physical activity/sedentary lifestyle ☐ Using tobacco ☐ Too much salt (sodium) in diet—salt intake
☐ *Genetic factors: Family history*	☐ Saturated fat and dietary fiber
☐ *Sex*	☐ Heavy alcohol consumption
	☐ Environmental stress
	☐ Socioeconomic status

134. Answer is a (It should actually measure what it is supposed to measure).
Ref: Park, 20th edition Pg 126.

- ***Validity*** refers to what extent the ***test accurately measures what it purports to measure.***
- In other words, validity expresses the ability of a test to separate or distinguish those who have the disease from those who do not.
- For example, glucosuria is a useful screening test for diabetes mellitus, but a more valid or accurate test is glucose tolerance test.
- Accuracy refers to the closeness with which measured values agree with true values.
- *Validity has two components sensitivity and specificity.*

135. Answer is b (2015).
Ref: Park, 20th edition Pg 27, Table 3; Pg 794.

- The ***Millennium Development Goals (MDGs)*** are ***eight goals to be achieved by 2015*** that respond to the world's main development challenges.
- The MDGs are drawn from the actions and targets contained in the Millennium Declaration that was adopted by 189 nations and signed by 147 heads of state and governments during the UN Millennium Summit in September 2000:
  - Goal 1: Eradicate extreme poverty and hunger
  - Goal 2: Achieve universal primary education
  - Goal 3: Promote gender equality and empower women
  - Goal 4: Reduce child mortality
  - Goal 5: Improve maternal health
  - Goal 6: Combat HIV/AIDS, malaria and other diseases
  - Goal 7: Ensure environmental sustainability
  - Goal 8: Develop a global partnership for development.

136. Answer is d (Incidence).
Ref: Park's, 20th edition Pg 57.

- ***Incidence rate*** is defined as the number of ***new cases*** occurring in a defined population during a specified period of time.
- Incidence rate refers:
  - ❖ Only to new cases
  - ❖ During a given period (usually 1 year)
  - ❖ In a specified population or 'population at risk'
  - ❖ It can also refer to new spells or episodes of a disease arising in a given period of time, per 100 population.

Also Know

- ☐ ***Prevalence*** is the number of events in a population at a designated time. The word prevalence usually denotes point prevalence ratio
- ☐ Prevalence depends upon two factors, the incidence and duration of illness. Given the assumption that population is stable and incidence and duration are not changing the relation between incidence and prevalence can be expressed as ***P = I X D***
- ☐ *Point prevalence* is the number of persons with a disease or attribute at a point in time
- ☐ *Period prevalence* is the number of persons who have had the disease or attribute at any time over a specified period.

137. Answer is a (Social assistance).
Ref: http://nsap.nic.in

- The ***National Social Assistance Program (NSAP)*** is a ***social assistance program*** for poor households and represents a significant step towards the fulfillment of the Directive principles in Articles 41 and 32 of the Constitution recognizing the concurrent responsibility of the Central and State Governments in the matter.
- NSAP was included in the Central Budget for 1995-96. The NSAP will include the following benefits as its components:
  - National Old Age Pension Scheme.
  - National Family Benefit Scheme.
  - National Maternity Benefit Scheme.
- The program came into effect on 15th August 1995.
- The scales of the benefit under NSAP is as below:
  - ***National Old Age Pension*** Scheme ₹75/- per month.
  - National Family Benefit Scheme ₹10,000/- in case of death of the primary bread winner to the bereaved household.
  - National Maternity Benefit Scheme ₹500/- per pregnancy up to two live births.

138. Answer is c (III).
Ref: RTNCP guidelines.

Diagnosis of extrapulmonary TB

- One culture positive specimen from extrapulmonary site

OR

- Histological evidence from extrapulmonary site

OR

- Strong clinical evidence consistent with active extrapulmonary TB followed by the doctor's decision to treat with a full course of TB therapy.

Treatment

- Seriously ill extrapulmonary TB cases: Category I.
- Not seriously ill extrapulmonary TB cases: Category III.

Seriously Ill	Not Seriously Ill
– TB meningitis	– Lymph node TB
– Disseminated TB	– Pleural effusion (unilateral)
– TB pericarditis	– Bone (excluding spine)

– B/L pleural effusion – Spinal TB – Genitourinary TB	– Peripheral joints

139. Answer is b (63 years).
Ref: Park, 20th edition Pg 417.

- The *life expectancy in India* was *63 years in 2002*.

DERMATOLOGY, ANESTHESIA, RADIOLOGY, PSYCHIATRY

140. Answer is c (Pancreatic carcinoma)
Ref: SRB's Manual of surgery by Sriram Bhat, 2nd edition Pg 437, Jaypee publishers.

Endoscopic retrograde cholangiopancreatography (ERCP) signs of pancreatic cancer:
- Abrupt obstruction of main duct
- Encasement of pancreatic duct
- Parenchymal filling with necrosis
- Double duct sign
- *Scrambled egg appearance*

Also Know

On barium meal in pancreatic carcinoma:
- Widened 'C' loop—*Pad sign*
- *Reverse '3' sign of Frostburg*—periampullary carcinoma.

141. Answer is c (Temperature).
Ref: Clinical Leprosy, by Virendra Sehgal, Illustrated 4th edition, Pg 76, 2004.

- In *leprosy, temperature is the first sensation that is lost*. Patients cannot sense extremes of hot or cold.
- The next sensation lost is light touch, then pain and finally deep pressure.
- These losses are especially apparent in the hands and feet; therefore, the chief complaint may be a burn or ulcer in an anesthetic extremity.

142. Answer is d (Atopic dermatitis).
Ref: Harrison's, 17th edition Pg 313.

Repeat Topic

- *Dennie-Morgan fold (atopic pleat)* or line below both lower eyelids caused by edema in *atopic dermatitis*.
- Refer *answer no. 71 in COMED-K 2008 answers* for detailed explanation.

143. Answer is b (Crohn's disease).
Ref: Robbins pathology, 7th edition Pg 849-50.

Repeat Topic

- See *answer no. 37 in COMED-K 2009 answers* for detailed explanation.

144. Answer is c (Multiple myeloma).
Ref: Radiology Secrets, 65.

Multiple Myeloma: Key Radiological Findings

- Bone scans are 'cold'
- Gross osteoporosis may be the only early sign
- Punched out lesions
- Vertebra plana or wrinkled vertebra is characteristic
- ***Raindrop skull*** (lytic myeloma defects—well-defined osteolytic areas are visible in the bone of the calvaria
- Pedicle sign of myeloma (preservation of pedicles of vertebrae) occur
- 'Moth eaten', permeative lesions
- Foggy cortical—medullary border

145. Answer is d (Pneumoperitoneum).

Ref: Chapman's Radiological D/D, 5th edition Pg 127.

- ***Rigler's sign***, (or ***'double wall sign'***) in pneumoperitoneum.
- Seen on an X-ray of the abdomen when air is present on both sides of the intestine, i.e. when air is present on the inside (lumenal side) and the outside (peritoneal side).

146. Answer is a (Pityriasis rosea).

Ref: Harrison, 17th edition Pg 315, Table 53-2.

□ **Presentation**	–	*Pityriasis* = fine scales; *rosea* = rose colored or pink
	–	*10–35 years age* range; MC in *women;* viral etiology has not been proved.
□ **Clinically**	–	First manifestation is a solitary, salmon-pink, annular plaque, 2–6 cm in diameter ***('Herald' or 'Mother' patch)***, usually on the *trunk*. This is followed in a few days by several small salmon-colored macules or patches mainly on the trunk, but also on the neck and thighs. A delicate peripheral (*trailing scale*—a collarette of scale that does not extend to the border of the lesion) scale (cigarette-paper scale) appears as the lesions evolve
	–	Lesions on the *back* are parallel to the ribs giving a ***'Christmas tree'*** distribution
	–	Lesions resemble that of *secondary syphilis* but unlike in syphilis, palms and soles are rarely involved in PR.
□ **Treatment**	–	The eruption tends to be moderately pruritic and is *self-limiting* in 4–10 weeks. Treatment is for alleviating the pruritus and consists of oral antihistamines and midpotency topical glucocorticoids.

147. Answer is d (Head lift for 3 seconds).

Ref: www.anesthesia-analgesia.org/content/111/1/3 ; http://www.anesthesia-analgesia.org/content/95/6/1656.full

- When used as an antagonist to non-depolarizing muscle relaxants, adequate recovery of voluntary respiration and neuromuscular transmission must be obtained prior to discontinuation of respiratory assistance and there should be continuous patient observation.
- Satisfactory recovery may be judged by *adequacy of skeletal muscle tone, respiratory measurements and by observation of the response to peripheral nerve stimulation*.
- A patent airway should be maintained and manual or mechanical ventilation should be continued until complete recovery of normal respiration is assured.
- ***Head lift for*** 5 s has been ***used clinically for the assessment of residual block***.

148. Answer is c (Nihilistic delusion).

Ref: Niraj Ahuja's Psychiatry, 6th edition Pg 77; Davdison's, 20th edition Pg 232.

- A ***delusion*** is ***a belief that is clearly false*** and that indicates an ***abnormality in the affected person's content of thought***.
- The false belief is ***not accounted for by the person's cultural or religious background*** or his or her ***level of intelligence***; a person with a delusion will ***hold firmly to the belief regardless of evidence to the contrary***.

☑ In A Nutshell

Types of Delusions

1. Nihilistic delusions	• ***Nihilistic*** is the root of the word '***annihilate***' and means ***destruction or death*** • People experiencing nihilistic delusions believe things like they are decomposing, their bodies do not work, their internal organs are rotten or solidifying or even that they are actually dead (e.g, ***Cotard's syndrome*** in ***severe depression***)
2. Delusions of reference	• Seen in ***schizophrenia*** • These delusions are concerned with ideas that objects, events or people, have a personal significance to the patient, e.g. a radio play about homosexuals is thought to have been broadcast in order to tell the patient that everyone knows he is a homosexual
3. Delusions of grandeur	• Occur in ***mania*** and *schizophrenia* • Beliefs of exaggerated self-importance. Patient may think himself to be a king and wealthy
4. Delusions of guilt	• Found most often in ***depressive illness*** (also delusions of worthlessness)
5. Delusions of jealousy	• MC in *men* • When the content of delusion is mainly jealousy (infidelity) involving the spouse, it is called ***Othello's syndrome*** (conjugal paranoia, morbid jealousy). Morbid jealousy is more common among ***alcoholics***
6. Sexual or erotic delusions	• Rare and MC in *women* • A woman believes that a man, who is inaccessible, of a higher social status and, to whom she has never spoken, loves her; a prominent feature of ***de Clérambault's syndrome***
7. Delusions of control	• Strongly suggest ***schizophrenia*** (e.g. the patient believes that his thoughts are controlled by an outside agency)
8. Induced delusional disorder	• This is characterized by ***sharing of delusions*** between two persons (***folie a deux***) or occasionally more persons (*folie a trois, folie a quatrae, folie a familie*) who usually have closely knit ***emotional bond***. Treatment is geographical and ***separation*** works very well • For example, a 20-year-old woman whose psychotic mother believes that aliens are coming to kidnap her now begins to believe the same thing. The belief disappears when her mother moves to another city
9. Capgras syndrome: Delusion of doubles	• MC in *women*, MC in ***paranoid schizophrenia***, also seen in delusional disorders, Lewy body dementia • ***Illusion des sosies***: The person sees a familiar person as a stranger who is imposing as the familiar person • ***Illusion de Fregoli***: The person falsely identifies strangers as familiar persons

149. Answer is b (Extrovert with excessive emotionality and attention seeking).
Ref: Niraj Ahuja's Psychiatry, 6th edition Pg 112, 126.

Simple Summary

Features of Personality Disorders

CLUSTER 'A' (Odd/Eccentric = 'Weird')	
Paranoid	Suspicious of fidelity of spouse, excessively sensitive, distrustful, bearing grudges, attributes responsibility for own problems to others, self-important, reading negative meaning into remarks, hypersensitivity to rebuffs, grandiose sense of personal rights, reluctance to confide, argumentative, stubborn.
Schizoid	Emotionally cold, voluntary social withdrawal without psychosis, restricted range of emotional expression, little interest in sex, lacking confidence, indifference to praise or criticism, aloofness and insensitivity to social norms, humorless, introspective.
Schizotypal	Inappropriate/Constricted affect, ideas (not delusions) of reference, magical thinking, unusual perceptions (e.g. bodily illusions), odd ideas (about telepathy), suspiciousness, circumstantial/tangential thinking, eccentricity and excess social anxiety. This type of personality disorder is more common in relatives of people with SZ and is more closely related to SZ than the schizoid type.
CLUSTER 'B' (Flamboyant, dramatic = 'Wild')	
Antisocial (psychopathic, sociopathic)	Callous disregard for the rights or safety of others, failure to maintain enduring relationships, low frustration tolerance and aggressive threshold, incapacity to experience guilt or profit from adverse experiences (e.g. punishment), proneness to blame others.
Borderline (impulsive)	Unstable relationships, impulsive behavior (reckless spending, binge eating or sex), variable moods, lack of control of anger, recurrent suicidal threats or behavior, identity confusion, chronic anhedonia and feelings of emptiness, transient paranoid ideation and frantic efforts to avoid real or imagined abandonment.
Histrionic (narcissistic)	Self-dramatization, excessive shallow (dramatic) emotionality, ***attention seeking***, suggestibility (easily influenced by others), vain, self-centered, short-lived ***enthusiasms***, inappropriate sexual seductiveness, but frigidity and immaturity, narcissism.
CLUSTER 'C' (Fearful/anxious = 'Worrying and Wimpy')	
Avoidant (anxious)	Persistent feelings of tension and inadequacy, social inhibition, introvert, restriction in lifestyle to maintain physical security. This disorder is an epitome of what is called as inferiority complex.
Dependent (asthenic)	Allowing others to make most of one's important life decisions, undue compliance with others wishes, feeling helpless when alone, limited capacity to make everyday decisions without others advice.
Obsessive-Compulsive (*anankastic*)	Rigidity of thinking; perfectionism; preoccupation with rules, order and schedules. Major depressive episodes are frequent. These are egosyntonic life traits with no obvious onset (*Note*: Obsessive compulsive disorder is egodystonic).

150. Answer is b (Anankastic).
Ref: Niraj Ahuja's psychiatry, 6th edition Pg 103, 128.

Repeat Topic

- Refer table in ***previous answer no. 150*** above for detailed explanation.

151. Answer is c (End tidal CO_2).
Ref: Lee's anesthesia, 13th edition Pg 339; Urology secrets, Martin Resnick, Andrew Novick, 3rd edition Pg 123.

Repeat Topic

- Refer ***answer no. 16 in COMED-K 2009 answers*** for detailed explanation.

152. Answer is d (Hallucination).
Ref: Niraj Ahuja's psychiatry, 6th edition Pg 51, 60.

Disorders of Perception

Illusions	Hallucinations
• Illusions are *misconceptions* of external stimuli, e.g. at dusk, a common illusion is to perceive the outline of a bush as that of a man.	• A perception experienced in the absence of external stimulus to the sense organs. A few normal people also experience them during transition between sleep and waking (when tired); they are called *hypnagogic,* if experienced while falling asleep and *hypnopompic* if experienced during awakening.

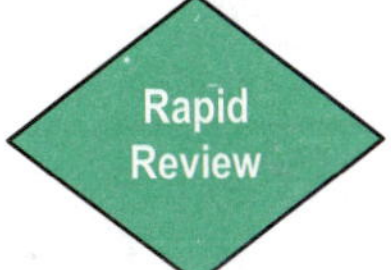

TYPES OF HALLUCINATIONS

<u>According To Complexity</u>

1. *Elementary hallucinations:* Bangs, whistles, flashes of light.
2. *Complex hallucinations*: Hearing voices or music, or seeing faces and scenes.

<u>According to Sensory Modality</u>

1. ***Auditory hallucinations:***
   - Voices, music or noises; common in non-organic psychiatric disorders.
   - Voices addressing the patient (second-person hallucinations and voices talking to one another ***referring to the patient) (third person hallucinations)*** seen commonly in ***schizophrenia***.
   - Sometimes voices seem to anticipate what the patient thinks a few moments later or speak his own thoughts as he speaks them (*Gedankenlautwerden*) or repeat his thoughts immediately after he has thought of them (*echo de la pensee*).
2. ***Visual hallucinations:***
   - These may be elementary or complex; common in *organic mental disorders* also seen in hysteria, severe affective disorders.
   - ***Extracampine***: Visual hallucinations are experienced as located outside the field of vision, i.e. behind the head.
3. ***Olfactory and gustatory hallucinations:***
   - Frequently experienced together, often as unpleasant smell or tastes; may suggest severe depressive disorders, schizophrenia, ***temporal lobe epilepsy,*** irritation of the olfactory bulb by a tumor.
4. ***Tactile (haptic) hallucinations:***
   - Experienced as insects crawling on the body or under the skin; occurs with ***cocaine abuse (Magnan's symptoms)***, amphetamine abuse, delirium tremens, opioid withdrawal and occasionally in schizophrenics.
5. ***Autoscopic hallucination:***
   - The experience of seeing one's own body projected into space, usually in front of oneself for short periods. This experience may convince the person that he has a double (***doppelganger***); this is a rare phenomenon encountered mainly in a small minority of patients with ***temporal lobe epilepsy or other organic brain disorders***.

153. Answer is c (Psoriasis).

Ref: Robbins pathology, 7th edition Pg 1257.

Types of Microabscesses

– ***Munro's microabscesses*** are composed of degenerated polymorphonuclear leukocytes in the horny layer and are seen in ***psoriasis and seborrhoeic dermatitis***

– ***Spongiform pustules of Kagoj:*** These are multilocular pustules in the upper stratum malpighii (spinosum) within a sponge-like network made up of flattened keratinocytes; seen in *psoriasis, Reiter's disease and geographic tongue and rarely in candidiasis*

– *Pautrier microabscesses:* These are collections of 3 or more atypical mononuclear cells within the epidermis in ***mycosis fungoides***

154. Answer is b (Perceptual anomalies).
Ref: Niraj Ahuja's Psychiatry, 6th edition Pg 103; Davidson's, 20th edition Pg 240.

Obsessive Compulsive Disorder (OCD)

- Patients with obsessions experience recurring intrusive feelings, thoughts and images (***obsessions***) that cause anxiety that is relieved in part by performing repetitive actions (***compulsions***).
- ***MC obsessions*** are concerned with ***contamination*** and ***handwashing is the MC compulsion***.

- Other obsessions
  - Seeing form of *images* (vivid, morbid or violent scenes)
  - *Ruminations* (continuous pondering, thoughts, doubts)
  - Obsessional *slowness*
  - *Arithmomania* (counting)
  - *Onomatomania* (urge to utter a forbidden word)
  - *Folie de pourquoi* (irresistible habit of seeking explanations for common place facts by asking perpetual questions)

- The obsessional urge is recognized as alien to the personality (***egodystonic* or *ego-alien***) and failure to resist this causes marked distress to the patient (i.e. ***they have insight***).
- ***Serotonin*** appears to be a closely related neurotransmitter in the etiology of OCD.
- Common ***complication*** of OCD is ***depression*** and abuse of anxiolytics.
- Psychoanalytic theory explains OCD as a defensive regression to ***anal-sadistic phase of Freudian stage*** of development.
- ***Undoing*** is the mechanism, which leads to compulsions.
- ***Behavior therapy*** has a success rate of about 80% for the compulsive acts.
- Antidepressants such as ***Clomipramine*** and the selective serotonin reuptake inhibitors (***SSRIs***) are effective in drug treatment of OCD (*even* in the absence of coexistent depression).
- Obsessional content does not seem to relate to prognosis.

Factors indicating poorer prognosis in OCD	Factors indicating a good prognosis in OCD
➢ Lack of resistance to compulsions ➢ Childhood onset ➢ Coexisting depressive disorder ➢ Delusional beliefs or overvalued ideas ➢ Personality disorder	➢ Good social and occupational adjustment ➢ A clear precipitating event ➢ Episodic symptoms

155. Answer is b (Isoflurane).
Ref: Lee's Anesthesia, 13th edition Pg 219.

- ***Isoflurane*** is a ***powerful systemic and coronary arterial dilator***. The effect on systemic arterial pressure is easily controlled in the normal healthy patient and has ***been used specifically as a means of inducing hypotension***.
- However, the phenomenon of 'coronary steal' means that isoflurane should be used with caution in patients with coronary artery disease.

156. Answer is b (Bupivacaine).
Ref: KD Tripathi, 6th edition Pg 355.

157. Answer is c (It will be the same)
Ref: Ganong's, 20th edition Pg 566.

- The pressure in any vessel below the level of the heart is increased and that in any vessel above the heart level is decreased by the effect of gravity.
- In the given question, the patient is lying flat, so the blood pressure ***will be same in all the vessels***, as the gravity will be same throughout the plane.

158. Answer is c (Related to underlying carcinoma in the body).
Ref: Harrison's, 17th edition Pg 2182, 2183.

- ***Hypertrophic osteoarthropathy (HOA)*** is characterized by ***clubbing of digits*** and, in more advanced stages, by periosteal new bone formation and synovial effusions. HOA occurs in primary or familial form and usually begins in childhood. The secondary form of HOA is associated with ***intrathoracic malignancies***, suppurative lung disease, congenital heart disease and a variety of other disorders, and is more common in adults. Clubbing is almost always a feature of HOA but can occur as an isolated manifestation.
- In HOA, the bone changes in the distal extremities begin as periostitis followed by new bone formation. Initially, the process of periosteal new bone formation involves the proximal and distal diaphyses of the tibia, fibula, radius and ulna and, ***less frequently, the femur***, humerus, metacarpals, metatarsals and phalanges. Occasionally, scapulae, clavicles, ribs and pelvic bones are also affected.
- However, the symptoms and signs of PHPO may **disappear completely** with removal or effective chemotherapy of a tumor.

ANATOMY, PHYSIOLOGY, BIOCHEMISTRY

159. Answer is c (Ventricular filling).
Ref: Ganong's, 23rd edition Pg 512.

Heart Sounds

Sound	Mechanism	Other features
S1	• Due to mitral and tricuspid valve closure • Occurs at onset of systole • Loudest at mitral area	• Loud S1 in hyperdynamic circulation (anemia, pregnancy, thyrotoxicosis), mitral stenosis • Soft S1 in heart failure, mitral regurgitation
S2	• Due to aortic and pulmonary valve closure • Occurs at end of systole • Loudest at left sternal border	• S2 splitting occurs since aortic valve closes before pulmonic (a < p); Inspiration ↑ S2 splIt • ***Fixed wide splitting*** a/w ***ASD*** • Variable wide splitting a/w pulmonic stenosis, RBBB • Reversed/Paradoxical splitting a/w aortic stenosis, LBBB
S3	• From ventricular wall due to abrupt cessation of rapid filling • Occurs early in diastole • Low pitched, often heard as 'gallop'	• May be physiological in young people, pregnancy • Pathological in heart failure, mitral regurgitation
S4	• Due to high atrial pressure and ***ventricular filling*** • Occurs at end of diastole	• S4 = 'atrial kick' • Always pathological— a/w severe LV hypertrophy (e.g. HOCM) • Absent in atrial fibrillation

160. Answer is b (Amytal).
Ref: Vasudevan's Biochemistry, 5th edition Pg 234, Table 20.5.

☐ **Cytochrome oxidase (complex IV)** carries out the following irreversible reaction:

$$O2 + 4\ H+ + 4\ e- \rightarrow 2\ H2O$$

- ☐ ***Cyanide, sulfide, azide and carbon monoxide** all bind to cytochrome c oxidase, thus inhibiting* the protein from functioning, which results in chemical asphyxiation of cells.

161. Answer is a (Resting tremor).
Ref: Davidson's, 20th edition Pg 1219; Harrison's, 17th edition Pg 2550.

Repeat Topic

- Refer ***answer no. 180 below in the same COMED-K 2007 answers*** for detailed explanation of cerebellar lesion manifestations.
- Three cardinal signs of ***Parkinson's disease—rest tremor, rigidity and bradykinesia.***
- ***Rest tremor,*** at a frequency of 4–6 Hz, typically appears unilaterally, first distally, involving the digits and wrist, where it may have a 'pill-rolling' character.
- Tremor usually spreads proximally and occasionally to the ipsilateral leg before appearing on the other side after a year or more. It may appear later in the lips, tongue and jaw, but spares the head and neck.

162. Answer is c (Bicarbonate).
Ref: Ganong's physiology, 23rd edition Pg 613.

- Carbon dioxide is transported in the blood in three forms
  - Dissolved in plasma—10%
  - Chemically bound to hemoglobin—10% is carried in RBCs as carbaminohemoglobin
  - ***Bicarbonate*** ion in plasma—***80%*** is transported as bicarbonate.

163. Answer is c (Long flexors of fingers).
Ref: Last's Anatomy, 11th edition Pg 94.

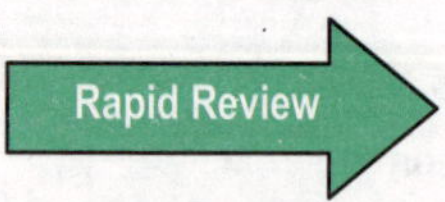

Types of Grips

- ***Power grip**: Depends on the long flexors of the fingers,* with opposition of the thumb assisting the whole hand to give a tight grip. Synergic contraction of wrist extensors is also essential for a firm grip of this kind; flexion of the wrist weakens the grip. Example: Holding a heavy hammer for banging in a nail.
- ***Hook grip***: The long flexors are in action, but wrist extension and opposition may not be necessary accompaniments, e.g. for carrying a suitcase.
- ***Precision grip*** for dealing with small objects requires wrist stability, but opposition of the thumb to finger pads, especially of the index and middle fingers are the essential features and here the small muscles of the hands are of prime importance.

164. Answer is d (Posterior cricoarytenoid).
Ref: BD Chaurasia, Vol 3, Pg 152.

Repeat Question

- Refer ***answer no. 171 in COMED-K 2008 answers*** for detailed explanation.

165. Answer is c (Radial).
Ref: BD Chaurasia, 3rd edition, Vol 1. Pg 134.

- ***Profunda brachii*** artery is a ***branch of the brachial artery.***
- Branches:
  - Ascending branch: Anastomoses with descending branch of posterior circumflex humeral of third part of axillary artery. Participate in *collateral circulation around shoulder joint*

  - Descending branch: Divides into middle and radial collateral arteries. Participate in *collateral circulation around the elbow*
  - Middle branch: Descend *behind* lateral humeral epicondyle
  - Radial branch: Descend in *front* lateral humeral epicondyle
- ***Important relation***: Passes laterally behind the humerus, ***associated with the radial nerve in the radial groove***.

166. Answer is c (Closure of aortic valve).
Ref: Ganong's physiology, 23rd edition Pg 512.

- The ***dicrotic notch***, a small oscillation on the falling phase of the pulse wave caused by vibrations set up when the ***aortic valve snaps shut*** is visible if the pressure wave is recorded, but is not palpable at the wrist.
- The pulmonary artery curve also has a dicrotic notch produced by closure of the pulmonary valves.

167. Answer is a (Lesser petrosal nerve).
Ref: BD Chaurasia, Vol 1 Pg 133.

Innervation of the parotid
- ***Preganglionic parasympathetic*** portion of the gland, beginning in the *inferior salivatory nucleus* and passing via the ***glossopharyngeal nerve, the tympanic plexus and the lesser petrosal nerve*** to the ***otic ganglion***.
- ***Postganglionic fibers*** travel along the ***auriculotemporal nerve*** and into the parotid gland, where they control glandular secretions.
- ***Preganglionic sympathetic*** fibers originate in the *first and second thoracic segments* and synapse in the *cervical sympathetic ganglia*.
- ***Postganglionic sympathetic*** fibers travel along the external carotid artery to the superficial temporal artery and the transverse facial artery and terminate in the *sweat glands*.

168. Answer is c (Superior mesenteric artery).
Ref: BD Chaurasia, vol2, Pg 213.

- **Blood supply of stomach** is from:
  - *Left gastric artery* from *celiac trunk*
  - *Splenic artery* and *left gastroepiploic artery*
  - *Common hepatic artery* through the *right gastroepiploic artery and gastroduodenal artery*.

169. Answer is d (LMN VII nerve).
Ref: Davdison's, 20th edition Pg 1249.

- ***Bell's palsy is a LMN paralysis of facial nerve (CN VII)*** in which there is an abolition of both voluntary and reflex movements of the facial muscles
- On the ***ipsilateral side, the face is mask like*** and the ***forehead immobile***
- Patient is ***unable to blink or close the eyelid***
- ***Lacrimation*** on the lesion side ***may be impaired (greater petrosal nerve)***
- There may be a ***reduction of saliva (chorda tympani nerve)***
- ***Taste is lost*** on the ***ipsilateral anterior two third of the tongue (chorda tympani***
- Ear pain
- There can be an ***increased acuity to sound (hyperacusis)*** due to ***paralysis of the stapedius muscle***
- When a lesion occurs at the location where VII emerges from the pons, as the patient opens his mouth, his eyes close (jaw-winking phenomenon).

170. Answer is b (Distal end of femur).
Ref: Narayan Reddy's FMT, 23rd edition Pg 48.

- The ossification centers used for age estimation of the fetus are:
  - Lower end of femur
  - Upper end of tibia
  - Sternum
  - Bones of the foot

171. Answer is c (Endothelial cells).
Ref: Harrison's, 17th edition Pg 722 and Fig 109-4.

- ***von Willebrand factor (vWF)*** is a large multimeric glycoprotein present in blood plasma and produced constitutively in ***endothelium*** (in the Weibel-Palade bodies) and subendothelial connective tissue.
- vWF serves two roles:
  - ☐ As the major ***adhesion molecule*** that tethers the platelet to the exposed subendothelium
  - ☐ As the ***binding protein for FVIII***, resulting in significant prolongation of the FVIII half-life in circulation.

172. Answer is d (A delta).
Ref: Ganong's Physiology, 23rd edition Pg 89.

Repeat Topic

- Refer ***answer no. 160 in COMED-K 2008*** answers for detailed explanation.

173. Answer is a (Pyruvate kinase).
Ref: Vasudevan's biochemistry, 5th edition Pg 146, 96.

- In starvation, the ***activities of the key gluconeogenic enzymes, increase markedly***, indicating compensatory ***gluconeogenesis***:
  - *Glucose-6-phosphatase*
  - *Fructose-1,6-diphosphatase*
  - *Pyruvate carboxylase and*
  - *Phosphoenolpyruvate carboxykinase.*

174. Answer is d (Increase calcium and phosphate excretion).
Ref: KD Tripathi, 6th edition Pg 331.

- Cholecalciferol is vitamin D_3; active form of cholecalciferol is calcitriol.
- Calcitriol ***stimulates the production of a protein*** in the digestive system called calbindin that allows the body to absorb calcium from the digestive system into the blood stream.
- Calcitriol ***enhances tubular reabsorption of calcium and phosphate*** in the kidney.
- Calcitriol indirectly ***helps in bone mineralization by induction of osteocalcin.***
- Vitamin D plays an important role in ***regulation of PTH secretion.***

175. Answer is a (Sympathetic adrenergic nerves).
Ref: Textbook of Human Physiology for Dental Students, Indu Khurana, 2007 edition Pg 257.

Nerve Supply of Cutaneous Vessels

- ***Sympathetic vasoconstrictor nerves*** supplying the cutaneous vessels exhibit a sympathetic constrictor discharge under set conditions. The sympathetic tonic discharge is more marked on A-V anastamoses vessels than other vessels.
- Parasympathetic dilator vessels DO NOT supply the cutaneous blood vessels vasodilation of cutaneous vessels results due to:
  - Reduction of sympathetic vasoconstrictor effect
  - Local production of bradykinin (a potent vasodilator polypeptide) in sweat glands
  - Production of other local vasodilator substances.

176. Answer is a (Muscular dystrophy).
Ref: Vasudevan's Biochemistry, 5th edition Pg 54, Table 6.2.

Isoenzymes of creatine kinase

Isoenzyme	Found in	Increased in
CK-BB (CK-1)	Brain	–
CK-MB (CK-2)	Heart	Myocardial infarction
CK-MM (CK-3)	Skeletal muscle	Muscular dystrophy, severe exercise, polymyositis

177. Answer is a (Lysyl oxidase).
Ref: Harrison's, 17th edition Pg 449.

- ***Copper*** is a ***cofactor*** for ***lysyl oxidase***, the enzyme that forms cross-links between ***collagen*** in connective tissue.
- ***Dietary sources of copper*** include shellfish, liver, nuts, legumes, bran and organ meats.
- Copper is also a component of ***ferroprotein***, a transport protein involved in the basolateral transfer of iron during absorption from the enterocyte.

Copper is an integral part of numerous enzyme systems including	Copper plays a role in
☐ Amine oxidases	☐ Iron metabolism
☐ Ferroxidase (ceruloplasmin)	☐ Melanin synthesis
☐ Cytochrome c oxidase	☐ Energy production
☐ Superoxide dismutase and	☐ Neurotransmitter synthesis and CNS function
☐ Dopamine hydroxylase	☐ Synthesis and cross-linking of elastin and collagen
	☐ Scavenging of superoxide radicals

178. Answer is b (Bell-Magendie law).
Ref: Ganong's physiology, 23rd edition Pg 157.

- ***Bell-Magendie law***: The anterior spinal nerve roots (ventral roots) contain only motor fibers and posterior roots (dorsal roots) only sensory fibers.

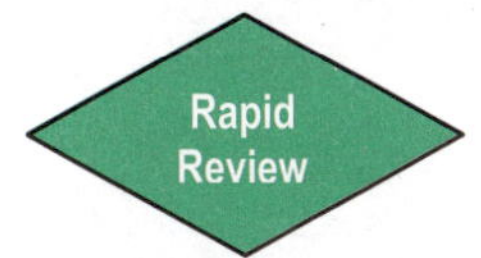

- ☐ **Muller's doctrine of specific nerve energies**: When the nerve pathways from a particular sense organ are stimulated, the sensation evoked is that for which the receptor is specialized no matter how or where along the pathway the activity is initiated.
- ☐ **Law of projection**: No matter where a particular sensory pathway is stimulated along its course to the cortex, the conscious sensation produced is referred to the location of the receptor, e.g. in phantom limb.
- ☐ **Weber-Fechner law**: The magnitude of the sensation felt is proportional to the log of the intensity of the stimulus (intensity discrimination).
- ☐ **Bainbridge reflex**: Rapid infusion of blood or saline in anesthetized animals sometimes produces a rise in heart rate, if the initial rate is low. It appears to be true reflex rather than a response to local stretch.
- ☐ **Cushing reflex**: When intracranial pressure is increased, the blood supply to the vasomotor area is compromised and the local hypoxia and hypercapnia increase its discharge. The resultant rise in systemic arterial pressure tends to restore blood flow to the medulla. The rise in blood pressure causes a reflex decrease in heart rate via the arterial baroreceptors and this is why bradycardia, rather than tachycardia is characteristically seen in patients with increased intracranial pressure. *Cushing's triad* = bradycardia, hypertension, respiratory depression.

- ☐ **Monro-Kellie hypothesis:** Under normal conditions, the three components of the skull (i.e. blood, brain, CSF) are in equilibrium and the intracranial pressure is the sum of the pressure exerted by each of them.

179. Answer is b (Adoptive immunity).
Ref: Textbook of Microbiology, CP Baveja, 3rd edition Pg 93.

- *Adoptive immunity*: Immunity to disease or infection conferred on a previously non-immune individual by ***transferring lymphocytes*** from a previously immune individual to the non-immune individual.

QuickLook

- ☐ ***Innate immunity*** is present from birth by virtue of his genetic and constitutional makeup.
- ☐ ***Acquired immunity*** is acquired during a person's lifetime by:
  - ***Active immunity***: Arises only after an infection (natural) or immunization (artificial)
  - ***Passive immunity***: Through transplacental maternal IgG antibodies (natural) or through antiserum injection (artificial).

180. Answer is c (Ataxia).
Ref: Ganong's physiology, 23rd edition Pg 258.

Clinical features of cerebellar disease:

- ***Truncal ataxia*** (of gait): Unsteadiness with a wide base, body sway and an inability to walk on tandem (heel to toe); (if ataxia worsens on eye closure, lesion is in the dorsal columns, not cerebellum)
- ***Dysarthria (dyssynergia)*** refers to a decomposition of movement instead of a smooth, continuous movement; it is associated with a tendency to miss a target and worsens when approaching the target
- ***Dysmetria*** (the misjudging of distance), with its characteristic overshooting and undershooting of a target *(past-pointing)*
- ***Intentional tremor***
- ***Dysdiadochokinesia*** *(inability to perform rapidly coordinated movements such as pronation and supination of hands)*
- ***Nystagmus***
- ***Scanning speech***
- ***Hypotonia***
- ***Decomposition of movements***

Must Know

Features of Localized Cerebral Lesions

☐ **Temporal Lobe**	Seizures; *hallucinations* (smell, taste, sound, déja-vu); complex partial with automatisms; dysphasia; field defect (contralateral superior quadrantanopia, *'pie in the sky'*); forgetfulness; functional psychosis; *fear/rage*; *hypersexuality*.
☐ **Frontal Lobe**	Hemiparesis; fits (contralateral movement); personality changes (indecent, indolent, indiscreet, *disinhibition*); *positive primitive reflexes* (grasp reflex) – significant only if unilateral; dysphasia (Broca's area); *loss of smell* unilaterally.
☐ **Parietal Lobe**	Hemisensory loss; ↓↓ *2-point discrimination*; *astereognosis* (☐☐ability to recognize object held in hand by touch lone); field defect (contralateral inferior quadrantanopia, *'pie on the floor'*); *sensory inattention*; dysphasia; *Gerstmann's syndrome* (finger agnosia, right/left disorientation, dysgraphia and acalculia = dominant parietal lesion). *Hemispatial neglect* (ignoring one side of body), trouble with *dressing* (non-dominant parietal lobe lesion).

☐ **Occipital lobe**	*Contralateral congruous homonymous hemianopia*, visual hallucinations.
☐ **Cerebellopontine angle**	Usually vestibular schwannoma; *ipsilateral deafness*; nystagmus; *reduced corneal reflex, VII and V nerve palsies*; ipsilateral cerebellar signs.
☐ **Corpus callosum (rare site for lesions)**	Usually *severe rapid intellectual deterioration* with focal signs of adjacent lobes; signs of loss of communication between lobes (e.g. left hand unable to carry out verbal commands).
☐ **Midbrain**	*Unequal pupils*; inability to direct eyes up or down; *amnesia for recent events with confabulation; somnolence.*

NOTES

COMED-K 2006

COMED-K 2006 QUESTIONS

MEDICINE

1. **White lung is due to**
   (a) Congenital syphilis
   (b) Toxoplasmosis
   (c) Congenital TB
   (d) Silicosis

2. **Lifetime risk of TB in HIV patients**
   (a) 20%
   (b) 50%
   (c) 10%
   (d) 5%

3. **The following are preventable risk factors for dementia**
   (a) Hypertension
   (b) APO E4
   (c) Age
   (d) Lowered homocysteine

4. **Patients with protracted vomiting can develop**
   (a) Hypokalemic hypochloremic alkalosis
   (b) Hyperkalemic hypochloremic acidosis
   (c) Hypokalemic hyperchloremic alkalosis
   (d) Hypokalemic hypochloremic acidosis

5. **All of the following are changes in an ECG that can be seen in patients with hyperkalemia *EXCEPT***
   (a) Peaked T waves
   (b) Prolongation of PR interval
   (c) Slurring of QRS
   (d) Terminal broad ventricular bradycardia

6. **All the following are features of adult polycystic kidney disease *EXCEPT***
   (a) Autosomal recessive trait
   (b) Present as renal mass
   (c) Hematuria
   (d) Renal failure

7. **All of the following are macrovascular complications of DM *EXCEPT***
   (a) Abnormality of coronary circulation
   (b) Cerebral circulation
   (c) Peripheral circulation
   (d) Retinopathy

8. **Adult respiratory distress syndrome is defined by all *EXCEPT***
   (a) PCW > 18 cm of H_2O
   (b) $PaO_2/FiO_2 < 200$
   (c) Diffuse B/l air space edema on Co X-ray
   (d) All of the above

9. **All of the following are components of nephrotic syndrome *EXCEPT***
   (a) Edema
   (b) Hypercoagulability
   (c) Hypocholesteremia
   (d) Infection

10. **A rise in 1% glycosylated Hb corresponds to rise in BLD glucose con**
    (a) 2 mmol/L
    (b) 3 mmol/L
    (c) 4 mmol/L
    (d) 5 mmol/L

11. **In syndrome X, patients have all of the following *EXCEPT***
    (a) Angina-like chest pain
    (b) Ischemic ST segment depression
    (c) Abnormal coronary arteriogram
    (d) Excellent prognosis

12. **Signs of UMN lesion are all *EXCEPT***
    (a) Fasciculation
    (b) Spasticity
    (c) Hyperactive tendon reflexes
    (d) Babinski's sign positive

13. **Serum ascites albumin gradient > 1.1 g/dL is seen in**
    (a) Nephrosis
    (b) Cirrhosis
    (c) Pancreatic ascites
    (d) Neoplasm

14. **Cockcroft-Gault formula to estimate creatinine clearance in women is**
    (a) (140 – age) × lean body wt (kg), plasma CR (mg/dL) × 72
    (b) (140 – age) × 0.85
    (c) (140 – age) × total body wt × 0.85/72 × plasma CR
    (d) (140 – age) × lean body wt × plasma CR × 72

15. The classic and most common HIV associated glomerulopathy is
(a) Focal segment glomerulosclerosis
(b) Diffuse proliferative glomerulonephritis
(c) Mesangioproliferative nephritis
(d) Pauci-immune necrotizing glomerulonephritis

16. Synthetic selective factor Xa inhibitor is
(a) Enoxaparin
(b) Dalteparin
(c) Fondaparinux
(d) Heparin

17. Nephrolithiasis occurs with the toxicity is
(a) Ritonavir
(b) Saquinavir
(c) Indinavir
(d) Nelfinavir

18. Mitral orifice area is
(a) 4–6 cm^2
(b) 2–4 cm^2
(c) 1–2 cm^2
(d) 0.5 cm^2

19. Most common organism for causing RHD in native valve
(a) *Streptococcus viridans*
(b) Enterococci
(c) Staphylococci
(d) Gram +ve bacilli

20. All the following produce exudative pleural effusion *EXCEPT*
(a) TB
(b) Malignancy
(c) Collagen diseases
(d) Cardiac failure

21. Pulmonary TB is more common association in the following diseases *EXCEPT*
(a) AIDS
(b) Type I + II DM
(c) CRF
(d) MS

22. Coronary heart diseases may manifest as all *EXCEPT*
(a) Angina on effort
(b) Cardiomyopathies
(c) MI
(d) Sudden death

23. LDH1:LDH2 in acute MI is
(a) > 1.0
(b) > 1.5
(c) > 2.0
(d) > 2.5

24. A 10-year-old boy presents with mucosal bleeding of 1 week duration the IOC that will be most useful in him is
(a) PT
(b) CT
(c) APTT
(d) Platelet

25. Syndrome of inappropriate ADH secretion (SIADH) is treated with
(a) Demeclocycline
(b) Morphine
(c) Carbamazepine
(d) Thiazide diuretics

SURGERY

26. Which of the following is not associated with left side portal hypertension?
(a) Secondary to pancreatic inflammation
(b) Normal superior mesenteric and portal venous pressure
(c) Easily reversed by splenectomy
(d) Isolated esophageal varices present

27. In the Forrest classification for bleeding peptic ulcer with a visible vessel it is classified as
(a) F I
(b) F IIa
(c) F IIb
(d) F IIc

28. In which of the following types of Ca breast, comedo growth pattern is seen?
(a) Ductal carcinoma in situ
(b) Medullary carcinoma
(c) Lobular CIS
(d) Infiltrating lobular carcinoma

29. Which of the following operations was first described by Orringer?
(a) En bloc esophagectomy
(b) Transhiatal esophagectomy
(c) Thoracoscopic esophagectomy
(d) Transthoracic esophagectomy

30. All the following are true for follicular ca thyroid *EXCEPT*
(a) Vascular invasion is common
(b) Younger pts. have good prognosis
(c) Lymph node involvement is rare
(d) Diagnosis is by fine needle aspiration

31. Triangle of vertebral artery is formed by the following *EXCEPT*
(a) Longus colli
(b) Scalenus anterior
(c) Scalenus medius
(d) Subclavian artery

32. All the following cranial nerves are at risk during removal of submandibular gland *EXCEPT*
(a) Lingual nerves
(b) Hypoglossal nerves
(c) Marginal mandibular branch of facial nerve
(d) Buccal branch of facial nerve

33. Kidney transplantation is an
(a) Allograft
(b) Isograft
(c) Xenograft
(d) Syngenic graft

34. Garrod's pads refer to thickened skin pads over
(a) Tip of finger
(b) Dorsum of wrist
(c) Palm
(d) Dorsum of PIP joint

35. The procedure of choice for elective removal of CBD stone is
(a) Open choledocholithotomy
(b) Endoscopic choledocholithotomy
(c) Laparoscopic choledocholithotomy
(d) Medical treatment

36. Contraindications to major hepatic resection for metastatic disease include all the following *EXCEPT*
(a) Total hepatic involvement
(b) Advanced cirrhosis
(c) Extrahepatic tumor
(d) Jaundice from extrinsic ductal obstruction

37. Following are the tumors of posterior mediastinum *EXCEPT*
(a) Neuroblastoma
(b) Ganglioneuroma
(c) Thymic tumor
(d) All

38. All are features of APKD *EXCEPT*
(a) AR trait
(b) Presents as renal mass
(c) Hematuria
(d) Renal failure

39. All the following are predisposing factors for torsion of testis *EXCEPT*
(a) Inversion of testis
(b) Low investment of tunica vaginalis
(c) 10–25 years age group
(d) Separation of epididymis

40. Ménétrier's disease—all are true *EXCEPT*
(a) Giant folds in pyloric antrum
(b) Foveolar hyperplasia
(c) Hypoalbuminemia
(d) Hypochlorhydria

41. In Clark's classification of level of tumor invasion for malignant melanoma, level 3 refers to
(a) All tumors above basement membrane
(b) Invasion into reticular dermis
(c) Invasion into loose connective tissue of papillary dermis
(d) Tumor cells at the junction of reticular and papillary dermis

42. Eradication of *Helicobacter pylori* has been proved to be beneficial in which of the following disorders of the stomach?
(a) Low-grade malt lymphoma
(b) Erosive gastrics
(c) Carcinoma stomach
(d) Gastroesophageal disease

43. Most common presentation of renal adenocarcinoma is
(a) Hematuria
(b) Local pain
(c) Mass
(d) Fever

44. Ogilvie's syndrome results from the denervation of the colon distal to the SURG
(a) Hepatic flexure
(b) Mid-transverse colon
(c) Splenic flexure
(d) Descending colon

45. Which of the following drugs has been found to increase the survival in locally advanced pancreatic cancer?
(a) Doxorubicin
(b) Streptozocin
(c) Gemcitabine
(d) Paclitaxel

46. Most commonly, aircraft accident takes place during
(a) Take off
(b) Flight
(c) Landing
(d) Acceleration

OBSTETRICS AND GYNECOLOGY

47. Variable deceleration in electronic fetal monitoring in a woman who is in labor indicates
(a) Congenital heart disease
(b) Compression of head
(c) Administration of sympathomimetic drugs to the mother
(d) Umbilical cord compression

48. The commonest cause for spontaneous abortion during the first trimester is
(a) Chromosomal aberrations
(b) Maternal infection
(c) Maternal DM
(d) Uterine malformations

49. Oligohydramnios is associated with the following *EXCEPT*
(a) B/L renal agenesis
(b) Premature rupture membranes
(c) Postmaturity
(d) Esophageal atresia

50. Deep transverse arrest is usually seen in
(a) Gynecoid pelvis
(b) Android pelvis
(c) Platypelloid pelvis
(d) Anthropoid pelvis

51. The most common cause of secondary PPH is
(a) Vaginal lacerations
(b) Coagulation failure
(c) Retained placental bits
(d) Submucous fibroid

52. CI for ventouse delivery include all the following *EXCEPT*
(a) Fetal coagulopathies
(b) Extreme prematurity
(c) Mentotransverse
(d) Occipitotransverse

53. In a C/O primary amenorrhea chromosomal study revealing XY chromosome and absence of Barr bodies is diagnostic of
(a) Turner's syndrome
(b) Androgen insensitivity syndrome
(c) Andrenogenital syndrome
(d) Klinefelter's syndrome

54. Presence of clue cells in vaginal discharge indicates
(a) Gardnerella vaginosis
(b) Moniliasis
(c) Trichomoniasis
(d) Senile vaginitis

55. Cystic glandular hyperplasia is associated with
(a) Theca cell tumor
(b) Hilus cell tumor
(c) Gynandroblastoma
(d) Dysgerminoma

56. Diethylstilbestrol therapy in pregnant mothers lead to one of the following cancers in their children
(a) Squamous cell carcinoma
(b) Embryonal carcinoma
(c) Clear cell adenocarcinoma
(d) Transitional cell carcinoma

57. Amniocentesis for prenatal diagnosis of genetic disorders can be carried out as early as
(a) 6–7 weeks of gestation
(b) 8–9 weeks of gestation
(c) 10–12 weeks of gestation
(d) 14–16 weeks of gestation

58. Krukenberg adenocarcinoma of ovary can occur as a result of metastesis from all, but
(a) Stomach
(b) Breast
(c) Liver
(d) Pancreas

PEDIATRICS

59. Surfactant synthesis starts after about
(a) 26 weeks of fetal life
(b) 20 weeks of fetal life
(c) 30 weeks of fetal life
(d) 18 weeks of fetal life

60. Pseudoparalysis in an infant is suggestive of
(a) Acute rheumatic fever
(b) Vitamin B_6 deficiency
(c) Vitamin E deficiency
(d) Vitamin C deficiency

61. Which one of the following suggest development of pulmonary edema in a child with VSD?
(a) Cyanosis
(b) Ejection murmur at left sternal border
(c) Initial resolution of symptoms of heart failure
(d) Inverted T wave in V1

62. Which one of the following is not true regarding Noonan syndrome?
(a) Affects male and females
(b) Short stature
(c) Chromosomal abnormality
(d) Congenital heart disease – ASD

63. Which one of the following antibacterial antibiotics are not recommended for lactating mother?
(a) Cephalosporins
(b) ATT
(c) Quinolones
(d) Aminoglycosides

64. Iron supplementation in a healthy term breastfed baby should be started at the age of
(a) 2 months
(b) 4 months
(c) 8 months
(d) 6 months

65. Each of the following features is considered for evaluation of APGAR score *EXCEPT*
(a) Heart rate
(b) Color
(c) Muscle tone
(d) Cry

66. Rapid antigen test for meningitis organisms in a child can be done on the following specimen *EXCEPT*
(a) Blood
(b) CSF
(c) Urine
(d) Throat swab

67. Gonadal sex of the fetus is determined by
(a) Secretion of testosterone
(b) Secretion of anti-Mullerian hormones
(c) Sex determine in a region on 'Y' chromosome
(d) Secretion of estrogens

68. Ligamentum teres is formed after
(a) Obliteration of umbilical vein
(b) Obliteration of ductus venosus
(c) Obliteration of ductus arteriosus
(d) Obliteration of hypogastric artery

69. All of the following are biochemical abnormalities in an infant with salt losing type of congenital adrenal hyperplasia *EXCEPT*
(a) Low-plasma sodium
(b) High-plasma potassium
(c) Metabolic alkalosis
(d) Hypoglycemia

70. At which of the following ages a child can remove front opening garment?
(a) 24 months
(b) 36 months
(c) 48 months
(d) 60 months

71. Most common congenital heart disease is
(a) ASD
(b) PDA
(c) VSD
(d) TOF

ORTHOPEDICS

72. One of the following is traction apophysitis
(a) Pellegrini-Stieda disease
(b) Osgood-Schlatter disease
(c) Albers-Schönberg disease
(d) Marble bone disease

73. **Ewing's sarcoma is best treated by**
(a) Radiotherapy and chemotherapy
(b) Radiotherapy, chemotherapy and surgery
(c) Surgery alone
(d) None of the above

74. **Best example for type IV epiphyseal injury**
(a) Lateral condyle of humerus
(b) Distal radial epiphyseal
(c) Proximal humeral fracture
(d) None of the above

75. **Type III acromioclavicular dislocation is best treated by acromioclavicular**
(a) Supervised neglect
(b) Cuff and collar
(c) Physiotherapy
(d) Coracoclavicular screw

76. **Lumbar disk prolapse is best diagnosed by**
(a) Plain X-ray
(b) CT scan
(c) MRI
(d) All of the above

77. **Ortolani's test is done for**
(a) Congenital dislocation of hip
(b) Dislocation of patellae
(c) Perthes' disease
(d) Ligamentous injury of the knee

78. **In carpal tunnel syndrome nerve affected is**
(a) Ulnar nerve
(b) Radial nerve
(c) Median nerve
(d) Posterior interosseous nerve

OPHTHALMOLOGY

79. **The mesoderm of primary optic vesicle gives rise to**
(a) Smooth muscle of iris
(b) Sclera
(c) Crystalline lens
(d) Ciliary epithelium

80. **Aqueous flare in iridocyclitis is due to**
(a) Lymphocytes
(b) Pigments
(c) RBCs
(d) Proteins

81. **Mannitol decreases the intraocular pressure by**
(a) Withdrawing water from vitreous
(b) Increasing uveoscleral outflow
(c) Increasing aqueous outflow through trabecular meshwork
(d) Inhibiting the enzyme carbonic anhydrase in the ciliary body

82. **Cyclitic membrane gives rise to**
(a) Exudative retinal detachment
(b) Rhegmatogenous retinal detachment
(c) Solid retinal detachment
(d) Tractional retinal detachment

83. **Ulcer serpens in cornea is caused by**
(a) *Moraxella*
(b) *Pseudomonas*
(c) *Pneumococcus*
(d) *Staphylococcus*

84. **Shafer's sign is seen in early cases of**
(a) Glaucoma
(b) Retinal detachment
(c) Corneal edema
(d) Anterior uveitis

85. **Smooth muscle of iris is developed from**
(a) Surface ectoderm
(b) Mesoderm
(c) Neural crest
(d) Neural ectoderm

86. **In retinoscopy examination, the observer's eye is at 1 meter in front of observed eye and observed is 1D myopic. Where is the far point situated?**
(a) In front of retina
(b) Behind the retina
(c) At infinity
(d) Observer's eye

87. **Visual angle is the angle subtended by the object at**
(a) Midpoint of posterior pole of the eye
(b) Fovea in the retina
(c) Nodal point of the lens
(d) Center of the retina

88. **Slit-lamp biomicroscopy is constructed on the principle of**
(a) Diffuse illumination
(b) Focal illumination
(c) Retroillumination
(d) Direct illumination

ENT

89. Isshiki thyroplasty type I is
(a) Lateralization of vocal cord
(b) Medialization of vocal cord
(c) Shortening of vocal cord
(d) Lengthening of vocal cord

90. Bezold's abscess following suppurative otitis media is seen in
(a) Postaural region
(b) Posterior wall of external auditory meatus
(c) In the neck
(d) In subdural space

91. Periodicity is characteristic of which sinus infection?
(a) Maxillary sinus infection
(b) Frontal
(c) Sphenoid
(d) Ethmoid

PHARMACOLOGY

92. Aspirin inhibits which of the following enzyme?
(a) Lipoprotein lipase
(b) Lipoxygenase
(c) Phospholipase A_2
(d) Cyclooxygenase

93. The most important target of chlorambucil is
(a) Myeloid tissue
(b) Lymphoid tissue
(c) Neural tissue
(d) Skin

94. Which of the following is the function of nitric oxide?
(a) Vasodilation
(b) Platelet inhibition
(c) Immune regulation
(d) All of the above

95. Which of the following is not a microsomal enzyme inhibitor?
(a) Chloramphenicol
(b) Ciprofloxacin
(c) Rifampicin
(d) Metronidazole

96. Which of the following is not a non-opioid analgesic drug?
(a) Meloxicam
(b) Methadone
(c) Nimesulide
(d) Nabumetone

97. Which of the following statements about domperidone is not correct?
(a) Prokinetic drug
(b) Antiemetic
(c) 5 HT antagonist
(d) Acts on CTZ

98. Carbamazepine in elderly causes
(a) Hypernatremia
(b) Hyponatremia
(c) Hyperkalemia
(d) Hypokalemia

99. Which anticonvulsants do not produce any fetal abnormalities?
(a) Eptoin
(b) Phenobarbitone
(c) Valproate
(d) Gabapentin

100. 5-LO (lipoxygenase) synthesis inhibitor is
(a) Zileuton
(b) Zafirlukast
(c) Montelukast
(d) All of the above

101. Orphan receptors have the following characteristics *EXCEPT*
(a) These are putative receptors
(b) These are identified by their similarity with other known receptors
(c) May elucidate entirely new therapeutic targets
(d) Their native ligands are identified

PATHOLOGY

102. Christmas disease is due to
(a) Deficiency of factor VIII
(b) Deficiency of factor IX
(c) Deficiency of factor X
(d) Deficiency of vWF

103. Autosplenectomy is seen in one of the following hemolytic anemias
(a) Hereditary spherocytosis
(b) Sickle cell anemia
(c) Thalassemia
(d) Immunohemolytic anemia

104. All of the following are inflammatory mediators produce vasoconstriction *EXCEPT*
(a) Leukotrienes
(b) Bradykinin
(c) Thromboxane A_2
(d) Platelet activating factor

105. In the diagnosis of idiopathic thrombocytopenic purpura, one of the following statements is true
(a) In the bone marrow there is increased megakaryocytes
(b) In the bone marrow there is decreased megakaryocytes
(c) PT is prolonged
(d) PTT is prolonged

106. Warm antibody immunohemolytic anemia is seen in all *EXCEPT*
(a) SLE
(b) Methyldopa ingestion
(c) Quinidine
(d) Infectious mononucleosis

107. Steroid sulfatase deficiency is seen in
(a) Ichthyosis vulgaris
(b) Lamellar ichthyosis
(c) X-linked recessive ichthyosis
(d) None of the above

108. The most common form of thyroid cancer is
(a) Papillary carcinoma
(b) Anaplastic carcinoma
(c) Follicular carcinoma
(d) Medullary carcinoma

109. Seminoma of testis has all the following tumor markers *EXCEPT*
(a) AFP
(b) hCG
(c) LDH
(d) Alkaline phosphatase

110. 'Creola bodies' in sputum are pathognomonic of
(a) Bronchial asthma
(b) Chronic bronchitis
(c) Bronchogenic carcinoma
(d) Pulmonary TB

MICROBIOLOGY

111. The string of pearl colonies on nutrient agar is produced by
(a) *Klebsiella*
(b) *Proteus*
(c) Anthracis
(d) *Salmonella*

112. Chancroid is caused by
(a) *Haemophilus ducreyi*
(b) *Yersinia pestis*
(c) Mycobacteria
(d) *B. pertussis*

113. Sabin-Feldman dye test is used to diagnose
(a) Toxoplasmosis
(b) Trypanosomiasis
(c) Trichinellosis
(d) Trichuriasis

114. Reynolds-Braude phenomenon is seen in which of the following fungus?
(a) *Cryptococcus neoformans*
(b) *C. albicans*
(c) *Geotrichum candidum*
(d) *Trichosporon*

115. Epstein-Barr virus is a
(a) Coronavirus
(b) Arbovirus
(c) Herpes virus
(d) Slow virus

116. The following is not a component of innate immunity
(a) Epithelial surfaces
(b) Antibody
(c) Lysozyme
(d) Sebum

117. **Negri bodies are commonly found in**
(a) Hippocampus
(b) Hypothalamus
(c) Medulla
(d) Midbrain

118. **"Plant penicillin" is the term used for**
(a) Organophosphorus compound
(b) Endrin
(c) Arsenious oxide
(d) Cyanide

119. **Which of the following is NOT a source of antibody diversity?**
(a) Germline repertoire
(b) Gene amplification
(c) Somatic recombination
(d) Somatic hypermutation

120. **All of the following are DNA oncogenic viruses *EXCEPT***
(a) Epstein-Barr virus
(b) Hepatitis B virus
(c) Adult T-cell leukemia/lymphoma virus
(d) Kaposi sarcoma herpesvirus

FORENSIC MEDICINE

121. **Abrasion collar is seen in fire arm injury**
(a) Entry wound only
(b) Exit wound only
(c) Both entry and exit wound
(d) None of the above

122. **Milky juice obtained by incising the leaves and stalk of the plant and fed for female infanticide**
(a) Madar juice
(b) Avanti juice
(c) Nopalea juice
(d) Rati juice

123. **Method of age estimation of adult over 21 years from the physiological age changes in each of the dental tissue is known as**
(a) Hadder's method
(b) Kpogmans method
(c) Trotter's method
(d) Gustafson's method

124. **In deep incised wounds Langers lines determine**
(a) Healing
(b) Shelving
(c) Gaping
(d) Direction

PREVENTIVE AND SOCIAL MEDICINE

125. **Crude death rate summarizes**
(a) Population and age-specific deaths
(b) Population and total deaths
(c) Population and cause of death
(d) Total death and age-specific deaths

126. **In doubtful cases, the presence of which organism confirms the fecal contamination of water?**
(a) Protozoa
(b) Yeast
(c) *Cl. perfringens*
(d) Fungi

127. **What percentage of khesari dal in diet causes lathyrism in 2–6 months?**
(a) 10%
(b) 20%
(c) 30%
(d) 73%

128. **Orthotolidine arsenite test determines**
(a) Free residual chlorine
(b) Combined chlorine
(c) Free and combined chlorine separately
(d) Free and combined chlorine together

129. **Systematic observation and recording activities carried out at intervals is**
(a) Systems analysis
(b) Input-output analysis
(c) Network analysis
(d) Work sampling

130. **Triage is**
(a) Classification of cases and treating them accordingly
(b) Treating moribund cases with higher priority
(c) Treating pediatric patients
(d) Treating geriatric patients

131. **Purpose of sentinel surveillance is**
(a) To know total number of cases
(b) Health planning

(c) Prevention of disease
(d) To know natural history of disease

132. Pyrethrum kills mosquitoes by
(a) Contact
(b) Residual action
(c) Repellent action
(d) Knockdown action

133. Antirabies vaccine is prepared from
(a) Wild virus
(b) Live attenuated virus
(c) Street virus
(d) Fixed virus

134. Immunity among a community to a particular disease is
(a) Passive immunity
(b) Humoral immunity
(c) Active immunity
(d) Herd immunity

135. Following are characteristics of an eradicable disease *EXCEPT*
(a) Persons with subclinical infection transmit the disease
(b) No known animal reservoir
(c) Highly effective vaccine available
(d) Lifelong immunity after recovery from disease

136. In epidemiology, observational studies include all *EXCEPT*
(a) Case-control studies
(b) Migration studies
(c) Randomized control studies
(d) Cohort studies

137. Which one of the statements is wrong about oral typhoid vaccine?
(a) Clinical trials in Chile and Egypt proven safety of Ty21a
(b) It contains not less than 109 viable organisms of *S. typhi*
(c) It can be administrated even in immunodeficiency persons
(d) Dosage schedule is 1 capsule on days 1, 3, 5

PSYCHIATRY

138. Which of the following symptoms are more frequent with agoraphobia?
(a) Panic attacks
(b) Adjustment problems
(c) Personality changes
(d) Depression

139. Which of the following is the range of IQ in mild mental retardations?
(a) 20–34
(b) Less than 20
(c) 35–49
(d) 50–69

140. In mental state examination on intelligence is measured by
(a) Fund of knowledge
(b) Forward and reverse
(c) Serial subtraction
(d) The degree of awareness and understanding of illness

141. Which one of the following is a Schneider's first rank symptom ?
(a) Persecutory delusion
(b) Thought insertion
(c) Loosening of association
(d) Autism

RADIOLOGY

142. Water lily sign is the radiological sign of the disease
(a) Hydatid cyst
(b) Bronchial cyst
(c) Dermoid cyst
(d) Pericardial cyst

143. The most characteristic radiographic sign in a child with leukemia is
(a) Osteosclerosis of the metaphysis
(b) Metaphyseal translucencies
(c) Periosteal reaction
(d) Osteolytic lesion

144. The most common cause of a focal expansile rib lesion is
(a) Myeloma
(b) Metastasis
(c) Histiocytosis
(d) Fibrous dysplasia

145. **Following are tumors of posterior mediastinum *EXCEPT***
(a) Neuroblastoma
(b) Ganglioneuroma
(c) Paravertebral
(d) Thymic tumor

146. **Following are tumors of posterior mediastinum *EXCEPT***
(a) Neuroblastoma
(b) Ganglioneuroma
(c) Paravertebral
(d) Thymic tumor

147. **The following are true of Cushing's disease *EXCEPT***
(a) Exuberant callus formation
(b) Osteoporosis
(c) Avascular necrosis
(d) Prognathism

148. **Cotton-wool appearance or ground-glass appearance of expanded bone is characteristic of**
(a) Fluorosis
(b) Melorheostosis
(c) Fibrous dysplasia
(d) All of the above

149. **Picture frame vertebrae is seen in**
(a) Ankylosing spondylitis
(b) Paget's disease
(c) Multiple myeloma
(d) Histiocytosis

150. **Syndesmophytes seen in ankylosing spondylitis is due to ossification of**
(a) Annulus fibrosis
(b) Anterior spinal ligament
(c) Posterior spinal ligament
(d) Interspinous ligament

ANESTHESIA

151. **Site for body temperature monitoring in patients under going GA is**
(a) Peripheries
(b) Skin
(c) Axilla
(d) Esophagus

152. **First Doc for an anaphylactic reaction is**
(a) Dexamethasone
(b) Adrenaline
(c) Hydrocortisone
(d) Dopamine

153. **Disadvantage of one of the following anesthetics is flammability**
(a) Halothane
(b) Enflurane
(c) Trichloroethylene
(d) Diethyl ether

154. **Spinal anesthesia is administered in an adult by performing LP between**
(a) C6 and C7
(b) T2 and T3
(c) L3 and L4
(d) T12 and L1

155. **What is the concentration of hyperbaric lignocaine used for SA?**
(a) 5%
(b) 10%
(c) 15%
(d) 20%

156. **What is the cardiovascular effect of spinal anesthesia?**
(a) Hypertension
(b) Hypotension
(c) Malignant hypertension
(d) Norm tension

DERMATOLOGY

157. **Erythema multiforme is most often related to**
(a) Herpes zoster infection
(b) Herpes simplex infection
(c) Molluscum contagiosum infection
(d) Human papilloma virus infection

158. **Drug-induced pemphigus is most commonly caused by**
(a) Penicillamine
(b) Phenytoin sodium
(c) Carbamazepine
(d) Penicillin

159. All the following statements regarding cutaneous anthrax are true *EXCEPT*
(a) It is often located on exposure areas
(b) The edema is brawny and non-pitting
(c) The lesions is very painful
(d) The regional lymph nodes may be enlarged

160. Shingles is the other name for
(a) Herpes simplex
(b) Varicella
(c) Herpes zoster
(d) Herpes labialis

ANATOMY, PHYSIOLOGY AND BIOCHEMISTRY

161. The following are branches of internal carotid artery *EXCEPT*
(a) Anterior cerebral artery
(b) Posterior cerebral artery
(c) Ophthalmic artery
(d) Middle cerebral artery

162. Eversion of foot is produced by
(a) Tibialis anterior
(b) Tibialis posterior
(c) Peroneus tertius
(d) Peroneus longus

163. Structure found between two layers of lesser omentum is
(a) Left gastric artery
(b) Short gastric artery
(c) Left gastroepiploic artery
(d) Right gastroepiploic artery

164. Deep circumflex iliac artery is a branch of
(a) Femoral artery
(b) Profunda femoris artery
(c) Lateral circumflex femoral artery
(d) External iliac artery

165. Vocalis muscle is a part of
(a) Thyroarytenoids
(b) Transverse arytenoids
(c) Cricothyroid
(d) Posterior cricoarytenoid

166. All the following hormones use cyclic AMP as a second messenger *EXCEPT*
(a) Glucagon
(b) Estrogen
(c) Epinephrine
(d) Luteinizing hormone

167. The amplitude of action potential in a neuron is about
(a) 125 mV
(b) 105 mV
(c) 90 mV
(d) 70 mV

168. Conduction velocity (m/s) of nerve fibers carrying fast pain is about
(a) 120
(b) 70
(c) 30
(d) 2

169. The intravesical pressure rises abruptly when the bladder volume is about
(a) 400 mL
(b) 300 mL
(c) 200 mL
(d) 100 mL

170. Peristaltic wave of small intestine is due to
(a) Extrinsic innervations
(b) Aboral orientation of VIP secreting neurons
(c) Aboral orientation of substance P secreting neurons
(d) Oral orientation of VIP secreting neurons

171. The 'C' type nerve fibers are highly susceptible to
(a) Hypoxia
(b) Pressure
(c) Local anesthesia
(d) All of the above

172. Amplitude of action potential is predominantly determined by
(a) Equilibrium potential of Na^+
(b) Equilibrium potential of K^+
(c) Equilibrium potential of Cl^+
(d) Equilibrium potential of HCO_3

173. Excitatory effects of acetylcholine are mediated by
(a) M2 receptors
(b) Nm receptors
(c) Both
(d) None

174. Which of the following is a polyamine?
(a) Histidine
(b) Spermidine
(c) Serotonin
(d) Tyramine

175. The alpha helix is an example of
(a) Primary structure of proteins
(b) Secondary structure of proteins
(c) Tertiary structure of proteins
(d) Quaternary structure of protein

176. Consumption of raw egg may lead to deficiency of
(a) Biotin
(b) Riboflavin
(c) Avidin
(d) Thiamine

177. The key regulatory enzyme of pentose phosphate pathway is positively regulated by
(a) NADH
(b) NADP
(c) ADP
(d) FADH

178. Lack of alpha oxidation of fatty acids lead to
(a) Accumulation of phytanic acid
(b) Formation of dicarboxylic acid
(c) Formation of propionic acid
(d) Oxidation of branched chain fatty acid

179. Which of the following arteries is least involved in atherosclerosis?
(a) Internal mammary
(b) Coeliac
(c) Anterior cerebral
(d) Intercostals

180. Plasticity of smooth muscle refers to
(a) Variability of tension at a given length of muscle fiber
(b) Increased force of contraction with increased length
(c) Increased force of contraction with decreased length
(d) Constancy of tension irrespective of length of muscle fiber

COMED-K 2006

ANSWERS AND EXPLANATIONS

MEDICINE

1. **Answer is a (Congenital syphilis).**
Ref: Thurlbeck's Pathology of the Lung, 2005 edition Pg 198.
http://www.ncbi.nlm.nih.gov/pmc/articles/PMC1019150/pdf/thorax00026-0013.pdf

Repeat Topic

- ***Pneumonia alba*** is also called the white lung of congenital syphilis
- See ***answer no. 51 in COMED-K 2009 answers*** for detailed table on manifestations of congenital syphilis.

2. **Answer is b (50%).**
Ref: HIV and AIDS: Basic Elements and Priorities, by S Karthikeyan, RN Bhamal, RP Tiwari, 2007 edition Pg 191.

Direct quote:

"Among those infected by *M. tuberculosis,* it is estimated that the ***lifetime risk of progression from latent to clinically active TB is about 50% (i.e. about 10 times higher) in HIV positive individuals*** as compared to the lifetime risk of 5–10% faced by their HIV negative counterparts (Harries et al 1004)".

Also *as per Park, 20th edition Pg 369:*

- ❖ HIV is the most powerful risk factor for the progression of TB infection to TB disease.
- ❖ This is substantiated by the fact that ***an HIV-positive TB infected person has a 50–60% lifetime risk of developing TB disease*** compared to an HIV-negative TB infected person, who has a 10% lifetime risk of developing TB disease.

3. **Answer is a (Hypertension).**
Ref: Evidence Based Dementia Practice, by Nawab Q, Jeffrey Kaye, 2002 edition Pg 797; GCP Mind Body Power for Active and Healthy Living, Parris M Kidd, Pg 34.

- As seen from below comprehensive table ***HTN is the only preventable risk factor among the choices given***.

Risk factors for dementia

Very likely risk factors	Likely risk factors
– Prior brain injury	– Long-term coronary heart disease
– Homozygosity of apolipoprotein E4	– Emotional stress
– Advanced age	– Smoking
– Family history of dementia or Parkinson's disease	– Pollutant solvents, herbicides, pesticides
– Down syndrome	– Nutrient deficiencies
– Alcohol abuse	– Metabolic deficits
– Depression	– HTN
– Stroke	– Underactivity (mental or physical)
– Reduced blood flow to brain	– Low-educational level
– Increased plasma homocysteine level	

4. **Answer is A (Hypokalemic hypochloremic alkalosis).**
Ref: Davidson's, 20th edition Pg 439, Fig 16.12.

- ***Protracted vomiting*** can lead to
  - ❖ ***Hypo****chloremic*
  - ❖ ***Hypo****kalemic*

- ❖ *Hyponatremic*
- ❖ ***Metabolic alkalosis.***

5. **Answer is d (Terminal broad ventricular bradycardia).**
Ref: Harrison's, 17th edition Pg 284.

- The ***earliest ECG changes = peaked T waves.***
- More severe degrees of hyperkalemia result in
  - ☐ ***Prolonged PR interval and QRS*** duration
  - ☐ ***AV conduction delay***
  - ☐ ***Loss of P waves***
  - ☐ Progressive widening of the QRS complex and merging with the T wave produces a ***sine wave pattern***
  - ☐ The *terminal event* = ***ventricular fibrillation or asystole.***

6. **Answer is a (Autosomal recessive trait).**
Ref: Harrison's, 17th edition Pg 1798.

Repeat Topic

- See ***answer no. 33 in COMED-K 2010 answers*** for detailed explanation.

7. **Answer is d (Retinopathy).**
Ref: Harrison's, 17th edition Pg 2285-86, Table 338-7.

Repeat Topic

- See flowchart in ***answer no. 1 COMED-K 2010 answers*** for detailed explanation.

8. **Answer is a (PCW > 18 cm of H_2O).**
Ref: Harrison's, 17th edition Pg 1680, Table 262-2.

- ***Acute respiratory distress syndrome (ARDS)*** is a clinical syndrome of severe dyspnea of rapid onset, hypoxemia and diffuse pulmonary infiltrates leading to respiratory failure. ARDS is caused by diffuse lung injury from many underlying medical and surgical disorders. The lung injury may be direct, as occurs in toxic inhalation or indirect, as occurs in sepsis.
- ***Edema fluid*** that is rich in protein accumulates in the interstitial and alveolar spaces. Alveolar edema predominantly involves *dependent* portions of the lung, leading to diminished aeration and atelectasis.
- The ***clinical features of ARDS*** are listed in Table below.

Diagnostic Criteria for ARDS

Oxygenation	Onset	Chest X-ray	Absence of left atrial HTN
$PaO_2/FiO_2 \leq 200$ mm Hg	Acute	Bilateral alveolar or interstitial infiltrates	PCWP ≤ 18 mm Hg *or* no clinical evidence of increased left atrial pressure

9. **Answer is c (Hypocholesteremia).**
Ref: Harrison's, 17th edition Pg 1785-86.

Features of nephrotic syndrome

- ❖ Heavy proteinuria (> 3.0 g/24 h)
- ❖ Hypertension
- ❖ Hypercholesterolemia
- ❖ Hypoalbuminemia and edema/anasarca
- ❖ Microscopic hematuria

10. **Answer is a (2 mmol/L).**
Ref: Harrison's, 17th edition Pg 2296.

- In standardized assays, the HbA1C (glycated hemoglobin) approximates the following mean plasma glucose values:
  - An A1C of 6% is 7.5 mmol/L (135 mg/dL)
  - 7% is 9.5 mmol/L (170 mg/dL)
  - 8% is 11.5 mmol/L (205 mg/dL), etc.
- [A ***1% rise in the A1C translates into a 2.0 mmol/L*** (35 mg/dL) increase in the mean glucose.]

Note:

❖ Measurement of ***glycated hemoglobin*** is the standard method for assessing long-term glycemic control.

❖ When plasma glucose is consistently elevated, there is an increase in ***non-enzymatic glycation of hemoglobin***; this alteration reflects the glycemic history over the previous 2–3 months, since erythrocytes have an average life span of ***120 days***.

11. **Answer is c (Abnormal coronary arteriogram).**
Ref: The ESC Textbook of Cardiovascular Medicine, John Camm, Thomas FL, 2006 edition Blackwell publishers Pg 417.

Features of Cardiac Syndrome X

- Angina typically on effort and severe enough to suggest IHD
- 'Ischemia-like' ST-segment depression during angina or provocation tests
- Normal coronary arteries at angiography
- Absence of epicardial arterial spasm and of known causes of microvascular dysfunction
- Excellent prognosis and no increase in risk of major cardiac events.

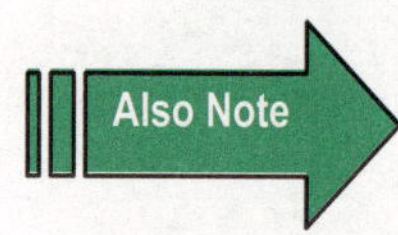

❖ The 'other (non-cardiac)' metabolic syndrome is described below.

❖ ***Metabolic syndrome*** = Insulin resistance syndrome = Syndrome X = Reaven's syndrome = all synonyms.

❖ This syndrome is strongly a/w atherosclerosis and is manifested by macrovascular disease (coronary, cerebral, peripheral) and an excess mortality.

Features of the "Metabolic Syndrome"

- Central (visceral) obesity
- Hyperinsulinemia
- Type 2 diabetes mellitus or impaired glucose tolerance
- Low HDL cholesterol; elevated triglycerides
- Hypertension
- Microalbuminuria
- Increased fibrinogen
- Increased plasminogen activator inhibitor-1
- Increased sympathetic neural activity
- Elevated plasma uric acid

12. **Answer is a (Fasciculation).**
Ref: Davidson's, 20th edition Pg 1179, Table 26.33.

UMN VS LMN LESIONS

	UMN lesions	**LMN lesions**
■ Anatomy	The corticospinal tract path extending from the brain down to but not including the anterior horn cells of the spinal cord ('CNS lesions')	Extending from the anterior horn cells of the spinal cord to the peripheral nerve ('PNS lesions')
■ Paresis	Affects upper extremity extensors more than flexors and the lower extremity flexors more than extensors	Distribution of motor neurons, dermatome and root. Affects the trunk, cord or nerves
■ Tone	↑, Spasticity	↓, Flaccidity
■ Deep tendon reflexes	↑	↓ or absent

■ Plantar reflexes	Upgoing (+ Babinski's)	Downgoing (normal)
■ Wasting/Atrophy	Absent	Present
■ Fasciculations	Absent	Present
■ Examples	Lesions in the cerebrum, basal ganglia, brainstem, cerebellum or spinal cord strokes, TIA, brain tumors, head trauma, AIDS, MS	Guillain-Barré syndrome, neuropathies, myopathies, myasthenia gravis, Bell's palsy, herpes zoster
■ Mnemonic	**Upper** MN = everything **Up** (tone, DTR, toes)	**Lower** MN = everything **lowere**d/down (tone, DTR, downgoing toes, less muscle mass)

13. **Answer is b (Cirrhosis)**
Ref: GI/Liver Secrets, by Peter R McNally, 3rd edition.

- ***Serum-ascites albumin gradient (SAAG)*** is more useful than the total protein concentration of ascetic fluid in the classification of ascites.
- This gradient is physiologically based on oncotic hydrostatic balance and is related directly to portal pressure.
- ***SAAG is calculated by*** subtracting albumin concentration of ascitic fluid from albumin concentration of serum obtained on the same day.

SAAG = albumin (serum) – albumin (ascites)

SAAG ≥ 1.1 g/dL	SAAG ≤ 1.1 g/dL
➢ ***Cirrhosis*** (MC cause) leading to ***Portal HTN*** ➢ Portal HTN from any cause (alcoholic hepatitis, cardiac ascites, massive liver metastases, fulminant hepatic failure, Budd-Chiari syndrome, portal vein thrombosis, veno-occlusive disease, myxedema, fatty liver of pregnancy, 'mixed' ascites)	➢ Normal portal pressure ➢ ***Peritoneal disease*** (peritoneal carcinomatosis—MC cause) ➢ Others—TB peritonitis, pancreatic disease, biliary ascites, nephrotic syndrome, serositis and bowel obstruction or infarction)

14. **Answer is c [(140 – age) × total body wt × 0.85/72 × Plasma CR].**
Ref: The chemotherapy sourcebook, by Micheal Clinton Perry, Pg 225.

Cockcroft-Gault equation

- It is a creatinine clearance measuring equation and hence, systematically overestimates GFR because of tubular secretion of creatinine.
- The values are not adjusted for body surface area, hence values are skewed for obese/edematous individuals.

CCr (mL/min) = (140 – age) × weight × 0.85 (if female)/(72 × Serum creatinine)

15. **Answer is a (Focal segment glomerulosclerosis).**
Ref: Harrison's, 17th edition Pg 1177.

HIV associated nephropathy (HIVAN):

- ***Early*** manifestation seen more in Africans and Hispanics, also in children
- ***Proteinuria*** is hallmark
- Edema and hypertension are ***rare***
- Diagnosis is by renal biopsy, characteristically shows ***focal segmental glomerulosclerosis***
- ***Treat with*** antiretrovirals and prednisolone.

16. **Answer is c (Fondaparinux).**
Ref: Harrison's, 17th edition Pg 721, 743; KD Tripathi, 6th edition Pg 599.

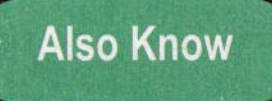

- ***Fondaparinux*** is the first ***synthetic selective factor Xa inhibitor***.
- *Fondaparinux*, which is an *exclusive factor Xa inhibitor*, compared with enoxaparin, which inhibits factors Xa and IIa in a ratio of 4:1.
- Also see ***answer no. 127 in COMED-K 2008 answers***.

17. Answer is c (Indinavir).
Ref: Harrison's, 17th edition Pg 1199.

Direct quote:

"The ***main side effects of indinavir are nephrolithiasis*** (seen in 4% of patients) and asymptomatic ***indirect hyperbilirubinemia*** (seen in 10%)".

Also Know

ANTIRETROVIRAL DRUGS (ANTI-HIV AGENTS)

1. **Nucleoside Reverse Transcriptase Inhibitors (NRTIs)**	– Drugs: Lamivudine, Emtricitabine, Abacavir, Zalcitabine, Zidovudine, Tenofovir, Didanosine, Stavudine – Mechanism: NRTIs inhibit the reverse transcriptase enzyme; prevent incorporation of viral genome into host DNA
2. **Non-nucleoside Reverse Transcriptase Inhibitors (NNRTIs)**	– Drugs: Etravirine, Delavirdine, Efavirenz, Nevirapine – Mechanism: NNRTIs inhibit the reverse transcriptase enzyme; prevent incorporation of viral genome into host DNA
3. Protease Inhibitors (PIs)	– Drugs: Saquinavir, Ritonavir, Indinavir, Nelfinavir, Amprenavir, Tipranavir, Lopinavir, Fosamprenavir, Darunavir, Atazanavir – Mechanism: Inhibit assembly of new virus by blocking protease in progeny virions
4. Fusion Inhibitors	– Drug: Enfuvirtide – Mechanism: Bind viral gp41 subunit; inhibit conformational change required for fusion with CD4 cells, therefore block entry and subsequent replication – Clinical use: In patients with persistent viral replication in spite of antiretroviral therapy; used in combination with other drugs
5. **Entry Inhibitors - CCR5 antagonists**	– Drug: Maraviroc – Mechanism: Specifically, maraviroc blocks the chemokine receptor CCR5, which HIV uses as a coreceptor to bind and enter a human helper T cell, because HIV can also use another coreceptor, CXCR4, an HIV tropism test such as a Trofile assay must be performed to determine if the drug will be effective
6. Integrase Inhibitors	– Drug: Raltegravir – Mechanism: Raltegravir inhibits integrase and prevents the integration of viral genetic material into human chromosomes—also called strand transfer inhibitors (this refers to the process of DNA strand transfer from the viral genome to the host genome); the drug is metabolized away via glucuronidation

ADVERSE EFFECTS OF ANTIRETROVIRAL DRUGS

- **Nucleoside Reverse Transcriptase Inhibitors (NRTIs):** These are associated with **lactic acidosis, hepatic steatosis and body fat redistribution (lipodystrophy)**. Most drugs need dose adjustment for renal failure.

1. **Zidovudine**	**Anemia (macrocytosis), neutropenia, skeletal and cardiac myopathy, bone marrow suppression**, GID,	Twice-daily dosing preferred over thrice-daily dosing. Fatigue, nausea, headache and myalgia usually resolve 2–4 weeks after

		hyperpigmentation of skin and nails, insomnia	initiation.
2.	**Didanosine**	**Pancreatitis**, PN, GID, dry mouth, hyperuricemia, renal failure, rash, seizures	Concomitant alcohol use may increase risk of pancreatitis.
3.	**Lamivudine**	**Headache**, rash, dry mouth, abdominal pain, pancreatitis, PN rare	Active against hepatitis B virus.
4.	**Stavudine**	**PN**, pancreatitis, dyslipidemia, diarrhea, hepatitis, neutropenia	Of the NRTIs, stavudine has greatest risk of lipodystrophy and other mitochondrial toxicity.
5.	**Emtricitabine**	**Headache, nausea**, insomnia Hyperpigmentation of palms and soles (MC in dark skinned people)	Active against hepatitis B virus.
6.	**Abacavir**	**Hypersensitivity syndrome** (can be fatal), rash, headache, GID	Risk of hypersensitivity related to certain genetic factors, particularly HLA B5701.
7.	**Tenofovir**	**Acute and chronic renal insufficiency**, Fanconi syndrome	Active against hepatitis B Gastrointestinal symptoms may be worse in lactose-intolerant patients; tenofovir is formulated with lactose.

- **Non-nucleoside Reverse Transcriptase Inhibitors (NNRTIs):** These are a/w **rash** and may cause Stevens-Johnson syndrome and toxic epidermal necrolysis. All NNRTIs may have significant interactions with other drugs; dosage adjustment of interacting agents may be required.

1.	**Delavirdine**	**Rash**, Fatigue, ↑ LFTs, hepatitis, GID	100 mg tablets can be dissolved in water. Seldom used; less potent than other NNRTIs.
2.	**Efavirenz**	↑ in LFTs, hyperlipidemia , **CNS symptoms** – abnormal dreams, drowsiness, dizziness, confusion	Teratogenic in animal studies; contraindicated during pregnancy.
3.	**Nevirapine**	Rash, ↑ LFTs, hepatitis, liver failure	Hepatotoxicity may be life-threatening. It is more common at higher CD4 cell counts in women and in patients with hepatitis B or C.

- **Protease Inhibitors:** All PIs are associated with metabolic abnormalities including **dyslipidemia, hyperglycemia, insulin resistance and body fat redistribution (lipodystrophy)**. (Atazanavir is less likely to cause dyslipidemia.); PIs may increase the risk of bleeding in hemophiliacs; PIs may have significant interactions with other drugs; dosage adjustment of interacting agents may be required.

1.	**Saquinavir**	GID, ↑ LFTs, headache, oral ulcerations	Must be used in combination with low-dose ritonavir.
2.	**Ritonavir**	GID, ↑ LFTs, fatigue, perioral paresthesia, taste perversion, hyperuricemia	Potent P-450 inhibitor; avoid combining oral solution with metronidazole or disulfiram - may cause disulfiram-like reaction.
3.	**Indinavir**	**Nephrolithiasis**, flank pain, hyperbilirubinemia, ↑ LFTs, alopecia, dry skin, ingrown nails, insomnia, taste distortion	To reduce risk of nephrolithiasis, patients should drink at least 1.5 liters of fluid daily.
4.	**Amprenavir**	GID, ↑ LFTs, rash, perioral paresthesia	May cause rash in patients sensitive to or intolerant of sulfonamides. The oral solution should not be combined with metronidazole or disulfiram; it contains propylene glycol and may cause disulfiram-like reaction.

5.	**Atazanavir**	**Hyperbilirubinemia**, jaundice, ↑ LFTs, PR interval prolongation	Proton pump inhibitors and other antacid medications and H2 blockers interfere with atazanavir absorption and are contraindicated/should be used with caution for use by patients receiving atazanavir.
6.	**Fosamprenavir**	GID, ↑ LFTs, rash	Prodrug of amprenavir. May cause rash in patients sensitive to or intolerant of sulfonamides.
7.	**Lopinavir/ ritonavir**	GID, dyslipidemia, ↑ LFTs, taste perversion, perioral paresthesia	Oral solution contains 42% alcohol. Avoid combining oral solution with metronidazole or disulfiram – cause disulfiram-like reaction.
8.	**Tipranavir**	Intracranial hemorrhage , GID, ↑ LFTs, rash	Must be coadministered with ritonavir; should never be used without ritonavir boosting.

- **Fusion Inhibitors**

1.	**Enfuvirtide**	Injection site reactions: erythema, cysts and nodules at injection sites; neutropenia, ↑ frequency of bacterial pneumonia	Requires extensive patient counseling on injection technique, adherence and management of possible side effects.

- **Chemokine Coreceptor Antagonists**

1.	**Maraviroc**	GID, ↑ LFTs, hepatitis, **nasopharyngitis**, fatigue, dizziness, headache, joint pain, muscle pain	Many drug-drug interactions; dose adjustment needed with many other antiretrovirals and/or other medications.

- **Integrase Inhibitors**

1.	**Raltegravir**	**GID**, ↑ in amylase and LFTs, headache, dizziness, abnormal dreams, pruritus, **rash**, fatigue, muscle pain	

Key: GID = Gastrointestinal distress, PN = Peripheral neuropathy, LFT = Liver function tests, CNS = Central nervous system.

18. Answer is a (4–6 cm²).
Ref: Harrison's, 17th edition Pg 1465.

❖ *Normal* area of the mitral valve orifice	= 4–6 cm^2 (in normal adults)
❖ *Significant* obstruction	= orifice area is reduced to < ~2 cm^2
❖ "*Severe*" stenosis	= orifice area is reduced to < 1 cm^2

19. Answer is c (Staphylococci).
Ref: CMDT 2013, Pg 1435.

- **Author's comments**: "The question should have asked you about "infective endocarditis and not RHD since we know that RHD is an immune phenomenon following streptococcal pharyngitis"
- ***Staphylococcus aureus*** is the MC cause of ***native valve endocarditis*** (both community acquired and healthcare associated).
- *Streptococcus viridans* causes endocarditis usually on *prosthetic valves in late cases (> 2 months); IN early cases* (< 2 *months),* ***Staphylococcus aureus is till the MC cause.***

20. Answer is d (Cardiac failure).
Ref: Harrison's, 17th edition Pg 1658, Davidson's, 20th edition Pg 664.

Must Know

	Transudative pleural effusion	Exudative pleural effusion
Mechanism	Due to either increased hydrostatic pressure or decreased osmotic pressure—due to systemic factors	Increased microvascular pressure due to disease of the pleura itself or injury in the adjacent lung—local factors
Causes	Left ventricular failure Cirrhosis and nephrosis	TB Bacterial pneumonia Malignancy Viral infection Pulmonary infarction/embolism

21. Answer is d (MS).
Ref: Harrison's, 17th edition Pg 1008.

Risk factors for active TB among persons who have been infected with TB bacilli

- Recent infection (< 1 year)
- Fibrotic lesions (spontaneously healed)
- Comorbidity
  - HIV infection
  - Silicosis
  - Chronic renal failure/hemodialysis
  - Diabetes
  - Intravenous drug use
  - Immunosuppressive treatment
  - Gastrectomy
  - Jejunoileal bypass
  - Post-transplantation period (renal, cardiac)
- Malnutrition and severe underweight

22. Answer is b (Cardiomyopathies).
Ref: Park, 20th edition Pg 317.

Manifestations of coronary heart disease

- Angina pectoris on effort
- Myocardial infarction
- Irregularities of the heart
- Cardiac failure
- Sudden death

23. Answer is a (> 1.0).
Ref: Cardiology Secrets, 2nd edition 2001, Pg 106.

- ***Lactate dehydrogenase*** **(LDH)** rises in ***acute MI*** beginning at 25–48 hours, peaking in 3–5 days and normalizing in 10 days.
- A ratio of isoenzymes ***LDH1/LDH2 of > 1.0 is sensitive for MI***.

24. Answer is d (Platelet).
Ref: Harrison's, 17th edition Pg 366.

- ***Mucosal bleeding symptoms*** are more suggestive of ***underlying platelet disorders*** or von Willebrand disease (vWD), termed *disorders of primary hemostasis or platelet plug formation*.
- ***Spontaneous hemarthroses*** are a hallmark of moderate and severe ***factors VIII and IX deficiency,*** and in rare circumstances of other clotting factor deficiencies.

25. Answer is a (Demeclocycline).
Ref: Harrison's, 17th edition Pg 2223.

- In ***chronic, persistent SIADH***, the hyponatremia can be corrected by treatment with ***demeclocycline or fludrocortisone***.
- The effect of the demeclocycline manifests in 7–14 days and is *due to production of a reversible form of nephrogenic DI.*
- Potential side effects include *phototoxicity and azotemia*.

SURGERY

26. Answer is d (Isolated esophageal varices present).
Ref: Essentials of General Surgery, Peter Lawrence, 4th edition Pg 374.

- ***Left sided (sinistral) portal hypertension*** is an uncommon, but relatively straightforward cause of portal hypertension.
- In this disorder, ***thrombosis of the splenic vein*** (usually caused by ***pancreatitis*** or ***pancreatic tumor***) leads to increased pressure in the spleen which cause splenomegaly and secondary hypersplenism.
- Another consequence of this disorder is the development of ***isolated gastric varices confined to the upper part of the stomach***, because of the return of splenic flow to the portal vein through the short gastrics, the submucosal veins of the stomach and the coronary vein.
- ***Splenectomy*** cures this compartmentalized form of portal hypertension.

27. Answer is b (F IIa).
Ref: General Surgery, Principles and International Practice, Vol 1, Kirby I Bland, 2008 edition Pg 535, Table 50-1.

Forrest Classification Of Upper GI Hemorrhage/Bleeding peptic ulcer

Acute hemorrhage	
F Ia	Arterial, spurting hemorrhage
F Ib	Oozing hemorrhage, non-spurting
Signs of recent hemorrhage	
F IIa; **g = vessel < 2 mm; G= vessel > 2 mm**	Non-bleeding "visible vessel"
F IIb	Adherent overlying clot
F IIc	Hematin covered lesion
Lesions without active bleeding	
F III	Clean ulcer base with No signs of recent hemorrhage

<u>**Author's Comments**</u>: *"The question should probably have been "non-bleeding visible vessel" since me mention of "bleeding visible vessel" is there in the classification".*

28. **Answer is a (Ductal carcinoma in situ).**
Ref: Robbin's 7th edition Pg 1139.

- Historically, ***ductal carcinoma in situ*** (intraductal carcinoma) has been divided into five architectural subtypes: ***comedocarcinoma***, solid, cribriform, papillary and micropapillary.
- ***Comedocarcinoma*** is characterized by solid sheets of pleomorphic cells with high grade nuclei and central necrosis.
- The necrotic cell membranes commonly calcify and are detected on mammography as clusters of linear and branching microcalcifications.

29. **Answer is b (Transhiatal esophagectomy).**
Ref: Bailey and Love, 25th edition Pg 1034.

- **Transhiatal esophagectomy (without thoracotomy):** This technique was popularized by ***Orringer*** in USA and ***Pinotti*** in Brazil.

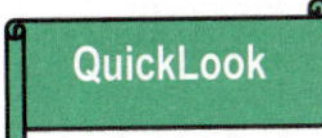

Few named surgeries

Surgery/Surgeon name	Performed for
Heller's myotomy	Achalasia cardia
Thiersch's, Delorome's, Altemier's operation	Full thickness prolapse of the rectum
Lord's and Jaboulay's	Hydrocele
Whipple's	Pancreaticoduodenectomy for Ca head of pancreas
Billroth I and II	Gastrectomy for peptic ulcers
Kasai procedure	Extrahepatic biliary atresia, type 2 and 3
Notaras	Lateral anal sphincterotomy for anal fissure

30. **Answer is d (Diagnosis is by fine needle aspiration).**
Ref: Bailey and Love, 25th edition Pg 780, 794-95.

- ***FNAC*** is investigation of choice in discrete thyroid swellings. Thyroid conditions that may be diagnosed by FNAC include colloid nodules, thyroiditis, ***papillary carcinoma, medullary carcinoma, anaplastic carcinoma*** and ***lymphoma***. FNAC cannot distinguish between benign follicular adenoma and follicular carcinoma, as this distinction is dependant not on cytology, but on histologic criteria, which include capsular and vascular invasion.
- ***Papillary carcinoma*** spreads to ***lymph nodes*** more commonly (35%).
- ***Vascular invasion*** is more common in ***follicular carcinoma*** (60%).
- Younger patients, ***age < 45 years*** at presentation have ***better prognosis***.

31. **Answer is c (Scaleneus medius).**
Ref: Chaurasia BD, Vol 3, Pg 168.

- ***Vertebral artery*** arises from the ***subclavian artery***.
- Vertebral artery has four parts:
  - ***First part***: Extends from the origin to the transverse process of 6th cervical vertebra. This part of the artery runs upwards and backwards in the triangular space between the ***scalenus anterior and longus colli*** muscles.
  - ***Second part***: Runs through the foramina tranverarium of upper 6th cervical vertebra.
  - ***Third part***: Lies in the suboccipital triangle.
  - ***Fourth part***: It extends from the posterior atlantooccipital membrane to the lower border of pons.

32. **Answer is d (Buccal branch of facial nerve).**
Ref: Bailey and Love, 25th edition Pg 758-59.

- Three ***cranial nerves are at risk during removal of the submandibular*** gland
  - Marginal mandibular branch of facial nerve
  - Lingual nerve
  - Hypoglossal nerve.

33. Answer is a (Allograft).
Ref: Textbook of Microbiology, CP Baveja, 3rd edition Pg 163.

TYPES OF GRAFTS

Autograft	From self
Syngeneic graft /Isograft	From identical twin or clone (i.e. genetically identical with recipient)
Allograft /Homograft	From non-identical member of same species
Xenograft	From different species

34. Answer is d (Dorsum of PIP joint).
Ref: Oxford Handbook of Clinical Surgery, 3rd edition Pg 542.

Extraplanar manifestations of Dupuytren's contracture:
- Garrod's pads: Thickening over dorsal aspect of PIPs
- Peyronie's disease: Thickened plaques in shaft of tibia
- Ledderhose's disease: Thickened plantar fascia, but no contractures

35. Answer is b (Endoscopic choledocholithotomy).
Ref: Bailey and Love's 25th edition Pg 1126 and Fig 63.34.

- ***Endoscopic papillotomy*** is the ***preferred first technique with sphincterotomy*** for removal of CBD stone using a Dormia basket or the placement of a stent if stone removal is not possible.
- If this technique fails, percutaneous transhepatic cholangiography can be performed to provide drainage and subsequent percutaneous choledochoscopy.
- Surgery in the form of ***choledochotomy, is now rarely used*** for this situation, as most patients can be managed by minimally invasive techniques.

36. Answer is c (Extrahepatic tumor).
Ref: *Bailey and Love, 24th edition Pg 1180-81.*

Must Know

☐ **Liver-general**	Largest **gland** in the body, weighs 1.5 kg, covered by a fibrous capsule – **Glisson's** capsule.
☐ **Anatomical lobes of liver**	4 lobes, right (largest), left, caudate and quadrate. Riedel's lobe is a tongue-shaped projection from the right lobe.
☐ **Surgical lobes of the liver**	The right and left are separated by a plane connecting the gallbladder and inferior vena cava.
☐ **Couinaud's segments**	8 functional segments of liver are present, each demarcated by the vascular and biliary drainage (based on the position of the hepatic veins and biliary ducts).
☐ **Blood flow to the liver**	Is **1,500 mL/min,** of this 75% of afferent blood is conveyed by **portal vein** and **25%** is conveyed by **hepatic artery**.
☐ **Bare area of the liver**	A triangular area devoid of peritoneal covering, it is limited by the upper and lower layers of the coronary ligament and the triangular ligament, clinically important because it represents a site where infection can spread from the abdominal cavity to the thoracic cavity.
☐ **Morrison's pouch**	Hepatorenal pouch, right subhepatic space is the **commonest site** of **subphrenic** abscess.
☐ **Porta hepatis contains**	Right and left hepatic ducts Right and left branches of hepatic artery Portal vein Hepatic lymph nodes.

☐ **Sinusoids of liver**	Irregular "capillaries" with fenestrated endothelium (pores 100–200 nm in diameter). No basement membrane. Allow macromolecules of plasma full access to basal surface of hepatocytes through perisinusoidal space (Space of Disse).
☐ **Space of Disse**	Contain cells of Ito (vitamin A synthesis) and Kupffer cells (liver macrophages) Apical surface of hepatocytes faces bile canaliculi. Basolateral surface faces sinusoids.
☐ **Portal acinus**	Is divided into 3 zones Zone 1—periportal zone—affected 1st by viral hepatitis Zone 2—intermediate zone Zone 3—pericentral vein (centrilobular) zone: contains P 450 system, affected 1st by ischemia, most susceptible to toxic injury, alcoholic hepatitis.

37. Answer is c (Thymic tumor).

Ref: Robbins Pathology, 7th edition Pg 707; Bailey and Love, 25th edition Pg 892.

- ***Thymoma*** is the commonest tumor of the anterior mediastinum and is locally invasive in 30–50% of cases
- ***Thymoma*** is also the most common mediastinal tumor accounting for ***25% of the total***.

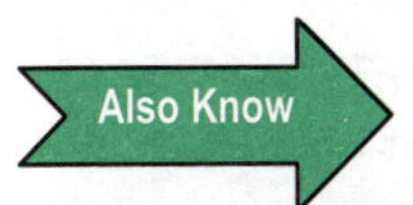

Anterior mediastinum	Middle mediastinum	Posterior mediastinum
– Thymic tumor – Retrosternal goiter – Pericardial cyst – Germ cell tumor	– Lymphoma – Cystic (bronchogenic cyst and pericardial cyst) – Mesenchymal tumor	– Neurogenic tumors (ganglioneuroma, neuroblastoma, pheochromocytoma) – Paravertebral abscess – Esophageal lesion

38. Answer is a (AR trait).

Ref: Harrison's, 17th edition Pg 1798.

Repeat Topic

- See ***answer no. 33 in COMED-K 2010 answers*** for detailed explanation.

39. Answer is b (Low investment of tunica vaginalis).

Ref: Bailey and Love, 25th edition Pg 1379.

Predisposing factors for testicular torsion:

❖ Inversion of testis (MC)
❖ High investment of tunica vaginalis
❖ Separation of epididymis from body of testis.

Difference Between Testicular Torsion and Epididymitis

	Testicular torsion	Epididymitis
Age	10–25 years (usually prepubertal)	> 30 years
Appearance	Testes may be elevated into the inguinal canal; swelling	Swollen testis, overlying erythema, urethral discharge/urethritis, prostatitis
Prehn's sign	Pain stays the same or worsens	Pain decreases with testicular elevation
Treatment	Immediate surgery to salvage testis; surgical orchiopexy for both testis	Antibiotics (co-trimoxazole or ciprofloxacin)

40. Answer is a (Giant folds in pyloric antrum).

Ref: Harrison's, 17th edition Pg 1871; Current Diagnosis and Treatment, Surgery, 2009, Pg 505.

Ménétrier's disease (Hypertrophic gastritis):

- ***Giant hypertrophy*** of gastric ***rugae prominently in body and fundus.***
- High, normal or low acid secretion.
- Excessive loss of protein from the thickened mucosa into the gut → ***hypoproteinemia (hypoalbuminemia) and edema, diarrhea, anorexia, weight loss, skin rash and chronic blood loss*** *may also occur.*
- Histologically, ***massive foveolar hyperplasia*** (hyperplasia of surface and glandular mucous cells) is noted, which replaces most of the chief and parietal cells. This hyperplasia produces the prominent folds observed.
- Etiology: Altered expression of ***TNF alpha***.
- Medical treatment: Antacids, atropine (for protein leak).
- Surgery indicated for severe intractable hypoproteinemia, anemia or to rule out cancer.
- ***Increased risk of adenocarcinoma*** of stomach in adults with Ménétrier's disease.

41. Answer is c (Invasion into loose connective tissue of papillary dermis).
Ref: http://www.cancer.gov/cancertopics/pdq/treatment/melanoma/HealthProfessional/page3

Clark's Classification of malignant melanoma (anatomic level of invasion)

- Level I: Lesions involving only the epidermis (in situ melanoma); not an invasive lesion
- Level II: Invasion of the papillary dermis, but does not reach the papillary-reticular dermal interface
- Level III: Invasion fills and expands the papillary dermis, but does not penetrate the reticular dermis
- Level IV: Invasion into the reticular dermis but not into the subcutaneous tissue
- Level V: Invasion through the reticular dermis into the subcutaneous tissue.

42. Answer is a (Low-grade malt lymphoma).
Ref: Davidson's, 20th edition Pg 785, 791.

Indications for *H. pylori* Eradication		
Definite	Not indicated	Uncertain
Peptic ulcer (duodenal and gastric ulcer) MALToma	Asymptomatic Gastroesophageal reflux disease	Family history of gastric Ca Non-ulcer dyspepsia Long-term NSAID users

43. Answer is a (Hematuria).
Ref: Harrison's 17th edition Pg 592; Bailey and Love, 25th edition Pg 1310.

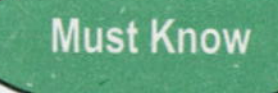

Renal Cell Carcinoma (RCC) – (syn: *Hypernephroma, Grawitz Tumor)*

• *Risk factors* ➢ Cigarette smoking ➢ Acquired cystic disease of the kidney a/w end stage renal disease ➢ Tuberous sclerosis ➢ Polycystic kidney disease ➢ von-Hippel-Lindau disease	• ***M:F = 2:1*** • ***Originates from proximal tubule cells*** • ***MC adenocarcinoma*** • ***MC*** occurs at the ***upper pole of kidney***

- 5 variants are clear cell tumors (75%); chromophilic tumors; chromophobic tumors; oncocytic tumors and collecting duct or Bellini duct tumors.

Clinical features	Paraneoplastic syndromes
• ***Hematuria (40%)*** • Flank ***pain (40%)*** • Flank ***mass (25%)***	• Erythrocytosis • Hypercalcemia • ***Stauffer's syndrome***: Non-metastatic reversible

• ***Fever (20%)*** • Weight loss • ***Anemia*** • ***Varicocele—left*** sided *(as left renal vein is more often compressed)*	hepatic dysfunction • Acquired dysfibrinogenemia • Nephrotic syndrome

- Spread: It is ***prone to grow into the renal vein***; may also be seen in the lungs as ***cannonball metastases***.
- ***CT scanning*** is the ***most valuable*** imaging test for renal cell carcinoma. It confirms the character of the mass and further stages the lesion with respect to regional lymph nodes, renal vein or hepatic involvement. It also gives valuable information on the contralateral kidney (function, bilaterality of neoplasm).
- *MRI and duplex Doppler ultrasonography* are excellent methods of assessing for the presence and extent of tumor thrombus within the renal vein or vena cava in selected patients.

- **Robson system** is used for staging renal cell carcinoma.
  - ***Stage I***: Tumors are confined to the kidney
  - ***Stage II***: Tumors extend through the renal capsule but are confined by Gerota's fascia
  - ***Stage III***: Tumors involve the renal vein or vena cava (stage IIIA) or the hilar lymph nodes (stage IIIB)
  - ***Stage IV***: Tumors that are locally invasive to adjacent organs (excluding the adrenal gland) or distant metastases

- The standard management for stage I and stage II tumors and selected cases of stage III disease is radical nephrectomy.
- Responds poorly to chemotherapy and radiotherapy; ***Vinblastine*** is the single most effective agent, with short-term partial response rates of 15%. Alpha ***interferon*** and ***interleukin-2*** have shown promising results.
- RCC is one of the several tumors in which ***spontaneous regressions*** *have been reported anecdotally*.

Note:
- ***Bellini duct carcinomas*** are *very rare*; believed to arise from collecting ducts in renal medulla; affect *younger patients* and have a *very aggressive* clinical course.

44. Answer is c (Splenic flexure).
Ref: Bailey and love, 25th edition Pg 1202; http://www.emedmag.com/html/pre/gic/consults/041504.asp

Acute colonic pseudo-obstruction is called ***Ogilvie's syndrome***.
- Diagnosis of ***Ogilvie's syndrome*** is made based upon the presentation of massive dilatation of colon usually predominantly the right and transverse colon.
- The right colon is distended with cutoff at the splenic flexure.

45. Answer is c (Gemcitabine).
Ref: Harrison's, 17th edition Pg 588-89.

- ***Advanced Pancreatic Cancer***: These patients have metastatic or locally advanced inoperable disease and are the majority with newly diagnosed disease.
- Debulking surgery or partial resections have no role, as these procedures are associated with the same risks as a curative resection, but are unlikely to improve survival.
- The deoxycytidine analogue gemcitabine, given as a single agent has been the preferred treatment for these patients since it was shown to yield clinical benefit (a composite parameter for evaluating symptomatic benefit of treatment used in some trials of this disease) and improved survival compared to 5- fluorouracil.

46. Answer is c (Landing).
Ref: http://news.rediff.com/report/2010/may/22/one-in-every-four-air-crashes-was-during-landing.html

Author's comments: "Couldn't find a routine medical textbook reference for this, however following the recent aircraft crash in Mangalore, the above internet link posted an article, which clearly gives the answer—read this article if you are interested".

OBSTETRICS AND GYNECOLOGY

47. Answer is d (Umbilical cord compression).
Ref: Dutta's Obstetrics, 6th edition Pg 110.

- Decelerations of fetal heart rate and their relationship to uterine contractions may be indicative of normal activity during labor or fetal distress.

Type of fetal heart rate decelerations

Type of deceleration	Description	Cause/Treatment
1. EArly decelerations	Deceleration begins and ends with uterine contractions	Due to fetal *hEAd compression* (no fetal distress), no treatment required
2. Late decelerations	Deceleration begins after uterine contraction and persist until after the contraction has finished	Indicates *fetal hypoxia* and chronic *uteroplacental insufficiency*. If late decelerations are recurrent, immediate delivery is necessary
3. Variable decelerations	Inconsistent onset, duration and degree of decelerations	Due to *umbilical cord compression*. Change the mothers position

48. Answer is a (Chromosomal aberrations).
Ref: Dutta's Obstetrics, 6th edition Pg 158-59.

- ***Spontaneous abortion*** (miscarriage) is the expulsion or extraction from its mother of an embryo or fetus weighing ***500 g or less*** when it is not capable of independent survival (WHO).
- 75% abortions occur before the 16th week and of these, 75% occur before the 8th week of pregnancy.
- ***Majority (50%) of spontaneous abortions*** are due to ***chromosomal abnormality*** in the conceptus (autosomal trisomy 16 is commonest).

49. Answer is d (Esophageal atresia).
Ref: Dutta's Obstetrics, 6th edition Pg 218.

Oligohydramnios	Polyhydramnios
❖ < 200 mL of amniotic fluid at term	❖ > 2 L of amniotic fluid
❖ Amniotic fluid index (AFI) ≤ 5 cm on U/S	❖ AFI ≥ 25 cm on U/S
❖ A/w – Fetal urinary tract abnormalities (bilateral renal agenesis, polycystic kidneys, posterior urethral valves) and resultant inability to excrete urine. – Drugs: PG inhibitors, ACE inhibitors – Fetal chromosomal anomalies – Intrauterine infection – IUGR a/w placental insufficiency – Amnion nodosum – Postmaturity – Can give rise to Potter's syndrome	❖ A/w anencephaly; open spina bifida; esophageal/duodenal atresia; hydrops fetalis due to Rh isoimmunization; cardiothoracic anomalies and fetal cirrhosis
❖ Complications: Cord compression → fetal hypoxia; IUGR, pulmonary hypoplasia, musculoskeletal abnormalities (clubfoot)	❖ Complications: Preterm labor, abruptio placentae, fetal malposition, cord prolapse

50. Answer is b (Android pelvis).
Ref: Dutta's Obstetrics, 6th edition Pg 346.

- The ***android*** or male type of pelvis.
  - The inlet is wedge-shaped with convergent side walls
  - The ischial spines are prominent
  - The subpubic arch is narrowed
  - The sacrum is inclined anteriorly in its lower third.
- The android pelvis is associated with ***persistent occiput posterior position*** and ***deep transverse arrest***.

51. Answer is c (Retained placental bits).
Ref: Dutta's Obstetrics, 6th edition Pg 418.

- ***Secondary postpartum hemorrhage***: Bleeding occurs beyond 24 hours postpartum and within puerperium usually, between 8th–14th day after delivery. Causes are:
  - ***Retained bits*** of cotyledon or membrane (***commonest***)
  - Infection and separation of slough over a deep cervicovaginal laceration
  - Endometritis and subinvolution of the placental site—delayed healing
  - Secondary hemorrhage from C/S wound.

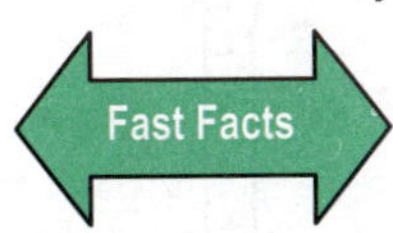

- ***Primary postpartum hemorrhage***: Occurs within 24 hours of birth of baby. Causes are given below.
- ***Atonic (commonest)***:
  - Grand multipara
  - Overdistension of uterus (large baby, multiple pregnancy, hydramnios)
  - Malnutrition and anemia
  - Antepartum hemorrhage
  - Prolonged labor
  - Anesthesia
  - Oxytocin usage
  - Persistent uterine distension
  - Uterine malformations
  - Uterine fibroids
  - Mismanaged third stage of labor
  - Constriction ring
  - Precipitate labor
- Traumatic (20%)
- Mixed (atonic + traumatic)
- Blood coagulation disorders.

52. Answer is d (Occipitotransverse).
Ref: Dutta's Obstetrics, 6th edition Pg 580.

Contraindications for ventouse delivery
- Any presentation other than vertex (face, brow, breech); mentotransverse is a type of face presentation and hence a contraindication for ventouse
- Preterm fetus (< 34 weeks); chance of scalp avulsion or aponeurotic hemorrhage
- Suspected fetal coagulation disorder
- Suspected fetal macrosomia (≥ 4 kg).

53. Answer is b (Androgen insensitivity syndrome).
Ref: Shaw's Gynecology, 14th edition Pg 100.

Direct quote:

"Chromosomal study reveals ***XY chromosomes and Barr bodies are absent*** (in testicular feminizing syndrome or androgen insensitivity syndrome)."

- ***Female phenotype, testes present*** (often abdominally), ***ovaries absent, uterus absent, blind vagina.***
- Remove testes, rear as female, vaginoplasty needed.

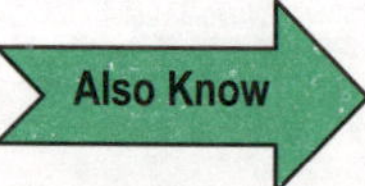

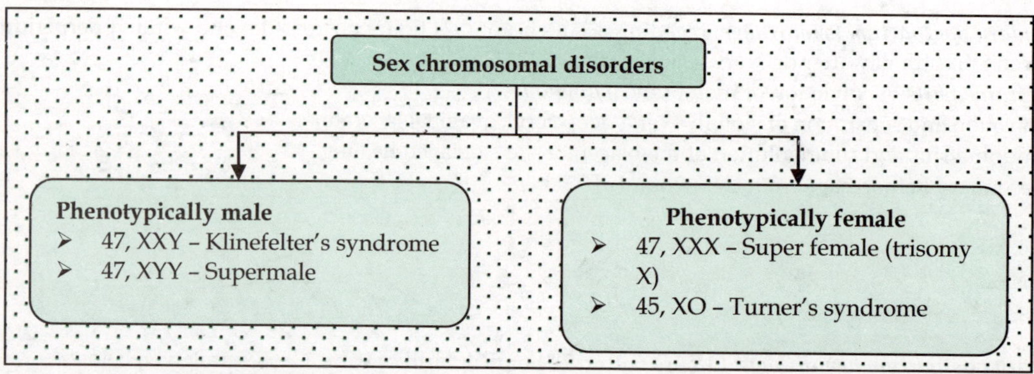

54. Answer is a (Gardnerella vaginosis).
Ref: Shaw's Gynecology, 14th edition Pg 117-18.

Repeat Topic

- See ***answer no. 51 in COMED-K 2010 answers*** for detailed explanation.

55. Answer is a (Theca cell tumor).
Ref: Shaw's Gynecology, 14th edition Pg 340, Fig 28.12.

- ***Theca cell tumor*** usually arises after menopause.
- It is nearly always unilateral and forms a solid mass.
- The tumor is ***intensely estrogenic*** and causes *postmenopausal hemorrhage* – effect on the endometrium closely resembled that of *metropathia hemorrhagica – cystic glandular hyperplasia.*
- It has been shown that both granulosa cell tumors and theca cell tumors may show luteinization of their cells with the result that progesterone is secreted and secretory hypertrophy can be demonstrated in the endometrium.

56. Answer is c (Clear cell adenocarcinoma).
Ref: Shaw's Gynecology, 14th edition Pg 357.

Direct quote:

"An unusual tumor, clear cell adenocarcinoma was seen in younger women who were themselves exposed to diethylstilbestrol (DES) in utero."

57. Answer is d (14–16 weeks of gestation).
Ref: Dutta's Obstetrics, 6th edition Pg 642.

- ***Amniocentesis*** is the deliberate puncture of the amniotic fluid sac per abdomen.

☐ **Indications**

■ ***Diagnostic***

❖ Early months (14–16 weeks): For antenatal diagnosis of chromosomal and genetic disorders
  - Sex-linked disorders
  - Inborn errors of metabolism
  - Karyotyping
  - Neural tube defects

- ❖ Later months
  - Fetal maturity
  - Degree of fetal Hb in Rh sensitized mother
  - Meconium staining of liquor: as e/o fetal distress
  - Amniography or fetography
- ■ ***Therapeutic***
- ❖ First half:
  - Induction of abortion
  - Repeated decompression of uterus in acute hydramnios
- ❖ Second half:
  - Amnioinfusion.

58. Answer is c (Liver).
Ref: Robbins Pathology, 7th edition Pg 826; Shaw's Gynecology, 14th edition Pg 381.

- **Krukenberg tumors** are secondary growths in the ovary and ***most commonly arise from a primary Ca of the stomach (70%)***, large bowel (15%), breast (6%), pancreas or gallbladder (*Robbins/7th/826*).
- **Krukenberg tumor** should be diagnosed ONLY if it conforms to the following pattern:
  - ❖ Almost always ***bilateral***
  - ❖ ***Smooth surfaces,*** which may be slightly bossed and these are ***freely movable in the pelvis***
  - ❖ ***NO tendency to form adhesions*** with neighboring viscera and ***NO infiltration through the capsule***
  - ❖ Tumor ***retains the shape of the normal ovary*** and has a peculiar solid waxy consistency although cystic spaces due to degeneration of the growth are common
  - ❖ Histologically the tumor has a cellular or myxomatous stroma against which are scattered numerous ***large signet ring cells.***
  - ❖ The tumors almost certainly arise by ***retrograde lymphatic spread.***

PEDIATRICS

59. Answer is a (20 weeks of fetal life).
Ref: Rudolph Pediatrics, 22nd edition. Pg 236; Respiratory Care Sciences: An Integrated Approac, By William W, Pg 503.

- ***Synthesis and storage of surfactant*** *begins at about 16 weeks' gestation*, and lung homogenates have high concentrations of surfactant by ***20 weeks***.
- Various other textbooks also mention 20 weeks as the answer… however the answer key in 2006 in previous edition gave "26 weeks" as the answer. IN case this question gets repeated the above references should be handy for you to challenge this question.

60. Answer is d (Vitamin C deficiency).
Ref: OP Ghai, 7th edition Pg 91.

- ***Scurvy (Barlow's disease)*** occurs due to ***vitamin C deficiency***
- Onset at 6 months to 2 years; rare in adults
- In infants: anorexia, diarrhea, irritability, increased susceptibility to infections
- ***Subperiosteal hemorrhages*** and ***long bone tenderness*** (***pseudoparalysis of lower extremities***) can occur
- In older children—*bleeding of gums, conjunctiva and GIT.*

Radiology of scurvy:

- ❖ Earliest signs are seen at the knees.
- ❖ ***Wimberger's line/ring***: Sclerotic ring around epiphysis indicating loss of epiphyseal density.
- ❖ Dense zone of provisional calcification due to excessive calcification of osteoid—↑ density at the ends of long bones seen as ***"white line of Frenkel"***.
- ❖ Zone of rarefaction proximal to white line (most important sign) —***Trummerfeld zone***—metaphyseal lucency.

- *Pelkan spur*: Metaphyseal corner fractures through the weakened lucent metaphysis.
- Ground glass appearance of shaft of diaphysis.
- Periosteal reaction due to subperiosteal hematoma.
- *Osteoporosis* (usually the only sign seen in *adults*).

61. Answer is c (Initial resolution of symptoms of heart failure).
Ref: Nelson's, 17th edition Pg 1508, 1509; Perloff's Congenital Heart Disease, 4th edition Pg 402, 406.

- In *VSD*, the pulmonary vascularity and heart size decreases when pulmonary resistance exceeds the systemic levels with reversal of shunt, a condition known as ***Eisenmenger's complex***.
- During this phase, the patient will have ***improvement in his clinical symptoms*** with rest and digitalis.

62. Answer is c (Chromosomal abnormality).
Ref: http://emedicine.medscape.com/article/947504-overview

- ***Noonan syndrome*** occurs in either a ***sporadic or autosomal dominant*** fashion.
- In either case, ***males and females are equally affected***.
- Cardinal features of Noonan syndrome include:
  - Unusual ***facies*** (i.e. hypertelorism, down-slanting eyes, webbed neck)
  - ***Congenital heart disease*** (in 50% – stenotic pulmonic valve, atrial septal defect, HOCM)
  - ***Short stature*** (80%)
  - Chest deformity
  - Mental retardation (25%)
  - Bleeding diathesis.

63. Answer is d (Aminoglycosides).
Ref: Dutta's Obstetrics, 6th edition Pg 512; KD Tripathi, 6th edition Pg 689.

- ***Aminoglycosides*** are contraindicated in pregnancy and lactation due to risk of fetal and neonatal ***ototoxicity***.

<u>Note</u>:
- Although quinolones are known to cause cartilage damage in animal studies, ***ciprofloxacin has been safely administered to millions of children*** in India.

Other drugs having effect on fetus due to transfer through breast milk are:
- ***Chloramphenicol***: ***Gray baby*** syndrome (peripheral vascular collapse)
- ***Tetracyclines***: Dental ***yellow*** discoloration and deformity; inhibition of bone growth
- Long acting ***sulfonamides***: ***Neonatal hemolysis***, jaundice, kernicterus
- ***Nitrofurantoin***: Hemolysis ***in newborn with G-6 PD deficiency*** is used at term.

64. Answer is b (4 months).
Ref: Nelson's 17th edition Pg 158.

- I feel options should be in months and NOT in weeks – however, I have given the correct answer below.
- The iron content of breast milk is somewhat low.
- However, most normal infants have sufficient iron stores for the first 6 months of life.
- Moreover, human milk iron is well-absorbed.
- Nonetheless, ***by 4–6 months of age***, the breastfed infants diet should be ***supplemented with iron*** fortified complementary foods or ferrous iron preparation.

65. Answer is d (Cry).
Ref: OP Ghai, 7th edition Pg 97, 107.

APGAR SCORE

	0	1	2
Appearance (Color)	Blue or pale	Body pink, extremities blue	Pink

Pulse (Heart rate)	0	< 100	> 100
Grimace to catheter in nose (Reflex stimulation)	No response	Grimace	Cries, coughs or sneezes
Activity (Muscle tone)	Flaccid	Some flexion	Actively moving extremities
Respiratory *effort (not rate)*	0	Slow irregular	Good crying

- Normal APGAR score = 8–10 at minute after birth; < 7 indicates asphyxia.

66. Answer is D (Throat swab).

Ref: Nelson's, 17th edition Pg 835.

- Several rapid antigen detection tests for bacterial pathogens are commercially available and widely used.
- These include latex agglutination (LA test), for detection of group A streptococci in pharynx and *H. influenzae;* group B streptococci and *N. meningitidis* in ***CSF***.
- Routinely performed LA test on CSF is expensive and offers no advantage over properly performed Gram stain.
- Their use is best reserved for patients with CSF pleocytosis who have received antibiotics.
- A rapid and sensitive test for the detection of *Streptococcus pneumoniae* antigen in ***urine*** of patients with invasive pneumococcal disease has become available in USA.
- A major limitation of the urine test is that approximately half of all well-children who are nasopharyngeal carriers of pneumococci also test positive.

67. Answer is c (Sex determine in a region on 'Y' chromosome).

Ref: Ganong, 23rd edition Pg 395-96, Fig. 25-6 and Pg 404; OP Ghai, 7th edition Pg 505.

- ***Gonadal differentiation.***
  - ❖ Germ cells arise from the coelomic epithelium of the hindgut and migrate to the gonadal ridge at 4–6 weeks of gestation. These cells combine with the somatic cells to give rise to the bipotential gonad.
  - ❖ A transcriptional factor present on Y chromosome called ***sex determining region of the Y chromosome (SRY)***, is one of the ***most important regulators of sexual differentiation***. SRY acts in conjunction with other genes such as Wilms tumor gene *WT-1, SOX-9* and *DAX-1* to induce testicular development.
  - ❖ In the absence of SRY, the bipotential gonad develops into ovary.
- Following development of testis, ***Sertoli cells*** secrete ***Müllerian inhibiting substance (MIS)*** and induce regression of Mullerian ducts. Dihydrotestosterone produced by action of 5-alpha reductase on testosterone is responsible for male external genital development (scrotal fusion, and development of penile corpus spongiosum and cavernosa).
- ***Leydig cells*** of fetal testis secretes ***testosterone***.
- In the ***normal male fetus (XY)***, the ***Wolffian duct*** system on each side develops into ***epididymis and vas deferens.***
- ***In the female fetus (XX), i.e. in the absence of MIS*** and testosterone Müllerian ducts develop into female external genitalia.
- Sertoli cells secretes ***androgen binding protein, which probably functions to maintain a high stable supply of androgens*** in the tubular fluid.

68. Answer is a (Obliteration of umbilical vein).

Ref: IB Singh's Embryology, Pg 144.

REMNANTS OF

- Ductus arteriosus : Ligamentum arteriosum
- Ductus venosus : Ligamentum venosum
- **L**eft umbilical vein : **L**igamentum teres of **L**iver
- Right umbilical vein : Disappears
- Vitello intestinal duct : Meckel's diverticulum
- Urachus : Median umbilical ligament
- Proximal part of umbilical A : Superior vesical A
- Distal part of umbilical A : Lateral umbilical ligament
- Left common cardinal vein : Oblique vein of left atrium

69. Answer is c (Metabolic alkalosis).
Ref: CPDT, 16th edition Pg 866.

- ***21-alpha-hydroxylase deficiency*** is the MC form of congenital adrenal hyperplasia – leads to salt wasting.
- Electrolyte abnormalities are:
  - Hyponatremia
  - Hyperkalemia
  - Low chlorides
  - Low bicarbonates (metabolic acidosis)
  - Normal blood urea
  - Normal creatinine.
- ***Symptoms*** are: vomiting, poor feeding, loose stools.

70. Answer is c (48 months).
Ref: OP Ghai, 7th edition Pg 28.

Dressing skills development

- *1 year*: Pulls off mittens and caps
- *18 months*: Can unzip but fumbles with buttons
- *2 years*: Can put on shoes or socks and can undress completely
- *3 years*: Can dress and undress fully ***if helped*** with buttons
- *5 years*: Can ties shoelaces.

71. Answer is c (VSD).
Ref: OP Ghai, 7th edition Pg 403.

- ***VSD is the commonest congenital cardiac disease*** accounting for 27% of cases
- About 90% of defects are located in membranous part of interventricular septum.

ORTHOPEDICS

72. Answer is b (Osgood-Schlatter disease).
Ref: John Ebnezer's Orthopedics, 4th edition Pg 428; Maheshwari, 3rd edition Pg 269.

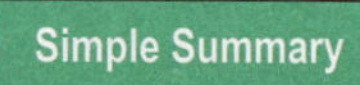

Types of Osteochondritis

Crushing (due to avascular necrosis)	
• HiP joint	Perthe's
• **Metatarsal**	**Freiberg (Fried Meat)**
• Navicu**LAR**	Koh**LER**
• Lunate	Kienbock **(Keen lunatic)**
• Thoracic Spine	*Scheuer*mann's **(Sure man, nice T Shirt)**
• Capitulum	Panner's **(PanCap)**
Traction epiphysitis (chronic strain injuries)	
• Tibial Tuberosity	Osgood-SchlaTTer
• Calcaneum	Sever **(Severely Calculative Calcaneum!)**
• Lower pole of patella	Sinding-Larsen's
Splitting (osteochondritis dissecans)	
• Femoral condyles	
• Elbow (capitulum)	
• Ankle (talus)	

73. Answer is b (Radiotherapy, chemotherapy and surgery).
Ref: John Ebnezer's Orthopedics, 4th edition Pg 635.

- ***Ewing's sarcoma*** is ***highly radiosensitive***, disappears with radiation only to recur (melts like snow).
- Hence, a ***combination of local radiotherapy with systemic chemotherapy*** brings down the recurrence rate dramatically.
- Nevertheless, even this treatment has a recurrence rate of 20–30% and because of the possibility of radiation-induced sarcomas; ***surgical resection of the primary lesion*** is being used.
- Combination of ***radiotherapy, chemotherapy and surgery has improved 2-year survival rate.***

74. Answer is a (Lateral condyle of humerus).
Ref: Maheshwari, 3rd edition Pg 85, 86.

- ***Fracture lateral condyle of the humerus*** is a common fracture in children resulting from varus injury to the elbow
- It is ***Salter and Harris type IV epiphyseal injury*** and hence accurate reduction is important.

Salter and Harris Classification of Epiphyseal (Growth Plate) Injuries

Type	**Injury**	**Treatment and Prognosis**
I	Separation of epiphysis from metaphysis, but without fracture	Closed reduction; Good prognosis
II	Separation, but with fracture of a small triangular piece of metaphysis	Closed reduction; Good prognosis
III	Intra-articular fracture extending from joint surface through growth plate with separation of the portion	Open reduction and internal fixation; Growth disturbance can occur
IV	Intra-articular fracture, the line going through the plate *and* through part of the metaphysis (*Thurston-Holland sign)*	Open reduction and internal fixation; Growth disturbance common
V	Severe end-on crush	Conservative; Growth disturbance always

75. Answer is d (Coracoclavicular screw).
Ref: Maheshwari, 3rd edition Pg 74.

- Dislocation of acromioclavicular joint is an uncommon injury caused by fall on the outer prominence of the shoulder.

Grades of acromioclavicular injury

Grade	**Pathoanatomy**
I	Minimal strain to acromioclavicular ligament and capsule
II	Rupture of acromioclavicular ligament and capsule
III	Rupture of acromioclavicular ligament, joint capsule and coracoclavicular ligaments

Treatment
- Grade I and II = rest in triangular sling and analgesics
- Grade III = surgical repair (coracoclavicular screw).

76. Answer is c (MRI).
Ref: Maheshwari, 3rd edition Pg 231.

- ***MRI*** is the investigation of choice for ***disk prolapse***
- It *shows the prolapsed disk, theca, nerve roots, etc. very clearly.*

77. **Answer is a (Congenital dislocation of hip).**
Ref: Essential Orthopedics, Maheshwari, Pg 200.

Tests Done to Diagnose Congenital Dislocation of Hip (CDH)
- Barlow's test
- Ortolani's test (positive)
- Galeazzi's sign
- Trendlenburg's test (positive)
- Telescopy test (positive)

78. **Answer is c (Median nerve).**
Ref: Maheshwari, 3rd edition Pg 258.

Carpal Tunnel Syndrome

- Causes: Rheumatoid arthritis; Wrist OA; Colles'; Myxedema; Acromegaly; Dislocation of lunate bone; Pregnancy, cardiac failure, premenstrual.
- Compression of ***median*** *N* as it passes beneath the flexor retinaculum; tingling and numbness in the radial two and half fingers more prominent during sleep; in later stages wasting of thenar eminence and decreased sensation over lateral 3 and half fingers; lateral palmar sensation is spared.
- Phalen's sign—Holding the wrist hyperflexed for 1–2 mins reproduces the symptoms and symptoms will disappear as soon as the wrist is straightened.
- Tinel's test: Tapping over the tunnel to produce paresthesia.
- Phalen's Phlexing, Tinel's Tapping!

OPHTHALMOLOGY

79. **Answer is b (Sclera).**
Ref: Parson's, 20th edition Pg 5.

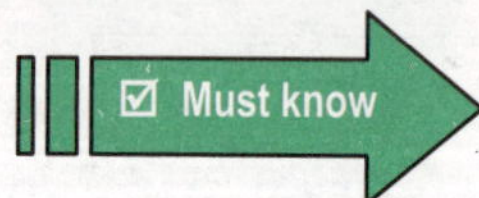

Embryology of Ocular Structures

Surface ectoderm	Mesoderm	Neural ectoderm
❖ Conjunctival Epithelium ❖ Corneal Epithelium ❖ Crystalline lens ❖ Lacrimal glands ❖ Tarsal glands (Meibomian, Zeis, Moll) ❖ Skin of eyelids and eyelashes	❖ Extraocular muscles ❖ Ciliary muscles and choroids ❖ Corneal stroma and endothelium ❖ Iris stroma ❖ Sclera ❖ Choroid ❖ Bony orbit ❖ Vitreous ❖ Vascular endothelium of eye and orbit	❖ Smooth muscle of the iris ❖ Retina and retinal pigment epithelium ❖ Iris and Ciliary body epithelium ❖ Optic N ❖ Sphincter and Dilator pupillae ❖ Melanocytes ❖ Optic vesicle and cup

- Eyelids and zonules: Both from surface ectoderm and mesoderm
- Bruch's membrane: neural ectoderm and mesoderm.

80. **Answer is d (Proteins).**
Ref: Parson's, 20th edition Pg 117-18.

- ***Protein transudation*** from the iris or ciliary vessels produces and opalescence of the aqueous, an *aqueous flare*, which may be visible on slit lamp, when its beam is narrowed to 2 × 1 mm.

Grading of aqueous flare

Grade	Flare
0	Absent
1 +	Faint, barely detectable
2 +	Moderate, iris and lens details clear
3 +	Marked, iris and lens details hazy
4 +	Intense flare, fibrinous aqueous

81. Answer is a (Withdrawing water from vitreous).
Ref: Kanski's, Clinical Ophthalmology, 6th edition Pg 436.

- ***Osmotic pressure*** is dependent on the number rather than the size of the particles in a solution.
- Lower molecular weight solutes therefore exert a greater osmotic effect per gram.
- ***Osmotic agents such as mannitol*** and glycerol remain intravascular, this increases blood osmolality.
- These lower intraocular pressure by creating an ***osmotic gradient*** between blood and vitreous so that ***water is 'drawn out' from the vitreous***.
- The higher the gradient the greater the reduction of IOP.
- To be effective in the eye, an osmotic agent must therefore be unable to penetrate the blood aqueous barrier.
- Osmotic agents are therefore of *limited value in the treatment of inflammatory glaucomas* in which the blood aqueous barrier is compromised.

82. Answer is d (Tractional retinal detachment).
Ref: Age Related Changes in Human Eye, Carlo C, Luciano C, Pg 169, 2008 edition.

- ***Cyclitic membranes*** are often sequelae to endophthalmitis, uveitis or anterior segment trauma.
- When mature, the membrane extends from the ciliary body centrally to occlude the visual axis like a diaphragm.
- Typically well-endowed with ***fibroblasts and thick bundles of collagen, cyclitic membranes have powerful contractile properties***.
- ***Myofiroblasts*** within the membrane contribute to its contractile strength that may secondarily ***cause peripheral tractional retinal detachment***, displace the crystalline lens or PCIOL and promote uveal effusion and hypotony.

83. Answer is c (*Pneumococcus*).
Ref: Parson's, 20th edition Pg 192.

- In adults, the ***hypopyon ulcer caused by pneumococci*** is characteristic and called ***ulcus serpens*** due to its tendency to creep over the cornea in a ***serpiginous fashion***.
- The typical ulcus serpens is a grayish-white or yellowish disk-like lesion near the center of the cornea.
- The opacity is greater at its edges than at the center and is particularly well-marked in one special direction.
- A cloudy gray cornea made up of fine lines, surrounds the disk.
- There is a violent iritis and there may be a definite hypopyon varying in size from hour to hour.

84. Answer is b (Retinal detachment).
Ref: Kanski's, Clinical Ophthalmology, 6th edition Pg 710-712.

- ***Shafer's sign***—anterior vitreous pigments in rhegmatogenous retinal detachment also described as ***"Tobacco dust"*** in vitreous.

Retinal Detachment

❖ RHEGMATOGENOUS RD	– MC type; Due to tear/break in retina; MC in myopes due to frequent lattice degeneration – Photopsia/Flashes (more temporally) and floaters present. Loss of vision like a "curtain coming across field of vision". Shafer's sign—"Tobacco dust" in vitreous (anterior vitreous pigments)

❖ TRACTIONAL RD	–	(2nd MC type) Due to proliferative vitreoretinopathy – mechanical pull on the retina, MC in diabetics
❖ EXUDATIVE RD	–	No tear/break; Causes are – choroidal tumors, toxemia of pregnancy, malignant hypertension, Harada's disease
	–	No photopsiae/floaters
	–	Shifting of subretinal fluid is the hallmark

85. Answer is d (Neural ectoderm).
Ref: Parson's, 20th edition Pg 5.

- See table in ***answer no. 79 above*** for detailed explanation.

86. Answer is d (Observer's eye).
Ref: Parson's, 20th edition Pg 62, Fig 7.4.

- If the observer's eye is 1 m in front of the observed eye and the latter has a 1D of myopia, the far point of the observed eye will be ***at the situation of the observer's eye***
- See above reference for complete explanation of the optics involved in this question.

87. Answer is c (Nodal point of the lens).
Ref: Parson's, 20th edition Pg 52, Fig 6.2.

- The ***nodal point N,*** lies in the ***posterior part of the crystalline lens***
- The ***visual angle is the angle subtended by the object at the nodal point.***

88. Answer is b (Focal illumination).
Ref: Parson's, 20th edition Pg 111.

- The ***slit lamp*** is a more sophisticated instrument and is essential for a thorough examination of the eye.
- It ***employs the same principles of focal illumination,*** in which a brilliant light is brought to focus as a slit or a point by an optical system supported by a movable arm and observations are made through a binocular microscope.

ENT

89. Answer is b (Medialization of vocal cord).
Ref: Scott Brown's, 6th edition Pg 5, 6, 20, 21.

- ***Thyroplasty*** (or laryngoplasty, ***Isshiki***) is most often performed to correct incompetent larynx (glottic or voice incompetence) caused by vocal cord paralysis, atrophy or scarring and for voice alteration. The types of thyroplasty are:

Vocal cord medialization (most often performed procedure)	**Type I**
Vocal cord lateralization	**Type II**
Anterior commissure set back (shortening vocal cord)	**Type III**
Cricothyroid approximation and anterior commissure advancement Arytenoid adduction (lengthening vocal cord)	**Type IV**

90. Answer is c (In the neck).
Ref: Maqbool's ENT, 11th edition Pg 73.

- ***Subperiosteal abscesses*** occurring as a complication of CSOM are:
  i. ***Postauricular*** is the ***MC type*** of subperiosteal abscess; lies over the mastoid temporal bone, *common in children.* Postauricular *sulcus is deepened.*

ii. ***Bezold's abscess***: Pus, after erosion of the mastoid tip or inner surface may give rise to an abscess in the *sternomastoid muscle* within its sheath.

iii. ***Zygomatic abscess***: If the abscess tracks along the zygomatic process of the mastoid, it produces a swelling above and in front of the external canal.

iv. ***Luc's abscess***: The abscess bursts through the anterior wall of the mastoid and leads to sagging of the posterior wall of the external auditory meatus.

v. ***Citelli's abscess***: The abscess spreads to *digastric triangle* along the posterior belly of digastric muscle.

91. Answer is b (Frontal).
Ref: Bhargava's ENT, 4th edition Pg 239.

- ***Acute frontal sinusitis*** presents with frontal tenderness—vacuum headache due to absorption of air in the sinus when the frontonasal duct gets blocked.
- ***Periodicity is much more common in acute frontal sinus infection***—pain is maximum in the morning and gradually subsides during the course of the day, as the drainage of secretions occurs in the vertical position.

PHARMACOLOGY

92. Answer is d (Cyclooxygenase).
Ref: Harrison's, 17th edition Pg 736.

- ***Aspirin*** produces its antithrombotic effect by ***irreversibly acetylating and inhibiting platelet cyclooxygenase (COX)-1***, a critical enzyme in the biosynthesis of thromboxane A_2.
- At ***high doses (~1 g/d), aspirin also inhibits COX-2***, an inducible COX isoform found in endothelial cells and inflammatory cells.
- Aspirin is widely ***used for secondary prevention of cardiovascular events*** in patients with coronary artery, cerebrovascular or peripheral vascular disease.
- Compared with placebo, ***aspirin produces a 25% reduction in the risk of cardiovascular death, MI or stroke***.
- Most common side effects are gastrointestinal and range from ***dyspepsia*** to ***erosive gastritis*** or ***peptic ulcers with bleeding*** and perforation.

93. Answer is b (Lymphoid tissue).
Ref: KD Tripathi, 6th edition Pg 822.

- ***Chlorambucil*** is a very slow acting alkylating agent e***specially active on lymphoid tissue***
- Myeloid tissue is largely spared
- It is ***drug of choice*** for long-term maintenance therapy of ***CLL and Hodgkin's disease***.

94. Answer is d (All of the above).
Ref: Robbins Pathology, 7th edition Pg 73.

- ***Nitric oxide*** (NO) is synthesized ***from L-arginine*** by the enzyme nitric oxide synthase.
- Properties of NO are:
  - ➲ Potent ***vasodilator*** (hence called endothelium-derived relaxing factor)
  - ➲ ***Reduces platelet aggregation*** and adhesion
  - ➲ Mediator of ***host defense against infection***.

95. Answer is c (Rifampicin).
Ref: KD Tripathi, 6th edition Pg 27.

Hepatic microsomal enzyme inducers

• Alcohol (chronic use)	• Phenytoin
• Barbiturates: Phenobarbitone, phentobarbitone, secobarbitone	• Primidone
	• ***Rifampin***
• Carbamazepine	• Sulfinpyrazone

- Glutethimide
- Griseofulvin
- Marijuana smoke
- Meprobamate
- Tobacco smoke

96. Answer is b (Methadone).
Ref: KD Tripathi, 6th edition Pg 184, 453.

Opioid analgesics

- ☐ Natural opium alkaloids: ***Morphine, Codeine***
- ☐ Semisynthetic opiates: Diacetylmorphine (***heroin***), pholcodine
- ☐ Synthetic opioids: ***Pethidine*** (meperidine), ***fentanyl, methadone, dextropropoxyphene, tramadol***

97. Answer is c (5 HT antagonist).
Ref: KD Tripathi, 6th edition Pg 641, 645.

- Domperidone is an ***antiemetic; prokinetic drug;*** a **D2 antagonist**
- Domperidone *crosses blood brain barrier poorly;* accordingly extrapyramidal side effects are rare, but hyperprolactinemia can occur
- However it **DOES ACT *on* CTZ** which is not protected by blood brain barrier.

Note:
❖ Antiemetics, which are 5 HT3 antagonists are ondansetron and granisetron.

98. Answer is b (Hyponatremia).
Ref: Harrison's, 17th edition Pg 2308, Table 353-9; KD Tripathi, 6th edition Pg 406.

Side effects of Carbamazepine

Neurologic	Systemic
➲ Ataxia	➲ Aplastic anemia
➲ Dizziness	➲ Leukopenia
➲ Diplopia	➲ Gastrointestinal irritation
➲ Vertigo	➲ Hepatotoxicity
	➲ ***Hyponatremia and water retention in elderly*** (it enhances ADH action)

99. Answer is b (Phenobarbitone).
Ref: Harrison's, 17th edition Pg 405, 406, 407.

- ***Teratogenic effects*** of antiepileptic drugs increases with the number of medications used.
  - ➲ ***Phenytoin***: Fetal hydantoin syndrome: Facial dysmorphism, cleft lip, cleft palate, cardiac defects, digital hypoplasia and nail dysplasia was originally ascribed to phenytoin, but now known to occur with valproic acid and carbamazepine as well.
  - ➲ ***Valproic acid and carbamazepine***: Neural tube defects and spina bifida, also now known to cause fetal hydantoin syndrome.
  - ➲ ***Lamotrigine*** = higher incidence of cleft lip.

100. Answer is a (Zileuton).
Ref: KD Tripathi, 6th edition Pg 175, 223.

- ***Zileuton*** is a ***5-LO (lipoxygenase) inhibitor,*** blocks LTC4/D4 as well as LTB4 synthesis
- Zileuton was used in asthma but duration of action is short and also is hepatotoxic
- Montelukast and Zafirlukast are leukotriene receptor (cysLT4) antagonists.

101. Answer is d (Their native ligands are identified).
http://en.wikipedia.org/wiki/Orphan_receptor

- An ***orphan receptor*** is a ***putative receptor*** that has a ***similar structure to other identified receptors,*** but ***whose endogenous ligand has NOT YET been identified***
- If a ligand for an orphan receptor is later discovered, the receptor is referred to as an "adopted orphan".

PATHOLOGY

102. Answer is b (Deficiency of factor IX).
Ref: Robbins Pathology, 7th edition Pg 656.

- ***Hemophilia A = Factor VIII*** deficiency
- ***Hemophilia B = Factor IX*** deficiency = ***Christmas disease.***

103. Answer is b (Sickle cell anemia).
Ref: Robbins Pathology, 7th edition Pg 630.

- In children, during the ***early phase of sickle cell disease,*** the spleen is commonly enlarged up to 500 g
- On histologic examination, there is marked congestion of the red pulp, mainly due to trapping of sickled red cells in the splenic cords and sinuses
- This erythrostasis in the spleen leads to marked tissue hypoxia, thrombosis, infarction and fibrosis
- Continued scarring causes progressive ***shrinkage of the spleen*** so that *by adolescence or early adulthood, only a small nubbin of fibrous tissue is left;* this process is called ***autosplenectomy.***

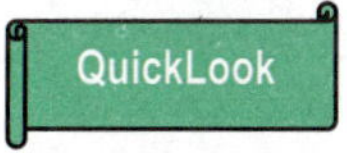

Sickle Cell Disease

- *AR* disease; defect in the β-globin chain of Hb (*glutamic acid replaced by valine* at position 6) leads to the production of HbS, a form of Hb that is poorly soluble when deoxygenated.
- *Heterozygotes* are relatively *malaria resistant.*
- *Acidosis, hypoxia and dehydration* → polymerization of HbS → distortion of RBCs into a sickle shape that is susceptible to hemolysis and vascular clumping.
- *Risk factors*: African or Latin American heritage.
- Clinically:
  - Patients may be *asymptomatic between crises* or may note bone pain
  - Stressful events (e.g. infection, illness, trauma) incite sickle cell crises characterized by *severe bone pain, chest pain, pain and swelling of the hands and feet (dactylitis), dyspnea and priapism*
  - Physical examination: decreased growth velocity, jaundice or pallor, splenomegaly, fever, possible leg ulcers.
- ***Tests***:
  - ↓Hb and ↑ reticulocytes; ↑ WBCs
  - ↓ serum haptoglobin; ↑ indirect bilirubin
  - No HbA, ↑ HbF and presence of HbS (normally not present) on electrophoresis
  - Solubility tests (e.g. SICKLEDEX, Streck, Omaha, Nebraska) can detect Hgb abnormalities but cannot differentiate between the carrier trait and homozygous disease states
  - Blood smear shows target cells, sickle cells and nucleated RBCs
  - X-rays may show *"fish-mouth" vertebrae, "H-shaped" vertebrae* and *avascular necrosis* of bony regions with a tenuous blood supply (e.g. femoral head).
- ***Treatment***:
  - Sickle cell crises are treated with hydration, supplemental oxygen and narcotic pain control
  - Transfusions, exchange transfusions and hydroxyurea are frequently useful to shorten crises or to decrease the number of crises in patients with frequent recurrences

- Bone marrow transplantation has demonstrated success as a curative therapy, but due to the appreciable mortality and morbidity rates it is currently reserved for patients with severe disease and multiple complications.

- *Complications*
  - Chronic anemia, pulmonary HTN, heart failure due to cardiac stresses, vascular insufficiency, renal failure and infections; *Salmonella* osteomyelitis (however even in sickle cells patients also *S. aureus* is the MC cause).
  - An *aplastic crisis* may follow *parvovirus B19* infection.
  - Acute chest syndrome is severe chest pain due to pneumonia, embolization or pulmonary infarction and requires pain control and respiratory support.
  - *Autosplenectomy*, stroke, osteonecrosis of the femoral or humeral head and multiorgan ischemia may result from vascular occlusion.
  - Increased risk of infection by encapsulated organisms (e.g. *Streptococcus pneumoniae, Haemophilus influenzae, Neisseria meningitidis, Klebsiella*)—keep pneumococcal vaccination up-to-date.
  - Despite the multiple potential complications, survival at 18 years of age is 86%.

104. Answer is b (Bradykinin).
Ref: Robbins Pathology, 7th edition Pg 65, 69, 70.

- ***Bradykinin*** increases vascular permeability and causes contraction of smooth muscle, ***dilation of blood vessels*** and pain when injected into the skin.

Note:
Vasoconstriction is caused by
- PAF (bronchoconstriction also)
- Thromboxane A_2
- Leukotrienes C4, D4 and E4.

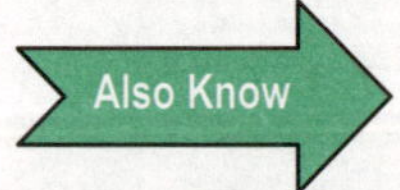

Role of mediators in different reactions of inflammation

Vasodilation	Prostaglandins Nitric oxide Histamine
Increased vascular permeability	Vasoactive amines C3 and C5a (through liberating amines) Bradykinin Leukotrienes C4, D4 and E4 PAF Substance P
Chematoxis. Leukocyte recruitment and activation	C5a Leukotriene B4 Chemokines **IL-1, TNF** Bacterial products
Fever	Il-1, TNF Prostaglandins
Pain	Prostaglandins Bradykinin
Tissue damage	Neutrophil and macrophage lysosomal enzymes O_2 metabolites Nitric oxide

105. Answer is a (In the bone marrow there is increased megakaryocytes).
Ref: Robbins Pathology, 7th edition Pg 651-52.

- ***Idiopathic thrombocytopenic purpura (ITP)*** is a severe thrombocytopenia due to ***antiplatelet IgG antibodies*** (against platelet membrane glycoproteins IIb–IIIa or Ib-IX)
- Peripheral platelet destruction occurs
- ↑ ***megakaryocytes*** in bone marrow
- ***Normal spleen*** size
- ***Bleeding time is prolonged*** but *PT and PTT are normal*
- Treat with prednisolone and if unresponsive splenectomy.

106. Answer is d (Infectious mononucleosis).
Ref: Robbins Pathology, 7th edition Pg 637, Table 13-4.

Classification of Autoimmune Hemolytic Anemias

☐ **Warm Antibody Type**	– Ig**G** mediated; active at 37°C. – Chronic anemia seen with SLE, Drugs (α-methyldopa, penicillamine, quinidine, cephalosporins); Lymphoma and Leukemias and other neoplastic diseases **Warm** weather is **G**reat!
☐ **Cold Agglutinin Type**	– Ig**M** mediated**; complement** mediated; acute anemia triggered by cold; may be – Acute (**M**ycoplasma infection, infectious **M**ononucleosis) or Chronic (a/w lymphoma, Blackwater fever, Trypanosomiasis, Syphilis). **MMM**……..my **compliments** for your **Cold** ice cream!

107. Answer is c (X-linked recessive ichthyosis).
Ref: Robbins Pathology, 7th edition Pg 1251-52.

TYPES OF ICHTHYOSIS

❖ Etiology	– A *scale* is an aggregate of horny cells that have failed to separate from one another in the horizontal plane and the condition of hyperkeratosis is an exaggeration of the problem.
❖ Types of ichthyosis	– ***Ichthyosis vulgaris***: AD, MC and develops around puberty as scaly lesions on the extensor surfaces of extremities (spares the flexures); palms and soles are involved; mild dry skin with follicular accentuation (keratosis pilaris). – ***Sex-linked ichthyosis: XLR***, begins shortly after birth; the generalized scaling is more severe and affects extensor as well as flexor surfaces but palms and soles are spared; a/w cryptorchidism, testicular cancer and cataract/corneal opacities; ***due to deficiency of steroid sulfatase***; a/w history of postmature pregnancies and difficult labor. – Histology: Hyperkeratosis.
❖ Treatment	– Topical emollients and keratolytic preparations (salicylic acid); topical tretinoin may be used, oral retinoids (acitretin, isotretinoin) are effective, but relapses are common. Oral liarozole fumarate, a cytochrome P450 inhibitor was shown efficacious in treatment of ichthyosis in one study.
❖ Ichthyosis presenting in neonatal period	– *Congenital Ichthyosiform Erythroderma (CIE):* Neonate may appear diffusely red with a fine, white scale. – *Epidermolytic hyperkeratosis:* Presents with widespread denuded areas and bullae - hence its older name bullous CIE; the hyperkeratotic component develops later. – ***Collodion baby****:* Baby is born covered by a shiny transparent membrane, which gradually peels off after a week or so, the peel looking like '*collodion*' (a gluey

	solution of nitrated cotton in alcohol an ether used in surgery and photography). – *Harlequin fetus:* Child is born encased in thick abnormal, fissured, hyperkeratotic skin and is associated with rudimentary ears, ectropion and eclabium. Child rarely survives beyond the first week.

108. Answer is a (Papillary carcinoma).
Ref: Robbins Pathology, 7th edition Pg 1176.

Relative frequencies of thyroid carcinomas

- ❖ ***Papillary Ca (75–85%)***
- ❖ Follicular Ca (10–20%)
- ❖ Medullary Ca (5%)
- ❖ Anaplastic Ca (< 5%)

109. Answer is a (AFP).
Ref: The Essentials of Clinical Oncology, Robert de Marsh, J Samuel, Pg 324, 2007 edition.

- AFP is a glycoprotein produced by fetal yolk sac and the liver
- ***AFP is NOT elevated*** in ***pure seminoma*** or choriocarcinoma
- So, a testicular tumor with raised AFP suggests a non-seminomatous histology
- ***Pure seminoma can have elevations of:***
  - ☐ ***Beta-hCG*** (elevated in 7% with pure seminoma)
  - ☐ ***LDH-1*** (correlates with volume of tumor, elevated in bulky testicular tumor of any histology including seminomas)
  - ☐ ***Placental alkaline phosphatase*** (sensitive for metastatic seminomas).

110. Answer is a (Bronchial asthma).
Ref: http://en.wikipedia.org/wiki/Creola_bodies

- **Creola bodies** are a histopathologic finding indicative of ***asthma***
- It is found in a patient's sputum, these are ***ciliated columnar cells sloughed from the bronchial mucosa*** of a patient with asthma
- *Also know*: ***Curschmann's spirals*** are seen in asthma.

MICROBIOLOGY

111. Answer is c (Anthracis).
Ref: Textbook of Microbiology, CP Baveja, 3rd edition Pg 219.

Colony appearance in culture	Organism
❖ Bamboo stick; medusa head; inverted fir tree appearance; string of pearls	*Bacillus anthracis*
❖ Thumbprint appearance, bisected pearls or mercury drops, aluminum paint appearance	*Bordetella pertussis*
❖ School of redfish	*Haemophilus ducreyi*
❖ Satellitism	*Haemophilus influenzae*

❖ Nagler's reaction	*Clostridium perfringens*
❖ Fried egg colony	*Mycoplasma*
❖ Lenticular-shaped	*Neisseria meningitidis*
❖ Draughtsman (concentric rings) appearance	*Pneumococcus*
❖ Swarming growth (fishy, seminal smell)	*Proteus*
❖ Oil paint appearance	*Staphylococcus*
❖ Stalactite growth in ghee broth	*Yersinia pestis*
❖ Daisy head colony	*C. diphtheriae* (gravis)
❖ Frog's egg colony	*C. diphtheriae* (intermedius)
❖ Poached egg colony	*C. diphtheriae* (mitis)

112. Answer is a *(Haemophilus ducreyi).*
Ref: Textbook of Microbiology, CP Baveja, 3rd edition Pg 314.

- ***Haemophilus ducreyi* is a** Gram-negative coccobacillus; growth requires factor X (hematin).
- It causes ***chancroid (soft chancre or soft sore)***, an STD—painful multiple genital ulcers, which bleed easily and tender inguinal lymphadenopathy *(bubo)*.
- Treat with azithromycin, ceftriaxone, ciprofloxacin.

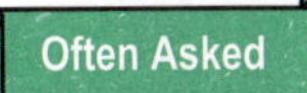

Highlights of other sexually transmitted diseases

Disease	Clinical features	Organism
Primary syphilis	***Painless chancre*** (***hard chancre***)	*Treponema pallidum*, treat with penicillin
Secondary syphilis	Fever, lymphadenopathy, skin rashes, condyloma lata	
Tertiary syphilis	Gummas, tabes dorsalis, Argyll Robertson pupil, general paresis, aortitis	
Granuloma inguinale (donovanosis)	Subcutaneous nodules breaks down to give ***painless*** genital ulcers, '***Pseudobubo***'. Treat with azithromycin, ceftriaxone, ciprofloxacin	*Klebsiella granulomatis* (earlier *Calymmatobacterium granulomatis)*
Lymphogranuloma venereum (LGV)	***Painless genital ulcer***, BUT ***tender lymphadenopathy*** (***bubo, sign of groove***), rectal strictures. Treat with doxycycline or erythromycin	*Chlamydia trachomatis* L1-3

113. Answer is a (Toxoplasmosis).
Ref: Chatterjee Parasitology, Pg 103.

- ***Toxoplasma gondii*** is an *obligate intracellular protozoan*
- Infection results from ingestion of cysts in meat or cat feces or transplacentally
- ***Sabin Feldman dye test*** was used for toxoplasmosis
- Treatment: *Sulfadiazine* + *pyrimethamine* + folinic acid
- Toxoplasmosis in *pregnancy—spiramycin* is drug of choice.

114. Answer is b (*C. albicans*).
Ref: Textbook of Microbiology, CP Baveja, 3rd edition Pg 546.

- ***Candida albicans*** is a common normal flora, but opportunistic pathogen; budding yeast with pseudohyphae in culture at 20°C; germ tube formation at 37°C diagnostic—***Reynolds-Braude phenomenon***
- Transmission occurs by inhalation of spores. No person-to-person spread
- Causes

- Oral Thrush, *perleche* (at angle of mouth), esophagitis in immunocompromised (neonates, steroids, diabetes, AIDS)
- Vulvovaginitis (high pH, pregnancy, diabetes, use of antibiotics)
- Chronic mucocutaneous candidiasis (ass. with T-cell deficiency)
- Endocarditis in IV drug users (caused by *Candida parapsilosis* and *Candida tropicalis)*, paronychia
- Disseminated candidiasis (to any organ)
- Intertrigo in skin folds

• Treatment: nystatin for superficial infection; amphotericin B for serious systemic infection.

115. Answer is c (Herpes virus).
Ref: Textbook of Microbiology, CP Baveja, 3rd edition Pg 437.

Summary of Herpes Viruses

Virus	Infection
• Varicella zoster virus (VZV) • α herpes virus	Chickenpox Shingles (herpes zoster)
• Cytomegalovirus (CMV), • β herpes virus	Congenital infection In AIDS: pneumonitis, retinitis (cottage cheese in tomato ketchup retinopathy, Pizza pie retinopathy), enteritis, generalized infection
• Epstein-Barr virus (EBV), • γ herpes virus	Infectious mononucleosis Burkitt's lymphoma Nasopharyngeal carcinoma Oral hairy leukoplakia (AIDS patients)
α, β, γ are Very Cunning Entities	
• Herpes simplex virus 1 (HSV 1)	Herpes labialis (cold sores) Keratoconjunctivitis Finger infections (whitlow) Encephalitis Gingivostomatitis Genital infections
• HSV 2	Genital infections Neonatal infections (acquired during vaginal delivery)
• Human herpes virus 6 (HHV-6) and HHV-7	Exanthem subitum disease in immunocompromised patients
• HHV-8	Associated with Kaposi's sarcoma

Tzanck test: A smear of an opened skin vesicle to detect multinucleated giant cells. Used to assay for HSV-1, HSV-2 and VZV. Infected cells also have intranuclear Cowdry A inclusions.

116. Answer is b (Antibody).
Ref: Textbook of Microbiology, CP Baveja, 3rd edition Pg 89-93.

Repeat Topic

• See *answer no. 179 in COMED-K 2007 answers* for detailed on different types of immunity.

Mechanisms of innate immunity

- *Epithelial surfaces*
  - Skin (including sweat, *sebaceous* secretions)
  - Respiratory tract
  - Intestinal tract
  - Conjunctiva
  - Genitourinary tract
- Antibacterial substances (properdin, complement, *lysozyme*, β-lysine, interferons)
- Cellular factors

- Chemotaxis
- Attachment
- Ingestion
- Intracellular killing

- Inflammation
- Fever
- Acute phase proteins

Note:

- Acquired immunity is associated with antibody formation.

117. Answer is a (Hippocampus).
Ref: Harrison's, 17th edition Pg 1222, 1224 (Fig 188-2).

- The most characteristic pathologic finding in ***rabies*** is the ***Negri body***.
- Negri bodies are eosinophilic ***cytoplasmic inclusions*** in brain neurons and are composed of randomly oriented rabies virus ***nucleocapsids*** embedded in an amorphous substance or matrix.
- These inclusions occur in a minority of infected cells, are most commonly present in ***Purkinje cells of the cerebellum*** and in ***pyramidal cells in the hippocampus*** and are less frequently seen in cortical neurons and in the brainstem.
- For obscure reasons, Negri bodies are rarely produced in infections caused by laboratory variants of rabies virus, whereas wild, or "street," rabies infection results in Negri bodies in ~80% of cases. Thus, the absence of Negri bodies does not exclude the diagnosis.

118. Answer is b (Endrin).
Ref: Narayan Reddy's FMT, 23rd edition Pg 257.

- ***Endrin*** is also called ***plant penicillin*** because of its broad spectrum of activity against various insect pests.

119. Answer is b (Gene amplification).
Ref: Harper's Illustrated Biochemistry, 26th edition Pg 593.

- ***Antibody diversity*** depends on ***gene rearrangement***.
- The generation of such immense antibody diversity depends upon a number or factors including existence of multiple gene segments (*VCJ* and *D* regions) their recombinations, the combinations of different L and H chains, a high frequency of somatic mutations in immunoglobulin gene and junctional diversity.
- The latter reflects addition or deletion of nucleotides when certain gene segments are joined together and introducing and additional degree of diversity.

120. Answer is c (Adult T cell leukemia/lymphoma virus).
Ref: Textbook of Microbiology, CP Baveja, 3rd edition Pg 527, Table 65.3.

Human Oncogenic Viruses

Virus	Associated Cancers
DNA viruses	
Human Papilloma virus	Genital (cervical, vulvar, penile) warts may progress to carcinoma
Epstein-Barr virus (EBV)	Nasopharyngeal carcinoma, Burkitt's lymphoma
Human Herpes Virus 8 (HHV 8)	Kaposi's sarcoma
Hepatitis B virus	Primary hepatocellular carcinoma
RNA viruses	
Human T cell leukemia virus (HTLV 1)	T cell leukemia/lymphoma
Hepatitis C virus	Primary hepatocellular carcinoma

FORENSIC MEDICINE

121. Answer is a (Entry wound only).
Ref: Narayan Reddy's, FMT, 23rd edition Pg 117-18.

- **Abrasion collar and contusion collar** are *two main proofs of an entry wound.*
  - As the bullet strikes the skin, it first indents and then stretches the skin surface, so that perforation takes place through a tense area.
  - After the bullet has perforated the skin, the elasticity of the skin causes the defect to contract.
  - The skin is abraded (abrasion collar) around the hole due to rubbing of the gyrating body of the bullet against the inverted epidermis.
  - Abrasion collar is reddish at first, but becomes brown and brownish-black as it dries.
  - Some contusion is also present in the abraded collar and as such it is also called ***contusion collar***.
  - The abrasion/contusion collar is *1-3 mm wide.*
  - Abrasion collar *may be absent* when the tissues are soft and yielding (*abdomen or buttocks*).
- **Grease or dirt collar (bullet wipe)**
  - A black narrow ring of skin lining the defect and is sharply outlined.
  - This results *from the removal of substances from the bullet* as it passes through the skin, i.e. bullet lubrication, gun oil, lead from surface of the bullet, barrel debris, etc. Soot is dark in the center and fades towards the periphery. The *abrasion collar surrounds the dirt collar.*

122. Answer is a (Madar juice).
Ref: Narayan Reddy's FMT, 23rd edition Pg 276.

- ***Calotropis gigantea*** (***akdo, madar***) has purple flowers and *Calotropis procera* has white flowers
- They grow wild throughout India
- The leaves and stem when incised yield thick milky juice
- It has been used for ***infanticide*** and sometimes for suicide.

123. Answer is d (Gustafson's method).
Ref: Narayan Reddy's, FMT, 23rd edition Pg 39.

- ***Gustafson's method***—the age estimation of adult ***over 21 years*** depends on the physiological changes in each of the dental tissues
- ***Transparency*** of root is not seen until about ***30 years*** of age. It is the most reliable of all criteria.

124. Answer is c (Gaping).
Ref: Narayan Reddy's, FMT, 23rd edition Pg 105, Fig 8-11. Apurba Nandy, Essentials of Forensic medicine, 3rd edition Pg 362.

- The pattern of fiber arrangement of the dense feltwork of intimately intermingled dermal collagen and elastic fibers is called cleavage direction lines or lines of cleavage of the skin and their linear representation on the skin are called ***Langer's lines***, which are almost same in all persons.
- If incision is perpendicular to Langer's lines the elastic fibers recoil resulting in ***more gaping,*** whereas if incision is parallel to Langer's line, then wound would be less wide.
- Thus deeply incised wound made across the Langer's lines gape more leading to false estimate of width of the weapon.

PREVENTIVE AND SOCIAL MEDICINE

125. Answer is b (Population and total deaths).
Ref: Park, 20th edition Pg 24, 53.

- ***Crude death rate***: It is the simplest measure of mortality. It is defined as ***'the number of deaths (from all causes) per 1,000 estimated midyear population in 1 year in a given place'.***

126. Answer is c *(Cl. perfringens).*
Ref: Park, 20th edition Pg 630.

- The primary bacterial indicator recommended for water quality is the coliform group of organisms as a whole.
- Supplementary indicator organism such as fecal streptococci and sulfate reducing clostridia may be useful in determining the origin of fecal pollution as well as in assessing the efficacy of water treatment process.
- ***Clostridium perfringens*** usually resists chlorination at doses normally used in water works practices.
- The ***presence of spores of clostridium perfringens in natural water suggests that fecal contamination*** has occurred and their presence, in the absence of coliform group, suggests that fecal contamination occurred at some remote time.

127. Answer is c (30%).
Ref: Park, 20th edition Pg 558.

- Lathyrism is a paralyzing disease referred to as neurolathyrism because it affects the nervous system and in animals as osteolathyrism.
- ***Neurolathyrism*** is a crippling disease of nervous system characterized by gradually developing spastic paralysis of lower limbs.
- Occurs MC in adults consuming the pulse *Lathyrus sativus*.
- Also known as ***'khesari dal'*** studies have shown that diets containing ***over 30%*** of this dal if taken ***over 2–6 months*** will result in neurolathyrism.
- The toxin is ***beta-oxalyl-amino-alanine*** (BOAA).
  - Removal of toxin is by
  - Stepping method
  - Parboiling
  - Education
  - Genetic approach
  - Socioeconomic change to root out lathyrism.

128. Answer is c (Free and combined chlorine separately).
Ref: Park, 20th edition Pg 626.

Repeat Topic

- See ***answer no. 132 in COMED-K 2007 answers*** for detailed explanation.

129. Answer is d (Work sampling).
Ref: Park, 20th edition Pg 774.

- ***Work sampling*** is ***systematic recording and observation of activities*** of one or more individuals carried out at predetermined or random intervals.
- It provides ***quantitative measurement*** of various activities.
- Work sampling permits judgments to the appropriateness of current staff, job description and training.
- It helps in standardizing the methods of performing jobs and determining the manpower needs in any organization.

130. Answer is a (Classification of cases and treating them accordingly).
Ref: Park, 20th edition Pg 701.

Repeat Topic

- See ***answer no. 121 in COMED-K 2007 answers*** for detailed explanation.

131. Answer is a (To know total number of cases).
Ref: Park, 20th edition Pg 38.

- No routine notification system can identify all cases of infection or disease. A method for ***identifying the missing cases*** and thereby ***supplementing the notified cases*** is required. This is known as ***'sentinel surveillance'***.
- The sentinel data is extrapolated to the entire population to estimate the disease ***prevalence in the total population.***

- The advantages of such a system are that the *reporting biases are minimized* and the feedback of information to the providers is issued.

132. Answer is a (Contact).
Ref: Park, 20th edition Pg 689.

- ***Pyrethrum*** is an insecticide of vegetable origin
- Extracted from *Chrysanthemum*
- Pyrethrum is an excellent space spray
- It ***kills mosquitoes instantly on mere contact***
- It does NOT possess residual action.

133. Answer is d (Fixed virus).
Ref: Park, 20th edition Pg 241.

Vaccines for rabies

Nervous tissue vaccines	Duck-embryo vaccines	Cell culture vaccines
• Prepared from ***fixed virus*** grown in the brain of adult sheep (Semple type) or other animals. • Crude products capable of causing severe/fatal reactions. • Large number of doses are required. • Suckling mouse brain vaccine: devoid of neuroparalytic effects. • Government of India has stopped nervous tissue vaccine from 2004.	• Inactivated vaccine with reduced neuroparalytic effects. Allergy to egg proteins is a risk factor. • Purified DEV available in India as VaxiRab.	• Human diploid cell culture vaccines—prepared in human diploid fibroblast cells; safe; highly potent; routinely used in India. • 'Second generation' tissue culture vaccines—derived from non-human sources based on either primary cell substrates (e.g. fetal, bovine kidney, chick embryo fiboblast, dog kidney cells, hamster kidney cells, etc.) or non-tumorigenic continuous cell lines (e.g. vero cells). • Cheaper, potent, WHO recommended.

134. Answer is d (Herd immunity).
Ref: Park, 20th edition Pg 97.

- ***Herd immunity*** is the level of ***resistance of a group or community of people to a particular disease.***
- According to another source, herd immunity implies group protection beyond that afforded by the protection of immunized individuals.
- Herd immunity provides an immunological barrier to the spread of the disease in the human herd. For example, when an infectious disease is introduced into a "virgin" population, i.e. a population with a very low or no immunity, the attack and case fatality rates tend to be very high involving practically all susceptibles as it had happened in the very severe measles epidemic in the Faroe islands in 1854, where the population had no previous experience of measles.
- ***Elements which contribute to herd immunity are:***
  - Occurrence of clinical and subclinical infection in the herd
  - Immunization of the herd
  - Herd structure (is never constant).
- If the herd immunity is sufficiently high, the occurrence of an epidemic is regarded as highly unlikely. If that high level of immunity is maintained by an ongoing program, to the point where susceptible persons are reduced to a small proportion of the population, it may lead to elimination of the disease in due course. This has been achieved in such diseases as diphtheria and poliomyelitis. In smallpox however, it may be mentioned that it was not herd immunity that played a crucial role in its eradication, but elimination of the source of infection by surveillance and containment measures.
- In case of tetanus, herd immunity does not protect the individual.
- Herd immunity may be determined by serological surveys.

135. Answer is a (Persons with subclinical infection transmit the disease).
Ref: Park, 20th edition Pg 90.

- ***Eradication***: Termination of all transmission of infection by extermination of the infectious agent through surveillance and containment.
- Eradication is an absolute process, an "all or none" phenomenon, restricted to termination of infection from the whole world.
- It implies that disease will no longer occur in a population.
- ***To-date only one disease has been eradicated, i.e. smallpox.***

In the state of our present knowledge diseases that are amenable to eradication are *(MDPG)*
- ➢ Measles
- ➢ Diphtheria
- ➢ Polio
- ➢ Guinea worm.

136. Answer is c (Randomized control studies).
Ref: Park, 20th edition Pg 59.

- ***Epidemiologic studies*** can be classified as observational studies and experimental studies with further division as below.

Observational studies	Experimental studies
• Descriptive studies	• Randomized control trials
• Analytical studies	• Field trials
– Ecological	• Community trials
– Cross-sectional	
– Case control	
– Cohort	

137. Answer is c (It can be administrated even in immunodeficiency persons).
Ref: Park, 20th edition Pg 206.

Live oral Ty21a vaccine
- Based on results of ***Chile and Egypt trials***, Ty21a vaccine is registered in more than 50 countries including India
- Typhoral is an enteric coated capsule of lyophilized vaccine
- It contains ***not less than 10^9 viable attenuated organisms*** *(Salmonella typhi* strain Ty21a)
- Indicated for immunization in adults and children over 6 years
- One capsule is administered on ***day 1, 3, 5*** irrespective of age, 1 hour before meal with cold milk or water
- Protection commences 2 weeks after taking the last capsule and lasts up to 3 years
- ***Not recommended for immunodeficiency*** states.

Note
❖ All ***live vaccines are contraindicated in immunodeficient*** states.

PSYCHIATRY

138. Answer is a (Panic attacks).
Ref: Niraj Ahuja's Psychiatry, 6th edition Pg 98-100.

Repeat Topic

- See *answer no. 123 in COMED-K 2010 answers* for detailed explanation.

139. Answer is d (50–69).
Ref: Niraj Ahuja's Psychiatry, 6th edition Pg 169, Table 13.2.

- Intelligence quotient (IQ) = Mental age (MA) divided by chronological age (CA) multiplied by 100; i.e. IQ = MA/CA × 100; according to Stanford-Binet.
- Stanford-Binet and Wechsler are the most famous test of IQ.

Classification of Mental Retardation	
Grade	**IQ**
Mild	50–69
Moderate	35–49
Severe	20–34
Profound	< 20

140. Answer is a (Fund of knowledge).
Ref: Kaplan and Sadock's Psychiatry, 7th edition Pg 660.

Mental status examination on intelligence is measured by
- ☐ Alertness
- ☐ Orientation
- ☐ Concentration
- ☐ Memory
- ☐ Calculation
- ☐ ***Fund of knowledge***
- ☐ Abstract thinking
- ☐ Insight
- ☐ Judgment.

141. Answer is b (Thought insertion).
Ref: Niraj Ahuja's Psychiatry, 6th edition Pg 59-60.

Kurt Schneider's first rank symptoms in schizophrenia

- ❖ ***Auditory hallucinations***: Audible thoughts (thought echo); voices discussing the subject in third person; voices commenting on his/her action.
- ❖ ***Thought withdrawal***, thought ***insertion***, thought ***diffusion*** or ***broadcasting***.
- ❖ 'Made' affect, impulses or actions.
- ❖ Delusional perception.
- ❖ Somatic passivity.

RADIOLOGY

142. Answer is a (Hydatid cyst).
Ref: www.ajronline.org/doi/pdf/10.2214/ajr.145.3.639

Repeat Topic

- See *answer no. 41 in COMED-K 2010 answers* for detailed explanation.

143. Answer is b (Metaphyseal translucencies).
Ref: Sutton, 6th edition Pg 464.

Important features of leukemia on X-ray

- Metaphyseal translucencies—affects maximum growth—distal femur, proximal tibia and distal radius
- Diffuse destruction of bones
- Osteolytic lesions of diaphysis of long bones
- Transverse line of dark band below the growth plate.

144. Answer is d (Fibrous dysplasia).
Ref: Chapman's Radiological D/D, 5th edition Pg 422.

- In ***fibrous dysplasia***, medullary bone is replaced by fibrous tissue.
- Most frequent sites are femur, pelvis, skull, mandible, ***ribs*** (***most common cause of a focal expansile rib lesion***) and humerus.
- ***McCune-Albright syndrome*** = polyostotic fibrous dysplasia + sexual precocity + skin pigmentation.

145. Answer is d (Thymic tumor).
Ref: Davidson's, 20th edition Pg 712.

- See ***answer no. 37 above*** for detailed explanation.

146. Answer is d (Thymic tumor).
Ref: Davidson's, 20th edition Pg 712.

- This is not a printing mistake by us BUT the question was actually repeated again in the original question paper with the same options!

147. Answer is d (Prognathism).
Ref: Chapman's Radiological D/D, 5th edition Pg 417.

Skeletal features of Cushing's disease are:

- ***Growth retardation*** in children
- ***Osteoporosis***
- Pathological fractures, which show ***excessive callus formation*** during healing; vertebral end plate fractures, in particular show prominent bone condensation
- ***Avascular necrosis*** of bone
- Increased incidence of ***infection***—including osteomyelitis and septic arthritis (knee affected most frequently).

More About

- Clinical features of ***Cushing's syndrome*** follow logically from the known action of corticosteroids:

'Moon' facies	Easy bruisability
'Buffalo hump'	Hypertension
'Truncal' obesity	Hyperglycemia
Muscle weakness	Acne
Fatigability	Hirsutism
Broad violaceous striae	Amenorrhea

- Occasionally ***hypokalemia***, hypochloremia and metabolic alkalosis are present, particularly with ectopic production of ACTH.

148. Answer is c (Fibrous dysplasia).
Ref: Chapman's Radiological D/D, 5th edition Pg 422.

Radiological changes in fibrous dysplasia include:

- A cyst-like lesion in the diaphysis or metaphysic with endosteal scalloping ± bone scalloping
- No periosteal new bone
- The epiphysis is only involved after fusion
- Thick sclerotic border: 'Rind sign'
- Internally the lesion shows a ground glass appearance ± Irregular calcifications together with irregular sclerotic areas
- Bone deformity: Shepherd's crook deformity of proximal femur
- Growth disparity
- Accelerated bone maturation
- Skull shows mixed lucency and sclerosis, mainly on the convexity of the calvarium and the floor of the anterior fossa
- Leontiasis ossea is a sclerosing form affecting the face ± the skull base and producing leonine facies.

149. Answer is b (Paget's disease).
Ref: Harrison's, 17th edition Pg 2409.

Paget's Disease (Osteitis Deformans)

- Abnormal bone architecture caused by ↑ in both osteoblastic and osteoclastic activity. Possibly viral in origin.
- Serum calcium, phosphorus and PTH levels are normal. ↑ ***serum ALP***. Mosaic bone pattern; long bone chalk stick fractures.
- ↑ blood flow from ↑ arteriovenous shunts may cause ***high output CHF***.
- *Age* > 40 y; M:F = 2:1.
- *Skull*: ***Osteoporosis circumscripta*** (outer table destroyed only), ***"cotton wool"*** areas of sclerotic bone, ↑ ***hat size!*** (facial bones not commonly affected, cf. fibrous dysplasia); ***hearing loss*** common due to auditory foramen narrowing.
- *Spine*: Especially lumbar spine. Enlargement of vertebrae and coarsened trabeculae and cortical thickening produces the ***"picture frame" vertebral body***.
- *Pelvis*: Cortical thickening, enlargement of pubis/ischium, coarse trabecular pattern, ***"brim sign"***.
- *Extremities*: Leading edge of the lytic phase of the disease has a ***"Blade of grass"*** appearance; ***"banana fractures"*** (incomplete pathologic fractures).
- *Complications:* Pathological fractures (usually femur = ***"Shepherd's crook"*** deformity), sarcomatous change in 1% (usually ***osteosarcoma*** or less commonly fibrosarcoma).

150. Answer is a (Annulus fibrosis).
Ref: Harrison's, 17th edition Pg 2110.

- In ankylosing spondylitis, in the spine, early in the process there is inflammatory granulation tissue at the ***junction of annulus fibrosus and vertebral bone***.
- The outer annular fibers are eroded and eventually replaced by bone, forming the beginning of a ***bony syndesmophyte***, which then grows by continued endochondral ossification, ultimately bridging the adjacent vertebral bodies.

ANESTHESIA

151. Answer is d (Esophagus).
Ref: Basics of Anesthesia, Robert K Stoelting, Ronald D Miller, 6th edition Pg 315, 2007.

- The ***best core temperature monitors*** are the ***pulmonary artery catheter***, which measures blood temperature within the pulmonary artery and the ***tympanic membrane monitor***, which measures blood temperature within the carotid artery.
- ***Bladder fluid temperature*** is closer to core temperature, whereas rectal temperature is a poor substitute.

- Many anesthesiologists use and ***esophageal temperature monitor***, but it may be better used to indicate the trend of heat gain or loss.
- ***Axillary and*** skin temperature monitors are ***highly prone to artifact***.

152. Answer is b (Adrenaline).
Ref: Harrison's, 17th edition Pg 2064; Davidson's, 20th edition Pg 86-87.

- Anaphylactic shock is precipitated in sensitized individual by parenteral exposure to
  - Blood and blood products
  - Vaccines
  - Drugs
  - Heparin
  - Insect stings: Bee and wasp, snake venom
  - Oral exposure: Peanuts and shellfish.
- Clinically
  - Laryngeal edema
  - Bronchospasm
  - Hypotension.
- Treatment
  - Early recognition of an ***anaphylactic reaction*** is mandatory, since ***death occurs within minutes to hours*** after the first symptoms.
  - 1:1000 (1.0 mg/mL) ***epinephrine*** SC or IM, with repeated doses as required at 5–20 min intervals for a severe reaction.
  - An IV infusion of ***epinephrine***, diluted 1:10,000, at 5–10 min intervals and volume expanders such as normal saline and vasopressor agents such as ***dopamine if intractable hypotension occurs***.
  - Epinephrine provides both α- and β-adrenergic effects, resulting in vasoconstriction, bronchial smooth muscle relaxation and attenuation of enhanced venular permeability.
  - Replacement of intravascular volume due to postcapillary venular leakage may require several liters of saline.
  - ***Oxygen*** alone via a nasal catheter or with nebulized albuterol may be helpful, but either endotracheal intubation or a tracheostomy is mandatory for oxygen delivery if progressive hypoxia develops.
  - Ancillary agents such as the ***antihistamine diphenhydramine*** and aminophylline, 0.25–0.5 g IV, are appropriate for urticaria-angioedema and bronchospasm, respectively.
  - ***Intravenous glucocorticoids***, 0.5–1.0 mg/kg of medrol, are ***not effective for the acute event***, but may alleviate later recurrence of bronchospasm, hypotension or urticaria.

Author's comments: *"From the above explanation it can be seen that epinephrine is the primary drug of utmost importance in anaphylaxis".*

153. Answer is d (Diethylether).
Ref: KD Tripathi, 6th edition Pg 370-71.

ETHER

Pharmacology

- ***WTG Morton*** of Boston demonstrated its effects in ***Boston*** on ***16th October 1846***, its anesthetic properties become known worldwide.
- It is stored in ***dark bottles*** with corks/caps as light may decompose it. If it is taken to high altitude its boiling point is lowered.
- Ether is ***explosive when mixed with oxygen and is inflammable in air***. Diathermy used along with ether has caused explosions.

Advantages

- Ether stimulates respiration and blood flow due to its sympathomimetic effect mediated by adrenaline release. When too much ether is given respiration becomes depressed before the heart. These effects make ether a *"safe"* anesthetic agent. It is a bronchodilator and produces analgesia. It may be used as the sole anesthetic agent and is capable of producing good abdominal muscle relaxation. It is the ***safest anesthetic in unskilled hands***.

- It is the volatile agent of choice when general anesthesia is needed, but no oxygen is available.

Disadvantages

- Ether is associated with a slow onset and a slow recovery; it stimulates salivation; has a pungent odor; the incidence of nausea and vomiting is higher with ether than with other agents.

154. Answer is c (L3–L4).
Ref: KD Tripathi, 6th edition Pg 359-61.

SPINAL ANESTHESIA

☐ **Site**	– Given in L3–L4 space in adults and L4–L5 space in children.
☐ **Structures that the needle will pierce**	– Skin/Subcutaneous fat, fascia. – Supraspinous ligament. – Interspinous ligament. – Ligamentum flavum. – Epidural space. – Dura mater. – Arachnoid mater. – Subarachnoid space—CSF.
☐ **Baricity**	– Local anesthetic agents are either heavier (*hyperbaric*), lighter (*hypobaric*) or have the same specific gravity (*isobaric*) as the CSF. Hyperbaric solutions tend to spread below the level of the injection, while isobaric solutions are not influenced in this way. It is *easier to predict* the spread of spinal anesthesia when using a hyperbaric agent.
☐ **Drugs**	– ***Bupivacaine: 0.5% hyperbaric (heavy) bupivacaine*** is the best agent to use; it lasts longer than most other spinal anesthetics (usually 2–3 hours). – ***Lignocaine: 5% hyperbaric (heavy) lignocaine gives best results***, which lasts 45–90 minutes. 2% lignocaine can also be used, but it has a much shorter duration of action. If 0.2 mL of adrenaline 1:1,000 is added to the lignocaine, it will usefully prolong its duration of action. Lignocaine from multidose vials should *not* be used for intrathecal injection as it contains potentially harmful preservatives.
☐ **Factors affecting height or level of block**	– Volume of drug—more volume, more the height of block. – Height of patient—in tall patients more drug is required. – Obesity, ascites, pregnancy.
☐ **Complications**	– *Hypotension* (MC complication). ➢ Prophylactic: Treat by preloading with 1.5 L Ringer lactate solution. ➢ Curative: Head low position, fluids, vasopressors (ephedrine, mephentermine), inotropes (dopamine) and oxygen inhalation. – ***Postspinal headache*** ➢ Usually occipital, relieved on lying down, lasting for 7–10 days. ➢ Prophylactic: Use small bore needle, adequate hydration, avoid sitting position postoperatively. ➢ Curative: Lie supine, analgesia, abdominal binder, epidural blood patch.

155. Answer is a (5%).
Ref: KD Tripathi, 6th edition Pg 359-61.

- See summary of spinal anesthesia under ***answer no. 154*** for detailed explanation.

156. Answer is b (Hypotension).
Ref: KD Tripathi, 6th edition Pg 359-61.

- See summary of spinal anesthesia under ***answer no. 154 above*** for detailed explanation.

DERMATOLOGY

157. Answer is b (Herpes simplex infection).
Ref: Harrison's, 17th edition Pg 311, Fig 52.9; 328.

Erythema Multiforme

❖ **Precipitating Factors**	– *Herpes simplex*, Orf, *Mycoplasma* infections; bacterial infections; *drugs* (sulfonamides, penicillin, barbiturates); *internal malignancy* or its *treatment with radiotherapy*.
❖ **Presentation**	– 'Bull's eye' or 'target' or 'iris' lesions are seen. – EM minor due to herpes simplex virus (HSV); and – EM major (Stevens-Johnson syndrome) due to HSV, *Mycoplasma pneumoniae* or rarely drugs. Severe bullous erythema multiforme (EM) with emphasis on mucosal involvement including the mouth, eyes and genitals with accompanying constitutional disturbance. – Toxic epidermal necrolysis is a severe variant of EM.
❖ **Treatment**	– Severe cases are usually managed with tapering courses of systemic corticosteroids after treatment, if possible of the primary cause.

158. Answer is a (Penicillamine).
Ref: Harrison's, 17th edition Pg 338.

- ***Drugs containing a thiol group*** in their chemical structure (e.g. ***penicillamine, captopril, enalapril***) are ***most commonly associated with drug-induced pemphigus***.
- Non-thiol drugs linked to pemphigus include penicillins, cephalosporins and piroxicam.
- It has been suggested that thiol- and non-thiol-containing drugs induce pemphigus via biochemical and immunologic mechanisms, respectively.
- Hence, the *better prognosis upon drug withdrawal in cases of pemphigus induced by thiol-containing medications.*
- Some cases of drug-induced pemphigus are durable and require treatment with systemic glucocorticoids and/or immunosuppressive agents.
- *Drug-induced pemphigus* usually *resembles pemphigus foliaceus* rather than pemphigus vulgaris.

159. Answer is c (The lesion is very painful).
Ref: Ananthnarayan and Panicker, 7th edition Pg 244.

- The cutaneous lesion in anthrax also known as ***malignant pustule*** is most often found on exposed areas of skin.
- Within days, after inoculation, a small red macule appears.
- During next week, the lesion typically progresses through papular and vesicular or pustular stages to form an ulcer with a characteristic blackened necrotic eschar surrounded by a highly characteristic expanding zone of brawny edema.
- The early lesion may be pruritic and the ***fully developed lesion is painless***.
- ***Spontaneous healing occurs in 80–90%*** of untreated cases.
- In 10–20% cases, bacteremia develops and is often associated with high fever and rapid death.

More About *Bacillus anthracis*

- ❖ Is first bacterium to be observed under microscope
- ❖ Is first communicable disease shown to be transmitted by inoculation of blood
- ❖ Is first bacilli to be purely isolated in culture
- ❖ Is first bacterium used for preparation of attenuated vaccine
- ❖ Appearances
  - ➢ Bamboo stick or boxcar appearance

- ➢ Medusa head appearance
- ➢ String of pearls appearance
- ➢ Inverted fir tree appearance
- ➢ McFadyen's reaction.

160. Answer is c (Herpes zoster).
Ref: Harrison's, 17th edition Pg 1102.

- Varicella-zoster virus (VZV) causes two distinct clinical entities:
  - ☐ Varicella (chickenpox)
  - ☐ Herpes zoster (shingles).

More About Shingles

- This is due to *reactivation* of the varicella-zoster virus *lying latent in the posterior root ganglion* of a spinal nerve.
- If a patient without immunity to chickenpox contacts a patient with shingles, he/she may develop chickenpox.
- Mostly affects those *past 50 years* of age and also *AIDS* patients.
- Shingles is characterized by *unilateral vesicular eruption within a dermatome*, often associated with *severe pain*. The dermatomes from T3 to L3 are most frequently involved.
- If the *ophthalmic branch of the trigeminal* nerve is involved, *zoster ophthalmicus* results.
- In *Ramsay-Hunt syndrome*, *pain and vesicles* appear in the *external auditory canal* and there is *loss of taste* sensation in the *anterior two thirds* of the tongue while developing *ipsilateral facial palsy*. The *geniculate ganglion* of the *sensory branch* of the *facial nerve* is involved.
- About 25–30% of patients with shingles continue to suffer from pain and paresthesia in the area long after the skin lesions have disappeared *(postherpetic neuralgia)*.

ANATOMY, PHYSIOLOGY AND BICOHEMISTRY

161. Answer is b (Posterior cerebral artery).
Ref: BD Chaurasia, Vol 1. Pg 219.

Branches of Internal Carotid Artery

1. Cervical part: No branch arises from internal carotid A. in the neck.
2. Petrous part: Caroticotympanic and pterygoid branch.
3. Cavernous part: Branch to trigeminal ganglion, superior and inferior hypophyseal branches.
4. Cerebral part
   I. ***Ophthalmic A.***: Accompanies optic N. and gives central retinal A.
   II. ***Anterior cerebral A.***:
   – Supplies the medial surface of the frontal and parietal cortex (medial surface of brain), leg-foot area of motor and sensory cortices.
   – Recurrent branch of the anterior cerebral A. (A. of Huebner) enters the anterior perforated substance.
   III. ***Middle cerebral A.***:
   – Supplies greater part of superolateral surface of brain, auditory area, trunk-arm-face area of motor and sensory cortices.
   – Lateral *striate branch* – "artery of stroke, *Charcot's Artery of Cerebral Hemorrhage*" → supplies internal capsule, caudate, putamen, globus pallidus.
   IV. ***Posterior communicating A.***: Common area of aneurysm that causes CNIII palsy.
   V. ***Anterior choroidal A.***: Enters inferior horn of lateral ventricle through choroidal fissure.

Note:

- ■ At the lower border of the pons vertebral A. unites with its fellow of the opposite side to form the Basilar A. This artery in turn ends at upper border of pons by dividing into the right and left Posterior Cerebral A.

162. Answer is d (Peroneus longus).
Ref: BD Chaurasia, Vol 2. Pg 79.

- Movements at the intertarsal joint (particularly talocalcaneonavicular) are:
  - ☐ **Inversion**: Tibialis anterior and posterior
  - ☐ **Eversion**: Peroneus longus and brevis.

163. Answer is a (Left gastric artery).
Ref: BD Chaurasia, 3rd edition Vol 2. Pg 194.

- **Contents of lesser omentum**
- ***The right free margin of lesser omentum contains***
  - The hepatic artery proper
  - Portal vein
  - Bile duct
  - Lymph nodes and lymphatics
  - Hepatic plexus of nerves.
- ***Along the lesser curvature of the stomach and along the upper border of the adjoining part of the duodenum contains***
  - Right gastric vessels
  - Left gastric vessels
  - Gastric group of lymph nodes and lymphatics
  - Branches from gastric nerves.

164. Answer is d (External iliac artery).
Ref: BD Chaurasia, Vol 2, Pg 139.

Continuing Course of External Iliac Artery and Their Respective Branches

Artery	Branches
External iliac A. ↓	– Inferior epigastric – *Deep circumflex iliac* – Branches to psoas major
Femoral A. ↓	– Superficial epigastric A. – Superficial external pudendal A. – Deep external pudendal A. – Profunda femoris A. – Descending genicular A.
Popliteal A. ↓	– Cutaneous and muscular branches – Superior, middle and inferior genicular A. – Sural A. (2 in number)
Anterior tibial A. ↓	– Anterior and posterior tibial recurrent A. – Anterior medial and lateral malleolar A. – Dorsalis pedis A.
Posterior tibial A.	– Circumflex fibular A – Peroneal A. – Nutrient A. of tibia – Calcaneal A. – Medial and lateral plantar A.

165. Answer is a (Thyroarytenoids).
Ref: BD Chaurasia, Vol 3, Pg 152.

Repeat Topic

- See *answer no. 171 in COMED-K 2008 answers* for detailed explanation.

166. Answer is b (Estrogen).
Ref: Textbook of Biochemistry, Vasudevan, 5th edition Pg 380, Table 36.1.

Repeat Topic

- See *answer no. 122 in COMED-K 2007 answers* for detailed explanation.

167. Answer is b (105 mV).
Ref: Ganong's Physiology, 23rd edition Pg 87-89.

- In neurons the ***resting membrane potential*** is about ***-70 mV***.
- The first manifestation of the approaching action potential is a beginning depolarization of the membrane.
- After an initial 15 mV of depolarization, the rate of depolarization increases.
- Thereafter, the tracing on the oscilloscope rapidly reaches and overshoots the zero potential line to approximately *+35 mV*. It then reverses and falls rapidly towards resting level.

168. Answer is c (30).
Ref: Ganong's Physiology, 23rd edition Pg 89, Table 4-1.

Nerve fiber types in mammalian nerve

Fiber type	Function	Conduction velocity (m/s)
A		
α	Proprioception, somatic motor	70–120
β	Touch, pressure	30–70
γ	Motor to muscle spindles	15–30
δ	Pain, cold, touch	12–30
B	Preganglionic autonomic	3–15
C		
Dorsal root	Pain, temperature, some mechanoreception	0.5–2
Sympathetic	Postganglionic sympathetic	0.7–2.3

- Thus from the above table, it can be seen that ***Aδ fibers carrying pain sensation*** have a velocity of ***12–30 m/s***.

169. Answer is a (400 mL).
Ref: Ganong's Physiology, 23rd edition Pg 661.

- A plot of the intravesical pressure against the volume of fluid in the urinary blader is called ***cystometrogram***
- The first urge to void is felt at a bladder volume of about 150 mL and a ***marked sense of fullness at about 400 mL***.

170. Answer is c (Aboral orientation of substance P secreting neurons).
Ref: Harrison's, 17th edition Pg 237, 240.

- Peristaltic activity can be increased or decreased by the autonomic input to the gut, but its occurrence is indepenedent of extrinsic innervations.
- Peristalsis is an excellent example of integrated activity of extrinsic nerve system.
- Local stretch releases serotonin, which activates sensory nerves that activates the myenteric plexus.
- Cholinergic neurons passing in a ***retrograde direction in the plexus*** activate neurons that release ***substance P and acetylcholine*** causing smooth muscle contraction.

171. Answer is c (Local anesthesia).
Ref: Ganong's Physiology, 23rd edition Pg 90, Table 4-3.

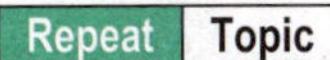

- See ***answer no. 158 in COMED-K 2010 answers*** for detailed explanation.

172. Answer is a (Equilibrium potential of Na^+).
Ref: Ganong's Physiology, 23rd edition Pg 83-85.

- The cell membrane of nerves has different types of ion channels.
- It is the behavior of these channels particularly Na^+ and K^+ that explains electrical events.
- At the beginning of depolarization, ***voltage gated Na^+ channels*** become active and when firing level is reached, K^+ channels are activated and the spike potential results.

173. Answer is c (Both).
Ref: KD Tripathi, 6th edition Pg 95-96.

- See ***tables no. 7.3 and 7.4*** at the above reference for detailed explanation.

174. Answer is b (Spermidine).
Ref: Vasudevan's Biochemistry, 5th edition Pg 200.

Polyamines are:
- Spermidine
- Spermine
- Putrescine

Also Know

- ***Polyamines*** are aliphatic amines synthesized from ***ornithine***.
- ***DFMO*** (difluoromethylornithine) is a powerful inhibitor of polyamine synthesis. It is an example of *suicide inhibition*.
- Key enzyme of polyamine synthesis is ***ornithine decarboxylase***; it requires ***pyridoxal phosphate***.
- Polyamines are involved in cell proliferation, stabilization of ribosomes and DNA, synthesis of DNA and RNA, protection of DNA against depurination, etc.
- Polyamine concentration is *increased in cancer tissues*.
- *Polyamines are growth factors* in cell culture systems.

175. Answer is b (Secondary structure of proteins).
Ref: Vasudevan's Biochemistry, 5th edition Pg 26.

- ***Secondary structure*** of protein is the steric relationship of amino acids, close to each other.
- Secondary structure of proteins consists of:
  - ***Alpha helix***
  - ***Beta pleated*** sheet
  - Collagen helix.
- The alpha helix is the most common and stable conformation of a polypeptide chain.

176. Answer is a (Biotin).
Ref: Harrison's, 17th edition Pg 446.

- ***Biotin*** is a water-soluble vitamin that plays a role in
  - Gene expression
  - Gluconeogenesis and
  - Fatty acid synthesis
  - Catabolism of specific amino acids (e.g. leucine).
- Serves as a CO_2 carrier on the surface of both cytosolic and mitochondrial carboxylase enzymes.
- Excellent *food sources* of biotin include organ meat such as liver or kidney, soybeans, yeast and egg yolks.
- However, ***egg white contains the protein avidin, which strongly binds biotin*** and reduces its bioavailability. ***Biotin deficiency has been induced by experimental feeding of egg white diets*** and in patients with short bowels who received biotin-free parenteral nutrition.
- ***Biotin deficiency***

- *In adults*: Mental changes (depression, hallucinations), paresthesia, anorexia and nausea. A scaling, seborrheic and erythematous rash may occur around the eyes, nose and mouth as well as on the extremities.
- *In infants*: Hypotonia, lethargy and apathy. In addition, the infant may develop alopecia and a characteristic rash that includes the ears.

177. Answer is b (NADP).
Ref: Vasudevan, 5th edition Pg 120.

- The HMP shunt (pentose phosphate pathway) is mainly regulated by the level of NADP+.
- The first reaction catalyzed by GDP is the rate limiting step and it is inhibited by NADPH.
- The oxidative phase is therefore controlled by the level of NADP+ and non-oxidative phase by the requirement of pentoses.
- Insulin will induce GPD and therefore will increase the overall pathway.

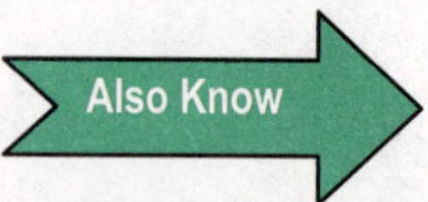

- ***HMP shunt*** takes place in ***cytoplasm*** (muscles, liver, fat cells, thyroid, lactating mammals and erythrocytes)
- Consists of two branches—***oxidative*** and ***non-oxidative***
- The net result is the production of 12 NADPH, 6 CO_2 and 1 glyceraldehyde-3-phosphate molecule for each glucose-6-phosphate molecule passing through the pathway
- Main function
  - Provides reducing equivalents which helps in the synthesis of fatty acids, cholesterol
  - Sources of pentoses
  - Oxidizes glucose to CO_2
  - Maintenance of integrity of RBC membrane.

178. Answer is a (Accumulation of phytanic acid).
Ref: Vasudevan's Biochemistry, 5th edition Pg 137.

- ***Refsum's disease*** is a metabolic disorder due to lack of alpha-hydroxylase (phytanic acid hydroxylase) so that ***alpha oxidation does not occur and phytanic acid accumulates in tissues***.
- Clinically: Palpable peripheral nerves, polyneuropathy, retinitis pigmentosa, nerve deafness and cerebellar ataxia.
- ***Milk*** is a good source of phytanic acid, which ***should be avoided***.

179. Answer is a (Internal mammary).
Ref: Robbins Pathology, 7th edition Pg 517; Bailey and Love, 25th edition Pg 856.

- ***MC involved artery in atherosclerosis = abdominal aorta*** > thoracic aorta.
- ***Next MC involved*** are coronary arteries > popliteal arteries > internal carotid arteries > vessels of the circle of Willis.
- Spared vessels = vessels of the upper extremities, mesenteric and renal arteries.
- The ***internal mammary artery is the conduit of choice for coronary artery bypass grafting*** (CABG) since it ***remains patent in 90% of cases***.

180. Answer is a (Variability of tension at a given length of muscle fiber).
Ref: Physiology-Prep Manual for Undergraduates, Vijaya D Joshi, 4th edition Pg 467; Textbook of Medical Physiology, Indu Khuarana, Pg 125.

- ***Smooth muscle*** exerts ***variable tension at any given length***. This is called ***plasticity***.
- If a piece of smooth muscle is stretched, it first exerts increased tension.
- However, if the muscle is held at greater length after stretching, tension gradually decrease. It is consequently impossible to correlate length and develop tension accurately and no resting length can be assigned.
- Thus the ***smooth muscle defies the usual length tension relationship*** that is valid for striated muscles (skeletal as well as cardiac muscles).

COMED-K 2005

COMED-K 2005 QUESTIONS

MEDICINE

1. **The drug of choice for persistent unstable ventricular arrhythmia is**
   (a) Procainamide
   (b) Verapamil
   (c) Amiodarone
   (d) Milrinone

2. **In idiopathic precocious puberty, the parents should be warned that**
   (a) Final height will be less than that of peers
   (b) Premature heterosexual activities is common
   (c) Future reproductive potential is adversely affected
   (d) Mental capacity may also be affected

3. **The drug used for eradication of meningococcal carrier state is (*KDT 5th edition 78*)**
   (a) Streptomycin
   (b) Tobramycin
   (c) Doxycycline
   (d) Minocycline

4. **All of the following are signs of cerebellar disease *EXCEPT (Kumar and Clark 1147*)**
   (a) Resting tremors
   (b) Past-pointing
   (c) Nystagmus
   (d) Ataxic gait

5. **Pseudomembranous colitis is associated with**
   (a) *Campylobacter*
   (b) *Clostridium difficile*
   (c) *Clostridium rettgeri*
   (d) *Salmonella typhi*

6. **Which of the following conditions is the most common complication of radioiodine treatment of Graves' diseases?**
   (a) Thyroid storm
   (b) Subacute thyroiditis
   (c) Thyroid cancer
   (d) Hypothyroidism

7. **All are predisposing causes of cerebral venous thrombosis *EXCEPT***
   (a) Hypotension
   (b) Oral contraceptives
   (c) Pregnancy
   (d) Sickle cell anemia

8. **In diabetes mellitus, cataract formation is facilitated by the interaction of blood glucose with**
   (a) Glucose oxidase
   (b) NADPH-dependent aldose reductase
   (c) Glucokinase
   (d) Glucose-6-phosphate dehydrogenase

9. **The 'opening snap' of mitral stenosis**
   (a) Denotes valve mobility
   (b) Disappears, if atrial fibrillation occurs
   (c) Is usually best heard at the apex
   (d) Replaces the third heart sound

10. **All of the following are cardiac causes of clubbing *EXCEPT***
    (a) Tricuspid atresia
    (b) Patent ductus arteriosus
    (c) Bacterial endocarditis
    (d) Eisenmenger's syndrome

11. **In nephrotic syndrome, the following features indicate poor prognosis *EXCEPT***
    (a) Selective proteinuria
    (b) Hematuria
    (c) Hypertension
    (d) Membranoproliferative histopathology

12. **Sarcoidosis is mimicked by chronic poisoning with**
    (a) Mercury
    (b) Beryllium
    (c) Aluminum
    (d) Lead

13. **Excessive production of aldosterone results in which of the following clinical features?**
    (a) Metabolic acidosis
    (b) Hypotension
    (c) Hyperkalemia
    (d) Renin suppression

14. **All these conditions can produce metabolic acidosis *EXCEPT***
    (a) Uncontrolled diabetes mellitus
    (b) Aspirin poisoning
    (c) Gastroenteritis with dehydration
    (d) Congenital hypertrophic pyloric stenosis

15. **Common presenting symptoms of pneumocystis pneumonia is**
(a) Cavity on X-ray
(b) Hemoptysis
(c) Breathlessness
(d) Purulent sputum

16. **Which one of the following is not associated with rheumatoid arthritis?**
(a) Pleural effusion
(b) Pulmonary hypertension
(c) Cricoarytenoid arthritis
(d) Fibrosing alveolitis

17. **Ramsay Hunt syndrome is seen in infection caused by**
(a) Mumps virus
(b) Varicella zoster
(c) Newcastle virus
(d) Orthomyxovirus

18. **In triage, green color indicates**
(a) Ambulatory patients
(b) Dead/Moribund patients
(c) High priority treatment or transfer
(d) Medium priority or transfer

19. **Diagnosis of organophosphate poisoning can be achieved by**
(a) Measuring serum creatinine
(b) Measuring RBC cholinesterase
(c) Performing ferric chloride test
(d) Estimating aminolevulinic acid level in the urine

20. **Early systolic murmur is heard in all *EXCEPT***
(a) Acute mitral regurgitation
(b) Small ventricular septal defect
(c) Mitral valve prolapse with mitral regurgitation
(d) Large ventricular septal defect with pulmonary hypertension

21. **A 'flea-bitten' kidney is seen in**
(a) Renal tuberculosis
(b) Malignant hypertension
(c) Renal amyloidosis
(d) Leptospirosis

SURGERY

22. **Mondor's disease is superficial thrombophlebitis of**
(a) Axillary vein
(b) Long saphenous vein
(c) Veins of the breast
(d) Internal mammary vein

23. **Gardner's syndrome has all of the following *EXCEPT***
(a) Colonic polyps
(b) Multiple epidermal cysts
(c) Bony exostosis
(d) Giant gastric folds

24. **Carcinoma of the colon develops in all patients with**
(a) Juvenile polyposis
(b) Hamartomatous polyp
(c) Inflammatory polyp
(d) Familial adenomatous polyposis

25. **Familial polyposis of the colon is most often associated with which of the following conditions?**
(a) Carcinoma of the pancreas
(b) Carcinoma of the colon
(c) Granulomatous disease of the colon
(d) Pneumatosis cystoides intestinalis

26. **Ectopia vesicae includes all *EXCEPT:***
(a) Hypospadias
(b) Exstrophy of bladder
(c) Defective abdominal wall
(d) Bifid clitoris

27. **Middle mediastinal masses include all of the following *EXCEPT***
(a) Bronchogenic cyst
(b) Lymphoma
(c) Pericardial cyst
(d) Ganglioneuroma

28. **Horner's syndrome is associated with**
(a) Bronchial carcinoid
(b) Pancoast's tumor
(c) Lymphangitis carcinomatosa
(d) Oat cell carcinoma

29. **The commonest cause of massive upper gastro-intestinal bleeding is**
(a) Esophageal varices
(b) Erosive gastritis
(c) Gastric carcinoma
(d) Peptic ulcer

30. **All are features of irritable bowel syndrome *EXCEPT***
(a) Vomiting
(b) Abdomen pain
(c) Diarrhea
(d) Constipation

31. **In a critically ill blunt abdominal trauma patient, the most accurate diagnostic modality is**
(a) CT scan
(b) MRI scan
(c) Ultrasound of abdomen
(d) Direct peritoneal lavage

32. **Poorest prognosis in lung cancer is associated with**
(a) Small cell carcinoma
(b) Adenocarcinoma
(c) Squamous cell carcinoma
(d) Adenosquamous carcinoma

33. **Regarding premalignant oral lesions**
(a) Leukoplakia should be proved by biopsy
(b) Leukoplakia does not disappear even after cessation of smoking
(c) Erythroplakia has a higher risk for malignancy
(d) Oral submucous fibrosis is seen in all parts of the world

34. **Surgically used suture material—polydioxanone (PDS)**
(a) Is nonabsorbable and remains encapsulated
(b) Undergoes hydrolysis and complete absorption
(c) Undergoes phagocytosis and enzymatic degradation
(d) Is specially used for heart valves or synthetic grafts

35. **The commonest cause of water intoxication in surgical patients is due to**
(a) Colorectal wash with plain water
(b) Syndrome of inappropriate secretion of ADH
(c) Irrigation during transurethral resection of prostate
(d) Excessive infusion of 5% glucose

36. **'Cobblestone' appearance seen on colonoscope is characteristic of the following disease**
(a) Crohn's disease
(b) Ulcerative colitis
(c) TB colitis
(d) Irritable bowel syndrome

37. **Major complication of cystogastrostomy for pseudopancreatic cyst is**
(a) Infection
(b) Obstruction
(c) Fistula
(d) Hemorrhage

38. **All of the following is true of testicular torsion *EXCEPT***
(a) Common in age 10–25
(b) Duplex scan in diagnostic
(c) Malignancy is the underlying cause
(d) Epididymo-orchitis is an important differential diagnosis

OBSTETRICS AND GYNECOLOGY

39. **Which of the following could be responsible for a persistent vaginal discharge in a pediatric patient?**
(a) Foreign body
(b) Pin worms
(c) Illicit drug use
(d) Vaginal laceration

40. **All of the following factors are associated with an increased risk of pelvic inflammatory disease (PID) *EXCEPT***
(a) Intrauterine contraceptive device
(b) An elective abortion
(c) Oral contraceptive
(d) Hysterosalpingography

41. **Mucinous cystadenoma of the ovary arises from**
(a) Cystic teratoma
(b) Surface coelomic epithelium
(c) Sex cord stromal cells
(d) Ectopic mucin-secreting glands

42. **Assessment of progress of labor is best done by**
(a) Station of head
(b) Rupture of membranes
(c) Uterine contractions
(d) Partogram

43. **Oligohydramnios is associated with which fetal abnormality?**
(a) Spina bifida
(b) Esophageal atresia
(c) Renal agenesis
(d) Amphalocele

44. **Which of the following structures is intact in a third-degree perineal tear?**
(a) Anal sphincter
(b) Perineal body
(c) Perineal muscles
(d) Rectal mucosa

45. **The best predictor of ovulation is**
(a) Estrogen peak
(b) Follicle-stimulating hormone surge
(c) Onset of the luteinizing hormone surge
(d) Preovulatory rise in progesterone

PEDIATRICS

46. **At what age does an infant discriminate strangers?**
(a) 4 months
(b) 7 months
(c) 12 months
(d) 20 months

47. **The age by which most of the normal babies know their gender is**
(a) 1 year
(b) 2 years
(c) 3 years
(d) 4 years

48. **Coarctation of the aorta may be associated with**
(a) Ventricular septal defect
(b) Atrial valvular defect
(c) Tricuspid stenosis
(d) Pulmonary stenosis

49. **In a neonate who has asphyxia, all of the following sequelae could be expected to develop *EXCEPT***
(a) Sustained rise in blood pressure
(b) Cardiomegaly and heart failure
(c) Cerebral edema and seizures
(d) Electrolyte abnormalities

50. **Wide open anterior fontanel is found in following diseases *EXCEPT***
(a) Rickets
(b) Cretinism
(c) Osteogenesis imperfecta
(d) Craniosynostosis

51. **To induce vomiting at home in a child who has ingested a poison, the recommended agent of choice would be**
(a) Oral rehydration solution
(b) Mustard in warm water
(c) Apomorphine
(d) Syrup of ipecac

52. **Common cause for epiglottitis in children is**
(a) *Haemophilus influenzae*
(b) *Pneumococcus*
(c) *Staphylococcus aureus*
(d) *Streptococcus hemolyticus*

53. **'Weight (kg)/Height (m^2)'is referred to as**
(a) Ponderal index
(b) Broca's index
(c) Body mass index
(d) Corpulence index

54. **Which of the following condition is commonly encountered in the newborn female and usually requires no therapy?**
(a) Enlarged clitoris
(b) Labial fusion
(c) Mucoid vaginal discharge
(d) Prolapsed urethra

ORTHOPEDICS

55. **Kocher's maneuver is used in reduction of**
(a) Hip
(b) Shoulder
(c) Ankle
(d) Elbow

56. **Ward triangle is significant in**
(a) TB hip
(b) Fracture
(c) Osteoporosis
(d) Congenital dislocation of hip

57. **The deformities seen in rheumatoid hand are all *EXCEPT***
(a) Swan-neck deformity
(b) Boutonniere deformity
(c) Radial deviation
(d) Adduction, external rotation, flexion

58. **All the statements regarding congenital radioulnar synostosis are true *EXCEPT***
(a) Fusion of both ends of the radius and ulna
(b) Fixed in midprone position
(c) Pulled elbow is a differential diagnosis
(d) Even with operative treatment prognosis is guarded

59. **Ape thumb deformity is seen in**
(a) Ulnar nerve injury
(b) Radial nerve injury
(c) Median nerve injury
(d) All of the above

60. **The following is a characteristic of osteomalacia in adults *EXCEPT***
(a) Bowing of the tibia
(b) Pseudofractures
(c) Long bone pain
(d) Proximal muscle weakness

OPHTHALMOLOGY AND ENT

61. **Posterior polar cataract is formed due to**
(a) Persistence of vascular sheath of the lens
(b) Delayed formation of posterior chamber
(c) Shrinkage of the vitreous
(d) Vitreous touch syndrome

62. **'A' wave in electroretinogram corresponds to activity in**
(a) Rods and cones
(b) Pigment epithelium
(c) Ganglion cell layer
(d) Nerve fiber layer

63. **An indirect ophthalmoscope will project**
(a) Virtual image
(b) Real image
(c) Upright image
(d) Flat image

64. **Coloboma of the lid is common in**
(a) Lateral half of the lower lid
(b) Medial half of the lower lid
(c) Medial half of the upper lid
(d) Lateral half of the upper lid

65. **Lid muscle supplied by sympathetic nerve is**
(a) Superior rectus
(b) Superior oblique
(c) Müller's muscle
(d) Inferior oblique

66. **Ophthalmia nodosa in seen in**
(a) Leprosy
(b) Tuberculosis
(c) Granulomatous uveitis
(d) Caterpillar hair in the eye

67. **Which of the following statements about congenital nasolacrimal duct obstruction is correct?**
(a) Should be treated with long-term antibiotics
(b) Probing must be performed as early as possible
(c) Probing is usually advised around the age 12–18 months
(d) Results of probing are not good

68. **Reduced corneal sensation is typically associated with**
(a) Adenoviral keratitis
(b) Acanthamoeba keratitis
(c) Herpes simplex keratitis
(d) Molluscum keratitis

69. **Scleritis is most frequently associated with**
(a) Polyarteritis nodosa
(b) Rheumatoid arthritis
(c) Wegener's granulomatosis
(d) Diabetes mellitus

70. **'Trotters triad' is seen in**
(a) Orbital tumor
(b) Middle ear malignancy
(c) Nasopharyngeal carcinoma
(d) Cavernous sinus thrombosis

71. **Which of the following venous sinuses is more likely to be affected with thrombosis in 'chronic otitis media'?**
(a) Cavernous
(b) Intercavernous
(c) Sigmoid
(d) Superior petrosal

72. **When a patient hears better in noisy surroundings the condition is**
(a) Hyperacusis
(b) Hypoacusis
(c) Presbycusis
(d) Paracusis

73. **Amyl nitrate inhalation test is used to detect**
(a) Carcinoma esophagus
(b) Achalasia cardia
(c) Esophageal diverticulum
(d) Tracheoesophageal fistula

DERMATOLOGY, ANESTHESIA, RADIOLOGY AND PSYCHIATRY

74. **Skin blister resulting from a burn is an example of**
(a) Serous inflammation
(b) Catarrhal inflammation
(c) Suppurative inflammation
(d) Fibrinous inflammation

75. **Which of the following is associated with pruritus?**
(a) Lichen planus
(b) White patches
(c) Ichthyosis
(d) Secondary syphilis

76. **Koebner phenomenon is seen typically with**
(a) Psoriasis
(b) Eczema
(c) Scabies
(d) Lupus vulgaris

77. **Ringworm infection affects**
(a) Dermis
(b) Papillary layer
(c) Stratum corneum
(d) Prickle cell layer

78. **Depression of level of consciousness in hypothermia starts when the core body temperature is below**
(a) 36°C
(b) 34°C
(c) 33°C
(d) 32°C

79. **Pulse oximeter works on the following principle**
(a) Beer-Lambert law
(b) Raman scattering effect

(c) Venturi principle
(d) Mass spectrometry

80. **Halothane hepatitis is more common in**
(a) Aged patients
(b) Patients with previous exposure to halothane
(c) Patients with history of cholecystitis
(d) Prolonged anesthesia

81. **Depolarizing neuromuscular blockade is associated with**
(a) Fasciculations
(b) Fade on titanic stimulation
(c) Enhancement by volatile anesthetic agents
(d) Antagonized by anticholinesterases

82. **The most important determination of resistance to laminar gas flow through a tube is the**
(a) Length of the tube
(b) Radius of the tube
(c) Viscosity of the gas
(d) Density of the gas

83. **Which of the following mechanism is most frequently responsible for hypoxia in the recovery room?**
(a) Ventilation/Perfusion mismatch
(b) Hypoventilation
(c) Hypoxic gas mixture
(d) Intracardiac shunt

84. **If thiopental is injected accidentally into an artery, treatment should include immediate dilution with**
(a) Norepinephrine
(b) Lidocaine
(c) Propranolol
(d) Physostigmine

85. **'Candle wax' appearance is seen in**
(a) Osteogenesis imperfecta
(b) Melorheostosis
(c) Diaphyseal dysplasia
(d) Exostosis

86. **Hypertranslucency of lung unilaterally is seen on all *EXCEPT***
(a) Pneumothorax
(b) Resection of mammary gland
(c) Pulmonary artery obstruction
(d) Pneumonectomy

87. **Banana sign seen in the fetal brain suggests**
(a) Renal agenesis
(b) Encephalocele
(c) Spina bifida
(d) Porencephaly

88. **Worm-like filling defect is seen in**
(a) Erosive gastritis
(b) Esophageal varices
(c) Esophagus carcinoma
(d) Schatzki ring

89. **Radionuclide used in pheochromocytoma is**
(a) Radioactive iodine–131
(b) Technetium pertechnetate
(c) Radiolabeled chromium
(d) ^{123}I metaiodobenzylguanidine

90. **Water-lily appearance in a chest radiogram suggests**
(a) Loculated pyopneumothorax
(b) Cavitating metastasis
(c) Necrotizing pneumonia
(d) Ruptured hydatid cyst

91. **For treatment of cognitive symptoms of dementia, the drug most effective is**
(a) Serotonergic drugs
(b) Dopaminergic drugs
(c) Catecholamines
(d) Cholinesterase inhibitors

92. **The drug of choice for attention deficit hyperactivity disorders is**
(a) Haloperidol
(b) Imipramine
(c) Methylphenidate
(d) Lecithin

93. **Which of the following antipsychotic drugs is the best in treatment of resistant schizophrenia?**
(a) Olanzapine
(b) Clozapine
(c) Risperidone
(d) Doxepin

94. **Panic disorder is often associated with the following condition**
(a) Night terrors
(b) Agoraphobia
(c) Tic disorder
(d) Bipolar affective disorder

PHARMACOLOGY

95. **Which of the following statements about stavudine is accurate?**
(a) Bone marrow suppression is dose limiting
(b) It causes marked neurotoxicity
(c) It inhibits HIV protease
(d) It is a non-nucleoside reverse transcriptase inhibitor

96. **A new drug that reduces craving for alcohol is**
(a) Naltrexone
(b) Buspirone
(c) Trazodone
(d) Phenindamine

97. **Hyperuricemia is a side effect of this antitubercular drug**
(a) Pyrazinamide
(b) Isoniazid
(c) Capreomycin
(d) Ethambutol

98. **The antagonism of leukotriene by terbutaline is an example of**
(a) Pharmacological antagonism
(b) Physical antagonism
(c) Physiological (functional) antagonism
(d) Chemical antagonism

99. **Orlistat is effective in obesity by**
(a) Reduction of food intake
(b) Beta-1 adrenoreceptor agonist activity
(c) Inhibition of pancreatic lipase
(d) 5-HT receptor agonist activity

100. **The most appropriate drug of emergency contraception is**
(a) Misoprostol
(b) Ethinyl estradiol
(c) Levonorgestrel
(d) Mifepristone

101. **Reticulocytopenia is a dose-dependent side effect of**
(a) Azithromycin
(b) Chloramphenicol
(c) Clindamycin
(d) Doxycycline

102. **Amphotericin should be administered in**
(a) Glucose infusion
(b) Mannitol infusion
(c) Saline infusion
(d) Ringer lactate infusion

103. **Which one of the following drugs is most suitable for management of essential tremors?**
(a) Diazepam
(b) Levodopa
(c) Metoprolol
(d) Propranolol

104. **All of the following drugs are used in management of peptic ulcer *EXCEPT***
(a) Alginic acid
(b) Sucralfate
(c) Misoprostol
(d) Ipratropium

105. **Most common drug resistance for tuberculosis in India is found for**
(a) INH
(b) Rifampin
(c) Streptomycin
(d) Ethambutol

106. **Which of the following is a potentiator of toxicity due to digoxin?**
(a) Quinidine
(b) Hyperkalemia
(c) Hypocalcemia
(d) Hypermagnesemia

107. **Which of the following ACE inhibitor is *not* a pro-drug?**
(a) Enalapril
(b) Captopril
(c) Perindopril
(d) Ramipril

108. **Inhaled glucocorticoids used in asthma include the following *EXCEPT***
(a) Betamethasone
(b) Budesonide
(c) Fluticasone
(d) Beclomethasone

109. **The following drugs can cause systemic lupus erythematosus-like syndrome *EXCEPT***
(a) Isoniazid
(b) Gatifloxacin
(c) Hydralazine
(d) Procainamide

110. **An untoward effect of prolonged phenothiazines therapy is**
(a) A marked increase in blood pressure
(b) Rigidity and tremor at rest
(c) Suppression of prolactin
(d) Nausea

MICROBIOLOGY

111. **The main infectious agent associated with cystic fibrosis is**
(a) *Mycoplasma*
(b) *Pseudomonas*
(c) *Pneumocystis carinii*
(d) *Aspergillus*

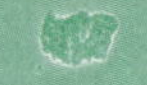

112. **Which organism causes a highly contagious pneumonia that is transmitted from human to human?**
(a) *Klebsiella pneumoniae*
(b) *Listeria monocytogenes*
(c) *Mycoplasma pneumoniae*
(d) *Nocardia asteroides*

113. **The bacteria producing a picture resembling 'pseudohemoptysis' in sputum sample due to *prodigiosin* production is**
(a) *Serratia marcescens*
(b) *Erwinia herbicola*
(c) *Ehrlichia sennetsu*
(d) *Legionella pneumophila*

114. **The bacteria frequently used as an immunomodulator is**
(a) *Corynebacterium parvum*
(b) *Mycobacterium marinum*
(c) *Chromobacterium violaceum*
(d) *Flavobacterium meningosepticum*

115. **Epsilometer test is done to detect**
(a) Bacterial motility
(b) Rate of bacterial growth
(c) Antibiotic susceptibility
(d) Coliform count

116. **Causative organism of molluscum contagiosum is**
(a) Papovavirus
(b) Poxvirus
(c) Orthomyxovirus
(d) Parvovirus

117. **Which of this immunoglobulin is associated with allergic disorders?**
(a) IgG
(b) IgM
(c) IgA
(d) IgE

118. **The reservoir in balantidium coli infection is**
(a) Dogs
(b) Pigs
(c) Cats
(d) Bats

119. **Following are acid-fast bacilli *EXCEPT***
(a) *Actinomyces israelii*
(b) *Mycobacterium avium* intracellulare
(c) *Mycobacterium leprae*
(d) *Nocardia*

120. **'Larva currens' occurs in infection caused by**
(a) *Toxocara canis*
(b) *Ancylostoma duodenale*
(c) *Gnathostoma spinigerum*
(d) *Strongyloides stercoralis*

121. **During the induction of an immune response, which cell is thought to process the initiating antigen?**
(a) Eosinophil
(b) Basophil
(c) Macrophage
(d) T cell

PATHOLOGY

122. **Malakoplakia of the urinary bladder is considered to be associated with**
(a) Tuberculosis
(b) Urothelial carcinoma
(c) Schistosomiasis
(d) Defects in phagocytosis

123. **Downey cell is seen in**
(a) Myeloma
(b) Chronic myeloid leukemia
(c) Hairy cell leukemia
(d) Infectious mononucleosis

124. **The following tumors secrete human chorionic gonadotropin *EXCEPT***
(a) Choriocarcinoma
(b) Polyembryoma
(c) Endodermal sinus tumor
(d) Embryonal cell carcinoma

125. **Glioblastoma multiforme is a variant of**
(a) Medulloblastoma
(b) Meningioma
(c) Astrocytoma
(d) Neuroblastoma

126. **Which of the following occur in epiphysis?**
(a) Chondroblastoma
(b) Osteochondroma
(c) Ewing sarcoma
(d) Chondrosarcoma

127. **A high maternal level of alpha-fetoprotein is noted in most cases of**
(a) Spina bifida
(b) Gaucher's disease
(c) Tay-Sachs disease
(d) Down syndrome

128. **Virchow lepra cells are seen in**
(a) Tuberculoid leprosy
(b) Indeterminate leprosy
(c) Borderline tuberculoid leprosy
(d) Lepromatous leprosy

129. **Which of the following manifestation is more likely to be found in the diffuse form of systemic sclerosis than in the CREST variant?**
(a) Esophageal motility dysfunction
(b) Pulmonary involvement
(c) Distal skin thickening
(d) Renal disease

130. **The transformation of a fibroblast to produce bone is an example of**
(a) Dysplasia
(b) Neoplasia
(c) Anaplasia
(d) Metaplasia

131. **'Microcytic anemia' is present in all the following conditions *EXCEPT* in**
(a) Folic acid deficiency
(b) Thalassemia trait
(c) Pyridoxine deficiency
(d) Copper deficiency

132. **'Chicken wire' pattern is characteristic of**
(a) Osteosarcoma
(b) Fibrosarcoma
(c) Angiosarcoma
(d) Chondroblastoma

133. **Increased levels of hemoglobin A2 are characteristic of which of the following disorders?**
(a) Sickle cell trait
(b) Beta-thalassemia trait
(c) Glucose-6-phosphate dehydrogenase (G6PD) deficiency
(d) Unstable hemoglobin disease

134. **Renal papillary necrosis is seen in**
(a) Sickle cell anemia
(b) Gouty nephropathy
(c) Chronic glomerulonephritis
(d) Hypercalcemia

135. **Rheumatoid factor (RA factor) is**
(a) IgM antibody against IgG
(b) IgE antibody against IgM
(c) Complement protein
(d) Cytokines

136. **Thrombocytopenia due to increased platelet destruction occurs in**
(a) Aplastic anemia
(b) Chemotherapy for cancer
(c) Acute lymphatic leukemia
(d) Systemic lupus erythematosus

137. **In myasthenia gravis, the antibodies are present against**
(a) Muscarinic receptor proteins
(b) Nicotinic receptor proteins
(c) Protein actin
(d) Protein myosin

138. **Most common manifestation of cardiac lupus is**
(a) Myocarditis
(b) Libman-Sacks endocarditis
(c) Pericarditis
(d) Aortic regurgitation

FORENSIC MEDICINE

139. **The powers of Chief Judicial Magistrate are**
(a) Death sentence
(b) Imprisonment for life
(c) Imprisonment up to 3 years
(d) Imprisonment up to 7 years

140. **Tattooing is seen surrounding the wound of entrance from a revolver or pistol, if the weapon is discharged up to distance of**
(a) 10 cm
(b) 30 cm
(c) 50 cm
(d) 90 cm

141. **Vegetable stains can be differentiated from blood stains by the presence of**
(a) Iron
(b) Tannin
(c) Copper
(d) Vitamin A

142. **The internal organ, which resists putrefaction for a longer time is**
(a) Heart
(b) Kidneys
(c) Liver
(d) Prostate

143. **Microscopic examination of the contused area, 2–3 months after infliction of injury shows the presence of**
(a) Histiocytes
(b) Monocytes
(c) Crystals of hemosiderin
(d) Crystals of hematoidin

PREVENTIVE AND SOCIAL MEDICINE

144. To find out whether the water has been properly chlorinated, the test used is
(a) Horrock's test
(b) Orthotolidine test
(c) Presumptive coliform test
(d) Coliform test

145. Disinfection of water is not required, if the source is from
(a) Tube well
(b) Step well
(c) Draw well
(d) River

146. A freshly prepared oral rehydration solution should not be used after
(a) 4 hours
(b) 6 hours
(c) 12 hours
(d) 24 hours

147. The gap in time between the onset of primary case and the secondary case is called
(a) Serial interval
(b) Incubation period
(c) Communicable period
(d) Prodromal period

148. The principal cause of blindness in India today is
(a) Glaucoma
(b) Retinitis pigmentosa
(c) Cataract
(d) Trachoma

149. The occurrence of a group of illness of similar nature at a rate above the expected number is called
(a) Hyperendemic
(b) Epidemic
(c) Endemic
(d) Pandemic

150. Following index measures average achievements in basic dimensions of human development
(a) Human poverty index
(b) Human development index
(c) Gender empowerment index
(d) Life expectancy at birth

151. Factor which is associated both with exposure and disease is called
(a) Confounding factor
(b) Risk factor
(c) Proximal risk factor
(d) Case

152. The person, animal, object or substance from which an infectious substance passes, or is disseminated to a susceptible host is called
(a) Reservoir
(b) Source
(c) Carrier
(d) Homologous reservoir

153. Validity of an indicator means
(a) It should actually measure what it is supposed to measure
(b) The answer should be same if measured by different persons in similar circumstances
(c) Indicator should reflect changes in the situation concealed
(d) Indicator should have ability to obtain data needed

154. The current maternal mortality rate per 100,000 live births in India is around
(a) 200
(b) 400
(c) 600
(d) 800

155. Panel discussion can be defined as
(a) Series of speeches
(b) Discussion by 4–8 qualified persons
(c) Groups describing individual experiences
(d) Stagewise-formatted teaching

ANATOMY, PHYSIOLOGY AND BIOCHEMISTRY

156. Skin at the level of umbilicus is supplied by the spinal nerve
(a) T9
(b) T10
(c) T11
(d) T12

157. Tooth is fixed in its socket by the
(a) Cementocytes
(b) Periodontal membrane
(c) Cement
(d) Dentin

158. Ligamentum denticulatum is from
(a) Dura mater
(b) Pia mater
(c) Arachnoid mater
(d) Spinal cord

159. The main antagonistic muscle of rectus abdominis muscle is
(a) Psoas major
(b) Latissimus dorsi

(c) Quadratus lumborum
(d) Erector spinae

160. The forward displacement of tibia on the femur is prevented by
(a) Anterior cruciate ligament
(b) Posterior cruciate ligament
(c) Medical collateral ligament
(d) Lateral collateral ligament

161. Circumvallate papillae are supplied by
(a) Lingual nerve
(b) Glossopharyngeal nerve
(c) Hypoglossal nerve
(d) Vagus nerve

162. The functions of the neocerebellum are
(a) Maintenance of equilibrium
(b) Servocorrection of voluntary movements
(c) Planning and programming of voluntary movements
(d) Maintenance of muscle tone

163. The earliest 'paranasal sinus' to develop is
(a) Ethmoid
(b) Sphenoid
(c) Frontal
(d) Maxillary

164. Carotid sinus massage sometimes stops supraventicular tachycardia because
(a) It decreases sympathetic discharge to the SA node
(b) It increases vagal discharge to the conducting tissue between the atria and the ventricles
(c) It increases vagal tone to the SA node
(d) It decreases sympathetic discharge to the conducting tissue between the atria and the ventricles

165. The oxygen buffer function of hemoglobin is related to
(a) Dissociation curve shape
(b) Haldane effect
(c) Bohr effect
(d) Respiratory exchange ratio

166. Podocytes are seen in
(a) Bowman's capsule
(b) Proximal convoluted tubule
(c) Distal convoluted tubule
(d) Collecting tubule of the kidney

167. The lower esophageal sphincter pressure is increased by
(a) Glucagon
(b) Gastrin
(c) Emptying of the stomach
(d) Chocolate

168. In which of the following tissues is glucose transport into the cell enhanced by insulin?
(a) Brain
(b) Lens
(c) Red blood cells
(d) Adipose tissue

169. Which of the following statements about the action of the somatomedins is true?
(a) They inhibit protein synthesis
(b) They antagonize the effect of insulin
(c) They promote growth of bone and cartilage
(d) They mediate the local effects of somatostatin

170. Mass movement of the colon would be abolished by
(a) Extrinsic denervation
(b) Distention of the colon
(c) Gastrocolic reflex
(d) Destruction of Auerbach's plexus

171. In the mucosal cells, triglycerides are formed primarily in the
(a) Rough endoplasmic reticulum
(b) Smooth endoplasmic reticulum
(c) Golgi apparatus
(d) Ribosomes

172. In a standard electrocardiogram, an augmented limb lead measures the electrical potential difference between
(a) Two limbs
(b) One limb and two other limbs
(c) One limb and neutral (zero)
(d) Two limbs and neutral (zero)

173. Functions of spleen include all *EXCEPT*
(a) Response to antigenic challenge
(b) Destruction of abnormal RBCs
(c) Production of platelet
(d) Erythrocyte production

174. The most important source of reducing equivalents for fatty acid synthesis in the liver is
(a) Oxidation of acetyl coenzyme A
(b) Glycolysis
(c) The citric acid cycle
(d) The pentose phosphate pathway

175. 'Hereditary fructose intolerance' is a condition caused by deficiency of
(a) Phosphofructokinase
(b) Fructokinase

(c) Fructose 1-phosphate aldolase B
(d) Fructose-1, 6-bisphosphate aldolase

176. Mucopolysaccharidoses are caused by
(a) An increased rate of synthesis of proteoglycans
(b) Defects in the degradation of proteoglycans
(c) The synthesis of polysaccharides with an altered structure
(d) An insufficient amount of proteolytic enzymes

177. The rate limiting step in catecholamines biosynthesis is
(a) The hydroxylation of tyrosine
(b) The hydroxylation of phenylalanine
(c) The formation of dopamine
(d) The reduction of dihydrobiopterin

178. A membrane phospholipid that does *not* contain glycerol is
(a) Lecithin
(b) Sphingomyelin
(c) Cardiolipin
(d) Ceramide

COMED-K 2005

ANSWERS AND EXPLANATIONS

MEDICINE

1. **Answer is c (Amiodarone).**
Ref: CMDT 2009, Pg 366.

Sustained ventricular tachycardia (arrhythmia)
- Several trials including the antiarrhythmic drugs versus implantable defibrillator, strongly suggests that these patients should be managed with implantable cardioverter defibrillator devices (ICDs).
- In those with preserved LV function, the mortality is lowered and treatment with amiodarone optimally in combination with beta blockers may be adequate.

Also Know

❖ ***Side effects of amiodarone***: Tremor, peripheral neuropathy, pulmonary inflammation, hypothyroidism and hyperthyroidism, photosensitivity and corneal deposits.

2. **Answer is a (Final height will be less than that of peers).**
Ref: Nelson's Pediatrics, 17th edition Pg 1863.

- ***Precocious puberty*** is defined as puberty before 8 years in girls or before 9 years in boys and menstruation before 10 years.
- The increased rate of bone maturation results in ***early closure of the epiphysis*** and ***ultimate stature is less than it would have been otherwise***.
- About one third of girls and boys achieve a height less than 5th percentile as adults
- Human growth hormone with GnRH agonists will improve the height.

3. **Answer is d (Minocycline).**
Ref: Remington: The science and practice of pharmacy, Pg 1440 Park, 20th edition Pg 151.

- Treatment with ***penicillin does not*** eradicate the carrier state of meningococci.
- ***Rifampicin*** is the ***drug of choice***.
- ***Minocycline***, but ***not other tetracyclines*** appear to be effective in the treatment of meningococcal carrier state.

4. **Answer is a (Resting tremors).**
Ref: Ganong's physiology, 23rd edition Pg 258.

Repeat Topic
- Refer ***answer no. 180 in COMED-K 2007 answers*** for detailed explanation.

5. **Answer is b (*Clostridium difficile*).**
Ref: Davidson's, 20th edition Pg 931.

- ***Antibiotic-associated diarrhea***, antibiotic-associated colitis and ***pseudomembranous enterocolitis*** are part of the same disease spectrum, which results from disturbance of the normal intestinal flora. ***Clostridium difficile*** is thought to be the cause in most cases.

- Metronidazole and vancomycin are the drugs of choice.
- HOWEVER **remember**: ***Metronidazole*** is more effective, less toxic and more convenient and therefore, preferred over vancomycin (*KD Tripathi, 6th/799*).

6. **Answer is d (Hypothyroidism).**
Ref: Harrison's, 17th edition Pg 2232, 2236.

How does radioactive iodine (RAI) act?

➢ RAI treatment decreases the activity of the overactive thyroid gland by destroying thyroid cells. The RAI is administered orally as a capsule or in water. The radioactive iodine becomes concentrated in the thyroid gland, where it emits radiation causing inflammation and necrosis of the cells in the gland.

What are the pretreatment precautions?

➢ Antecedent treatment with antithyroid drugs should be considered for all elderly patients or for those with cardiac problems to deplete thyroid hormone stores before administration of radioiodine.

➢ *Carbimazole or methimazole* must be *stopped at least 3 days before radioiodine* administration to achieve optimum iodine uptake.

➢ *Propylthiouracil* has a prolonged radioprotective effect and *should be stopped several weeks before radioiodine is* given or a larger dose of radioiodine will be necessary.

What are the side effects?

➢ In the first 3–4 months after radioiodine treatment, transient ***hypothyroidism*** may occur due to reversible radiation damage.

What are the contraindications?

➢ Absolute: Pregnancy.

➢ Relative: Ophthalmopathy (RAI can aggravate thyroid eye disease).

7. **Answer is a (Hypotension).**
Ref: Harrison's, 17th edition Pg 2517, Table 364-2.

Quick Look

Disorders Associated with Thrombosis

Acquired	Inherited
Diseases or syndromes	**Coagulation factor deficiencies**
• Lupus anticoagulant	• Factor V Leiden
• Malignancy	• Protein C deficiency
• Myeloproliferative disorder	• Protein S deficiency
• Thrombotic thrombocytopenic purpura	• Antithrombin III deficiency
• Estrogen/OCP treatment	**Impaired clot lysis**
• Nephrotic syndrome	• Dysfibrinogenemia
• Hyperlipidemia	• Plasminogen deficiency
• Hyperviscosity	• TPA deficiency
• Diabetes mellitus	• PAI-1 excess
• Congestive heart failure	**Uncertain mechanism**
• Paroxysmal nocturnal hemoglobinuria	• Homocystinuria
• Sickle cell anemia	
• β-thalassemia	
Physiologic states	
• Pregnancy	
• Obesity	
• Postoperative stage	
• Immobilization	
• Old age	

<u>Note</u>: On ***CT scan,*** cerebral venous thrombosis shows ***empty delta sign***.

8. **Answer is b (NADPH-dependent aldose reductase).**
Ref: Vasudevan's biochemistry, 5th edition Pg 123.

- In ***diabetes mellitus***, the lens glucose is converted to ***sorbitol by NADPH-dependant aldose reductase*** → diabetic cataract.
- ***Aldose reductase*** inhibitors are being studied to prevent diabetic cataract.

9. **Answer is a (Denotes valve mobility).**
Ref: Harrison's, 17th edition Pg 1676; Davidson's, 20th edition Pg 619.

- A ***characteristic finding of rheumatic mitral stenosis*** is an ***opening snap following S2*** due to the stiff mitral valve.
- Opening snap (OS) of the mitral valve is most readily audible in expiration at or just medial to the cardiac apex.
- This sound generally follows the sound of aortic valve closure (A2) by 0.05–0.12 second. The time interval between A2 and OS varies inversely with the severity of the MS.
- The *intensity of the mitral opening snap* ***correlates well with the mobility of the valve***. A loud opening snap is found in mobile stenotic valves with good excursions, whereas the opening snap is absent with severe calcific fixation of the valve.

10. **Answer is b (Patent ductus arteriosus).**
Ref: Harrison's, 17th edition Pg 1382.

- Central cyanosis often associated with clubbing of the fingers and toes indicates right-to-left cardiac or extracardiac shunting or inadequate oxygenation of blood by the lungs.
- Cardiac causes of clubbing include:
  - ❖ ***Infective endocarditis***
  - ❖ PDA with reversal of shunt (***Eisenmenger's syndrome***)
  - ❖ ***Tricuspid atresia.***

  ✈ Note: Clubbing is typically seen in cyanotic congenital heart disease. PDA by itself is an acyanotic congenital heart disease.

11. **Answer is a (Selective proteinuria).**
Ref: Harrison's, 17th edition Pg 1790; OP Ghai, 7th edition Pg 451.

- In children, the abnormal urine principally contains albumin with minimal amounts of higher molecular weight proteins and is sometimes called ***selective proteinuria***. The determination of urinary protein selectivity, however, is of ***generally little clinical importance***.
- Poor prognostic factors include:
  - ➲ Hematuria
  - ➲ Hypertension
  - ➲ Steroid resistance
  - ➲ Membranoproliferative histology.

12. **Answer is b (Beryllium).**
Ref: Harrison's, 17th edition Pg 1615.

Repeat Topic

- Refer ***answer no. 130 in COMED-K 2010 answers*** for detailed explanation.

13. **Answer is d (Renin suppression).**
Ref: Harrison's, 17th edition Pg 2260.

- The criteria for the diagnosis of ***primary hyperaldosteronism*** are:
  - ➢ Diastolic hypertension without edema
  - ➢ ***Hyposecretion of renin*** (as judged by low plasma renin activity levels) that fails to increase appropriately during volume depletion (upright posture, sodium depletion)
  - ➢ Hypersecretion of aldosterone that does not suppress appropriately in response to volume expansion.

- ***Hypokalemia may be severe*** (< 3 mmol/L) and reflects body potassium depletion, usually > 300 mmol. In mild forms of primary aldosteronism, potassium levels may be normal.
- ***Hypernatremia is infrequent,*** but may be caused by sodium retention, concomitant water loss from polyuria and resetting of the osmostat.
- ***Metabolic alkalosis*** and elevation of serum bicarbonate are caused by hydrogen ion loss into the urine and migration into potassium-depleted cells.

14. Answer is d (Congenital hypertrophic pyloric stenosis).
Ref: Harrison's 17th edition Pg 290, 292.

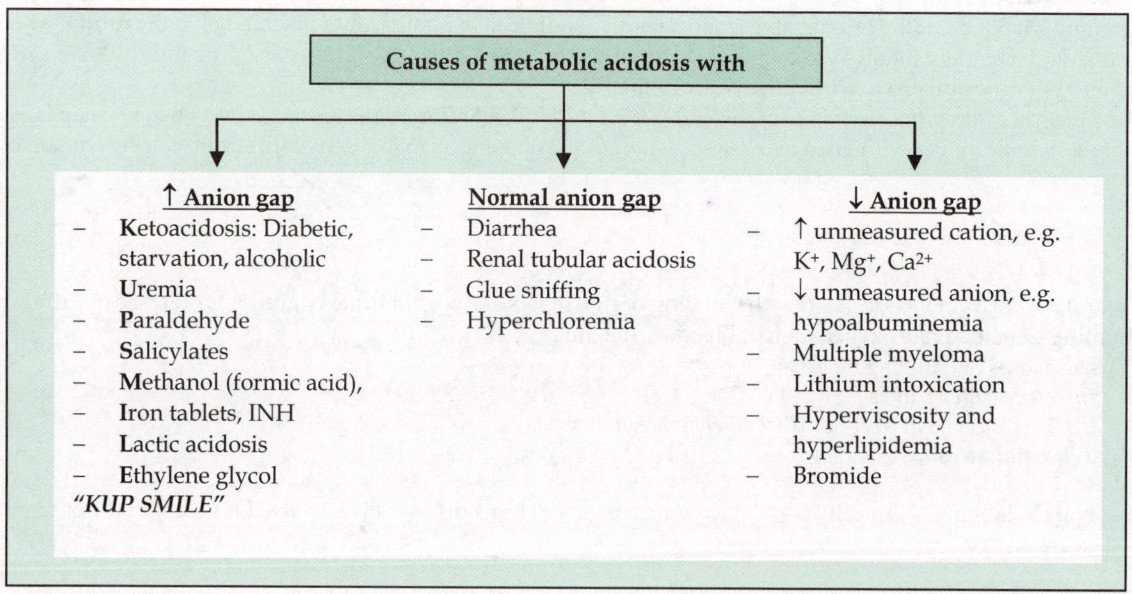

Causes of metabolic acidosis with

↑ Anion gap	Normal anion gap	↓ Anion gap
– Ketoacidosis: Diabetic, starvation, alcoholic	– Diarrhea	– ↑ unmeasured cation, e.g. K^+, Mg^+, Ca^{2+}
– Uremia	– Renal tubular acidosis	– ↓ unmeasured anion, e.g. hypoalbuminemia
– Paraldehyde	– Glue sniffing	– Multiple myeloma
– Salicylates	– Hyperchloremia	– Lithium intoxication
– Methanol (formic acid),		– Hyperviscosity and hyperlipidemia
– Iron tablets, INH		– Bromide
– Lactic acidosis		
– Ethylene glycol		
"KUP SMILE"		

Note:

❖ ***Congenital hypertrophic pyloric stenosis*** classically causes ***hypochloremic hypokalemic metabolic alkalosis*** – frequently asked MCQ in each and every entrance examination.

15. Answer is c (Breathlessness).
Ref: Davidson's, 20th edition Pg 390, Box 14.14.

Clinical features of *Pneumocystis carinii (jiroveci) pneumonia*

- 2–3 weeks history
- Fever with dry cough
- *Disproportionate breathlessness*
- Chest X-ray normal or perihilar ground-glass infiltrate
- No response to standard antibiotics
- Few signs on auscultation
- Exercise-related desaturation.

16. Answer is d (Fibrosing alveolitis).
Ref: Harrison's, 17th edition Pg 2087.

Author's comments: *"Harrison's 18th edition also does not mention the word "fibrosing alveolitis" under pulmonary manifestations of RA. However there are many many articles on pubmed about association of fibrosing alveolitis and RA (it IS associated in 2% of cases of RA); hence if this question is repeated in 2015- "none" will be the best answer ! and for challenging the answer key the pubmed links maybe used".*

Pulmonary manifestations of RA

- Pleurisy with or without effusion
- Interstitial Lung Disease (ILD) in up to 20% of cases
- Necrobiotic nodules (non-pneumoconiotic intrapulmonary rheumatoid nodules) with or without cavities
- Caplan's syndrome (rheumatoid coal worker's pneumoconiosis)
- Pulmonary hypertension secondary to rheumatoid pulmonary vasculitis
- Bronchiolitis obliterans with organizing pneumonia (BOOP)
- Upper airway obstruction due to cricoarytenoid arthritis

17. Answer is b (Varicella zoster).
Ref: Harrison's, 17th edition Pg 1103.

Ramsay Hunt syndrome

- Caused by *VZV*
- *Pain and vesicles appear in the external auditory canal*
- Patients *lose their sense of taste in the anterior two-thirds of the tongue*
- Develop *ipsilateral facial palsy*
- *Geniculate ganglion of the sensory branch of the facial nerve* is involved

QuickLook

- *Herpes zoster* (also called shingles) is a sporadic disease that results from reactivation of latent VZV from dorsal root ganglia.
- Herpes zoster is characterized by a unilateral vesicular eruption within a dermatome, often associated with severe pain.
- The dermatomes from T3 to L3 are most frequently involved.
- If the ophthalmic branch of the trigeminal nerve is involved, *zoster ophthalmicus* results.

18. Answer is a (Ambulatory patients).
Ref: Park, 20th edition Pg 701.

Repeat Topic

- Refer *answer no. 129 in COMED-K 2007 answers* for detailed explanation.

19. Answer is b (Measuring RBC cholinesterase).
Ref: Narayan Reddy's FMT, 23rd edition Pg 254.

- Diagnosis of OP poisoning is by *estimation of cholinesterase enzyme in the blood.*
- Normal value in RBC is 77–142 nmol/dL and in plasma is 41–140 nmol/dL.
- The *plasma cholinesterase levels fall more rapidly than RBCs level*. So *plasma cholinesterase is more sensitive* in diagnosis of OP poisoning.
- Diagnosis can be confirmed by giving 2 mg of atropine; in normal patient it will cause marked atropinization and in OP poisoning symptoms are relieved.

20. Answer is c (Mitral valve prolapse with mitral regurgitation).
Ref: Harrison's, 17th edition Pg 1387.

- *Early systolic murmurs* begin with the first heart sound and end in midsystole. It is seen in:
  1. *Large VSD with pulmonary hypertension.*
  2. Very small *muscular VSD.*
  3. *Tricuspid regurgitation occurring in the absence of pulmonary hypertension* (common in narcotics abusers).
  4. *Acute mitral regurgitation* into a noncompliant left atrium and a large *v* wave.

Note:

- ***Late systolic murmurs*** following midsystolic clicks are due to late systolic *mitral regurgitation caused by prolapse of the mitral valve into the left atrium.*

21. **Answer is b (Malignant hypertension).**
Ref: Harsh Mohan's Pathology, 4th edition Pg 357.

➲ **Flea bitten kidney**: Petechial hemorrhages on the renal surface grossly look like fleas have bitten the entire kidney. Seen in:
- *Malignant hypertension*
- Henoch-Schönlein purpura (HSP)
- Subacute bacterial endocarditis (SABE)
- Acute poststreptococcal glomerulonephritis (APGN)
- Rapidly progressive GN (RPGN)
- Hemolytic uremic syndrome (HUS)
- Thrombotic thrombocytopenic purpura (TTP)
- Leukemia, lymphoma, myeloma.

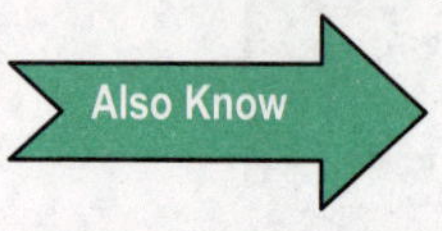

➲ **Large kidney**	– Diabetic nephropathy – Amyloidosis – Scleroderma – Polycystic disease – Medullary cystic/sponge kidney – Acute glomerulonephritis
➲ **Small contracted kidney**	– Chronic GN – Chronic pyelonephritis – Benign nephrosclerosis

SURGERY

22. **Answer is c (Veins of the breast).**
Ref: Bailey and Love, 25th edition Pg 833.

- ***Mondor's disease*** is ***thrombophlebitis of the superficial veins of the breast*** and anterior chest wall, although it has also been encountered in the arm.
- Cause is obscure. ***Pathognomonic feature*** is ***thrombosed subcutaneous cord***, usually attached to the skin.
- The only *treatment required is restricted movements of the arm* and in any case, the ***condition subsides within a few months*** without recurrence, complications or deformity.

Fast Facts

❖ ***Amazia***: Congenital absence of one or both breasts, more common in males; root of the word 'Amazon'.
❖ ***Poland's syndrome***: Congenital absence of the breast (amazia) associated with absence of sternal portion of pectoralis major.
❖ ***Polymazia***: Accessory breasts, MC in axilla.

23. **Answer is d (Giant gastric folds).**
Ref: Harrison's, 17th edition Pg 575, Table 87-5.

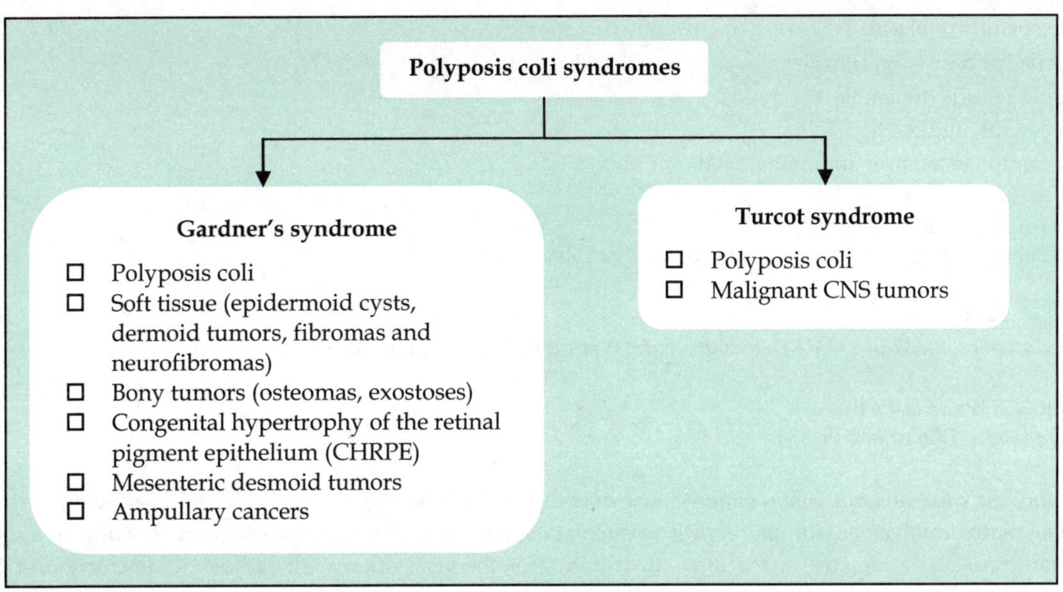

24. **Answer is d (Familial adenomatous polyposis).**
Ref: Harrison's, 17th edition Pg 575.

- ***Polyposis coli*** (***familial polyposis of the colon***) are a rare condition characterized by the appearance of thousands of adenomatous polyps throughout the large bowel.
- It is transmitted as an ***autosomal dominant***, chromosome ***5p-, APC gene***.
- The colonic polyps in all these conditions are rarely present before puberty, but are generally evident in affected individuals by age 25.
- If the polyposis is not treated surgically, ***colorectal cancer will develop in almost all patients before age 40***.

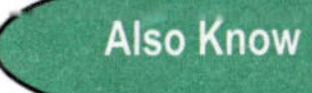

Risk factors for development of colorectal cancer

- Diet: Animal fat
- Hereditary syndromes (autosomal dominant inheritance)
  - Polyposis coli
  - Non-polyposis syndrome (Lynch syndrome)
- Inflammatory bowel disease
- *Streptococcus bovis* bacteremia
- Ureterosigmoidostomy
- Tobacco use

25. **Answer is b (Carcinoma of the colon).**
Ref: Harrison's, 17th edition Pg 575.

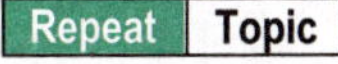

- Refer ***above answer*** for detailed explanation.

26. **Answer is a (Hypospadias).**
Ref: Bailey and Love, 25th edition Pg 1314, Fig. 72.2.

Ectopia vesicae

- Exstrophy of bladder
- Broad short penis (in males)
- Bifid clitoris (in females)
- Bilateral inguinal hernia
- Incomplete anterior abdominal wall.

27. Answer is d (Ganglioneuroma).
Ref: Robbins Pathology, 7th edition Pg 707; Bailey and Love, 25th edition Pg 892.

Repeat Topic

- See ***answer no. 37 in COMED-K 2006 answers*** for detailed explanation.

28. Answer is b (Pancoast's tumor).
Ref: Harrison's, 17th edition Pg 554.

- ***Pancoast's* (or *superior sulcus tumor*) *syndrome*** results from local extension of a tumor growing in the ***apex of the lung*** with involvement of the ***eighth cervical and first and second thoracic nerves,*** with shoulder pain that characteristically radiates in the ulnar distribution of the arm, often with radiologic destruction of the first and second ribs.
- Often ***Horner's syndrome and Pancoast's syndrome coexist.***
- ***Horner's syndrome*** = Sympathetic nerve paralysis with enophthalmos, ptosis, miosis and ipsilateral loss of sweating.

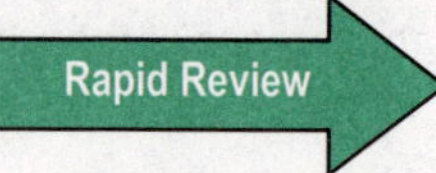

- Regional spread of lung tumor in the thorax (by contiguous growth or by metastasis to regional lymph nodes) may cause:
  - *Tracheal obstruction*
  - Esophageal compression with *dysphagia*
  - Recurrent laryngeal nerve paralysis with *hoarseness*
  - *Phrenic nerve paralysis* with elevation of the hemidiaphragm and dyspnea
  - *Horner's* syndrome.

29. Answer is d (Peptic ulcer).
Ref: Harrison's, 17th edition Pg 257; Davidson's, 20th edition Pg 866, 868.

- MC of ***Upper GI Bleeding = Peptic ulcers*** (accounts for up to ~50% of cases)
- MC cause of lower GI bleeding = Diverticular disease

- ***Ligament of Treitz*** is a fibromuscular band, which suspends and supports the duodenojejunal flexure.
- Ligament of Treitz is an important landmark; *bleeding from proximal to this ligament is called upper GI bleeding* whereas *distal to it is called lower GI bleeding.*

30. Answer is a (Vomiting).
Ref: Harrison's, 17th edition Pg 1899.

Clinical features of irritable bowel syndrome are:

- ***Abdominal pain*** or discomfort.
- Altered bowel habits (most consistent feature); most common pattern is ***constipation alternating with diarrhea,*** usually with one of these symptoms predominating.
- Upper gastrointestinal symptoms: Dyspepsia, heartburn, nausea and ***vomiting*** (25–50%).

31. Answer is c (Ultrasound of abdomen).
Ref: Mastery of Surgery, Vol 1, Josef E Fischer, Pg 177, 2007 edition.

- Use of the ***focused abdominal sonography for trauma (FAST) examination*** has blossomed during the last decade and is ***replacing diagnostic peritoneal lavage in most trauma centers.***
- The primary indication is to diagnose free intraperitoneal fluid in the setting of blunt trauma.
- Although CT scans provide better solid organ resolution, ***US is quicker, less expensive and portable to the bedside, obviating transportation of tenuous (weak, critically ill patients).***
- Diagnostic peritoneal lavage is more sensitive for detection of blood, but is invasive and NOT applicable to all patients (i.e. pregnancy or prior abdominal operations).
- ***Overall ultrasound*** is more portable, quicker, reproducible and less expensive.

32. Answer is a (Small cell carcinoma).
Ref: Harrison's, 17th edition Pg 551, Table 85-1.

- Four major cell types make up 88% of all primary lung neoplasms according to the WHO classification as below:

Cancer	5-year survival rate
Squamous or epidermoid carcinoma	15%
Small cell (also called oat cell) carcinoma	5%
Adenocarcinoma	17%
Large cell carcinoma	11%

33. Answer is c (Erythroplakia has a higher risk for malignancy).
Ref: Harrison's, 17th edition Pg 218, Table 32-3; Bailey and Love's 25th edition Pg 735, 737.

Smoker's leukoplakia and smokeless tobacco lesions

- ☐ Location: Any area of oral mucosa, sometimes related to location of habit.
- ☐ Clinically: White patch that may become firm, rough or red fissured and ulcerated; may become sore and painful, but usually painless; a purely descriptive term with NO histological correlation. So obviously ***biopsy is not necessary to call a lesion as leukoplakia.***
- ☐ Course: ***May or may not resolve with cessation of habit***; 2% develop squamous cell carcinoma (speckled leukoplakia has highest risk); early biopsy essential.

Erythroplakia with or without white patches

- ☐ Location: Floor of mouth, common in men; tongue and buccal mucosa in women.
- ☐ Clinically: ***Velvety, reddish plaque***; occasionally mixed with white patches or smooth red areas.
- ☐ Course: ***High risk of squamous cell cancer***; early biopsy essential.

Oral submucous fibrosis

- ☐ Location: Fibrous bands form beneath oral mucosa.
- ☐ Clinically: Scarring produces contracture resulting in limited mouth opening and restricted tongue movement.
- ☐ ***Almost entirely confined to Asian population***; a/w ***pan masala areca nut*** with/without concurrent alcohol use.
- ☐ Course: Treat with intralesional steroids or surgical excision and skin grafts.

34. Answer is b (Undergoes hydrolysis and complete absorption).
Ref: Bailey and Love, 25th edition Pg 236-239, Table 18.2.

- Suture materials absorb in one of two ways:
  - ➢ Catgut and collagen get absorbed by enzymatic digestion.

- The other method is one of preliminary hydrolysis, which is the effect of water on suture materials. Once a suture has been broken up by hydrolysis, polymorphonuclear cells and other macrophage (giant cells) digest. This type of suture degradation is seen in polydioxanone (PDS).

- PDS is not used in a/w heart valves or synthetic grafts, or in situations in which prolonged tissue approximation under stress is required.

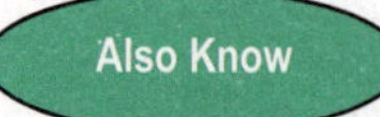

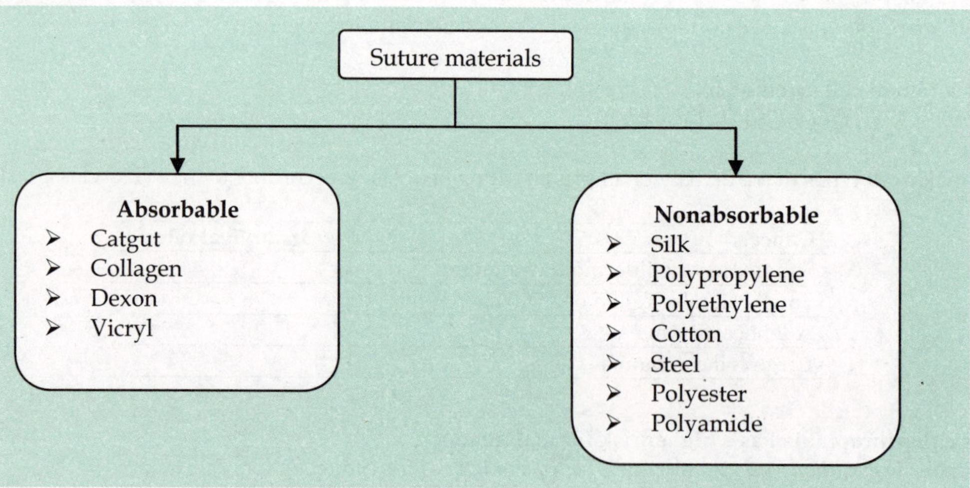

35. Answer is d (Excessive infusion of 5% glucose).
Ref: http://surgeryonline.wordpress.com/tag/fluid-intake/

Direct quote

- The ***commonest cause of water intoxication in surgical wards is the over prescribing of intravenous 5% glucose solutions*** to ***postoperative patients***.
- Colorectal washouts with plain water, instead of saline, have caused water intoxication during total bowel wash-through prior to colonic surgery.
- A major component of the TURP (transurethral resection of the prostate) syndrome is the water intoxication caused by excessive uptake of water (and glycine) from irrigation fluid.

Author's Comments: *"The direct quote for the above question is found at the above internet reference; however this has been verified from various textbooks that excess of 5% dextrose causes water intoxication".*

36. Answer is a (Crohn's disease).
Ref: Robbins Pathology, 7th edition Pg 849-50.

Repeat Topic

- Refer *answer no. 37 in COMED-K 2009 answers* for detailed explanation.

37. Answer is d (Hemorrhage).
Ref: CSDT, 13th edition Pg 544.

Direct quote:

"***Serious postoperative hemorrhage*** occurs from the cyst most often after ***cystogastrostomy***".

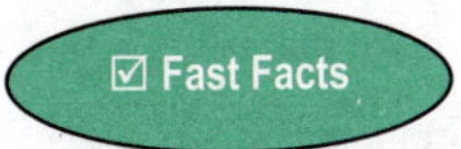

Pseudopancreatic cysts of > 6 cm size, > 6 weeks duration and symptomatic cysts of any size require intervention.

- Cyst in head: Cystogastrostomy
- Cyst in body: Cystojejunostomy
- Cyst in tail: Distal pancreatectomy.

38. **Answer is c (Malignancy is the underlying cause).**
Ref: Harrison's, 17th edition Pg 824.

Repeat Topic

- Refer ***answer no. 42 in COMED-K 2010 answers*** for detailed explanation.

OBSTETRICS AND GYNECOLOGY

39. **Answer is a (Foreign body).**
Ref: Shaw's Gynecology, 14th edition Pg 119.

- The possibility of a ***foreign body inserted into the vagina***, the variety of which baffles enumeration, must not be forgotten as a cause of vulvovaginitis in children.
- This primitive Freudian urge accounts for many otherwise inexplicable ***vaginal discharge in young children***.

40. **Answer is c (Oral contraceptive).**
Ref: Harrison's, 17th edition Pg 829; Park, 20th edition Pg 430.

Direct quote:

"Women using ***oral contraceptives appear to be at decreased risk of symptomatic PID*** and tubal sterilization reduces the risk of salpingitis by preventing intraluminal spread of infection into the tubes."

Beneficial effects of OCPs: Protection against at least 6 diseases

- ❖ Benign breast disorders including fibrocystic breast disease and fibroadenoma
- ❖ Ovarian cysts and ovarian cancer
- ❖ Endometrial cancer
- ❖ Ectopic pregnancy
- ❖ Pelvic inflammatory disease
- ❖ Iron deficiency anemia

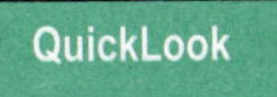

Important risk factors for acute PID include:

- ❖ The presence of endocervical infection or bacterial vaginosis
- ❖ A history of salpingitis or of recent vaginal douching
- ❖ The use of an IUD (especially among nulliparous women, during the first few months after IUD insertion and among women with multiple sex partners)
- ❖ Dilatation and curettage or cesarean section.

41. **Answer is b (Surface coelomic epithelium).**
Ref: Robbins Pathology, 7th edition Pg 1094, Fig. 22-37.

Derivation of various ovarian tumors

Origin	Surface epithelial cells	Germ cell	Sex cord stroma	Metastases to ovaries
Overall frequency	65–70%	15–20%	5–10%	5%
Proportion of malignant ovarian tumors	90%	3–5%	2–3%	5%
Age group affected	20+ years	0–25+ years	All ages	Variable
Types	Serous tumor Mucinous tumor Endometrioid tumor Clear cell tumor Brenner tumor Cystadenofibroma	Teratoma Dysgerminoma Endodermal sinus tumor Choriocarcinoma	Fibroma Granulosa-theca cell tumors Sertoli-Leydig cell tumor	

42. Answer is d (Partogram).
Ref: Dutta's Obstetrics, 6th edition Pg 529, 403.

- ***Partogram*** is a ***composite graphical record of cervical dilatation*** in centimeters and ***descent of head against duration of labor in hours.***
- In a partograph, the labor process is divided into:
  - ➢ ***Latent phase,*** that ends when the cervix is 3 cm dilated
  - ➢ ***Active phase*** starts with cervical dilation of 3 cm. Cervix should dilate at least 1 cm/hour in this active phase.
- ***Cervical dilation rate (cerviograph)*** is plotted in relation to alert line and action line.
- ***Alert line*** starts at the end of latent phase (3 cm cervical dilation) and ends with full dilation of the cervix (10 cm) in 7 hours (1 cm/hour dilation rate).
- ***Action line*** is drawn 4 hours to the right of the alert line. An interval of 4 hours is allowed to diagnose delay in active phase and then appropriate intervention is done.

Note:

- ***Labor is considered abnormal*** when ***cerviograph crosses the alert line and falls on zone 2***
- ***Intervention is required when it crosses the action line and falls on zone 3.***

43. Answer is c (Renal agenesis).
Ref: Dutta's Obstetrics, 6th edition Pg 218.

Repeat Topic

- Refer ***answer no. 49 in COMED-K 2006 answers*** for detailed explanation.

44. Answer is d (Rectal mucosa).
Ref: Dutta's textbook of Obstetrics, 6th edition Pg 423.

Degrees of perineal tear

• **First degree**	Lacerations of hymen, the fourchette, lower part of the vagina and the perineal skin, but the perineal body remains intact
• **Second degree**	Lacerations of the posterior vaginal wall and varying degrees of tear of the perineal body excluding the anal sphincter
• **Third degree (complete)**	Involves major lacerations of the posterior vaginal wall and tear of the perineal body including the anal sphincter with or without involvement of the anal canal or even the rectum

45. Answer is c (Onset of the luteinizing hormone surge).
Ref: Ganong's Physiology, 23rd edition Pg 414.

Direct quote:
"A surge in LH secretion triggers ovulation and ovulation normally occurs about 9 h after the peak of the LH surge at midcycle."

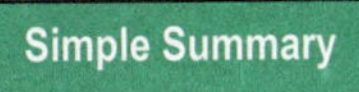

Other tests for ovulation

Basal body temperature test (BBT)
- BBT falls by about 0.5°F at the time of ovulation.
- Subsequently ***during the progestational half of the cycle, the temperature is slightly raised*** above the preovulatory level and the rise is of the order of 0.5–1°F.
- If the patient conceives, the temperature remains elevated at this level and does not fall as it would during a menstrual cycle.
- This phenomenon is due to the thermogenic action of progesterone and hence presumptive evidence of a functioning corpus luteum and hence ovulation.

Fern test
- During estrogenic phase, the cervical mucus shows ***ferning due to effect of NaCl secreted under estrogen*** influence.
- This ferning disappears after ovulation and if previously present, is presumptive evidence of a corpus luteum activity.

Ultrasound
- Ultrasound has now become the ***standard procedure for monitoring maturation of the Graafian follicle*** and in ***detecting imminent ovulation in in vitro fertilization*** and timing intercourse.

PEDIATRICS

46. **Answer is b (7 months).**
Ref: OP Ghai, 7th edition Pg 30.

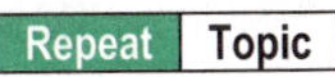

- ***At 6 months***: Child ***recognizes strangers/stranger anxiety*** appears.
- For more on developmental milestones see detailed table – ***answer no. 65 in COMED-K 2007 answers***.

47. **Answer is c (3 years).**
Ref: Nelson's, 17th edition Pg 39.

- A ***child knows his/her age and sex by the age of 3 years***.
- For more on developmental milestones see detailed table – ***answer no. 65 in COMED-K 2007 answers***.

48. **Answer is a (Ventricular septal defect).**
Ref: Essential revision notes for MRCP, Philip A Kalra, 2004 edition Pg 26.

Associations of coarctation

Cardiac	Noncardiac
– Bicuspid aortic valve (an thus AS ± AR) in 10%–20% – PDA – VSD – Mitral valve disease	– Berry aneurysms – Turner's syndrome – Renal abnormalities

49. **Answer is a (Sustained rise in blood pressure).**
Ref: Nelson's Pediatrics, 17th edition Pg 56.

- ***Sustained rise in BP*** is seen usually in ***renal parenchymal disease***.

Effects of asphyxia

System	Effects
CNS	Hypoxic ischemic encephalopathy, intracranial hemorrhage, infarction, seizures, cerebral edema, hypotonia, hypertonia
CVS	Myocardial ischemia, poor contractility, tricuspid insufficiency, hypotension
Renal	ATN and acute cortical necrosis
Respiratory	Pulmonary HTN, pulmonary hemorrhage, RDS
Adrenal	Hemorrhage
GIT	Perforation, ulceration
Metabolic	SIADH, decreased sodium, glucose and calcium, myoglobinuria
Blood	DIC

50. Answer is d (Craniosynostosis).
Ref: Nelson's, 17th edition Pg 525.

Disorders a/w wide open anterior fontanel

– Achondroplasia	– IUGR
– Apert syndrome	– Kenny syndrome
– Athyrotic hypothyroidism	– Osteogenesis imperfecta
– Cleidocranial dysostosis	– Prematurity
– Congenital rubella syndrome	– Pykn dystrophy
– Hallermann syndrome	– Russell syndrome
– Hydrocephalus	– Trisomies
– Hypophosphatasia	– Vitamin D deficiency
	– Rickets

51. Answer is b (Mustard in warm water).
Ref: Narayan Reddy's, 23rd edition Pg 251.

Household emetics

- A tablespoon of mustard powder in warm water; efficient emetic (supported by many other reference books).
- Two tablespoonful of common salt in a tumbler of warm water.

Note:
Ref: First aid, CPR and AED, Alton LT et al. American Academy of Orthopedic Surgeons. Pg 242 says – "Since 1965, syrup of ipecac ***HAD BEEN recommended*** by poison centers for most swallowed poisons. When taken by mouth it can induce vomiting. In November 2003, the American Academy of Pediatrics (AAP) announced its new guideline on syrup of ipecac saying that it NO longer has a place in the home management of poisoning cases since it has not been associated with improvement in victim outcome".

52. Answer is a (*Haemophilus influenzae*).
Ref: OP Ghai, 7th edition Pg 340.

	Croup (laryngotracheobronchitis)	Acute epiglottitis
Etiology	**MC** *parainfluenza virus*; **also by RSV**	MC by ***H. influenzae type b***
Presenting age	3 months to 3 years	3–7 years
Clinically	Prodrome with URI symptoms for 1–7 days; low grade fever, inspiratory stridor that worsens with agitation; hoarseness of voice, barking cough	Rapid onset (4–12 hour); high fever, dysphagia, drooling, muffled voice, stridor; patients may be in 'sniffing' position with neck hyperextended and chin protruding
X-ray	***'Steeple sign'*** on lateral neck film	**'Thumb sign'** on lateral neck film
Treatment	Mist therapy, oxygen, aerosolized racemic epinephrine, dexamethasone	Call anesthesia, transfer to operation theater, ***endotracheal intubation*** and IV antibiotics

53. Answer is c (Body mass index).
Ref: Davidson's, 20th edition Pg 113, Table 5.23.

- ***Body mass index (BMI)*** = Weight/height^2 (in kg/m^2).
- Although not a direct measure of adiposity it is the ***most widely used method to gauge obesity.***

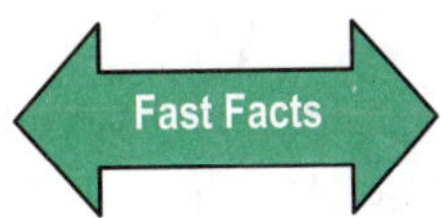

BMI	Classification
18.5–24.9	Normal range
25.0–29.9	Overweight
> 30	Obese
30.0–34.9	Class I
35.0–39.9	Class II
> 40.0	Class III

54. Answer is c (Mucoid vaginal discharge).
Ref: Nelson's, 17th edition Pg 1829.

- ***Thick, white, viscid, vaginal discharge*** is seen during ***early neonatal period*** because of estrogen. It should not be confused with purulent discharge and requires ***no treatment.***

Note:
- ***Labial fusion***: Commonly seen in patients younger than 6 years and is often asymptomatic and a/w local inflammation and hypoestrogenic states.
- Topical estrogen applied each evening for 1 week is the treatment of choice and is effective in 90% of cases.

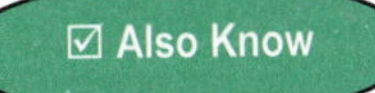

Minor clinical problems observed in normal neonate during 1st week of life

– Milia	– Breast engorgement
– Erythema toxicum	– Epithelial pearls
– Mongolian spots	– Vaginal bleeding
– Stork bite	– Phimosis
– Peeling of skin	– Cephalohematoma
– Subconjunctival hemorrhage	– Predeciduous teeth

ORTHOPEDICS

55. Answer is b (Shoulder).
Ref: Maheshwari, 3rd edition Pg 75.

Treatment of shoulder dislocation:
- *Kocher's maneuver for* reduction of dislocation = **Tr**action, **E**xternal **R**otation, **Add**uction, **I**nternal **R**otation; *"**TR**eat **ER**rors with **ADDI**tional **R**esponsibility"*.
- *Hippocrates maneuver* (with foot in axilla).
- Treat recurrent dislocation with surgery (*Putti Platt operation, Bankart operation*).

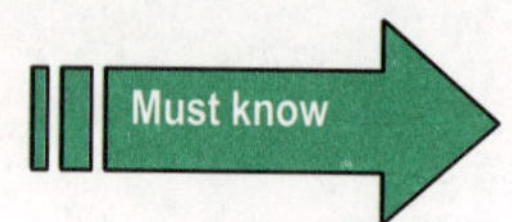

Shoulder Dislocation

- ***MC joint in human body to dislocate;*** *MC in* ***adults; anterior dislocation*** *MC: MC joint to undergo* ***recurrent dislocation.***
- Fall on outstretched hand with shoulder externally rotated is common mechanism of anterior dislocation (ADL).
- ***Posterior dislocation*** may result from ***electric shock or epileptic convulsion***; luxatio erecta is rare type where the head of humerus lies in subglenoid position.
- Pathologically ***Bankart*** lesion, ***Hill-Sack*** lesion occur in ADL.
- Clinically, patient enters casualty with shoulder abducted and elbow supported with opposite hand; ***Dugas' test*** - inability to touch opposite shoulder; ***Hamilton ruler test***—it is possible to place a ruler on the lateral side of the arm touching the acromion and lateral condyle of humerus simultaneously due to flattening of shoulder; ***Callaway's test***—increased vertical circumference of axilla compared to normal side.
- ***Early complication***—injury to axillary N; ***late complication***—recurrent dislocation.

COMED-K 2005 ANSWERS

56. **Answer is c (Osteoporosis).**

Ref: Bone Densitometry in Clinical Practice, Application and Interpretation, Vol 1, Sydney Lou Bonnick, 2004 edition Pg 6; http://www.gemm-therapy.com/eng/conditions_osteoporosis.php.

- ***Ward's triangle*** was first described by FO Ward in Outlines of Human Osteology, London, Henry Renshaw, 1838.
- It is a triangular region created by the ***intersection of three groups of trabeculae in the femoral neck***.
- 1 year mortality rate following hip fracture due to osteoporosis is around 20%.
- ***Ward's triangle*** is the area generated by the ***DEXA scan*** as the area having the **lowest *BMD*** in the femoral head.
- Therefore it has a key importance in patients with hip fracture risk due to ***osteoporosis***.

57. **Answer is d (Adduction, external rotation, flexion).**

Ref: Harrison's, 17th edition Pg 2086-87.

Characteristic changes of the rheumatoid hand

- ***Radial deviation*** at the wrist with ulnar deviation of the digits, often with palmar subluxation of the proximal phalanges (***'Z' deformity***).
- Hyperextension of the proximal interphalangeal joints, with compensatory flexion of the distal interphalangeal joints (***Swan-neck deformity***).
- Flexion contracture of the proximal interphalangeal joints and extension of the distal interphalangeal joints (***boutonnière deformity***).
- Hyperextension of the first interphalangeal joint and flexion of the first metacarpophalangeal joint with a consequent loss of thumb mobility and pinch.

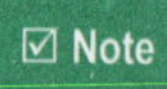

Typical joint changes in **rheumatoid feet** include:

- Eversion at the hindfoot (subtalar joint)
- Plantar subluxation of the metatarsal heads
- Widening of the forefoot
- Hallux valgus
- Lateral deviation and dorsal subluxation of the toes.

58. **Answer is a (Fusion of both ends of the radius and ulna).**

Ref: Sharad Pediatric Orthopedics, Pg 279; Turek's Orthopedics, 4th edition Pg 291.

- The term ***primary radioulnar synostosis*** is applied to that condition where there is usually a bilateral synostosis at ***upper end of forearm.***
- A/w absence of supinator muscles of the forearm such as pronator teres and quadratus. The forearm is held in fixed pronation. It is a/w anterior and posterior dislocation of the elbow.
- Treatment is limited to osteotomy. No fully satisfactory operation is yet devised.
- ***Pulled elbow*** is a differential diagnosis.

59. **Answer is c (Median nerve injury).**
Ref: Maheshwari, 3rd edition Pg 54.

Median nerve palsy tested by:
- ***Ape thumb*** (simian deformity)
- ***Pointing index*** (Ochsner's clasping test)—flexor digitorum superficialis and flexor digitorum profundus of the index finger are paralyzed
- ***Pen test***— tests the abductor pollicis brevis.

60. **Answer is a (Bowing of the tibia).**
Ref: Davidson's, 20th edition Pg 1076, Box 25.5; Pg 1127; Essential Orthopedics, Maheshwari, 3rd edition Pg 263.

- ***Osteomalacia,*** literally means 'softening of bones'; is the adult counterpart of rickets.
- The hypocalcemia and hypophosphatemia that accompany ***vitamin D deficiency*** result in impaired mineralization of bone matrix proteins → osteomalacia.
- Proximal myopathy is a striking feature of severe vitamin D deficiency, both in children and in adults.
- X-rays appear to be of ***'poor quality',*** i.e. not sharply defined.
- Diffuse ***rarefaction*** of bones.
- ***Looser's zones*** (*pseudofractures*): Radiolucent zones occurring at fracture sites; MC pubic ram, axillary border of scapula, ribs and medial cortex of neck of femur.
- ***Triradiate pelvis*** in females.
- ***Protrusio acetabuli.***
- ***Milkman's fractures.***
- ***Bowlegs*** are a feature in the growing skeleton and ***NOT*** seen in adults.

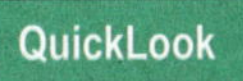

Laboratory diagnosis of vitamin D deficient osteomalacia

- Low or low-normal serum Ca^{2+} and P^{+}
- ***Raised serum alkaline phosphatase***
- Low 25(OH)D
- Raised parathormone (PTH)

OPHTHALMOLOGY AND ENT

61. **Answer is a (Persistence of vascular sheath of the lens).**
Ref: Nema, 2nd edition Pg 174.

- ***Posterior polar cataract*** is the presence of an ***opacity at the central posterior lens capsule.***
- It is commonly a/w remnants of the hyaloid artery or the posterior fibrovascular sheath of the lens.
- The remnants may range in size from tiny Mittendorf's dot to persistent hyperplastic primary vitreous.

Often Asked

Types of cataract

Type of cataract	Comment
■ Blue dot cataract	MC Congenital cataract; no significant visual symptoms
■ Radiation cataract	Posterior subcapsular cataract
■ Steroid induced cataract	Posterior subcapsular cataract
■ Sunflower cataract	Chalcosis (excess copper accumulation in lens)
■ Traumatic cataract	Rosette cataract, Vossius ring (pigments on anterior lens capsule due to constricted pupil striking lens during blunt trauma)
■ After cataract	Posterior capsule opacification, Elschnig's pearls, Soemmering's ring
■ Anterior lenticonus	ALport's syndrome
■ Complicated cataract	Due to any disease process in eye (e.g. uveitis), polychromatic lustre, bread crumb appearance
■ Christmas tree cataract	Myotonic dystrophy
■ Glassblowers' cataract	Heat cataract, infrared rays
■ Posterior subcapsular cataract	Even in the early stages, vision is usually impaired owing to the position of the opacity near the nodal point of the eye; more blurring in bright sunlight and headlights of oncoming cars
■ Nuclear cataract	'Second sight' due to induced myopia – person who was using glasses to read earlier will be able to read better without glasses
■ Oil drop cataract	Galactosemia
■ Posterior polar	Early visual impairment since located at nodal point of the eye; high risk of posterior capsule rupture during surgery
■ Zonular (lamellar) cataract	Hypocalcemia, riders are seen
■ Snowflake cataract	Diabetes mellitus
■ Diabetic cataract	In diabetes mellitus, in the lens glucose is converted to sorbitol by aldose reductase → diabetic cataract. Aldose reductase inhibitors are being studied to prevent diabetic cataract

62. Answer is a (Rods and cones).
Ref: Parson's, 20th edition Pg 107,110.

Electroretinogram (ERG)

'a' wave = Photoreceptor (rods and cones) activity
'b' wave = Response of bipolar cells
'c' wave = Generated by retinal pigment epithelium and related to retinal metabolism

63. Answer is b (Real image).
Ref: Parson's, 20th edition Pg 126-134.

Comparison of ophthalmoscopy

Direct ophthalmoscopy	Indirect ophthalmoscopy
Distant direct: From 25 cm distance Near direct ophthalmoscopy: From very close to patient's eye (within 1–2 cm)	From about 1 m distance
Handheld instrument	Worn on the head with head band
Erect, virtual image	***Inverted, real*** image
Magnified *15 times*	Magnified *5 times*

Useful to see posterior pole, i.e. optic disk and macula/fovea, cannot see periphery	Useful to see periphery, ora serrata, vitreous base (posterior pole also), especially in retinal detachments and degenerations
Less illumination, difficult to use when cataract is present	Bright illumination, can see through cataracts
No stereopsis	Good stereopsis (i.e. depth perception)—elevations/depressions (as in retinal detachments) can be made out

64. Answer is c (Medial half of the upper lid).
Ref: Kanski, 5th edition Pg 42; Nema, 2nd edition Pg 250.

- ***Coloboma*** is an uncommon ***congenital partial or full thickness eyelid defect***—especially at the junction of the ***middle third and medial third of the upper lid***.

65. Answer is c (Müller's muscle).
Ref: Snell's anatomy, 6th edition Pg 713.

- The ***muscle of Müller*** is a thin layer of smooth muscle that bridges the inferior orbital fissure. It is ***supplied by sympathetic nerve*** and its function is unknown.

Note:
- ***Levator palpebrae superioris*** is supplied by ***sympathetic nerves*** from ***superior cervical ganglion***.

66. Answer is d (Caterpillar hair in the eye).
Ref: Parson's, 20th edition Pg 170.

- ***Ophthalmia nodosa*** is a nodular conjunctivitis and may be mistaken for TB due to irritation caused by caterpillar hair.
- ***Treatment***: Nodules should be excised and the conjunctivitis treated.

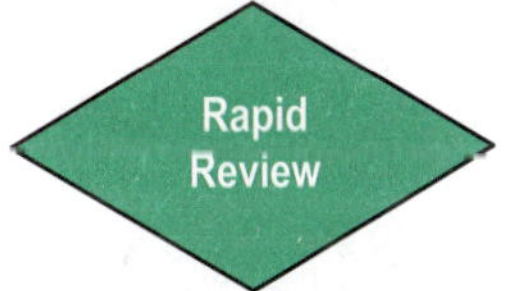

Conjunctivitis

❖ **Bacterial conjunctivitis**	*Staphylococcus aureus, Streptococcus pneumoniae, H. influenzae* Mucopurulent discharge, sticky eyes, matted eyelashes, papillae	Topical antibiotic drops and ointments
❖ **Viral conjunctivitis**	Adenovirus (pink eye), herpes simplex, picornavirus Watery discharge, subconjunctival hemorrhages, follicles, preauricular lymphadenopathy, lasts for longer time	Cold compresses, lubricant eyedrops, antibiotic drops to prevent bacterial superinfection
❖ **Ligneous conjunctivitis**	MC in children/young adults; unknown etiology 'woody' membrane over conjunctiva,	Surgical removal of membranes—tends to recur; topical cyclosporine, hyaluronidase or corticosteroids
❖ **Angular conjunctivitis**	*Staphylococcus aureus* MC, classically described as due to *Moraxella lacunata*	Treat with zinc oxide containing eye drops
❖ **Phlyctenular conjunctivitis**	Type IV hypersensitivity reaction to endogenous tuberculoprotein or to staphylococcal blepharitis; small pinkish nodule on conjunctiva	Treat with topical antibiotic ointment; corticosteroid drops

❖ **Giant papillary conjunctivitis**	Due to mechanical trauma (exposed sutures, prosthesis) or hypersensitivity to contact lens wear (soft 10%, rigid 1%); 'giant' papillae > 0.3 mm diameter	Remove mechanical irritation; change/refit contact lenses; topical antiallergics or topical corticosteroids
❖ **Vernal conjunctivitis (spring catarrh)**	Affects children/young adults; type I hypersensitivity reaction due to external allergens; intense itching, mucoid 'stringy/ropy' discharge (Maxwell Lyon sign); cobblestone papillae on undersurface of upper eyelid; Horner Trantas spots at limbus; corneal 'shield ulcer' may be seen; pseudogerontoxon	Mast cell stabilizers (sodium cromoglycate, olopatadine); limited topical corticosteroids; topical cyclosporine; cool compress

67. **Answer is c (Probing is usually advised around the age 12–18 months).**
Ref: Kanski, 5th edition Pg 50, 51.

- ***Congenital NLD obstruction*** is perhaps better termed delayed canalization of the NLD, since it often resolves spontaneously. The lower part of the NLD is the last part of the lacrimal duct to canalize.
- ***Signs***: Epiphora, matted lashes.
- ***Treatment***: Massage the lacrimal sac accompanied by lid hygiene. However topical antibiotics should be reserved for superadded conjunctivitis.
- ***Probing*** should be delayed until age of ***12 months*** because spontaneous closure occurs in 95% of cases. Results of probing are good.

68. **Answer is c (Herpes simplex keratitis).**
Ref: Parson's, 20th edition Pg 193-94.

- ***Corneal sensation*** is ***characteristically reduced in herpes simplex keratitis***; also ***dendritic figures*** are seen.

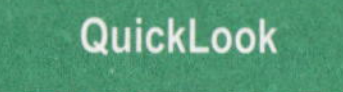

Causes of reduced corneal sensation

- Herpes simplex and herpes zoster keratitis
- Leprosy
- Diabetes mellitus
- Riley-Day syndrome
- Congenital sensitivity to pain
- Section of trigeminal nerve

<u>**Note:**</u>
- Reduced corneal sensation causes = Neuro***trophic*** keratitis
- Facial (7th) nerve palsy causes = Neuro***paralytic*** keratitis

69. **Answer is b (Rheumatoid arthritis).**
Ref: http://www.ncbi.nlm.nih.gov/pubmed/8035992 [Ophthalmology. 1994 Jul;101(7):1281-6; discussion 1287-8]

"Scleritis associated with rheumatoid arthritis and with other systemic immune-mediated diseases".

Direct quote:
"<u>Rheumatoid arthritis is the most common systemic immune-mediated condition associated with scleritis</u>".

- *Harrison's, 17th edition Pg 185*: *Scleritis* refers to a deeper, more severe inflammatory process of the sclera, frequently associated with a connective tissue disease such as rheumatoid arthritis, lupus erythematosus, polyarteritis nodosa, Wegener's granulomatosis or relapsing polychondritis.

70. Answer is c (Nasopharyngeal carcinoma).
Ref: Maqbool's ENT textbook, 11th edition Pg 416.

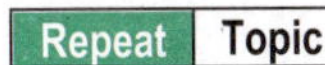

- Refer ***answer no. 59 in COMED-K 2008 answers*** for detailed explanation.

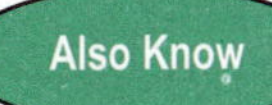

- ***Petrositis and Gradenigo's syndrome:*** Deep temporal headache and retro-orbital pain; diplopia (paralysis of abducens nerve) and presence of ear discharge and mastoiditis.
- ***Griesinger's sign:*** An indurated tender area over the upper part of the internal jugular vein and mastoid region may be palpated due to extension of sigmoid sinus thrombosis.

71. Answer is c (Sigmoid).
Ref: Dhingra's, 3rd edition Pg 109.

- ***Lateral (sigmoid) sinus thrombosis*** is an inflammation of inner wall of lateral sinus with formation of a thrombus.
- It occurs as a ***complication of acute adolescent mastoiditis, masked mastoiditis or CSOM and cholesteatoma***.
- ***Griesinger's sign:*** An indurated tender area over the upper part of the internal jugular vein and mastoid region maybe palpated due to extension of sigmoid sinus thrombosis.
- ***Tests done in lateral sinus thrombosis*** are:
  - Tobey-Ayer test
  - Crowe-Beck test.

72. Answer is d (Paracusis).
Ref: Dhingra, 3rd edition Pg 115.

- ***Paracusis*** is the ability to hear better in noisy surroundings.
- Seen in ***otosclerosis***.
- This is because a normal person raises his voice in noisy surroundings.

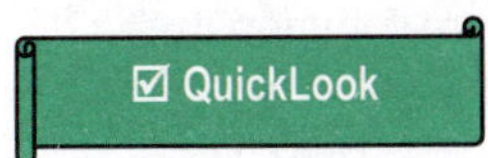

- ***Presbycusis***: Sensorineural deafness a/w physiological aging and manifests after 65 years.
- ***Hyperacusis***: Seen in facial nerve palsy due to stapedius muscle palsy.

73. Answer is b (Achalasia cardia).
Ref: http://www.ajronline.org/cgi/content/abstract/146/1/21

- In a simple radiologic test, amyl nitrite inhalation seems to distinguish patients with pseudoachalasia from those with idiopathic achalasia.
- In three pseudoachalasia patients with tumor infiltration of the distal esophagus, the narrow lower esophageal sphincter segment was unaffected by the smooth-muscle relaxant effect of amyl nitrite.
- In contrast, ***amyl nitrite caused a measurable increase of 2 mm or more in sphincter diameter in 9 patients with idiopathic achalasia***.

DERMATOLOGY, ANESTHESIA, RADIOLOGY AND PSYCHIATRY

74. Answer is a (Serous inflammation).
Ref: Harsh Mohan's pathology, 4th edition Pg 130.

Types of exudation

- ***Serous***: When the fluid exudates resemble serum or is watery, e.g. pleural effusion in TB, blister formation in burns.
- ***Fibrinous***: When the fibrin content of the fluid exudates is high, e.g. in pneumococcal and rheumatic pericarditis.
- ***Purulent/Suppurative***: Formation of pus as in infection with pyogenic bacteria, e.g. abscess.
- ***Hemorrhagic***: When there is vascular damage, e.g. hemorrhagic pneumonia in influenza.
- ***Catarrhal***: When the surface inflammation of epithelium produces increased secretion of mucus, e.g. common rhinitis.

75. Answer is a (Lichen planus).
Ref: Harrison's, 17th edition Pg 315, Table 53-2.

- ***Lichen planus*** is marked by ***severe pruritus***.

About the other choices

- Secondary syphilis affect palms and soles with scaling red brown papules—nonpruritic.
- White patches (vitiligo) is nonpruritic.
- Ichthyosis.

All about lichen planus

❖ **Presentation**	– 5Ps = Lesions are Pruritic (itchy), Plain (flat) topped, Polygonal, Purple (violaceous), Papules.
❖ **Etiology**	– Cell-mediated immune response of unknown origin.
❖ **Clinically**	– *Common sites*: Inner aspects of *wrists and ankles*, flexor aspect of *forearms*, *shins*, lower back (*lumbar region*), *genitalia* (as annular white lesion), *oral mucosa* (as white netlike/lacelike eruption). – *Wickham's striae*: Fine network of gray/white lines on the lesions. – *Koebner's phenomenon*: New lesions may appear at the site of trauma. – *Lichen planopilaris*: LP affecting hairy areas such as the scalp more common in women and is more likely to have ungual and erosive mucosal involvement. A *scarring alopecia* may result. – *Nail changes*: Seen in 10% of cases and include nail plate thinning causing longitudinal grooving and ridging. *Hyperpigmentation, subungual hyperkeratosis, onycholysis, 20-nail dystrophy and longitudinal melanonychia* can result from LP. Rarely, the matrix can be permanently destroyed with prominent *pterygium* formation. – *Malignant* transformation has been reported in *ulcerative oral lesions* in men. – *Vulvar* lesions can be *pruritic* and *painful*. – Hypertrophic lesions are often chronic; *residual pigmentation* and *scarring* can occur.
❖ **Histology**	– There is *hyperkeratosis*, a prominent granular layer, basal cell degeneration (forming "*colloid*" or *Civatte* bodies in the epidermis), '*liquefactive degeneration*' of the basal layer and a heavy T-lymphocyte infiltration in the upper dermis. – The T-cell basal cell interaction leaves a '*saw tooth*' dermoepidermal junction. – *IgM* on the colloid body surface gives "*bunch of grapes*" immunofluorescent pattern. Confirmation of diagnosis is by skin biopsy.

❖ **Associations**	– *Hepatitis C infection, autoimmune diseases* (ulcerative colitis, vitiligo, myasthenia gravis, alopecia areata, dermatomyositis, morphea, lichen sclerosus). – Cutaneous lesions resembling LP have been seen after usage of *drugs* like gold, antimalarials, diuretics, penicillamine, phenothiazines and in patients with skin lesions of *chronic graft-versus-host disease.*
❖ **Treatment**	– *Spontaneous resolution* occurs in 6 months to 2 years. – If needed *topical glucocorticoids* are the mainstay of therapy, antihistamines are used for pruritus. – Oral lichen planus is more difficult to treat and typically lasts longer than skin lichen planus.

76. Answer is a (Psoriasis).
Ref: Harrison's, 17th edition Pg 316.

- ***Koebner/Isomorphic phenomenon***: Traumatized areas (scratching, wounds, hat band pressure, sunburn) often develop lesions of ***psoriasis***.
- Also seen in ***lichen planus***.

77. Answer is c (Stratum corneum).
Ref: Fitzpatrick's Dermatology, 5th edition Pg 2340.

- The presence of a suitable environment on host skin is of critical importance in the development of clinical dermatophytosis (ringworm)
- They usually affect stratum corneum layer of the skin.

Also Know

Dermatophytes
– *Trichophyton* (affects skin, hair, nails) – *Microsporum* (affects hair and skin) – *Epidermophyton* (affects skin and nails)
Infections (by location)
– *Tinea pedis* (athlete's foot) is MC – *Tinea capitis* (hair and scalp) – *Tinea barbae* (beard) – *Tinea manuum* (hands) – *Tinea unguium* (nails) – *Tinea corporis* (trunk, glabrous skin) – *Tinea cruris* (jock itch, groin or perianal region)

78. Answer is d (32°C).
Ref: Harrison's, 17th edition Pg 135-36.

Severity	Body Temp	CNS	CVS	Respiratory	Renal and endocrine	Neuromuscular
Mild	35°C (95°F)–32.2°C (90°F)	Depression of cerebral metabolism; *amnesia; apathy; dysarthria;*	Tachycardia, then progressive bradycardia; cardiac cycle prolongation;	Tachypnea, then progressive decrease in respiratory minute volume;	Diuresis; increase in catecholamines, adrenal steroids,	Increased preshivering muscle tone, then fatiguing

		impaired judgment	vasoconstriction; ***increase*** in cardiac output and BP	declining oxygen consumption; bronchorrhea; bronchospasm	triiodothyronine and thyroxine; increase in metabolism with shivering	
Moderate	< 32.2°C (90°F)–28°C (82.4°F)	EEG abnormalities; progressive ***depression of level of consciousness***; ***pupillary dilation***; ***paradoxical undressing***; hallucinations	Progressive ***decrease*** in pulse and cardiac output; atrial and ventricular arrhythmias; ***suggestive (Osborne J-wave) ECG changes***	***Hypoventilation***; 50% decrease in carbon dioxide production per 8°C drop in temperature; absence of protective airway reflexes	50% increase in renal blood flow; renal autoregulation ***intact***; impaired insulin action	Hyporeflexia; reduced shivering-induced thermogenesis; rigidity
Severe	< 28°C (82.4°F)	Loss of cerebrovascular autoregulation; decline in cerebral blood flow; ***coma***; loss of ocular reflexes; progressive decrease in EEG	Progressive decrease in BP, heart rate, and cardiac output; re-entrant dysrhythmias; maximum risk of ***ventricular fibrillation***; asystole	Pulmonic congestion and edema; 75% decrease in oxygen consumption; apnea	Decrease in renal blood flow parallels decrease in cardiac output; extreme oliguria; poikilothermia; 80% decrease in basal metabolism	No motion; decreased nerve-conduction velocity; peripheral areflexia; no corneal or oculocephalic reflexes

79. Answer is a (Beer-Lambart law).

Ref: http://www.newbornwhocc.org/pdf/pulse.pdf

- The ***concept of pulse-oximetry is based*** on the ***Beer-Lambert law***, which states that the concentration of an unknown solute in a solvent can be determined by light absorption, i.e.

$$L\ (out) = L\ (in) - (DCa)$$

where,

L = Intensity of light
C = Concentration of solution
D = Distance that light travels through the solution
a = Absorption coefficient of solute.

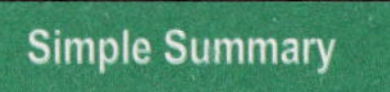

PULSE OXIMETRY

- Pulse oximetry is a simple non-invasive method of monitoring the *oxygen* saturation of blood (% of Hb saturated with oxygen).
- Normal oxygen saturation = *97–100%*.
- *How does an oximeter work?* A source of light originates from the probe at two wavelengths *(650 nm and 805 nm)*. The light is partly absorbed by hemoglobin, by amounts, which differ depending on whether it is saturated or desaturated with oxygen. By calculating the absorption at the two wavelengths, the processor can compute the proportion of hemoglobin, which is oxygenated. The oximeter is dependant on a pulsatile flow and produces a graph of the quality of flow. Where flow is sluggish (e.g. hypovolemia or vasoconstriction), the pulse oximeter may be unable to function. The computer within the oximeter is capable of distinguishing pulsatile flow from other more static signals (such as tissue or venous signals) to display only the arterial flow.

- It is *accurate in the range of* oxygen saturations of 70–100% (± 2%), but *less accurate under 70%*.
- Pulse oximeter shows error in the following, carboxyhemoglobinemia, methemoglobinemia, hypovolemia and vasoconstriction, nail polish, shivering and motion.

80. **Answer is b (Patients with previous exposure to halothane).**
Ref: KD Tripathi, 6th edition Pg 370-72.

HALOTHANE (FLUOTHANE)

• **Pharmacology**	– Chemical structure contains *fluorine, chlorine and bromine*. The carbon-fluoride bonds are responsible for its non-flammable and non-explosive nature. – ***Colorless, volatile liquid***, pleasant odor. – Halothane contains thymol as a stabilizing agent and is stored in dark bottles as it is decomposed by ultraviolet light. The vapor is absorbed by rubber. – It has *no analgesic* action. It can be used with soda lime in a circle system.
• **Systemic Effects**	– ***Decreased BP*** due to ***myocardial depression*** and vasodilation. – Sensitizes the myocardium to adrenaline-induced arrhythmias. – Causes depression of ventilation and the ventilatory response to both hypercarbia and hypoxia is lost. – ***Slight bronchial dilation, non-irritant to respiratory tract.*** – ↑↑ ***cerebral blood flow*** and the ICT. – Relaxation of skeletal and smooth muscle including the pregnant uterus, which may increase blood loss during cesarean section. – Shivering ***('halothane shakes')*** and tremor are common in the immediate postoperative period following halothane anesthesia. – Repeated doses of halothane cause hepatotoxicity (***'halothane hepatitis'***—do not use halothane twice within a 6-month period) and it can trigger ***malignant hyperpyrexia***.

81. **Answer is a (Fasciculations).**
Ref: KD Tripathi, 6th edition Pg 342.

- ***Decamethonium and succinylcholine*** have affinity as well as NM cholinergic receptors.
- They depolarize muscle end plate by opening Na+ channels and produce ***twitch and fasciculations***.

82. **Answer is b (Radius of the tube).**
Ref: Ganong's physiology, 23rd edition Pg 541-42.

- ***Poiseuille's law***: Of laminar flow through tubes.
- The rate is directly proportional to the perfusion pressure and proportional to 4th power of diameter and inversely proportional to viscosity and length of the tube.
- Because flow varies directly and resistance inversely with the fourth power of the radius, blood flow and resistance in vivo are markedly affected by ***small changes in the caliber of the vessels***.
- Thus for example, ***flow through a vessel is doubled by only a 19% increase in its radius*** and when the ***radius is doubled, resistance is reduced to 6%*** of its previous value.

83. **Answer is a (Ventilation/Perfusion mismatch).**
Ref: Textbook of Anesthesia by Alan and David, 4th edition Pg 530.

Functional classification of hypoxemia in the postop period is:

❖ Reduced inspired oxygen

- Ventilation perfusion abnormalities
- Shunts
- Hypoventilation
- Diffusion defects
- Diffusion hypoxia after nitrous oxide anesthesia.

- Among all the above causes, ***MC cause is ventilation perfusion mismatch***. Cardiac output and pulmonary arterial pressure may be reduced after GA or regional anesthesia causing impaired perfusion of some areas of lungs.

84. Answer is b (Lidocaine).
Ref: Lee's Anesthesia, 13th edition Pg 155-156.

Accidental Intra-arterial Thiopentone Injection

- This causes ***immediate pain and blanching***; ***arterial obstruction*** is due to vascular spasm and obstruction by thiopentone crystals.

Treatment

- Leave needle in place; irrigate with ***saline***
- Commence ***anticoagulation*** with heparin and then warfarin for 2 weeks
- Give 10 mL of ***1% procaine*** to buffer thiopentone and act as local anesthetic
- Consider ***papaverine*** 40 mg, ***phenoxybenzamine*** 0.5 mg or ***urokinase***
- ***Sympathetic block***, e.g. brachial plexus block
- Keep limb warm and elevated and continue with GA to dilate vessels.

85. Answer is b (Melorheostosis).
Ref: Chapman's Radiological D/D, 5th edition Pg 6.

Melorheostosis

- ***Cortical and periosteal new bone*** giving the appearance of ***molten wax flowing down a burning candle***.
- The ***hyperostosis*** tends to extend from one bone to the next.
- Usually affects ***one limb***, but both limbs on one side can be affected.
- Skull, spine and ribs are seldom affected.

Also Know

• **Strip**ed bone disease	= Osteopathia **striata**
• **Spot**ted bone disease	= Osteo**poi**kilosis
• Marble bone disease	**= Osteopetrosis**

86. Answer is d (Pneumonectomy).
Ref: Chapman's Radiological D/D, 5th edition Pg 63, 66.

Unilateral, hypertransradiant hemithorax

Rotation of patient – Poor technique – Scoliosis **Chest wall** – Mastectomy: Absent breast, absent pectoral muscle shadows	**Lung** – Compensatory emphysema – Airway obstruction – Unilateral bullae – Swyer-James syndrome (Mcleod's syndrome): Late sequel of childhood bronchiolitis

– Poliomyelitis: Atrophy of pectoral muscles – Poland syndrome: Unilateral amazia with syndactyly (in 10%) **Pleura** – Pneumothorax	– Congenital lobar emphysema **Pulmonary vessels** – Pulmonary embolism to a major pulmonary artery

Note:
– ***Postpneumonectomy***: ***Dense hemithorax*** is seen.

87. **Answer is c (Spina bifida).**
Ref: Sutton's Radiology, 7th edition Pg 1052, 1121.

Ultrasound findings of spina bifida are:

- ***Banana sign***: Cerebellum is stretched around brainstem with effacement of cisterna magna.
- ***Lemon sign***: Flattening of frontal bones.
- Foot deformity like pes cavus.
- Bony defects of spine.
- Hydrocephalus with ventriculomegaly.

88. **Answer is b (Esophageal varices).**
Ref: Wolfgang's Radiology, 2nd edition Pg 509.

Esophageal varices on ultrasound shows:
- Thickened sinus, interrupted mucosal folds (earliest sign)
- Tortuous radiolucencies of variable size
- ***Worm-eaten*** lobulated filling defects.

89. **Answer is d (^{123}I metaiodobenzylguanidine).**
Ref: Harrison's, 17th edition Pg 2271.

Pheochromocytoma can be localized using radioactive tracers including:
- ^{131}I or ^{123}I-metaiodobenzylguanidine (*MIBG*)
- ^{111}In-somatostatin analogues
- ^{18}F-dopa (or dopamine) positron-emission tomography (PET)

90. **Answer is d (Ruptured hydatid cyst).**
Ref: www.ajronline.org/cgi/reprint/145/3/639.pdf (article titled "The radiology of hydatid disease)".

Repeat Topic
- Refer ***answer no. 41 in COMED-K 2010 answers*** for detailed explanation.

91. **Answer is d (Cholinesterase inhibitors).**
Ref: Harrison's, 17th edition Pg 2543.

FDA-approved drugs for treatment of Alzheimer's Dementia
- Donepezil
- Rivastigmine
- Galantamine
- Memantine
- Tacrine (due to hepatotoxicity, no longer used)

- The pharmacologic action of donepezil, rivastigmine and galantamine is ***inhibition of cholinesterase***, with a resulting ***increase in cerebral levels of acetylcholine***.
- Memantine appears to act by blocking overexcited N-methyl-D-aspartate (NMDA) channels.
- Double blind, placebo controlled, crossover studies with ***cholinesterase inhibitors and memantine*** have shown them to be associated with improved caregiver ratings of patients' functioning and with an apparent ***decreased rate of decline in cognitive test scores over periods of up to 3 years***—slows cognitive deterioration.

92. Answer is c (Methylphenidate).
Ref: OP Ghai, 7th edition Pg 39.

Attention Deficit Hyperactivity Disorder (Hyperkinetic Syndrome)

Example: A 7-year-old boy frequently gets into trouble at school because he interrupts the teacher, disturbs the other students and cannot seem to sit still in class.

- Described first by *Heinrich Hoff*, also called *Strauss syndrome*.
- Characterized by an early onset (*usually 3–8 years*) of short attention span, distractibility, overactivity, impulsivity, clumsiness and language delay, which last longer than 6 months.
- MC in *boys* present in two or more settings (school, home, work) and is often associated with antisocial behavior/conduct disorder; 50% continue to have ADHD into adulthood.
- Etiologic factors include genetic loading, poverty, parental alcohol abuse, dietary constituents (lead, tartrazine) and exposure to tranquilizers (barbiturates).
- Treatment (CNS stimulants) is given only when severe and includes the drug of choice ***methylphenidate***; others like amphetamine derivatives (pemoline and dextroamphetamine) are also tried.
- *Adverse effects* of CNS stimulants in children include failure to gain weight and inhibition of growth. *Barbiturates* are contraindicated as they *increase hyperactivity*.
- Pemoline and imipramine should *not* be given before 6 years of age.

93. Answer is b (Clozapine).
Ref: Davidson's, 20th edition Pg 243; Ref: Harrison's, 17th edition Pg 2722.

Repeat Topic

- Refer ***answer no. 124 in COMED-K 2010 answers*** for detailed explanation.

94. Answer is b (Agoraphobia).
Ref: Niraj Ahuja's Psychiatry, 6th edition Pg 97.

Repeat Topic

- Refer ***answer no. 125 in COMED-K 2010 answers*** for detailed explanation.

PHARMACOLOGY

95. Answer is b (It causes marked neurotoxicity).
Ref: KD Tripathi, 6th edition Pg 771.

- ***Stavudine*** is a ***nucleoside reverse transcriptase inhibitor (NRTI)***.
- Of the NRTIs, stavudine has greatest risk of ***lipodystrophy and other mitochondrial toxicity***.
- ***Peripheral neuropathy and pancreatitis*** are main side effects, which have ***limited its use***.
- Refer ***answer no. 17 in COMED-K 2006 answers*** for detailed table on antiretroviral drugs.

96. Answer is a (Naltrexone).
Ref: KD Tripathi, 6th edition Pg 385.

- ***Naltrexone*** helps prevent relapse of alcoholism in trials among postaddicts.

- It *reduces alcohol craving*, number of drinking days and chances of resumed heavy drinking.
- ***Naltrexone is being used in India*** in most deaddiction centres after the individual has undergone withdrawal and is motivated.
- ***Acamprosate*** is rated comparable to naltrexone and is used in Europe.

97. Answer is a (Pyrazinamide).

Ref: Harrison's, 17th edition Pg 1033, Table 161-3.

Firstline Anti-TB Drugs

Drugs	Mechanism of action	Side effects	Remarks
Isoniazid (INH)	Inhibits mycolic acid cell wall synthesis via oxygen-dependent pathways. INH resistance is a/w ↓ catalase and peroxidase activity in the bacterium.	Peripheral neuritis (MC in slow acetylators) and neurotoxicity (seizures); hepatitis, optic neuritis, hemolysis in G6PD deficiency, SLE-like syndrome.	Bactericidal to both extra- and intra-cellular organisms. Pyridoxine, 10 mg orally daily as prophylaxis for neuritis. INH is Hepatotoxic and Neurotoxic.
Rifampicin (R)	Blocks RNA synthesis by inhibiting DNA dependent RNA polymerase.	Hepatotoxicity and P-450 drug interactions; orange-colored urine and sweat (harmless); 'respiratory' and 'abdominal' syn.	Bactericidal to all subpopulations of TB bacilli, but acts best on intermittently dividing bacilli (spurters).
Pyrazinamide (P)	Derivative of isonicotinic acid; inhibits mycolic acid synthesis, but by interacting with a different fatty acid synthase encoding gene. More active at pH < 6; good penetration into CSF.	Hepatotoxicity (less in Indians) and ***Hyperuricemia.***	Bactericidal to slowly dividing intracellular bacilli and those within caseous granuloma (acidic pH at these sites).
Ethambutol (E)	Inhibits arabinosyl transferases involved in arabinogalactan synthesis and interferes with mycolic acid incorporation into mycobacterial cell wall.	Optic neuritis, color vision disturbance (red green). Ethambutol affects Eyes.	Bacteriostatic; fast multiplying bacilli are more susceptible as are many atypical mycobacteria; least potent of the first-line drugs.
Streptomycin (S)	Bind to 30S ribosomal subunit; freeze initiation of protein synthesis and cause misreading of the mRNA code.	Ototoxicity and nephrotoxicity.	Bactericidal to extracellular bacilli only.

☑ Also Know

Medications with Uricosuric Activity

Acetohexamide	Glyceryl guaiacolate
ACTH	Glycopyrrolate
Ascorbic acid	Halofenate
Azauridine	Losartan
Benzbromarone	Meclofenamate
Calcitonin	Phenolsulfonphthalein

Chlorprothixene	Phenylbutazone
Citrate	Probenecid
Dicumarol	Radiographic contrast agents
Diflunisal	Salicylates (> 2 g/2d)
Estrogens	Sulfinpyrazone
Fenofibrate	Tetracycline that is outdated
Glucocorticoids	Zoxazolamine

98. Answer is c [Physiological (functional) antagonism].
Ref: KD Tripathi, 6th edition Pg 56-58.

Drug antagonism types are:

- ***Physical antagonism***: Based on physical property of drug, e.g. charcoal absorbs alkaloids and prevents their absorption.
- ***Chemical antagonism***: Two drugs react chemically and form an inactive product, e.g. chelation of metals by BAL.
- ***Physiological/Functional antagonism***: Two drugs act on different receptors or different mechanisms, but have opposite overt effect on the same physiological function, e.g. histamine and adrenaline on bronchial muscle and BP; ***leukotrienes and terbutaline*** on respiratory mucosa.
- ***Receptor antagonism***: Interferes with binding of agonist, e.g. acetylcholine with atropine.

99. Answer is c (Inhibition of pancreatic lipase).
Ref: Harrison's, 17th edition Pg 472.

- ***Orlistat (Xenical)*** is a synthetic hydrogenated derivative of a naturally occurring lipase inhibitor, lipostatin, produced by the mold *Streptomyces toxytricini*.
- Orlistat is a ***potent, slowly reversible inhibitor of pancreatic, gastric and carboxyl ester lipases and phospholipase A2***, which are required for the hydrolysis of dietary fat into fatty acids and monoacylglycerols.
- The drug acts in the lumen of the stomach and small intestine by forming a covalent bond with the active site of these lipases.
- Taken at a therapeutic dose of 120 mg tid, orlistat blocks the digestion and absorption of about 30% of dietary fat. After discontinuation of the drug, fecal fat usually returns to normal concentrations within 48–72 hours.
- SE: Diarrhea, gas and cramping, reduced absorption of fat-soluble vitamins.

Appetite-suppressing Drugs (Antiobesity Drugs)

Drug	Comments
Noradrenergic agents: Increase extraneuronal noradrenaline by enhancing its release	
Amphetamine	High abuse potential
Mazindol	Nonamphetamine, indole derivative, long acting, has additional peripheral effect of increasing the metabolic rate
Phentermine	Available as resin also
Diethylpropion	Short half-life of 4–6 hours
Phenylpropanolamine	Blocks NA uptake by inhibiting □1 adrenergic receptors
Serotonergic agents: Release serotonin and block its reuptake	
Fenfluramine, Dexfenfluramine	SE: Valvular heart defects, pulmonary hypertension, sudden deaths, echocardiographic abnormalities
Newer drugs	
Sibutramine	Blocks uptake of both serotonin and NA in the CNS. SE: Dry mouth, anorexia, constipation, insomnia and dizziness. In some (< 5%) patients it markedly increases BP
Orlistat	Refer answer above

100. Answer is c (levonorgestrel).
Ref: http://www.who.int/mediacentre/factsheets/fs244/en/

- ***WHO recommends levonorgestrel*** for emergency contraceptive pill use. Ideally, this progestogen-only method should be taken as a single dose (1.5 mg) within 5 days (120 hours) of unprotected intercourse. Alternatively, a woman can take the levonorgestrel in two doses (0.75 mg each; 12 hours apart).
- Levonorgestrel emergency contraceptive pills prevent pregnancy by preventing or delaying ovulation. They may also work to prevent fertilization of an egg by affecting the cervical mucus or the ability of sperm to bind to the egg.

101. Answer is b (Chloramphenicol).
Ref: KD Tripathi, 6th edition Pg 717; Griffith's Hematology, Pg 134.

Hematologic Toxicity of Chloramphenicol

- ***Chloramphenicol*** affects the hematopoietic system (bone marrow) in two ways:
- ☐ By a ***non-dose-related idiosyncratic*** response manifested by ***aplastic anemia***, leading in many cases to ***fatal pancytopenia***.
- ☐ By a ***dose and duration of therapy-related myelosuppression***—a direct toxic effect, predictable and probably due to inhibition of mitochondrial enzyme synthesis. The clinical picture is marked initially by ***reticulocytopenia***, which occurs ***5–7 days after the initiation of therapy***, followed by a *decrease in hemoglobin*, an *increase in plasma iron*, *cytoplasmic vacuolation of early erythroid forms* and granulocyte precursors and *normoblastosis* with a shift to early erythrocyte forms.

102. Answer is a (Glucose infusion).
Ref: KD Tripathi, 6th edition Pg 758-59.

Repeat Topic

- Refer ***answer no. 13 in COMED-K 2007 answers*** for detailed explanation.

103. Answer is d (Propranolol).
Ref: Harrison's, 17th edition Pg 2560, Davidson's, 20th edition Pg 1182, KD Tripathi, 6th edition Pg 143.

- ***Essential tremor (ET)*** is the most common involuntary movement disorder.
- It is a progressive disorder, which can present in childhood, but dramatically increases in prevalence over the age of 70.
- ET is characterized by a ***high-frequency tremor*** (up to 11 Hz) that ***predominantly affects the upper extremities***.
- The tremor is most prominent when trying to maintain a posture (postural tremor) or perform an action such as touching the finger to an object (kinetic tremor).
- It is typically ***bilateral and symmetric***.
- ***Non-selective beta blockers like propranolol*** (20–80 mg/d) are the ***standard drug therapy***.

104. Answer is d (Ipratropium).
Ref: KD Tripathi, 6th edition Pg 636-37.

- ***Alginates (alginic acid)*** are combined with antacids for use in reflux esophagitis, since they are believed to increase adherence of mucosa to esophageal mucosa.
- PG analogues such as ***misoprostol*** are useful in drug-induced gastritis.
- ***Sucralfate*** is an ulcer protective drug.
- Anticholinergics such as ***pirenzepine*** are used in peptic ulcer treatment, but **NOT** ipratropium.

105. Answer is a (INH).
Ref: Park, 20th edition Pg 173.

Repeat Topic

- Refer *answer no. 127 in COMED-K 2007 answers* for detailed explanation.

106. Answer is a (Quinidine).
Ref: KD Tripathi, 6th edition Pg 480.

Digoxin toxicity can be potentiated by:

- *Quinidine*: Reduces binding of digoxin to tissue proteins as well as its renal and biliary clearance; plasma concentration of digoxin is doubled.
- *Calcium*: Synergizes with digitalis.
- *Verapamil, diltiazem, captopril and amiodarone*: Increase plasma concentration of digoxin.
- *Atropinic drugs* and *tricyclic antidepressants*: Delay gastric emptying and increase digoxin absorption.
- *Erythromycin, omeprazole and tetracyclines*: Increase bioavailability of digoxin.

107. Answer is b (Captopril).
Ref: KD Tripathi, 6th edition Pg 483-84.

- *Captopril and lisinopril* are *active drugs.*

Also Know

Prodrugs	Active forms
Enalapril	Enalaprilat
Perindopril	Perindoprilat
Ramipril	Ramiprilat
Levodopa	Dopamine
Dipivefrine	Epinephrine
Sulindac	Sulfide metabolite
Bacampicillin	Ampicillin
Cyclophosphamide	Aldophosphamide
Prednisone	Prednisolone

108. Answer is a (Betamethasone).
Ref: KD Tripathi, 6th edition Pg 227.

Inhaled corticosteroids for asthma (beclomethasone, flunisolide, budesonide)	*MOA*: Inhibit synthesis of virtually all cytokines. Inactivate NF-κB, the transcription factor that induces the production of TNF-α	*Role*: Mild persistent or worse cases; frequently combined with β_2-agonist, use for chronic asthma

109. Answer is b (Gatifloxacin).
Ref: Harrison's, 17th edition Pg 2083.

Substances that can induce lupus-like disease

Antiarrhythmics	**Antihypertensives**	**Antibiotics**
– Procainamide	– Hydralazine	– Isoniazid
– Disopyramide	– ACE inhibitors	– Minocycline
– Propafenone	– Beta blockers	– Macrodantin
Anticonvulsants	**Antipsychotics**	**Antihyperlipidemics**
– Carbamazepine	– Chlorpromazine	– Lovastatin
– Phenytoin	– Lithium	– Simvastatin

Antirheumatic	Diuretic	Antithyroid
– Sulfasalazine	– Hydrochlorothiazide	– Propylthiouracil
Interferons and TNF inhibitors		

110. Answer is b (Rigidity and tremor at rest).
Ref: KD Tripathi, 6th edition Pg 430-432.

Adverse effects of phenothiazines

- Extrapyramidal side effects with timing of evolution:

– 4 hour	***Acute dystonia*** (MC in young men, girls < 10 years, especially after IV/IM, muscle spasm, stiffness, oculogyric crisis)
– 4 day	Akinesia (***Parkinsonian symptoms—rigidity, tremors***, etc.)
– 4 week	***Akathisia*** (MC side effects, restlessness with a compelling desire to move about, but without anxiety)
– 4 month	***Tardive dyskinesias*** (stereotypical orofacial movements, ***Rabbit syndrome***)

- Anticholinergic: Dry mouth, blurred near vision, urinary retention.
- Antiadrenergic: Sedation, postural ***hypotension*** and sexual dysfunction.
- Endocrine: Dopamine receptor blocking → ***hyperprolactinemia*** → galactorrhea, amenorrhea.
- Idiosyncratic reactions: Cholestatic jaundice, agranulocytosis, skin rashes, urticaria, contact dermatitis, photosensitivity.
- ***Neuroleptic malignant syndrome***: Rigidity, myoglobinuria, autonomic instability, hyperpyrexia; treated with dantrolene and dopamine antagonists (bromocriptine, amantadine).

MICROBIOLOGY

111. Answer is b (*Pseudomonas*).
Ref: Harrison's, 17th edition Pg 949-50, 1633.

- ***P. aeruginosa***, the major pathogen of the group, is mainly associated with infections in hospitalized patients and in patients with ***cystic fibrosis***.
- The predisposition of CF airways to chronic infection by *Staphylococcus aureus* and ***Pseudomonas aeruginosa*** is consistent with failure to clear mucus.
- Indeed, both mucus stasis and mucus hypoxia may contribute to the propensity for ***Pseudomonas to grow in biofilm colonies*** within mucus plaques adherent to CF airway surfaces.

112. Answer is c (*Mycoplasma pneumoniae*).
Ref: Harrison's, 17th edition Pg 1068.

- ***M. pneumoniae (Eaton agent)*** causes ***upper and lower respiratory tract infection in all ages*** with ***highest attack rate*** in 5–20 years age group.
- The infection is acquired by inhalation of aerosols.
- Clinically: Fever, headache, cough, bullous myringitis, etc.
- On auscultation findings may be normal despite strikingly abnormal chest X-ray.
- Chest X-ray shows pleural effusion (20%) and patchy or lobar consolidation with hilar lymphadenopathy.

113. Answer is a (*Serratia marcescens*).
Ref: Ananthanarayan and Panicker, 6th edition Pg 259.

- ***Serratia*** forms pink, red or magenta ***non-diffusible pigment called prodigiosin,*** which is formed optimally at room temperature.

- It *may grow in sputum after collection and may suggest hemoptysis* because of pigment formed (***pseudohemoptysis***).
- *Serratia* is pleomorphic with minute coccobacilli.
- It is a saprophyte found in water, soil and food.

☑ More About

Other pseudos U should know

- ☐ Pseudoparalysis – vitamin C deficiency
- ☐ Pseudofractures – osteomalacia
- ☐ Pseudodementia – depression
- ☐ Pseudocommunity – paranoid states
- ☐ Pseudolymphoma – Sjögren's syndrome
- ☐ Pseudotabes – diabetic foot
- ☐ Pseudocoxalgia – Perthe's disease

114. Answer is a (*Corynebacterium parvum*).
Ref: Ananthanarayan, 6th edition Pg 222.

- ***Corynebacterium parvum,*** which is frequently used as an ***immunomodulator*** is a mixture of *Propionibacterium* species.

115. Answer is c (Antibiotic susceptibility).
Ref: Ananthanarayan and Panicker, 6th edition Pg 581.

- Antibiotic susceptibility test includes:
  1. Diffusion test.
  2. Dilution test.
  3. Antibiotic assays in body fluids.
- In diffusion tests, the drug is allowed to diffuse through the solid medium so that a gradient is established and the zone of inhibition of bacterial growth is measured.
- A recent modification of agar diffusion sensitivity test employing a quantitative diffusion gradient is known as ***epsilometer or E-test.***
- Types of diffusion tests:
  - ➲ Mueller-Hinton agar
  - ➲ Kirby Baner.

116. Answer is b (Poxvirus).
Ref: Harrson's, 17th edition Pg 1113, Table 176-1.

Poxviruses and Human Infections

Genus	Species	Human diseases
Orthopoxvirus	Variola	Smallpox, systemic
	Monkeypox	Smallpox-like, systemic
	Vaccinia	Local pox lesion, occasionally systemic
	Cowpox	Local pox lesions
Molluscipoxvirus	Molluscum contagiosum	Molluscum contagiosum, multiple cutaneous lesions
Parapoxvirus	Orf	Contagious pustular dermatitis, local pox lesions
	Pseudocowpox	Milker's nodule, local pox lesions
Yatapoxvirus	Tanapox	Local pox lesions

117. Answer is d (IgE).
Ref: Harrison's, 17th edition Pg 2036.

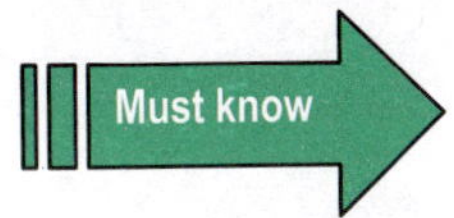

Biological properties of immunoglobulins

IgG	: Placental transfer, secondary Ab for most antipathogen responses
IgA	: Secretory immunoglobulin
IgM	: Primary Ab responses, complement activation
IgD	: Marker for mature B cells
IgE	: *Allergy*, antiparasite responses, reaginic hypersensitivity

118. Answer is b (Pigs).
Ref: Harrison's, 17th edition Pg 1314; Parasitology, Cahtterjee, 12th edition Pg 92-93.

- ***B. coli*** is the ***largest protozoan parasite*** inhabiting the large intestine of man.
- It is also found in pigs and monkeys.
- The ***pig is the common reservoir of infection***.
- Clinical features: Blood and mucus diarrhea.
- Diagnosis: Stool microscopy and demonstrate trophozoites.
- ***Treatment***: ***Tetracycline*** or doxycycline.

119. Answer is a (*Actinomyces israelii*).
Ref: Ananthanarayan and Panicker, 6th edition Pg 369.

Acid-fast organisms are:
- TB
- Leprosy
- *Brucella*
- *Nocardia*
- *Rhodococcus*
- Spores

120. Answer is d (*Strongyloides stercoralis*).
Ref: Harrison's, 17th edition Pg 1322.

- In uncomplicated ***strongyloidiasis***, many patients are asymptomatic or have mild cutaneous and/or abdominal symptoms.
- ***Recurrent urticaria***, often involving the buttocks and wrists, is the ***most common cutaneous manifestation***.
- ***Migrating larvae*** can elicit a ***pathognomonic serpiginous eruption, larva currens ("running larva")***.
- This pruritic, raised, erythematous lesion advances as rapidly as 10 cm/h along the course of larval migration.

121. Answer is c (Macrophage).
Ref: Textbook of Microbiology, CP Baveja, 3rd edition Pg 71.

- ***Antigen presenting cells (APCs)*** include specialized cells called ***dendritic cells*** in the lymph nodes and spleen and the ***Langerhans*** dendritic cells in the skin.
- ***Macrophages*** and ***B cells*** themselves and likely many other cell types, can also function as APCs.

PATHOLOGY

122. Answer is d (Defects in phagocytosis).
Ref: Robbins Pathology, 7th edition Pg 1027-28.

- ***Malakoplakia*** refers to a peculiar pattern of ***urinary bladder inflammatory reaction*** characterized macroscopically by soft, yellow, slightly raised mucosal plaque of 3–4 cm in diameter.
- Plaque is made up of foamy macrophage with occasional giant cells and interspersed lymphocytes.
- In addition, laminated mineralized concretions known as ***Michaelis-Gutmann bodies*** are typically present.
- ***Genesis of malakoplakia*** lesions is still uncertain. Current opinion favors the hypothesis that *unusual appearing macrophages and giant phagosomes* result from ***defect in phagocytic and degradation process***.

123. Answer is d (Infectious mononucleosis).
Ref: Harsh Mohan's Pathology, 4th edition Pg 380.

- ***In infectious mononucleosis***, blood picture shows a moderate rise in total WBCs with absolute lymphocytes.
- The lymphocytosis is due to rise in normal as well as ***atypical T-lymphocytes***.
- Essential to diagnose IM is the presence of 10–12% atypical T cells.
- The mononucleosis cells are of variable appearance and classified as ***Downey type I, II, III*** of which ***type I are found more frequently***.

124. Answer is c (Endodermal sinus tumor).
Ref: Davidson's, 20th edition Pg 259.

- ***Endodermal sinus tumors*** secrete ***AFP and alpha-1 antitrypsin*** as tumor markers.

TUMOR MARKERS

Tumor marker	Cancer	Non-neoplastic conditions
Hormones		
Human chorionic gonadotropin	Gestational trophoblastic disease, Gonadal germ cell tumor, embryonal carcinoma, polyembryoma	Pregnancy
Calcitonin	Medullary thyroid Ca	
Catecholamines (Epinephrine, norepinephrine)	Pheochromocytoma	
Oncofetal antigens		
Alpha-fetoprotein (AFP)	Hepatocellular Ca, gonadal germ cell tumor (NOT pure seminoma)	Cirrhosis, hepatitis
Carcinoembryonic antigen (CEA)	Colon cancer Others – pancreas, lung, breast, ovary	Pancreatitis, hepatitis, IBD, smoking
Enzymes		
Prostatic acid phosphatase	Prostate cancer	Prostatitis, prostatic hypertrophy
Neuron-specific enolase	Small cell Ca of the lung, neuroblastoma	
Lactate dehydrogenase	Lymphoma, Ewing's sarcoma	Hepatitis hemolytic anemia
Alkaline phosphatase	Osteosarcoma	
Placental alkaline phosphatase	Ca ovary, seminoma	Pregnancy, smoking

Tumor-associated proteins		
Prostate specific antigen (PSA)	Prostate cancer	Prostatitis, prostatic hypertrophy
Monoclonal immunoglobulin	Multiple Myeloma	Infection
Bladder tumor antigen (BTA)	Bladder cancer	Kidney stones, UTI
CA-15-3	Breast cancer	
CA 27.29	Breast	
CA-125 (a glycoprotein)	Ovarian cancer Other cancers - breast, hepatoma, lymphomas	Menstruation, peritonitis, pregnancy, cirrhosis
CA-19-9 (a carbohydrate)	Pancreatic, colon, cancer	Pancreatitis, ulcerative colitis
CD30	Hodgkin's disease, anaplastic large cell lymphoma	
CD25	Hairy cell leukemia, adult T-cell leukemia/lymphoma	
S-100	Melanoma, CNS and nerve tumors	
Intermediate filaments		
Keratins	Carcinomas, mesotheliomas	
Desmin	Muscle tumors	
Vimentin	Sarcomas	
Others		
Factor VIII	Kaposi's sarcoma, angiosarcoma	
Serum ferritin	Hepatoma	
Thyroglobulin	Thyroid cancer and thyroid disorders	

125. Answer is c (Astrocytoma).
Ref: Robbins Pathology, 7th edition Pg 1401.

- *Astrocytoma*: Includes several different categories of tumors derived from astrocytes including:
  - ☐ Fibrillary astrocytoma
  - ☐ Glioblastoma multiforme (GBM)
  - ☐ Pilocytic astrocytoma
  - ☐ Pleomorphic xanthoastrocytoma.
- GBM accounts for 80% of adult primary brain tumors usually found in cerebral hemisphere, cerebellum, brainstem, spinal cord; most often seen in 4th–6th decade.
- Histopathology shows necrosis and vascular or endothelial cell proliferation, tufts of piled up vascular cells that bulge into the vascular lumen—glomeruloid body.

126. Answer is a (Chondroblastoma).
Ref: Essential of Orthopedics, Maheshwari, 4th edition Pg 221.

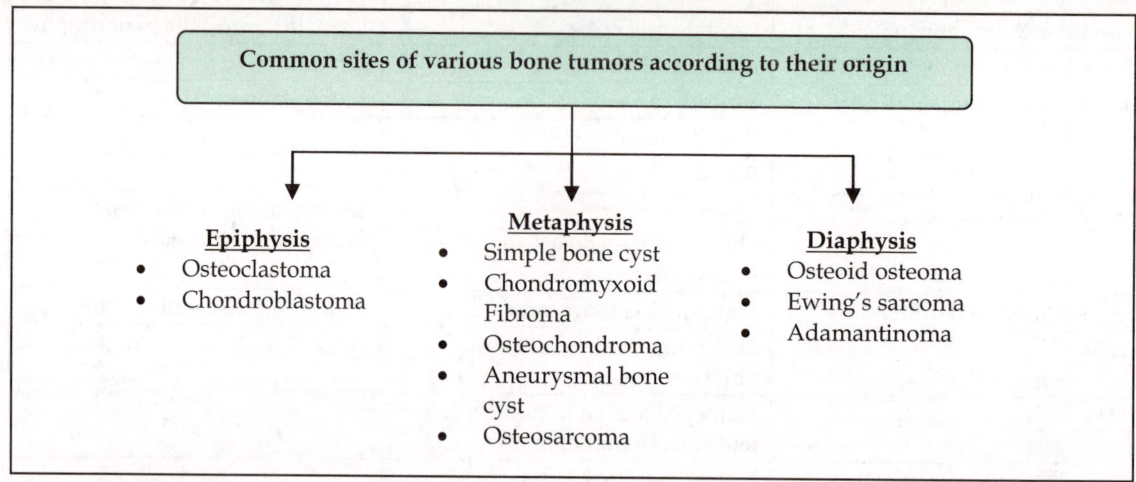

127. Answer is a (Spina bifida).

Ref: Dutta's Obstetrics, 6th edition Pg 107, 494.

Maternal Serum Alpha-fetoprotein Levels (MSAFP)

Raised MSAFP levels

- ***Fetal causes***
  - Neural tube defects: Open spina bifida, anencephaly and others
  - GI obstruction, exomphalos and gastroschisis
  - Renal: Nephrosis (polycystic/absent kidney), posterior urethral valve
  - Aplasia cutis, amniotic band disruption
  - IUGR
  - Meckel's syndrome
  - Osteogenesis imperfecta
  - Placental and umbilical cord tumors, preterm labor
  - Teratoma (sacrococcygeal), Turner's syndrome (cystic hygroma), twins
- ***Maternal causes***
  - Low maternal weight
  - Underestimated gestational age
  - Maternal diseases like hepatocellular Ca, viral hepatitis and SLE

Low MSAFP levels

- Down syndrome
- Fetal cystic fibrosis
- Fetal hydrocephalus
- ↑ maternal weight
- Overestimated gestational age

128. Answer is d (Lepromatous leprosy).

Ref: Harsh Mohan's Pathology, 4th edition Pg 145, 534.

- In the dermis there is proliferation of macrophages with foamy changes, particularly around the blood vessels, nerves and dermal appendages.
- The *foamy macrophages are called lepra cells or Virchow cells*—these are heavily laden with acid fast bacilli—seen in *lepromatous leprosy*.
- Also *subepidermal clear zone is seen in lepromatous leprosy*.

129. Answer is b (Pulmonary involvement).

Ref: Harrison's, 17th edition Pg 2097 and Table 316-2 and Table 316-3.

- ***Diffuse cutaneous SSc (dcSSc)*** presents with progressive skin induration, starting in the fingers and ascending from distal to proximal extremities, the face and the trunk.
- ***dcSSc*** patients are at risk for ***early pulmonary fibrosis and acute renal involvement***.
- In ***limited cutaneous SSc (lcSSc),*** patients generally have long-standing Raynaud's phenomenon before other manifestations of SSc appear. Skin induration is limited to the fingers (sclerodactyly), distal extremities and face and the trunk is not affected.
- A subset of patients with lcSSc have *CREST syndrome*:
  - ☐ Calcinosis cutis
  - ☐ Raynaud's phenomenon
  - ☐ Esophageal dysmotility
  - ☐ Sclerodactyly
  - ☐ Telangiectasia.

Features	Limited Cutaneous SSc	Diffuse Cutaneous SSc
Skin involvement	Limited to fingers, distal to elbows, face; slow progression	Diffuse: fingers, extremities, face, trunk; rapid progression
Raynaud's phenomenon	Precedes skin involvement; associated with critical ischemia	Onset contemporaneous with skin involvement
Pulmonary fibrosis	May occur, moderate (35%)	***Frequent, early and severe (65%)***
Pulmonary arterial hypertension	Frequent, late, may be isolated	May occur, associated with pulmonary fibrosis
Scleroderma renal crisis	Very rare (2%)	Occurs in 15%; early
Calcinosis cutis	Frequent, prominent	May occur, mild
Autoantibodies	Anticentromere	Antitopoisomerase I (Scl-70)

130. Answer is d (Metaplasia).

Ref: Robbins Pathology, 7th edition Pg 10-11.

***-PLASIA* DEFINITIONS**

Reversible	
Hyperplasia	↑ in number of cells
Metaplasia	One adult cell type is replaced by another; often 2° to irritation and/or environmental exposure – can revert back to normal after removal of stimulus
Dysplasia	Abnormal growth with loss of cellular orientation, shape and size in comparison to normal tissue maturation; commonly preneoplastic
Carcinoma in situ	When dysplasia involves the entire thickness of the epithelium
Irreversible	
Anaplasia	Abnormal cells lacking differentiation; like primitive cells of same tissue, often equated with undifferentiated malignant neoplasms
Desmoplasia	Fibrous tissue formation in response to neoplasm
Neoplasia	A clonal proliferation of cells that is uncontrolled and excessive

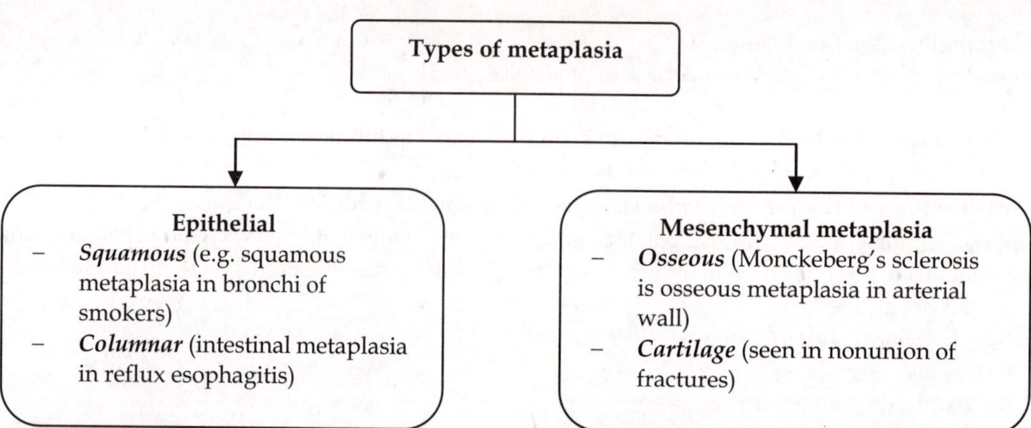

131. Answer is a (Folic acid deficiency).

Ref: Blueprints in Pediatrics, 2008 edition Pg 119; Harrison's, 17th edition Pg 632, Table 98-4.

- ***Folic acid deficiency*** causes ***megaloblastic anemia.***

Causes of microcytic hypochromic anemia:

- Iron deficiency
- Thalassemia
- Sideroblastic anemia
- Chronic inflammation (maybe normocytic also)
- Lead poisoning
- Copper deficiency
- Pyridoxine deficiency.

132. Answer is d (Chondroblastoma).

Ref: http://emedicine.medscape.com/article/1254949-diagnosis.

- One of the ***most characteristic findings in the histologic examination of chondroblastomas*** is linear deposition of calcification surrounding individual chondroblasts, creating a ***chicken-wire pattern.***
- Calcification may be so extensive that the chondrocytes in the area are not viable.

133. Answer is b (Beta-thalassemia trait).

Ref: Harrison's, 17th edition Pg 637.

- ***HbA2 is frequently elevated in β-thalassemia trait*** and *depressed in iron deficiency.*
- ***Beta-thalassemia minor (i.e. thalassemia trait)*** usually presents as ***profound microcytosis and hypochromia with target cells,*** but only *minimal or mild anemia.*
- The mean corpuscular volume is rarely > 75 f L;
- the hematocrit is rarely < 30–33%.
- Hemoglobin electrophoresis classically reveals an ***elevated HbA2 (3.5–7.5%).***

Note:

- HbF is elevated in HPFH, some β-thalassemia syndromes and occasional periods of erythroid stress or marrow dysplasia.

Normal Human Hemoglobins

Form	% of normal adult Hb	% of Hb at birth	Globin structure
HbA	97	25	$\alpha 2\beta 2$
HbA_2	2.4	Traces	$\alpha 2\delta 2$
HbF (fetal)	0.5	75	$\alpha 2\gamma 2$

134. Answer is a (Sickle cell anemia).
Ref: Harrison's, 17th edition Pg 1814.

- ***Sickle cell disease*** causes renal complications as a result of sickling of red blood cells in the microvasculature.
- The hypertonic and relatively hypoxic environment of the renal medulla, coupled with the slow blood flow in the vasa recta, favors sickling of red blood cells, with resultant ***local infarction*** (***papillary necrosis***).
- ***"Hyperfiltration nephropathy"***, namely, ***focal segmental glomerular sclerosis*** occurs.

☑ More About

☐ A ***"ring sign"*** on the ***pyelogram is pathognomonic of papillary necrosis*** and represents the radiolucent sloughed papilla surrounded by the radiodense contrast material in the calyx.

Causes of renal papillary necrosis (mnemonic—'ADIPOSE')
- Analgesics—phenacetin and aspirin
- Diabetes (MC cause)
- Infants in shock
- Pyelonephritis
- Obstruction
- Sickle cell disease
- Ethanol

135. Answer is a (IgM antibody against IgG).
Ref: Harrison's, 17th edition Pg 2088.

Rheumatoid factor (RF)

- ***RF = IgM autoantibodies*** reactive with the ***Fc portion of IgG.***
- RF is found in ***> 2/3 of adults*** with ***Rheumatoid arthritis*** (RA).
- The presence of RF is ***not specific for RA,*** as RF is found in 5% of healthy persons. RF in the general population increases with age > 65 years.
- The presence of RF ***does not establish the diagnosis of RA*** as the predictive value of the presence of rheumatoid factor in determining a diagnosis of RA is poor. Therefore, the ***RF test is not useful as a screening procedure.***
- However, the ***presence of RF can be of prognostic significance because*** patients with high titers tend to have more severe and progressive disease with extra-articular manifestations. RF is uniformly found in patients with nodules or vasculitis.
- ***In summary,*** a test for the presence of rheumatoid factor can be employed to confirm a diagnosis in individuals with a suggestive clinical presentation and, if present in high titer, to designate patients at risk for severe systemic disease.

More About

Rheumatoid Factor (RF) is also present in:
- Connective tissue diseases: SLE, Sjögren's syndrome
- Lung disease: Sarcoidosis, interstitial pulmonary fibrosis
- Chronic Liver disease
- Infections: Infectious mononucleosis, hepatitis B, tuberculosis, leprosy, syphilis, subacute bacterial endocarditis
- Parasitic: Visceral leishmaniasis, schistosomiasis and malaria
- Transiently in normal individuals after vaccination or transfusion and may also be found in relatives of individuals with RA

Above conditions can be remembered as the mnemonic: "HIT LIST" *(see below)*

Hepatitis B	SLE
Infectious mononucleosis	Sjögren's syndrome
Tuberculosis	Sarcoidosis
Leprosy	Syphilis
Leishmaniasis (Visceral)	Subacute bacterial endocarditis
Liver disease (chronic)	Schistosomiasis
Infections-malaria	Transiently after vaccination (in normals) or after Transfusion

136. Answer is d (Systemic lupus erythematosus).
Ref: Davidson's, 20th edition Pg 1017, 1056.

Repeat Topic

- Refer ***answer no. 11 in COMED-K 2008 answers*** for detailed explanation.

137. Answer is b (Nicotinic receptor proteins).
Ref: Ganong's physiology, 23rd edition Pg 126.

- ***Myasthenia gravis*** is a serious and sometimes fatal disease in which skeletal muscles are weak and tire easily.
- It is caused by formation of circulating ***antibodies to nicotinic acetylcholine receptors***.
- These antibodies destroy some receptors, trigger their removal by endocytosis.

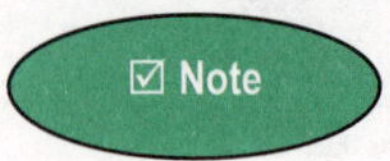

☐ ***Lambert Eaton myasthenic syndrome*** (LEMS) is due to antibodies against ***voltage gated calcium channels***. This decreases the Ca^{2+} influx that causes acetylcholine release.

138. Answer is c (Pericarditis).
Ref: Harrison's, 17th edition Pg 2079.

- ***Pericarditis*** is the ***most frequent cardiac manifestation***; it usually responds to anti-inflammatory therapy and infrequently leads to tamponade.
- More serious cardiac manifestations are myocarditis and fibrinous endocarditis of Libman-Sacks.
- The endocardial involvement can lead to valvular insufficiencies, most commonly of the mitral or aortic valves, or to embolic events.

FORENSIC MEDICINE

139. Answer is d (Imprisonment up to 7 years).
Ref: Narayan Reddy's FMT, 23rd edition Pg 3, Table (2-1).

Powers of magistrate (S.29 Cr.P.C)

Class of magistrate	Imprisonment	Fine
Chief judicial magistrate	Up to 7 years	Unlimited
I class judicial magistrate	Up to 3 years	Rs. 5,000
II class judicial magistrate	Up to 1 year	Rs. 1,000

140. Answer is b (30 cm).

Ref: Narayan Reddy's FMT, 23rd edition Pg 114.

- In ***close range gunshot wounds within a distance of 30 cm***, tissues surrounding the world are signed by flame and blackened by smoke and ***tattooed*** by unburnt or partially burnt powder.

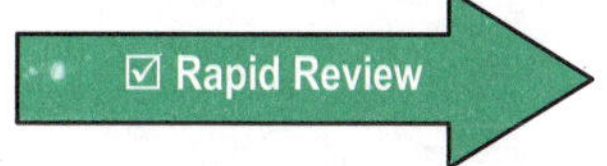

FORENSIC BALLISTICS

Entry wound from rifle

☐ Abrasion collar is seen in entry wound from rifled bullet and it surrounds the dirt collar.

Entry wounds from shotgun

☐ Wound from shotgun depends upon distance from which weapon is discharged
☐ Smoke effect (blackening) is seen with shot from up to 1 foot (30 cm)
☐ Flame/Burning/Scratching seen with shot from up to 1.5 feet (45 cm)
☐ Powder residue effect up to (unburnt and partially burnt powder/tattooing effect) seen with shot from up to 2–3 feet (60–90 cm).

Entry wounds from revolvers and automatic pistols

Contact shot

☐ There may be no burning, no soot, no tattooing around entrance wound
☐ It produces split wound, stellate/cruciate wound over bone (like skull). But other usual contact wounds are oval.

Close shot

☐ Tissue may be signed by flame, blackened by smoke and tattooed by unburnt/partially burnt-particles (smudging/fouling/blackening effect seen)
☐ Entry wound in a close shot is classically circular and inverted, but it may be irregular if gases build up
☐ ***Tattooing*** is seen surrounding the wound of entrance from a revolver or pistol, if the weapon is discharged up to a distance to ***90 cm.***

Distant shot

☐ Clubbed hairs
☐ Unburnt powder embedded into skin producing tattooing (stippling/pipering).

MISCELLANEOUS

❖ ***Gun powder residue*** on hands can be detected by ***dermal nitrate test (Paraffin test).***
❖ Pyrodex is a mixture of black powder and pot. Perchlorate, sodium, benzoate, dicyandiamide, dextrin wax and graphite.
❖ In firearm injury blackening of entry wound is d/to fine carbon particles in smoke.
❖ Blackening represents a near range of discharge, while smudging may be present in distant ranges.
❖ ***Caliber or Gauge***: Of a firearm is measured by internal dimension of barrel and is given in decimals of inch or mm.
❖ ***Paradox Guns***: There are some shotguns, which have small portion of their bore near the muzzle end rifled, which are called paradox guns.
❖ ***Detonator cap*** is present at the base of the cartridge.
❖ Air rifle—in this compressed air is used to fire lead slugs.
❖ ***Dum Dum bullet*** is one, which fragments extensively upon striking.
❖ ***Incendiary bullets*** contain phosphorus.
❖ At a distance of 2 m, the shot mass begins to spread and individual pellet holes maybe detected, which are usually round and show a rim of abrasion at their margins.

- In the skull, *entry* wound shows bevelling of *inner* table and *exit* wound shows bevelling of *outer table*.
- *Doubt* as to whether a wound is an *entry wound or exit wound* is called *Kennedy phenomenon*.

141. Answer is b (Tannin).
Ref: Narayan Reddy's FMT, 23rd edition Pg 213-214.

- ***Vegetable stains*** can ***resemble blood stains***.
- Certain fruits, e.g. *mulberry, gooseberry, currants, jam bands,* etc. produce such stains.
- On microscopic examination, vegetable cells are seen.
- *Henna, catechu, pan juice, tobacco* and the bark of some trees such as babool and gab produce red stains.
- Most of them contain ***tannin, which becomes black if a drop of ferric chloride*** is added.
- For more on ***blood stains*** see ***answer no. 127 in COMED-K 2010*** answers.

☑ More About

Tests for seminal stains

- Acid phosphatase test
- Fluorescence test—detects choline
- Barberio's test—detects spermine.

142. Answer is d (Prostate).
Ref: Narayan Reddy's FMT, 23rd edition Pg 85.

- ***Last organ to putrefy in male is prostate; in female is virgin uterus.***

PUTREFACTION

- This is the final stage following death produced mainly by the ***action of bacterial enzymes***, mostly *anaerobic organisms derived from the bowel*. Due to putrefaction, vessel walls stain purplish red giving marbled appearance.
- The ***first external sign of putrefaction*** in a body lying in air is usually a ***greenish discoloration of skin over the region of the cecum (right iliac fossa)***. Color is due to sulfhemoglobin formed by the hydrogen sulfide formed in the large intestine.
- The ***first internal sign*** of putrefaction is greenish discoloration of undersurface of liver.
- Rate of Putrefaction is maximum in air > water > soil/earth.
- ***Early putrefaction*** is seen after death due to septicemia, peritonitis, asphyxia, moisture.
- ***Delayed putrefaction*** is seen after death due to wasting disease, anemia, debility; poisoning by carbolic acid, zinc chloride, strychnine and chronic heavy metal poisoning.

143. Answer is c (Crystals of hemosiderin).
Ref: Narayan Reddy's FMT, 23rd edition Pg 95.

- When bruising is extensive and deep, the color takes a long time to appear externally.
- Towards the end of the healing process, large histiocytes containing coarse granules of hemosiderin pigment can be seen microscopically in a section of contused area.
- The site of bruise may contain ***crystals of hemosiderin for a long period after injury***.

PREVENTIVE AND SOCIAL MEDICINE

144. Answer is b (Orthotolidine test).
Ref: Park, 20th edition Pg 626.

Repeat Topic

- Refer ***answer no. 132 in COMED-K 2007 answers*** for detailed explanation.

145. Answer is a (Tube well).
Ref: Park, 20th edition Pg 620.

- ***Tube wells (borewells)*** are successful as a source of drinking water in many parts of India.
- They yield ***water, which is bacteriologically safe*** and also cheap in comparison to other sources of water supply.
- The yield is normally very high and does not depend upon direct rainfall.

146. Answer is d (24 hours).
Ref: Park, 20th edition Pg 198.

- The ORS solution should be ***made freshly daily and used within 24 hours***. It should not be boiled or sterilized.
- WHO and UNICEF now recommend to use ORS (citrate) whenever feasible.

ORS bicarbonate	ORS citrate
NaCl 3.5 g $NaHCO_3$ 2.5 g KCl 1.5 g Glucose 20 g Potable water 1 L	NaCl 3.5 g Trisodium citrate 2.9 g KCl 1.5 g Glucose 20 g Potable water 1 L

147. Answer is a (Serial interval).
Ref: Park, 20th edition Pg 94, 95.

- ***Serial interval***: The ***gap in time between the onset of the primary case and the secondary case*** is called serial interval.
- In actual practice we seldom know the incubation period of a disease. But we know when an outbreak of disease occurs, say in a family, which is the smallest group and also a closed group, there is an initial primary case. The primary case is followed by 2 or 3 secondary cases within short time.
- By collecting information about a series of such onsets, we get a distribution of secondary cases from which we can guess the incubation period of the disease.

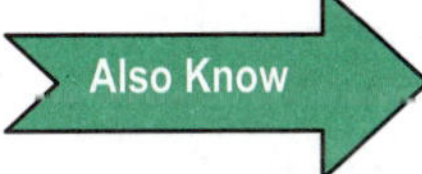

- ***Latent period*** is *equivalent of incubation period* in infectious diseases. It is used in non-communicable disease and is defined as the period from disease initiation to disease detection.
- ***Generation time*** is defined as "*the interval of time between receipt of infection by a host and maximal infectivity of the host*". In general, generation time is roughly equal to the incubation period. However, these two terms are not the same. Incubation period can be applied to infections that result in manifest disease, whereas generation time refers to transmissions of infection, whether subclinical or clinical.
- ***Communicable period*** is defined as "*the time during which an infectious agent may be transmitted directly or indirectly from an infected person to another person, from an infected animal to a man, or from an infected person to an animal including arthropods*".

148. Answer is c (Cataract).
Ref: Park, 20th edition Pg 351, Table-3.

National survey on blindness	
Cataract	62.6%
Refractive error	19.7%
Glaucoma	5.8%
Posterior segment pathology	4.7%
Corneal opacity	0.9%
Other causes	6.2%

149. Answer is b (Epidemic).
Ref: Park, 20th edition Pg 88.

- *Epidemic*: Occurrence of a group of illness of similar nature at a rate above the expected number.

☑ Also Know

- *Endemic*: Is a disease, which is constantly present in the community.
- *Pandemic*: Is an epidemic affecting a large population.
- *Hyperendemic*: Is a term that expresses the disease is constantly present at a higher incidence.
- *Sporadic*: Is the case that occurs irregularly, haphazardly from time to time and generally infrequently.

150. Answer is b (Human development index).
Ref: Park, 20th edition Pg 16.

■ **Human development index (HDI)**	• Longevity (life expectancy at birth) • Income (real GDP per capita or purchasing power) • Knowledge/Education (adult literacy rate and mean years of schooling) *"LIKE"* • High HDI ≥ 0.800; Medium HDI 0.500–0.799; Low HDI < 0.500 • HDI for India is 0.545 (***medium HDI*** category); ***rank 132***

☑ Simple Summary

Summary of "Indicators"

■ **Physical quality of life index (PQLI)**	• Infant mortality rate • Life expectancy at age 1 • Literacy *"ILL"* • PQLI in India is 43
■ **Sullivan's index**	• Expectation of life ***free of disability*** • Computed by subtracting from the life expectancy the probable duration of bed disability and inability to perform major activities • One of the most advanced indicators currently available
■ **Disability adjusted life year (DALY)**	• It expresses years of life lost to premature death and years lived with disability adjusted for the severity of the disability. One DALY is one lost year of healthy life • ***Measure used to express global burden of disease***
■ **Health adjusted life expectancy (HALE)**	• It is based on life expectancy at birth, but includes an adjustment for time spent in poor health. It means equivalent number of years in full health that a newborn can expect to live based on current rates of ill health and mortality

151. Answer is a (Confounding factor).
Ref: Park, 20th edition Pg 68.

- *"Confounding factor"* is defined as the one, which is associated with both exposure and disease and is distributed unequally in study and control group.
- More specifically a "confounding factor" is one that although associated with 'exposure' under study, it itself, independently of any such association is a "risk factor" of the disease.
- The confounding factor ***can be eliminated by matching***.

152. Answer is b (Source).
Ref: Park, 20th edition Pg 90.

Source: "The person, animal, objects or substance from which an infectious agent passes or is disseminated to a host".

Reservoir: "Any person, animal, arthropod, soil, plant or substance (or combination of these) in which an infectious agent lives and multiplies on which it depends primarily for survival and where it reproduces in such manner that it can be transmitted to a susceptible host."

Carrier: "An infected person or animal that harbors a specific infectious agent in the absence of discernible clinical disease and serves as a potential source of infection for others."

153. Answer is a (It should actually measure what it is supposed to measure).
Ref: Park, 20th edition Pg 126.

Repeat Topic

- Refer ***answer no. 134 in COMED-K 2007 answers*** for detailed explanation.

154. Answer is b (400).
Ref: Park, 20th edition Pg 134.

- ***Maternal mortality rate*** is total number of female deaths due to complications of pregnancy, childbirth or within 42 days of delivery from puerperal causes in an area during a given year.
- According to ***2000 census, MMR is 4.07 or 407 per 100,000 live births***.
- Target is to bring down MMR to 200 by 2007 and 100 per 100,000 by 2012.

155. Answer is b (Discussion by 4–8 qualified persons).
Ref: Park, 20th edition Pg 768.

Panel discussion
- ***4–8 people*** who are ***qualified to talk about the topic*** and secussa given problem.
- There is no specific agenda, no set order, no set speeches.
- Panel discussion is extremely effective method of education provided it is properly planned and guided.

Group discussion
- It is effective when the group contains 6–12 members, all sit in a circle and discuss.

Symposium
- A series of speeches on a selected topic. There is no discussion among the members.

ANATOMY, PHYSIOLOGY AND BIOCHEMISTRY

156. Answer is b (T10).
Ref: BD Chaurasia, Vol 2, 3rd edition Pg 166.

- The skin of the anterior abdominal wall is supplied by lower six thoracic nerves and by 1st lumbar nerve.
- ***T10 at level of umbilicus.***
- T7 at level of xiphoid process.

157. Answer is b (Periodontal membrane).
Ref: Wheater's functional histology, 4th edition Pg 238.

- Each tooth may be divided into 2 segments: The ***crown and the root***.
- The ***crown*** is the portion, which projects into the oral cavity and is protected by a layer of highly mineralized enamel, which covers it entirely.
- The bulk of tooth is made up of ***dentine***, a mineralized tissue, which has a similar chemical composition as bone.

- The dentin has a central ***pulp cavity*** containing dental pulp, which contains a specialized supporting tissue containing many sensory nerve fibers.
- The tooth is embedded in a bony ridge on the jaw called ***alveolar ridge***.
- The tooth socket is known as ***alveolus***.
- The root of the teeth is invested by a thin layer of ***cementum,*** which is connected to bone of socket by a thin fibrous layer called ***periodontal ligament*** or ***periodontal membrane***.

158. Answer is b (Pia mater).
Ref: Grey's anatomy, 38th edition Pg 1216.

- ***Ligamenta denticulata*** are two ***ribbon like lateral extensions of the pia mater*** situated between the dorsal and ventral nerve roots.

☑ In A Nutshell

- ❖ Deltoid ligament: Ligament on medial side of the ankle
- ❖ Spring ligament: Calcaneonavicular ligament
- ❖ Poupart's ligament: Inguinal ligament
- ❖ Copper ligament: Pectinate ligament
- ❖ Bigelow ligament: Iliofemoral ligament
- ❖ Mackenrodt's ligament: Transverse cervical ligament
- ❖ Ligament of Berry: Suspensory ligament of thyroid gland.

159. Answer is d (Erector spinae).
Ref: Grey's aatomy, 38th edition Pg 786; BD Chaurasia, Vol 2, 3rd edition Pg 276.

- Action of ***rectus abdominis*** muscle is flexion, lateral flexion of lumbar spine.
- Quadratus lumborum fixes the last ribs during inspiration, lateral flexion of vertebral column and extension of lumbar vertebra.
- ***Erector spinae*** stabilizes the spine and helps in deep inspiration, and it is the chief extensor of the vertebral column.

160. Answer is a (Anterior cruciate ligament).
Ref: BD Chaurasia, Vol 2, 3rd edition Pg 127.

- ***Cruciate ligaments*** are very thick strong fibrous bands, which act as direct bonds of union between the femur and tibia.
- They give the anteroposterior stability of the knee joint; ***anterior cruciate ligament (ACL) prevents forward displacement of tibia on the femur***.
- ACL injuries are due to twisting force on a semiflexed knee.
- Tests to diagnose ACL tear are anterior drawer test and Lachman test.

161. Answer is b (Glossopharyngeal nerve).
Ref: BD Chaurasia's, Vol 3, 3rd edition Pg 214; Snell's anatomy, 6th edition Pg 737.

Nerve supply of tongue

Anterior 2/3	Nerve of general sensation: Lingual nerve. Nerve of taste: chorda tympani branch of facial nerve.
Posterior 1/3 (including circumvallate papillae)	Nerve of general sensation and taste: Glossopharyngeal nerve.
Posterior most part	Vagus through internal laryngeal nerve.

162. Answer is c (Planning and programming of voluntary movements).
Ref: Principles of Physiology, Debasis pramanik, Academic publishers, Pg 437.

Phylogenetic divisions of the cerebellum

Archicerebellum (vestibulocerebellum):	– ***Most primitive*** parts of the cerebellum. – Consist of lingula and flocculonodular lobe. – Mainly concerned with ***balance and maintaining equilibrium.***
Paleocerebellum (spinocerebellar):	– Consist of entire anterior lobe except the lingula including the pyramis and uvula of the posterior lobe. – Mainly concerned with maintaining ***tone and posture*** of the body.
Neocerebellum (cerebrocerebellum):	– ***Most recent part*** of the cerebellum. – Mainly concerned with ***planning and programming of voluntary movements*** through its connections with the highly developed neocortex.

163. Answer is d (Maxillary).

Ref: Essential Otolaryngology: head and neck surgery, Kaet Jin Lee, 8th edition Pg 682.

Paranasal sinus embryology

1. **Maxillary sinuses**
   - Grow laterally from a middle meatal infundibulum at about ***3 months gestation*** and are ***about 7 X 7 mm at birth.***
   - Visible on plain X-ray at about 5–6 months.
   - ***Earliest sinus to develop.***

2. **Ethmoid sinuses**
   - Appear as middle meatal outgrowths at about 3rd to 4th month gestation.
   - *Several are present at birth.*
   - Visible on plain X-ray only at 1 year.

3. **Frontal sinuses**
   - Develop from anterior ethmoid air cells and are usually **NOT** present at birth.
   - Not visible on plain X-ray until after age 1 year.

4. **Sphenoid sinuses**
   - Paired sinuses develop at about 4 months gestation.
   - Only ***minimal size at birth.***

164. Answer is c (It increases vagal tone to the SA node).

Ref: Davidson's, 20th edition Pg 553, 565.

- An attack of ***supraventricular tachycardia (SVT)*** may be terminated by ***carotid sinus pressure or other measures that increase vagal tone (Valsalva maneuver).***
- ***IV adenosine or verapamil*** will restore sinus rhythm in most cases.
- Suitable alternative drugs include beta blockers, flecainide and digoxin.
- In an emergency, when there is severe hemodynamic compromise, the tachycardia should be terminated by DC cardioversion.

165. Answer is a (Dissociation curve shape).

Ref: Ganong's Physiology, 22nd edition Pg 732.

- Buffering system of hemoglobin is due to dissociation of the imidazole groups of the histidine residue in hemoglobin.

COMED-K 2005 ANSWERS

Also Know

- ☐ Haldane effect: Binding of O_2 to Hb reduces its affinity for CO_2.
- ☐ Bohr effect: Decrease in O_2 affinity to Hb when the pH of blood falls.

166. Answer is a (Bowman's capsule).
Ref: Harrison's, 17th edition Pg 1782 and Fig. 277-1.

- Two human kidneys harbor nearly 1.8 million glomerular capillary tufts.
- Each ***glomerular tuft resides within Bowman's space***.
- The ***Bowman's capsule*** circumscribing this space is lined by parietal epithelial cells that transition into tubular epithelia forming the proximal nephron.
- The glomerular capillary tuft derives from an afferent arteriole that forms a branching capillary bed embedded in mesangial matrix.
- This capillary network funnels into an efferent arteriole, which passes filtered blood into cortical peritubular capillaries or medullary vasa recta that supply and exchange with a folded tubular architecture.
- Hence, the glomerular capillary tuft, fed and drained by arterioles, represents an arterial portal system.
- Fenestrated endothelial cells resting on a glomerular basement membrane (GBM) line glomerular capillaries.
- ***Delicate foot processes extending from epithelial podocytes shroud the outer surface of these capillaries*** and podocytes interconnect to each other by slit-pore membranes forming a selective filtration barrier.

167. Answer is b (Gastrin).
Ref: Harrison's, 17th edition Pg 1847.

Lower Esophageal Sphincter Pressure

Increased by	Decreased by
– Muscarinic M2 and M3 receptor agonists	– Fatty meals
– α-adrenergic agonists	– Smoking
– Gastrin	– Beverages with high xanthine content (tea, coffee, cola)
– Substance P	– Gastric dilatation
– Prostaglandin F2α	
– Nicotine	
– β-adrenergic agonists	
– Dopamine	
– Cholecystokinin	
– Secretin	
– Vasoactive intestinal peptide (VIP)	
– Calcitonin gene-related peptide	
– Adenosine	
– Prostaglandin E	
– Nitric oxide donors such as nitrates	
– Inhibitors of phosphodiesterase-5 (sildenafil)	

168. Answer is d (Adipose tissue).
Ref: KD Tripathi, 6th edition Pg 257.

- *L-BRICK (don't need insulin for glucose uptake)* = **L**iver, **B**rain, **R**BCs. **I**ntestine, **C**ornea, **K**idneys.

169. Answer is c (They promote growth of bone and cartilage).
Ref: Ganong's physiology, 23rd edition Pg 383.

- The effects of growth hormone on growth, cartilage and protein metabolism depend on an interaction between growth hormone and ***somatomedins***, which are polypeptide growth factors secreted by the liver and other tissues.

- The principal circulating somatomedins are ***insulin-like growth factor-I (IGF-I, somatomedin C)*** and ***insulin-like growth factor-II (IGF-II)***.
- Somatomedins are helpful in ***incorporation of sulfate into cartilage*** and also stimulate ***collagen formation***.

170. Answer is d (Destruction of Auerbach's plexus).
Ref: Khurana TB of medical physiology, 2006 edition Pg 651.

- There are two major networks of fibers that are intrinsic to GIT
- ***Auerbach'c myenteric plexus***: Between the outer longitudinal and middle circular fibers
- ***Meissner's submucosal plexus***: Between the middle circular layer and mucosa
- The ***mass movements*** are a special type of peristaltic contraction, which are observed in colon only.
- These occur 3–4 times/day generally after meals and each contraction lasts for about 3 minutes.
- ***Mass movement can be initiated*** by:
  - Gastrocolic or duodenocolic reflex
  - Overdistension of a segment of colon
  - Intense stimulation of the parasympathetic nerves.

171. Answer is b (Smooth endoplasmic reticulum).
Ref: Ganong's Physiology, old 19th edition Pg 453; The Pleura in health and disease, Jacques C, 1985 edition Pg 288.

Repeat Topic

- Refer ***answer no. 179 in COMED-K 2008 answers*** for detailed explanation.

172. Answer is b (One limb and two other limbs).
Ref: Ganong's physiology, 23rd edition Pg 494; Harrison's, 17th edition Pg 1389.

Direct quote:
"Augmented limb leads designated by the letter a (aVR, aVL, aVF) are generally used. The augmented leads are ***recordings between one limb and other two limbs****. This increases the size of the potentials by 50% without any change in configuration from the non-augmented record".*

- The ***12 conventional ECG leads*** record the difference in potential between electrodes placed on the surface of the body.
- These leads are divided into two groups:
  - 6 limb (extremity) leads
  - 6 chest (precordial) leads.
- The limb leads record potentials transmitted onto the *frontal plane* and the chest leads record potentials transmitted onto the *horizontal plane* (Fig. 221-3B).
- The six limb leads are further subdivided into:
  - 3 standard *"bipolar" leads* (I, II and III)
  - 3 augmented *"unipolar" leads* (aVR, aVL and aVF).
- Each **standard bipolar lead** ***measures the difference in potential between electrodes at two extremities***: Lead I = left arm-right arm voltages, lead II = left leg-right arm and lead III = left leg-left arm.
- The **augmented unipolar leads** ***measure the voltage (V) at one locus relative to an electrode (called the central terminal or indifferent electrode)*** that has ***approximately zero potential***.
- Thus, aVR = right arm, aVL = left arm and aVF = left leg (foot).
- The lowercase *a* indicates that these unipolar potentials are electrically augmented by 50%.
- The ***right leg electrode functions as a ground***.

☑ Note

❖ The ***six chest leads*** are unipolar recordings obtained by electrodes in the following positions: Lead V1, fourth intercostal space, just to the right of the sternum; lead V2, fourth intercostal space, just to the left of the sternum; lead V3, midway between V2 and V4; lead V4, midclavicular line, fifth intercostal space; lead V5, anterior axillary line, same level as V4; and lead V6, midaxillary line, same level as V4 and V5.

173. Answer is c (Production of platelet).
Ref: Harrison's, 17th edition Pg 372.

Area of spleen	Composition	Function
1. Red pulp	• 'Sinuses' (or 'sinusoids'), which are filled with blood • 'Splenic cords' of reticular fibers • 'Marginal zone' bordering on white pulp	• ***Destruction of abnormally shaped and rigid red cells*** by **culling and pitting**
2. White pulp	Composed of nodules, called Malpighian corpuscles. These are composed of: • 'Lymphoid follicles' rich in B-lymphocytes • 'Periarteriolar lymphoid sheaths' (PALS), rich in T-lymphocytes	• Helps fight infections

Other functions of spleen are:
- ***Erythrocyte production***—up to 5th month of gestation
- ***Synthesis of antibodies*** in the white pulp
- The removal of antibody-coated bacteria and antibody-coated blood cells from the circulation
- ***Phagocytosis*** of foreign substances
- ***Platelet reservoir***—spleen normally contains 30–40% of platelets.

174. Answer is d (The pentose phosphate pathway).
Ref: Vasudevan, 5th edition Pg 120.

Repeat Topic

- Refer ***answer no. 177 in COMED-K 2006 answers*** for detailed explanation.

175. Answer is c (Fructose 1-phosphate aldolase B).
Ref: Harrison's, 17th edition Pg 2458, 356-1.

Disease	Enzyme defect	Clinically	Comments
Essential fructosuria	Fructokinase	Asymptomatic, positive urine-reducing substance	Benign
Hereditary fructose intolerance	Fructose 1-phosphate aldolase B	Vomiting, lethargy, failure to thrive, hepatic failure	Prognosis good with early diagnosis and fructose restriction
Fructose 1,6-diphosphatase deficiency	Fructose 1,6-diphosphatase	Episodic hypoglycemia and lactic acidosis	Avoid fasting, good prognosis

176. Answer is b (Defects in the degradation of proteoglycans).
Ref: Harper's illustrated biochemistry, 26th edition Pg 45, 546; Vasudevan's biochemistry, 5th edition Pg 129.

- ***Mucopolysaccharidoses*** is due to ***deficiency of enzymes that degrade glycosaminoglycans (GAGs)*** and result in accumulation in various tissues in the body.
- GAGs as well as their oligosaccharides are excreted in the urine.

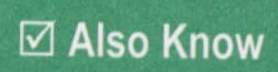

Mucopolysaccharidoses

Disease	Deficient enzyme	Clinical findings
1. **Hurler's (type 1), AR**	α-L-iduronidase	Severe mental retardation, skeletal deformity, coarse face, thick skin (gargoylism), corneal opacity, dermatan sulfate and heparan sulfate in urine

2. **Hunter's (type 2), XR** **Hunter's aim for the 'X' = XR**	Iduronate sulfatase	Mild Hurler's + aggressive behavior, deafness, NO corneal opacity. Hunter cannot hunt if he has corneal opacity, so **NO** corneal opacity for Hunter!

177. Answer is a (The hydroxylation of tyrosine).
Ref: KD Tripathi, 6th edition Pg 117.

Repeat Topic

- Refer ***answer no. 163 in COMED-K 2010 answers*** for detailed explanation.

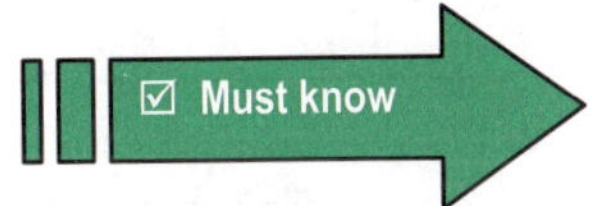

RATE LIMITING ENZYMES OF METABOLIC PROCESSES

Process	Enzyme
• Glycogenesis	Glycogen synthetase
• Glycogenolysis	Phosphorylase
• Glycolysis	Phosphofructokinase-1 (PFK-1)
• Gluconeogenesis	Phosphoenolpyruvate carboxykinase
• Fatty acid synthesis	Acetyl-CoA carboxylase
• Cholesterol synthesis	HMG-CoA reductase
• Bile acid synthesis	7-α-hydroxylase
• Urea synthesis	Carbamoyl phosphate synthetase, ornithine transcarbamylase
• Porphyrin synthesis	δ-aminolevulinate synthase
• Uric acid synthesis	Xanthine oxidase
• Purine biosynthesis	Phosphoribosyl pyrophosphate synthetase
• HMP shunt	Glucose-6-phosphate dehydrogenase
• TCA cycle	Isocitrate dehydrogenase
• Fatty acid oxidation	Carnitine acyltransferase-1

178. Answer is d (Ceramide).
Ref: Vasudevan's biochemistry, 5th edition Pg 78, 170.

- ***Phospholipids***: They contain glycerol, fatty acids and a nitrogen base.
- ***Glycolipids*** (glycosphingolipids): Widely distributed in nervous system; does not contain phosphoric acid, instead contains carbohydrates and ceramides.
- ***Cardiolipin***: Formed by reaction between diacylglycerol and glycerol-3-phosphate.
- ***Sphingomyelins***: The only sphingolipid that contains phosphate and no sugar moiety.

NOTES

COMED-K 2004

COMED-K 2004 QUESTIONS

MEDICINE

1. **Indicators of internal malignancy are all *EXCEPT***
   (a) Acanthosis nigricans
   (b) Generalized pruritus
   (c) Deep thrombophlebitis
   (d) Dermatomyositis

2. **Which is true in porphyria?**
   (a) Porphyria cutanea tarda is autosomal recessive
   (b) Protoporphyrin oxidase is a cytosolic coenzyme
   (c) ALA synthase requires TPP
   (d) Variegate protoporphyrinogen oxidase abnormality

3. **In a HIV+ person, AIDS develops when CD4+ count is**
   (a) < 200
   (b) 50–100
   (c) 500
   (d) 1,000

4. **Most severe complication of LGV is**
   (a) Urethral stricture
   (b) Rectal stricture
   (c) Inguinal swelling
   (d) Severe spiking fever

5. **Drugs used in CML are all *EXCEPT***
   (a) Busulfan
   (b) Alpha-interferon
   (c) Melphalan
   (d) Hydroxyurea

6. **All are true regarding drug-induced lupus *EXCEPT***
   (a) Acetylation makes a change
   (b) Anti-ds DNA is rare
   (c) Can resolve spontaneously
   (d) Renal manifestation is common

7. **About sarcoidosis all are true *EXCEPT***
   (a) Bilateral lymphadenopathy is present
   (b) Increased angiotensin-converting enzyme is present
   (c) Tuberculin is strongly positive
   (d) Egg shell calcification of X-ray chest

8. **Drug contraindicated in chronic renal failure**
   (a) Calcium carbonate with meal
   (b) Aluminum hydroxide before meal
   (c) Magnesium hydroxide with meal
   (d) All of the above

9. **Drug contraindicated in A/C MI**
   (a) Nifedipine
   (b) ACE inhibitors
   (c) Metoprolol
   (d) Aspirin

10. **Hypokalemia is a feature of**
   (a) Vomiting
   (b) Diarrhea
   (c) Diuretics
   (d) All the above

11. **Decreased O_2 carrying capacity and normal PO_2 is a feature of**
   (a) Anemic hypoxia
   (b) Histotoxic hypoxia
   (c) Stagnant hypoxia
   (d) Hypoxic hypoxia

12. **Cause of decreased cardiac output is**
   (a) Decreased venous return
   (b) Decreased end diastolic volume
   (c) Increased sympathetic stimulation
   (d) Decreased vagal tone

13. **Normal anion gap is a feature of**
   (a) Lactic acidosis
   (b) Diarrhea
   (c) Metabolic acidosis
   (d) Respiratory acidosis

14. **Abelson murine leukemia virus implicated in**
   (a) AML
   (b) CML
   (c) ALL
   (d) CLL

15. **Systemic necrotizing vasculitis is a feature of**
   (a) Wegener's granulomatosis
   (b) Takayasu's arteritis
   (c) PAN
   (d) Systemic sclerosis

16. **In Turner's syndrome, all the following are true *EXCEPT***
   (a) Amenorrhea
   (b) Mental retardation
   (c) Short stature
   (d) Coarctation of aorta

17. The Philadelphia chromosome most commonly associated with
(a) ALL
(b) CML
(c) AML
(d) All the above

18. DOC for resistant gonococcal infection is
(a) Erythromycin
(b) Benzathine penicillin
(c) Ciprofloxacin
(d) Ceftriaxone

19. By which procedures RNA is extracted?
(a) Northern blot
(b) Southern blot
(c) Eastern blot
(d) Western blot

20. Depolarization of the heart from the SA node to the ventricle is seen on the ECG as
(a) QT interval
(b) PR interval
(c) RS interval
(d) QRS complex

21. Hyperkalemia with acidosis is a feature of
(a) RTA type I
(b) RTA type II
(c) RTA type IV
(d) ARF

22. Drug of choice for *Toxoplasma* infections
(a) Tinidazole
(b) Co-trimoxazole
(c) Penicillin
(d) Ciprofloxacin

23. 'Mitsuda reaction' indicates
(a) Patient has leprosy
(b) Patient does not have leprosy
(c) CMI is intact
(d) Patient had leprosy in the past

24. A patient develops prebreakfast hyperglycemia. Next step of management is
(a) Start oral hypoglycemic in morning
(b) Monitor overnight blood glucose levels
(c) Start a dose of short-acting insulin at bedtime
(d) Start early morning insulin therapy

SURGERY

25. Meleney's gangrene is
(a) Abdominal wall synergistic gangrene caused by *E. coli* and anaerobic streptococci
(b) Synergistic gangrene of the scrotum
(c) Gangrene due to clostridia
(d) Idiopathic in nature

26. Risk factors of Ca stomach are all *EXCEPT*
(a) *H. pylori*
(b) Pernicious anemia
(c) Peptic ulcer surgeries
(d) Hyperplastic pyloric stenosis

27. Commonest esophageal benign tumor
(a) Fibrovascular polyps
(b) Epithelial polyps
(c) Leiomyoma
(d) Angioma

28. Features of De Quervain's thyroiditis are all *EXCEPT*
(a) Due to viral infection
(b) Raised ESR is a feature
(c) Thyroid antibodies absent
(d) Causes lymphoma

29. Peau d'orange is associated with
(a) Acute lymphedema
(b) Orange-puckered skin
(c) Inflammatory CA
(d) All the above

30. Drug used in isolated limb perfusion is done in malignant melanoma
(a) Cytosine
(b) Cyclophosphamide
(c) Methotrexate
(d) Melphalan

31. Commonest surgical complication of enteric fever is
(a) Intestinal perforation
(b) Intestinal bleeding
(c) Stricture formation
(d) Peritonitis

32. Commonest site of urethral injury
(a) Membranous
(b) Bulbar
(c) Prostatic
(d) Panvel

33. Ligation of ________ artery of abdomen leads to immediate death of the patient
(a) Superior mesenteric artery
(b) Inferior mesenteric artery
(c) Inferior vena cava
(d) Internal iliac artery

34. Strangulated hernia is commonly seen in which of the following?
(a) Direct inguinal hernia
(b) Indirect inguinal hernia
(c) Femoral hernia
(d) Obturator hernia

35. Butcher's thigh would refer to
(a) Penetrating wound through femoral artery
(b) Vertical cut across popliteal artery
(c) Penetrating wound through major vessels of thigh
(d) Cut in external iliac artery

36. Calot's triangle is in relation to all *EXCEPT*
(a) Gallbladder and cystic duct
(b) Common hepatic duct
(c) Right gastric artery
(d) Right lobe of liver

37. Commonest benign tumor of esophagus
(a) Epithelial polyp
(b) Leiomyoma
(c) Carcinoid tumor
(d) Fibrovascular polyp

38. In Clarke's classification of malignant melanoma, which type indicates lesion has reached the dermis?
(a) Level 1
(b) Level 2
(c) Level 3
(d) Level 4

39. Potato tumor is
(a) Sternocleidomastoid tumor
(b) Carotid body tumor
(c) Cystic tumor
(d) Sublingual dermoid

40. True regarding Meckel's diverticulum
(a) All the 3 layers of intestine are present in it
(b) Present at antimesenteric border
(c) Diverticulectomy and invagination done during appendicectomy
(d) All the above

41. A feature of DVT
(a) No symptoms
(b) Fever
(c) Cyanosis
(d) None of above

42. Features of duodenal atresia
(a) Bile not seen in vomitus
(b) Bile present in vomitus
(c) There is no vomiting
(d) Loose stools present

OBSTETRICS AND GYNECOLOGY

43. Blood supply to the uterus at term is
(a) 1,000 mL/min
(b) 50 mL/min
(c) 500 mL/min
(d) 750 mL/min

44. 'Physiological chills' is seen in
(a) 1st stage
(b) 2nd stage
(c) 3rd stage
(d) 4th stage

45. Biophysical profile is composed of all *EXCEPT*
(a) Amniotic fluid volume
(b) NST
(c) Fetal breathing and movement
(d) Placental maturity

46. Which of the following is not a primary tumor of ovaries?
(a) Teratoma
(b) Struma ovarii
(c) Krukenberg's
(d) Dysgerminoma

47. Genital tuberculosis primarily affects
(a) Uterus
(b) Ovary
(c) Fallopian tubes
(d) Cervix

48. Not a benign neoplasm of ovary
(a) Follicular cyst
(b) Granulosa cell thecomas
(c) Dermoid cyst
(d) Cystadenoma

49. Drug useful in last stage of endometrial carcinoma is
(a) Danazol
(b) OC pills
(c) Cisplatin
(d) Levonorgestrel

50. All the following hormones cross the placenta *EXCEPT*
(a) Insulin
(b) PTH
(c) Adrenal hormone
(d) Thyroxine

51. Which of the following ovarian tumor is associated with genital complication?
(a) Theca cell
(b) Granulosa cell
(c) Dysgerminoma
(d) Choriocarcinoma

52. AFP can be used to determine all *EXCEPT*
(a) Down syndrome
(b) Preterm labor
(c) Fetal distress
(d) Open neural tube defects

53. Litzmans obliquity is
(a) Posterior asynclitism
(b) Anterior asynclitism
(c) Same as neagles obliquity
(d) None of the above

ENT

54. Cause of refractor hoarseness in smokers
(a) Leukoplakia of vocal cords
(b) Malignancy of vocal cord
(c) Laryngitis
(d) None of the above

55. All are true regarding ozaena *EXCEPT*
(a) A feature of atrophic rhinitis
(b) More common in females
(c) Greenish foul smelling crust seen
(d) Patient complains of foul smell

56. Ossicular leverage ratio
(a) 1.1:1
(b) 1.2:1
(c) 1.3:1
(d) 1:1.3

OPHTHALMOLOGY

57. Keratomalacia is due to
(a) Hypovitaminosis D
(b) Hypovitaminosis A
(c) Hypovitaminosis E
(d) B-complex deficiency

58. False about background diabetic retinopathy
(a) Dot and blot hemorrhages seen
(b) Microaneurysms present
(c) Flame hemorrhages seen
(d) Gunn's sign is a feature

59. Cherry red spot is a feature of
(a) CRAO
(b) Retinal detachment
(c) Diabetic retinopathy
(d) Glaucoma

60. Cobble stone appearance is a feature of
(a) Vernal Catarrh
(b) Trachoma
(c) Phlyctenular conjunctivitis
(d) Angular conjunctivitis

61. In myopia, correction is done with lenses
(a) Convex
(b) Concave
(c) Cylindrical
(d) Elliptical

62. Angle of anterior chamber is examined with the help of
(a) Gonioscope
(b) Fundusope
(c) Ophthalmoscope
(d) Bulls' lamp

63. Hypovitaminosis D causes
(a) Zonular cataract
(b) Blue-dot cataract
(c) Rosette cataract
(d) Cupuliform cataract

64. Resolving power of direct ophthalmoscope
(a) 20–30 microns
(b) 30–40 microns
(c) 40–50 microns
(d) 70–80 microns

65. Pathology of retinal detachment
(a) Effusion of fluid into the suprachoroidal space
(b) Retinoschisis
(c) Separation of sensory retina from pigment epithelium
(d) None of the above

PEDIATRICS

66. Newborn with neonatal tetanus shows
(a) Risus sardonicus
(b) Opisthotonos
(c) Poor feeding and rigidity
(d) Trismus and lockjaw

67. **Complications of Fallot's tetralogy are all *EXCEPT***
(a) Infective endocarditis
(b) Paradoxical embolism
(c) Cerebral infarction
(d) Hypertensive crisis

68. **A child who presented with twitching movements of the face and the upper extremities, most probably has lesion would be in**
(a) Precentral gyrus
(b) Postcentral gyrus
(c) Caudate nucleus
(d) Frontal lobe

69. **Commonest cause of secondary hypertension in a child**
(a) Renal artery stenosis
(b) Adrenal tumors
(c) Renal disease
(d) Coarctation of aorta

70. **Congenital stridor is caused by**
(a) Small size of the larynx
(b) Loose submucosal connective tissue around the glottic region
(c) Rigid cricoid cartilage encircling the subglottic zone
(d) All the above

71. **Wide anterior fontanel is not a feature of**
(a) Craniosynostosis
(b) Rubella
(c) Achondroplasia
(d) Hydrocephalus

72. **Breastfeeding prevents which of the following infections?**
(a) Ocular
(b) Dermatological
(c) Urinary
(d) Enteric

73. **Child rides a tricycle by**
(a) 2–3 years
(b) 1–2 years
(c) 4–5 years
(d) 5–6 years

74. **Vitamin B_6 deficiency causes anemia**
(a) Microcytic hypochromic
(b) Spherocytic
(c) Megaloblastic
(d) Normocytic

ORTHOPEDICS

75. **Most common site of ganglion is**
(a) Dorsum of wrist
(b) Volar aspect of wrist
(c) Elbow
(d) Metacarpophalangeal joint

76. **Bunion refers to**
(a) Exostosis of the base of the 1st metatarsal bone
(b) Bursa at the base of the metatarsal bone
(c) Inflamed adventitial bursa at the base of the 1st metatarsal bone
(d) Exostosis at the head of the 1st metatarsal bone

77. **Earliest change in TB spine on X-ray is**
(a) Erosion of pedicle
(b) Narrowing of disk space
(c) Abscess with soft tissue swelling
(d) Disc collapse

78. **Criteria for rheumatoid arthritis include all the following *EXCEPT***
(a) Morning stiffness for 15 min
(b) Symmetrical
(c) Hand joints involved
(d) 3 joint swelling for 6 weeks

79. **Lytic lesion on metaphysis is a feature of**
(a) Osteosarcoma
(b) Osteoid osteoma
(c) Osteoclastoma
(d) Osteochondroma

80. **Osteomyelitis is commonly a complication of**
(a) Frontal sinusitis
(b) Ethmoid sinusitis
(c) Sphenoid sinusitis
(d) Maxillary sinusitis

PHARMACOLOGY

81. **Site of action of ACE inhibitors**
(a) Proximal tubules
(b) Distal tubules
(c) Henle's loop
(d) Collecting ducts

82. **True regarding phenylephrine are all *EXCEPT***
(a) Used as a nasal decongestant
(b) Causes reflex bradycardia
(c) Causes hypotension
(d) Causes mydriasis

83. **Mechanism of action of moricizine**
(a) Prolongs action potential duration
(b) Shortens action potential duration
(c) No change in AP
(d) None of the above

84. **Antiandrogen drug used in prostatic carcinoma**
(a) Fosfestrol
(b) Finasteride
(c) Stilboestrol
(d) Cyproterone

85. **DOC for meningococcal meningitis is**
(a) Penicillin
(b) Rifampin
(c) Ciprofloxacin
(d) Ceftriaxone

86. **MOA of adenosine is by**
(a) Increase K^+ efflux and decreasing Ca^{++} release in heart muscle
(b) Inhibiting K^+ channels
(c) Inhibiting Na^+-K^+-ATPase
(d) Increase Ca^+ influx

87. **Chlamydial infection can be treated by**
(a) Tetracycline
(b) Chloramphenicol
(c) Amoxicillin
(d) Penicillin

88. **Dry cough is an adverse effect seen in administration of which of the following?**
(a) Nifedipine
(b) Enalapril
(c) Prazosin
(d) Furosemide

MICROBIOLOGY

89. **Hepatitis D virus**
(a) Transmitted by fecal-oral route
(b) Is a DNA virus
(c) Has independent existence
(d) Resembles some plant viruses

90. **An example of heterophile reaction**
(a) Weil-Felix
(b) Paul-Bunnell test
(c) Cold agglutinin test
(d) All of the above

91. **Cannot be cultured in Sabouraud agar**
(a) *Blastomyces*
(b) *Coccidioides*
(c) *Sporotrichum*
(d) *Rhinosporidium seeberi*

92. **Long-lasting immunity in hepatitis infection is due to**
(a) IgA
(b) IgG
(c) IgM
(d) IgE

93. **Visceral larva migrans is secondary to**
(a) *Toxocara canis*
(b) *Toxoplasma*
(c) *Toxocara cati*
(d) *Ascaris*

94. **Addition of detergent does not cause disruption of phospholipid membrane in**
(a) Polio virus
(b) Vaccinia
(c) Variola
(d) Eastern equine encephalitis virus

95. **Koch's postulates**
(a) The bacteria should be associated with the lesions of the disease
(b) It should be possible to isolate the bacteria in pure culture from lesions
(c) Specific antibodies to the bacteria should be demonstrated in serum
(d) All the above

PATHOLOGY

96. **True about CA bronchus are all *EXCEPT***
(a) Incidence is low in non-smoking women
(b) Sq cell CA is the commonest type and arises from the periphery
(c) Adenocarcinoma arises from the periphery
(d) Smokers have 10 times more risk of developing CA bronchus than non-smokers

97. **Aortic valves with friable vegetations and destruction of its cusps is seen in**
(a) *Streptococcus* endocarditis
(b) *Candida* endocarditis
(c) *Staphylococcus aureus* endocarditis
(d) Viral endocarditis

98. **Eosinophilia is a feature of**
(a) Worm infestations
(b) PAN
(c) Hodgkin's lymphoma
(d) All the above

99. **The test commonly used to follow-up patients to check for response of treatment in syphilis is**
(a) FTA Abs
(b) VDRL
(c) Microhemagglutination
(d) TPI

100. **In a 40-year-old patient, there was pleural fluid analysis and this fluid showed a protein level of 22g/L and a LDH level of 125 U/L. The most probable diagnosis is**
(a) TB
(b) Congestive cardiac failure
(c) Sarcoidosis
(d) Pulmonary infarction

101. **True regarding ESR**
(a) Increased in polycythemia
(b) Increased in sickle cell anemia
(c) Useful in monitoring the treatment response in giant cell arteritis
(d) Decreased in pregnancy

102. **Features of ulcerative colitis are all *EXCEPT***
(a) Pinpoint ulcers
(b) Crypt abscess
(c) Stricture
(d) Pseudopolyposis

103. **Edward's syndrome is**
(a) Chromosome 13 defect
(b) Chromosome 18 defect
(c) Chromosome 11 defect
(d) Chromosome 21 defect

104. **In AML, the M4 stage is known as**
(a) Acute myelocytic leukemia
(b) Acute myelomonoblastic leukemia
(c) Acute myelomonocytic leukemia
(d) Acute monoblastic leukemia

105. **Causative microorganism of 'Burkitt's lymphoma'.**
(a) EB virus
(b) Arbovirus
(c) Human papilloma virus
(d) Human immunodeficiency virus

106. **Philadelphia chromosomes**
(a) t21:8
(b) t9:22
(c) t22:8
(d) t9:21

107. **Chromosome 5 defect causes**
(a) Myotonic dystrophy
(b) Wilm's tumor
(c) CML
(d) Familial adenomatous polyposis

FORENSIC MEDICINE

108. **All are true about gunshot entry wound *EXCEPT***
(a) Entry wound is smaller than exit wound
(b) Entry wound is surrounded with cornea
(c) Entry wound is everted
(d) Entry wound is inverted

109. **Stomach wash is absolutely contraindicated in**
(a) Corrosive poisoning
(b) Convulsant poisoning
(c) Comatose patients
(d) Hypothermia

110. **Which of the following is a 'Somniferous toxin'?**
(a) Datura
(b) Opium
(c) Belladonna
(d) Cannabis

111. **Death penalty can be passed in which judicial court?**
(a) High Court
(b) Supreme Court
(c) Sessions Court
(d) Assistant Sessions Court

112. **Feature of 'Antemortem drowning'**
(a) Fine froth from mouth and nostrils
(b) Cutis anserina
(c) Weeds and grass in hand
(d) Water in stomach

113. **Double Barr bodies are seen in**
(a) XXX
(b) XO
(c) Androgen resistance
(d) Male pseudohermaphroditism

PREVENTIVE AND SOCIAL MEDICINE

114. **Most efficient mode of transmission of HIV**
(a) Hematogenous spread
(b) Unprotected sexual intercourse
(c) Infected syringes
(d) Mother-to-child transmission

115. **Predictive value of a negative test is**
(a) d/(c + d) × 100
(b) d/(a + d) × 100
(c) a/(c + d) × 100
(d) a/(a + c) × 100

116. **PQLI takes into consideration**
(a) Literacy, infant mortality, life expectancy at 1 year
(b) Literacy, infant mortality, life expectancy at birth
(c) Per capita income, infant mortality, life expectancy at 1 year
(d) Per capita income, infant mortality, life expectancy at birth

117. **Recommended iodine concentrations at consumer level should be**
(a) 10,000 ppm
(b) 50 ppm
(c) 30 ppm
(d) 15 ppm

118. **Iron content in human milk is**
(a) 0.1 mg
(b) 0.3 mg
(c) 0.5 mg
(d) Negligible

119. **Road to health chart was given by**
(a) John Snow
(b) David Morley
(c) Koch
(d) Henry Dunant

120. **Global eradication of smallpox was done on**
(a) 11th Sept 1985
(b) 8th May 1980
(c) 5th July 1975
(d) 4th April 1974

121. **World Health Day is on**
(a) 7th April
(b) 4th April
(c) 5th April
(d) 6th April

122. **Path of longest duration in network analysis is**
(a) Limiting path method
(b) Critical path method
(c) a and b
(d) Neither a nor b

123. **KFD is transmitted by**
(a) Soft tick
(b) Hard tick
(c) Mosquito
(d) Sand fly

124. **Mid-day meal contains**
(a) 1/2 proteins and 1/2 calories
(b) 1/2 proteins and 1/3 calories
(c) 1/3 proteins and 1/3 calories
(d) 2/3 calories and 1/3 proteins

125. **The optimum protein requirement for your body should be**
(a) 1 g/kg
(b) 5 g/kg
(c) 3 g/kg
(d) 7 g/kg

126. **Prevention of disease by immunization comes under which category?**
(a) Primordial prevention
(b) Primary prevention
(c) Secondary prevention
(d) Tertiary prevention

127. **A positive tuberculin test is indicative of**
(a) Active infection
(b) Past infection
(c) Both a and b
(d) Neither a nor b

128. **Conventional contraceptives are**
(a) IUCD
(b) OCP
(c) Coitus interruptus
(d) Condom

PSYCHIATRY

129. **Regarding anorexia nervosa, all are true *EXCEPT***
(a) Usually occurs in teenage girls
(b) It is an attempt to use food and weight to deal with emotional problems
(c) Patients eat huge amounts of food, but they throw up soon after eating
(d) Treatment involves more than changing the person's eating habits

130. **Uncinate fits are commonly associated with**
(a) Visual hallucinations
(b) Unpleasant olfactory sensations
(c) Feeling of unreality
(d) Auditory hallucinations

DERMATOLOGY

131. **'Erythema marginatum' is a feature of**
(a) Measles
(b) Chickenpox
(c) Rheumatic fever
(d) Rubella pox

132. The most common type of skin cancer is
(a) Basal cell CA
(b) Squamous cell CA
(c) Melanoma
(d) Keratosis

133. Uses of 'Calcipotriol' is in
(a) Lichen planus
(b) Psoriasis
(c) Acne vulgaris
(d) Erythema multiforme

134. Norwegian scabies is seen in
(a) Infants
(b) Elderly
(c) Females
(d) Immunocompromised and mentally retarded

135. Treatment for tinea unguium
(a) Griseofulvin + Ketoconazole
(b) Amphotericin B
(c) Zinc oxide
(d) Nystatin

RADIOLOGY

136. In USG, double bubble sign is seen in
(a) Duodenal atresia
(b) Encephalocele
(c) Umbilical hernia
(d) Posturethral valve

ANESTHESIA

137. Laryngeal mask is contraindicated in
(a) Full stomach
(b) Elderly
(c) Empty stomach
(d) Esophageal varices

138. Local anesthetics with adrenaline are not used in dirty wound because
(a) They cannot act in acidic pH
(b) They spread the infection
(c) Both of the above
(d) None of the above

139. Saddle block anesthesia is
(a) Hyperbaric solution injected in spinal canal
(b) Another name of epidural anesthesia
(c) Used for perineal and rectal surgeries
(d) Inferior gluteal nerve block

140. Best muscle relaxant effect can be obtained by which of the following?
(a) Halothane
(b) Nitrous oxide
(c) Ether
(d) Theophylline

141. *False* about halothane
(a) Bronchoconstriction and ↑ respiratory secretions
(b) Volatile liquid non-inflammable
(c) Myocardial depressant
(d) Hypotension

ANATOMY

142. All are true about trigeminal nerve *EXCEPT*
(a) Mesencephalic nucleus is proprioceptive
(b) Supplies buccinator muscle
(c) Supplies medial pterygoid
(d) Supplies masseter muscle

143. Which of the following are not correct?
(a) Vermis Plans: The limb movement
(b) Cerebrocerebellum: Communicates via pontine nucleus with cerebral cortex
(c) Spinocerebellum: Regulation of muscle tone
(d) Vestibulocerebellum: Controls eye movements

144. In dislocation of 5th and 6th cervical vertebra, which of the following spinal nerve is injured?
(a) VI
(b) V
(c) IV
(d) III

145. The muscle that crosses both shoulder and elbow joint
(a) Coracobrachialis
(b) Medial head of triceps
(c) Biceps brachii
(d) Brachialis

146. Fecal fistula at umbilicus is due to
(a) Persistent vitellointestinal duct
(b) Persistent patent urachus
(c) Persistent remnant of urachus
(d) Ligamentum arteriosum

147. Muscle causing 'Depression of mandible'
(a) Medial pterygoid
(b) Lateral pterygoid
(c) Masseter
(d) Buccinator

148. Length of the fallopian tube is
(a) 5 cm
(b) 7 cm

(c) 8.5 cm
(d) 10 cm

PHYSIOLOGY

149. During moderate exercise, there is
(a) Decrease in blood flow to brain
(b) Decrease in blood flow to heart
(c) Decrease in blood flow to skeletal muscles
(d) Decrease in total peripheral resistance

150. Insulin-like growth factor synthesized in
(a) Liver
(b) Pituitary
(c) Placenta
(d) Kidneys

151. Transport of long-chain fatty acids across the inner mitochondrial membrane is facilitated by
(a) Carnitine
(b) Epinephrine
(c) Pyruvate kinase
(d) NADPH

152. Not a function of saliva
(a) Lubrication
(b) Taste sensation
(c) Digestion of carbohydrates
(d) Digestion of proteins

153. Normal testicular development requires which of the following chromosomes?
(a) XY
(b) XX
(c) Y chromosome
(d) X chromosome

154. The olfactory tract ends at the cortex by passing through which of the following?
(a) Medial olfactory striae
(b) Lateral olfactory striae
(c) Diagonal band of Broca
(d) All of the above

155. Regarding surfactant, false is
(a) Composed of phosphosphingolipids
(b) It causes decreased compliance
(c) Secreted by type II cells
(d) Prevents lung collapse

156. All are true regarding tendon jerk *EXCEPT*
(a) Deep proprioceptive reflexes
(b) Monosynaptic reflex
(c) Fractionated stretch reflexes
(d) None of the above

BIOCHEMISTRY

157. Anaerobic glycolysis yields
(a) 2 lactate + 2 ATP
(b) 2 lactate + 2 NADPH + 2 ATP
(c) 4 lactate + 6 ATP
(d) 2 lactate + 6 NADPH + 6 ATP

158. Which one of the enzyme deficiency is correctly paired?
(a) Fabry's – alpha galactosidase
(b) Gaucher's – beta glucosidase
(c) Cystic fibrosis – glucuronidase
(d) Chronic bronchitis – alpha 1 antitrypsin

159. The enzyme used in recombinant DNA technology
(a) Restriction endonuclease
(b) Pyridoxine dehydrogenase
(c) RNA polymerase II
(d) DNA ligase

160. For single carbon transfer, which coenzyme is responsible
(a) Acetyl coenzyme A
(b) Biotin
(c) THFA
(d) Pyridoxine

161. NH_4 is released by
(a) Arginase
(b) Glutamate dehydrogenase
(c) Glutaminase
(d) All of the above

162. The sequence in respiratory chain in the mitochondria is
(a) C-cl-b-a-a3
(b) Cl-c-b-bl-a3-a
(c) B-cl-c-a-a3
(d) A-a3-b-c-cl

163. Anion gap means
(a) Gap in anion molecule
(b) Difference between high and normal anion gap acidosis

(c) Unmeasured ions
(d) Primary deficit of anions

164. After a 2 days fast the substance likely to be involved in the formation of energy would be
(a) Muscle glycogen
(b) Liver glycogen
(c) Amino acid
(d) Acetoacetate

165. Meroanencephaly is due to
(a) Non-closure of rostral neuropore
(b) Non-closure of caudal neuropore
(c) Early closure of rostral neuropore
(d) Early closure of caudal neuropore

This is a memory-based recall paper (only YEAR 2004–rest are direct from the official question papers issued out to the candidates' hands at the end of exam).

COMED-K 2004

ANSWERS AND EXPLANATIONS

MEDICINE

1. **Answer is b (Generalized pruritus).**
Ref: Fitzpatrick's dermatology, 2nd edition Pg 132.

Cutaneous Markers of Internal Malignancy

1. **Acanthosis nigricans**	– Velvety hyperpigmented thickened skin lesion, prominent on the dorsum of the neck and major flexures (axillae or groin). – MC a/w adenocarcinoma stomach; also other GIT malignancies. – Also a/w obesity, acromegaly, Cushing's syndrome, polycystic ovary syndrome, type 2 DM and drugs (diethylstilbestrol, nicotinic acid, glucocorticoids).
2. **Seborrheic keratoses**	– Sign of Leser Trélat (sudden appearance of large number of seborrheic keratoses).
3. **Necrolytic Migratory erythema**	– Migratory erythema with erosions; favors lower extremities and girdle area. Seen in glucagonoma syndrome.
4. **Dermatomyositis**	– Maybe associated with malignancy of lung, ovary, breast, GIT, lymphoproliferative and nasopharynx.
5. **Erythema gyratum repens**	– Hundreds of mobile concentric arcs and wavefronts that resemble the grain in wood. Associated with Carcinoma bronchus.
6. **Acquired ichthyosis**	– When generalized scaling without erythema starts for the first time in adulthood there is a strong likelihood of an underlying neoplasm.
7. **Thrombophlebitis migrans**	– Successive crops of tender nodules affecting blood vessels throughout the body, associated with Carcinoma pancreas (especially body and tail tumors).
8. **Bullous Pemphigoid**	– Controversial.
9. **Pyoderma gangrenosum**	– Rarely associated with leukemia.
10. **Bazex syndrome**	– Paraneoplastic acrokeratosis.
11. **Bowen's disease**	– Intraepidermal carcinoma.
12. **Others**	– Sudden appearance of lanugo hair (hypertrichosis lanuginosa), multiple papillomata. – Cowden's disease (multiple hamartoma syndrome).

2. **Answer is d (Variegate protoporphyrinogen oxidase abnormality).**
Ref: Vasudevan's biochemistry, 5th edition Pg 260; Cecil's internal medicine, Pg 361.

PORPHYRIAS

- **Porphyrias** are a group of inherited or acquired disorders of certain enzymes in the heme biosynthetic pathway (also called porphyrin pathway). Based on the site of the overproduction and accumulation of the porphyrins (or their chemical precursors), porphyrias are broadly classified as acute (hepatic) porphyrias cutaneous (erythropoietic) porphyrias.
- Hepatic porphyrias are characterized by acute neurological attacks (seizures, psychosis, extreme back and abdominal pain and an acute polyneuropathy).
- Erythropoietic porphyrias present with skin problems, usually a light-sensitive blistering rash and increased hair growth.
- Variegate porphyria (mixed porphyria), has both neurological and skin features.

- "Porphyrias = **Disease of 5Ps** = Pain abdomen, Psychological disturbances, Polyneuropathy, Purple urine, Precipitated by Pills".

Classification of human porphyrias

Condition	Enzyme defect
Hepatic porphyrias	
Acute intermittent porphyria (AD)	Porphobilinogen deaminase
Porphyria cutanea tarda (AD), MC	Uroporphyrinogen decarboxylase
Hereditary coproporphyria (AD)	Coproporphyrinogen oxidase
Erythropoietic porphyria	
Congenital erythropoietic porphyria (Günther's disease) (AR)	Uroporphyrinogen cosynthase
Erythropoietic protoporphyria (AD)	Ferrochelatase
Mixed	
Variegate porphyria (AD)	Protoporphyrinogen oxidase

3. **Answer is a (< 200).**
Ref: Harrison's, 17th edition Pg 1138 and Table 182-1; Davidson's, 20th edition Pg 384, Box 14.7

- The current ***CDC classification system for HIV-infected*** adolescents and adults categorizes persons on the basis of clinical conditions associated with HIV infection and CD4+ T lymphocyte counts.
- The system is based on three ranges of CD4+ T lymphocyte counts and three clinical categories and is represented by a matrix of nine mutually exclusive categories.
- Using this system, ***any HIV-infected individual with a CD4+ T cell count of < 200/μL has AIDS*** by definition, regardless of the presence of symptoms or opportunistic diseases.

1993 Revised Classification System for HIV Infection and Expanded Aids Surveillance Case Definition for Adolescents and Adults

	Clinical Categories		
CD4+ T Cell Categories	**A Asymptomatic, Acute (Primary)** HIV or PGL	**B Symptomatic, Not A or C** Conditions	**C AIDS Indicator Conditions**
>500/μL	A1	B1	C1
200–499/μL	A2	B2	C2
<200/μL	A3	B3	C3

PGL = Persistent Generalized Lymphadenopathy

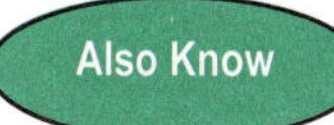

Correlation between CD4 count and HIV-associated diseases

> 500 cells/mm³	• Acute primary infection • Recurrent vaginal candidiasis • Persistent generalized lymphadenopathy
< 500 cells/mm³	• Pulmonary TB • Pneumococcal pneumonia • Herpes Zoster • Oropharyngeal candidiasis

	• Oral hairy leukoplakia • Extraintestinal salmonellosis • Kaposi's sarcoma • HIV-associated ITP • Cervical intraepithelial neoplasia II–III • Lymphoid interstitial pneumonitis
< 200 cells/mm³	• *Pneumocystis jiroveci* (carinii) pneumonia • Mucocutaneous herpes simplex
< 100 cells/mm³	• Cryptosporidium • Microsporidium • Esophageal candidiasis • Military/extrapulmonary TB • HIV associated wasting • Peripheral neuropathy
< 50 cells/mm³	• CMV retinitis/GI disease • Disseminated MAC infection

4. Answer is b (Rectal stricture).
Ref: Adolescent Health Care: A Practical Guide Issue 414, Pg 786.

- In LGV, ***the most common severe morbidity results from rectal involvement***; ***rectal stricture*** may result from 1 to 10 years after infection.

<u>Note</u>:

- ☐ *LGV is more symptomatic in men*, but *late complications are more common in women.*

5. Answer is c (Melphalan).
Ref: Harrison's, 17th edition Pg 686.

- ***Imatinib mesylate*** (Gleevec) ***currently the first line therapy for CML*** specifically targets and inhibits Bcr-Abl tyrosine kinase and eliminates the CML clone—leads to 90% hematological remission.
- Before imatinib, when allogeneic SCT was not feasible, Interferon (***IFN-alpha) therapy*** was the treatment of choice.
- ***Hydroxyurea***, a ribonucleotide reductase inhibitor, induces rapid disease control. Unfortunately, cytogenetic remissions with hydroxyurea are uncommon.
- ***Busulfan***, an alkylating agent that acts on early progenitor cells, has a more prolonged effect. However, serious side effects include unexpected and occasionally fatal, myelosuppression in 5–10% of patients; pulmonary, endocardial and marrow fibrosis; and an Addison-like wasting syndrome.

<u>Note</u>:

- ***Allogeneic bone marrow transplantation*** (BMT) is the ***only curative therapy for CML*** and when feasible is the treatment of choice.
- ***Melphalan*** shows variable oral bioavailability and undergoes extensive binding to albumin and α1-acidic glycoprotein. Mucositis appears more prominently; however, it has prominent activity in multiple myeloma.

6. Answer is d (Renal manifestation is common).
Ref: Rheumatology, diagnosis and therapeutics, John J Cush, 2005 edition Pg 162.

- Patients who are ***slow acetylators are at higher risk*** for adverse effects including drug induced SLE because of the potential for accumulation of the active drug.
- ***Anti-dSDNA are rare***, but ***antihistone*** antibodies are typical.
- ***CNS and renal findings*** are **RARE** in drug induced lupus.
- With discontinuation of drug treatment, ***symptoms invariably resolve over weeks to months***.

7. Answer is c (Tuberculin is strongly positive).
Ref: Harrison's, 17th edition Pg 2138-2140.

Sarcoidosis

- Microscopically: N***on-caseating granulomas; also called 'naked' granulomas*** since they only have a ***sparse lymphocytic infiltrate*** at the margins; granulomas contain inclusions such as:
  - ***Schaumann bodies*** (concentric calcified concretion conchlike).
  - ***Asteroid bodies*** (stellate structures).
  - ***Residual bodies*** (refractile calcium-containing inclusions).
- Clinically, two syndromes in sarcoidosis are:
  - ***Lofgren's syn***: Erythema nodosum, bilateral hilar adenopathy, arthritis.
  - ***Heerfordt-Waldenström syn*** *(uveoparotid fever)*: Fever, parotid enlargement, anterior uveitis and facial N. palsy.
  - ***Lungs*** almost always involved (interstitial lung disease); ***lymphadenopathy*** (paratracheal commonly, also mediastinal, cervical); skin (***lupus pernio***).
- Diagnosis: Is by biopsy, ↑ ***ACE levels***, hypercalcemia, lymphocytopenia.
- *Chest X-ray:* Stage I disease shows ***bilateral hilar lymphadenopathy (BHL)***. Stage II disease shows BHL plus pulmonary infiltrates. Stage III disease shows pulmonary infiltrates without BHL. Stage IV disease shows pulmonary fibrosis. However now, except for epidemiological purposes this classification is only of historical interest.
- *CT of the thorax:* May demonstrate lymphadenopathy or granulomatous infiltration.
- *Whole body gallium-67 scanning:* Two common findings seen in sarcoidosis are the lambda and panda patterns. *Lambda pattern* is produced by uptake of right paratracheal and bilateral hilar lymph nodes. *'Panda image'* is produced by symmetric uptake by lacrimal and parotid glands.
- ***Kveim test***: It is the *most specific test* for sarcoidosis—involves *intradermal injection* of tissue from spleen or lymph node of a patient with sarcoidosis. The area is *biopsied 4–6 weeks after* injection and histologically examined for non-caseating granuloma formation, which, if found, means a positive result.
- *Tuberculin skin test:* Two-third patients will have ***cutaneous anergy to tuberculin*** skin test.
- ***Bronchoalveolar lavage*** with a CD4/CD8 ratio: ***CD4/CD8 ratio of*** **> 3.5** has a *94% specificity* for sarcoidosis.
- Treatment: DOC for sarcoidosis is ***glucocorticoids***.

8. Answer is b (Aluminum hydroxide before meal).
Ref: Kumar and Clarke, Pg 649-50.

- ***Aluminum-containing gut phosphate binders*** have the disadvantage that absorption of aluminum poses the risk of ***aluminum bone disease and development of cognitive impairment***.

9. Answer is a (Nifedipine).
Ref: Harrison's, 17th edition Pg 1534-36.

Direct quote:
"Unlike beta-blockers, ***calcium antagonists are of little value in the acute setting*** and there is evidence that ***short-acting dihydropyridines (nifedipine) may be associated with an increased mortality risk***.

Treatment of myocardial infarction BeMOAN:
- **Be**ta-blockers (metoprolol),
- **M**orphine,
- **O**xygen,
- **A**spirin and ACE inhibitor,
- **N**itroglycerin.

10. Answer is d (All the above).
Ref: Harrison's, 17th edition Pg 281, Table 46-3.

CAUSES OF HYPOKALEMIA

I. Decreased intake	III. Increased loss
A. Starvation	A. Non-renal
B. Clay ingestion	1. Gastrointestinal loss (diarrhea, vomiting)
II. Redistribution into cells	2. Integumentary loss (sweat)

A. Acid-base 1. Metabolic alkalosis B. Hormonal 1. Insulin 2. β2-adrenergic agonists (endogenous or exogenous) 3. α-adrenergic antagonists C. Anabolic state 1. Vitamin B12 or folic acid (red blood cell production) 2. Granulocyte-macrophage colony stimulating factor (white blood cell production) 3. Total parenteral nutrition D. Other 1. Pseudohypokalemia 2. Hypothermia 3. Hypokalemic periodic paralysis 4. Barium toxicity	B. Renal 1. Increased distal flow: Diuretics, osmotic diuresis, salt-wasting nephropathies 2. Increased secretion of potassium a. Mineralocorticoid excess: Primary hyperaldosteronism, secondary hyperaldosteronism (malignant hypertension, renin-secreting tumors, renal artery stenosis, hypovolemia), apparent mineralocorticoid excess (licorice, chewing tobacco, carbenoxolone), congenital adrenal hyperplasia, Cushing's syndrome, Bartter's syndrome b. Distal delivery of non-reabsorbed anions: Vomiting, nasogastric suction, proximal (type 2) renal tubular acidosis, diabetic ketoacidosis, glue-sniffing (toluene abuse), penicillin derivatives c. Other: Amphotericin B, Liddle's syndrome, hypomagnesemia

11. Answer is a (Anemic hypoxia).
Ref: Ganong's physiology, 23rd edition Pg 513.

TYPES OF HYPOXIA

1.	**Hypoxic hypoxia (anoxic anoxia)**	↓ PO_2 of the arterial blood
2.	**Anemic hypoxia**	↓ O_2 carrying capacity of blood (amount of Hb available to carry O_2 is ↓); arterial PO_2 is normal.
3.	**Stagnant hypoxia (ischemic hypoxia)**	↓ Rate of blood flow to tissue so that adequate O_2 is not delivered to it despite a normal arterial PO_2 and Hb concentration (CCF)
4.	**Histotoxic hypoxia**	↓ Utilization of O_2 by tissues; the amount of O_2 delivered to a tissue is adequate but because of the action of a toxic agent (e.g. cyanide), the cells cannot make use of the O_2 supplied to them

12. Answer is a (Decreased venous return).
Ref: Guyton's physiology, Pg 134.

- Three fundamental factors, which influence the cardiac output are:
  - Cardiac inflow: Greater the venous return, greater will be the end diastolic fiber length of the ventricle and (provided it remains within physiological limits) greater will be the force of contraction due to Frank Starling's law.
  - Contractility of heart.
  - Heart rate.

13. Answer is b (Diarrhea).
Ref: Harrison's, 17th edition Pg 290, 292.

- See ***answer no. 14 in COMED-K 2005 answers*** for detailed explanation and causes of ***normal anion gap metabolic acidosis***.

14. Answer is b (CML).
Ref: Harrison's, 17th edition Pg 683.

- The diagnosis of ***CML*** is established by identifying a clonal expansion of a hematopoietic stem cell possessing a reciprocal translocation between chromosomes 9 and 22.
- This translocation results in the head-to-tail fusion of the breakpoint cluster region (*BCR*) gene on chromosome 22q11 with the ***ABL (named after the abelson murine leukemia virus) gene located on chromosome 9q34***.
- Untreated, the disease is characterized by the inevitable transition from a chronic phase to an accelerated phase and on to blast crisis in a median time of 4 years.

15. Answer is c (PAN).
Ref: Harrison's, 17th edition Pg 2124.

- *PAN*, also referred to as *classic PAN*, was described in 1866 by Kussmaul and Maier.
- It is a ***multisystem, necrotizing vasculitis*** of small and medium-sized muscular arteries in which involvement of the renal and visceral arteries is characteristic.
- PAN does NOT involve pulmonary arteries, although bronchial vessels may be involved; granulomas, significant eosinophilia and an allergic diathesis are not observed.

16. Answer is b (Mental retardation).
Ref: OP Ghai, 7th edition Pg 456.

Turner's syndrome

- 45 XO, i.e. no sex chromatin body; due to non-disjunction of sex chromosomes.
- Clinical features:

❖ Phenotypically female ❖ Short stature ❖ Wide carrying angle ❖ Webbing of neck ❖ Lymphedema of dorsum of hands and feet ❖ Short metacarpals (retarded bone age) ❖ Shield-like chest with widely spaced nipples ❖ Scanty pubic and axillary hair	❖ Primary amenorrhea, high gonadotropin levels, low estrogen level ❖ ***Slight*** intellectual defect (NO mental retardation) ❖ Coarctation of aorta ❖ Renal anomalies (horseshoe kidney, double or cleft renal pelvis) ❖ Sensorineural hearing loss

17. Answer is b (CML).
Ref: Robbins pathology, 7th edition Pg 696, 697.

- See ***answer no. 103 and answer no. 106 below*** for detailed explanation.

18. Answer is d (Ceftriaxone).
Ref: Harrison's, 17th edition Pg 916.

- ***Penicillin, ampicillin and tetracycline*** are NO LONGER RELIABLE for the treatment of gonorrhea and should not be used.
- ***Third-generation cephalosporins have remained highly effective as single-dose therapy*** for gonorrhea.
- Even though the minimal inhibitory concentrations (MICs) of ceftriaxone for certain strains may reach 0.015–0.125 mg/L (higher than the MICs of 0.0001–0.008 mg/L for fully susceptible strains), these levels are greatly exceeded in the blood, the urethra and the cervix when the routinely recommended ceftriaxone and cefixime regimens are administered.
- These regimens ALMOST ALWAYS RESULT IN AN EFFECTIVE CURE.

19. Answer is a (Northern blot).
Ref: Lippincott's illustrated biochemistry, Pg 10.

- Northern blot = RNA
- Southern blot = DNA

20. Answer is b (PR interval).
Ref: Harrison's, 17th edition Pg 1388-91.

Normal ECG

☐ **P wave**	A
☐ **PR interval**	: Conduction through AV node (< 0.2 s)
☐ **QRS complex**	: Ventricular depolarization (< 0.12 s)
☐ **QT interval**	: Mechanical contraction of ventricles
☐ **T wave**	: Ventricular repolarization
☐ **ST segment**	: Isoelectric ventricular contraction
☐ **U wave**	: Caused by hypokalemia, bradycardia

21. Answer is c (RTA type IV).
Ref: Harrison's, 17th edition Pg 1802, 1805, 1816.

Renal Tubular Acidosis (RTA)

- There are 4 types, only 3 are clinically important. Type 3 is uncommon and seen only in children. It is a non-anion gap metabolic acidosis.

❖ **Type 1 (distal) RTA**	Hypokalemic hyperchloremic metabolic acidosis and is due to selective **deficiency in** H^+ **secretion** in the **distal** nephron Despite acidosis, **urinary pH cannot be acidified** and is always above 5.5; ↓ K^+ *Etiology*: Renal stones, hereditary, amphotericin, cirrhosis, collagen vascular disease (SLE, Sjögren's, chronic active hepatitis) Treatment: Potassium citrate Complications: Nephrolithiasis "Type **ONE** = St**ONE**"
❖ **Type 2 (proximal) RTA**	Hypokalemic hyperchloremic metabolic acidosis due to a selective **defect in the proximal tubule's ability to adequately reabsorb filtered** HCO_3^-; ↓ K^+ *Etiology*: Carbonic anhydrase inhibitors (acetazolamide, **Di**amox); hereditary; ***Fan**coni's* syndrome (defects of absorption in the proximal tubule, resulting in glucosuria, aminoaciduria, phosphaturia and uric aciduria). *Treatment*: Potassium citrate *Complications*: Rickets, osteomalacia **"Di**-hard **Fan** of **type 2"**
❖ **Type 4 (hyperkalemic distal) RTA**	MC type of RTA Hyporeninemic hypoaldosteronism → defects in Na^+ absorption, H^+ and K^+ excretion, ↓ ammoniagenesis; ↑ $\mathbf{K^+}$ *Etiology*: MC found in diabetic nephropathy, tubulointerstitial renal diseases, hypertensive nephrosclerosis, drugs (ACE inhibitors, NSAIDs and heparin) and AIDS; *acquired* disorder *Treatment*: Furosemide, kayexalate *Complications*: Hyperkalemia

22. Answer is b (Co-trimoxazole).
Ref: Harrison's, 17th edition Pg 1310.

Infection in Immunocompetent Patients

- Immunologically competent adults and older children who have only lymphadenopathy do not require specific therapy unless they have persistent, severe symptoms.
- Patients with ocular toxoplasmosis should be treated for 1 month with pyrimethamine plus either sulfadiazine or clindamycin.

Infection in Immunocompromised Patients

- Of the currently available agents, ***trimethoprim-sulfamethoxazole (TMP-SMX)*** appears to be an effective alternative for Toxoplasmic encephalitis (TE) in resource-poor settings where the preferred combination of pyrimethamine plus sulfadiazine is not available.
- The daily dose of TMP-SMX recommended as the preferred regimen for PcP prophylaxis ***(one double-strength tablet)*** is effective against TE.
- If patients cannot tolerate TMP-SMX, the recommended alternative is dapsone-pyrimethamine, which is also effective against PcP.
- Atovaquone with or without pyrimethamine also can be considered.
- Prophylactic monotherapy with dapsone, pyrimethamine, azithromycin, clarithromycin, or aerosolized pentamidine is probably insufficient.

23. Answer is c (CMI is intact).
Ref: Fitzpatrick's dermatology, 2nd edition Pg 1314.

Lepromin test

- ***Mitsuda*** lepromin (integral lepromin) contained tissue particles and lipids in addition to the bacilli.
- ***Dharmendra*** lepromin is a 'defatted' bacillary suspension.
- The reactions are of two types: ***Early Fernandez reaction*** (read at 48 hours); ***Late Mitsuda reaction*** (read at 21 days).
- The *early reactions* is induced by the *soluble constituents* if the leprosy bacilli and the *late reaction* by the *bacillary component* of the antigen.
- It is a ***useful tool in evaluating the immune status (CMI) of leprosy patients***; Lepromin test is ***not a diagnostic test***; it is unique among all tests for CMI in that ***it not only measures pre-existing CMI, but is in fact a mini-dose vaccine***.
- It is of great value in estimating ***prognosis*** in leprosy of all types.

24. Answer is b (Monitor overnight blood glucose levels).
Ref: Harrison's, 17th edition Pg 2298.

- Moving the long-acting insulin from before the evening meal to bedtime may avoid nocturnal hypoglycemia and provide more insulin ***as glucose levels rise in the early morning*** (so-called ***dawn phenomenon***).

SURGERY

25. Answer is a (Abdominal wall synergistic gangrene caused by *E. coli* and anaerobic streptococci).
Ref: Lecture notes in general surgery, Harold Ellis and Roy Claine, 2006 edition Pg 28.

- ***Synergistic spreading gangrene***, also known as ***progressive bacterial gangrene***, is caused by the synergistic action of two or more organisms, commonly aerobic hemolytic *Staphylococcus* and microaerophilic non-hemolytic *Streptococcus*.
- Abdominal wall infections are known as ***Meleney's gangrene*** and scrotal infection as ***Fournier's gangrene***.

26. Answer is d (Hyperplastic pyloric stenosis).
Ref: Harrison's, 17th edition Pg 571-72.

Risk Factors for Gastric Cancer
❖ *H. pylori* infection ❖ Chronic Atrophic gastritis ❖ Blood group A

- Pernicious **A**nemia
- **A**denomatous polyps
- Smoking and **A**lcohol
- Nitrosamines in smoked fish
- Menetrier's disease
- Postantrectomy – 15–20 years after Billroth II anastomosis

27. Answer is c (Leiomyoma).
Ref: General thoracic surgery, Thomas W Shields, 2009 edition Pg 1976.

- **Esophageal *leiomyomas*** are benign smooth muscle *tumors* arising from the muscularis propria and represent by far the *most* common benign esophageal tumor (> 70% of all benign tumors).

28. Answer is d (Causes lymphoma).
Ref: Harrison's, 17th edition Pg 2238.

	Grave's disease	**Subacute thyroiditis (de Quervain's)**	**Hashimoto's disease**
Etiopathology	Antibody to TSH receptor, mc in females	Viral (possibly Coxsackievirus or Mumps)	Autoimmune
Clinically	Hyperthyroidism; diffuse painless goiter; ophthalmic (proptosis, lid lag, conjunctival injection); pretibial myxedema	Hyperthyroidism → hypothyroidism. Painful tender thyroid gland; jaw pain, granulomatous inflammation	Hypothyroidism; painless thyroid enlargement; slow course, lymphocyte infiltrate with germinal centers, Hurthle cells on histology; may lead to lymphoma
Diagnosis	↑ RAIU	↓ RAIU, ↑ ESR, thyroid antibodies are negative	Antimicrosomal and antithyroglobulin antibodies
Treatment	Propylthiouracil, methimazole, thyroid ablation with I 131	NSAIDs, steroids if pain severe	Levothyroxine

29. Answer is d (All the above).
Ref: Robbins pathology, 7th edition Pg 122.

- ***"Inflammatory Breast Cancer"*** is a hot, tender breast with ***skin looking like an orange peel, called "peau d'orange"*** and almost always has spread to the axilla.

30. Answer is d (Melphalan).
Ref: Harrison's, 17th edition Pg 545.

- Patients who have ***advanced regional disease (malignant melanoma)*** limited to a limb may benefit from ***hyperthermic limb perfusion with melphalan.***
- High complete response rates have been reported and responses are associated with significant palliation of symptoms.

31. Answer is b (Intestinal bleeding).
Ref: TB of surgery, Das, 1st edition Pg 929.

Complications of typhoid fever

- ***Intestinal hemorrhage*** (10–20%)
- Perforation (2%)

- ❖ Paralytic ileus
- ❖ Cholecystitis
- ❖ Osteomyelitis.

32. Answer is b (Bulbar).
Ref: Bailey and Love's surgery, 25th edition Pg 1363-65.

- ***Rupture of bulbar urethra*** is the *most common type of urethral injury*.
- Urethra angulates in the perineum where it gets injured.
- ***Possible situations***: Workers losing footing on scaffolding, cycling, gymnasium accidents, loose manhole covers.

33. Answer is a (Superior mesenteric artery).
Ref: TB of surgery, Das, 1st edition Pg 627.

- ***Superior mesenteric artery*** supplies the ***entire midgut*** starting from the duodenojejunal flexure to right one third of the transverse colon and it is an end artery.
- As a result of thrombosis, the entire small bowel and portion of the large bowel becomes gangrenous (if there is a thrombus at the origin of superior mesenteric artery) and leads to ***immediate death of the patient***.

34. Answer is c (Femoral hernia).
Ref: Bailey and Love's, 25th edition Pg 969.

- ***Femoral hernia*** although less common in incidence than ***inguinal hernia***, is more likely to strangulate due to ***narrowness of the neck and its rigid surroundings***.

35. Answer is c (Penetrating wound through major vessels of thigh).
Ref: Bailey and Love, 23rd edition Pg 40.

- ***Butcher's thigh*** = bleeding from the ***great vessels of the thigh, i.e. mainly femoral vessels***.

36. Answer is c (Right gastric artery).
Ref: http://en.wikipedia.org/wiki/Cystohepatic_triangle

- The ***hepatobiliary triangle*** (or ***cystohepatic triangle***) is an anatomic space bordered by the:
  - Common hepatic duct medially
  - The cystic duct inferiorly
  - Inferior edge of the liver superiorly.
- Another name used to refer to this region is **Calot's Triangle**. It is named for *Jean-François Calot*
- The ***cystic artery normally passes through the triangle***; this anatomic feature is important during laparoscopic cholecystectomies.

Note:

- The ***lymph node located within the triangle, Calot's node***. This is frequently enlarged due to inflammation of the gallbladder (e.g. cholecystitis) or the biliary tract (e.g. cholangitis) and may be removed along with the gallbladder during surgical treatment (cholecystectomy).

37. Answer is b (Leiomyoma).
Ref: General Thoracic Surgery By Thomas W shields, 2009 edition Pg 1976.

Repeat Topic

- See ***answer no. 27 above***—repeated question in the same paper.

38. Answer is b (Level 2).
Ref: http://www.cancerpage.com/articles/default.asp?id=2&subarea=Your_Illness

- See ***answer no. 41 in COMED-K 2006 answers*** for detailed explanation.

39. Answer is b (Carotid body tumor).
Ref: Bailey and Love's 25th edition Pg 732.

- *Carotid body tumor = potato tumor = chemodectoma*
- *Benign tumor* arising from chemoreceptors in the carotid body
- Situated in tunica adventitia at the bifurcation of common carotid artery, hence tumor is called chemodectoma
- Consistency is form to hard, hence called *potato tumor*.

40. Answer is d (All the above).
Ref: Bailey and Love's, 25th edition Pg 1158.

Repeat Topic

- ***Meckel's diverticulum*** is the ***MC congenital abnormality of the small intestine***; it is caused by an ***incomplete obliteration of the vitelline duct (i.e. omphalomesenteric duct),*** i.e. it represents the patent intestinal end of the vitellointestinal duct.

Fast Facts

Rule of 2's – Meckel's diverticulum

❖ It is present in about 2% of subjects
❖ Its length is about 2 *inches*
❖ Usually 2 ***feet (60 cm)*** proximal to the ileocecal valve and occurs on the ***antimesenteric border*** of the ileum
❖ ***Present in*** 2% of the population

- Meckel's diverticulum is typically lined by ileal mucosa, but *other tissue types are also found* with varying frequency, ***ectopic gastric mucosa*** in about 50%.
- A Meckel's diverticulum ***possesses all 3 coats of the intestinal wall*** and ***has its own blood supply***. It is therefore ***vulnerable to infection*** and ***obstruction*** in the same way as the appendix.

41. Answer is b (Fever).
Ref: NMS Board review series, surgery, Pg 38.

- **Signs and symptoms of DVT include:**
  - ☐ Lower extremity swelling
  - ☐ ***Fever***
  - ☐ ***Pain***
  - ☐ ***Homan's sign***: Calf pain on dorsiflexion
  - ☐ ***Phlegmasia alba dolens*** (white leg): Occurs when thrombus extends from calf region to iliofemoral vein an there is generalized edema and lymphatic obstruction
  - ☐ ***Phlegmasia cerulea dolens (blue leg):*** Occurs when deep veins get blocked and skin becomes congested and blue (*should not be mistaken for cyanosis*).

42. Answer is b (Bile present in vomiting).
Ref: TB of surgery, Das, Pg 680.

- ***Bilious vomiting*** is a feature of ***duodenal atresia***
- A newborn with this deformity may or may not pass meconium
- On X-ray and USG ***'double bubble'*** is seen.

OBSTETRICS AND GYNECOLOGY

43. Answer is d (750 mL/min).
Ref: Dutta's obstetrics, 6th edition Pg 53.

- Uterine blood flow is increased from ***50 mL/min in non-pregnant state to about 750 mL near term.***

44. Answer is D (4th stage).
Ref: Dutta's obstetrics, 6th edition Pg 133.

- There may be chills and occasional shivering in fourth stage of labor.

45. Answer is d (Placental maturity).
Ref: Dutta's obstetrics, 6th edition Pg 110, 464.

Biophysical Profile (Manning's Score)

- The 5 components measured by real time ultrasound are:

1. Fetal **T**one
2. Fetal **B**reathing
3. Fetal **M**ovement
4. **A**mniotic fluid volume
5. **N**on-stress test.

Mnemonic: **T**est the **Ba**by **MAN!**

- A score of 2 (normal) or 0 (abnormal) is assigned to each component. Reassuring score = 8–10; low score < 6 = fetal distress.

Also Know

Non-stress test (NST)

- Fetal heart rate (FHR) is monitored externally by Doppler with mother lying in left lateral decubitus position and mother reports the fetal movements. Effects of fetal movement on heart rate are noted—Fetal Cardiotocography.
- A normal ('reactive') test is considered to be 2 or more ≥ 15 beats per minute accelerations over baseline of the FHR that lasts ≥ 15 seconds during a 20 minute monitoring period.
- A *non-reactive* (abnormal) NST should prompt the performance of a biophysical profile (BPP) or contraction stress test as below.
- A non-reactive NST can be due to fetal sleep cycle, gestational age < 30 weeks, a fetal CNS anomaly or maternal sedative/narcotic use.

Contraction stress test (CST)

- Used to assess uteroplacental dysfunction
- Fetal heart rate is monitored during spontaneous or induced contractions
- Beat to beat variability, long-term heart rate variability and occasional heart rate accelerations are reassuring signs
- Decelerations of fetal heart rate and their relationship to uterine contractions may be indicative of normal activity during labor or fetal distress.

Type of fetal heart rate decelerations

Type of deceleration	Description	Cause/Treatment
1. EArly decelerations	Deceleration begins and ends with uterine contractions	Due to fetal *hEAd compression* (no fetal distress), no treatment required
2. Late decelerations	Deceleration begins after uterine contraction and persist until after the contraction has finished	Indicates *fetal hypoxia* and chronic *uteroplacental insufficiency*. If late decelerations are recurrent, immediate delivery is necessary
3. Variable decelerations	Inconsistent onset, duration and degree of decelerations	Due to *umbilical cord compression*. Change the mother's position

46. Answer is c (Krukenberg's).
Ref: Robbins pathology, 7th edition Pg 826; Shaw's gynecology, 14th edition Pg 381.

- See ***answer no. 58 in COMED-K 2006 answers*** for detailed explanation.

47. Answer is c (Fallopian tubes).
Ref: Shaw's gynecology, 14th edition Pg 137.

- ***Fallopian tube*** is the most frequently involved part of the genital tract in ***90% of cases***.

48. Answer is b (Granulosa cell thecomas).
Ref: Robbins pathology, 7th edition Pg 1102.

- ***Granulosa-theca cell tumors*** have clinical importance or the two reasons
  - Their potential elaboration of large amounts of estrogen
  - The ***small, but distinct hazard of malignancy in the granulosa cell forms***.

49. Answer is c (Cisplatin).
Ref: Shaw's gynecology, 14th edition Pg 376.

- ***Stage III*** endometrial cancer is ***inoperable***
- ***Doxorubicin with cisplatin and paclitaxel*** is employed
- ***Medroxyprogesterone acetate*** 1 g weekly IM is ***adjuvant*** to chemotherapy.

50. Answer is b (PTH).
Ref: Dutta's obstetrics, 6th edition Pg 58-60.

- **Hormones that cross the placenta are:**
  - Insulin
  - Steroids from adrenals
  - Thyroid
  - Chorionic gonadotropin or placental lactogen
- **Neither** parathormone nor calcitonin crosses the placenta.

51. Answer is c (Dysgerminoma).
Ref: Shaw's gynecology, 13th edition Pg 313.

- ***Dysgerminoma*** is the ***commonest malignant germ cell tumor***
- It is ***often a/w gonadal dysgenesis*** or ***androgen insensitivity syndrome*** or ***true hermaphroditism***.

52. Answer is c (Fetal distress).
Ref: Dutta's obstetrics, 6th edition Pg 107, 494.

Repeat Topic

- See *answer no. 129 in COMED-K 2005 answers* for detailed explanation.

53. Answer is a (Posterior asynclitism).
Ref: Willaim's obstetrics, 22nd edition Pg 112.

- When the sagittal suture lies near the symphysis, the posterior parietal bone becomes the leading presenting part
- It is the termed, ***posterior parietal presentation or posterior asynclitism (Litzmann's obliquity)***
- When the sagittal suture is near the sacral promontory, an anterior parietal presentation results. This is termed ***anterior asynclitism or Naegele's obliquity***
- Moderate degrees of asynclitism are the rule in labor.

ENT

54. Answer is b (Malignancy of vocal cords).
Ref: Logan Turner's ENT, 9th edition Pg 451.

55. Answer is D (Patient complains of foul smell).
Ref: Logan Turner's ENT, 9th edition Pg 355.

Atrophic Rhinitis

• Etiology	– ***Klebsiella ozaenae*** (*Perez bacillus*), ↓ estrogen levels (begins in pubertal females).
• Clinically	– Most characteristic symptom is the ***foul odor detected by others*** while the ***patient himself/herself is anosmic*** (***merciful anosmia***). – In severe atrophic rhinitis when there is ***extensive crusting and fetor***, the condition is known as ***ozaena***. – Atrophied mucosa, ***roomy nasal cavities*** are seen, middle turbinate involved earliest.
• Treatment	– Medical: Alkaline nasal douches, local estrogen spray, human placental extract, Kemicctinc antiozaena solution. – Surgical: ***Young's operation*** consists of closure of the anterior nares or narrowing of the anterior nares (modified Young's). ***Lauten Langer's operation*** aimed at medializing the lateral nasal wall.

56. Answer is c (1.3:1).
Ref: Scott Brown's otolaryngology, vol 2, Pg 132.

- The eardrum is 14 times the size of the footplate (areal or hydraulic ratio). The ratio of the malleus handle to that of the lenticular process of the incus is ***1.3:1 (ossicular leverage ratio)***.
- These two factors (14 × 1.3 = 18.2) reduce the amplitude of the vibrations, but increase the force of sound 18 times (***transformer action***).

OPHTHALMOLOGY

57. Answer is b (Hypovitaminosis A).
Ref: Park, 20th edition Pg 532, 555.

WHO GRADING OF XEROPHTHALMIA (Vitamin A deficiency)

- **XN** = Night blindness
- **X1** = Conjunctival xerosis (X1A) with Bitot spot (X1B)

- **X2** = Corneal xerosis
- **X3** = Corneal ulceration (***keratomalacia***) < one third (X3A); > one third (X3B)
  - ***Keratomalacia,*** sterile corneal melting by colliquative necrosis (absence of inflammation)
- **XS** = Corneal scar
- **XF** = Xerophthalmic fundus (Uyemura's fundus).

58. Answer is d (Gunn's sign is a feature).
Ref: Parson's, 20th edition Pg 295-96.

- ***Marcus Gunn pupil (relative afferent pupillary defect, RAPD)*** is a feature of ***optic neuritis*** and is not seen in background diabetic retinopathy.

DIABETIC RETINOPATHY

– **Classification**	Non-proliferative DR (mild, moderate, severe), Proliferative DR and Macular edema – CSME (clinically significant macular edema) now accepted classification
– **Clinically**	***Microaneurysms, Hard exudates, retinal hemorrhages*** Other ocular features of DM: corneal hypoesthesia, recurrent corneal erosions, POAG, cataracts, neovascular glaucoma, pupil sparing III CN palsy, orbital mucormycosis
– **Treatment**	Treatment consist of laser photocoagulation ETDRS stands for Early Treatment Diabetic Retinopathy Study

59. Answer is a (CRAO).
Ref: Parson's, 20th edition Pg 302, Fig 20.16.

D/D of Cherry Red Spot

1. Central retinal artery occlusion (CRAO)
2. Berlins edema of the macula (commotio retinae)
3. Macular hemorrhage
4. Macular hole with surrounding retinal detachment
5. Quinine toxicity
6. Sphingolipidoses
   - Niemann Pick's disease
   - Tay-Sach's disease
   - Sandhoff's disease
   - Infantile Metachromatic Leukodystrophy
   - Sialidosis (Cherry-red spot myoclonus syn)
   - GM1 gangliosidoses.

60. Answer is a (Vernal Catarrh).
Ref: Parson's, 20th edition Pg 172.

Repeat Topic

- See topic of ***vernal conjunctivitis in table under answer no. 68 in COMED-K 2005 answers.***

61. Answer is b (Concave).
Ref: Parson's, 20th edition Pg 73.

- ***In myopia, eyeball is longer*** and ***image is formed anterior (in front of) to the retina.*** Hence by ***using a concave lens (minus lens)*** the rays diverge further before converging and can be brought to focus on the retina.
- In ***hypermetropia, plus (convex) lenses*** are used for correction.

62. Answer is a (Gonioscope).
Ref: Parson's 20th edition Pg 121-22.

Repeat Topic

- See ***answer no. 69 in COMED-K 2008 answers*** for detailed explanation.

63. Answer is a (Zonular cataract).
Ref: Parson's 20th edition Pg 256.

- ***Lack of vitamin D and hypocalcemia*** are potent risk factors for development of ***zonular type of congenital cataract***.
- ***Riders*** are seen in zonular cataract.

64. Answer is d (70–80 microns).
Ref: Ocular Therapeutics Handbook: A Clinical Manual, Bruce EO et al. 2nd edition, Pg 52. 2005.

Resolving power

- ***Direct*** ophthalmoscope = ***70*** microns
- ***Indirect*** ophthalmoscope = ***200*** microns

65. Answer is c (Separation of sensory retina from pigment epithelium).
Ref: Parson's, 20th edition Pg 311.

- ***Retinal detachment*** occurs when ***subretinal fluid accumulates in the potential space between the neurosensory retina and the retinal pigment epithelium***.

PEDIATRICS

66. Answer is c (Poor feeding and rigidity).
Ref: NMS pediatrics, Pg 231.

- Neonatal tetanus usually occurs as the generalized form and is fatal if left untreated.
- It develops in children born to inadequately immunized mothers, frequently after ***unsterile treatment of the umbilical stump***.
- Onset is during the ***first 2 weeks*** of life.
- ***Poor feeding, rigidity and spasms*** are the typical features.

67. Answer is d (Hypertensive crisis).
Ref: OP Ghai, 7th edition Pg 409, 410.

Complications of Fallot's tetralogy

- Erythrocytosis/Polycythemia
- Brain abscess
- Infective endocarditis
- Neurological: Cerebrovascular thrombosis, hemiplegia, paradoxical embolism to CNS
- Acute gouty arthritis, delayed puberty
- *Congestive cardiac failure does not commonly occur in tetralogy of Fallot (Ref: Pediatrics By Shyam bhaktavatsala, Tim Newson, 3rd edition Pg 97)*
- Anemia reduces the exercise tolerance and can result in cardiac enlargement and CCF making the diagnosis difficult *(OP Ghai, 7th edition Pg 410)*.

68. Answer is c (Caudate nucleus).
Ref: NMS pediatrics, Pg 412.

- Child is suffering from ***Huntington's chorea***.

69. Answer is c (Renal disease).
Ref: NMS pediatrics, Pg 112.

- Most cases of HTN in children are secondary to underlying cause
- Londe (1978) cited literature to show that:
  - ***78% were related to renal disease***
  - 12% to disease of renal arteries
  - 2% had coarctation
  - 0.5% had pheochromocytoma.

70. Answer is d (All the above).
Ref: OP Ghai, 7th edition Pg 312.

- Stridor indicates URT obstruction and is usually accompanied by hoarseness, brassy cough, dyspnea, retraction of the chest during inspiration and restlessness. Accessory muscle sof respiration are usually working.
- Congenital stridor is frequently seen in infants and is often attributed to:
  - Small size of the larynx
  - Loose submucosal connective tissue around the glottic region
  - Rigid cricoid cartilage encircling the subglottic zone.

71. Answer is a (Craniosynostosis).
Ref: Nelson's, 17th edition Pg 525.

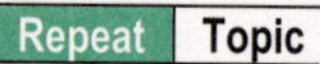

- See ***answer no. 52 in COMED-K 2005 answers*** for detailed explanation.

72. Answer is d (Enteric).
Ref: OP Ghai, 7th edition Pg 216.

- ***Breast milk contains antimicrobial factors*** such as macrophages, lymphocytes, secretory IgA, antistreptococcal factor, lysozyme and lactoferrin, which provide considerable ***protection not only against diarrheal diseases and necrotizing enterocolitis,*** but also against respiratory infections in the early months of life.

73. Answer is a (2–3 years).
Ref: OP Ghai, 7th edition Pg 30.

- For more on developmental milestones see detailed table – ***answer no.65 in COMED-K 2007 answers***.

74. Answer is a (Microcytic hypochromic).
Ref: Harrison's, 17th edition Pg 442, 444, Table 71.1.

Manifestations of Vitamin B_6 deficiency

- Seborrhea
- Glossitis
- Convulsions
- Neuropathy
- Depression
- Confusion
- Microcytic anemia.

- Contributing factors: Alcoholism, isoniazid
- ***Microcytic, hypochromic anemia*** is due to diminished hemoglobin synthesis, since the first enzyme involved in heme biosynthesis (aminolevulinate synthase) requires PLP (***Pyridoxal 5′-phosphate***) as a cofactor.

ORTHOPEDICS

75. Answer is a (Dorsal of wrist).
Ref: Maheshwari, 3rd edition Pg 258.

- ***Ganglion*** is a smooth multilocular jelly-like swellings that is a bulge of synovium (***most commonly on dorsum of wrist***)
- They communicate with joint capsules or tendon sheaths
- Asymptomatic and treatment usually not needed
- If painful, aspiration needed.

76. Answer is c (Inflamed adventitial bursa at the base of the 1st metatarsal bone).
Ref: Maheshwari, 3rd edition Pg 256.

COMMON BURSITIS

• Prepatellar Bursitis	Housemaid's knee
• Infrapatellar bursitis	Clergyman's knee or Vicar's knee
• Ischial bursitis	Weaver's bottom
• On lateral malleolus	Tailor's ankle
• On great Toe	Bunion
• Popliteal cyst	Morrant Baker's cyst

77. Answer is b (Narrowing of disk space).
Ref: Maheshwari, 3rd edition Pg 175.

- ***Reduction of disk space*** is the ***earliest radiological sign*** in the commoner ***paradiscal type of spinal TB*** (Pott's disease).

78. Answer is d (3 joint swelling for 6 weeks).
Ref: Cecil's internal medicine, Pg 230.

American Rheumatism Association criteria for rheumatoid arthritis

- Morning stiffness
- Pain in one joint
- Swelling in one joint for 6 weeks
- Swelling in another joint for 3 months
- Symmetrical joint involvement
- Positive agglutination test
- Involvement of hand joints.

79. Answer is a (Osteosarcoma).
Ref: Maheshwari, 3rd edition Pg 218.

Osteosarcoma

- 2nd MC primary malignant bone tumor (after multiple myeloma)
- Peak at 15–25 years
- Affects ***metaphysis of long bones***, lower femur, upper tibia (knee)
- Present with pain and swelling of few weeks to months present
- X-ray:
  - ***Lytic lesion with moth eaten*** appearance
  - Spiculated periosteal reaction—***Sunburst*** appearance

- Cuff of periosteal new bone formation at margin of soft tissue mass – ***Codman's triangle***
- New bone formation.

- ***Increased alkaline phosphatase*** (ALP)
- Preop chemotherapy with limb sparing surgery with postop chemotherapy is standard
- Extremely radioresistant
- Poor prognosis
- ***Predisposing factors***:
  - Paget's disease (adult osteosarcoma)
  - Familial Retinoblastoma
  - Bone infarcts
  - Radiotherapy.

80. Answer is a (Frontal sinusitis).
Ref: Maqbool's ENT textbook, 10th edition Pg 123.

- ***Pott's puffy tumor – Osteomyelitis of the frontal bone*** as a complication of ***frontal sinusitis***.

PHARMACOLOGY

81. Answer is a (Proximal tubules).
Ref: KD Tripathi, 6th edition Pg 483-88.

- Mechanism of action of ACE inhibitors is in the ***proximal tubule*** of the nephrons.

82. Answer is c (Causes hypotension).
Ref: KD Tripathi, 6th edition Pg 120, 125, 127, 129.

- ***Phenylephrine*** is a selective alpha-1 agonist, has negligible beta action
- It ***raises BP*** by causing vasoconstriction
- Because it has little cardiac action, ***reflex bradycardia*** is prominent
- It is used ***commonly as a mydriatic*** when cycloplegia is not required
- It is a frequent component of ***orally administered nasal decongestant*** medications.

83. Answer is a (Prolongs action potential duration).
Ref: KD Tripathi, 6th edition Pg 511, 513.

- ***Moricizine*** belongs to ***subclass IA*** of antiarrhythmic drugs
- It is an open state Na channel blocker with moderate delay in channel recovery (1–10s)
- It suppresses A-V conduction and ***prolongs*** PR, QRS, QT and ***action potential duration***.

84. Answer is b (Finasteride).
Ref: Harrison's, 17th edition Pg 598.

- ***In metastatic prostate cancer***, medical therapies that lower testosterone levels include the gonadotropin-releasing hormone (GnRH) analogues, estrogens and progestational agents.
- ***Estrogens*** such as ***diethylstilbestrol*** and ***fosfestrol*** have fallen out of favor due to the risk of vascular complications such as fluid retention, phlebitis, emboli and stroke.
- GnRH analogs include leuprolide acetate and goserelin acetate.
- Finasteride (10 mg/d PO) and other 5α-reductase inhibitors are antiandrogens that block the conversion of testosterone to dihydrotestosterone decrease prostate size, increase urine flow rates, for palliation in advanced prostate cancer.

85. Answer is a (Penicillin).
Ref: Davidson's, 20th edition Pg 1127, Table 26.99.

- ***Benzylpenicillin*** is the ***drug of choice*** for ***meningococcal meningitis***
- For ***carriers, rifampicin is the drug of choice.***

86. Answer is a (Increase K^+ efflux and decreasing Ca^{++} release in heart muscle).
Ref: KD Tripathi, 6th edition Pg 511, 518, 519.

- Administered by ***rapid IV injection, adenosine terminates*** within 30 seconds, ***more than 90% episodes of PSVT*** involving the AV node.
- ***Mechanism of action***: It activates Ach sensitive K^+ channels and causes membrane hyperpolarization through interaction with AI type of G protein coupled adenosine receptors on SA node (pacemaker depression bradycardia), AV node (prolongation of ERP—slowing of conduction) and atrium (shortening of AP, reduced excitability).

87. Answer is a (Tetracycline).
Ref: Harrison's, 17th edition Pg 1075.

- The ***first line of treatment for Chlamydia is azithromycin***
- ***Tetracyclines*** are the *second line of treatment.*

88. Answer is b (Enalapril).
Ref: KD Tripathi, 6th edition Pg 484, 485.

Side effects of ACE inhibitors (including enalapril)

- *Dry* **C***ough*
- **A***ngioedema* rarely
- **P**roteinuria
- **T**aste alteration and rash (MC with *captopril*)
- Hyp**O**tension
- **P**regnancy (CI due to teratogenicity)
- **R**enal dysfunction (azotemia)
- *Hyperkalemia* (Increased **K**$^+$)
- **CI in** and bilateral renal artery stenosis.

MICROBIOLOGY

89. Answer is d (Resembles some plant viruses).
Ref: CP Baveja, TB of microbiology, 3rd edition, Pg 496.

- ***Hepatitis D virus (delta)*** is a ***defective RNA virus*** dependent upon hepatitis B virus or its replication and expression.
- Therefore it has ***no independent existence*** and can survive and replicate only as long as HBV infection persists in the host.
- It ***resembles some plant viruses*** such as viroids or satellite viruses.

90. Answer is d (All of the above).
Ref: TB of microbiology, 3rd edition CP Baveja, Pg 97.

- ***Heterophile specificity***: The same or closely related antigens may sometimes occur in different biological species, classes and kingdoms.
- These are known as heterogenetic or heterophile antigens.
- The best known example of such heterophile antigens is the ***Forssman antigen,*** which is a lipid carbohydrate complex widely distributed in human beings, animals, birds, plants and bacteria.
- The ***Weil-Felix reaction for typhus fever, Paul-Bunnell test for infectious mononucleosis*** and the ***cold agglutination test for primary atypical pneumonia*** are examples for this reaction.

91. Answer is d (*Rhinosporidium seeberi*).
Ref: CP Baveja, TB of microbiology, 3rd edition, Pg 541.

- ***Rhinosporidium*** has been successfully cultivated in epithelial cell culture.

92. Answer is b (IgG).
Ref: CP Baveja, TB of microbiology, 3rd edition, Pg 492.

Hepatitis B Serology

• HBsAg	First virologic marker detectable in serum after infection with HBV (even before elevation of serum aminotransferase and clinical symptoms appear). Indicates active hepatitis B infection, either acute or chronic (> 6 months)
• Anti-HBs	***IgG Antibody to HbsAg. Provides immunity to hepatitis B. Persists for years***
• HBcAg	Not routinely detectable in blood
• Anti-HBc	Positive during the window period. IgM anti-HBc is an indicator of recent disease, IgG anti-HBc signifies chronic disease
• HB**e**Ag	Indicates active viral replication and high infectivity **(Beware!)**
• Anti-HBe	When present in HBsAg carrier, blood is potentially less infectious

93. Answer is a (*Toxocara canis*).
Ref: Harrison's, 17th edition Pg 1317.

- ***Visceral larva migrans*** is a syndrome caused by ***nematodes*** that are normally parasitic for non-human host species.
- In humans, the nematode larvae do not develop into adult worms, but instead ***migrate through host tissues and elicit eosinophilic inflammation***.
- The ***more common form of visceral larva migrans is toxocariasis due to larvae of the canine ascarid Toxocara canis,*** less commonly to the feline ascarid *T. cati* and even less commonly to the pig ascarid *Ascaris suum.*
- Rare cases with eosinophilic meningoencephalitis have been caused by the raccoon ascarid *Baylisascaris procyonis.*

94. Answer is a (Poliovirus).
Ref: CP Baveja, TB of microbiology, 3rd edition, Pg 449, 451.

- Poliovirus is resistant to ether, chloroform, bile, proteolytic enzymes of the intestinal contents and detergents.

95. Answer is a (The bacteria should be associated with the lesions of the disease) and b (It should be possible to isolate the bacteria in pure culture from lesions).
Ref: CP Baveja, TB of microbiology, 3rd edition, Pg 5.

- According to ***Koch's postulates,*** a microorganism can be accepted as the causative agent of an infection only, if it satisfies the following criteria:
  - The bacterium should be ***constantly a/w lesions*** of the disease
  - It should be possible to ***isolate the bacterium in pure culture*** from the lesions
  - ***Inoculation*** of such pure culture into suitable laboratory animals should reproduce the lesions of the disease
  - It should be possible to ***reisolate the bacterium in pure culture*** from the lesions produced in experimental animals.

PATHOLOGY

96. Answer is b (Sq cell CA is the commonest type and arises from the periphery).
Ref: see below.

Regarding options a and d—see points below,

❖ *Harrison's, 17th/552* – "The relative risk of developing lung cancer is increased about thirteen fold by active smoking and about 1.5-fold by long-term passive exposure to cigarette smoke".

❖ *Harrison's, 17th/552* – "About 15% of lung cancers occur in individuals who have never smoked. The majority of these are found in women. The reason for this sex difference is not known, but may be related to hormonal factors".

Regarding options b and c see comprehensive table below (derived from Robbin's, Bailey and Harrison's)

LUNG CANCER

- Presents with cough, hemoptysis, bronchial obstruction, wheezing, pneumonic 'coin' lesions on X-ray film
- Risk factors: Tobacco/smoking, asbestos.

Type	*Characteristics*
Squamous cell Ca	• Central location • MC lung cancer in **C**igarette smokers • Hilar-mass arising from bronchus; **C**avitation; direct extension to hilar lymph nodes • PN: Parathyroid like activity (PTHrP)—hyper**C**alcemia; dermatomyositis • Histology: Keratin Pearls and Intercellular Bridges • MC Lung Ca detected by positive sputum **C**ytology • MC Lung Ca leading to Pan**C**oast tumor • **C**avitating, **C**entral, **C**igarette, hyper**C**alcemia • *Best prognosis* • Treatment: Surgery
Adeno Ca	• ***Peripheral*** • MC lung cancer in ***non-smokers and females*** • Develops in site of prior pulmonary inflammation or injury • Wide metastases, *a/w asbestosis*; pleural effusions show ↑ hyaluronidase levels • 2 types are bronchial and bronchioloalveolar • Histology: Clara cells, type 2 pneumocytes • PN: *DIC, thrombophlebitis, microangiopathic hemolytic anemia* • *Good prognosis*
Small cell (oat cell) Ca	• Central • *Rapidly growing*, early distant metastases • PN: *SIADH, Ectopic GH and ACTH secretion, peripheral neuropathy, Eaton-Lambert syndrome* • MC lung Ca causing *SVC syndrome* • Neoplasm of neuroendocrine Kulchitsky cells, Small blue round cell tumor • Responsive to *chemotherapy* (cisplatin and etoposide)
Large cell Ca	• *Peripheral* • Highly undifferentiated *anaplastic* tumor • *Poor prognosis* • Less tendency to metastasis • PN: *Gynecomastia* • Less responsive to chemotherapy • Treat surgically

PN = Paraneoplastic syndrome; SVC = Superior vena cava; SIADH = Syndrome of inappropriate secretion of ADH; DIC = Disseminated intravascular coagulation.

1. **Pancoast tumor**: Carcinoma that occurs in the apex of the lung and may affect cervical sympathetic plexus causing Horner's syndrome.
2. **SVC syndrome**: Characterized by swelling of face and arm, most often on the right side and elevated JVP. Treated with radiation therapy.
3. **Trousseau's syndrome**: A hypercoagulable state seen MC with adenocarcinoma.
4. **Eaton-Lambert syndrome**: Autoantibodies against calcium channels, clinically similar to myasthenia, except that muscle fatigue improves with repeated stimulation).

97. Answer is c (*Staphylococcus aureus* endocarditis).
Ref: Harshmohan, 3rd edition Pg 303.

- *Staphylococcus aureus* causes acute endocarditis, which affects previously normal valves
- Mitral valve MC affected, than aortic valve
- Leads to ***extensive friable vegetations,*** which are single/multiple and irregular in appearance.

98. Answer is d (All the above).
Ref: Davidson's, 20th edition Pg 297, Box 13.20, 13.21, 13.22; Harrison's, 17th edition Pg 383.

Parasitic infections causing eosinophilia	Tropical infections not a/w eosinophilia
• Strongyloides • Hookworm • Ascariasis • Toxocariasis • Schistosomiasis • Filariasis (loiasis, *W. bancrofti, B. malayi, M. perstans,* Onchocerciasis) • Cysticercosis *(T. saginata* and *T. solium)* • *Echinococcus* (Hydatid disease) • Liver flukes *(Fasciola hepatica, Clonorchis sinensis* and *O. felineus)*	• Leprosy • Tuberculosis • *Bruce*llosis (*Bruce*) • *Lei*shmaniasis (*Lee*) • *Trypanosomiasis* (*Trip*) • *Enter*ic fever (*Entered*) • *Ame*biasis (*Ame*rican) • *Ma*l***aria*** (*Male*) • *Gard*iasis (*Garden*) • Arboviral infections • Tapeworms other than cysticercosis

Mnemonic: "Bruce Lee's Trip Entered American Male Garden"; remember that from 1st MBBS you have never read anywhere that leprosy or TB cause eosinophilia.

Author's comments: *"Best source for the answer is in Davidson's at the above mentioned reference; easier to remember the infections not a/w eosinophilia; use the above mnemonic or make your own – however ridiculous associations (like above mnemonic) is a proven method of remembering (ex: imagine a horse carrying a flower vase in its mouth to remember that 'flower vase' appearance in IVU is seen in 'horseshoe kidney'!)."*

In A Nutshell

- ***Eosinophilia*** is the presence of **> *500 eosinophils per µL of blood*** and is common in many settings besides parasite infection. Significant tissue eosinophilia can occur without an elevated blood count.
- ***Non-infectious causes of eosinophilia:***
  - ***Allergic reaction to drugs*** (iodides, aspirin, sulfonamides, nitrofurantoin, penicillins and cephalosporins).
  - ***Allergies***: Hay fever, asthma, eczema, serum sickness, allergic vasculitis and pemphigus.
  - ***Collagen vascular diseases*** (e.g. rheumatoid arthritis, eosinophilic fasciitis, allergic angiitis and ***polyarteritis nodosa***).
  - ***Malignancies*** (e.g. ***Hodgkin's disease***; mycosis fungoides; chronic myeloid leukemia and cancer of the lung, stomach, pancreas, ovary or uterus)
  - ***Job's*** syndrome and *Chronic Granulomatous Disease.*

Clinical features a/w helminthic infections and eosinophilia

Urticarial rash	Myositis
• Strongyloides, Onchocerca, Fasciola, Hydatid, Trichinosis	• Trichinosis, cysticercosis
Cutaneous larva migrans	**Lymphatic orchitis**
• Ancylostoma braziliense	• Lymphatic filariasis
Dermatitis	**Febrile hepatosplenomegaly**
• Onchocerca	• Schistosoma, toxocara

Migratory subcutaneous swellings	Pneumonitis
• Loa loa (calabar swellings), gnathostomiasis	• Migratory stage of larval helminths (Loeffler's syndrome); lymphatic filariasis (tropical pulmonary eosinophilia)
Enteritis and colitis	**Meningitis**
• Strongyloides, capillariasis, trichinella	• Angiostrongyliasis, strongyloides

99. Answer is b (VDRL).
Ref: Harrison's, 17th edition Pg 1043.

For practical purposes, most clinicians need to be familiar with the three uses of serologic tests for syphilis:

(1) ***Screening*** or diagnostic purposes ***(RPR or VDRL).***
(2) Quantitative measurement of antibody to assess clinical syphilis activity or ***to monitor response to therapy (RPR or VDRL).***
(3) ***Confirmation of a syphilis*** diagnosis *in a patient with a reactive RPR or VDRL test* ***(FTA-ABS or Serodia TP-PA).***

100. Answer is b (Congestive cardiac failure).
Ref: Harrisons, 17th edition Pg 1658.

101. Answer is c (Useful in monitoring the treatment response in giant cell arteritis).
Ref: Kanski's 4th edition Pg 456.

102. Answer is c (Stricture).
Ref: Robbins pathology, 7th edition Pg 849-50.

Repeat Topic

- See ***answer no. 37 in COMED-K 2009 answers*** for detailed explanation.

103. Answer is b (Chromosome 18 defect).
Ref: Robbins pathology, 7th edition Pg 176.

Gene location of certain diseases on chromosomes

Chromosome	Diseases
• Chromosome 1	**Contains the most** known genetic diseases (890 total) of any human chromosome. Alzheimer disease, Charcot-Marie-Tooth disease, galactosemia, Gaucher disease, Homocystinuria, Prostate cancer.
• Chromosome 2	Genes on chromosome 2 may play an important role in **human intelligence**. Alport's syndrome, Amyotrophic lateral sclerosis, Ehlers-Danlos syndrome
• Chromosome 3	Alkaptonuria, Myotonic dystrophy, von Hippel-Lindau syndrome, susceptibility/resistance to HIV infection.
• Chromosome 4	Achondroplasia, Huntington's disease.
• Chromosome 5	Familial Adenomatous Polyposis is caused by a deletion of the **APC tumor suppressor gene** on 5q. Cri-du-**chat** syndrome is caused by partial deletion of 5p (5p-) **5** pussy **c**(h)**ats**.
• Chromosome 6	It contains the Major Histocompatibility Complex **(MHC)**. AR polycystic kidney disease, porphyria cutanea tarda.
• Chromosome 7	Contains the Homeobox A gene cluster. **Cyst**ic fibrosis (**7q**); "**7** qute **cyst**ers"Williams syndrome (7q).
• Chromosome 8	Burkitt's lymphoma (**B** looks like **8**).
• Chromosome 9	Friedreich ataxia, tuberous sclerosis.

COMED-K 2004 ANSWERS

• Chromosome 10	Hirschsprung's disease.
• Chromosome 11	More than 40% of **olfactory receptor genes** are located here. Ataxia-telangiectasia, Beckwith-Wiedemann syndrome, multiple endocrine neoplasia type 1.
• Chromosome 12	Contains the Homebox C gene cluster. Tyrosinemia, Noonan syndrome
• Chromosome 13	**Retinoblastoma (13q14),** Wilson disease, Trisomy 13 (Patau's syn).
• Chromosome 14	α-1 antitrypsin deficiency.
• Chromosome 15	*Angelman syndrome* and *Prader-Willi syndrome* result from a loss of gene activity in a specific part of chromosome 15, the 15q11-q13 region.
• Chromosome 16	AD polycystic kidney disease, pseudoxanthoma elasticum, Autism.
• Chromosome 17	Contains the Homeobox B gene cluster. **LI-Fraumeni syndrome** (**LI** inverted = **17**), Neurofibromatosis type 1.
• Chromosome 18	Trisomy 18 (Edward's syndrome = Eighteen).
• Chromosome 19	Peutz-Jeghers syndrome (AD).
• Chromosome 20	Adenosine deaminase deficiency, Alagille syndrp,e
• Chromosome 21	**Smallest human chromosome**, was the *second* human chromosome to be fully sequenced. Translocations of genetic material between chromosome 21 and other chromosomes have been a/w several types of cancer. For example, acute lymphoblastic leukemia (ALL) has been a/w a translocation between chromosomes 12 and 21. Acute myeloid leukemia (AML), has been a/w a translocation between chromosomes 8 and 21. **Trisomy 21** – Down syndrome extra chromosome 21 due to *non-disjunction.*
• Chromosome 22	**First human chromosome** to be **fully sequenced**. **Philadelphia chromosome** is a/w *chronic myelogenous leukemia* (CML); due to reciprocal translocation between chromosome 9 and 22 and is specifically designated t(9;22)(q34;q11). The presence of this translocation is a highly sensitive test for CML, since 95% of people with CML have this abnormality. It persists during remission and the prognosis is worse, if absent. Also reported to occur in myelofibrosis and polycythemia rubra vera. Catch 22 syndrome (microdeletions of 22).

104. Answer is c (Acute myelomonocytic leukemia).
Ref: Robbins pathology, 7th edition Pg 692.

Revised FAB Classification of AML

MO Minimally differentiated AML	Immature morphology
M1 AML without differentiation	
M2 AML with maturation	t(8;21) – favorable prognosis, chloromas
M3 Acute Promyelocytic leukemia (APML)	Patients are younger; Multiple Auer rods (peroxidase + cytoplasmic inclusions), t(15;17) is characteristic; excellent response to tretinoin; treatment can release Auer rods → often develop DIC
M4 Acute myelomonocytic leukemia	inv (16), good prognosis, lymphadenopathy, CNS involvement
M5 Acute Monocytic leukemia	Stomatitis, gingival hypertrophy, rectal fissures, Non-specific esterase +
M6 Acute erythroleukemia	Di Guglielmo's disease
M7 Acute megakaryocytic leukemia	Megakaryoblasts > 30% of all nucleated cells

105. Answer is a (EB virus).
Ref: Robbins pathology, 7th edition Pg 326, 677.

Burkitt's lymphoma

- Affects most often children
- B cell type
- t(8;14) *c-myc* gene moves next to heavy chain *Ig* gene
- 'Starry sky' appearance (sheets of lymphocytes with interspersed macrophages)
- a/w EB Virus infection
- Jaw lesion in endemic form in African
- Pelvis or abdomen in sporadic form

☑ Also Know

Epstein-Barr virus (EBV), γ herpes virus causes:
- Infectious mononucleosis
- Burkitt's lymphoma
- Nasopharyngeal carcinoma
- Oral hairy leukoplakia (AIDS patients).

106. Answer is b (t9:22).
Ref: Robbins pathology, 7th edition Pg 696, 697.

- **Philadelphia chromosome—t(9:22),** *bcr-abl.*
- It persists during remission and the ***prognosis is worse if absent***.
- Characteristically seen in ***chronic myeloid leukemia (CML)***.
- Also reported to occur in *myelofibrosis and polycythemia rubra vera.*

☑ Also Know

Other Important Chromosomal Translocations

Translocation	Associated disorder
t(9;22)	CML (philadelphia chromosome)
t(15;17)	AML M3
t(8;14)	Burkitt's lymphoma (c-myc activation)
t(14;18)	Follicular lymphoma (bcl-2 activation)
t(11;14)	Mantle cell lymphoma
T(11;22)	Ewing's sarcoma
t(8;21)	AML M2

107. Answer is d (Familial adenomatous polyposis).
Ref: Harrison's, 17th edition Pg 575.

Repeat Topic
- See ***answer no. 24 in COMED-K 2005 answers*** for detailed explanation.
- Also see ***table in answer no. 103 above*** for chromosomal associations of diseases.

FORENSIC MEDICINE

108. Answer is c (Entry wound is everted).
Ref: Narayan Reddy's FMT, 23rd edition Pg 118, Table 8-8.

Difference between wounds of entry and exit

Trait	Entrance wound	Exit wound
Size	Smaller than diameter of bullet In close discharge, skin is torn	Bigger than bullet
Edges	Inverted	Everted, puckered or torn
Contusion, abrasion and grease collar	Present	Absent
Burning, blackening and tattooing	May be seen around the wound	Absent
Bleeding	Less	More
Fat	No protrusion	May protrude
Tissues within and around wound	May be cherry red due to Co or explosive gases	Absent
Lead ring and metal ring	May be seen around the wound by radiological exam	Absent
Fibers of clothing	Turned in and may be carried into the wound	Turned out
Spectrography	More metal is found around entrance wound, if bullet has only passed through soft tissues	Exit wound may contain more metal, if a bone is struck nearer to it

109. Answer is a (Corrosive poisoning).
Ref: Narayan Reddy's FMT, 23rd edition Pg 251.

- The ***only absolute contraindication for stomach wash is corrosive poisoning*** (except carbolic acid) owing to the danger of perforation.

110. Answer is b (Opium).
Ref: Narayan Reddy's FMT, 23rd edition Pg 291.

- ***Opium (afim)*** is the dried juice of poppy ***(Papaver somniferum),*** which is cultivated in India and other Eastern countries only under a license.
- Ripe and dry poppy capsules contain a trace of opium and are used for their ***narcotic and sedative action.***

111. Answer is c (Sessions Court).
Ref: Narayan Reddy's FMT, 23rd edition Pg 11.

- ***Sessions court*** is located at the district headquarters. It can only try cases, which have been committed to it by a magistrate.
- It can ***pass any sentence authorized by the law, but a sentence of death passed by it must be confirmed by the high court*** (S.366 Cr.P.C).
- An assistant sessions court can pass any sentence authorized by law except a sentence of death or imprisonment exceeding 10 years.

112. Answer is a (Fine froth from mouth and nostrils).
Ref: Narayan Reddy's FMT, 23rd edition Pg 171.

- In drowning, a ***fine, white, lathery froth*** is seen at the mouth and nostrils, which is one of the most ***characteristic external signs*** of drowning.
- Vigorous agitation of the seromucoid secretion and the surfactant with aspirated water and retained air by the violent respiratory efforts converts the mixture of endogenous secretions and drowning medium not froth.
- Froth is usually NOT stained with blood.
- If wiped away it reappears.

- *Cutis anserina* (gooseflesh) due to spasm of erector pili muscles may also be seen after death.
- *Weeds and grass in hand* are only rarely seen—suggestive of antemortem drowning.

113. Answer is a (XXX).
Ref: Harsh Mohan's pathology, 4th edition Pg 7.

- ***Barr body is the inactive X chromosome*** in a female cell or the inactive Z in a male. The Barr body chromosome is generally considered to be inert, but in fact a small number of genes remain active and expressed in some species. These genes are generally those which are present on the other sex chromosome (Y or W).
- Condensed X chromosomes called Barr bodies are visible using ordinary light microscopy.
- Normal males do not have Barr bodies since they have only on X chromosome.

Condition	No. of Barr bodies
Normal male	0
Normal female	1
XXX female	2
XXXX female	3
XXY (Klinefelter male)	1

PREVENTIVE AND SOCIAL MEDICINE

114. Answer is a (Hematogenous spread).
Ref: HIV and AIDS, Dr A Benjamin, WSIC books ltd. Pg 2 and a little bit of common sense also ☺.

- The ***most efficient mode of HIV transmission is to introduce HIV into the bloodstream***—particularly through transfusion of infected blood (the questions says most efficient and Not most common).
- Most blood-to-blood transmission now occurs due to multiple use of contaminated syringes in IV drug abusers.

Note:

- Worldwide, the ***most common mode of infection in AIDS***, particularly in developing countries, is ***clearly heterosexual transmission***.
- Most efficient method of transmission during sexual intercourse is by receptive anal intercourse.

115. Answer is a [d / (c + d) × 100].
Ref: Park, 20th edition Pg 128.

Repeat Topic

- See ***answer no. 180 in COMED-K 2010 answers*** for detailed explanation.

116. Answer is a (Literacy, infant mortality, life expectancy at 1 year).
Ref: Park, 20th edition Pg 16.

Repeat Topic

- See table under ***answer no. 152 in COMED-K 2005 answers*** for detailed explanation.

117. Answer is d (15 ppm).
Ref: Park, 20th edition Pg 557.

Repeat Topic

- See ***answer no. 145 in COMED-K 2008 answers*** for detailed explanation.

118. Answer is d (Negligible).
Ref: Park, 20th edition Pg 545.

- ***Milk*** contains almost all known minerals needed by the body such as calcium, phosphorus, sodium, potassium, magnesium, cobalt, copper, iodine, etc.
- Milk is particularly ***rich in calcium***, however it is a ***poor source of iron***.

119. Answer is b (David Morley).
Ref: Park, 20th edition Pg 460.

- The growth or 'road to health' chart (first designed by David Morley) and later modified by WHO is a visible display of the child's physical growth, and development.
- It is designed primarily for the longitudinal follow up (growth monitoring) of a child, so that changes over time can be interpreted.

120. Answer is b (8th May 1980).
Ref: Park, 20th edition Pg 131.

- On ***8th May 1980***, the ***WHO declared that the global eradication of smallpox*** had been achieved.

121. Answer is a (7th April).
Ref: Park, 20th edition Pg 817.

- The constitution of the WHO came into force on ***7th April 1948*** and hence 7th April is celebrated as the World Health Day.

122. Answer is b (Critical path method).
Ref: Park, 20th edition Pg 775.

- The ***path of longest duration is called the critical path***.
- If any activity along the critical path is delayed the entire project will be delayed.

123. Answer is b (Hard tick).
Ref: Harrison's 17th edition Pg 1236, Table 189-4; Park, 20th edition Pg 685; Haemaphysalis ticks of India By G Geevarghese, AC Mishra, 2011 edition Pg 6.

Kyasanur forest disease (KFD)

- ❖ KFD is a ***tick borne, viral hemorrhagic fever*** found in ***Karnataka, India and Western Siberia***.
- ❖ Named after Kyasanur forest area in ***Shimoga district, Karnataka*** where cases were first reported.
- ❖ KFD is seen in monkeys and humans and is genetically rekated to RSSE (Russian spring summer encephalitis).
- ❖ ***Reservoir hosts***: Forest birds and small mammals.
- ❖ ***Amplifier hosts: Monkeys.***
- ❖ ***Vector tick: H. spinigera (HARD tick—MC in India and H. spinigera is a hard tick***—*some books give soft tick also for KFD, but most MCQ answers will hold good with hard tick as answer – refer book on Haemophysalis tick in India given under ref. above)*.
- ❖ Major outbreak: In 1982 in Belthangady taluk, South Canara, 1142 human cases were reported with 104 deaths.
- ❖ Russian counterpart of KFD is *Omsk hemorrhagic fever*.

Soft ticks transmit	*Hard ticks* transmit
♦ Q fever ♦ Relapsing fever ♦ KFD also	♦ Tick typhus ♦ Viral encephalitis ♦ Viral hemorrhagic fevers (KFD in India) ♦ Tularemia ♦ Tick paralysis ♦ Human babesiosis

124. Answer is b (1/2 proteins and 1/3 calories).
Ref: Park, 20th edition Pg 500.

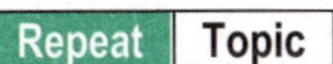

- See *answer no. 134 in COMED-K 2010 answers* for detailed explanation.

125. Answer is a (1 g/kg).
Ref: Park, 20th edition Pg 528.

- The Indian council of medical research (ICMR) in 1989 recommended 1 gram protein/kg body weight for an Indian adult, assuming an NPU of 65 for the dietary proteins.

126. Answer is b (Primary prevention).
Ref: Park, 20th edition Pg 39.

Primordial prevention

- New concept receiving special attention in the prevention of chronic diseases (obesity, hypertension).
- This is primary prevention in its purest sense, i.e. prevention of the emergence or the development of risk factors in countries or population groups in which they have not yet appeared.
- In primordial prevention efforts are directed towards discouraging children from adopting harmful lifestyles.
- The main intervention is through *individual and mass education*.

Primary prevention

- Defined as "action taken prior to he onset of disease, which removes the possibility that a disease will ever occur."
- It signifies intervention in the prepathogenesis phase of a disease or health problem. It includes the concept of positive health.
- The concept of primary prevention is being applied to the prevention of chronic diseases such as coronary heart disease, hypertension and cancer based on elimination or modification of risk factors of disease.

Secondary prevention

- Action, which halts the progress of a disease at its incipient stage and prevents complications.
- The specific interventions are early diagnosis (screening tests, case finding programs) and adequate treatment.
- Secondary domain is largely the domain of clinical medicine—*early diagnosis and treatment*.

Tertiary prevention

- All measures available to limit or reduce impairments and disabilities, minimize suffering caused by existing departures from good health and to promote the patients adjustment to irremediable conditions (includes *rehabilitation*).
- It signifies interventions in the late pathogenesis phase.

127. Answer is b (Past infection).
Ref: Park, 20th edition Pg 164.

- ***A positive tuberculin test*** (reaction of 10 mm or more to 1 TU PPD) indicates that the ***person is infected with M. tuberculosis***; it ***does not prove that the person is suffering*** from the disease.
- If a child below 2 years is found to be tuberculin positive, it is an indirect evidence of an active tuberculous lesion in the body even if it is not manifest.

128. Answer is d (Condom).
Ref: Park, 20th edition Pg 424.

- The term ***conventional contraceptives*** is used to denote ***those methods that require action at the time of sexual intercourse***, e.g. ***condoms, spermicides***, etc.

PSYCHIATRY

129. Answer is c (Patients eat huge amounts of food, but they throw up soon after eating).
Ref: Niraj Ahuja's psychiatry, 6th edition Pg 78.

	Anorexia nervosa	**Bulimia**
• Method of weight control	Restriction of intake	Vomiting
• Binge eating	Uncommon	Common
• Weight at diagnosis	Markedly decreased	Near normal
• Ritualized exercise	Usual	Rare
• Amenorrhea	100%	50%
• Other endocrine changes	Common	Uncommon
• Antisocial behavior	Rare	Frequent
• Cardiovascular changes (bradycardia, hypotension)	Common	Uncommon
• Skin changes (lanugo hair, carotenemia, dryness)	Usual	Rare
• Hypothermia	Usual	Rare
• Medical complications	Hypokalemia, cardiac arrhythmias, aspiration of gastric contents, esophageal or gastric rupture	Hypokalemia, cardiac arrhythmias

Anorexia nervosa

- Psychological characteristics: ***Excessive dieting; refusal to eat despite normal appetite*** ('anorexia' is a misnomer); *abnormal behavior dealing with food* (e.g. cutting food into very small pieces; simulating eating; collecting recipes and cooking for others).
- Treatment: Most effective form of psychotherapy is ***family therapy***. Behavior therapy consists of ***positive reinforcement***. Amitriptyline and cyproheptadine are given to patients whose body weight is not dangerously low.

Note

- The salient feature of *anorexia nervosa* (AN) is a refusal to maintain a minimally normal body weight.
- ***Bulimia nervosa*** (BN) is characterized by ***recurrent episodes of binge eating followed by abnormal compensatory behaviors, such as self-induced vomiting.***
- In the current diagnostic system, the critical distinction between AN and BN depends on body weight: patients with AN are, by definition, significantly underweight, whereas patients with BN have body weights in the normal range or above.

130. Answer is b (*Unpleasant olfactory sensations*).
Ref: linkinghub.elsevier.com/retrieve/pii/S0967586809001386-

- Olfactory hallucinations, also known as uncinate fits, consist of sudden and unexplained ***perceptions of smell, usually described as unpleasant.***

DERMATOLOGY

131. Answer is c (Rheumatic fever).
Ref: Harrison's, 17th edition Pg 323.

- ***Erythema marginatum*** is seen in patients with rheumatic fever, primarily on the ***trunk***.
- Lesions are ***pink-red*** in color, flat to mildly elevated and ***transient***.

☑ Also Know

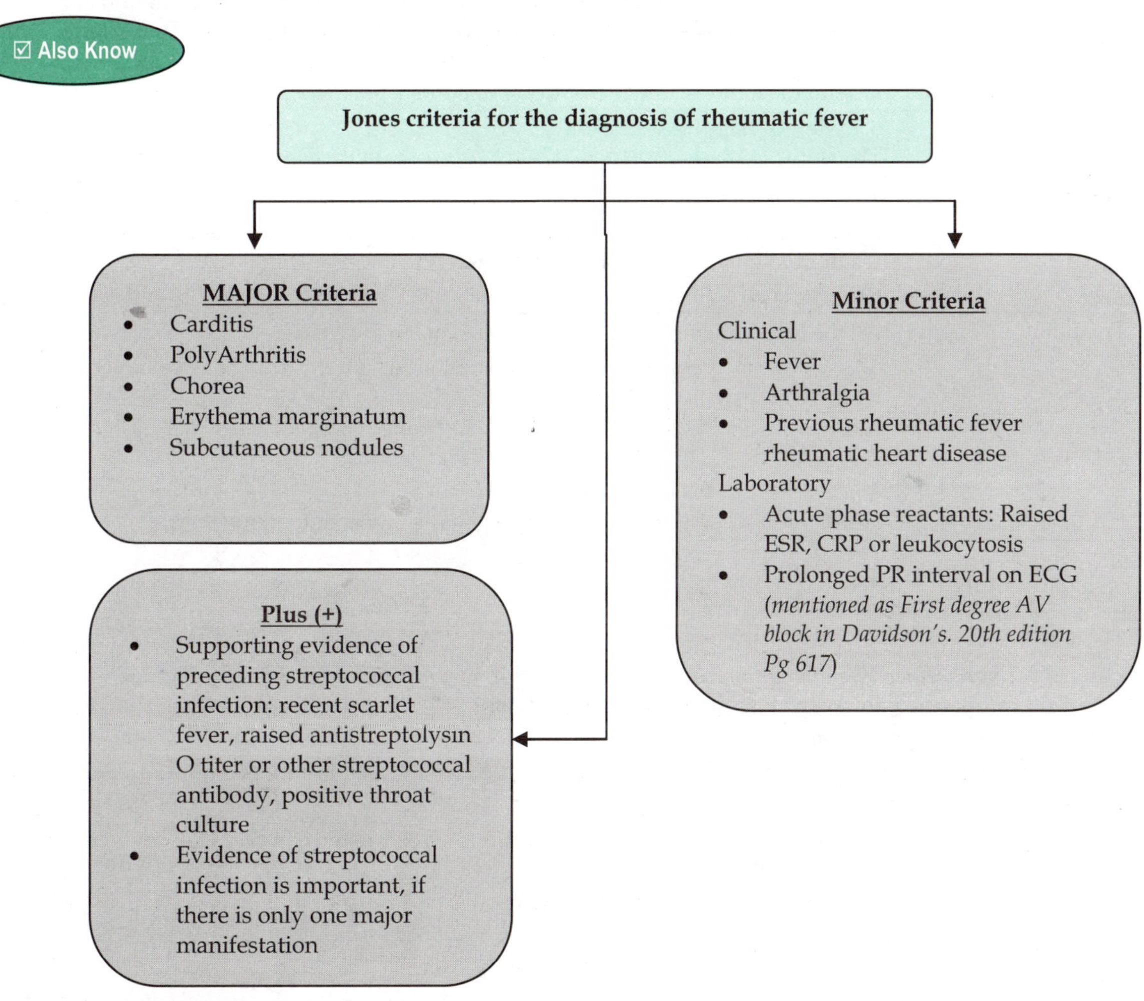

132. Answer is a (Basal cell CA).
Ref: Robbins pathology, 7th edition Pg 1242.

- ***Most common type of skin cancer*** is ***basal cell carcinoma*** followed by squamous cell carcinoma.

133. Answer is b (Psoriasis).
Ref: KD Tripathi, 6th edition Pg 850.

- ***Calcipotriol*** is a synthetic non-hypercalcemic vitamin D analogue effective topically in plaque type psoriasis.
- It binds to the ***intracellular vitamin D receptors in epidermal keratinocytes*** and suppresses their proliferation, while enhancing differentiation.

134. Answer is d (Immunocompromised and mentally retarded).
Ref: Harrison's, 17th edition Pg 2748.

Scabies

■ **Etiology and spread**	– Caused by *itch mite, Sarcoptes scabiei;* spread through *contact* (sexual promiscuity, crowding, uncleanliness) with infected individuals, spread is common in families.
■ **Presentation**	– Intense pruritus (itching) that *worsens* at *night* and *after a hot shower* – Burrows appear as dark wavy lines in the epidermis that measure 3–15 mm and end in a small pearly bleb that contains the female mite. Such lesions are seen on *interdigital webs, flexor aspects of wrists,* the elbows, anterior axillary folds, around the nipples, umbilicus, lower abdomen, genitalia, buttocks, medial aspects of thighs, legs and feet. – The *face, scalp, neck, palms and soles* are *spared except in children.*
■ **Varieties of scabies**	– *Scabies incognito*: Occurs in persons treated with steroids. – *Norwegian scabies*: Hyper infestation with thousands or millions of mites, may result from glucocorticoid use, immunodeficiency or AIDS. – *Sarcoptic mange*: Animal scabies.
■ **Treatment**	– All the family members should be treated at the *same time.* – *5% permethrin* cream applied from the neck down after bathing and removed 8 h later with soap and water. – Alternatives include *benzyl benzoate, sulfur ointments, topical crotamiton cream, ivermectin.* – *Lindane solution* was used earlier, but it causes *neurotoxicity* (seizures) and *aplastic anemia.* Contraindicated in pregnant women and infants.

135. Answer is a (Griseofulvin + Ketoconazole).
Ref: Harrison's, 17th edition Pg 318.

- ***Infection of the nails (tinea unguium or onychomycosis)*** occurs in many patients with tinea pedis and is characterized by opacified, thickened nails and subungual debris.
- The distal-lateral variant is most common.
- Proximal subungual onychomycosis may be a marker for HIV infection or other immunocompromised states.
- Treatment:
  - Oral antifungal agents are required for dermatophyte infections involving the hair and nails and for other infections unresponsive to topical therapy.
  - ***Griseofulvin is the only oral agent approved*** in the United States for dermatophyte infections involving the skin, hair or nails.
  - ***Oral itraconazole and terbinafine*** are approved for ***onychomycosis***.
  - Itraconazole—fingernails require 2 months of continuous therapy or two pulses. Toenails require 3 months of continuous therapy or three pulse.
  - Terbinafine (250 mg/d) is also effective for onychomycosis.
  - Therapy with terbinafine is continued for 6 weeks for fingernail infections and 12 weeks for toenail infections.

RADIOLOGY

136. Answer is a (Duodenal atresia).
Ref: Chapman's radiological D/D, 5th edition Pg 363.

- ***Duodenal atresia*** shows marked dilatation of the proximal duodenum with the double bubble sign, which may also be seen by ***ultrasound of the fetus***.
- *A/w Down syndrome.*

ANESTHESIA

137. Answer is a (Full stomach).
Ref: http://www.anesthesia.utoronto.ca/edu/cme/courses/m01/m01p04.htm

Absolute Contraindications for laryngeal mask airway

- Full stomach/significant aspiration risk (including hiatus hernia)
- Morbidly obese patients
- Untrained in LMA use
- Oropharyngeal pathology very likely to result in a poor mask fit (e.g. radiotherapy for hypopharynx/larynx)
- Glottic surgery.

138. Answer is c (Both of the above).
Ref: KD Tripathi, 6th edition Pg 354.

- In an ***inflamed area, local anesthetic is less effective*** due to the high vascularity, rapid washout and low pH of the area.
- Injectable local anesthetics are not used on dirty wound for ***fear of spread of infection***. Wound healing may get delayed.

139. Answer is c (Used for perineal and rectal surgeries).
Ref: Lee's synopsis of anesthesia, 13th edition Pg 546, 552.

- ***Saddle block anesthesia***: A type of anesthesia produced by introducing the anesthetics agent into the fourth lumbar interspace.
- This ***anesthetizes the perineum and the buttocks area***.

140. Answer is c (Ether).
Ref: KD Tripathi, 6th edition Pg 371.

- ***Ether is a potent anesthetic***, produces ***good analgesia*** and *marked muscle relaxation* by reducing acetylcholine output from motor nerve endings—dose of competitive neuromuscular blockers should be reduced to one third.

141. Answer is a (Bronchoconstriction and ↑ respiratory secretions).
Ref: KD Tripathi, 6th edition Pg 370-72.

Repeat Topic

- See ***answer no. 82 in COMED-K 2005 answers*** for detailed explanation.

ANATOMY

142. Answer is b (Supplies buccinator muscle).
Ref: Snell's anatomy, 2nd edition Pg 145.

- The ***buccinator*** is supplied by the *buccal branch of the* ***facial nerve***.

143. Answer is a (Vermis Plans: The limb movement).
Ref: Principles of physiology, Debasis pramanik, Academic publishers, Pg 437.

Repeat Topic

- See ***answer no. 164 in COMED-K 2005 answers*** for detailed explanation.
- The vermis is a thin central part between the cerebellar hemispheres that controls our trunk (posterior vermis) and legs (anterior vermis).

144. Answer is a (VI).
Ref: Maheshwari, 3rd edition Pg 229.

- The nerve root affected in disc prolapse/vertebral dislocation is usually the one, which leaves the spinal canal ***below the next vertebra***.
- This is because the root at the level of the prolapsed disk leaves the canal in the upper half of the foramen.
- Thus the nerve root affected in 5th and 6th cervical vertebral dislocation is *C6*, although it is the C5 root, which exits at this level.

145. Answer is c (Biceps brachii).
Ref: BD Chaurasia, Vol 1. Pg 34.

Biceps brachii
- *Origin*
  - Long head from the supraglenoid tubercle of the scapula
  - Short head from the tip of coracoid process of scapule
  - The tendon of the long head crosses the humeral head within the capsule of the shoulder joint and emerges from the joint surrounded by a synovial sheath and lying in the bicipital groove of the humerus.
- *Insertion*
  - Into the posterior part of the tuberosity of the radius and by an aponeurotic band called the bicipital aponeurosis into the deep fascia on the medial aspect of forearm.

146. Answer is a (Persistent vitellointestinal duct).
Ref: IB singh, embryology, 2nd edition Pg 132.

Causes of umbilical fecal fistula
- *Congenital*
  - **Persistent vitellointestinal duct**—uncommon anomaly. If the fistula is all, it leads to mucoid discharge, but if it is large it results in ***omphaloenteric fecal fistula***.
- *Acquired*
  - Internal hollow viscus malignancies
  - TB peritonitis.

147. Answer is b (Lateral pterygoid).
Ref: BD Chaurasia, Vol 3, Pg 23.

- ***Lateral pterygoid*** causes ***depression of the mandible***.

148. Answer is d (10 cm).
Ref: Dutta's obstetrics, 6th edition Pg 8.

- The fallopian tube is about 10 cm long.
- It has four parts:
  - Infundibulum (funnel shaped lateral extreme)
  - Ampulla (widest part)
  - Isthmus (narrowest part)
  - Intramural part (within uterine wall).

PHYSIOLOGY

149. Answer is d (Decrease in total peripheral resistance).
Ref: Guyton's physiology, Pg 44.

150. Answer is a (Liver).
Ref: Harrison's, 17th edition Pg 2208.

- Although GH exerts direct effects in target tissues, many of its physiologic effects are mediated indirectly through ***Insulin-Like Growth Factor-I*** *(IGF-I)*, a potent growth and differentiation factor.
- The ***liver is the major source of circulating IGF-I***.
- In peripheral tissues, IGF-I exerts local paracrine actions that appear to be both dependent on and independent of GH. Thus, GH administration induces circulating IGF-I as well as stimulating IGF-I production in multiple tissues.

151. Answer is a (Carnitine).
Ref: Ganong's, 17th edition Pg 274.

152. Answer is d (Digestion of proteins).
Ref: Ganong's, 17th edition Pg 448-49.

153. Answer is c (Y chromosome).
Ref: Ganong's, 23rd edition Pg 395-96, Fig. 25-6 and Pg 404; OP Ghai, 7th edition Pg 505.

Repeat Topic

- See ***answer no. 67 in COMED-K 2006 answers*** for detailed explanation.

154. Answer is b (Lateral olfactory striae).
Ref: Chaudhuri's physiology, 2nd edition Pg 604.

155. Answer is b (It causes decreased compliance).
Ref: Ganong's, 23rd edition Pg 597.

Repeat Topic

- See ***answer no. 166 in COMED-K 2009 answers*** for detailed explanation.

156. Answer is d (None of the above).
Ref: Chaudhuri's physiology, 2nd edition Pg 411.

BIOCHEMISTRY

157. Answer is a (2 lactate + 2 ATP).
Ref: Lippincott's illustrated biochemistry, Pg 135.

158. Answer is a (Fabry's—alpha galactosidase).
Ref: Harrison's, 17th edition Pg 2453.

- See table below for explanation.
- Also know that cystic fibrosis is not due to enzyme defect, but autosomal recessive condition resulting from mutations in the gene that encodes the ***CF transmembrane conductance regulator (CFTR) protein located on chromosome*** *7*.
- ***Alpha-1-antitrypsin deficiency*** leads to ***COPD (esp. panacinar emphysema)***.

Lipid Storage Diseases or Sphingolipidoses

Disease	*Enzyme defect*	*Lipid accumulating*	*Salient features*
1. FAbry's disease (XLR); 'FAX'	α-galactosidase	Ceramide trihexoside	Angiokeratomas, kidney/heart failure, peripheral neuropathy of hands/feet
2. Gaucher's disease (AR), MC	β-glucocerebrosidase	Glucocerebroside	3 types—adult, infantile, juvenile Hepatosplenomegaly, osteoporosis, moderate

			anemia, 'crumpled tissue paper' macrophages – Gaucher's cells, aseptic necrosis of femur, bone crises
3. Niemann-Pick, AR,	**Sphing**omyelinase; No Man Picks (Niemann Pick) his nose with his **sphing**er	Sphingomyelin	CNS damage, MR, cherry red spot in macula, foam cells, fatal in early life, hepatosplenomegaly
4. Tay-Sach's disease, AR	Hexosaminidase A	Ganglioside (GM2)	CNS damage, MR, cherry red spot in macula, developmental delay, lysosomes with onion skin
5. Krabbe's, AR	β-galactocerebrosidase	Galactocerebroside	Severe MR; total absence of myelin in CNS, globoid bodies in white matter, optic atrophy, fatal in early life
6. Metachromatic leukodystrophy	Arylsulfatase A	Cerebroside sulfate	Central and peripheral demyelination with ataxia, dementia, nerves stain yellowish brown with cresyl violet (metachromasia), fatal in first decade
7. Sandhoff's disease, AR	Hexosaminidase A and B	Globoside	Same as Tay Sach's, but progresses rapidly

159. Answer is a (Restriction endonuclease).
Ref: Lippincott's illustrated biochemistry, Pg 509.

160. Answer is c (THFA).
Ref: Harrison's, 17th edition Pg 444, Fig. 71-1.

Folic acid

Sources	– Green leafy vegetables, dried beans and peas, lentils, liver. "FOLate from FOLiage".
Deficiency	– Macrocytic megaloblastic anemia.
Function	– ***Coenzyme for (single) 1-carbon transfers.*** – Involved in methylation reactions. – Required for synthesis of bases in DNA and RNA. – Supplementary folic acid in early pregnancy reduces neural tube defects.

161. Answer is c (Glutaminase).
Ref: Lippincott's illustrated biochemistry, Pg 199.

162. Answer is c (B-cl-c-a-a3).
Ref: Abbott's biochemistry, Pg 199.

163. Answer is c (Unmeasured ions).
Ref: Harrison's 17th edition Pg 290, 292.

Repeat Topic

- Routine serum electrolyte determination measures most of the cations, but only a few anions.
- This ***apparent disparity between the total cation and the total anion concentration*** is called the ***anion gap***.
- ***Anion gap*** = $[(Na^+) + (K^+)] - [(Cl^-) + (HCO_3^-)]$ = normally about 10–16 mmol/L.

164. Answer is d (Acetoacetate).
Ref: Vasudevan's biochemistry, 3rd edition Pg 132.

165. Answer is a (Non-closure of rostral neuropore).
Ref: The developing human, Keith L Moore, 4th edition Pg 344, 392.

- ***Meroanencephaly*** is ***congenital absence of part of the brain***, usually the ***forebrain and midbrain***.
- This malformation results from ***failure of the cranial end (rostral neuropore) of the neural tube to close*** during 4th week of intrauterine life.
- This defect causes subsequent failure of forming of calvaria.

NOTES